# SLEEP APNEA AND SNORING
## SURGICAL AND NON-SURGICAL THERAPY

*Commissioning Editor:* Scott Scheidt
*Development Editor:* Nani Clansey
*Project Manager:* Kathryn Mason
*Design:* Erik Bigland
*Illustration Manager:* Bruce Hogarth
*Illustrator:* Jim Millerick
*Marketing Manager:* Brenna Christensen

# SLEEP APNEA AND SNORING
## SURGICAL AND NON-SURGICAL THERAPY

**MICHAEL FRIEDMAN** MD, FACS

Professor of Otolaryngology
Chairman, Division of Sleep Surgery
Rush University Medical Center
Chairman of Otolaryngology
Advocate Illinois Masonic Medical Center
Advanced Center for Specialty Care
Chicago, IL
USA

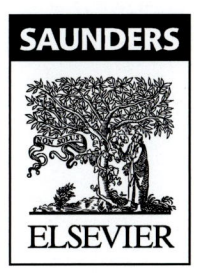

SAUNDERS
ELSEVIER

**SAUNDERS**
ELSEVIER

Saunders is an imprint of Elsevier Ltd

© 2009, Elsevier Inc. All rights reserved.

First published 2009

No part of this publication may be reproduced or transmitted in any form or by any means, electronic or mechanical, including photocopying, recording, or any information storage and retrieval system, without permission in writing from the publisher. Permissions may be sought directly from Elsevier's Rights Department: phone: (+1) 215 239 3804 (US) or (+44) 1865 843830 (UK); fax: (+44) 1865 853333; e-mail: healthpermissions@elsevier.com. You may also complete your request on-line via the Elsevier website at http://www.elsevier.com/permissions.

ISBN 978-1-4160-3112-3

**British Library Cataloguing in Publication Data**
Friedman, Michael, 1948–
   Sleep apnea and snoring : surgical and non-surgical therapy
   1. Sleep apnea syndromes – Treatment 2. Snoring –
   Prevention
   I. Title
   616.2'0906

**Library of Congress Cataloging in Publication Data**
A catalog record for this book is available from the Library of Congress

**Notice**
Medical knowledge is constantly changing. Standard safety precautions must be followed, but as new research and clinical experience broaden our knowledge, changes in treatment and drug therapy may become necessary or appropriate. Readers are advised to check the most current product information provided by the manufacturer of each drug to be administered to verify the recommended dose, the method and duration of administration, and contraindications. It is the responsibility of the practitioner, relying on experience and knowledge of the patient, to determine dosages and the best treatment for each individual patient. Neither the Publisher nor the author_assume any liability for any injury and/or damage to persons or property arising from this publication.   *The Publisher*

Printed in China
Last digit is the print number: 9 8 7 6 5 4 3 2 1

ELSEVIER  your source for books, journals and multimedia in the health sciences
www.elsevierhealth.com

Working together to grow libraries in developing countries
www.elsevier.com | www.bookaid.org | www.sabre.org
ELSEVIER   BOOK AID International   Sabre Foundation

The Publisher's policy is to use paper manufactured from sustainable forests

# Contents

Foreword  viii
Preface  x
List of Contributors  xi
Dedications  xvii

### SECTION A  INTRODUCTION

1. The role of otolaryngologist in the treatment of snoring and obstructive sleep apnea  1
*Michael Friedman*

### SECTION B  DIAGNOSIS

2. Signs and symptoms of obstructive sleep apnea and upper airway resistance syndrome  3
*Christian Guilleminault and Shanon Takaoka*
3. Airway evaluation in obstructive sleep apnea  11
*Boris A. Stuck and Joachim T. Maurer*
4. Clinical polysomnography  22
*Stephen Lund and Jon Freeman*
5. Practical considerations and clinical caveats in polysomnographic interpretation in sleep-related breathing disorder  33
*Michel A. Cramer Bornemann and Mark W. Mahowald*
6. Validity of sleep nasendoscopy in the investigation of sleep-related breathing disorder  42
*Sandeep Berry and Heikki B. Whittet*

### SECTION C  NON-SURGICAL TREATMENT OF OSA/HS

7. Obstructive sleep apnea: decision making and treatment algorithm  45
*Andrew N. Goldberg*
8. Obesity management  51
*Robert F. Kushner*
9. CPAP, APAP and BIPAP  60
*Terence M. Davidson*
10. Analysis of NCPAP failures  69
*Wietske Richard, Jantine Venker, Cindy den Herder, Dennis Kox and Nico de Vries*
11. Oral appliance and craniofacial problems of obstructive sleep apnea syndrome  72
*Soichiro Miyazaki and Makoto Kikuchi*

### SECTION D  SURGICAL TREATMENT OF OSA/HS

12. Rationale and indications for surgical treatment  80
*Donald M. Sesso, Robert W. Riley and Nelson B. Powell*
13. The impact of surgical treatment of OSA on cardiac risk factors  85
*Darius Bliznikas and Ho-Sheng Lin*

### SECTION E  ANESTHESIA FOR OSA/HS

14. Perioperative monitoring in obstructive sleep apnea hypopnea syndrome  88
*Samuel A. Mickelson*
15. Perioperative and anesthesia management  96
*Arthur J. Klowden, Usharani Nimmagadda and Benjamin Salter*

### SECTION F  TREATMENT SELECTION

16. Friedman tongue position and the staging of obstructive sleep apnea/ hypopnea syndrome  104
*Michael Friedman*
17. Multilevel surgery for obstructive sleep apnea/hypopnea syndrome  111
*Michael Friedman, Hsin-Ching Lin, T.K. Venkatesan and Berk Gurpinar*

### SECTION G  NASAL SURGERY FOR THE TREATMENT OF OSA/HS

18. Nasal obstruction and sleep-disordered breathing  120
*Kristin K. Egan, David Kim and Eric J. Kezirian*
19. Effects of nasal surgery on snoring and sleep apnea  124
*Michael Friedman and Paul Schalch*
20. Nasal valve repair  129
*Michael Friedman and Paul Schalch*
21. Correction of nasal obstruction due to nasal valve collapse  134
*Maria T. Messina-Doucet*
22. Radiofrequency volumetric reduction for hypertrophic turbinate  140
*Kasey K. Li*

23 Bipolar radiofrequency cold ablation turbinate reduction for obstructive inferior turbinate hypertrophy   143
*Neil Bhattacharyya*

## SECTION H  MINIMALLY INVASIVE PALATAL PROCEDURES

24 Laser-assisted uvulopalatoplasty: techniques and results   148
*Andrew N. Goldberg and Amol M. Bhatki*

25 Snare uvulectomy for upper airway resistance   154
*James Newman*

26 Cautery-assisted palatal stiffening operation   159
*Kenny P. Pang and David J. Terris*

27 Injection snoreplasty   165
*Scott E. Brietzke and Eric A. Mair*

28 Palatal implants for primary snoring: short- and long-term results of a new minimally invasive surgical technique   169
*Joachim T. Maurer*

## SECTION I  PALATAL SURGERY

29 Uvulopalatopharyngoplasty   176
*George P. Katsantonis*

30 Uvulopalatopharyngoplasty – effects on the airway   184
*Aaron E. Sher*

31 Uvulopalatopharyngoplasty – the Fairbanks technique   190
*David N.F. Fairbanks*

32 Submucosal uvulopalatopharyngoplasty   195
*Michael Friedman and Paul Schalch*

33 Zetapalatopharyngoplasty (ZPP)   201
*Michael Friedman and Paul Schalch*

34 The uvulopalatal flap   206
*Tod C. Huntley*

35 Modified uvulopalatopharyngoplasty with uvula preservation   211
*Han Demin, Ye Jingying and Wang Jun*

36 Transpalatal advancement pharyngoplasty   217
*B. Tucker Woodson*

37 Expansion sphincter pharyngoplasty   224
*Kenny P. Pang and B. Tucker Woodson*

38 Lateral pharyngoplasty   227
*Michel Burihan Cahali*

## SECTION J  MINIMALLY INVASIVE HYPOPHARYNGEAL PROCEDURES

39 Fundamentals of minimally invasive radiofrequency applications in ear, nose and throat medicine   233
*Kai Desinger*

40 Radiofrequency tongue base reduction in sleep-disordered breathing   243
*Robert J. Troell*

41 Minimally invasive submucosal glossectomy   248
*Sam Robinson*

42 A minimally invasive technique for tongue base stabilization   258
*B. Tucker Woodson*

43 Endoscopic coblation lingual tonsillectomy   265
*Peter G. Michaelson and Eric A. Mair*

## SECTION K  MULTILEVEL PHARYNGEAL SURGERY

44 Multilevel pharyngeal surgery for obstructive sleep apnea   268
*Kenny P. Pang and David J. Terris*

45 Open tongue base resection for OSA   279
*Tod C. Huntley*

46 Midline laser glossectomy with linguoplasty: treatment of obstructive sleep apnea   287
*Hsueh-Yu Li*

47 External submucosal glossectomy   292
*Sam Robinson*

48 Genioglossus advancement in sleep apnea surgery   301
*Kasey K. Li*

49 Hyoid suspension as the only procedure   305
*Nico de Vries and Cindy den Herder*

50 Multilevel surgery (hyoid suspension, radiofrequent ablation of the tongue base, uvulopalatopharyngoplasty) with/without genioglossal advancement   312
*Nico de Vries, Wietske Richard, Dennis Kox and Cindy den Herder*

51 Hyo–mandibular suspension and hyoid expansion for obstructive sleep apnea   321
*Yosef P. Krespi*

## SECTION L  MAXILLOFACIAL SURGICAL TECHNIQUES

52 Maxillofacial surgical techniques for hypopharyngeal obstruction in obstructive sleep apnea   326
*Donald M. Sesso, Robert W. Riley and Nelson B. Powell*

53 Modified maxillomandibular advancement technique   334
*Yau Hong Goh, Winston Tan and Mark Hon Wah Ignatius*

54 Distraction osteogenesis and obstructive sleep apnea syndrome   339
*Kasey K. Li*

## SECTION M  TRACHEOSTOMY FOR OSAHS

55 Tracheostomy for sleep apnea   343
*Robert H. Maisel*

56 Speech-ready, long-term, tube-free tracheostomy for obstructive sleep apnea   349
*Isaac Eliachar, Lee M. Akst and Robert R. Lorenz*

## SECTION N  POSTOPERATIVE MANAGEMENT AND COMPLICATIONS

57  The postoperative management of OSA patients after uvulopalatopharyngoplasty. inpatient or outpatient?   361
*Jeffrey H. Spiegel and Yanina Greenstein*

58  Multi-modality management of nasopharyngeal stenosis following uvulopalatoplasty   366
*Yosef P. Krespi and Ashutosh Kacker*

59  Current techniques for the treatment of velopharyngeal insufficiency   370
*Harlan R. Muntz*

60  Uvulopalatopharyngoplasty: analysis of failure   378
*Nico de Vries and Naomi Ketharanathan*

61  Salvage of failed palate procedures for sleep-disordered breathing   386
*David J. Terris and Manoj Kumar*

62  Revision uvulopalatopharyngoplasty (UPPP) by Z-palatoplasty (ZPP)   393
*Michael Friedman and Paul Schalch*

## SECTION O  PEDIATRIC OSAHS

63  Management of sleep-related breathing disorders in children   398
*David H. Darrow and Kaalan E. Johnson*

64  Obstructive sleep apnea in children with adenotonsillar hypertrophy   414
*Soichiro Miyazaki and Min Yin*

65  The effect of polysomnography on pediatric adenotonsillectomy postoperative management   420
*Anthony A. Rieder, Stacey L. Ishman and Valerie Flanary*

66  Current techniques of adenoidectomy   425
*Peter J. Koltai and Christopher M. Discolo*

67  Radiofrequency tonsil reduction: safety, morbidity and efficacy   429
*Michael Friedman and Paul Schalch*

68  Microdebrider-assisted tonsillectomy   434
*Peter J. Koltai and Christopher M. Discolo*

69  Laryngomalacia   437
*Peggy E. Kelley*

Index   445

# Foreword

Sleep disordered breathing is an extraordinarily common condition. Pharyngeal collapse during sleep as a consequence of abnormal structural anatomy and loss of muscle tone during sleep is the defining event. Obstruction is not airway stenosis but is instead airway instability occurring in a structurally vulnerable airway. Snoring is its cardinal sign. Not just an obnoxious noise, snoring represents flutter in a Starling resistor when collapsing pressures exceed dilating forces. Such a state is both abnormal and common affecting 30% or more of adults and a significant number of children. Social concerns about snoring likely predate recorded history since humans began to first congregate. More ominously, the spectrum of snoring includes pathologic obstruction and sleep disordered breathing which occurs in 10% to 20% of the population. Defined obstructive sleep apnea occurs in 2% to 4% of middle aged adults. Sleep apnea is associated with a wide variety of health concerns including a lower quality of life, neurocognitive disfunction, medical/cardiovascular morbidity especially related to cardiovascular outcomes, and increased mortality risks. A wide variety of therapies have been described to treat sleep disordered breathing. These range from modifying predisposing conditions, reducing medical risk factors (such as obesity), appliances (oral, nasal, and CPAP), and finally upper airway surgeries. Nasal CPAP is the most common medical treatment and has revolutionized treatment since its introduction by Sullivan in 1981. Many have been improved. However, it may be argued that many if not most patients with the disorder fail treatment. Even among the patients who are considered successful, long term treatment for a lifelong disease has yet to be demonstrated. There is a need for improved treatment options.

This book represents a major effort to bring together expertise in sleep surgery to describe the current state of the art. As a surgical atlas, it provides descriptions of a wide variety of specific techniques. These address multiple levels of the upper airway as is commonly required in the sleep disordered breathing patient. Distinct from other surgical books, this work presents the widest variety of surgical techniques. This variability is represented in 26 chapters directly addressing surgery of the soft palate, 8 chapters on pediatric sleep apnea, and 6 chapters relating to soft tissue techniques of the tongue. As much as possible it describes state of the technical art.

Many challenges exist in the field. Successful treatment requires a minimum of three steps. These include accurate diagnosis, correct selection of technique, and skillful application. Although, in children lymphoid hyperplasia contributes significantly to disease, defined upper airway pathology is uncommon in adults. Instead, upper airway anatomy tissue is normal but structurally disproportionate. As such, upper airway surgery for sleep disordered breathing is not excisional but is reconstructive. The primary goal of these procedures is to modify tissues and alter structure to improve and restore upper airway function. As a multifactoral disease, no single structure contributes and treating a single structure infrequently treats the disease adequately. Since many structures may contribute to sleep disordered breathing and most reconstructive procedures address only limited segments of the upper airway, few patients can be effectively treated using a cookie cutter, palate only algorithm. Instead, multiple pathologies require multiple techniques. Techniques also vary with surgeon's preferences and skills. Many techniques have been too morbid for patients with milder disease. This is now less so although major progress is needed. The wide variety of techniques makes assessment of effectiveness difficult. Most accept that multiple segments of the airway contribute to upper airway collapse, increased resistance and ventilatory instability, but how to treat is without concensus. Available data supports that isolated procedures offer far less benefit than more comprehensive treatment of the upper airway. Too often suboptimal treatment results from a failure to recognize or understand the structure and pathophysiology of the upper airway.

Some are critical of the wide variety of surgical procedures used for the disease. They state that variability is an indication that no surgical procedure works rather than acknowledging structural variability. Such a narrow bias is not supported when viewing airway structure, but current outcomes data provide little insight in evaluating individual techniques to treat this variability. In fact, some surgeons attempt to treat all with uniform techniques as if the airway structure were the same in all patients. Patient's anatomy and clinical needs for treatment vary. Therefore, procedures must vary. Furthermore, surgical variation is a mechanism leading to surgical evolutionary changes and improvements. Clinical studies are needed to guide surgical decision making. Major efforts are needed to evaluate procedures in controlled clinical trials. Studies claiming effectiveness without trials are no longer acceptable. However, those evaluating surgical trials must understand the extraordinary difficulty in performing surgical trials. Reviews of surgical effectiveness must be inclusive with outcomes reviewed in their totality. Highly focused reviews that methodologically exclude high level studies due to non-uniformity of metrics should also not be accepted. With an already limited data set, such an "ivory tower" approach seriously skews outcomes by eliminating well done studies showing benefit.

# FOREWORD

Lastly, surgery does not have a single role in the treatment of disease. For sleep disordered breathing, it may have the goal of preventing or curing disease, salvage and reducing disease severity after failure of other treatments, or ancillary treatment to augment other therapies. Currently, the opportunities to cure or prevent disease are infrequent. More commonly, surgery is to salvage after medical treatment failure and to act as ancillary treatment to improve outcomes with other therapy. As sleep disordered breathing is a chronic, presumably life long condition, the needs to adjust and modify therapies are inescapable. The future of surgery is to provide reconstructive techniques to manage the airway over a lifetime.

This book provides a unique single source reference of many techniques to better address the challenges of the upper airway.

**B. Tucker Woodson, MD, FACS**
Professor and Chief
Division of Sleep Medicine
Department of Otolaryngology & Communication Sciences
Medical College of Wisconsin
Milwaukee, Wisconsin
USA

# Preface

Surgical treatment of obstructive sleep apnea/hypopnea syndrome (OSAHS) is the most controversial, confusing and frustrating of all diseases that we treat as otolaryngologists. Although the majority of sleep medicine specialists deny the role of surgery in the treatment of this disease, we continue to introduce many new and innovative techniques that have proven beneficial to our patients. Clearly, no surgical treatment can compare to CPAP therapy with respect to morbidity and successful elimination of disease. Nevertheless, the reality is that approximately half of the patients with severe OSAHS cannot or will not use CPAP. In addition to those patients with severe OSAHS, more than 25% of the world's population has significant snoring, upper airway resistance syndrome or mild sleep apnea but refuse CPAP therapy. It is our responsibility to offer them alternatives that may palliate or possibly cure their symptoms.

We must understand that surgery is only salvage for those patients who fail noninvasive treatment. It is therefore crucial for every surgeon treating OSAHS to be an expert in its surgical and non-surgical treatment just as we are experts in the surgical and non-surgical treatment of sinusitis and head and neck cancer. Our approach must be comprehensive. This book therefore is comprehensive in presenting both surgical and non surgical treatment.

After a period of excitement when uvulopalatopharyngoplasty was introduced as a surgical treatment for OSAHS, there was tremendous disillusionment with the success rate. Similarly, LAUP and radiofrequency palatal reduction created initial excitement. As new procedures were developed most otolaryngologists remained unclear about two aspects of treatment:

1. When are surgical treatments appropriate and
2. Which treatment is appropriate for which patients

It is precisely these two questions that are answered by this book. Every leading sleep surgeon in the world was kind enough to give their time to help clarify their procedures with medical illustrations and algorithms to identify the role of that procedure in clinical practice. Most of these surgeons joined us for the first and second international conference on sleep and breathing. They then took the time to detail their techniques for this book.

This book also features outstanding illustrations by the artist James Millerick. Over the past 15 years, Jim has dedicated his skill and talents to illustrate new and innovative techniques in *Operative Techniques in Otolaryngology Head and Neck Surgery*. Thousands of our colleagues have complimented and benefited from his work. In this book, outstanding illustrations of complicated surgical techniques make each technique crystal clear and easy to follow. The book not only includes every published technique for OSAHS, but it focuses on the precise technique of each surgeon. Some procedures are presented more than once so that the reader can understand the technical nuances of each expert.

I believe that the combination of expert opinion complemented by clear illustrations help make this book a unique and useful guide for every sleep surgeon.

**Michael Friedman, MD, FACS**
August 2008

# List of Contributors

**Lee M. Akst, MD**
The Head and Neck Institute
The Cleveland Clinic Foundation
Cleveland, Ohio
USA

**Sandeep Berry, MD, FRCS, ORL-HNS**
Otolaryngologist
Department of Otorhinolaryngology, Head & Neck Surgery
Singleton Hospital
Swansea
UK

**Neil Bhattacharyya, MD, FACS**
Associate Professor of Otology & Laryngology
Division of Otolaryngology
Brigham and Women's Hospital, Boston;
Department of Otology & Laryngology
Harvard Medical School
Boston, Massachusetts
USA

**Amol M. Bhatki, MD**
Chief Resident
Department of Otolaryngology – Head and Neck Surgery
University of California – San Francisco
San Francisco, California
USA

**Darius Bliznikas, MD**
Resident
Department of Otolaryngology, Head and Neck Surgery
Wayne State University School of Medicine,
Detroit, Michigan
USA

**Michel A. Cramer Bornemann, MD, D-ABSM**
Co-Director, Minnesota Regional Sleep Disorders Center,
Hennepin County Medical Center;
Assistant Professor, Department of Neurology, University of Minnesota School of Medicine;
Faculty Instructor, Biomedical Engineering, University of Minnesota Graduate School, Twin Cities
Minneapolis, Minnesota
USA

**Scott E. Brietzke, MD, MPH**
Assistant Professor of Surgery
Uniformed Services University of the Health Sciences
Bethesda, MD;
Otolaryngology Service, Department of Surgery
Walter Reed Army Medical Center
Washington, District of Columbia
USA

**Michel Burihan Cahali, MD, PhD**
Professor of Otolaryngology
Department of Otolaryngology
Hospital das Clínicas, University of Sao Paulo Medical School
Hospital do Servidor Público Estadual, Sao Paulo
Sao Paulo, Sao Paulo
Brazil

**David H. Darrow, MD, DDS**
Professor
Department of Otolaryngology and Pediatrics
Eastern Virginia Medical School
Children's Hospital of The King's Daughters
Norfolk, Virginia
USA

**Terence M. Davidson, MD**
Professor of Surgery, Head and Neck Surgery
Associate Dean, Continuing Medical Education
University of California, San Diego School of Medicine
VA San Diego Healthcare System
La Jolla, California
USA

**Cindy den Herder, MD**
Resident
Department of Otolaryngology—Head and Neck Surgery
Academic Medical Centre
Amsterdam
The Netherlands

**Nico de Vries, MD, PhD**
Otorhinolaryngologist
Department of Otorhinolaryngology
St Lucas Andreas Hospital Amsterdam
Amsterdam
The Netherlands

# LIST OF CONTRIBUTORS

**Han Demin, MD, PhD**
Chairman, Chinese Society of Otolaryngology, Head & Neck Surgery
Department of Otolaryngology
Beijing Tongren Hospital
Capital University of Medical Science
Chairman, Chinese Medical Doctor Association ENT Branch;
Chairman, Council of World Chinese Otolaryngology, Head & Neck Surgery;
Director, Beijing Institute of Otolaryngology
Beijing
China

**Kai Desinger, MD**
CEO, Celon AG Medical Instruments
Teltow
Germany

**Christopher M. Discolo, MD**
Otorhinolaryngologist
Section of Pediatric Otolaryngology
Head and Neck Institute
Cleveland, Ohio
USA

**Kristin K. Egan, MD**
Resident
Department of Otolaryngology – Head and Neck Surgery
University of California San Francisco
San Francisco, California
USA

**Isaac Eliachar, MD, FACS, FICS**
Professor of Medicine (retired)
The Head and Neck Institute
The Cleveland Clinic Foundation
Cleveland, Ohio
USA

**David N.F. Fairbanks, MD**
Clinical Professor Surgery — Otolaryngology
George Washington University School of Medicine
Washington, District of Columbia
USA

**Valerie Flanary, MD**
Associate Professor
Division of Pediatric Otolaryngology
Department of Otolaryngology and Communication Sciences
Medical College of Wisconsin
Milwaukee, Wisconsin
USA

**Jon Freeman PhD, RPSGT**
Director of Laboratory Services
Clinilabs, Inc.
New York, New York
USA

**Michael Friedman, MD, FACS**
Professor of Otolaryngology
Chairman, Division of Sleep Surgery
Rush University Medical Center
Chairman of Otolaryngology
Advocate Illinois Masonic Medical Center
Advanced Center for Specialty Care
Chicago, IL
USA

**Andrew N. Goldberg, MD, MSCE, FACS**
Associate Professor
Department of Otolaryngology-Head and Neck Surgery
University of California, San Francisco
San Francisco, California
USA

**Yau Hong Goh, FRCS, FAMS (ORL)**
Consultant ENT, Head and Neck Surgeon
Mount Elizabeth Medical Centre
Singapore

**Christian Guilleminault, MD, DM, BiolD**
Professor, Sleep Medicine Program
Stanford University Sleep Disorders Clinic
Stanford, California
USA

**Berk Gurpinar, MD**
Assistant Professor
Department of Otolaryngology
Kasimpasa Military Hospital
Istanbul
Turkey

**Yanina Greenstein, BA**
Research Assistant
Department of Otolaryngology – Head and Neck Surgery
Boston University School of Medicine
Boston, Massachusetts
USA

**Tod C. Huntley, MD, FACS**
Otolaryngologist
Head & Neck Surgery Associates
The Center for Ear, Nose, Throat & Allergy
Indianapolis, Indiana
USA

**Mark Hon Wah Ignatius, FRCS, MMed (ORL)**
Associate Consultant
Department of Otolaryngology
Singapore General Hospital
Singapore

**Stacey L. Ishman, MD**
Assistant Professor
Department of Otolaryngology—Head and Neck Surgery
Johns Hopkins Medical Institutions
Baltimore, Maryland
USA

## LIST OF CONTRIBUTORS

**Ye Jingying, MD, PhD**
Director of Division of Pharyngolaryngeal Diseases and Sleep Center
Department of Otolaryngology
Beijing Tongren Hospital
Capital University of Medical Science
Beijing
China

**Kaalan E. Johnson, MD**
Resident Physician
Department of Otolaryngology—Head and Neck Surgery
Eastern Virginia Medical School
Norfolk, Virginia
USA

**Wang Jun, MD**
Vice Director of Division of Pharyngolaryngeal Diseases
Department of Otolaryngology
Beijing Tongren Hospital
Capital University of Medical Science
Beijing
China

**Ashutosh Kacker, MD**
Associate Professor
Department of Otolaryngology
Weill College of Medicine of Cornell University
New York, New York
USA

**George P. Katsantonis, MD, FACS**
Professor
Department of Otolaryngology
Head and Neck Surgery
St. Louis University School of Medicine
St. Louis, Missouri
USA

**Peggy E. Kelley, MD**
Associate Professor of Otolaryngology
Department of Otolaryngology
University of Colorado Health Sciences Center
Denver, Colorado
USA

**Naomi Ketharanathan, MD**
Resident
Department of Otolaryngology/Head and Neck Surgery
St Lucas Andreas Hospital
Amsterdam
The Netherlands

**Eric J. Kezirian, MD, MPH**
Assistant Professor
Department of Otolaryngology - Head and Neck Surgery
University of California San Francisco
San Francisco, California
USA

**Makoto Kikuchi, DDS, PhD**
President of Japanese Dental Sleep Medicine
Private Practice
Orthodontics and Dental Sleep Medicine
Narita
Chiba
Japan

**David Kim, MD**
Associate Professor
Director, Division of Facial Plastic and Reconstructive Surgery
Department of Otolaryngology - Head and Neck Surgery
University of California San Francisco
San Francisco, California
USA

**Arthur J. Klowden, MD**
Attending Anesthesiologist
Department of Anesthesiology
Advocate Illinois Masonic Medical Center
Chicago, Illinois
USA

**Peter J. Koltai, MD, FACS, FAAP**
Professor and Chief
Division of Pediatric Otolaryngology
Stanford University School of Medicine
Stanford, California
USA

**Dennis Kox, MD**
Resident
Department of Otolaryngology/Head and Neck Surgery
Leiden University Medical Centre
Leiden
The Netherlands

**Yosef P. Krespi, MD, FACS**
Chairman
Department of Otolaryngology
St. Luke's Roosevelt Hospital Center;
Professor of Clinical Otolaryngology
Columbia University
New York, New York
USA

**Manoj Kumar, MD**
Fellow
Department of Otolaryngology
Medical College of Georgia
Cortland, New York
USA

**Robert F. Kushner, MD**
Professor of Medicine
Northwestern University Feinberg School of Medicine
Chicago, Illinois
USA

## LIST OF CONTRIBUTORS

**Hsueh-Yu Li, MD**
Associate Professor
Department of Otolaryngology
Chang Gung Memorial Hospital, Chang Gung University
Taoyuan
Taiwan

**Kasey K. Li, MD, DDS, FACS**
Adjunct Associate Clinical Professor in Sleep Medicine
Department of Psychiatry;
Clinical Assistant Professor
Department of Otolaryngology
Stanford Sleep Disorders Clinic and Research Center
Palo Alto, California
USA

**Ho-Sheng Lin, MD, FACS**
Associate Professor
Department of Otolaryngology—Head and Neck Surgery
Wayne State University School of Medicine;
Chief, Section of Otolaryngology
Department of Surgery
John D. Dingell VA Medical Center
University Health Center
Detroit, Michigan
USA

**Hsin-Ching Lin, MD, FARS**
Associate Professor
Department of Otolaryngology
Chang Gung Memorial Hospital
Chang Gung University
Kaohsiung Medical Center
Taoynan
Taiwan

**Robert R. Lorenz, MD, FACS**
Section Head
The Head and Neck Institute
The Cleveland Clinic
Cleveland, Ohio
USA

**Stephen Lund, MD**
Co-Director, Sleep Disorders Institute
Director of Fellowship Training
Assistant Clinical Professor of Psychiatry
Columbia University College of Physicians and Surgeons
Sleep Disorders Institute
New York, New York
USA

**Mark W. Mahowald, MD, D-ABSM**
Director, Minnesota Regional Sleep Disorders Center
Chair, Department of Neurology
Hennepin County Medical Center
Professor, Department of Neurology
University of Minnesota School of Medicine

Minnesota Regional Sleep Disorders Center
Minneapolis, Minnesota
USA

**Eric A. Mair, MD, FAAP, COL (ret.), MC, USAF**
Adjunct Clinical Professor
Department of Otolaryngology—Head and Neck Surgery
University of North Carolina
Charlotte Eye, Ear, Nose and Throat Associates, PA
Charlotte, North Carolina
USA

**Robert H. Maisel, MD, FACS**
Interim Chairman and Professor
Department of Otolaryngology
University of Minnesota;
Chief, Department of Otolaryngology
Hennepin County Medical Center
Minneapolis, Minnesota
USA

**Joachim T. Maurer, MD**
Professor, Vice Chair
Department of Otorhinolaryngology, Head and Neck Surgery
University Hospital Mannheim
Mannheim
Germany

**Maria T. Messina-Doucet, MD**
Otolaryngologist
Lafayette, Louisiana
USA

**Peter G. Michaelson, MD, Major, USAF, MC, FS**
Chief
Department of Otolaryngology — Head and Neck Surgery
Wright Patterson AF Medical Center
Wright Patterson Air Force Base, Ohio
USA

**Samuel A. Mickelson, MD, FACS, ABSM**
Director, The Atlanta Snoring and Sleep Disorders Institute
Director, Advanced Sleep Center
Atlanta, Georgia
USA

**Soichiro Miyazaki MD, PhD**
Professor
Department of Sleep Medicine
Shiga University of Medical Science
Tsukiwa-Machi
Seta
Otsu
Japan

**Harlan R. Muntz, MD**
Director
Pediatric Otolaryngology
Primary Children's Medical Center
Salt Lake City, Utah
USA

# LIST OF CONTRIBUTORS

**James Newman MD, FACS**
Adjunct Assistant Professor
Department of Otolaryngology/Head and Neck Surgery
Stanford University Medical Center
San Mateo, California
USA

**Usharani Nimmagadda, MD**
Attending Anesthesiologist
Department of Anesthesiology
Advocate Illinois Masonic Medical Center
Chicago, Illinois
USA

**Kenny P. Pang FRCSEd, FRCSI(OTO), FAMS(ORL)**
Consultant
Director Sleep Surgery Service
Department of Otolaryngology
Tan Tock Seng Hospital
Singapore

**Nelson B. Powell, MD, DDS**
Adjunct Clinical Professor
Department of Otolaryngology—Head & Neck Surgery;
Adjunct Clinical Professor of Sleep Disorders Medicine
Department of Psychiatry and Behavioral Science
Stanford University School of Medicine
Palo Alto, California
USA

**Robert W. Riley, MD, DDS**
Adjunct Clinical Professor
Department of Otolaryngology—Head & Neck Surgery;
Adjunct Clinical Associate Professor of Sleep Disorders Medicine
Department of Psychiatry and Behavioral Science
Stanford University School of Medicine
Palo Alto, California
USA

**Anthony A. Rieder, MD**
Volunteer Clinical Faculty
Department of Otolaryngology and Communication Sciences
Medical College of Wisconsin
Wauwatosa, Wisconsin
USA

**Wietske Richard, MD**
Resident
Department of Otolaryngology—Head and Neck Surgery
Academic Medical Centre
Amsterdam
The Netherlands

**Sam Robinson, MD**
Clinical Instructor
Department of Otolaryngology
Tulane University;
Coastal ENT Associates, PLLC
Gulfport, Mississippi
USA

**Benjamin Salter, MD**
Resident
Department of Anesthesiology
Advocate Illinois Masonic Medical Center
Chicago, Illinois
USA

**Paul Schalch, MD**
Resident
Department of Otolaryngology—Head & Neck Surgery
University of California, Irvine Medical Center
Orange, California
USA

**Aaron E. Sher, MD, FACS, FAASM**
Medical Director, St. Peter's Sleep Disorders Center;
Capital Region Otolaryngology-Head and Neck Group, LLP;
Associate Clinical Professor, Otolaryngology-Head and Neck Surgery;
Associate Clinical Professor of Pediatrics
Albany Medical College;
Professor (adjunct), Neurocognitive Science Program (Psychology)
Graduate Center, City University of New York
Albany, New York
USA

**Donald M. Sesso, DO**
Attending Surgeon
Department of Otolaryngology/Head & Neck Surgery
Stanford University Medical Center
Facial Reconstructive Surgical and Medical Center
Palo Alto, California
USA

**Jeffrey H. Spiegel, MD, FACS**
Chief, Facial Plastic and Reconstructive Surgery;
Associate Professor
Department of Otolaryngology – Head and Neck Surgery
Boston University School of Medicine
Boston, Massachusetts
USA

**Boris A. Stuck, MD**
Professor, Sleep Disorders Center
Department of Otorhinolaryngology, Head and Neck Surgery
University Hospital Mannheim
Mannheim
Germany

**Winston Tan, FDSRCS, FAMS (OMS)**
Consultant Oral Maxillofacial Surgeon
Mount Elizabeth Medical Centre
Singapore

**Shanon Takaoka, MD**
Fellow, Sleep Medicine Program
Stanford University Sleep Disorders Clinic
Stanford, California
USA

# LIST OF CONTRIBUTORS

**David J. Terris, MD, FACS**
Porubsky Professor and Chairman
Department of Otolaryngology
Medical College of Georgia
Augusta, Georgia
USA

**Robert J. Troell, MD, FACS**
Director
The Center of Excellence for Facial, Plastic & Reconstructive Surgery
Las Vegas, Nevada
USA

**T.K. Venkatesan, MD**
Assistant Professor
Department of Otolaryngology
Rush University Medical Center
Advocate Illinois Masonic Medical Center
Advanced Center for Specialty Care
Chicago, Illinois
USA

**Jantine Venker, MD**
Resident
Department of Otolaryngology/Head and Neck Surgery
Leiden University Medical Center
Leiden
The Netherlands

**Heikki B. Whittet, MBBS, FRCSE**
Consultant Otorhinolaryngologist
Head & Neck Surgeon
Clinical Director
Department of Otorhinolaryngology—Head & Neck Surgery
Singleton Hospital
Swansea
UK

**B. Tucker Woodson, MD, FACS**
Professor and Chief Division of Sleep Medicine
Department of Otolaryngology and Communication Sciences
Medical College of Wisconsin
Milwaukee, Wisconsin
USA

**Min Yin, MD, PhD**
Associate Professor
Department of Otolaryngology
The First Affiliated Hospital of Nanjing Medical University
Nanjing
China

# Dedications

To my father, *z"l* – For teaching me the importance of integrity, precision, and the need to strive for perfection

To my mother, *z"l* – For teaching me that life is about giving to others

To my wife, Susan – For her devotion, understanding and support

To all my teachers – For teaching me that learning never ends

To all my fellows and residents, past and present – For making me truly learn and teach that which I thought I knew

To my surgical team, Jean Wurtz and Winnie Martinez, and surgical assistant, Pascuel Beltran – For helping me to help thousands of patients; their dedication and skills are unmatched

To my associate Dr. T. K. Venkatesan – For always being a loyal and dedicated colleague and friend

To all the authors – For sharing their expertise and time to make this book possible

To Jim Millerick – For illustrating this book with his unique talent and dedication

**Michael Friedman, MD, FACS**
August 2008

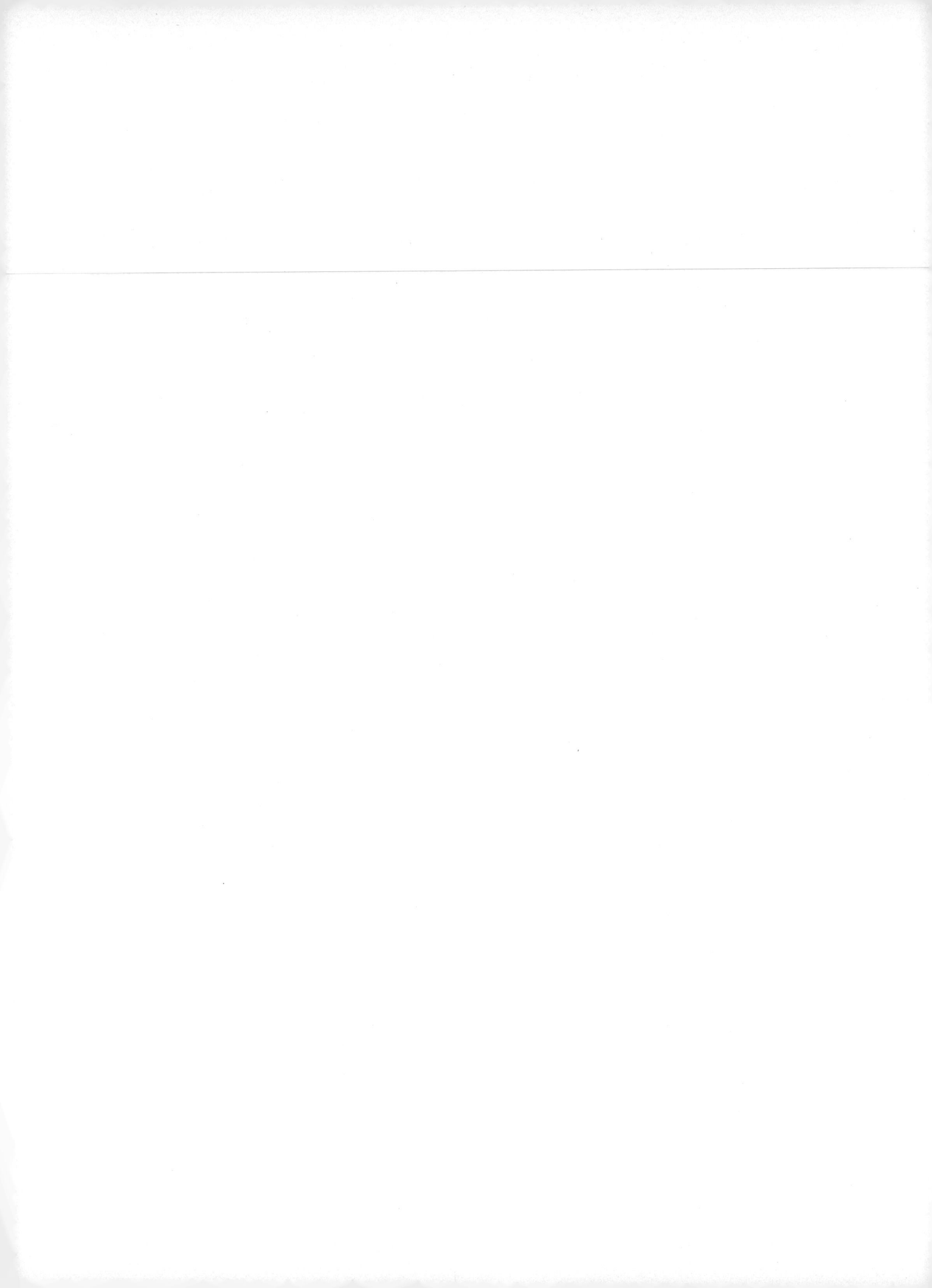

# SECTION A INTRODUCTION

## CHAPTER 1

# The role of the otolaryngologist in the treatment of snoring and obstructive sleep apnea

*Michael Friedman*

Sleep medicine is perhaps the youngest medical specialty recognized by the American Board of Medical Specialties (ABMS). The specialty has just recently been recognized and will offer its first qualifying board examinations in 2007. Prior to that time, the American Board of Sleep Medicine recognized itself and granted certification to its own members, but was never recognized as a medical specialty. People from medical and non-medical backgrounds interested in sleep medicine often took additional training and thus qualified to be certified in this field. Although the clinical and research people involved includes a large variety of different areas, the most common specialists have a background in pulmonary medicine or neurology. Otolaryngologists have played a distant role as consultants for the definitive treatment of sleep medicine.

Neurologists have training and expertise in interpretation of polysomnographic data, which overlaps with interpretation of electroencephalograms. Pulmonologists are experienced and trained in the use of continuous positive airway pressure (CPAP). Otolaryngologists are trained and have special expertise in the upper airway. For many years, otolaryngologists were not involved in the primary care of obstructive sleep apnea. We would often deal with obstructive sleep apnea/hypopnea syndrome (OSAHS) patients if they were specifically referred for surgery. Otolaryngology, however, is a specialty that deals with both surgical and non-surgical treatment of the upper airway. We have the expertise to obtain a proper history, to do a proper examination, and to assess dysfunction and disorders of the upper airway that no other specialist has. We, therefore, are the comprehensive treaters of such disorders as chronic rhinosinusitis and neoplasms of the upper airway. We do not wait for patients to be referred in for definitive treatment of these disorders.

We screen our patients for symptoms and we always include a thorough examination of the upper airway that would alert us to abnormalities that require additional history or diagnostic testing when it comes to problems with chronic rhinosinusitis or upper airway neoplasms. When diagnostic testing is ordered, we control those tests and independently evaluate the results even when other specialists – such as radiologists – interpret the examinations. After the evaluation, we help guide the patient to select the proper treatment.

We should take this approach for patients with OSAHS. OSAHS is extremely common and often overlooked by both patients and physicians. We should screen every patient for both symptoms and physical findings suggestive of OSAHS. This should be part of a thorough routine upper airway examination. We should have enough basic understanding of polysomnography to determine if the testing that is done is adequate. We should be able to offer our patients both surgical and non-surgical treatment.

Many patients seen by sleep specialists are never informed of surgical options. They are told that CPAP therapy is their only option. Although CPAP therapy is clearly safer and more effective than any surgical therapy, there is a huge number of patients who cannot or will not use CPAP.

Sleep medicine is a dynamic and rapidly growing field in which opportunities for physicians of many backgrounds abound. The newly recognized status of the field and the establishment of a certification examination by the

---

**Box 1.1  Symptoms associated with obstructive sleep apnea**

| Adults | Children |
|---|---|
| Heavy persistent snoring | Snoring |
| Excessive daytime sleepiness | Restless sleep |
| Apneas as observed by bed partner | Sleepiness |
| Choking sensations while waking up | Hyperactivity |
| Gastroesophageal reflux | Aggression and behavioral disturbance |
| Reduced ability to concentrate |  |
| Memory loss | Frequent colds or coughing |
| Personality changes | Odd sleeping positions |
| Mood swings |  |
| Night sweating |  |
| Nocturia |  |
| Dry mouth in the morning |  |
| Restless sleep |  |
| Morning headache |  |
| Impotence |  |

# SECTION A INTRODUCTION

ABMS will accelerate the growth of the field and increase the importance of board certification of practitioners. The public will increasingly expect that physicians who provide comprehensive sleep medicine services will have ABMS Sleep Medicine board certification. The new ABMS examination, starting in 2007, will be co-sponsored by the American Board of Internal Medicine, the American Board of Psychiatry and Neurology, the American Board of Pediatrics, and the American Board of Otolaryngology.

There are three pathways that qualify physicians to sit for the new examination: (1) certification by one of the primary sponsoring boards and the current ABMS; (2) certification by one of the primary sponsoring boards and completion of training in a 1-year sleep medicine fellowship program, not overlapping with any other residency or fellowship; and (3) clinical practice experience: this clinical practice experience pathway consists of a 5-year 'grandfathering' period open to physicians who are board certified in one of the sponsoring specialty boards and who can attest that he or she has the equivalent of 1 year of clinical experience in sleep medicine during the prior 5 years. This experience could, for example, be gained by an individual practitioner who has devoted one-third of his or her practice to sleep medicine over 3 years, or by someone who spent 25% of their practice in the field over the past 4 years. Physicians in the clinical practice pathway would also have to attest to a specified minimum number of patients seen and polysomnograms and multiple sleep latency tests read. At the end of this initial 5-year period, the only route to board eligibility will be through an accredited fellowship training program. This creates a one-time, unprecedented opportunity for pulmonologists, neurologists, psychiatrists, and other physicians already working in the field to sit for the board examination.

While no one knows the number of 'unboarded' sleep medicine practitioners, we are confident there are a considerable number of otolaryngologists and other specialists who practice sleep medicine who could, with a little work, become board certified in the next 5 years. The necessary work might include strategic use of continuing medical education activities in sleep medicine, reading review articles and texts, reviewing cases with experts, and board review courses. We believe a larger number of boarded sleep medicine physicians will be good for the field and, additionally, good for patient care, and will help address future workforce issues in sleep medicine.

Whether we choose to be boarded in sleep medicine or not, we are clearly the upper airway experts and, as such, should take the primary responsibility for treating this disorder. We can certainly consult with sleep specialists during the care of our patients. We should, however, be involved in the diagnosis, testing, and treatment in all areas.

SECTION B  DIAGNOSIS

CHAPTER 2

# Signs and symptoms of obstructive sleep apnea and upper airway resistance syndrome

*Christian Guilleminault and Shanon Takaoka*

## 1 INTRODUCTION

Obstructive sleep apnea (OSA) and upper airway resistance syndrome (UARS) represent two distinct but related entities in the spectrum of sleep-disordered breathing (SDB). OSA is characterized by repetitive partial or complete collapse of the upper airway during sleep, resulting in disruptions of normal sleep architecture and usually associated with arterial desaturations.[1] If these respiratory events occur more than five times per hour of sleep and are associated with symptoms, most commonly snoring, excessive daytime fatigue, and witnessed apneas, the term obstructive sleep apnea/hypopnea syndrome (OSAHS) is applied.[2] UARS is a more recent entity and describes patients with symptoms of OSA and polysomnographic evidence of sleep fragmentation but who have minimal obstructive apneas or hypopneas (Respiratory Disturbance Index < 5) and do not exhibit oxyhemoglobin desaturation.

Epidemiologically, OSAHS is estimated to affect 2–5% of the population.[3–5] Although it can occur at any age, OSAHS typically presents between the ages of 40 and 60 and increases with age.[6–8] Men are twice as likely to develop OSAHS with an estimated prevalence of 4% vs. 2% in women.[8] Other at-risk groups include postmenopausal women[9–11] who have a two to three-fold increase in prevalence of OSAHS, Pacific Islanders, Hispanic-Americans, and blacks.[5,12–15] Additionally, obesity and weight gain have been shown to be important risk factors in the development and progression of OSAHS in middle-aged adults.[8,16] UARS epidemiology is less well characterized, and to date, there has been no reliable assessment of its prevalence in the general population. Compared to OSAHS, there appears to be no gender bias,[17] and patients with UARS are commonly non-obese (mean Body Mass Index of 25 kg/m$^2$)[18,19] and are frequently younger (mean age of 37.5 years).[18]

OSAHS has been shown to be a gradually progressive disease, even in the absence of weight gain.[16,20] Some have attributed this slow progression to upper airway damage characterized by palatal denervation with a localized polyneuropathy and inflammatory cell infiltration of the soft palate thought to be caused by snoring-related vibrations and/or large intraluminal pressure oscillations in the setting of obstruction.[21,22] As OSAHS worsens in severity, it has been shown to be associated with the development of significant medical co-morbidities, including hypertension, cardiovascular disease, stroke, obesity, and insulin resistance. Furthermore, the presence of OSAHS has been linked to an increased risk of motor vehicle accidents,[23–25] impaired daytime performance and quality of life,[26,27] and increased mortality independent of co-morbidities.[28,29]

## 2 CLINICAL ASSESSMENT

A thorough history (with participation by the bedpartner if possible) and physical examination are integral to the initial evaluation of patients with suspected SDB. However, studies show that the predictive value of these clinical tools is poor. In an observational study of 594 patients, the sensitivity and specificity of subjective clinical impression in determining the presence of OSAHS were 60% and 63% respectively.[30] This study also showed that history, physical examination, and clinician impression were only able to predict OSAHS in about 50% of patients. Furthermore, none of the commonly reported symptoms alone has sufficient predictive value to provide an accurate diagnosis of OSAHS.[31] Diagnostic accuracy can be improved by identifying constellations of symptoms, such as snoring and witnessed apneas, which increase the sensitivity and specificity of OSAHS diagnosis to 78% and 67% respectively.[32,33] Ultimately, overnight polysomnography remains the gold standard in the initial diagnosis of SDB and the only means of distinguishing OSAHS from UARS. However, as such testing can be expensive, time-consuming, and may not always be readily available, a thorough history and physical examination remain important tools to identify those patients who need further evaluation by polysomnography.

# SECTION B  DIAGNOSIS

## 3 CLINICAL PRESENTATION OF OSA

### 3.1 SLEEP-RELATED (NOCTURNAL) SYMPTOMS

Snoring is the most frequently reported symptom in OSAHS and is found in 70–95% of such patients.[34] Typically, the snoring may have been present for many years but has increased with intensity over time and is further exacerbated by nighttime alcohol consumption, weight gain, sedative medications, sleep deprivation, or supine position. Snoring may become so loud as to be greatly disruptive to the bedpartner and is often a source of relationship discord; in one report, 46% of patients slept in a different room from their partners.[35] The characteristic snoring pattern associated with OSAHS is one of loud snores or brief gasps alternating with 20- to 30-second periods of silence. Because snoring is so common in the general population (35–45% in men, 15–28% in women[8,36]), it is a poor predictor of OSAHS; however, only 6% of patients with OSAHS do not report snoring and its absence makes OSAHS unlikely.[37] Corroboration with bedpartners is important as approximately 75% of patients who deny snoring are found to snore during objective measurement.[38]

Witnessed apneas are observed by up to 75% of bedpartners and are the second most common nocturnal symptom reported in OSAHS.[30,39] Occasional apneas are normal and do not cause symptoms; however, as the frequency of apneas increases, a certain threshold may be exceeded which results in symptomatic disease. This threshold is variable and unique to each patient such that some patients with a low Respiratory Disturbance Index (RDI) may be profoundly symptomatic while others with frequent respiratory events present with relatively few complaints.[40] Particularly in OSAHS of milder severity, the apneic episodes are usually associated with maintenance of respiratory movements and are terminated by loud snorts, gasps, moans, or other vocalizations and sometimes with brief awakenings and body movements. In more severe disease, cyanosis can occur along with the cessation of respiratory movement during the apnea which will often cause considerable distress to the bedpartner. Body movements at the time of arousals in severe OSAHS can be frequent and sometimes violent. Patients themselves are rarely aware of the apneas, vocalizations, frequent arousals, movements, or brief awakenings, although the elderly are particularly sensitive to the frequent nocturnal awakenings and will report insomnia and unrefreshing sleep.[1]

Nocturnal dyspnea, sometimes described by patients as a sensation of choking or suffocating, has been observed in 18–31% of patients with OSAHS.[35,41,42] These episodes typically occur with arousal, are associated with feelings of panic and anxiety, and generally subside within a few seconds. During apneas or hypopneas, greater negative intrathoracic pressures are generated as patients increase their inspiratory efforts to overcome the upper airway obstruction. This increases venous return to the heart and thus elevates pulmonary capillary wedge pressure which produces the sensation of dyspnea.[43,44] Other important causes of paroxysmal nocturnal dyspnea include left heart failure, nocturnal asthma, acute laryngeal stridor, or Cheyne–Stokes respirations; however, these episodes tend to be longer in duration and may also occur during the daytime.[39] Further investigation may be warranted to differentiate OSAHS from these other entities although they may also coexist.

Other common symptoms of OSAHS include drooling in about one-third and dry mouth in up to three-quarters of patients.[35] In one study of 668 patients with suspected SDB, dry mouth was observed in 31.4% of patients with confirmed OSA as compared to 16.4% in primary snorers and 3.2% in normal subjects.[45] Furthermore, there was a linear increase in prevalence of dry mouth as the severity of OSA increased. Sleep bruxism is also a common finding, occurring in 4.4% of the general population, with OSAHS patients being at higher risk (odds ratio 1.8) of reporting sleep bruxism.[46] In a small study of 21 patients, 54% of those with mild OSA and 40% of those with moderate disease were diagnosed with bruxism which was not observed to be directly associated with respiratory events but rather seemed to be related to sleep disruption and arousal.[47–49]

In addition to the common complaint of restless sleep and frequent awakenings, up to half of patients with OSAHS report nocturnal sweating that typically occurs in the neck and upper chest area.[41,42] This symptom is likely due to the increased work of breathing and respiratory effort in the setting of repetitive airway obstruction,[50] but may also be a manifestation of the autonomic instability observed in OSAHS. Similar to dyspnea, nocturnal diaphoresis is a highly non-specific symptom with a broad differential diagnosis, including perimenopausal state, thyroid disease, tuberculosis, lymphoma, and myriad other co-morbid conditions that warrant further investigation.[51]

Gastroesophageal reflux (GER) also occurs with greater frequency in patients with OSAHS with prevalence rates of 64–73%, but appears to be unrelated to the severity of SDB.[52,53] As GER and OSA share several risk factors, the exact relationship between the two entities has been difficult to characterize. However, it has been postulated that OSAHS may contribute to GER via the following mechanism: upper airway obstruction results in increased intraabdominal pressure combined with more negative intrathoracic pressure that produces an increased transdiaphragmatic pressure gradient, thereby promoting reflux of gastric contents into esophagus.[50] In a long-term study of 331 patients, treatment of OSAHS with nasal positive pressure resulted in a 48% decrease in the frequency of nocturnal GER symptoms with higher pressures being associated with greater improvement, suggesting that OSAHS may indeed be a causal factor in nocturnal gastroesophageal reflux.[54]

Nocturia has also been observed with increased frequency in OSAHS with a reported 28% of patients experiencing four to seven episodes nightly.[55] The presence and frequency of nocturia have been shown to be related to the severity of OSA,[55,56] and the proposed physiologic mechanisms include increased atrial natriuretic peptide secretion with a corresponding increase in total urine output,[57] or an increase in intraabdominal pressure. One study of 80 patients showed that although a majority of nocturnal awakenings were actually due to sleep-related phenomena (78.3% of 121 total awakenings), patients voluntarily urinated with each arousal and were only able to identify the correct source of the awakenings in five instances (4.9%).[58] These data show that patients mistakenly attributed their arousals to need to urinate when they were in fact due to SDB, suggesting that patient misperception may be a contributing factor to the increased frequency of reported nocturia in OSAHS.

## 3.2 DAYTIME SYMPTOMS

While the nocturnal symptoms of OSAHS are characteristic and tend to be more specific for the disease, the common daytime symptoms are less specific as they can result from abnormal sleep of any cause. Excessive daytime sleepiness (EDS) is the most common daytime complaint in patients with OSAHS;[30,35,41] however, as 30–50% of the general population also report moderate to severe sleepiness,[8,59] this symptom alone is a poor predictor of OSAHS. EDS is caused by sleep fragmentation leading to frequent arousals and insufficient sleep;[40] it is manifested by the inappropriate urge to sleep, particularly during relaxing, sedentary activities (i.e. watching television, reading). As it worsens, the inability to control sleepiness can result in dozing during meetings, active conversations, and at mealtimes. When severe, EDS can be a cause of motor vehicle and machinery accidents, poor school or job performance, and relationship discord.

Establishing the presence and severity of inappropriate daytime sleepiness can be challenging. EDS is often insidious, may be subtle, and is often confused with fatigue or lethargy. Patients themselves often have a poor perception of EDS severity and underestimate their level of impairment.[60] Co-morbidities such as chronic insomnia, depression, fibromyalgia, and other organic diseases, as well as medication use or substance abuse, may contribute to the symptom of inappropriate sleepiness. The clinician should focus on the urge to sleep in passive situations, since both physical and mental activity can mask underlying EDS.

The Epworth Sleepiness Scale (ESS) is a simple, self-administered questionnaire that is a quick and inexpensive tool with a high test–retest reliability,[2] and is thus a practical means of measuring the general level of daytime sleepiness. Patients are asked to assess their probability of falling asleep in eight situations commonly encountered in daily life, and a numeric score is tabulated. Higher Epworth scores, reflecting increased average sleep propensity, are able to distinguish patients with OSAHS from primary snorers and appear to correlate with severity of OSA as well as sleep latency measured objectively during multiple sleep latency testing.[35,61,62] The major disadvantage of the ESS is its reliance on subjective reporting by patients who may underestimate or intentionally underreport severity of daytime sleepiness.[39]

Morning or nocturnal headaches are reported in about half of patients with OSAHS, are typically dull and generalized, last 1 to 2 hours, and may require analgesics.[1,35] However, this symptom is non-specific as morning headaches occur in 5–8% of the general population and have been associated with many other entities, including other sleep disorders as well as depression, anxiety, and various medical conditions.[63,64] These headaches have been attributed to nocturnal episodes of oxygen desaturation, hypercapnia, cerebral vasodilatation with resultant increases in intracranial pressure, and impaired sleep quality with corresponding polysomnographic evidence of decreased total sleep time, sleep efficiency, and amount of REM sleep.[65,66] It has been observed that treatment of the underlying OSAHS results in disappearance of the morning headaches.

Neurocognitive impairment has also been observed in patients with OSAHS, although there is no practical method of quantifying such deficits in this setting. The processes most affected in OSAHS appear to be vigilance, executive functioning, and motor coordination.[67] Decreased vigilance is a result of sleep fragmentation, which can also lead to diminished concentration and memory (short term and long term). However, psychomotor impairment appears to be largely related to hypoxemia with more severe OSAHS potentially resulting in irreversible anoxic brain damage.[68–70] This hypothesis is supported by the observation that psychomotor deficits in patients with severe OSAHS are only partially reversible with treatment of the underlying sleep disorder with continuous positive airway pressure.[68,69]

Patients with OSAHS have a tendency to report decrements in their quality of life and often experience concomitant mood and personality changes. Depression is the most common mood symptom, and daytime sleepiness has been identified as a reliable predictor.[63,71] Other behavioral manifestations of OSAHS include anxiety, irritability, aggression, and emotional lability.[72] Treatment with continuous positive airway pressure has been shown to ameliorate symptoms of depression and thereby improve quality of life in some patients.[73,74] Sexual dysfunction, manifested primarily as erectile dysfunction and decreased libido, is also associated with OSAHS, and appears to be fully reversible with treatment of the underlying sleep disorder[75,76] (Table 2.1).

## 3.3 CLINICAL SIGNS

Physical examination of the patient with suspected OSAHS and UARS can reveal characteristic findings suggestive of

## SECTION B  DIAGNOSIS

| Table 2.1 Sleep and wake-related symptoms of OSAHS ||
|---|---|
| Nocturnal symptoms | Daytime symptoms |
| Snoring<br>Witnessed apneas<br>Dyspnea (choking/gasping)<br>Drooling<br>Dry mouth<br>Bruxism<br>Restless sleep/frequent arousals<br>Gastroesophageal reflux<br>Nocturia | Excessive daytime sleepiness<br>Morning headaches<br>Neurocognitive impairment:<br>  vigilance (secondary impact on<br>    concentration and memory)<br>  executive functioning<br>  motor coordination<br>Diminished quality of life<br>Mood and personality changes:<br>  Depression<br>  Anxiety<br>  Irritability<br>Sexual dysfunction:<br>  decreased libido<br>  impotence<br>  abnormal menses |

upper airway obstruction and associated SDB. Blood pressure should always be recorded as both hypertension and hypotension have been found in patients with SDB. Obesity has also been frequently associated with OSAHS,[8,37] particularly in women, and measurement of height and weight followed by calculation of Body Mass Index (kg/m$^2$) to define and quantify obesity are important components of the physical examination. Grunstein and colleagues demonstrated that a BMI of at least 25 kg/m$^2$ was associated with a 93% sensitivity and 74% specificity for OSAHS.[77] However, 18 to 40% of affected patients are less than 20% above ideal body weight,[35] and patients with UARS are typically non-obese.

Increased neck circumference has consistently been shown to be a more reliable clinical predictor of OSAHS and has been shown in one study to correlate with severity of disease.[30,78,79] Katz and colleagues showed that patients with OSAHS had an increased mean neck circumference (measured at the superior aspect of the cricothyroid membrane with the patient upright) of 43.7 cm ± 4.5 cm versus 39.6 cm ± 4.5 cm in control subjects ($P = 0.0001$).[80] Likewise, Kushida et al. found that neck circumference of 40 cm was associated with a sensitivity of 61% and specificity of 93% for OSAHS.[81] Thus, neck circumference should be routinely measured during physical examination, and if greater than 40 cm, underlying OSAHS must be considered and further investigated.

Examination of the upper airway is an essential component of the clinical evaluation of all patients with suspected SDB in order to identify potential areas of airway narrowing as well as to guide future therapies. The evaluation for both OSAHS and UARS is the same, and patients should be examined in both the upright and supine positions to optimize the detection of those anatomic features that predispose to SDB. The hallmark of both OSAHS and UARS is a crowded upper airway which is manifested by various characteristic morphologic abnormalities of the craniofacial, pharyngeal, dental, and nasal anatomy. Thorough inspection of these particular components of the upper airway, preferably with the aid of direct laryngoscopy, is essential in the evaluation of patients with suspected SDB.

The craniofacial abnormalities most commonly associated with airway narrowing and SDB are retrognathia[82] and high arched palate. Retrognathia, also known as mandibular retroposition, is a result of delayed growth of the mandible, maxilla, or both and is associated with posterior displacement of the tongue base.[81] Thus, the finding of retrognathia signifies a narrowed upper airway, particularly in the region of the retroglossal space. Patients with SDB are also commonly found to have high arched hard palates due to the early, forced expansion of the lateral palatine processes over the posteriorly displaced tongue prior to midline fusion. The significance of retrognathia and high arched palate in SDB was supported by Kushida et al., who described four craniofacial parameters indicative of airway narrowing: maxillary intermolar distance, mandibular intermolar distance, palatal height, and dental overjet (a sign of mandibular insufficiency).[81] Palpation of the temporomandibular joint with mouth opening may reveal varying degrees of dislocation (TMJ 'click') which confers greater risk of airway collapse in the supine patient due to posterior displacement during sleep.[50]

Examination of the pharyngeal structures may reveal further evidence of airway restriction and underlying SDB. These findings include macroglossia (often associated with lateral lingual scalloping by adjacent teeth), erythema and edema of the uvula due to snoring, and redundant lateral wall soft tissue with tonsillar pillar hypertrophy, and tonsillar enlargement (graded with 0–4 scale) which is a particularly significant cause of obstruction in children.[50] The degree of oropharyngeal crowding can be further characterized by the Friedman tongue position, formerly called the modified Mallampati score, which incorporates visual assessment of size, length, and height of the soft palate and uvula and is similar to the Friedman Tongue Index (further described in other sections of this text). These structures represent the anterior limit of the upper airway, and a low-lying, elongated, or enlarged soft palate/uvula decreases airway caliber and increases susceptibility to obstruction. This scoring system was initially developed to assess difficulty of airway intubation; a numeric grade from 1 to 4 is assigned depending on the relative size and positions of the soft palate, tip of the uvula, tongue, and tonsillar pillars. The Friedman tongue position has been shown to be an independent predictor of both the presence and severity of OSA with an average two-fold increase in odds of having OSA for every one point increase in the Friedman tongue position.[83] However, the gold standard in pharyngeal evaluation remains direct laryngoscopy as it is the most reliable means of identifying actual static and dynamic restriction of the retroglossal or retropalatal space, which are common sites of obstruction during sleep.

Abnormalities of dentition are often observed in patients with SDB and are typically reflective of maxillomandibular

# Signs and symptoms

## Table 2.2 Common physical findings in patients with OSAHS

| |
|---|
| *Craniofacial* |
| Retrognathia<br>High arched palate<br>Temporomandibular dislocation |
| *Pharyngeal* |
| Macroglossia<br>Erythema/edema of uvula<br>Elongated, low-lying soft palate<br>Tonsillar pillar hypertrophy<br>Tonsillar enlargement<br>Retropalatal, retroglossal space restriction |
| *Dental* |
| Overjet<br>Malocclusion<br>Bruxism<br>Orthodontia |
| *Nasal* |
| Asymmetric, small nares<br>Inspiratory collapse of alae and internal valves<br>Septal deviation<br>Inferior turbinate hypertrophy |

deficiencies and airway crowding. Patients with these physical features will frequently report previous wisdom teeth extraction and/or childhood orthodontia. Dental overjet is a common sign of underlying mandibular retroposition and refers to the forward extrusion of the upper incisors beyond the lower incisors by more than 2.2 mm. Findings of dental malocclusion and overlapping teeth indicate a restricted oral cavity that is prone to collapse. Because OSAHS has been associated with bruxism, evidence of teeth grinding should also be noted.

Examination of the nose is the last important component of the upper airway evaluation. Although nasal obstruction is rarely the sole cause of SDB, it appears to occur with higher frequency in OSAHS[84] and may contribute significantly to increased upper airway resistance and the development of UARS.[85] Furthermore nasal obstruction in children may cause chronic mouth breathing and secondarily result in abnormal craniofacial development. Inspection of the nose should note the size and symmetry of nares, collapsibility of internal/external valves and nasal alae with inspiration, evidence of septal deviation or prior nasal trauma, and hypertrophy of the inferior nasal turbinates.[50] Identifying nasal obstruction can be particularly important in patients with SBD who have difficulty tolerating nasal continuous positive airway pressure (CPAP) therapy as treatments such as septoplasty and turbinate reduction can decrease nasal resistance with resultant improvements in CPAP compliance and comfort (Table 2.2).

## 4 CLINICAL PRESENTATION OF UARS

UARS was first described in children in 1982,[86] although it was later observed that a population of adults with chronic daytime sleepiness but without typical polysomnographic evidence of OSA (apneas, hypopneas, or oxygen desaturations) exhibited increased inspiratory effort during sleep detected by esophageal manometry that resulted in transient, repetitive alpha EEG arousals.[18] Although these increases in upper airway resistance were not sufficient to cause detectable airflow abnormalities or oxyhemoglobin desaturation on routine sleep testing, the required increase in inspiratory work to overcome the elevated resistive load appeared to lead to recurrent arousals and sleep fragmentation and daytime hypersomnolence.

As such, there is considerable overlap between the symptoms of OSAHS and UARS, with excessive daytime sleepiness, snoring, and restless sleep being frequent complaints in UARS. However, key differences do exist, and recent data suggest that chronic insomnia is much more common in UARS than in OSAHS.[50] Many adult UARS patients report frequent nocturnal awakenings with an inability to fall back asleep (sleep maintenance insomnia) as well as difficulties with sleep initiation (sleep-onset insomnia). Chronic insomnia in UARS has been attributed to cognitive-behavioral conditioning resulting from frequent sleep disruptions.[87] Parasomnias are more prevalent in young patients with UARS, with sleepwalking with or without night terrors and associated confusional arousal being most common.[88] Treatment of UARS typically results in resolution of the parasomnias.

While daytime symptoms are also similar to those seen in OSAHS, adult patients with UARS are more likely to complain of daytime fatigue rather than sleepiness.[50] Cold hands and feet are described in half of UARS patients, and about a quarter (typically teenagers and young adults) will report symptoms of dizziness or orthostatic hypotension, with lightheadedness upon rapid change of positions.[89] This orthostatic intolerance may be related to the finding that roughly a fifth of UARS patients exhibit resting hypotension (systolic blood pressure < 105 mm Hg, diastolic < 65 mm Hg) as compared to OSAHS,[90] which is typically associated with hypertension.[91–93]

Lastly, Gold and colleagues observed that symptoms closely resembling those found in the functional somatic syndromes were more often reported by patients with UARS than by those with OSAHS.[17] Complaints such as headache, sleep-onset insomnia, and irritable bowel syndrome were more prevalent in UARS and decreased progressively as severity of SDB increased. Because of the frequency of these and other related non-specific somatic complaints such as fainting and myalgias, it is not uncommon for UARS to be misinterpreted as one of the many functional somatic syndromes, including chronic fatigue syndrome, fibromyalgia, irritable bowel syndrome, temporomandibular joint syndrome, or migraine/tension headache syndrome (Table 2.3).

SECTION B  DIAGNOSIS

Table 2.3  Major clinical features differentiating OSAHS and UARS

| OSAHS | UARS |
| --- | --- |
| Men > women | Men = women |
| Obese | Non-obese |
| Hypertension | Hypotension |
| Hypersomnia, excessive daytime sleepiness | Insomnia, fatigue |
| Rare somatic symptoms | Somatic symptoms |

## 5 SLEEP-DISORDERED BREATHING IN WOMEN

In the early descriptions of OSAHS, the vast majority of data came from studies performed on male subjects, and women were characterized as the 'forgotten gender.'[94] Preliminary observations of SDB in women appeared to suggest a strong correlation with obesity, resulting in a clear bias against the recognition of this entity in non-obese women (BMI < 30 kg/m$^2$), even in the presence of clinical and polysomnographic findings of OSAHS.[94,95] As a result, women experienced longer durations of symptoms and significant delays in appropriate referral and diagnosis compared to age-matched men.[94,96]

It is now recognized that women often present with different symptoms of SDB, report 'typical' symptoms less frequently, and may underestimate symptom severity as compared to men, which may be additional factors contributing to disease underrecognition in this population.[97] Symptoms more commonly observed in women include non-specific somatic complaints, such as insomnia, fatigue, myalgias, and morning headache.[17,98] Amenorrhea and dysmenorrhea have been reported in 43% of women with SDB.[94] Depression, anxiety, and social isolation occur with higher frequency in women as compared to men with SDB.[94,99] While women with OSAHS do tend to be more obese than men with similar disease severity, those with UARS are typically non-obese, younger, and have fewer witnessed apneas.[18,100]

## 6 SUMMARY

Although the understanding of sleep-disordered breathing continues to evolve, it is clear that both OSAHS and UARS are important causes of morbidity and mortality in a significant portion of the population. Snoring, excessive daytime sleepiness, and witnessed apneas are the hallmark symptoms of OSAHS, and although there is considerable overlap with UARS, there are several notable differences as well. Increased neck circumference and craniofacial characteristics suggesting airway crowding are also highly associated with SDB. Women tend to present with less typical complaints and may require a higher index of suspicion for diagnosis. Although it remains debatable whether OSAHS and UARS are distinct entities or represent ends of a continuum, the more clinically relevant task is the recognition that symptomatic patients without characteristic evidence of OSA may still have UARS, and thus warrant further evaluation with polysomnography.

## REFERENCES

1. American Academy of Sleep Medicine. Obstructive sleep apnea syndrome. In: The International Classification of Sleep Disorders Revised Diagnostic and Coding Manual; 2001, pp. 52–58.
2. American Academy of Sleep Medicine. Sleep related breathing disorders in adults: recommendations for syndrome definition and measurement techniques in clinical research. Sleep 1999;22:667–89.
3. Bresnitz EA, Goldberg R, Kosinski RM. Epidemiology of obstructive sleep apnea. Epidemiol Rev 1994;16:210–27.
4. Olson LG, King MT, Hensley MJ, et al. A community study of snoring and sleep-disordered breathing. Prevalence. Am J Respir Crit Care Med 1995;152:711–16.
5. Kripke DF, Ancoli-Israel S, Klauber MR, et al. Prevalence of sleep-disordered breathing in ages 40–64 years: a population-based survey. Sleep 1997;20:65–76.
6. Ancoli-Israel S. Epidemiology of sleep disorders. Clin Geriatr Med 1989;5.
7. Bixler EO, Vgontzas AN, Ten Have T, et al. Effects of age on sleep apnea in men: I. Prevalence and severity. Am J Respir Crit Care Med 1998;157:144–48.
8. Young T, Palta M, Dempsey J, et al. The occurrence of sleep-disordered breathing among middle-aged adults. N Engl J Med 1993;328:1230–35.
9. Bixler EO, Vgontzas AN, Lin HM, et al. Prevalence of sleep-disordered breathing in women: effects of gender. Am J Respir Crit Care Med 2001;163:608–13.
10. Young T. Menopausal status and sleep-disordered breathing in the Wisconsin Sleep Cohort Study. Am J Respir Crit Care Med 2003;167:1181–85.
11. Redline S, Kump K, Tishler PV, et al. Gender differences in sleep disordered breathing in a community-based sample. Am J Respir Crit Care Med 1994;149:722–26.
12. Grunstein RR, Lawrence S, Spies JM. Snoring in paradise – the Western Samoa Sleep Survey. Eur Respir J 1989;2(Suppl 5):4015.
13. Schmidt-Nowara WW, Coultas DB, Wiggins C, et al. Snoring in a Hispanic-American population. Risk factors and association with hypertension and other morbidity. Arch Intern Med 1990,150.597–601.
14. Friedman M, Bliznikas D, Klein M, et al. Comparison of the incidences of obstructive sleep apnea–hypopnea syndrome in African–Americans versus Caucasian–Americans. Otolaryngol Head Neck Surg 2006;134:545–50.
15. Ancoli-Israel S, Klauber MR, Stepnowsky C, et al. Sleep-disordered breathing in the African–American elderly. Am J Respir Crit Care Med 1995;152:1946–49.
16. Peppard PE, Young T, Palta M, et al. Longitudinal study of moderate weight change and sleep-disordered breathing. JAMA 2000;284:3015–21.
17. Gold AR, Dipalo F, Gold MS, et al. The symptoms and signs of upper airway resistance syndrome: a link to the functional somatic syndromes. Chest 2003;123:87–95.
18. Guilleminault C, Stoohs R, Clerk A, et al. A cause of daytime sleepiness: the upper airway resistance syndrome. Chest 1993;104:781–87.
19. Woodson BT. Upper airway resistance syndrome after uvulopalatopharyngoplasty for obstructive sleep apnea syndrome. Otolaryngol Head Neck Surg 1996;114:457–61.
20. Pendlebury ST, Pepin JL, Veale D, et al. Natural evolution of moderate sleep apnoea syndrome: significant progression over a mean of 17 months. Thorax 1997;52:872–78.

21. Boyd JH, Petrof BJ, Hamid Q, et al. Upper airway muscle inflammation and denervation changes in obstructive sleep apnea. Am J Respir Crit Care Med 2004;170:541–46.
22. Friberg D, Ansved T, Borg K, et al. Histological indications of a progressive snorers disease in an upper airway muscle. Am J Respir Crit Care Med 1998;157:586–93.
23. George CF, Nickerson PW, Hanly PJ, et al. Sleep apnoea patients have more automobile accidents. Lancet 1987;2:447.
24. Findley LJ, Weiss JW, Jabour ER. Drivers with untreated sleep apnea. A cause of death and serious injury. Arch Intern Med 1991;151:1451–52.
25. Young T, Blustein JF, et al. Sleep-disordered breathing and motor vehicle accidents in a populations-based sample of employed adults. Sleep 1997;20:608–13.
26. Chugh DK, Dinges DF. Mechanisms of sleepiness in obstructive sleep apnea. In: Sleep Apnea: Pathogenesis, Diagnosis, and Treatment, Lung Biology in Health and Disease. Pack AI, ed. New York: Marcel Dekker; 2002, pp. 265–85.
27. Jenkinson C, Stradling J, Petersen S. Comparison of three measures of quality of life outcome in the evaluation of continuous positive airways pressure therapy for sleep apnoea. J Sleep Res 1997;6:199–204.
28. Partinen MJ, Guilleminault C. Long-term outcome for obstructive sleep apnea syndrome patients. Mortality. Chest 1988;94:1200–4.
29. Yaggi HK, Concato J, Kernan WN, et al. Obstructive sleep apnea as a risk factor for stroke and death. N Engl J Med 2005;353:2034–41.
30. Hoffstein V, Szalai JP. Predictive value of clinical features in diagnosing obstructive sleep apnea. Sleep 1993;16:118–22.
31. Flemons WW, Whitelaw WA, Brant R, et al. Likelihood ratios for a sleep apnea clinical prediction rule. Am J Respir Crit Care Med 1994;150:1279–85.
32. Kapuniai LE, Andrew DJ, Crowell DH, et al. Identifying sleep apnea from self-reports. Sleep 1988;11:430–36.
33. Young T, Shahar E, Nieto FJ, et al. Predictors of sleep-disordered breathing in community-dwelling adults: the Sleep Heart Health Study. Arch Intern Med 2002;162:893–900.
34. Whyte KF, Allen MB, Jeffrey AA, et al. Clinical features of the sleep apnoea/hypopnoea syndrome. Q J Med 1989;72:659–66.
35. Kales A, Cadieux RJ, Bixler EO, et al. Severe obstructive sleep apnea. I: Onset, clinical course, and characteristics. J Chron Dis 1985;38:419–25.
36. Ohayon MM, Guilleminault C, Priest RG, et al. Snoring and breathing pauses during sleep: telephone interview survey of a United Kingdom population sample. BMJ 1997;314:860–63.
37. Strohl KP, Redline S. Recognition of obstructive sleep apnea. Am J Respir Crit Care Med 1996;154:279–89.
38. Hoffstein V, Mateika S, Anderson D. Snoring: is it in the ear of the beholder? Sleep 1994;17:522–26.
39. Schlosshan D, Elliott MW. Clinical presentation and diagnosis of the obstructive sleep apnoea hypopnoea syndrome. Thorax 2004;59:347–52.
40. Roehrs T, Zorick F, Wittig R, et al. Predictors of objective level of daytime sleepiness in patients with sleep-related disorders. Chest 1989;95:1202–6.
41. Maislin G, Pack AI, Kribbs NB, et al. A survey screen for prediction of apnea. Sleep 1995;18:158–66.
42. Coverdale SG, Read DJ, Woolcock AJ, et al. The importance of suspecting sleep apnoea as a common cause of excessive daytime sleepiness: further experience from the diagnosis and management of 19 patients. Aust NZ J Med 1980;10:284–88.
43. Buda AJ, Schroeder JS, Guilleminault C. Abnormalities of pulmonary artery wedge pressure in sleep-induced apnea. Int J Cardiol 1981;1:67–74.
44. Hetzel M, Kochs M, Marx N, et al. Pulmonary hemodynamics in obstructive sleep apnea: frequency and causes of pulmonary hypertension. Lung 2003;181:157–66.
45. Oksenberg A, Froom P, Melamed S. Dry mouth upon awakening in obstructive sleep apnea. J Sleep Res 2006;15:317–20.
46. Ohayon MM, Li KK, Guilleminault C. Risk factors for sleep bruxism in the general population. Chest 2001;119:53–61.
47. Sjoholm TT, Lowe AA, Miyamoto K, et al. Sleep bruxism in patients with sleep-disordered breathing. Arch Oral Biol 2000;45:889–96.
48. Macaluso GM, Guerra P, Di Giovanni G, et al. Sleep bruxism is a disorder related to periodic arousals during sleep. J Dent Res 1998;77:565–73.
49. Okeson JP, Phillips BA, Berry DT, et al. Nocturnal bruxing events in subjects with sleep-disordered breathing and control subjects. J Craniomandib Disord 1991;5:258–64.
50. Guilleminault C, Bassiri A. Clinical features and evaluation of obstructive sleep apnea–hypopnea syndrome and upper airway resistance syndrome. In: Principles and Practice of Sleep Medicine, 4th edn. Kryger MH, Roth T, Dement WC, eds. Philadelphia: Elsevier Saunders; 2005, pp. 1043–52.
51. Viera AJ, Bond MM, Yates SW. Diagnosing night sweats. Am Fam Physician 2003;67:1019–24.
52. Valipour A, Makker HK, Hardy R, et al. Symptomatic gastroesophageal reflux in subjects with a breathing sleep disorder. Chest 2002;121:1748–53.
53. Wise SK, Wise JC, DelGaudio JM. Gastroesophageal reflux and laryngopharyngeal reflux in patients with sleep-disordered breathing. Otolaryngol Head Neck Surg 2006;135:253–57.
54. Green BT, Broughton WA, O'Connor JB. Marked improvement in nocturnal gastroesophageal reflux in a large cohort of patients with obstructive sleep apnea treated with continuous positive airway pressure. Arch Intern Med 2003;163:41–5.
55. Hajduk IA, Strollo PJJ, Jasani RR, et al. Prevalence and predictors of nocturia in obstructive sleep apnea–hypopnea syndrome – a retrospective study. Sleep 2003;26:61–4.
56. Fitzgerald MP, Mulligan M, Parthasarathy S. Nocturic frequency is related to severity of obstructive sleep apnea, improves with continuous positive airways treatment. Am J Obstet Gynecol 2006;194:1399–403.
57. Umlauf MG, Chasens ER, Greevy RA, et al. Obstructive sleep apnea, nocturia and polyuria in older adults. Sleep 2004;27:139–44.
58. Pressman MR, Figueroa WG, Kendrick-Mohamed J, et al. Nocturia. A rarely recognized symptom of sleep apnea and other occult sleep disorders. Arch Intern Med 1996;156:545–50.
59. Duran J, Esnaola S, Rubio R, et al. Obstructive sleep apnea–hypopnea and related clinical features in a population-based sample of subjects aged 30 to 70 yr. Am J Respir Crit Care Med 2001;163:685–89.
60. Engleman HM, Hirst WS, Douglas NJ. Under reporting of sleepiness and driving impairment in patients with sleep apnoea/hypopnoea syndrome. J Sleep Res 1997;6:272–75.
61. Johns MW. Daytime sleepiness, snoring, and obstructive sleep apnea. The Epworth Sleepiness Scale. Chest 1993;103:30–36.
62. Johns MW. A new method for measuring daytime sleepiness: the Epworth sleepiness scale. Sleep 1991;14:540–45.
63. Ohayon MM. Prevalence and risk factors of morning headaches in the general population. Arch Intern Med 2004;164:97–102.
64. Ulfberg J, Carter N, Talback M, et al. Headache, snoring and sleep apnea. J Neurol 1996;243:621–25.
65. Goder R, Friege L, Fritzer G, et al. Morning headaches in patients with sleep disorders: a systematic polysomnographic study. Sleep Med 2003;4:385–91.
66. Provini F, Vetrugno R, Lugaresi E, et al. Sleep-related breathing disorders and headache. Neurol Sci 2006;27(Suppl 2):S149–S52.
67. Beebe DW, Groesz L, Wells C, et al. The neuropsychological effects of obstructive sleep apnea: a meta-analysis of norm-referenced and case-controlled data. Sleep 2003;26:298–307.
68. Ferini-Strambi L, Baietto C, Di Gioia MR, et al. Cognitive dysfunction in patients with obstructive sleep apnea (OSA): partial reversibility after continuous positive airway pressure (CPAP). Brain Res Bull 2003;61:87–92.
69. Montplaisir J, Bedard MA, Richer R, et al. Neurobehavioral manifestations in obstructive sleep apnea syndrome before and after treatment with continuous positive airway pressure. Sleep 1992;15(Suppl 6):S17–S19.
70. Naegele B, Thouvard V, Pepin JL, et al. Deficits of cognitive executive functions in patients with sleep apnea syndrome. Sleep 1995;18:43–52.
71. Kjelsberg FN, Ruud EA, Stavem K. Predictors of symptoms of anxiety and depression in obstructive sleep apnea. Sleep Med 2005;6:341–46.
72. Day R, Gerhardstein R, Lumley A, et al. The behavioral morbidity of obstructive sleep apnea. Prog Cardiovasc Dis 1999;41:341–54.

# SECTION B  DIAGNOSIS

73. Kawahara S, Akashiba T, Akahoshi T, et al. Nasal CPAP improves the quality of life and lessens the depressive symptoms in patients with obstructive sleep apnea syndrome. Intern Med 2005;44:422–27.
74. Schwartz DJ, Kohler WC, Karatinos G. Symptoms of depression in individuals with obstructive sleep apnea may be amenable to treatment with continuous positive airway pressure. Chest 2005;128:1304–9.
75. Goncalves MA, Guilleminault C, Ramos E, et al. Erectile dysfunction, obstructive sleep apnea syndrome and nasal CPAP treatment. Sleep Med 2005;6:333–39.
76. Teloken PE, Smith EB, Lodowsky C, et al. Defining association between sleep apnea syndrome and erectile dysfunction. Urology 2006;67:1033–37.
77. Grunstein R, Wilcox I, Yang TS, et al. Snoring and sleep apnoea in men: association with central obesity and hypertension. Int J Obes Relat Metab Disord 1993;17:533–40.
78. Davies RJ, Stradling JR. The relationship between neck circumference, radiographic pharyngeal anatomy, and the obstructive sleep apnoea syndrome. Eur Respir J 1990;3:509–14.
79. Stradling J, Crosby J. Predictors and prevalence of obstructive sleep apnoea and snoring in 1001 middle aged men. Thorax 1991;46:85.
80. Katz I, Stradling J, Slutsky AS, et al. Do patients with obstructive sleep apnea have thick necks?. Am Rev Respir Dis 1990;141:1228–31.
81. Kushida CA, Efron B, Guilleminault C. A predictive morphometric model for the obstructive sleep apnea syndrome. Ann Intern Med 1997;127:581–87.
82. Jamieson A, Guilleminault C, Partinen M, et al. Obstructive sleep apneic patients have craniomandibular abnormalities. Sleep 1986;9:469–77.
83. Nuckton TJ, Glidden DV, Browner WS, et al. Physical examination: Mallampati score as an independent predictor of obstructive sleep apnea. Sleep 2006;29:903–8.
84. Zonato AI, Bittencourt LR, Martinho FL, et al. Association of systematic head and neck physical examination with severity of obstructive sleep apnea–hypopnea syndrome. Laryngoscope 2003;113:973–80.
85. Guilleminault C, Kim YD, Stoohs RA. Upper airway resistance syndrome. Oral Maxillofac Surg Clin North Am 1995;7:397–406.
86. Guilleminault C, Winkle R, Korobkin R, et al. Children and nocturnal snoring: evaluation of the effects of sleep related respiratory resistive load and daytime functioning. Eur J Pediatr 1982;139:165–71.
87. Guilleminault C, Palombini L, Poyares D, et al. Chronic insomnia, post menopausal women, and SDB, part 2: comparison of non drug treatment trials in normal breathing and UARS post menopausal women complaining of insomnia. J Psychosom Res 2002;53:617–23.
88. Guilleminault C, Palombini L, Pelayo R, et al. Sleepwalking and sleep terrors in prepubertal children: what triggers them?. Pediatrics 2003;111:17–25.
89. Bao G, Guilleminault C. Upper airway resistance syndrome – one decade later. Curr Opin Pulm Med 2004;10:461–67.
90. Guilleminault C, Faul JL, Stoohs R. Sleep-disordered breathing and hypotension. Am J Respir Crit Care Med 2001;164:1242–47.
91. Bixler EO, Vgontzas AN, Lin HM, et al. Association of hypertension and sleep-disordered breathing. Arch Intern Med 2000;160:2289–95.
92. Nieto FJ, Young TB, Lind BK, et al. Association of sleep-disordered breathing, sleep apnea, and hypertension in a large community-based study. Sleep Heart Health Study. JAMA 2000;283:1829–36.
93. Peppard PE, Young T, Palta M, et al. Prospective study of the association between sleep-disordered breathing and hypertension. N Engl J Med 2000;342:1378–84.
94. Guilleminault C, Stoohs R, Kim YD, et al. Upper airway sleep disordered breathing in women. Ann Intern Med 1995;122:493–501.
95. Guilleminault C, Stoohs R, Clerk A, et al. Excessive daytime somnolence in women with abnormal respiratory effort during sleep. Sleep 1993;16:S137–S38.
96. Larsson LG, Lindberg A, Franklin KA, et al. Gender differences in symptoms related to sleep apnea in a general population and in relation to referral to sleep clinic. Chest 2003;124:204–11.
97. Kapsimalis F, Kryger MH. Gender and obstructive sleep apnea syndrome, Part 1: Clinical features. Sleep 2002;25:412–19.
98. Chervin RD. Sleepiness, fatigue, tiredness, and lack of energy in obstructive sleep apnea. Chest 2000;118:372–79.
99. Shepertycky MR, Banno K, Kryger MH, Differences between men and women in the clinical presentation of patients diagnosed with obstructive sleep apnea syndrome. 2005; 28:309–314
100. Quintana-Gallego E, Carmona-Bernal CC, et al. Gender differences in obstructive sleep apnea syndrome: a clinical study in 1166 patients. Respir Med 2004;98:984–89.

# SECTION B  DIAGNOSIS

## CHAPTER 3

# Airway evaluation in obstructive sleep apnea

*Boris A. Stuck and Joachim T. Maurer*

## 1 METHODS OF AIRWAY EVALUATION

As the interest in sleep-disordered breathing (SDB) has increased, various attempts have been made to assess upper airway anatomy in patients with this relatively frequent disorder. From the very beginning, researchers and clinicians used a multitude of different techniques not only to reveal potential differences in upper airway anatomy to better understand the origin and the pathophysiology of the disease but also to improve patient management and treatment success. While the value of thorough clinical assessment remains indubitable, the value of the Mueller maneuver has been questioned from the beginning. Static radiologic imaging techniques such as x-ray cephalometry, computed tomography (CT) scanning and magnetic resonance imaging (MRI) have been used mostly to detect differences in airway anatomy. Dynamic scanning protocols (e.g. ultrafast CT or cine MRI) and multiple pressure recordings have been used to gain insights into the mechanism and level of airway obstruction. Upper airway endoscopy has been inaugurated during sleep and sedated sleep to directly visualize airway obstruction, and the assessment of critical closing pressures has been used to quantify upper airway collapsibility.

## 2 CLINICAL EXAMINATION AND CLINICAL SCORES

A clinical examination including an endoscopy of the upper airway during wakefulness still constitutes the basis of every airway evaluation in snorers and obstructive sleep apnea (OSA) patients. Anatomic and static clinical findings were the first parameters to be evaluated in order to improve treatment success. The impact of enlarged palatine tonsils became evident in the surgical experiences with children. If performed simultaneously, tonsillectomy was described by most authors as a positive predictive factor for a successful uvulopalatopharyngoplasty (UPPP).

All the other anatomic parameters such as the size of the uvula, the existence of longitudinal pharyngeal folds and so forth did not show any relationship to the success rate of UPPP if evaluated separately. In contrast to the significant influence of enlarged tonsils in palatal obstruction, equivalent clinical finding for tongue base obstructions could not be detected. Woodson and Wooten only found hints that the oropharynx was normal in cases with retrolingual obstruction.[1]

Aware of this dilemma, Friedman et al. developed a clinical four degree staging system incorporating the tonsil size, the position of the soft palate, the tongue size, and the Body Mass Index (BMI).[2] This anatomic staging system predicted the success rate better than OSA severity did.[3] One may argue that the staging system merely reflects the clinical examination of an experienced sleep physician; nevertheless, such a system may be particularly helpful for less experienced observers.

Whether there are further predictive anatomic parameters for other surgical strategies has not been evaluated to date. The subjectivity of the assessment and the variability of the nomenclature of the clinical findings are significant limitations in this context.

## 3 THE MUELLER MANEUVER

Snoring as well as apneas can be simulated by most people and a direct effect of the Mueller Maneuver may be seen during wakefulness. Thus, snoring simulation and the effects of the Mueller Maneuver have been used in upper airway evaluation before surgical intervention in patients to predict surgical outcome and to improve patient selection. Nevertheless, the value of this relatively simple examination has been questioned repeatedly in the past.

### 3.1 TECHNIQUES OF THE MANEUVER

In order to be able to compare results between different investigators and patients as well as before and after an intervention, the Maneuver should be performed and documented in a standardized fashion. Due to its simplicity the classification according to Sher has been widely used to describe the finding obtained during the Maneuver.[3] In this classification, four degrees of airway obstruction at the different levels are defined, ranging from minimal to complete occlusion. Furthermore, any visible obstruction linked to the epiglottis is described. The reproducibility and inter-rater reliability of the results remain problematic. Taking all the available data into account, the reliability of the Mueller Maneuver remains highly questionable and the evaluation of the Maneuver seems highly subjective and hard to reproduce.

## 3.2 PREDICTING AIRWAY OBSTRUCTION DURING SLEEP AND SURGICAL SUCCESS

There is some evidence that the sites of obstruction detected with the Mueller Maneuver do not reliably reflect the sites of obstruction during sleep. This could be demonstrated through a comparison with videoendoscopy, multi-channel pressure recordings, and dynamic MRI during sleep. Table 3.1 shows the different sites of airway obstruction detected with the different methods of airway evaluation according to selected examples from the literature.

The impact of body position on the significance of the Mueller Maneuver remains unclear. During the Mueller Maneuver, healthy subjects may produce extreme negative pressures of −80 mbar without any signs of pharyngeal collapse.[4] This clearly demonstrates the significant differences in upper airway collapsibility during wakefulness and sleep. All the data given do not support the idea that the results obtained by the Mueller Maneuver may be transferred to natural sleep.

Various research groups were not able to better predict the success rates obtained with UPPP when using the Mueller Maneuver. Some authors considered an additional retrolingual collapse during the Mueller Maneuver as an exclusion criterion for a UPPP or performed a

**Table 3.1** Distribution of the sites of obstruction detected by different methods of airway evaluation (selected literature)

| Method | Author | Diagnosis | n | Palatal | Retrolingual | Combined | Epiglottis | No result |
|---|---|---|---|---|---|---|---|---|
| Mueller Maneuver | Petri et al. | OSAS | 30 | 8 | 0 | 22 | n.d. | 0/30 |
| | Sher et al. | OSAS | 171 | 101 | 56 | 14 | 2/101 | 0/171 |
| | Skatvedt | SBAS | 20 | 4 | 0 | 4 | n.d. | 0/20 |
| | Sum (mean value %) | | 221 | 113 (51%) | 56 (25%) | 40 (18%) | 2 (1%) | 0/221 (0%) |
| Endoscopy during sleep | Launois et al. | OSAS | 18 | 11 | 2 | 5 | n.d. | 8/26 |
| | Woodson and Wooten | OSAS | 11 | 5 | 6 | n.d. | n.d. | n.d. |
| | Sum (mean value %) | | 29 | 16 (55%) | 8 (28%) | 5 (17%) | | 8/26 (31%) |
| Endoscopy under sedation | Croft and Pringle | SBAS | 56 | 25 | n.d. | 31 | 0 | 15/71 |
| | Pringle and Croft | SBAS | 70 | 33 | 9 | 28 | 0 | 20/90 |
| | Camilleri et al. | SBAS | 25 | 17 | 0 | 8 | 0 | 2/27 |
| | Hessel et al. | SBAS | 340 | 111 | 8 | 221 | n.d. | n.d. |
| | Steinhart et al. | SBAS | 306 | 139 | 23 | 134 | 10 | 16/322 |
| | Den Herder et al. | SBAS | 127 | 65 | 15 | 47 | n.d. | n.d. |
| | Quinn et al. | Snoring | 50 | 35 | 4 | 5 | 6 | 4/54 |
| | Marais | Snoring | 168 | 101 | 52 | 13 | 2 | 37/205 |
| | El Badawey et al. | Snoring | 46 | 8 | 2 | 36 | n.d. | 5/55 |
| | Abdullah et al. | Snoring | 30 | 12 | 0 | 18 | 0 | n.d. |
| | Abdullah et al. | OSAS | 89 | 12 | 4 | 71 | 2 | 4/93 |
| | Sum (mean value %) | | 1307 | 558 (43%) | 117 (9%) | 612 (47%) | 20 (1.5%) | 103/917 (11%) |
| Pressure recordings during sleep | Hudgel | OSAS | 9 | 4 | 5 | 0 | n.d. | 0/9 |
| | Chaban et al. | OSAS | 10 | 5 | 5 | 0 | n.d. | n.d. |
| | Metes et al. | SBAS | 51 | 30 | 7 | n.d. | n.d. | 13/51 |
| | Tvinnereim and Miljeteig | OSAS | 12 | 6 | 2 | n.d. | 4 (?) | 0/12 |
| | | | 20 | 2 | 5 | 10 | n.d. | 0/20 |
| | Skatvedt | SBAS | 20 | 5 | 4 | 9 | 2 (?) | 0/20 |
| | Katsantonis et al. | OSAS | 11 | 8 | 3 | n.d. | n.d. | n.d. |
| | Woodson and Wooten | OSAS | | | | | | |
| | Sum (mean value %) | | 133 | 60 (47%) | 31 (23%) | 19 (14%) | 6 (4,5%?) | 13/112 (12%) |

SBAS, patients with primary snoring or OSAS; OSAS, only patients with OSAS; Palatal, nasopharynx, tonsils, soft palate and/or lateral pharyngeal wall; Retrolingual, tongue base and/or hypopharynx; Epiglottis, exclusively epiglottis; No result, either the method was not tolerated or the result was not utilizable. n.d.: not detected.

partial resection of the epiglottis in UPPP failure patients with laryngeal obstruction during the Mueller Maneuver by partial resection of the epiglottis.

## 3.3 SIGNIFICANCE OF THE MUELLER MANEUVER

The Mueller Maneuver is a safe and simple examination that does not exert relevant strain on the patient. The reliability of the Mueller Maneuver is insufficient and the results of the Mueller Maneuver cannot be transferred to natural sleep. A hypopharyngeal collapse may indicate the exclusion of patients from UPPP. Altogether, the Mueller Maneuver does not facilitate patient selection for the varying surgical interventions used in OSA patients.

## 4 X-RAY CEPHALOMETRY

Over the years, lateral x-ray cephalometry has become one of the standard diagnostic tools in patients with SDB, especially with regard to the evaluation of the skeletal craniofacial morphology. Not specifically developed for the fields of SDB, imaging techniques and standards for data analysis have been incorporated from the field of maxillofacial surgery, where it has already been used for decades.

## 4.1 PROVIDING INSIGHTS INTO THE PATHOPHYSIOLOGY OF SDB

Extensive literature is available comparing upper airway anatomy and dentofacial structures using x-ray cephalometry between OSA patients and healthy controls. In siblings a significantly longer distance from the hyoid bone to the mandibular plane has been documented in those affected by SDB.[5] Further differences were described by different working gropus. The concrete results are often difficult to compare, as the authors not only use different landmarks and parameters but also sometimes rather complex calculated indices and ratios to describe the differences they found. Therefore, the following findings in OSA patients can only be a selection: longer soft palates, reduced minimum palatal airway widths, increased thickness of the soft palate, differences in calculated craniofacial scores, increased pharyngeal lengths, retroposition of the mandible or the maxilla, micrognathia, increased mid-facial heights, and differences in hyoid bone position. In general, the differences are more pronounced in non-obese patients, suggesting that craniofacial changes play a dominant role in this subgroup. Furthermore, substantial differences in maxillofacial appearance of different ethnic groups need to be taken into account.

Various authors could demonstrate that the aberrations in craniofacial morphology they found in OSA patients were more pronounced in patients with severe OSA. Dempsey et al. demonstrated that in non-obese patients and in patients with narrow upper airway dimensions, four cephalometric dimensions were the dominant predictors of Apnea/Hypopnea Index (AHI) level, accounting for 50% of the variance.[6] Rose et al. questioned the diagnostic relevance of x-ray cephalometry for OSA, as they found no direct correlation between skeletal cephalometric findings and OSA severity; nevertheless, they also reported a correlation with hyoid bone position.[7]

## 4.2 X-RAY CEPHALOMETRY AND THERAPEUTIC INTERVENTIONS

One of the dominant indications for performing x-ray cephalometry has been treatment with oral appliances. Especially with regard to the evaluation of potential predictive parameters for treatment success and dental side effects, x-ray cephalometry has been the standard diagnostic tool. As early as 1995, Mayer and Meier-Ewert, two of the fathers of treatment with oral appliances in Europe, looked for cephalometric predictors of treatment success[8] and reported that specific cephalometric variables were indeed predictive for the therapeutic effect. Other authors have confirmed the existence of predictive cephalometric parameters, especially in relation to hyoid bone position and oropharyngeal airway dimension. Nevertheless, the problems related to different nomenclature and selection of airway parameters described above remain.

X-ray cephalometry has also been evaluated with regard to potential predictive parameters for postoperative results of UPPP alone or in combination with other approaches. To date there is no convincing evidence that skeletal measurements obtained with x-ray cephalometry could predict the outcome of UPPP. Nevertheless, lateral x-ray cephalometry is the standard tool in the preoperative evaluation of the craniofacial skeletal anatomy before maxillomandibular advancement surgery. It can be regarded as a mandatory procedure and its value is not questioned.[9]

## 4.3 X-RAY CEPHALOMETRY IN PATIENT MANAGEMENT

X-ray cephalometry has provided substantial insights into the pathophysiology of OSA, demonstrating significant craniofacial characteristics associated with this disease. Although the results are not easy to compare, specific cephalometric characteristics have been repeatedly mentioned as a risk factor for OSA and correlate with the severity of the disease. Selected cephalometric parameters indicate favorable results of mandibular advancement by oral appliances. Nevertheless, no cephalometric parameter exists that would reliably rule out treatment success with an oral appliance and surgical outcome cannot be predicted. This may explain why x-ray cephalometry has not become a routine procedure in the diagnostic work-up of OSA as long as maxillomandibular surgery is not planned.

## 5 CT SCANNING

Compared to lateral x-ray cephalometry, CT scanning significantly improves soft tissue contrast and allows precise measurements of cross-sectional areas at different levels as well as three-dimensional reconstruction and volumetric assessment. Fast scanning times and relatively quiet scanning conditions even allow a dynamic assessment of the airway during a respiratory cycle as well as measurements during natural sleep. Nevertheless, ionizing radiation remains problematic.

### 5.1 TECHNIQUES AND STANDARDS

Despite its widespread use in airway assessment in patients with SDB, no standardized scanning protocol exists for this indication and the nomenclature of the soft tissue structures is not uniform. In addition to a two-dimensional assessment of the upper airway, three-dimensional techniques were used to assess volumes of soft tissue structures and airway spaces. As early as 1987 ultrafast or dynamic CT was inaugurated in this field to evaluate dynamic changes of the upper airway dimensions during respiratory cycles. While the vast majority used CT imaging during wakefulness, several authors also used scanning protocols under hypnotic relaxation, sleep and sleep during apneas, and also used direct comparisons between wakefulness and sleep.

### 5.2 PROVIDING INSIGHTS INTO THE PATHOPHYSIOLOGY OF SDB

The majority of published data points to potential differences in upper airway structures and dimension between OSA patients and healthy controls or snorers. In general, the upper airway is described as smaller in apneic patients compared to controls, especially with regard to the retropalatal region. Cross-sectional areas were found to be significantly narrower in affected patients. Inversely, retropalatal tissue was described as being greater in OSA patients compared to controls and larger tongue and soft palates dimensions and volumes were found. Schwab et al. have pointed out the differences in upper airway configuration with an anterior–posterior configuration – a result that is in line with data obtained from magnetic resonance imaging.[10]

Different authors have described anatomic conditions that reflect the severity of the disease and have correlated their measurements with polysomnographic data. A high apnea index seems to be associated with large tongue and soft palate volumes, and a significant correlation of the retropalatal space and its lateral diameter with the Respiratory Disturbance Index was documented. A combination of the smallest cross-sectional area, the upper airway resistance, and the Body Mass Index was used to predict the severity of OSA and a narrower cross-sectional area and a thicker soft palate were found in severely affected patients compared to patients with only mild to moderate OSA.

With the help of dynamic and ultrafast CT further insights into airway obstruction were gained. In addition to the fact that the naso- and oropharyngeal airways were smaller in OSA patients compared to weight-matched controls, an increased collapsibility in affected patients was found. During a respiratory cycle, substantial changes in cross-sectional areas were seen in patients with SDB, the velopharyngeal segment being the narrowest and most collapsible region.[11] These results were essentially confirmed later, showing that patients with severe OSA have significantly narrower cross-sectional areas at the velopharyngeal level[12] (see Figure 3.1).

### 5.3 EVALUATING THE EFFECTS OF THERAPEUTIC INTERVENTION

Effects of therapeutic intervention have been assessed, mostly with regard to treatment with oral appliances and surgical intervention. While a decrease in the diameters at the retropalatal and retroglossal level was seen during apnea, these cross-sectional areas were significantly enlarged with the help of the appliance. With regard to surgical treatment effects, it has been demonstrated that the

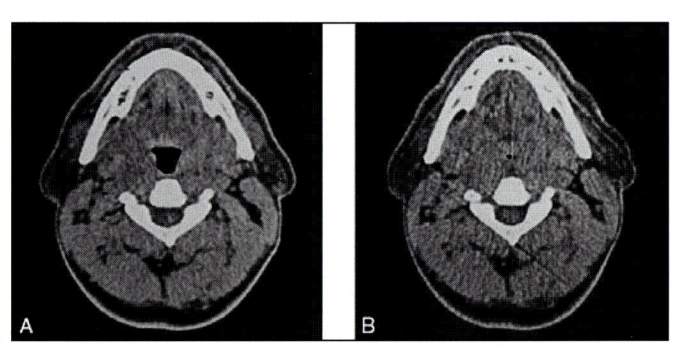

**Fig. 3.1** Upper airway narrowing during tidal breathing as assessed with CT scanning. A. Cross-sectional image of a patient at the level of uvula in tidal breathing. B. The significant narrowing at the same level in forced expiration is seen. The region of interest (*white line*) was used to assess total cross-sectional areas in each image (according to Yucel et al., 2005).[12]

upper airway increases after mandibular distraction osteogenesis in children and after maxillomandibular advancement in adults. Even more data are available for the effects of UPPP and its modifications, demonstrating that UPPP significantly increases the upper airway cross-sectional area and that the oropharyngeal enlargement seen in pharyngeal CT measures is associated with a good outcome in UPPP.

## 5.4 CT SCANNING IN PATIENT MANAGEMENT

CT scanning has provided valuable insights into the pathophysiology of SDB. In addition, it has often been stated that CT scanning does play or will play a major role in the management of patients with SDB. Nevertheless, CT scanning has not become part of the routine assessment of patients with SDB, especially not with regard to surgical treatment selection. The limited availability, associated costs, practical considerations and ionizing radiation remain problematic. Beneficial effects on treatment selection and thereby treatment outcome have been postulated repeatedly but could not be demonstrated to date.

## 6 MR IMAGING

Compared to lateral x-ray cephalometry or CT scanning magnetic resonance imaging (MRI) offers various advantages, such as excellent soft tissue contrast, three-dimensional assessments of tissue structures, and lack of ionizing radiation. The latter has made MR-imaging the imaging technique of choice in the assessment of children with SDB.

## 6.1 TECHNIQUES AND STANDARDS

Concerning their scientific or clinical use in the context of SDB, routine imaging techniques were initially applied following various protocols used in everyday clinical practice. For patients suffering from SDB it was attempted to determine anatomic preconditions and peculiarities for SDB. In this research, comparisons with healthy controls have been utilized, measuring two-dimensional distances and diameters of the upper airway or its related structures. In addition, three-dimensional data were obtained. Volumes were either calculated based on cross-sectional areas and slice thickness or established by various computerized models. Ultimately, ultrafast or dynamic imaging was used to visualize dynamic motion of the upper airway to assess upper airway collapse or differences in upper airway motion between patients with SDB and healthy controls. Subjects were either measured during wakefulness or during wakefulness and sleep; children were routinely scanned under sedation. Sleep in adults was either pharmacologically induced or spontaneous.

Only a small number of authors have attempted to establish distinct protocols for MRI of the upper airway in SDB; the results of the measurements were either validated with a phantom or tested for variability in repeated measures over time and with different investigators.[13] Validation and standardization of this imaging paradigm seem essential; nevertheless, in contrast to, for example, lateral x-ray cephalometry, hardly any consensual standards exist for this indication.

## 6.2 PROVIDING INSIGHTS INTO THE PATHOPHYSIOLOGY OF SDB

### 6.2.1 OSA IN CHILDREN

Especially in children, extensive research has been done with regard to the pathophysiology of OSA. Children with or without persistent OSA after tonsillectomy and adenoidectomy were compared and it was demonstrated that enlarged lingual tonsils were present in those children with persistent disease, especially in children with Down syndrome. Further findings were an airway restriction in the vicinity of both the adenoids and the tonsils and an enlarged soft palate in the affected group. Nevertheless, the airway restriction is not limited to these areas but seems to occur throughout the initial two thirds of the upper airway. Furthermore, a close dependency between the frequency of respiratory events and the size of the tonsils and the soft palate could be demonstrated and the upper airway narrowing was more pronounced in those children with a high number of respiratory events compared to the less affected group. With regard to dynamic airway evaluation, more pronounced fluctuations in airway area during tidal breathing[14] and significant differences in airway motion[15] were demonstrated in children with OSA compared to controls.

### 6.2.2 OSA IN ADULTS

As early as 1989, authors pointed out the significance of pharyngeal fat deposits in adult patients with OSA.[16] In this group, more fat is present in the areas surrounding the collapsible segment of the pharynx and fat deposition has been described even in non-obese patients with OSA. Some authors could demonstrate a trend for larger tongues or a significantly higher tongue volume in relation to the oral cavity volume in patients with OSA compared to controls. Other anatomic conditions associated with SDB were an elliptic horizontal cross-sectional area of the pharynx and large volumes of the lateral pharyngeal walls and total soft tissue surrounding the upper airway. Nevertheless, other authors did not find any significant differences in tongue volume, soft palates or pharyngeal walls, but pointed out specific anatomic factors of the mandible in OSA patients.

Numerous authors have demonstrated that the mechanism and level of airway obstruction can be visualized by MRI, even under natural sleep[17] (Figure 3.2). The fact that patients with OSA present multiple sites of pharyngeal abnormality was demonstrated by Suto et al. as early as 1993;[18] nevertheless, the authors pointed out that the levels of airway obstruction during wakefulness did not match those levels found during sleep. Other trials have shown that no pharyngeal airway narrowing was seen in the healthy subjects but a significant narrowing was seen in the OSA patients during wakefulness, and even more so during sleep. Moreover, it was demonstrated that apneic patients have a more circular occlusion, underlining the relevance of the lateral pharyngeal walls in the pathogenesis of airway obstruction.

## 6.3 EVALUATING THE EFFECTS OF THERAPEUTIC INTERVENTION

Finally, MRI has been used to assess the effects or side effects of various therapeutic interventions, including surgical and non-surgical strategies. Although potential anatomic criteria for successful treatment with mandibular advancement devices were reported, MRI has not become a routine procedure in the management of patients designated for treatment with a mandibular advancement device.

With regard to surgical treatment, MRI has been used to assess potential effects of surgery on upper airway anatomy. In radiofrequency surgery, imaging has been used to visualize immediate postoperative effects on the soft palate and the tongue base, the latter leading to concrete recommendations for the technical settings of this technique.[19] A standardized protocol has furthermore been used to study anatomic changes at the upper airway after radiofrequency surgery of the tongue base[20] and after hyoid suspension.[21]

## 6.4 MRI IN PATIENT MANAGEMENT

Static and dynamic MRI has substantially improved our understanding of the pathophysiology of SDB. Significant differences in upper airway anatomy and structure have been detected between patients with SDB and healthy subjects, and relevant insights have been gained in terms of the mechanisms and levels of airway obstruction. Nevertheless, MRI has not become a standard procedure either in the diagnostic work-up for patients with SDB or in the management of the disease in terms of surgical or non-surgical treatment, as a number of issues remain unresolved. MRI during sleep (especially spontaneous sleep) is possible but not easy to perform and measurements during wakefulness or induced sleep are, to a certain extent, artificial or may simply not reflect clinical conditions. Furthermore, the results of MRI, even when performed during sleep, can

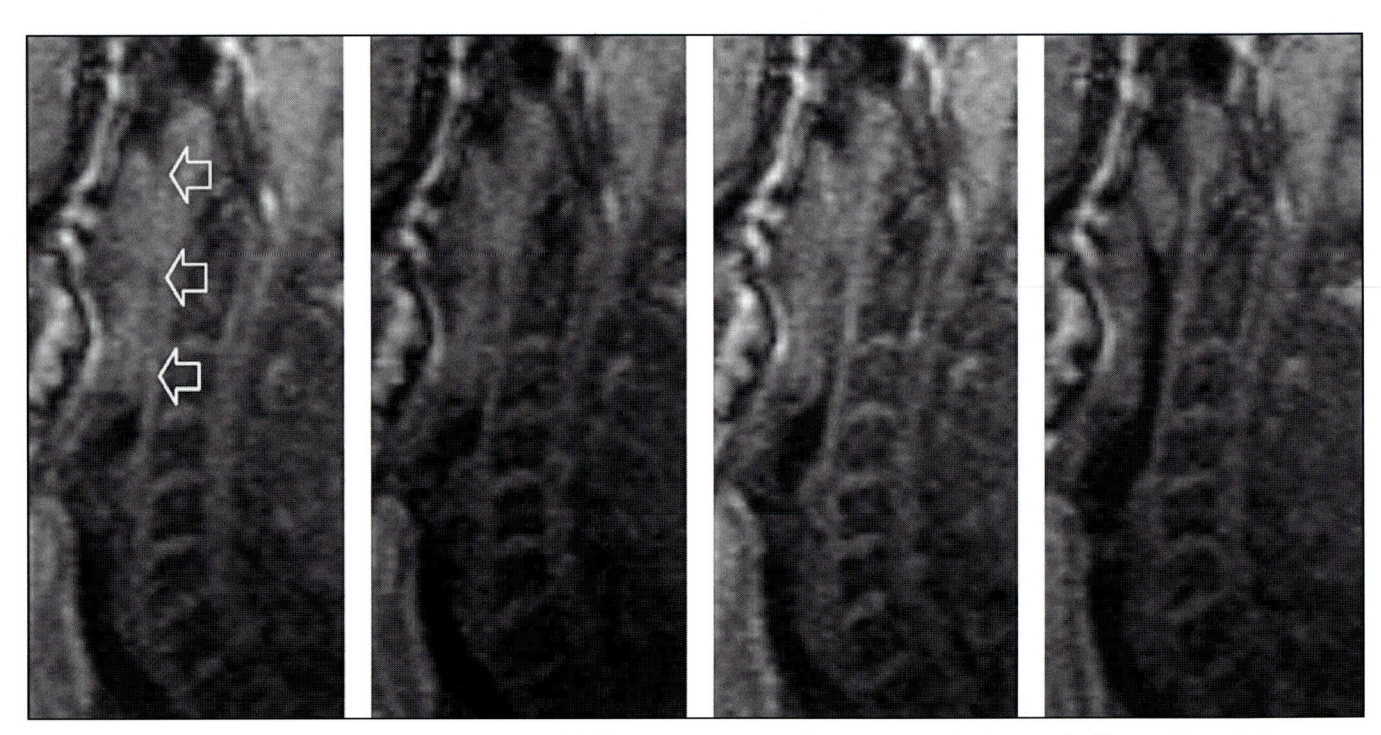

**Fig. 3.2** Complete pharyngeal collapse as detected with dynamic MRI during natural sleep. Dynamic single slice images of a 45 year old man during an apnea period. The first images show the complete naso-, oro- and hypopharyngeal obstruction; the arrows mark collapse of the different pharyngeal regions (according to Schoenberg et al. 2000).[17]

only provide information concerning a short period of time and are limited to the supine position. For routine clinical application, the limited availability and the associated costs are additional limiting factors.

## 7 VIDEOENDOSCOPY DURING SPONTANEOUS SLEEP

As early as 1978 the first report about videoendoscopic recordings of the pharynx and larynx during sleep was published. Borowiecki and colleagues described a palatopharyngeal collapse at the end of expiration and directly before inspiration in patients with OSA.[22] They described different degrees of airway obstruction, often associated with a medialization of the lateral pharyngeal walls. As there was no treatment other than tracheotomy available at this time for those patients, patient selection was not an issue.

Today videoendoscopy during spontaneous sleep is performed in order to improve patient selection for the different treatments available and may also be performed in combination with overnight sleep recordings. Because videoendoscopy during spontaneous sleep allows the assessment of the upper airway during different sleep stages and lacks the side effects of sedating drugs, this method may be considered superior to videoendoscopy under sedation. However, sleep videoendoscopy is rarely performed as it usually requires nightly measurements and puts additional strain on both patient and doctor.

## 8 VIDEOENDOSCOPY UNDER SEDATION

### 8.1 IMPACT OF VIDEOENDOSCOPY UNDER SEDATION ON SLEEP, BREATHING, AND SNORING

Videoendoscopy under sedation allows the visualization of the site and mechanism of snoring and airway obstruction in patients with SDB. Therefore it is mandatory that snoring and airway obstruction can be provoked in affected patients and that neither the endoscope itself nor the drugs used for sedation disturb or influence breathing patterns, snoring or airway obstruction during sedation. With this regard, statistically significant differences were found for the longest apnea and the portion of REM sleep as well as for acoustically analyzed snoring sounds when sleep under sedation was compared to natural sleep. Furthermore, it has to be mentioned that videoendoscopy during sedation is usually performed for 10 to 15 minutes due to practical considerations, and may therefore not reflect the conditions during an entire night of natural sleep.

Endoscopy under sedated sleep does not always succeed in inducing existing breathing disorders, and on the other hand, snoring may be provoked even in healthy patients. In a cohort study using propofol, Marais detected snoring sounds in 45% of 126 healthy, non-snoring controls.[23] When titrating propofol with target-controlled infusion, all snorers did snore reliably whereas not a single control person did at the same plasma level, amounting to a sensitivity and specificity of 100%.[24] Therefore, target-controlled infusion with propofol seems superior to manual titration.

### 8.2 DESCRIPTION OF FINDINGS

The patterns of snoring and airway obstruction that can be observed during videoendoscopy under sedation are multiform. Pringle and Croft were the first to standardize the findings according to their data obtained in a large series of patients.[25] Currently, different classifications coexist and, ultimately, none of them are feasible. They distinguish either between an isolated or a multisegmental obstruction, or they are modifications of existing classifications comprising the epiglottis. The majority of authors do not classify their findings but enumerate the various mechanisms and anatomic sites of snoring and obstruction. The obstructive patterns are described as being circular, antero-posterior and latero-lateral at the level of the soft palate, the tonsils, the tongue base, and the epiglottis. A combination of as many as five different concomitant sites of obstruction in primary snorers and even six in sleep apnea patients was described and an isolated site of obstruction was found in only 15% of OSA patients.

### 8.3 IMPACT ON CLINICAL DECISION MAKING

In clinical routine a large tongue – defined by a modified Mallampati score of 3 or 4 – is usually considered a negative predictive parameter for a successful UPPP. However, den Herder and co-workers could not demonstrate a correlation between videoendoscopy under sedation (retrolingual obstruction) and Mallampati index (tongue size).[26] Pringle and Croft compared their results of the Mueller Maneuver to those obtained by videoendoscopy under sedation in a group of 50 patients and could demonstrate that treatment recommendations were not identical based on these two investigation to a significant extent.[25] Other authors also reported substantial differences in treatment recommendation when adding sedated endoscopy to simply using the Mueller Maneuver. Taking the limited significance of the Mueller Maneuver into account, there seems to be a potential for an improvement in treatment selection based on sedated endoscopy.

# SECTION B  DIAGNOSIS

## 8.4 IMPACT ON THE SUCCESS RATE

Surprisingly enough, no prospective data are available to date comparing success rates of surgical intervention with and without the use of videoendoscopy under sedation. This is particularly confusing as there have been numerous advocates of sedated endoscopy presenting data and videos on countless patients with SDB, but they have not yet been able to demonstrate its usefulness with regard to surgical outcome. For example, no superiority was seen with regard to success rates compared to historic controls, despite using sedated endoscopy.[27] Yet an improved success rate was only found in those patients who did not even show the slightest involvement of structures other than the palate. Hessel and de Vries retrospectively reviewed snorers and sleep apnea patients after UPPP. In those patients where the soft palate was least involved in airway collapse during preoperative sedated videoendoscopy, the outcome was superior compared to the others.[28] In another retrospective analysis of 55 sleep apnea patients after UPPP, the same investigators did not find significantly different success rates for different sites of obstruction as revealed by videoendoscopy under sedation.

## 8.5 VIDEOENDOSCOPY UNDER SEDATION AND THE ROLE OF THE EPIGLOTTIS

According to our own experience videoendoscopy under sedation or in sleep is particularly helpful in detecting or excluding a possible glottic or supraglottic obstruction, most often described as a posterior movement of the epiglottis during inspiration. In those cases where an epiglottic collapse during sleep videoendoscopy was seen, a significant reduction of respiratory events may be achieved with partial epiglottectomy. Videoendoscopy under sedation or during sleep may be particularly helpful in cases of laryngeal collapse and failures of standard therapy.

## 8.6 SIGNIFICANCE OF VIDEOENDOSCOPY DURING SEDATION

Videoendoscopy under sedation is able to initiate snoring and upper airway obstruction during a short period of induced sleep, mostly restricted to the supine position. The severity of the underlying disorder appears comparable to natural sleep, although snoring sounds seem different and the short examination time is a significant limitation. The classification of findings can be reduced to isolated obstruction at the palate, the tongue base or the epiglottis or to combinations of these. There are subtle hints that videoendoscopy under sedation may change the indication for a limited number of surgical intervention. Nevertheless, there is not enough evidence to date that this procedure improves the outcome of snoring and sleep apnea surgery.

## 9 MULTI-CHANNEL PRESSURE MEASUREMENTS

Changes in inspiratory pressure in the upper airway during obstructive events can be measured with catheters. Different measuring points meaning different pressure transducers can be used from the nasopharynx through the oro- and hypopharynx down to the esophagus. Initially, pressure transducers were used mainly to investigate the mechanisms of airway obstruction in general; nowadays research is focused on the diagnostic potentials compared to standard polysomnography and on the assessment of obstruction level and its impact on the outcome of sleep apnea surgery.

## 9.1 TOLERABILITY OF THE PRESSURE CATHETERS

Initially, pressure recordings in the field of SDB were performed with balloon and open catheters, but esophageal balloon catheters irritated the patients significantly. The reliability of the results of micro-tip catheters was shown during wakefulness and sleep for the esophagus and for the pharynx. Well-designed studies demonstrated that catheters with no more than 2 mm diameter did not alter the sleep structure of patients suspected of SDB and the results obtained with or without catheters in place did not differ significantly.[29] In a large trial with 799 patients only 3% rejected the placement of the catheter and 1% refused further measurement during the night, while 96% tolerated the procedure.[30]

## 9.2 RELIABILITY OF MEASURING POINTS AND ASSESSMENT OF OBSTRUCTIVE EVENTS

Multi-channel pressure catheters require a reliable positioning of the measuring points in order to attribute the site of obstruction to the anatomically defined segment of the airway. Most investigators choose the oropharyngeal sensor as a reference to be placed under visual control at the free edge of the soft palate. The level of obstruction is usually described as an 'upper' or 'lower' obstruction, meaning an obstruction at the level of the soft palate or the level of the tongue base (an isolated collapse at the level of the epiglottis cannot be assessed with this method).

Pressure catheters also can be used to measure nasal and pharyngeal airflow. This implies that they are suitable to assess increased respiratory effort as well as the AHI. Tvinnereim et al. demonstrated that the absolute number of obstructive and mixed apneas during sleep can be assessed with these catheters with minimal deviation from the results obtained by polysomnography.[31] The overall sensitivity, specificity and negative predictive value for the detection of the different types of apneas and hypopneas may reach up to 100%. The data available indicate that multi-channel pressure recordings are suitable to assess the severity of SDB.

## 9.3 ASSESSING THE SITES OF AIRWAY OBSTRUCTION

When using only one measuring point placed at different levels of the upper airway it is difficult to identify a combined collapse at different levels of hypo- and oropharynx; therefore, catheters with five to six sensors are currently used. With those sensors a collapse extending over more than one segment may routinely be found, the segments may not even be adjacent and the site of obstruction may change during the night.

Investigations concerning night-to-night variability of the distribution of the obstructive sites showed that the predominant site of obstruction can be reproduced during the second night in more than 70% of the cases. Rollheim et al. compared the patterns of obstruction as obtained in the hospital with a recording at home. Although the mean AHI was significantly higher in the hospital than at home, the occurrence of palatal obstructions did not differ between both recordings.[32] In patients who had less than 40% or more than 60% palatal obstructions in the first recording, this relationship was reproduced in 90% of the cases during the second recording.

## 9.4 IMPACT ON THE SUCCESS RATE OF SURGERY FOR SDB

Metes et al. were the first to publish data concerning the impact of pharyngeal pressure measurements on the success rate of surgery.[33] They used a catheter with one measuring point only which was pulled through the pharynx and placed at several sites along the upper airway in order to record several obstructive events at each site. The obstruction they found in this way persisted in eight of 12 patients after UPPP. Nevertheless, the success rate of UPPP did not differ between patients with predominant palatal or tongue base obstruction. Skatvedt et al. selected 16 patients with different degrees of SDB and predominant palatal obstruction detected by multi-channel pressure transducers for laser-assisted uvulopalatoplasty.[34] While the rate of 'upper' obstructions dropped from 90% to 8.8% of all apneas, the number of upper hypopneas was reduced only minimally. Osnes et al. compared the efficacy of UPPP in patients with predominantly transpalatal and subpalatal obstructions.[35] After UPPP, transpalatal apneas and hypopneas were reduced by 81% whereas subpalatal events only dropped by 42%. The success rate in patients with transpalatal obstruction was significantly higher than in those with subpalatal obstruction. Multi-channel pressure recordings seem to be superior to single-channel pull-through techniques in predicting surgical success of soft palate surgery.

## 9.5 SIGNIFICANCE OF MULTI-CHANNEL PRESSURE RECORDINGS

Pressure catheters with a small diameter of not more than 2 mm are well tolerated and have only minimal impact on sleep quality and airway obstructions. The pressure curves allow a reliable detection of respiratory events. Positioning of the measuring points by means of pharyngeal inspection seems to be sufficiently accurate for the evaluation of the palatal airway segment. There are no data suggesting that obstructions at the hypopharynx and the epiglottis can be discriminated reliably. The data available support the idea that the success rate of soft palate surgery can be improved when using multi-channel pressure recordings for patient selection.

## 10 CRITICAL CLOSING PRESSURE

The severity of SDB is usually described by the AHI, representing the number of upper airway obstructions during sleep. Nevertheless, it has to be kept in mind that the AHI simply describes the frequency of upper airway obstructions, not the severity of the pharyngeal collapse itself. Furthermore, measuring the severity of upper airway collapse is believed to be important when estimating the forces needed to overcome these obstructions or to maintain upper airway stability. Schwartz et al.[36] and Smith et al.[37] first measured upper airway collapsibility. They assessed airflow and airway pressure using a special nasal continuous positive airway pressure (CPAP) device with integrated pneumotachograph and pressure sensor, being able to produce positive as well as negative pressure levels. A pressure flow diagram can be drawn at different levels of airway pressure and a regression line can be calculated. Smith defined the critical closing pressure ($P_{crit}$) as being the upper airway pressure when the regression line is crossing the zero line, indicating that airflow completely stops (see Figure 3.3). Patients with obstructive apneas have a $P_{crit}$ clearly above zero, in simple snorers it drops to $-3$ to $-12$ mbar, whereas in normal controls $P_{crit}$ is on average below $-8$ mbar.

## SECTION B — DIAGNOSIS

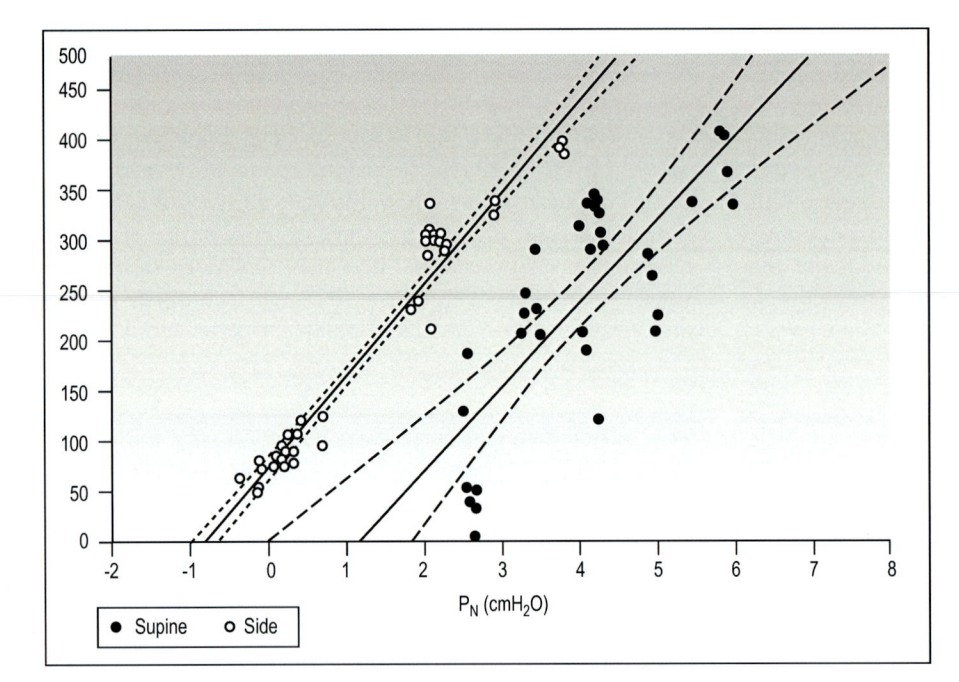

**Fig. 3.3** Representative pressure flow relationships in the lateral recumbent and supine positions for one subject in non-REM sleep. Maximal inspiratory airflow ($V_1$ max) vs nasal mask pressure ($P_N$) is illustrated for lateral recumbent (open circles) and supine (closed circles) positions with corresponding regression lines and confidence interval. Critical closing pressure is represented by the $P_N$ at which airflow becomes zero in each body position (according to Boudewyns et al. Chest 2000;118:1031–41).

### 10.1 IMPACT OF TREATMENT ON $P_{crit}$

Schwartz et al.[38] showed that substantial weight loss resulted in an improvement of $P_{crit}$ and a concomitant reduction of the AHI. They investigated the effect of UPPP on $P_{crit}$ in 13 patients and found a significant decrease for the entire group.[39] Even though a complete normalization of $P_{crit}$ could be demonstrated in the subgroup of responders in contrast to non-responders they could not find any preoperative predictor of response. An identical operation had individually varying effects on $P_{crit}$.

### 10.2 SIGNIFICANCE OF CRITICAL CLOSING PRESSURE

The assessment of the critical closing pressure is an important tool in the investigation of upper airway patency. It is the gold standard for the measurement of the overall collapsibility of the pharynx and is especially useful in research projects. Currently, there are no data concerning the benefit of a preoperative assessment of $P_{crit}$ for a better prediction of success of upper airway surgery. Together with the relatively complex assessment of $P_{crit}$ this may explain why $P_{crit}$ measurements have not become a routine procedure in clinical testing so far.

### 11 SUMMARY

The various techniques of airway evaluation presented in this chapter have significantly increased our insight into the pathophysiology of SDB. Nevertheless, potential benefits with regard to patient management or the superiority over simple clinical assessment remain under discussion and their significance in daily practice is limited. There is not enough evidence that these techniques are superior to the routine clinical assessment.

### ACKNOWLEDGMENTS

We want to thank Mr. J. Wich-Schwarz, PhD, for his editorial assistance.

### REFERENCES

1. Woodson BT, Wooten MR. Comparison of upper-airway evaluations during wakefulness and sleep. Laryngoscope 1994;104:821–8.
2. Friedman M, Ibrahim H, Bass L. Clinical staging for sleep-disordered breathing. Otolaryngol Head Neck Surg 2002;127:13–21.
3. Sher AE, Thorpy MJ, Shprintzen RJ, et al. Predictive value of Muller maneuver in selection of patients for uvulopalatopharyngoplasty. Laryngoscope 1985;95:1483–7.
4. Ritter CT, Trudo FJ, Goldberg AN, et al. Quantitative evaluation of the upper airway during nasopharyngoscopy with the Muller maneuver. Laryngoscope 1999;109:954–63.
5. Riha RL, Brander P, Vennelle M, et al. A cephalometric comparison of patients with the sleep apnea/hypopnea syndrome and their siblings. Sleep 2005;28:315–20.
6. Dempsey JA, Skatrud JB, Jacques AJ, et al. Anatomic determinants of sleep-disordered breathing across the spectrum of clinical and nonclinical male subjects. Chest 2002;122:840–51.
7. Rose EC, Staats R, Lehner M, et al. Cephalometric analysis in patients with obstructive sleep apnea. Part I: diagnostic value. J Orofac Orthop 2002;63:143–53.
8. Mayer G, Meier-Ewert K. Cephalometric predictors for orthopaedic mandibular advancement in obstructive sleep apnoea. Eur J Orthod 1995;17:35–43.

9. Hochban W, Brandenburg U, Peter JH. Surgical treatment of obstructive sleep apnea by maxillomandibular advancement. Sleep 1994;17:624–29.
10. Schwab RJ, Gefter WB, Hoffman EA, et al. Dynamic upper airway imaging during awake respiration in normal subjects and patients with sleep disordered breathing. Am Rev Respir Dis 1993;148:1385–400.
11. Shepard JW Jr., Stanson AW, Sheedy PF, et al. Fast-CT evaluation of the upper airway during wakefulness in patients with obstructive sleep apnea. Prog Clin Biol Res 1990;345:273–9.
12. Yucel A, Unlu M, Haktanir A, et al. Evaluation of the upper airway cross-sectional area changes in different degrees of severity of obstructive sleep apnea syndrome: cephalometric and dynamic CT study. AJNR Am J Neuroradiol 2005;26:2624–9.
13. Stuck BA, Kopke J, Maurer JT, et al. Evaluating the upper airway with standardized magnetic resonance imaging. Laryngoscope 2002;112:552–8.
14. Arens R, Sin S, McDonough JM, et al. Changes in upper airway size during tidal breathing in children with obstructive sleep apnea syndrome. Am J Respir Crit Care Med 2005;171:1298–304.
15. Donnelly LF, Surdulescu V, Chini BA, et al. Upper airway motion depicted at cine MR imaging performed during sleep: comparison between young patients with and those without obstructive sleep apnea. Radiology 2003;227:239–45.
16. Horner RL, Mohiaddin RH, Lowell DG, et al. Sites and sizes of fat deposits around the pharynx in obese patients with obstructive sleep apnoea and weight matched controls. Eur Respir J 1989;2:613–22.
17. Schoenberg SO, Floemer F, Kroeger H, et al. Combined assessment of obstructive sleep apnea syndrome with dynamic MRI and parallel EEG registration: initial results. Invest Radiol 2000;35:267–76.
18. Suto Y, Matsuo T, Kato T, et al. Evaluation of the pharyngeal airway in patients with sleep apnea: value of ultrafast MR imaging. AJR Am J Roentgenol 1993;160:311–14.
19. Stuck BA, Kopke J, Maurer JT, et al. Lesion formation in radiofrequency surgery of the tongue base. Laryngoscope 2003;113:1572–6.
20. Stuck BA, Kopke J, Hormann K, et al. Volumetric tissue reduction in radiofrequency surgery of the tongue base. Otolaryngol Head Neck Surg 2005;132:132–5.
21. Stuck BA, Neff W, Hormann K, et al. Anatomic changes after hyoid suspension for obstructive sleep apnea: an MRI study. Otolaryngol Head Neck Surg 2005;133:397–402.
22. Borowiecki B, Pollak CP, Weitzman ED, et al. Fibro-optic study of pharyngeal airway during sleep in patients with hypersomnia obstructive sleep-apnea syndrome. Laryngoscope 1978;88:1310–3.
23. Marais J. The value of sedation nasendoscopy: a comparison between snoring and non-snoring patients. Clin Otolaryngol Allied Sci 1998;23:74–6.
24. Berry S, Roblin G, Williams A, et al. Validity of sleep nasendoscopy in the investigation of sleep related breathing disorders. Laryngoscope 2005;115:538–40.
25. Pringle MB, Croft CB. A grading system for patients with obstructive sleep apnoea, based on sleep nasendoscopy. Clin Otolaryngol Allied Sci 1993;18:480–4.
26. den Herder C, van Tinteren H, de Vries N. Sleep endoscopy versus modified Mallampati score in OSA and snoring. Laryngoscope 2005;115:735–9.
27. Camilleri AE, Ramamurthy L, Jones PH. Sleep nasendoscopy: what benefit to the management of snorers? J Laryngol Otol 1995;109:1163–5.
28. Hessel NS, de Vries N. Results of uvulopalatopharyngoplasty after diagnostic workup with polysomnography and sleep endoscopy: a report of 136 snoring patients. Eur Arch Otorhinolaryngol 2003;260:91–5.
29. Skatvedt O, Akre H, Godtlibsen OB. Nocturnal polysomnography with and without continuous pharyngeal and esophageal pressure measurements. Sleep 1996;19:485–90.
30. Oeverland B, Akre H, Kvaerner KJ, et al. Patient discomfort in polysomnography with esophageal pressure measurements. Eur Arch Otorhinolaryngol 2005;262:241–5.
31. Tvinnereim M, Cole P, Haight JS, et al. Diagnostic airway pressure recording in sleep apnea syndrome. Acta Otolaryngol 1995;115:449–54.
32. Rollheim J, Tvinnereim M, Sitek J, et al. Repeatability of sites of sleep-induced upper airway obstruction. A 2-night study based on recordings of airway pressure and flow. Eur Arch Otorhinolaryngol 2001;258:259–64.
33. Metes A, Hoffstein V, Mateika S, et al. Site of airway obstruction in patients with obstructive sleep apnea before and after uvulopalatopharyngoplasty. Laryngoscope 1991;101:1102–8.
34. Skatvedt O, Akre H, Godtlibsen OB. Continuous pressure measurements in the evaluation of patients for laser assisted uvulopalatoplasty. Eur Arch Otorhinolaryngol 1996;253:390–4.
35. Osnes T, Rollheim J, Hartmann E. Effect of UPPP with respect to site of pharyngeal obstruction in sleep apnoea: follow-up at 18 months by overnight recording of airway pressure and flow. Clin Otolaryngol Allied Sci 2002;27:38–43.
36. Schwartz AR, Smith PL, Wise RA, et al. Induction of upper airway occlusion in sleeping individuals with subatmospheric nasal pressure. J Appl Physiol 1988;64:535–42.
37. Smith PL, Wise RA, Gold AR, et al. Upper airway pressure-flow relationships in obstructive sleep apnea. J Appl Physiol 1988;64:789–95.
38. Schwartz AR, Gold AR, Schubert N, et al. Effect of weight loss on upper airway collapsibility in obstructive sleep apnea. Am Rev Respir Dis 1991;144:494–8.
39. Schwartz AR, Schubert N, Rothman W, et al. Effect of uvulopalatopharyngoplasty on upper airway collapsibility in obstructive sleep apnea. Am Rev Respir Dis 1992;145:527–32.

# SECTION B  DIAGNOSIS

## CHAPTER 4

# Clinical polysomnography

*Stephen Lund and Jon Freeman*

## 1 INTRODUCTION

The field of sleep medicine has experienced an explosion of interest in recent years. This heightened focus on achieving an advanced understanding of sleep and its inherent pathologies is attributable, in large part, to significant improvement in the development of more suitable instrumentation. This, in turn, has led to more accurate measurement and comprehension of sleep processes and related parameters, although many questions regarding sleep mechanisms remain. The relative simplicity of instrumentation used by Hans Berger in the late 1920s to first describe the human electroencephalogram (EEG)[1] has been eclipsed by technology implemented today at sleep centers around the world where not only the EEG is recorded during polysomnography (PSG), but usually the electro-oculogram (EOG), electromyogram (EMG), electrocardiogram (ECG), respiratory effort, nasal/oral airflow, $SaO_2$ levels, snoring, and body position with video monitoring are as well. In a much less standardized manner, additional parameters may be measured depending upon the clinical presentation of the patient and the technical capabilities of the individual sleep center. Thus, end tidal $CO_2$ ($ETCO_2$) may be measured in a patient with chronic obstructive pulmonary disease (COPD) or the placement of an esophageal balloon may be considered in appropriate patients to clarify the diagnosis of upper airway resistance syndrome (UARS) by measuring esophageal pressures during sleep. We have seen a gradual transformation from the traditional, pen-and-paper recording of sleep to the current, state-of-the-art, digital acquisition and reviewing of sleep (see Figs 4.1–4.4). As our knowledge of sleep and its pathologies is refined, the inexorable demand for further advancements concerning instrumentation becomes more acute, as is true in many other areas of health science in general. This chapter will serve to clarify the types of sleep studies used in the evaluation process of sleep-related breathing disorders (SRBD), provide guidelines for their acquisition pre- and postoperatively, and present typical montages used during PSG with special attention paid to the measurement of nasal/oral airflow.

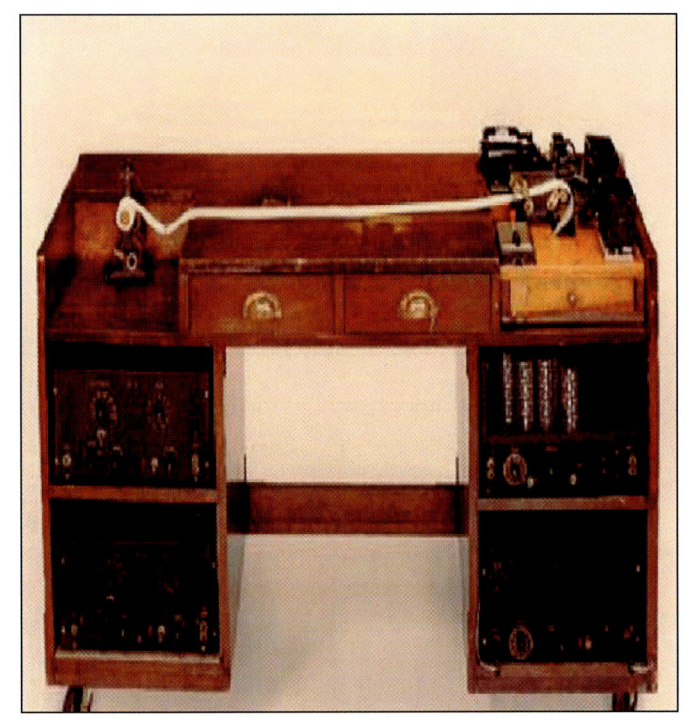

**Fig. 4.1** The Grass Model 1. A two-channel, analog recorder, based on the d'Arsnval galvanometer. Courtesy of Grass Technologies, An Astro-Med, Inc. Product Group.

## 2 SLEEP-RELATED BREATHING DISORDERS (SRBDs) AND RECOMMENDED TESTING

According to the American Academy of Sleep Medicine (AASM), when factors inclusive of sensitivity, specificity, likelihood ratios, and strength of evidence are analyzed, a categorization of four subtypes of sleep-monitoring procedures is the outcome.[2] Type 1 is the gold standard attended in-laboratory PSG, while the other three include *portable* monitoring methods inclusive of Type 2 (comprehensive), Type 3 (modified portable sleep apnea testing or cardiorespiratory sleep study), and Type 4 (continuous single recording, such as ambulatory overnight pulse oximetry, or

Clinical polysomnography | CHAPTER 4

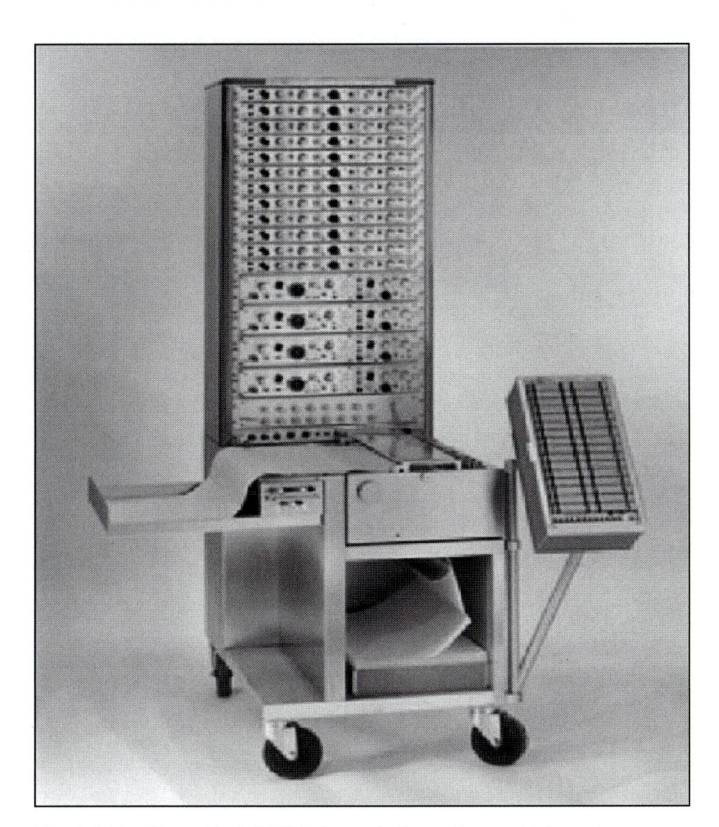

**Fig. 4.2** The Grass Model 78C Polygraph. An analog, multichannel, recorder. The first 12 rows (thin bands) are AC amplifiers and the following four rows (wider bands) are DC amplifiers. This polygraph stood around 6 feet tall and the number of channels was limited by the number of amplifiers/oscillographs that could be placed within the chassis. Courtesy of Grass Technologies, An Astro-Med, Inc. Product Group.

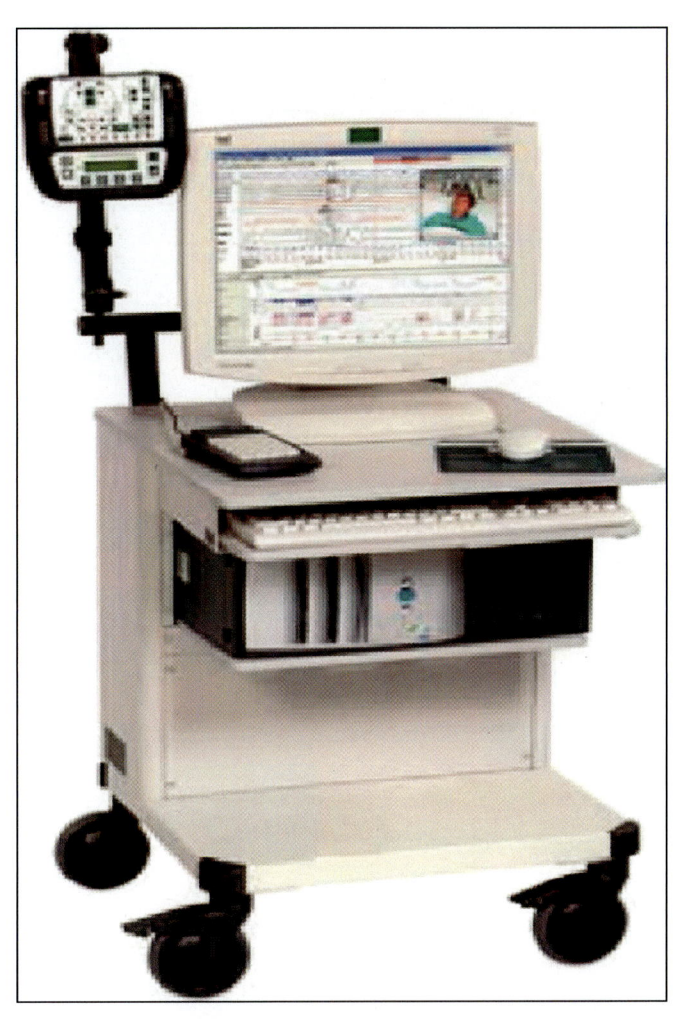

**Fig. 4.3** The Grass Comet® PSG system. The entire AC/DC amplifier apparatus is contained within the small black box to the upper-left of the monitor. This system is capable of recording up to 50 channels. Courtesy of Grass Technologies, An Astro-Med, Inc. Product Group.

dual bioparameter recording). Type 4 monitoring devices are considered unacceptable by the AASM for making the diagnosis of obstructive sleep apnea. Type 2 and 3 devices may be helpful in an *attended* setting used for patients without significant comorbid conditions, and if manually scored by trained personnel. It has been noted that the Type 3 devices have a tendency to underestimate the severity of OSA secondary to the absence of EEG monitoring in that arousals are not scored.[3] Furthermore, it is recommended by the AASM that symptomatic patients with negative *portable* studies undergo attended PSG for further clarification.[2] According to AASM standards, a full night PSG is routinely indicated for the diagnosis of SRBDs and for continuous positive airway pressure (CPAP) titration in patients with a documented diagnosis of a SRBD for whom PAP is warranted. Such patients include those with a Respiratory Disturbance Index (RDI) of at least 15 per hour of sleep regardless of their presenting symptomatology or those with a RDI of at least five per hour of sleep with excessive daytime sleepiness. Split-night PSGs (diagnostic segment followed by CPAP titration on the same night) are considered acceptable if the Apnea/Hypopnea Index (AHI) is at least 40 events per hour of sleep and is documented by means of at least 2 hours of diagnostic recording, or if the AHI is between 20 and 40 in the presence of repetitive lengthy obstructions and major desaturations. In addition, the CPAP titration must be carried out for more than 3 hours, and the PSG must document that CPAP eliminates the respiratory events during sleep, including REM sleep with the patient in the supine position.[2]

Excessive daytime somnolence is often part of the clinical presentation of patients with a SRBD. There are several means by which the degree of somnolence may be measured, both subjectively (e.g. Epworth Sleepiness Scale) and objectively. The Multiple Sleep Latency Test (MSLT) is a series of nap opportunities (usually four or five) scheduled 2 hours apart beginning 1.5–3 hours after the morning awakening following PSG, which are conducted under specified conditions using accepted protocols. Patients are asked to try to fall asleep during these nap opportunities. The procedures used to perform the Maintenance of Wakefulness Test (MWT) are similar to those utilized for

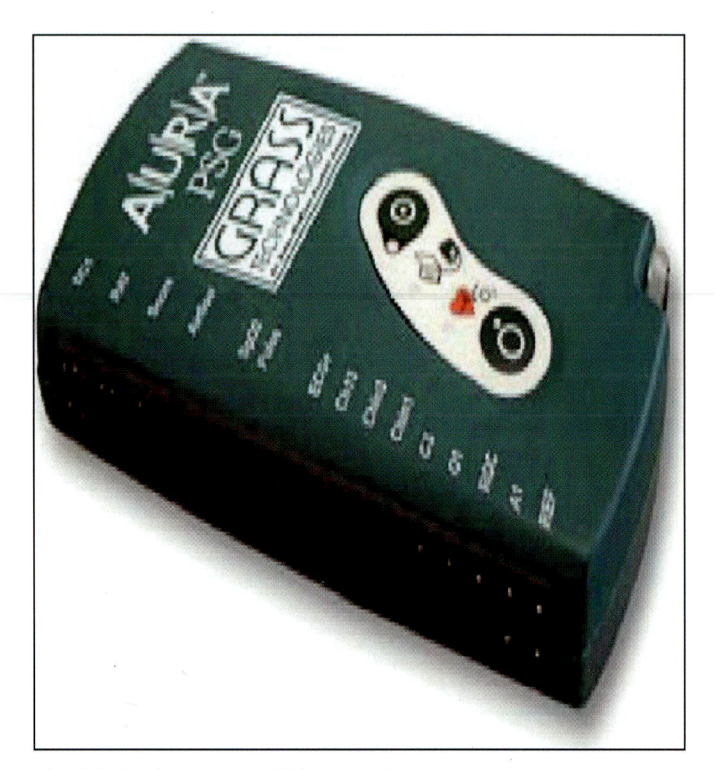

**Fig. 4.4** The Grass Aura® PSG system. This portable system contains all AC/DC amplifiers and is small enough to fit in a person's hand. This system is capable of recording up to 25, wireless, channels. Courtesy of Grass Technologies, An Astro-Med, Inc. Product Group.

the MSLT with the exception that the patient is asked to remain awake under the same soporific conditions utilized for the MSLT. The MSLT is a validated objective measure of the patient's ability or tendency to fall asleep while the MWT is a validated objective measure of the patient's ability to remain awake under soporific conditions. Although closely related, these two procedures serve to define a patient's sleepiness from different perspectives. The MSLT is not routinely indicated in the initial evaluation for a SRBD or in the assessment of change following treatment with nasal CPAP.[4] However, the MWT may be used to assess an individual's ability to remain awake if an inability to do so potentially constitutes a public or personal safety issue. Patients with a SRBD who are employed in occupations involving public transportation or safety may require assessment of their ability to remain awake. Although data regarding usefulness of the MSLT or the MWT are limited, using the MWT to assess ability to remain awake has been reported to have greater face validity than using the MSLT.[4] However, the predictive value of either test for assessing accident risk and safety within the context of real-life circumstances is not well established. The assessment of the patient's ability to remain awake and consequent safety risks should involve the integration of findings from the history, compliance with therapy, subjective rating scales, and in some cases, objective testing using the MWT.

## 3 PREOPERATIVE AND POSTOPERATIVE ASSESSMENTS

For patients undergoing upper airway surgery either for snoring or for a SRBD, the preoperative routine should be inclusive of PSG or an attended cardiorespiratory (Type 3) sleep study. In certain instances after the surgery has been completed, a follow-up PSG or attended cardiorespiratory (Type 3) sleep study is recommended. This should be considered following the surgical treatment of patients with moderate to severe OSA, to ensure satisfactory response, and in those whose clinical response is insufficient or when symptoms return despite a good initial response to CPAP treatment. In addition, follow-up PSG is indicated in other circumstances: (1) after substantial weight *loss* (e.g. 10% of body weight) in patients on CPAP for treatment of SRBDs to ascertain whether the pressure requirement has changed; (2) after substantial weight *gain* (e.g. 10% of body weight) in patients previously treated with CPAP successfully, who are again symptomatic despite the continued use of CPAP. In the latter case, the possibility of a pressure requirement change must also be entertained.

## 4 SPECIAL POPULATIONS

Patients with some specific medical conditions deserve mention. In general, those with a history of coronary artery disease, congestive heart failure, a history of stroke or transient ischemic attacks, significant tachyarrhythmias or bradyarrhythmias should be screened for signs and symptoms of a SRBD.[2] If there is a reasonable suspicion of these conditions, then a PSG is warranted. Furthermore, the application of CPAP at least during the perioperative period in many cases is prudent.

The pediatric population also merits attention. Although most children with obstructive sleep apnea present with a history of snoring and evidence of some difficulty breathing during sleep, not all of them snore. Paradoxical breathing is often prominent secondary to their very compliant rib cages. The scoring of respiratory events in adults requires a duration of at least 10 seconds, while the standard in children has been defined by a period of at least two respiratory cycles.[5] In children, these respiratory events may or may not be followed by EEG arousals. This often leads to fairly normal sleep architecture. The respiratory events occur predominantly in REM sleep. The ordering of PSG is indicated in neonates and infants when apnea of prematurity or of infancy is suspected, or following apparent life-threatening events (ALTEs). When severe gastroesophageal reflux is suspected, PSG is also indicated. The presence of a craniofacial congenital malformation involving the face, mouth, tongue, neck or chest, such as Treacher Collins syndrome or Pierre Robin syndrome, or following surgery on a child performed to correct these anatomical abnormalities, should also prompt a consideration for PSG. Other disorders which should urge the clinician to obtain PSG include suspected seizure disorders or any disorder which can cause hypotonia.[6]

## 5 UNDERSTANDING SLEEP MONTAGES

Polysomnography refers to the simultaneous recording of multiple neurophysiologic signals that are of interest to a clinician. For the purpose of sleep recording, these channels ought to reflect the information necessary to formulate an accurate diagnostic picture. A montage refers to the order in which channels are displayed. These channels can be any combination of bipolar AC or DC amplifiers although EEG, EOG and EMG signals are typically recorded with AC amplifiers and respiratory, $ETCO_2$ and $SaO_2$ channels are typically recorded through DC amplifiers.

AC amplifier recordings on pen and paper are, by definition, bipolar derivations. Since electrical potential is a relative measurement and is always calculated as the difference between two potential points,[7] each individual AC channel on the pen-and-paper recording represents a derivation of one channel being subtracted from another. Most typically, the EOG as measured by the left and right outer canthi (LOC/ROC) and EEG channels (i.e. C3/C4/O1/O2) are referenced to the contralateral mastoid (i.e. A1/A2) whereas EMG (i.e. mentalis–submentalis), left and right anterior tibialis (LAT/RAT) and ECG signals (i.e. left and right subclavicle) are typically referenced to themselves. This means that there are two electrodes applied to the same site. Through various combinations of analog capacitors and resistors, biological signals that are amplified are also filtered for unwanted electrical potentials (i.e. 60 cycle noise). Ultimately, what is written to paper is the final product of amplified and filtered, biological signals that are plotted as a function of time (e.g. paper speed). There is no way to alter the data once they are written.

Although pen-and-paper recordings were once considered the gold standard for recording sleep, numerous problems with recordings were relatively commonplace. It would not be uncommon, for example, to have an ink-well run dry or a pen clog during the recording. If the sleep technician was not alert to this, then data would be missing. Another common problem with this type of recording was that alterations to data collection (e.g. changing filter settings, changing amplifier gain settings, re-referencing derivations, inverting polarity, changing paper speed) required notation on the recording. If the sleep technician failed to do this, there was a chance that the data could be misinterpreted by the clinician who read the data. Lastly, if the polygraph had not been calibrated properly, data were potentially suspect. Often, each amplifier had to be calibrated before each recording and this was especially true for DC amplifiers.

Given these difficulties plus the recent advances in computing technology, digital PSGs are currently the standard for most sleep laboratories. Although digital sleep systems were originally designed to emulate the analog polygraphs, improvements in microprocessor speed and graphic cards have allowed digital systems to advance beyond the limitations of the analog systems. For example, analog PSG systems were limited by physical space; there were only so many oscillators (the magnet, coil and pen apparatus that allowed the biological signal to be written to paper) you could attach to the chassis of the polygraph. As is evidenced by the original standardized manual for recording and staging sleep,[8] only a limited number of channels were used to record sleep compared to today's standards. In contrast, today's digital sleep systems can easily allow for more than 32 channels of AC and DC channels.

Another important advance in digital PSG is the ability to perform referential recording. Referential recording, in contrast to bipolar recording, sends the signals from each biological input to a common reference (e.g. C3-Ref, LOC-Ref, Chin EMG-Ref). In other words, referential recording allows us to record the potential difference between a particular electrode and a reference electrode.[9] Frequently, the common reference is cephalic (e.g. Cz or FPz) although there are several examples of non-cephalic references (e.g. the nose). The advantage of this type of recording is that it allows the polysomnographer to re-reference electrodes, invert polarity, change montages and change filter settings after the PSG is complete.

Figure 4.5 shows a standard, referential sleep montage. In particular, channels 1–11 are referenced to a common reference (Cz) and channels 12–19 are bipolar in origin. Channels 1–19 are collected through an AC amplifier. The $SaO_2$ channel is collected through a DC amplifier. As is typically the case with referential data, there are no filters applied. Figure 4.6 shows the same epoch of data, but is correctly referenced as bipolar derivations (except the DC channel ($SaO_2$)) and appropriate filter settings are applied. In this case, EOG and EEG channels 1–6 are referenced to the contralateral mastoid and channels 8–15 are referenced to themselves.

## 6 UNDERSTANDING MONTAGE CHANNELS

In order to interpret and score sleep stages, a combination of EOG, EEG and Chin EMG channels are necessary. Some of the derivations are, by default, back-up channels[8] (e.g. C4/A1 and O2/A1) as a way of avoiding disruption of the patient's sleep should one of the leads become compromised. As is seen in Figure 4.5, there are three referential Chin EMG channels collected, with one of these leads always serving as a back-up. When displayed in its appropriate bipolar derivation, only one Chin EMG channel appears (see Fig. 4.6). The third chin lead can be re-referenced in case one of the other chin leads falls off. In order to interpret the impact of physiological events upon sleep architecture, other channels have been added to aid in the differential diagnosis of sleep disorders. In particular, these

# SECTION B  DIAGNOSIS

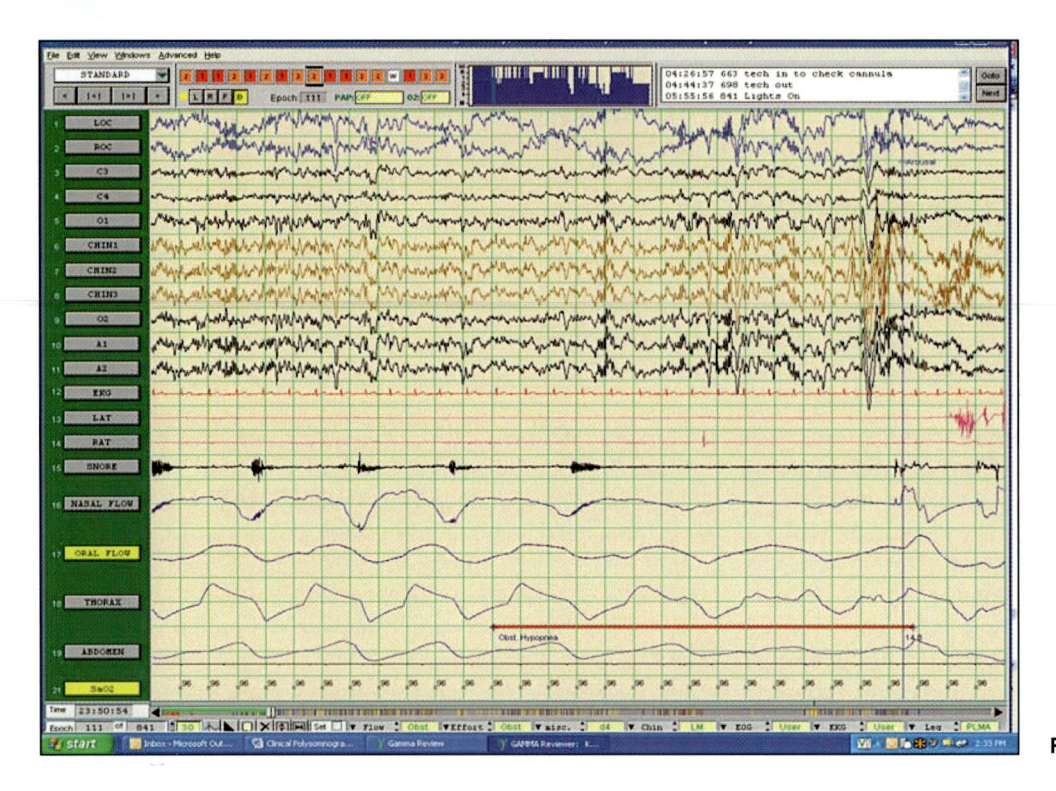

Fig. 4.5 Referential sleep montage.

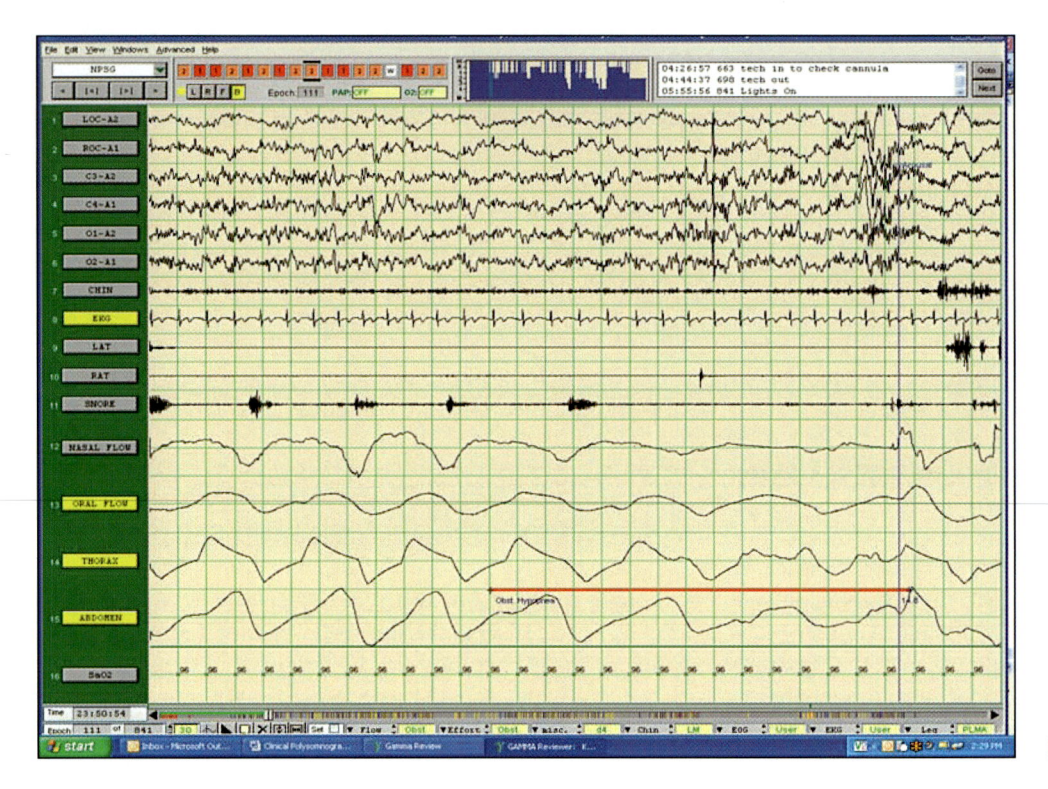

Fig. 4.6 Bipolar sleep montage.

channels are typically ECG, Leg EMG (LAT, RAT), a snore microphone, airflow from the nose and mouth, thoracic and abdominal deflections and pulse oximetry (SaO$_2$). It is also not uncommon in sleep recordings to see additional channels measuring capnometry (ETCO$_2$) and position sensors. Table 4.1 illustrates the types of channels that are most typically included in current digital recordings of sleep along with their appropriate labels, sample rates and filter setting ranges. Included in Table 4.1 are the traditional PSG sensitivity settings and their approximated, corresponding, digital, peak-to-peak (p-p) values. This is because analog and digital PSG systems differ regarding

### Table 4.1 Types of channel included in digital recordings of sleep

| Signal type | Channel labels | Sample rate (Hz) | Sensitivity (μV/mm) | p-p width (μV/mm) | LFF (Hz) | HFF (Hz) |
|---|---|---|---|---|---|---|
| EOG | LOC-A2<br>ROC-A1 | 100–256 | 5 | 150 | 0.3 | 35–70 |
| Chin EMG<br>Leg EMG<br>Microphone EMG | Chin1-Chin2<br>(Chin3)<br>LAT<br>RAT<br>Snore | 100–512 | 2 | 50 | 10 | 70–120 |
| EEG | C3-A2<br>C4-A1<br>O1-A2<br>O2-A1 | 100–256 | 5 | 150 | 0.3 | 35–70 |
| ECG | ECG | 100–1024 | 20 | | 1.0 | 70–120 |
| Airflow transducer<br>Airflow thermocouple or thermister | Nasal, oral or nasal/oral | | 7 | 300 | <0.1* | 15–35 |
| **Respiratory** | | | | | | |
| Piezo sensors<br>Inductive plethysmography<br>Pneumatic transducer | Thorax<br>Abdomen | n/a | 7 | 300 | <0.1* | 15–35 |
| Capnometer | ET CO$_2$ | n/a | n/a | n/a | n/a | n/a |
| Oximeter | SpO$_2$ | n/a | n/a | n/a | n/a | n/a |
| Miscellaneous | Position<br>Heart rate | n/a | n/a | n/a | n/a | n/a |

*The lower limit of most amplifier systems is 0.1 Hz. Some systems (i.e. Grass Gamma) have constructed amplifiers that are capable of recording near DC width (i.e. 0.01 Hz). As a general rule for AC amplifiers, the longer the time constant (lower LFF), the closer the reproduction to a DC channel.[11]

units of sensitivity: units of analog sensitivity are calculated as follows:

$$\text{Potential } (\mu V) = \text{height (mm)} \times \text{amplifier sensitivity } (\mu V/mm).[10]$$

Digital systems, in contrast, divide the display into the number of vertical pixels allowed for each channel that are expressed in peak-to-peak microvolts per channel.[10]

In contrast to the continuous, voltage-time display seen in analog data, digital data converts biological signals into discrete impulses, called quantizing. The finer the steps, the more accurately digital data represents the analog data.[12] This analog-to-digital (A–D) conversion is dependent upon two factors for accuracy: sampling frequency and bit depth. Sampling frequency, the number of digital samples taken per second, is modulated by Nyquist's theorem:

$$\text{Sample frequency} = 2 \times f_{max}$$

Nyquist's theory dictates that the fastest frequency signal that can be represented is one-half the sampling frequency. For example, a sampling frequency of 256 Hz accurately represents signal frequencies up to 128 Hz. Sampling below 2 $f_N$ ($f_N$ = Nyquist frequency) results in either aliasing or signal distortion due to folding of frequency components larger than $f_N$ onto lower frequencies.[13] Aliasing refers to the phenomenon where sinusoidal signals change frequency and phase during sampling (see Fig. 4.7). In either case, since the digital data are no longer uniquely related to a particular analog signal, unambiguous reconstruction is impossible.[13]

Bit depth (vertical resolution) designates the number of divisions into which the range of voltages can be represented. Each stepwise increase in bit depth increases the number of possible amplitude levels by a factor of two. For example, a bit depth of eight means that there are $2^8 = 256$ individual steps between the minimum and maximum allowable voltages. For PSG recordings, the full scale range should approximate 2000 μV. The lower limit of the dynamic range is set by amplifier noise which, in most commercial systems, is around 0.1 μV. Systems not capable of meeting this minimum dynamic range run the possibility of losing data or collecting inadequate data. Adding bits will tend to increase the precision of the measurement. It should be noted that most commercial systems are now capable of collecting data with a large enough dynamic range (+5000 μV) that data errors such as saturation, a process whereby the amplifier sends a signal greater in strength than the dynamic range (see Fig. 4.8), are highly unlikely.

## SECTION B DIAGNOSIS

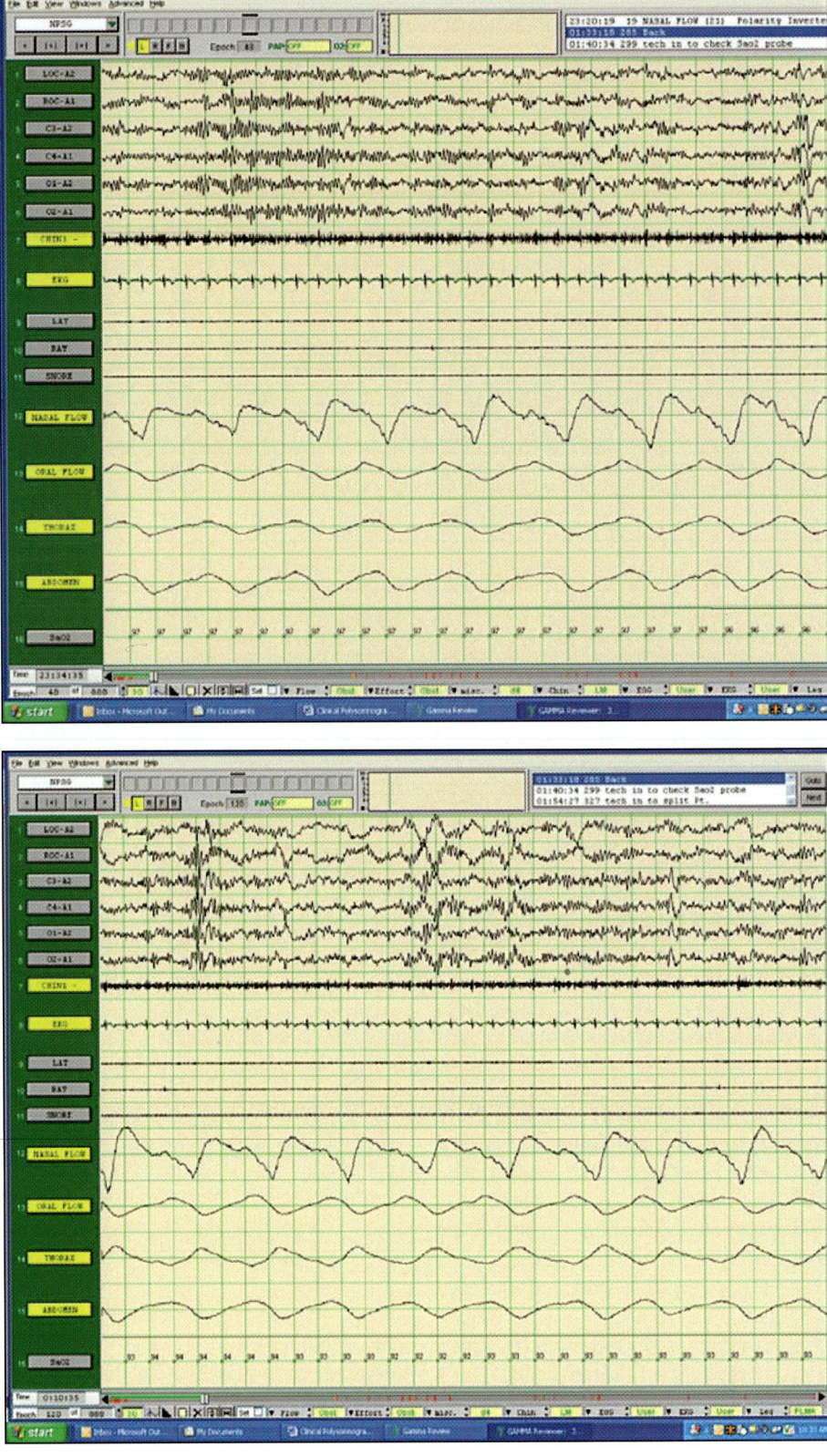

**Fig. 4.7** Aliasing. The NPSG on the top shows exactly what is expected. All respiratory signals are 'in-phase', meaning that all channels move in the same direction when a subject inhales and exhales. The phase of the signals is crucial for determination of obstructive versus central respiratory events. In contrast, the NPSG on the bottom (same patient, 36 minutes later) shows significant aliasing on the thorax channel. The phase of the thorax signal has randomly become inverted and suggests the patient is having paradoxical breathing when this is not the case. Paradoxical breathing is a hallmark of obstructive respiratory events. Respiratory channels were collected using piezo sensors and, compared to RIP sensors, Piezo sensors are prone to aliasing problems. Fortunately, since this is a referential montage, the polarity can be reversed.

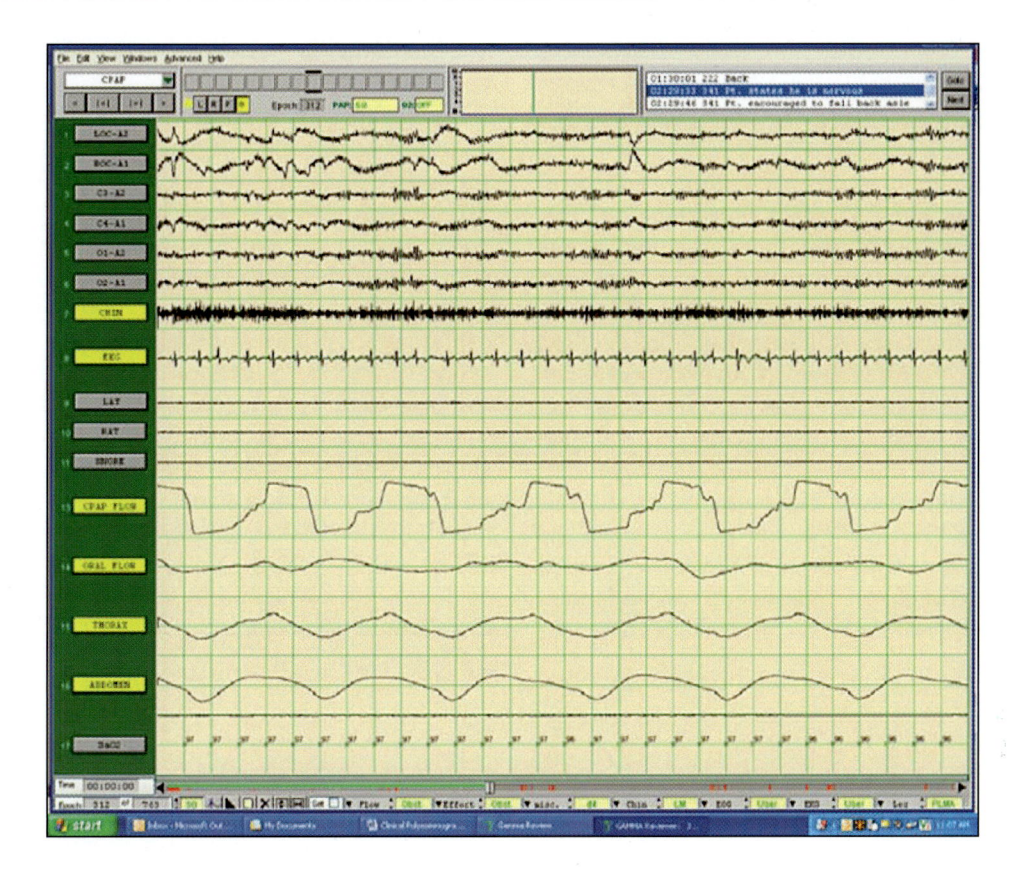

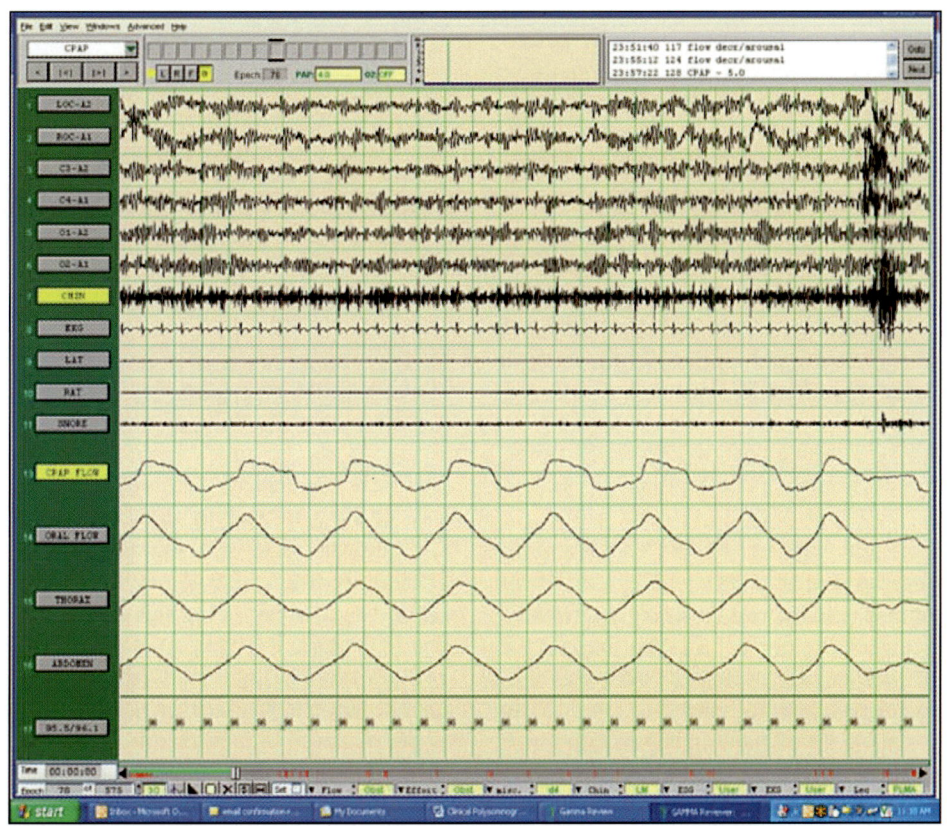

**Fig. 4.8** Saturation (amplifier pegging). The NPSG on the top demonstrates the error of saturation. In particular, the CPAP flow channel is notable for a flattened or blocked top and bottom. This occurred because the gain setting on the transducer channel was too high for the dynamic range of the digital recording. If this signal were misinterpreted as real, then the likelihood is that flow limitation would be improperly diagnosed. In contrast, the NPSG on the bottom demonstrates accurate flow limitation on the CPAP flow channel as is evidenced by the flattened contour of the inspiratory signal.

# SECTION B: DIAGNOSIS

## 7 ASSESSING AIRFLOW AND RESPIRATORY SIGNALS

The matters of aliasing and dynamic range are of no small consequence when assessing a patient's breathing and respiration. This is for the reason that the morphology of the airflow signals, in combination with the morphology and phase of the respiratory signals, is critical for determining the differential diagnoses of obstructive apnea (OSA) and hypopnea (OSH), central apnea (CSA) and hypopnea (CSH), upper airway resistance (UAR), flow limitation and primary snoring. An inaccurate representation of these signals due to errors in digital processing can have odious and potentially life-threatening consequences for the patient. For this reason, it is important to understand the properties of the sensors used to make these assessments. For the purpose of this chapter, discussion will be limited to the methods most commonly used to assess airflow and respiration.

### 7.1 THERMOCOUPLES AND THERMISTERS

For years, thermocouples and thermisters were the only available, non-invasive tools for assessing airflow. Thermocouples are made from two dissimilar metals with different coefficients of expansion.[14] The thermocouple is typically placed under the nares and over the mouth and rates of temperature change are expressed as a continuous, analog, sinusoidal signal. Thermisters also detect temperature changes between room air and expired air through use of a Wheatstone bridge circuit that acts as a DC converter.[14] The beads of the thermisters are placed in a nearly identical fashion to the thermocouple and signal output is also continuous and sinusoidal in nature. While these measures were adequate for detecting either the presence or absence of airflow, they were not designed to or not sensitive enough to detect subtle changes that were occurring in the upper airway.

### 7.2 NASAL PRESSURE TRANSDUCER

Even though the esophageal balloon is considered the gold standard for identifying respiratory effort and upper airway physiology, the insertion of the balloon is so highly invasive that this is an impractical technique for routine use. In the mid-1990s, however, it was determined that use of a nasal cannula connected to a pneumotachograph provided a very close approximation to the sensitivity of the esophageal balloon.[15] With the advent of this technology and its widespread usage, a number of differential diagnostic possibilities emerged in the assessment and treatment of SRBDs. In particular, UARS was introduced to the diagnostic lexicon and alternative treatment opportunities became available to patients with milder forms of OSA.

Nasal flow, as measured through a nasal cannula system, measures a pressure drop across a relatively constant resistance (nares). Even though nasal flow is not precisely quantifiable, the flow signal generated is approximately proportional to the pressure across the resistor.[11] The pressure across the resistor is noteworthy because some commercial nasal cannulas include an oral measurement component. This type of cannula recording system is flawed due to lack of resistance on the oral flow and, as a result, caution is warranted when interpreting data from this type of system. DC amplification is the preferred modality for the nasal cannula signal although amplifiers capable of long time constants (>5 seconds) will also work. Time constants shorter than 5 seconds will adversely affect the morphology of the inspiratory flow signal. Figure 4.9 shows an accurate representation of flow limitation during stage 1 sleep.

### 7.3 STRAIN GAUGES

The piezoelectric sensor is the most common method utilized to detect changes in lung volume. Its popularity is due to the relatively low cost and ease of application. This type of gauge is sensitive to changes in length since electrical current varies inversely to the length of the gauge,[16] although the signal is not easily quantifiable. Instead, the qualitative or morphological aspect of the signal is taken into account with the ideal respiratory signal appearing as a perfect sinusoid. Figure 4.5 shows an example of respiratory signals collected with piezoelectric sensors. One important caution is that since piezoelectric respiratory sensors typically sample at less than 2 $f_N$, there is an increased likelihood of aliasing errors (see Fig. 4.7).

### 7.4 RESPIRATORY INDUCTANCE PLETHYSMOGRAPHY (RIP)

Electrical conductors that, by definition, measure inductance can be applied to thoracic and abdominal sensors.[16] The changes in inductance can be measured electronically through frequency oscillators that are output to a demodulator unit that converts the signal into a scaled, analog form.[14] The advantage RIP sensors have over other methods of respiratory monitoring is that the RIP signal can be calibrated. As a result, the RIP sensor is considered the truest measure of paradoxical breathing and it has additionally been utilized as a way of assessing UARS. Disadvantages to this sensor include cost and artifact due to patient movement. For example, if a RIP sensor were to slide from its original position, the initial calibration would become less meaningful. As is seen in Figure 4.10, the output signal of the RIP sensors is qualitatively comparable to the piezoelectric sensors.

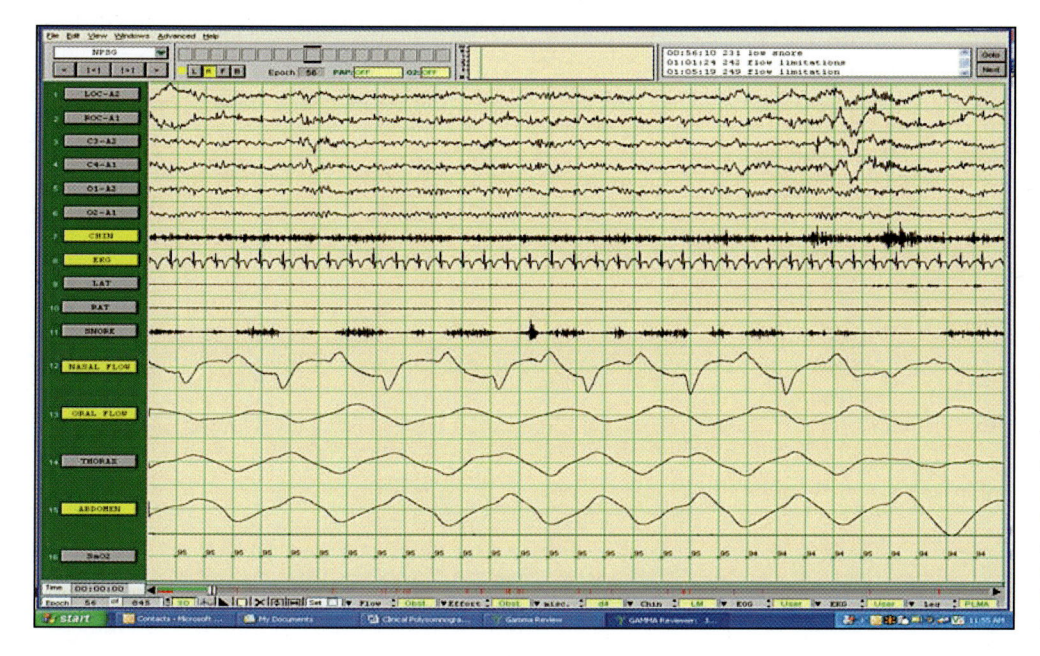

**Fig. 4.9** Flow limitation. This is nicely illustrated on the nasal flow channel. Nasal flow was assessed with a nasal cannula attached to a pressure transducer. Clear flattening of the contour is seen on the inspiratory portion of the nasal flow signal indicating a mild collapse of the upper airway. Snoring corresponds to the inspiratory (flattened) portion of the nasal flow signal. Oral flow was assessed with a thermocouple device.

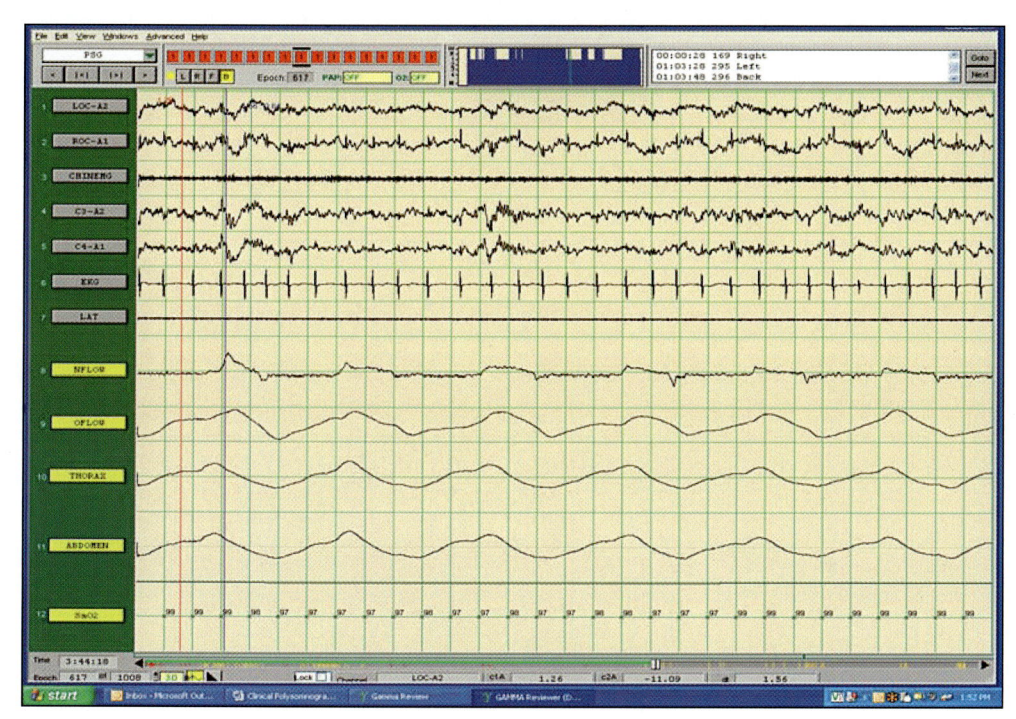

**Fig. 4.10** Respiratory inductance plethysmography (thorax and abdomen).

## 8 CONCLUSION

Prior to the development of suitable instrumentation, sleep apnea was viewed largely as a singular entity. Through recent advances in sleep assessment technologies, an expansion of our knowledge of sleep-related breathing disorders has taken place. In particular, advances in upper airway assessment as measured through a pressure transducer have allowed for a wider range of differential SRBD diagnoses including UARS. These recent advances in technology have prompted the fields of sleep medicine and otolaryngology to have greater interaction. It is when the sleep specialist and ENT work in concert that treatment outcome is maximized.

### REFERENCES

1. Berger H. Uber dar elektrenkephalogram des menschen. Arch Psychiat Nervenky 1929;87:527–70.
2. Kushida CA, Littner MR, Morgenthaler T, et al. Practice parameters for the indications for polysomnography and related procedures: an update for 2005. Sleep 2005;28(4):499–516.
3. Littner M, Hirshkowitz M, Shararfkhaneh A, et al. Nonlaboratory assessment of sleep-related breathing disorders. In: Sleep Medicine

4. Littner M, Kushida CA, Wise M, et al. Practice parameters for clinical use of the multiple sleep latency test and the maintenance of wakefulness test. Sleep 2005;28(1):113–21.
5. Rosen G, Carskadon M, Ferber R, et al. Pediatric obstructive sleep apnea. In: The International Classification of Sleep Disorders, 2nd edn. Sateia M, ed. Westchester, Illinois: American Academy of Sleep Medicine; 2005, pp. 56–59.
6. Sheldon S. Polysomnography in infants and children. In: Principles and Practice of Pediatric Sleep Medicine. Sheldon S, Ferber R, Kryger M, eds. Edinburgh: Elsevier Saunders; 2005, pp. 49–71.
7. Quigg M. Channels and montages. In: EEG Pearls. Quigg M, ed. The Pearls Series. Edinburgh: Mosby, Elsevier; 2006, pp. 21–23.
8. Rechtschaffen A, Kales A, eds. A Manual of Standardized Terminology: Techniques and Scoring System for Sleep Stages of Human Subjects. Los Angeles, CA: UCLA Brain Information Service/Brain Research Institute; 1968.
9. Rowan JA, Tolunsky E. Origin and technical aspects of the EEG. In: Primer of EEG with a Mini-Atlas. Philadelphia, PA: Butterworth-Heinemann; 2003, pp. 1–21.
10. Quigg M. Channels and montages. In: EEG Pearls. Quigg M, ed. The Pearls Series. Edinburgh: Mosby, Elsevier; 2006, pp. 11–12.
11. Norman RG, Ahmed MM, Walsleben JA, et al. Detection of respiratory events during NPSG: nasal cannula/pressure sensor versus thermistor. Sleep 1997;20:1175–84.
12. Quigg M. Channels and montages. In: EEG Pearls. Quigg M, ed. The Pearls Series. Edinburgh: Mosby, Elsevier; 2006, pp. 13–14.
13. Smith SW. The Scientist's and Engineer's Guide to Digital Signal Processing. 2nd edn. California Technical Publishing, CA; pp. 225–42.
14. Spriggs WH. Equipment and amplifiers. In: Principles of Polysomnography: A Complete Training Program for Sleep Technicians. Salt Lake City, UT: Sleep Ed, LLC, 2002; pp. 50–58.
15. Hosselet JJ, Norman RG, Ayappa I, et al. Detection of flow limitation with a nasal cannula/pressure transducer system. Am J Respir Crit Care Med 1998;157(5):1461–7.
16. Kryger MH. Monitoring respiratory and cardiac function. In: Principles and Practice of Sleep Medicine, 3rd edn. Kryger M, Roth T, Dement W, eds. Philadelphia: W.B. Saunders; 2000, pp. 1217–30.

## FURTHER READING

Bolliger CT. Sleep Apnea – Current Diagnosis and Treatment. Progress in Respiratory Research Series, vol. 35. Basel: Karger; 2006.

Butkov N. Atlas of Clinical Polysomnography, volumes 1 and 11. Ashland, OR: Synapse Media; 1996.

Kryger M, Roth T, Dement W. Principles and Practice of Sleep Medicine, 4th edn. Philadelphia: Elsevier Saunders; 2005.

McNicholas W, Phillipson E. Breathing Disorders in Sleep. Philadelphia: WB Saunders; 2002.

SECTION B    DIAGNOSIS

CHAPTER 5

# Practical considerations and clinical caveats in polysomnographic interpretation in sleep-related breathing disorder

*Michel A. Cramer Bornemann and Mark W. Mahowald*

Events of abnormal breathing in sleep are characterized by snoring, apneas, hypopneas, and respiratory effort-related arousals (RERAs). These events are the result of essentially three physiologic derangements that interact to create the characteristic findings that are seen, analyzed, and summarized in polysomnography (PSG). These derangements include upper airway obstruction or flow limitation, dysregulation of respiratory control, and hypoventilation. Though apneas, hypopneas, and RERAs are seen in normal sleepers, they are rather uncommon. Nevertheless, it is the frequency of these abnormal breathing events that is pathophysiologically linked to symptoms or adverse health outcomes. Taken together, abnormal breathing events during sleep associated with clinically significant sequelae comprise many syndromes that are part of the sleep-related breathing disorder (SRBD). Aside from obstructive sleep apnea syndrome that was first defined over 30 years ago, other syndromes within SRBD include upper airway resistance syndrome (UARS), central sleep apnea syndrome (CSA), Cheyne–Stokes respiration (CSR), and alveolar hypoventilation syndrome (AHS).

It has been well established that untreated OSA has been associated with poor-quality and non-restorative sleep, excessive daytime hypersomnolence, and cognitive impairment. Furthermore, untreated OSA can adversely affect quality of life and may compromise a patient's safety when operating machinery or driving a motor vehicle. The latter is undoubtedly fraught with both personal and public tragedy and its consequent legal ramifications should not be left unheeded. From retrospective and matched control studies, morbidity and mortality appear to be proportional to the severity of SRBD and are further influenced by underlying chronic medical conditions.

There is convincing evidence that SRBD likely plays an important causal or contributing role in the development and/or progression of hypertension, congestive heart failure (CHF), cardiac arrhythmias, stroke, and diabetes mellitus. Only a few studies have evaluated the association of SRBD in patients with coronary artery disease (CAD) with a normal percentage ejection fraction (%EF). OSA does appear to be associated with several factors that are known to contribute to the progression of CAD such as elevated sympathetic tone, increases in serum levels of inflammatory mediators (such as C-reactive protein, interleukin-6, and tumor necrosis factor-a), and a shift towards a more pro-coagulative state. Despite these striking findings, the clinical-based evidence supporting the association of SRBD with CAD is less compelling and studies that have utilized appropriate polysomnographic methodology and have attained statistical relevance have yet to be achieved.

In the last 15 years alone there has been a rapid technological evolution involving the means by which airflow and other cardiorespiratory parameters can be measured. Unfortunately, the development of many of these exquisitely sensitive physiologic monitors has yet to exhibit clinical relevance. In other words, as many sleep laboratories step up to maintain a competitive advantage by being on the 'cutting edge' as a technological leader, many of these new technologies are without substance as the clinical-based evidence supporting its use is often completely lacking. As such, there have been various definitions of apnea, hypopnea, and RERAs. Given that these abnormal breathing events are critical in determining the severity of SRBD, the American Academy of Sleep Medicine (AASM) has addressed this concern in its 2005 consensus guidelines on practice parameters for PSG. The recommended definitions for apneas, hypopneas, and RERAs are detailed in Table 5.1.

The use of PSG for evaluating SRBD requires a minimum of the following recording: electroencephalogram (EEG), electro-oculogram (EOG), chin electromyogram (EMG), airflow, respiratory effort, arterial oxygen saturation (SaO$_2$), and electrocardiogram (ECG) or heart rate. An anterior tibialis EMG is strongly encouraged to detect movement arousals and periodic limb movement. The AASM-recommended key items in PSG monitoring and summary reports are listed in Table 5.2. It must be noted that these recommendations are for hospital- or sleep laboratory-based PSGs. Currently, there is insufficient information from investigations using well-controlled clinical-based evidence to recommend or

SECTION B  DIAGNOSIS

Table 5.1  Clinical definitions of breathing events during sleep

| | |
|---|---|
| Obstructive apnea | Apnea is defined as a cessation of airflow for at least 10 seconds. The event is obstructive if during apnea there is effort to breath. |
| Central apnea | Apnea is defined as a cessation of airflow for at least 10 seconds. The event is central if during apnea there is no effort to breath. |
| Mixed apnea | Apnea is defined as a cessation of airflow for at least 10 seconds. The event is mixed if the apnea begins as a central apnea, but towards the end there is effort to breath without airflow. |
| Hypopnea | Several definitions of hypopnea are in clinical use but there is no clear consensus. The Centers for Medicare and Medicaid (CMS) have approved the definition of hypopnea as an abnormal respiratory event with at least a 30% reduction in thoracoabdominal movement or airflow as compared to baseline lasting at least 10 seconds, and with ≥4% oxygen desaturation. |
| Respiratory effort-related arousal (RERA) | *Clinical definition:* not agreed upon. *Research definition:* sequence of breaths with increasing respiratory effort leading to an arousal from sleep, as shown by progressively more negative esophageal pressure for at least 10 seconds preceding an arousal with resumption of more normal pressures. |

Table 5.2  Key items for polysomnography (PSG) data collection and reporting

| | |
|---|---|
| Recorded PSG parameters | Central monopolar recording<br>Occipital mono- or bipolar recording<br>Chin EMG<br>R/L anterior tibialis EMG<br>ROC and LOC<br>ECG (traditionally, single lead II)<br>Snoring microphone<br>Nasal/oral airflow<br>Thoracic effort<br>Abdominal effort<br>$SaO_2$ (peripheral pulse oximetry)<br>$pCO_2$, if clinically indicated:<br>• End-tidal $CO_2$<br>• Transcutaneous monitoring (TCM)<br>Body position |
| Lights out<br>Lights on<br>Total sleep time (TST)<br>Sleep efficiency index<br>Sleep latency<br>REM sleep latency<br>Wake after sleep onset (WASO) | |
| Sleep stages | Total time in each stage (I, II, III/IV, REM)<br>Percent of total sleep time |
| Number and index of apneic events:<br>• Obstructive<br>• Mixed<br>• Central<br>Number and index of RERAs<br>Apnea/hypopnea index<br>Respiratory arousal/disturbance index<br>Minimum oxygen saturation | *During sleep*<br>By body position<br>NREM vs. REM<br>Means and longest duration<br>Duration of $SaO_2$ in percentage ranges:<br>• Wake, NREM and REM<br>Mean, minimum, and maximum $SaO_2$:<br>• Wake, NREM and REM |
| Periodic limb movements (PLMs), with and without arousal | |
| Summary/impression | Diagnosis<br>Any EEG or ECG abnormalities<br>Unusual behavior observed during study |

support unattended home PSGs in the diagnosis and management of SRBD.

Awareness of sleep disorders has grown immensely. In 1990, there were an estimated 110,000 office visits for SRBD. By 1998, this had risen to 1.3 million visits per year. Though the health benefits of treating SRDB are well established, the potential cost savings to healthcare providers and insurers have only recently been explored. Patients with untreated SRBD are more likely to be hospitalized and incur higher healthcare costs than matched control subjects. One study revealed that the length of stay of hospitalized patients with untreated SRBD was increased 2.8-fold and incurred excess hospital costs of $100,000–200,000. The magnitude of the medical costs correlated with the severity of the SRBD. There is only one study that details the SRBD treatment benefit on healthcare costs and utilization. In this study, patients were followed for 2 years following their diagnosis and then compared to matched control subjects over the same period of time. The SRBD-treated patients when compared to control subjects revealed an overall decrease in physician costs of 33% and a decrease in the duration of consequent hospital stays. The improvement in physician costs and hospital stay was only significant in patients maintaining compliance with SRBD treatment. Lastly, there are also cost advantages in including attended hospital- or sleep laboratory-based PSGs in the diagnosis of SRBD. A recent cost analysis of the benefit of a PSG in the detection of SRBD demonstrated a cost saving of $9200–13,400 per quality-adjusted life-year gained. Compared to other outpatient diagnostic tests, the cost of a PSG to diagnose SRBD is favorable. For example, the cost of a diagnostic PSG is one-fourth the cost of a standard screening for carotid stenosis in an asymptomatic patient.

Practical considerations and clinical caveats in polysomnographic interpretation in sleep-related breathing disorder

CHAPTER 5

**Table 5.3 General algorithm for polysomnography (PSG) interpretation**

| | |
|---|---|
| 1. Review patient history for symptoms and presenting complaints. | What symptoms or complaints are you trying to confirm, account for, or rule out with the PSG? |
| 2. Review the subjective sleep diary (or log) and/or the objective actigraphy study report:<br>• Determine the patient's typical sleep pattern<br>• Estimate average total sleep time<br>• Characterize the number of arousals<br>• Determine the usual bedtime and wake time. | Review the patient's PM and AM sleep questionnaire that characterizes his/her experience during the PSG peri-monitoring period. |
| 3. Review the raw data in the PSG recording. | Review the sleep technologist's notes, observations, and assessments. |
| 4. Compare the values in the PSG to normative data and the patient's estimates. | Determine the age- and sex-related range of values thought to be normal, if available. |
| 5. Determine what values in the PSG summary are artifacts inherent in the sleep laboratory and what values are representative of the patient's usual sleep. | Consider the influence of:<br>• First night effect (FNE)<br>• Paradoxical first night effect (PFNE)<br>• Environment<br>• Medications<br>• Alcohol and illicit drugs. |
| 6. Review the recording for other features that may have clinical significance. | Explain any discrepancies.<br>Account for all non-breathing related EEG abnormalities, technical artifacts, and sources of interference. |
| 7. Review the audio and videotape for sleep-related behaviors, if indicated. | Consider referral to an appropriate neurology consultant, if indicated. |
| 8. Make a final statement as to the likely interpretation and diagnosis. | *Do the PSG findings explain the clinical picture?*<br>Arrange for treatment, management, and follow-up evaluation as clinically indicated. |

The diagnosis and treatment of SRBD are justifiable on the basis of its negative impact on the individual as well as the general public. Furthermore, there is now evidence that treatment of SRBD has a significant impact on improving short-term and lifetime healthcare utilization. Unfortunately, the assessment and interpretation of a PSG are often not straightforward and require the involvement of a physician who is formally trained in sleep medicine. A multidisciplinary approach is often effective as it is not uncommon to serendipitously encounter a physiological abnormality or behavior that is not directly related to the primary indication for the PSG. Thus, the diagnosis and management of SRBD are more efficiently accomplished by a comprehensive physician evaluation and formal sleep monitoring than either component done alone. A general algorithm for PSG interpretation and patient management has been outlined in Table 5.3.

## 1 POLYSOMNOGRAPHY CASE REVIEWS WITH CLINICAL CAVEATS

### 1.1 CASE 1: POSITION-DEPENDENT OSA

**Case description**
This 44-year-old Caucasian male has a past medical history significant for well-controlled hypertension and a family history significant for coronary artery disease. He has episodes of socially disruptive snoring and poor-quality non-restorative sleep. He is concerned about excessive daytime fatigue and sleepiness but denies any cognitive impairment. Physical examination is remarkable for a Friedman Tongue Position I oropharynx and a neck circumference less than 17 inches. There was no evidence for any signs of lower extremity edema. PSG was indicated to evaluate for suspected SRDB and for other possible causes of excessive daytime sleepiness.

**PSG findings**
The baseline PSG revealed a monitoring pre-treatment time of 195 minutes with a wake after sleep onset (WASO) time of 50 minutes. All stages of sleep were attained as reflected in the hypnogram (Fig. 5.1). The patient did exhibit marked snoring associated with episodes of apnea and hypopnea. He attained a lowest $SaO_2$ of 82%, compared with a wake baseline in the upper 90s. Given the Apnea/Hypopnea Index (AHI) was calculated to be only seven events/hour, one might conclude that this patient has mild OSA. However, the hypnogram revealed that OSA only occurred during a very discrete portion of the study (as noted by the arrows in Fig. 5.1).
Reviewing the sleep technologist's notes as well as reviewing the PSG video it became readily apparent that the patient only exhibited marked OSA while in a supine position. The sleep technologist's notes also revealed that

SECTION B  DIAGNOSIS

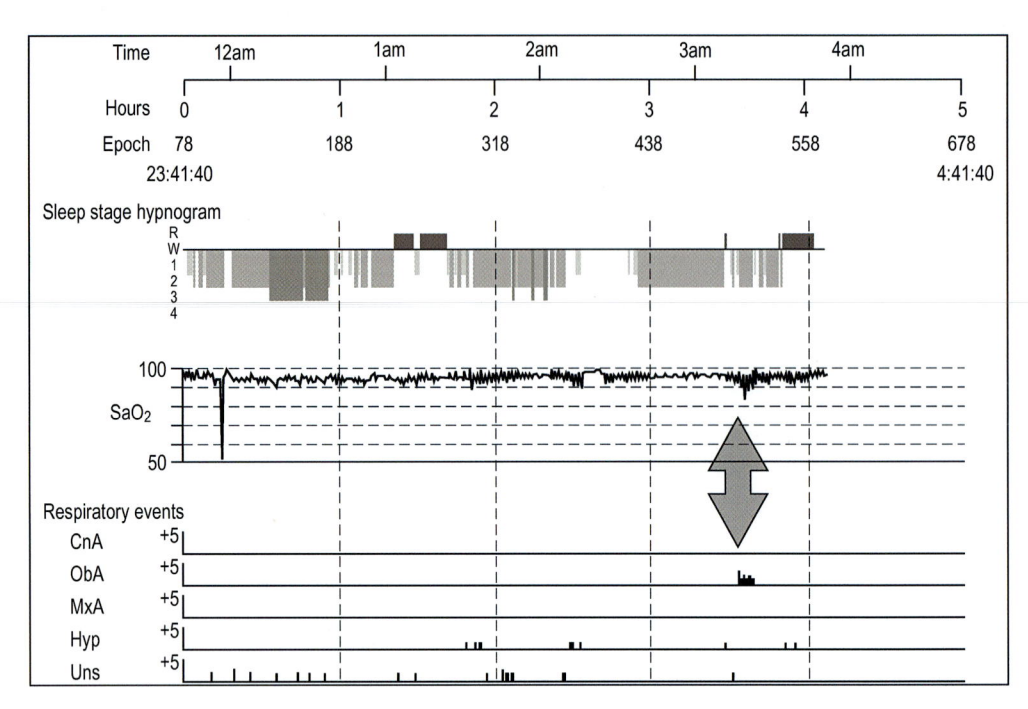

**Fig. 5.1** Baseline pre-treatment hypnogram with position-dependent OSA. Sleep stage hypnogram legend: Stages 1–4 = NREM sleep; R = REM sleep. SaO$_2$: percent arterial oxygen saturation using peripheral pulse oximetry. Respiratory events legend: Cn.A = Central sleep apnea; Ob.A = Obstructive sleep apnea; Mx.A = Mixed apnea; Uns = Unspecified respiratory event.

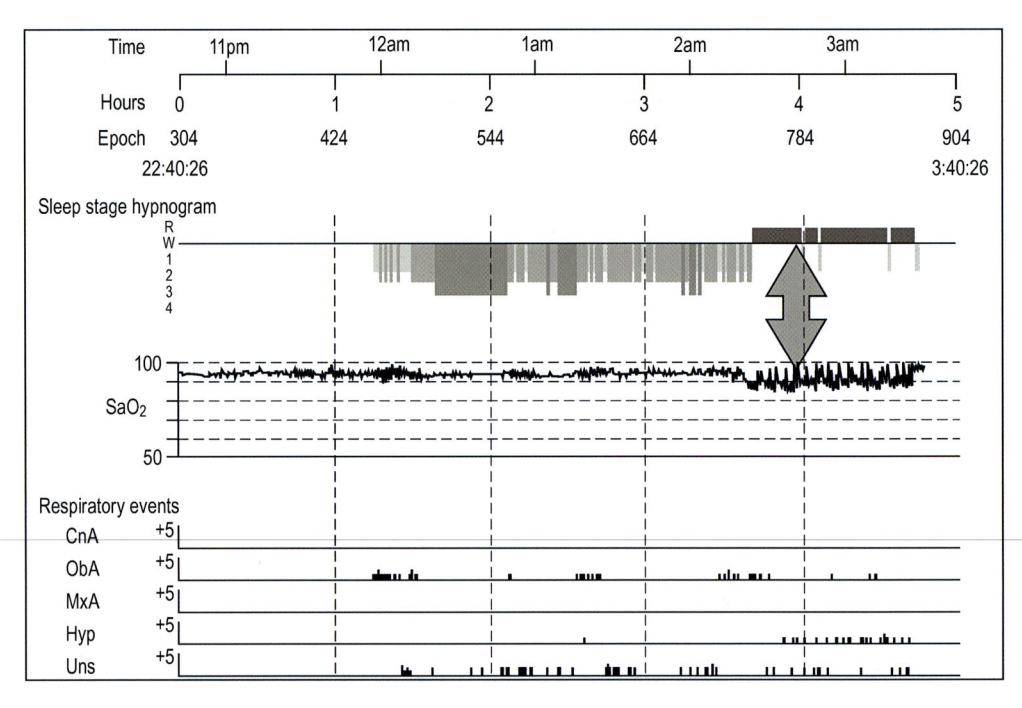

**Fig. 5.2** Baseline pre-treatment hypnogram with state-dependent OSA. Sleep stage hypnogram legend: Stages 1–4 = NREM sleep; R = REM sleep. SaO$_2$: percent arterial oxygen saturation using peripheral pulse oximetry. Respiratory events legend: Cn.A = Central Sleep Apnea; Ob.A = Obstructive sleep apnea; Mx.A = Mixed apnea; Uns = Unspecified respiratory event.

the patient only slept in that supine position during that brief isolated instance. Upon reviewing the patient's AM and PM sleep questionnaire, it was noted that he prefers to sleep in either a prone or supine position but due to a recent aggravation of his chronic low back condition the patient has opted to sleep in a lateral position. Thus, it would appear that the calculated AHI is an underestimation of the patient's OSA. The therapeutic portion the PSG which includes a titration of non-invasive positive pressure ventilation (NIPPV) should ensure that all positions of sleep have been attained to ensure optimal management for this patient.

### Clinical caveat

The expression and severity of SRBD have many influences. A complete diagnostic and therapeutic PSG should observe the patient in all positions of sleep. One should also remember that SRBD may be sleep state dependent. In this

**Practical considerations and clinical caveats in polysomnographic interpretation in sleep-related breathing disorder** | CHAPTER 5

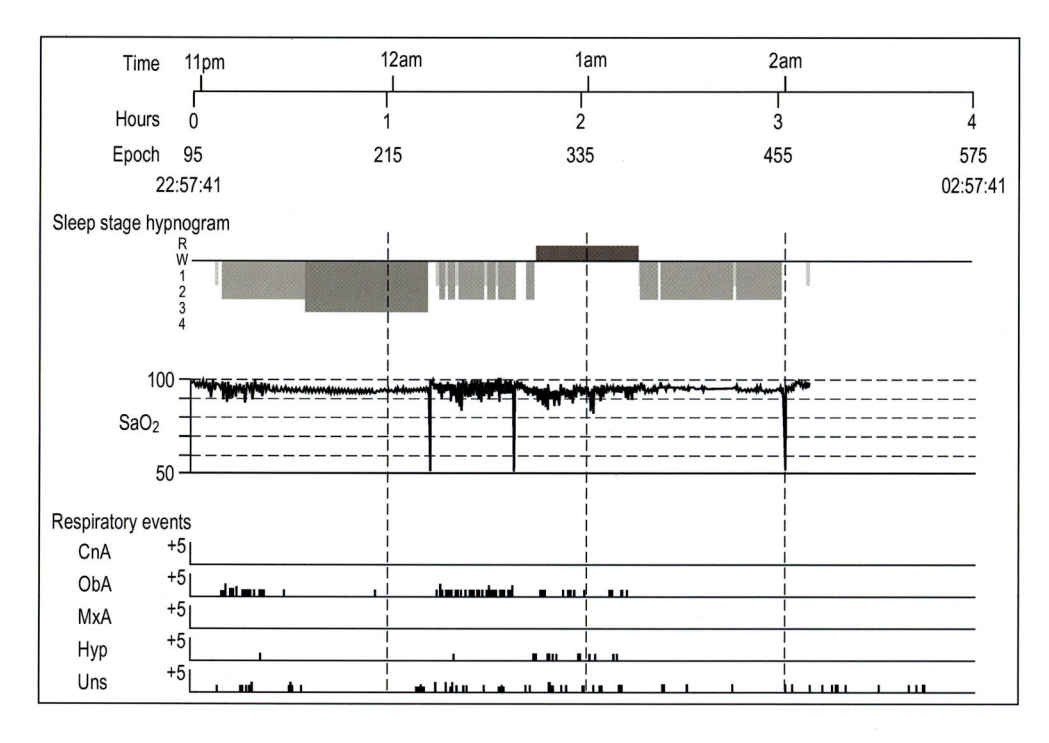

**Fig. 5.3** Baseline pre-treatment hypnogram with intact sleep architecture. Sleep stage hypnogram legend: Stages 1–4 = NREM sleep; R = REM sleep. $SaO_2$: percent arterial oxygen saturation using peripheral pulse oximetry. Respiratory events legend: Cn.A = Central sleep apnea; Ob.A = Obstructive sleep apnea; Mx.A = Mixed apnea; Uns = Unspecified respiratory event.

regard, REM sleep, with its generalized muscle atonia and predisposition for further upper airway collapse, appears to be a particularly vulnerable state for the progression of SRBD. REM sleep also is associated with increased respiratory rate variability, a mild increase in arterial $CO_2$ levels, and a decrease in minute ventilation. A clinical case of OSA that is further complicated during REM sleep is seen in Figure 5.2. In this case, note the accentuated $SaO_2$ desaturations and persistent downward trend in the $SaO_2$ baseline suggestive of REM hypoventilation.

Allow the patient the opportunity to express all influences that might impact sleep. Though this may be an inconvenience for sleep laboratory support staff who often work in shifts, this undoubtedly sets the foundation for optimal patient care. Furthermore, always review all the resources available including the patient's questionnaire and the sleep technologist's notes.

## 1.2 CASE 2: SEVERE OSA WITH INTACT SLEEP ARCHITECTURE

### Case description

This 39-year-old African-American male has had a significant weight gain of approximately 60 lb over the last 2 years and now has a Body Mass Index (BMI) of 37. Within the last 8–12 months his stentorian snoring has contributed to marital discord with his wife such that they now sleep in separate bedrooms. He does not have obvious episodes of observed apneas. Though the patient minimizes any daytime problems that might be associated with his non-restorative sleep, his wife is concerned that his daytime sleepiness leaves him unmotivated and unable to maintain his household duties. His physical examination was only remarkable for a Friedman Tongue Position II oropharynx and a neck circumference of $17\frac{1}{4}$ inches. A PSG was indicated for this patient with a high probability for moderate-to-severe SRBD.

### PSG findings

The baseline PSG confirmed the patient's severe OSA as supported by an AHI of 35 events/hour with an absolute $SaO_2$ nadir of 80%, compared with a wake $SaO_2$ baseline in the upper 90s. Surprisingly, the baseline hypnogram (see Fig. 5.3) revealed consolidated sleep with normal sleep stage progression and % sleep efficiency and % stage REM of 90% and 20%, respectively. Though the OSA was more pronounced in stage REM, this stage too exhibited apparent continuity without fragmentation.

Figure 5.4 exhibits episodes of obstructive apnea associated with $SaO_2$ desaturations into the low 80s. Using the majority of epoch (MOE) rule for sleep staging in 30-second increments, this 2-minute page exhibits uninterrupted Stage I sleep. However, this page also exhibits two types of arousals that might not be appreciated on a hypnogram or PSG summary report. Arrow A denotes a subcortical arousal as supported by a respiratory event that is associated with consequent increase in heart rate of at least 10 bpm within a 60-second interval. This segment reveals a heart rate increase from 62 to 76 bpm in less than 30 seconds. Arrow B denotes a microarousal with a generalized

SECTION B  DIAGNOSIS

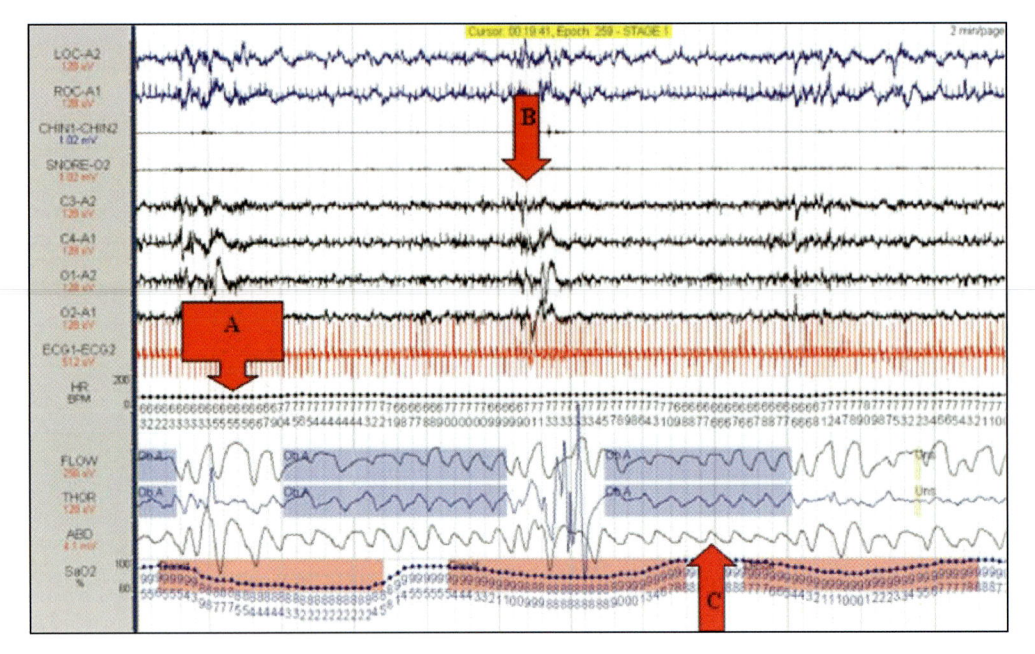

Fig. 5.4 Baseline stage I PSG epoch with OSA. PSG legend: LOC = Left eye; ROC = Right eye; Chin1-Chin2 = Chin EMG; Snore = microphone; C3-A2/C4-A1 = Left/right central EEG leads; O1-A2/O2-A1 = Left/right occipital EEG leads; ECG1-ECG2 = Electrocardiogram lead II; HR = heart rate in numeric read-out (beats per minute); FLOW = Airflow monitor; THOR = Thoracic respiratory effort; ABD = Abdominal respiratory effort; SaO$_2$ = peripheral pulse oximetry (arterial oxygen saturation) with numeric read-out.

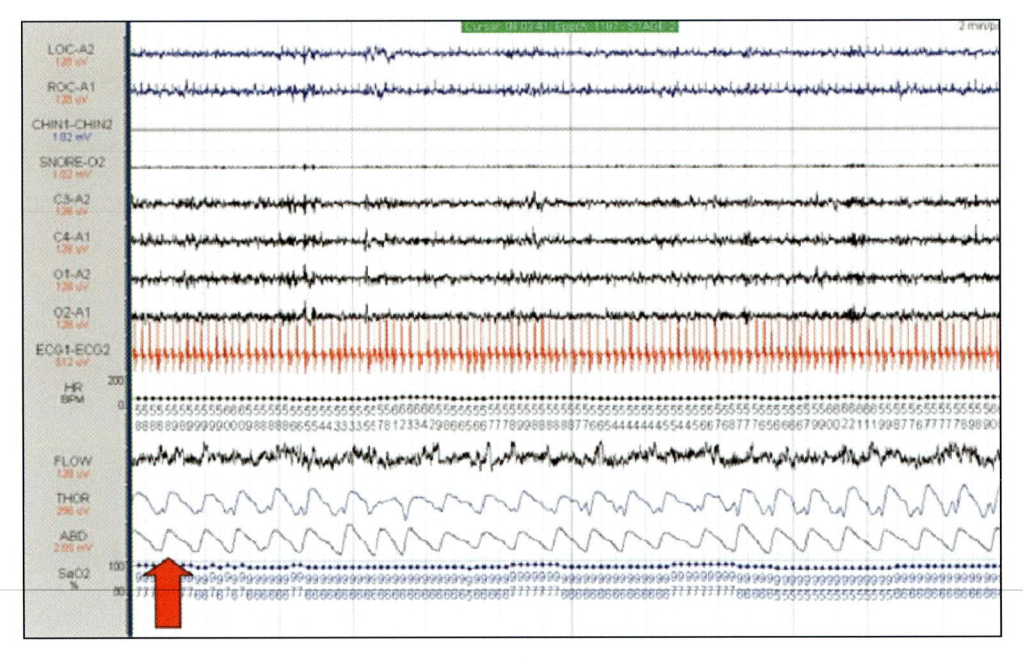

Fig. 5.5 Baseline stage I PSG epoch with OSA. PSG Legend: LOC = Left eye; ROC = Right eye; Chin1-Chin2 = Chin EMG, Snore = Microphone; C3-A2/C4-A1 = Left/right central EEG leads, O1-A2/O2-A1 = Left/right occipital EEG leads; ECG1-ECG2 = Electrocardiogram lead II; HR = Heart rate in numeric read-out (beats per minute); FLOW = Airflow monitor; THOR = Thoracic respiratory effort; ABD = Abdominal respiratory effort; SaO$_2$ = Peripheral pulse oximetry (arterial oxygen saturation) with numeric read-out.

increase in amplitude and frequency noted in the central and occipital EEG leads. Arrow C points to a paradoxical breathing pattern in the thoracic and abdominal respiratory monitors. Such an abnormal breathing pattern is often found with upper airway flow limitation. Lastly, when one takes into account the number of subcortical arousals and microarousals, this patient's sleep certainly would appear more fragmented than first appreciated and this might contribute to the perceived daytime inattentiveness.

Figure 5.5 is a representative example of the patient's sleep in Stage II after continuous positive airway pressure (CPAP) was titrated to an optimal setting of 9 cmH$_2$O with heated humidity applied for comfort. Note that the upper airway patency has been achieved as supported by the resolution of apneic episodes and the return of synchronized breathing in the thoracic and abdominal respiratory monitors (see arrow, Fig. 5.5). Also, oxygen desaturations have resolved and SaO$_2$ has normalized to the upper 90s while heart rate has declined appreciably and now exhibits a range with decreased variability over a 2-minute page. Finally, note that this stage in sleep truly does appear to be consolidated and an epoch-by-epoch review at 30 seconds/page does not reveal any evidence of subcortical arousals or microarousals.

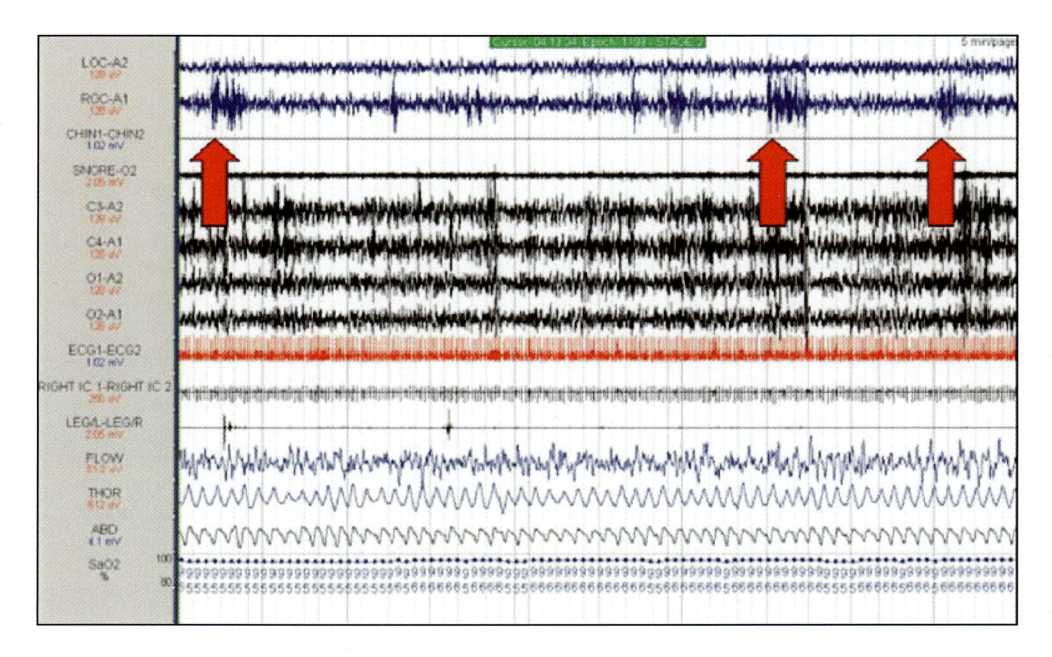

Practical considerations and clinical caveats in polysomnographic interpretation in sleep-related breathing disorder

CHAPTER 5

Fig. 5.6 Baseline stage II PSG Epoch 1199 at 5 minutes per page. PSG legend: LOC = Left eye; ROC = Right eye; Chin1-Chin2 = Chin EMG; Snore = Microphone; C3-A2/C4-A1 = Left/right central EEG leads; O1-A2/O2-A1 = Left/right occipital EEG leads; ECG1-ECG2 = Electrocardiogram lead II; HR = Heart rate in numeric read-out (beats per minute); FLOW = Airflow monitor; THOR = Thoracic respiratory effort; ABD = Abdominal respiratory effort; SaO$_2$ = Peripheral pulse oximetry (arterial oxygen saturation) with numeric read-out.

## Clinical caveat

The methodology for scoring sleep by Rechtshaffen and Kales and the majority of epoch (MOE) rule used at a speed of 30 seconds per page may be appropriate for staging sleep but one must bear in mind their limitations. Sleep staging and PSG summary reports often do not adequately reflect the extent of sleep fragmentation attributed to SRBD. In this particular case, the goals for optimal management for this patient's OSA using CPAP can be measured by: (1) complete resolution of apnea and/or hypopnea; (2) normalization of SaO$_2$; (3) resolution of a paradoxical breathing pattern; (4) the development of sleep maintenance and consolidation; and (5) the resolution of breathing-related arousals.

## 1.3 CASE 3: PEDIATRIC OSA WITH AN UNUSUAL EYE LEAD FINDING

### Case description

This 10-year-old Caucasian female underwent a craniopharyngioma resection approximately 4 years ago. The perioperative period included the temporary placement of a ventriculo-peritoneal shunt. The postoperative period was significant for a 6-week course of localized central nervous system (CNS) radiation therapy. As a result of the neurosurgical intervention the patient has required multiple hormone replacements including growth hormone. Within the last year, the patient has developed loud snoring that appears to be associated with observed episodes of both central and obstructive apneas. The patient has also developed an apparent prolonged sleep requirement and has become increasingly sleepy during the daytime with the resumption of regular naps in the afternoon. Her physical examination is remarkable only for a BMI of 33 and a Friedman Tongue Position I oropharynx. A PSG was indicated to assist in determining causes of daytime sleepiness and to characterize the extent of her presumed SRBD.

### PSG findings

The baseline PSG confirmed OSA with a calculated AHI of 13 events/hour. All stages of sleep were attained with % sleep efficiency and % REM at 81% and 4%, respectively. The patient attained a SaO$_2$ nadir of 77% during an apneic episode, compared with a wake SaO$_2$ baseline in the upper 90s. For a child this degree of apnea combined with such a SaO$_2$ desaturation would classify the patient with severe OSA. There was no evidence for central sleep apnea or a periodic breathing pattern. No abnormal motor activity of any kind was observed during the overnight study. However, when reviewing the PSG at a speed of 5 minutes per epoch, the conventional page speed when assessing respiratory pattern, frequent high-amplitude waves in discrete packets were noted in lead ROC-A1 (see Fig. 5.6). Given the other leads did not exhibit this wave pattern, it appears that these abnormal waves are coming from the right eye lead (ROC).

To further characterize and discern the cause of these abnormal waves, the epoch length was reduced to 30 seconds per page, the conventional epoch for staging sleep. Again, the same epoch was reviewed and the sharp wave activity was clearly seen in ROC-A1 (see Fig. 5.7). In Stage II sleep this activity would not be related to eye movements. The A1 lead is also linked to the EEG leads of C4 and O2, but neither of these leads exhibited the abnormal wave activity, thereby confirming the localization of the abnormality to the right eye lead. Without additional physiologic correlates or data, the PSG epochs of either 5 minutes or 30 seconds were unable to determine whether the abnormal waves were of any clinical relevance or whether they were related to technical or environmentally induced artifacts.

# SECTION B  DIAGNOSIS

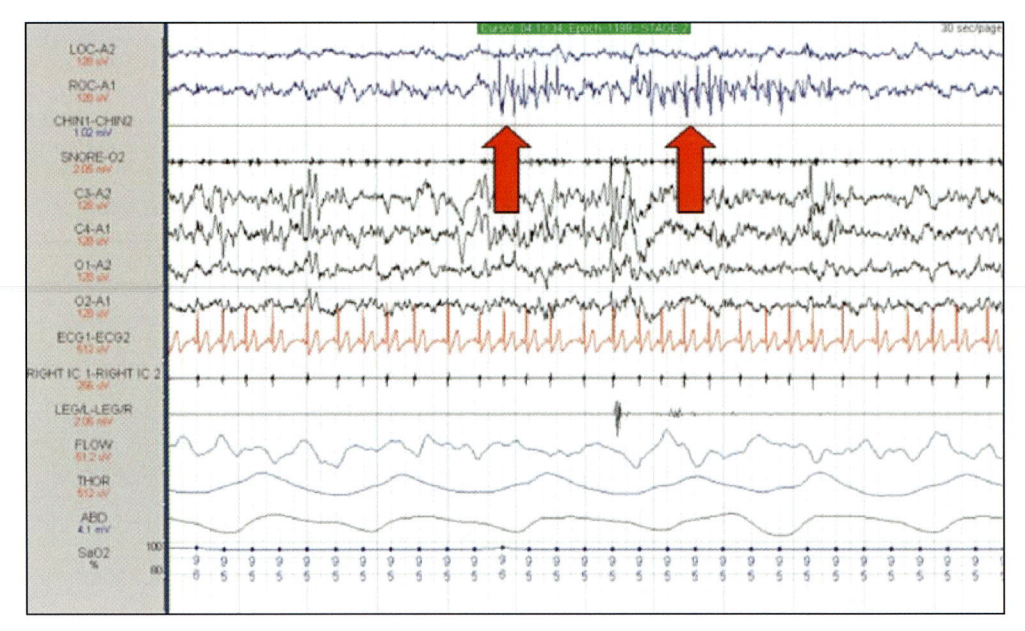

**Fig. 5.7** Baseline stage II PSG Epoch 1199 at 30 seconds per page. PSG legend: LOC = Left eye; ROC = Right eye; Chin1-Chin2 = Chin EMG; Snore = Microphone; C3-A2/C4-A1 = Left/right central EEG leads; O1-A2/O2-A1 = Left/right occipital EEG leads; ECG1-ECG2 = Electrocardiogram lead II; HR = Heart rate in numeric read-out (beats per minute); FLOW = Airflow monitor; THOR = Thoracic respiratory effort; ABD = Abdominal respiratory effort; SaO₂ = Peripheral pulse oximetry (arterial oxygen saturation) with numeric read-out.

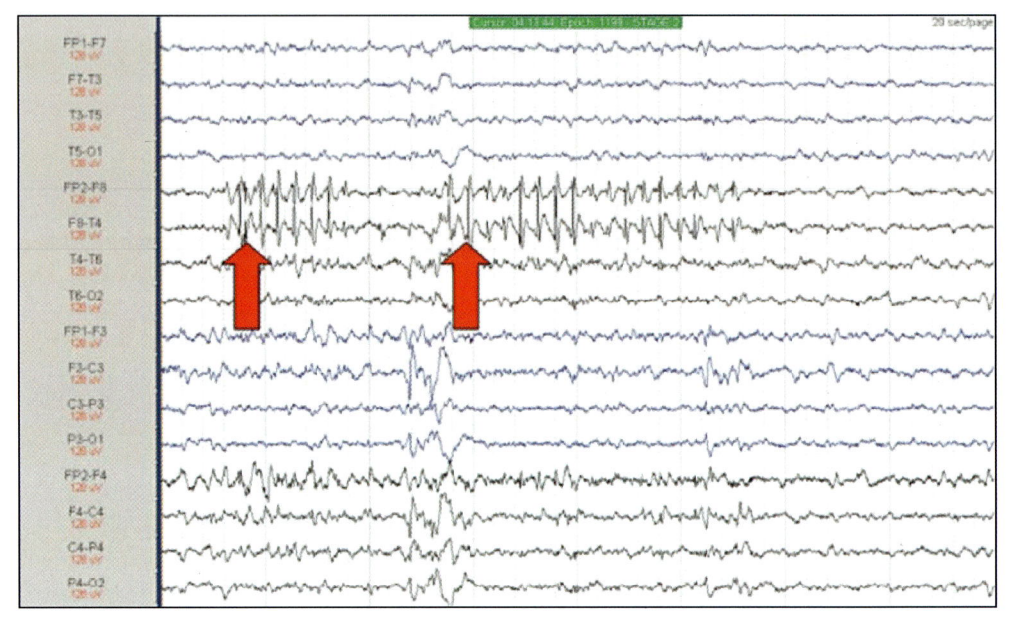

**Fig. 5.8** 20-20 EEG configuration revealing epileptiform activity in the right frontal hemisphere (F8). EEG legend: Left temporal region = FP1-F7, F7-T3, T3-T5, T5-O1; Right temporal region = FP2-F8, F8-T4, T4-T6, T6-O2; Left parasagittal region = FP1-F3, F3-C3, C3-P3, P3-O1; Right parasagittal region = FP2-F4, F4-C4, C4-P4, P4-O2.

Fortunately, given the patient's CNS pathology, the PSG was also complemented with a full 20-20 EEG configuration which is a standard montage used to evaluate nocturnal seizures. Though the patient did not exhibit any tonic–clonic or overt motor activity, the seizure montage clearly exhibited sharp wave activity along the right hemisphere. Such an activity is highlighted in Figure 5.8. Note the sharp wave activity and phase reversal in EEG leads FP2-F8 and F8-T4. This finding is consistent with epileptiform activity in the right frontal hemisphere as localized by EEG lead F8.

Clinical management for this patient involved a thorough discussion concerning the appropriate management for her OSA. This included discussions involving the role of non-invasive positive pressure ventilation, upper airway surgical intervention, and the possibility of a dental evaluation for the placement of a mandibular advancement device. Further discussion also involved a debate with a pediatric endocrinologist related to the risks and benefits of continued growth hormone therapy. Lastly the patient was also referred to a pediatric neurologist to determine whether the right hemispheric epileptiform activity was a contributor to her constellation of concerns.

## Clinical caveat

Especially in patients with a complex past medical history, it is not uncommon to serendipitously discover a non-breathing related clinically significant abnormality. All discrepancies and artifacts need to be accounted for and explained. EEG electrodes are amplified and filtered and do not distinguish whether the incoming electrical signal is reflective of real physiologic input or whether it is the result of external electrical or technical interference. An understanding of the physiology behind the EEG is helpful and the involvement of a neurologist skilled in interpreting both wake and sleep EEGs is often beneficial.

## 2 CONCLUSION

The interpretation of the PSG should not start with the review of the study's summary statistics and should not be done in isolation. It involves more than reviewing the respiratory variables at the compressed PSG rate of 5 minutes/epoch conventionally used to characterize anticipated SRBD. It also requires that the EEG data be completely reviewed at a rate of 20–30 seconds/epoch in order to confirm the sleep technologist's preliminary sleep staging and to account for any non-apneic discrepancies that might be clinically relevant. As non-apneic sleep disorders are often encountered in a PSG, *all of the patient's information needs to be reviewed by the interpreter*. This information should at least include: patient's past medical and psychiatric history; sleep laboratory orientation, monitoring calibration, and preparation of equipment; acquisition of 8–16 channels of physiological data; review of sleep diaries: lights out and lights on sleep laboratory questionnaires; and scoring of physiological data for sleep stages, respiration/ventilation, muscle tone or movements, and ECG/heart rate variability. The PSG is the culmination of a multi-faceted complex process. Only after such a comprehensive and detailed approach to the PSG has been undertaken can one attain efficient, individualized, optimal, and cost-effective medical management for the patient.

## FURTHER READING

AASM Position Statement. Cost justification for diagnosis and treatment of obstructive sleep apnea. Sleep 2000;23:1–2.

Butkov N. Atlas of Clinical Polysomnography, volumes I and II. Ashland, Oregon: Synapse Media; 1996.

Goldensohn ES, Legatt AD, Koszer S, Wolf SM. Goldensohn's EEG Interpretation: Problems of Overreading and Underreading, 2nd edn. New York: Futura; 1999.

Kreiger MH, Roth T, Dement WC. Principles and Practice of Sleep Medicine, 4th edn. Philadelphia: Elsevier Saunders; 2005.

Kushida CA, Littner MR, Morgenthaler T, et al. Practice parameters for the indications for polysomnography and related procedures: an update for 2005. Sleep 2005;28(4):499–521.

Pressman MR. Primer of Polysomnogram Interpretation. Boston: Butterworth-Heinemann; 2002.

Spriggs WH. Principles of Polysomnography: A Complete Training Program for Sleep Technicians. Salt Lake City: Sleep Ed LLC; 2002.

# SECTION B — DIAGNOSIS

## CHAPTER 6

# Validity of sleep nasendoscopy in the investigation of sleep-related breathing disorder

*Sandeep Berry and Heikki B. Whittet*

## 1 INTRODUCTION

Croft and Pringle introduced the technique of sleep nasendoscopy for use in the assessment of snoring to aid proper case selection for surgical intervention.[1]

The attraction of sleep nasendoscopy lies with its ability to provide a dynamic visualization of the anatomical areas responsible for the generation of noise (snoring) or obstruction, under conditions which mimic sleep. Prior to the introduction of sleep nasendoscopy various methods including lateral cephalometry, computerized tomography and the Mueller maneuver had been used in an attempt to achieve the above objective.[2]

Sleep nasendoscopy has been criticized for not being a true reflection of normal physiological sleep in view of the sedation process involved. Various techniques of sedation have been used.[3-5] Bolus injections of sedatives are commonly used and may lead to fluctuating blood, plasma and tissue levels leading in turn to fluctuating drug effects. The correct level of sedation is crucial to produce sufficient muscle relaxation to recreate snoring but not cause respiratory depression.[3] Roblin et al. adopted a computer-controlled infusion system that employs the concept of target controlled infusion (TCI)[2] using propofol as the sedating agent. Propofol has the attraction of possessing a rapid onset of action and recovery period, with minimal side effects.[6] In addition it allows for standardization and reproducibility between different operators.

## 2 PATIENT SELECTION

Sleep nasendoscopy has the potential to be a valuable investigation for making an accurate dynamic anatomical assessment in patients with snoring and obstructive features. Determination of the anatomical site of the obstruction in this way allows an appropriate or targeted choice of treatment options to be made.[1] Although commonly used, questions have been raised regarding the potential for false-positive results; that is, the production of symptoms (snoring/obstruction) in individuals with no history of sleep-disordered breathing.

During sleep endoscopy the correct level of sedation is vital to induce symptoms of snoring with or without obstruction but not cause respiratory depression.[3] This window of sedation can be narrow, may differ from patient to patient and be difficult to maintain for any length of time.

Sleep nasendoscopy is employed as a diagnostic tool for patients with snoring problems as well as those with obstructive sleep apnea (OSA) as selected by the sleep multidisciplinary team.

## 3 TECHNIQUE OF SLEEP NASENDOSCOPY

The procedure is carried out in the operating room. A size 14 G cannula is inserted into the patient's vein. The Diprifusor TCI system (Zeneca Pharma, Wilmslow, Cheshire, UK), incorporating an electronically tagged prefilled syringe of 1% propofol, is placed into a Graseby 3500 (Graseby Medical Ltd, Watford, Herts, UK) dedicated infusion pump. The sex and weight of the patient are entered on the pump and the pump connected to the cannula. Pulse oximetry, heart rate and blood pressure are closely monitored throughout the procedure. No local anesthesia is used in the nasal cavity to avoid any anesthesia in the pharynx.

A starting concentration of 2 µg/ml of propofol is chosen and the dual microprocessor component within the pump then determines the infusion rate required to attain the desired concentration by calculating the absorption, distribution and excretion of propofol. Immediately the pump will administer a bolus dose to fill the pharmacological central compartment followed initially by a high infusion rate to compensate for drug distribution and thereafter the infusion rate decreases with time.

The blood concentration level is increased in 2 µg/ml incremental doses and the system automatically adjusts the rate of propofol infusion to achieve the required blood concentration level. The flexible nasendoscope (Olympus

P4) is introduced when the patient begins to snore; if the patient obstructs the target concentration level is reduced. In the location of obstructive sites, attention is paid to the following levels:

1. Soft palate.
2. Lateral pharyngeal wall.
3. Palatine tonsil.
4. Tongue base/lingual tonsil.
5. Epiglottis.

A video and sound recording of the sleep nasendoscopy is carried out during the procedure.

The degree of obstruction is categorized as follows.

- **Simple palatal snoring.** In this group, the noise arises from the vibration of the soft palate, walls of velopharyngeal sphincter and upper oropharynx.
- **Lateral wall collapse.** The obstruction involves the oropharyngeal area (palatine tonsil when present).
- **Tongue base/epiglottis.** The velopharyngeal sphincter remains patent but the obstruction is at the tongue base level as a consequence of lower jaw regression or tongue base or lingual tonsil hypertrophy. The epiglottis may contribute to noise and/or obstruction in combination with tongue component or in isolation.
- **Multi-segmental collapse.** The obstruction appears to arise from all the areas above.

## 3.1 PHARMACOKINETICS OF PROPOFOL

Propofol is a white, sterile, odorless and isotonic oil in water emulsion, prepared by chemical synthesis. The emulsion vehicle contains soybean oil and purified egg phosphatide. Propofol is used as the sedating agent for target controlled infusion as it has a rapid onset of action, is metabolized quickly, giving a fast recovery phase, and has a low incidence of postoperative nausea, vomiting and headache. Propofol has the attraction of possessing a rapid onset of action and recovery period, with minimal side effects.[6] In addition, it allows for standardization and reproducibility between different operators.

The combination of target controlled infusion and propofol allows a more accurate and reproducible (between different operators) control of sedation during sleep nasendoscopy. The procedure is well tolerated by the patient and is performed as a day case. There are no known complications of sleep nasendoscopy.

## 4 SPECIFICITY AND SENSITIVITY OF SLEEP NASENDOSCOPY

Previous studies have questioned the value of sleep nasendoscopy because asymptomatic subjects could be induced to snore and obstruct. Marais[3] stated that although sleep nasendoscopy is a widely used investigation in patients with sleep-disordered breathing despite its non-physiological basis, there still remains a doubt of its validity as an investigative tool. Marais compared the presence or absence of snoring and its site of generation between a group of 205 snorers and another of 126 non-snorers. Snoring was produced at nasendoscopy in 45.3% of non-snorers but could not be produced in 18.1% of snorers. There was no significant difference in the site of sound production between the two groups and although the noise produced by the non-snoring group was quieter, this difference was not significant. Abdullah et al.[7] suggested that a clear establishment of the site of obstruction is crucial for subsequent treatment planning. Video sleep nasendoscopy (VSE) is probably the most accurate assessment of the situation and also helps in identifying the situation that needs correction.

Berry et al.[8] conducted a prospective cohort study involving 107 patients divided into two groups. The two groups of patients were matched for their Body Mass Index (BMI). The first group consisted of 53 patients with a history suggestive of obstructive sleep apnea. The second group consisted of 54 patients with a partner-confirmed history of no snoring. These patients were undergoing anesthesia for other reasons. Both groups of patients were free of associated otorhinolaryngological symptoms. The main outcome measure was assessment of production of snoring or obstruction in patients with no documented history of snoring when sedation was administered as part of general anesthesia using TCI with propofol.

The symptomatic group comprised 53 patients whereas 54 patients made up the non-symptomatic group. The various relevant characteristics are summarized in Table 6.1. Categorical variables (gender) were assessed using the chi-squared test whereas continuous variables (BMI and Epworth score) were analyzed using tests for normality; differences were compared by the paired $t$-test. Taking gender into account, both the groups are reasonably matched.

Both groups contained similar numbers of males and females but there was a predominance of males in the snoring group whereas females were predominant in the non-snoring group (Table 6.1). The mean age of the patients in the second group was 47.4 years whereas in the first group, it was 51.7 years.

There was a difference ($P = 0.046$) between the means of the Epworth score in the two groups: non-snorers 5.32 (with SD of 3.473) against snorers 7.36 (SD of 3.346). However, gender difference, whether considered alone or as a second factor, was not significantly different (Table 6.1).

Body Mass Index was effectively matched between the two groups overall, and between males and females within these groups. A difference ($P = 0.038$) between the means of the BMI values was observed in the two groups: non-snorers 27.11 (with SD 3.984) against snorers 28.83 (SD 4.462) and also, there was a difference ($P = 0.027$) between the means of the BMI values for men (mean 28.75, SD 3.902) and women (mean 26.91, SD 4.604) (Table 6.1).

### Table 6.1 Comparison of symptomatic and non-symptomatic patients

|  | Snoring group (symptomatic) |  | Non-snoring group (asymptomatic) |  | P-value |
| --- | --- | --- | --- | --- | --- |
| 1. Male/female |  | 42/11 |  | 19/35 | <.001 |
| 2. Age (n/mean/sd) | 53 | 51.7 (11.37) | 54 | 47.4 (14.09) | 0.088 |
| 3. BMI (n/mean/sd) |  |  |  |  |  |
| Overall | 53 | 28.83 (4.46) | 54 | 27.11 (3.98) | 0.038 |
| Males | 42 | 29.17 (4.28) | 19 | 27.84 (2.79) | 0.156 |
| Females | 11 | 27.55 (5.13) | 35 | 26.71 (4.49) | 0.607 |
| 4. Epworth score (n/mean/sd) |  |  |  |  |  |
| Overall | 22 | 7.36 (3.35) | 25 | 5.32 (3.47) | 0.046 |
| Males | 18 | 7.33 (3.55) | 9 | 6.22 (2.82) | 0.422 |
| Females | 4 | 7.50 (2.65) | 16 | 4.81 (3.78) | 0.200 |

### Table 6.2 Cumulative proportion of snoring

| Propofol conc. (μg/ml) | Snoring group (symptomatic) | Non-snoring group (asymptomatic) | P-value |
| --- | --- | --- | --- |
| 2 | 3/53 | 0/54 | 0.076 |
| 4 | 27/53 | 0/54 | <0.001 |
| 6 | 50/53 | 0/54 | <0.001 |
| 8 | 53/53 | 0/54 | <0.001 |

All patients in the symptomatic (snoring) group snored or obstructed at different concentrations of propofol (Table 6.2). There was no statistically significant difference ($P = 0.401$) in the distributions of concentrations of propofol at which snoring started between men and women.

In comparison, all patients in the asymptomatic (non-snoring) group could not be induced to snore or obstruct at incremental levels of propofol and this was clearly significant statistically ($P < 0.001$).

Earlier authors who have noted false-positive results with sleep endoscopy did not use this technique. Different individuals may have administered the sedating agent or agents used in these studies. The sedating agents indeed differed between operators in such studies, and no measure of sedation effect was used.[3-5] This difference in technique is perhaps an explanation for the encouraging and obvious differentiation of symptomatic from asymptomatic patients demonstrated in this study.

## 5 CONCLUSION

Sleep nasendoscopy allows for a targeted management of snoring or obstructive sleep apnea in suitable individuals by clarifying the underlying contributing anatomical sites. The procedure has previously been questioned for not being a true reflection of normal sleep in view of the sedation process required and for the possibility of inducing false-positive results.

This study does, however, confirm the authors' clinical impression that sleep nasendoscopy performed by a target controlled technique is a useful, specific and sensitive means of assessing patients with sleep-related breathing disorders. It should therefore perhaps be considered for a more prominent role in the investigation of such cases particularly when selection for surgical intervention may be assisted by the anatomical targeting information that may be provided. It may also prove helpful in individuals with OSA who have proved intolerant of nasal CPAP. Such cases may be further assisted by further judicial intervention dependent upon the anatomical information provided by sleep endoscopy.

The authors commend this technique to others involved in the management of such cases where there is appropriate anesthetic interest and availability.

### REFERENCES

1. Croft CB, Pringle M. Sleep nasendoscopy: a technique of assessment in snoring and obstructive sleep apnea. Clin Otolaryngol 1991;16:377–82.
2. Roblin G, Williams A, Whittet HB. Target controlled infusion in sleep endoscopy. Laryngoscope 2001;111:175–76.
3. Marais J. The value of sleep nasendoscopy: a comparison between snoring and non snoring patients. Clin Otolaryngol 1998;23:74–76.
4. Quin SJ, Huang L, Ellis PDM. Observation of the mechanism of snoring using sleep nasendoscopy. Clin Otolaryngol 1995;20:360–74.
5. Sadoka T, Kakitsuba N, Fujiwara Y, Kanai R, Takahashi H. The value of sleep nasendoscopy in he evaluation of patients with suspected sleep related breathing disorders. Clin Otolaryngol 1986;21:485–89.
6. Glen JB. The development of 'Diprifusor': a TCI system for Propofol. Anaesthesia 1985;53(Suppl 1):13–21.
7. Abdullah VJ, Wing YK, Van Hasselt CA. Video sleep nasendoscopy: the Hong Kong experience. Otolaryngol Clin North Am 2003;23:461–71.
8. Berry S, Roblin G, Williams A, Watkins A, Whittet HB. Validity of sleep nasendoscopy in the investigation of sleep related breathing disorders. Laryngoscope 2005;115(3):538–40.

SECTION C  NON-SURGICAL TREATMENT OF OSA/HS

CHAPTER 7

# Obstructive sleep apnea: decision making and treatment algorithm

*Andrew N. Goldberg*

## 1 INTRODUCTION

Numerous treatment options for obstructive sleep apnea (OSA) presently exist. These treatments range from non-invasive behavioral modifications to nightly use of positive airway pressure (PAP) devices to surgical treatments that alter airway anatomy. Selection of patients for these treatments is complex given the range of variability in patient anatomy and physiology, patient preference, disease severity, and controversy with regard to the effectiveness of available treatments. The threshold for treatment is also in flux with some arguing that symptoms of sleepiness are more important than measured disease severity in most patients.[1] What can result from this is a confusing array of treatment options and treatment guidelines which leave patients and physicians unsure as to what decision is most appropriate for the individual. This chapter seeks to provide a framework for these issues and a guide for synthesis and evaluation of treatment options in this disease.

While this chapter is dedicated to application of treatment guidelines, a more detailed description of the individual components of the evaluation and treatment of OSA patients is discussed in chapters fully dedicated to them. This includes making the diagnosis of OSA, physical examination, delivering positive airway pressure, oral appliances and individual surgical treatments. Furthermore, details of surgical procedure selection are also presented in chapters dedicated to this topic.

## 2 DEFINITIONS OF DISEASE

Sleep-disordered breathing can be viewed as a continuum from normal non-obstructed breathing at one end to a patient with sleep apnea and Pickwickian syndrome at the other (Table 7.1). The level of disease in an individual patient can improve or worsen, moving the patient up or down this continuum both over time and on a night-to-night

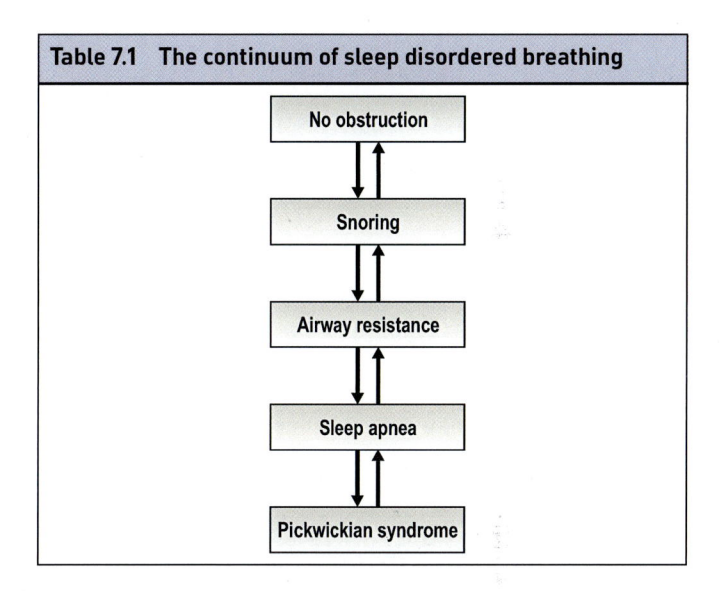

**Table 7.1 The continuum of sleep disordered breathing**

No obstruction ↕ Snoring ↕ Airway resistance ↕ Sleep apnea ↕ Pickwickian syndrome

basis. For instance, a normal patient who gains a significant amount of weight may begin to snore, develop arousals during the night and begin to move into a disease state. With additional weight gain, this patient may develop increased airway resistance or sleep apnea. A patient who consumes alcohol on a given night can also move on the scale in a similar fashion; as muscle tone decreases, obstruction increases. Similarly, a patient with sleep apnea who loses weight may develop less severe airway resistance, simple snoring, or even achieve a normal state of breathing at night. Thus, the number generated on a polysomnogram must be viewed in the context of the patient's overall disease and night-to-night variation of their sleep-disordered breathing.

Although there are numerous metrics to measure the severity of obstructive sleep apnea, disease severity is generally described in terms of the number of apneas plus hypopneas per hour of sleep, or via the Apnea Hypopnea Index (AHI) and $O_2$ saturation as measured on an overnight sleep study, or polysomnogram. The polysomnogram represents a snapshot in time which may not reflect a patient's level of disease over a long period of time, but it is still the best measure of disease severity available at present.

# SECTION C: NON-SURGICAL TREATMENT OF OSA/HS

Using polysomnography as our standard of determining disease severity, obstructive sleep apnea is represented by an AHI of greater than five events per hour and obstructive sleep apnea syndrome is defined as an AHI of greater than five events per hour with daytime and/or nighttime symptoms such as choking, gasping, snoring and daytime sleepiness. Patients can be further divided into a group with mild apnea with an AHI between five and 15, moderate apnea in patients with an AHI of 15 to 30, and severe apnea in patients who have an AHI of greater than 30. Many use $O_2$ desaturation nadir to modify the description of severity in sleep-disordered breathing. For instance, a patient with an AHI of 12 and $O_2$ desaturation to 70% may be referred to as a patient with moderate OSA. Similarly, a patient with an AHI of 25 and significant desaturation may be called a patient with severe apnea. Other factors on the sleep test such as the presence or absence of REM sleep, the presence or absence of delta sleep (Stage III and IV sleep), and the percentage of time spent with oxygen saturation below 90% may also be important as well. They may help explain the patient's symptoms and may serve as a guideline as to the success of a procedure if these parameters are improved post treatment.

Lastly, a respiratory effort-related arousal (RERA) is an event that occurs when a patient develops an arousal on electroencephalogram in conjunction with increasing inspiratory effort during sleep. RERAs can be added to apneas and hypopneas to create the Respiratory Disturbance Index (RDI) which many use to guide treatment.[2]

## 3 EFFECTS OF SLEEP APNEA AND TREATMENT THRESHOLDS

There are three principal manifestations of sleep-disordered breathing: *physiological*, *behavioral* and *social*.

The *physiological* manifestations are important and principally relate to cardiovascular consequences of OSA, though there are other physiological effects of disordered breathing during sleep, such as alterations in inflammatory biomarkers, which also occur. Cardiovascular consequences include associations with stroke, hypertension and myocardial infarction and are being studied rigorously in the Sleep Heart Health Study, which is longitudinally tracking a cohort of OSA patients with measures of OSA and medical outcomes.[3]

The *behavioral* effects of sleep disruption are commonly evident. These may manifest as tiredness in the morning or daytime, falling asleep in permissive situations such as watching TV or reading a book, an increased incidence of motor vehicle accidents, and losses of concentration and productivity. A simple patient self-report scale, the Epworth Sleepiness Scale, was designed to quantify this level of tiredness[4] though there are also objective measures of alertness such as the psychomotor vigilance test.[5] The behavioral effects of OSA can be variable among patients where a patient with snoring may have significant tiredness whereas a patient with an elevated AHI and greater nighttime obstruction may not display tiredness. This discrepancy appears to make behavioral measurement alone insufficient to fully characterize the disease or its treatment.

Lastly, *social* effects are principally related to snoring which may disrupt social harmony by disturbance of bedpartners and others in the home. Subjective measures are commonly used to measure this feature of the disease, such as bedpartner scoring. Snoring is a common reason why patients seek medical attention for obstructive sleep apnea, as it is one of the most obvious and disruptive outward manifestations of obstruction during sleep.

In light of the variability in the manifestation of OSA in patients and the gaps in our knowledge as to which patients will suffer cardiovascular consequences of this disease, significant controversy exists with respect to selection of patients for OSA treatment. In a review article on OSA, Ward Flemons writes, 'In the majority of patients without coexisting conditions … the primary reason to test for and treat sleep apnea is the potential to improve the quality of life.'[1] Studies vary in determining the magnitude of effects of mild to moderate OSA on hypertension and cardiovascular consequences. However, ongoing studies of large cohorts of patients such as the Sleep Heart Health Study are yielding important data that will provide guidelines for treatment in the future.[6] With information on physiological consequences of OSA such as effects on inflammatory and other biomarkers as well as data from the Sleep Heart Health Study emerging, our threshold and circumstances for intervention will certainly evolve.

Nevertheless, physicians are faced today with patients needing treatment and decisions must be made. The best available evidence is synthesized to assist with these decisions, and treatment thresholds developed. In an attempt to help delineate a treatment threshold, one oft-quoted study determined that patients with an Apnea Index (AI) of >20 were at increased cardiovascular risk.[7] Many use the cut-off of an AHI of 20 as the threshold for treatment (note the original cut-off of AI >20 has been subsequently adopted as AHI >20). While virtually all admit that patients with an AHI of >30 should be treated regardless of co-morbidity or behavioral effects, rigorous evidence for treatment of patients with an AHI of <30 is lacking.[2] However, patients with AHI <30 with significant co-morbidity or behavioral effects (e.g. tiredness, loss of concentration) are also considered candidates for treatment of OSA.

It is the opinion of the author that all patients with an AHI >30 should be treated for OSA and symptomatic patients with an AHI <30 should be treated. Patients with an AHI <30 may have other factors that bring them to treatment including medical co-morbidities or other parameters on the polysomnogram that mandate treatment (e.g. low oxygen saturation, arrhythmias).

## 4 EVALUATION FOR OSA

Proper evaluation and diagnosis of patients with OSA are critical for determining a suitable treatment plan. Clearly a patient whose depression is misdiagnosed as OSA, or conversely, a patient whose OSA is misdiagnosed as depression will receive a treatment plan inappropriate for the clinical condition. In the evaluation of a patient with suspected sleep-disordered breathing, the *history* and *physical examination*, various *adjunctive studies* and *consultations* are helpful to properly diagnose and therefore treat the patient.

### 4.1 HISTORY

A history of snoring, gasping, or witnessed apneas may be characteristic of sleep-disordered breathing, and the duration of the problem should be noted. Patients may be tired in the morning or daytime and may fall asleep in permissive situations. Patients should be generally questioned about their sleep habits and relevant history. Various questionnaires are available to evaluate the patient with sleep-disordered breathing. The Epworth Sleepiness Scale is particularly easy to administer, it is quantitative, and gives insight into the degree of sleepiness that the patient is experiencing.[4]

Other diagnoses besides sleep apnea must be considered in a patient who presents with symptoms of tiredness or sleep disturbance. These include narcolepsy, insomnia, sleep hygiene disorder, Pickwickian disorder, drug effects and depression. Specifically, a patient who awakes with a morning headache, is obese, with symptoms of sleep-disordered breathing should be considered for Pickwickian syndrome with appropriate blood gas measurements made and cardiovascular evaluation considered. In addition, depression screening is a routine part of the evaluation of a patient who complains of sleep disturbance.

### 4.2 PHYSICAL EXAMINATION

On physical examination, the patient's height and weight, height 1 year and 5 years ago, and neck circumference should be recorded. Examination of the nose, oral cavity, oropharynx, bony structure of the head and neck, and a fiberoptic examination should be undertaken. Sleep endoscopy has been used more commonly in the evaluation to further examine patients in a pharmacologically induced state of sleep.[8] Fiberoptic endoscopy is performed during pharmacologically induced sleep to determine the site of airway collapse, typically using propofol. It is hoped that use of this method will increase the accuracy in determining the site of obstruction in patients with OSA.

### 4.3 ADJUNCTIVE STUDIES

Adjunctive studies such as polysomnography are typically necessary if the patient's history and examination point toward sleep-disordered breathing as a possibility. The type of study may be a full-night diagnostic study, a split-night study with the CPAP trial, or a home study. In some patients, multiple sleep latency tests or arterial blood gases may be helpful in discerning the effects of sleep-disordered breathing or differentiating OSA from narcolepsy. Cephalometric radiography may help in delineating the bony structure of the patient by assessing craniofacial abnormalities that may guide treatment. Additional imaging studies, such as static and dynamic MRI and CT scanning, have been used in protocols for upper airway assessment, though no data support their clinical use at this point.[9]

### 4.4 CONSULTATIONS

Lastly, consultations with other medical professionals such as medical sleep specialists can augment the evaluation of a surgical sleep specialist particularly when issues of sleep hygiene, insomnia, narcolepsy and Pickwickian syndrome are in question. Psychological evaluation by the primary care physician, psychiatrist, or other mental health professional can be helpful in patients with a question of depression, while medical conditions that accompany OSA such as cardiac concerns, diabetes and restrictive lung disease may warrant consultation with the appropriate internal medicine specialist.

## 5 TREATMENT OPTIONS

There are three categories of treatment options available to treat patients with OSA: *behavioral modification*, *devices that can be worn* and *surgical options*. Every patient should be informed of the options available in each category and the treating physician and patient should review the appropriateness of treatments in each category based on individual considerations. Various brochures and informational material can be reviewed with the patient to insure that all treatment options are presented to the patient while providing an opportunity for questions to be answered.

### 5.1 BEHAVIORAL MODIFICATION

In general, all patients should be informed of behavioral modifications that can reduce or eliminate OSA without the need for medicines, device use, or surgery. In patients with moderate or severe OSA, these maneuvers are not likely to

# SECTION C: NON-SURGICAL TREATMENT OF OSA/HS

be effective as stand-alone therapy; however, they can help to mitigate some effects of OSA in these patients and can also assist in education of the patient in the pathogenesis of their disease (e.g. with regard to weight loss or sleep position).

Behavioral modifications include principally sleep position therapy, weight loss where appropriate, and avoidance of sedatives, alcohol, or large meals before bedtime. In sleep position therapy, the patient sleeps on their side or stomach as opposed to on the back, as most patients obstruct more in the supine position. Pillows or positioners can be helpful to assist in this type of postural therapy. Patients should be encouraged to lose weight if they are overweight or obese, as weight loss reduces the bulk of tissue in the neck which narrows the airway, and reduces airway collapse. As surgical intervention for obesity has become safer and more refined, recommendations for surgical treatment of obesity are becoming more common.[10] Patients should be counseled to avoid sedatives, including alcohol and other medications prior to bedtime, as sedatives may be important in causing loss of muscle tone and causing airway collapse during sleep. Eating a large or fatty meal or one replete with carbohydrates before bedtime can have the same effect by reducing muscle tone during sleep and should be avoided.

## 5.2 DEVICES THAT CAN BE WORN

Two devices are available to help maintain airway patency and reduce the incidence of sleep-disordered breathing. These include positive airway pressure (PAP) and an oral appliance (OA).

### Positive airway pressure (PAP)

Positive airway pressure is recognized as the most effective treatment for OSA in patients who can tolerate wearing the device, particularly moderate to severe OSA.

The delivery of positive airway pressure is available in many forms, such as continuous positive airway pressure (CPAP), bilevel positive airway pressure, automatically titrating positive airway pressure, and demand positive airway pressure. A description of each is beyond the scope of this chapter, but suffice it to say that each provides positive pressure to the airway through a device worn on the face, and serves as an internal pneumatic splint for the airway. CPAP, which is the most commonly used form of PAP, typically uses between 5 and 15 cm of water pressure to maintain airway patency. These devices have the advantage of a high rate of effectiveness in the laboratory setting in reversing sleep-disordered breathing. Unfortunately, not all patients are able to wear the device regularly in the home setting, making compliance a significant issue. Additionally, patients frequently misrepresent their PAP use as being more compliant, necessitating close follow-up and the use of covert monitoring that is integrated into the device.[11] Issues with regard to use of PAP such as desensitization of the patient to mask use at night, comfort and leaking at the mask interface, and claustrophobia must be reconciled and may require working with the patient intensively.

It is appropriate for every patient with moderate or severe OSA to gain exposure to PAP before undergoing surgical therapy. This allows them experience with a treatment option that is typically effective, reversible, associated with few side effects and widely available. As the effects of PAP are dependent on wearing the device during sleep and no 'training' of the airway occurs, compliance with wearing the device nightly is necessary and is the principal obstacle to use. If a patient can tolerate the device, it can sometimes provide diagnostic information as well. Relief of symptoms with PAP can help determine which symptoms are caused by OSA. Patients who tolerate the device for even one full night often awake more refreshed than they have for many years and realize the magnitude of the negative cognitive and behavioral effects sleep-disordered breathing has had. When patients feel the beneficial effects of normal sleep in the absence of sleep-disordered breathing there can be a positive change in their attitude towards treatment of the disease and to PAP as well. The prospect of lifelong use is typically less palatable in young patients who are faced with the prospect of wearing PAP for the remainder of their lives, but even in these patients, even short-term use of PAP can be enormously helpful to highlight the behavioral physiologic effects of OSA.

### Oral appliances

Oral appliances, principally a mandibular repositioning device, can also be used for sleep-disordered breathing.[12] Mandibular repositioning devices advance the mandible anteriorly, which brings forward the tongue and other muscles of the oropharynx and hypopharynx. The position of the palate is also changed with the mandibular repositioning device, likely through action of the palatoglossus muscle, and airway patency is typically improved. It is used principally for patients with simple snoring and mild apnea and has reduced effectiveness in patients with more severe disease.[12] Patients with pre-existing disorders of the temporomandibular joint and edentulous patients are not considered to be good candidates for this device. As with PAP, no training of the airway occurs, therefore nightly use is necessary for treatment effect.

## 5.3 SURGICAL THERAPY FOR OSA

Surgical therapy for OSA can be classified in three categories. The first category includes procedures on the upper airway which may improve PAP use and compliance. The second category includes surgery that improves OSA without surgically altering the upper airway such as tracheotomy and bariatric surgery. The third category includes surgery that directly alters the upper airway to reduce obstruction of breathing during sleep.

### Surgical procedures to improve PAP use
Patients who tolerate PAP and whose sleep-disordered breathing is abolished by PAP do not typically need surgery. However, there is a significant number of patients who do not tolerate PAP because of the need for elevated pressures or because of nasal obstruction. In selected patients with elevated pressures, surgery on the upper airway can reduce PAP pressures and improve compliance. Examples include patients with large tonsils, adenoid hypertrophy or nasal obstruction. If medical treatment of these issues fails, surgical treatment including tonsillectomy, adenoidectomy, or nasal surgery may help reduce PAP pressures and/or improve compliance.[13] Obstruction from turbinate hypertrophy, deviated septum, or nasal polyps, for example, may benefit from surgical correction.

### Non-upper airway surgery for OSA
Despite its efficacy in bypassing upper airway obstruction, tracheotomy is rarely considered as a sole treatment for patients with OSA.[14] More commonly, tracheotomy is used on a temporary basis in the perioperative period for patients undergoing upper airway surgery for OSA. The need for an opening in the neck with its associated hygiene and social burdens appropriately limits its routine use. Tracheotomy is typically reserved for morbidly obese patients who are unable to tolerate PAP, morbidly obese patients with Pickwickian syndrome who require upper airway bypass *and* nocturnal ventilation, and patients who are unable to tolerate PAP with significant co-morbidities in whom other treatment options have failed.[14]

Since a significant number of patients with OSA are obese and obesity is a major cause of OSA, bariatric surgery has the potential to significantly reduce a patient's weight and improve sleep-disordered breathing. Bariatric surgery should be considered in patients with a BMI >40 or patients with a BMI >35 with significant medical co-morbidities.[10] Patients who fall into this category should preferably be referred to an appropriate center for bariatric surgery for evaluation. This therapy has the significant advantage of treating other co-morbidities associated with obesity such as diabetes and cardiovascular disease in addition to OSA.[10]

### Upper airway surgery for OSA
In selecting patients for surgical treatment in obstructive sleep apnea, one needs to take into account: (1) OSA severity; (2) individual patient anatomy; (3) the patient's desires; and (4) associated co-morbidities. Specific recommendations for evaluating site of obstruction and procedure choice are discussed elsewhere in this book. General guidelines for application of these procedures follow.

Patients with a higher AHI are generally in greater need for intervention, as the severity of the disease is greater. Individual anatomy plays a significant role in formulating recommendations for treatment of OSA as specific surgical treatments are targeted at areas of obstruction. In discussing the surgical options with the patient, patient expectations and desires should be explicitly discussed, including the patient's feelings on cure of their snoring, apnea and symptoms of tiredness that they might have. Lastly, patients with OSA may have significant medical co-morbidities such as cardiovascular issues which must be taken into account when considering a patient for upper airway surgery. As in all surgical procedures, a frank discussion of the surgery including the types of surgery that are available, pain, complication rates, expected consequences, morbidity and costs should be undertaken so that the patient has a full understanding of the treatment plan. The need for evaluation of the patient after the surgical procedure and possible need for subsequent surgeries should be discussed as well, as these are commonly important parts of the treatment plan. As noted above, first-line treatment for patients with moderate or severe OSA is PAP for the reasons stated.

## 6 ALGORITHM FOR TREATMENT OF OSA AND TREATMENT GOALS

Decision making by the patient and physician is predicated on a thorough history and physical examination. Individual anatomy, disease severity and patient preferences play a central role in the selection of treatment, as not all treatments can be effectively applied to all patients. The choice of treatment and degree of invasiveness of the treatments chosen remain in the hands of doctor and patient.

The goal for treatment for OSA is to alleviate sleep-disordered breathing completely when possible manage the disease if complete cure is not possible. Re-evaluation after a treatment has been instituted is critical to determining treatment success. If one cannot normalize a patient completely, one attempts, at minimum, to move the patient into a less severe disease state through behavioral treatments, application of positive airway pressure, or surgery.

---

**Disease severity\***

*Mild (5 < AHI < 15)*
No symptoms
Behavioral modification
Symptoms
Behavioral modification
- Consider oral appliance
- Consider PAP
- Consider surgical intervention

*Moderate (15 < AHI < 30)*
No symptoms

Behavioral modification
- Consider PAP
- Consider oral appliance
- Consider surgical intervention

Symptoms
Behavioral modification
PAP
Surgical intervention for PAP failures
- Consider oral appliance

*Severe (AHI > 30)*
Symptoms or no symptoms
Behavioral modification (rarely sufficient alone)
PAP
Surgical intervention for PAP failures

- Consider tracheotomy if other treatments fail and significant symptoms or co-morbidities exist.
- Co-morbidities should also be taken into account when discussing the strength of recommendations.
- Patients with BMI >35 and co-morbidities or BMI >40 should be considered for bariatric surgery.
- Interventions should typically be applied in the order listed. Proceed down the list until success is reached.
- Interventions listed as 'consider' should be discussed and applied based on an individual basis.

*Additional parameters from the polysomnogram, such as oxygen desaturation nadir, RERAs, and time spent below oxygen saturation of 90%, can also be used to guide treatment, as these can shift a patient into a higher category of disease severity.

## 7 CONCLUSION

All causes of a patient's sleep disturbance, including non-obstructive causes, should be identified when evaluating a patient for a sleep disorder. Only then can they be appropriately treated, with the proper cause of the patient's symptoms identified. For patients with OSA, a thorough history and examination, with special attention to the upper airway, is critical to guide medical and surgical choices. Decisions on treatment arise from evaluation of the patient's history, anatomy, disease severity, symptoms and co-morbidities in conjunction with input from the patient.

All appropriate treatments should be discussed and should include behavioral treatments, use of oral appliances, PAP and surgical therapy while providing realistic expectations for success and a realistic description of treatment burdens. Follow-up after medical and surgical intervention is critical to insure the patient has benefited from the chosen treatment and to provide an opportunity to implement further recommendations in case of incomplete treatment response.

## REFERENCES

1. Flemons WW. Obstructive sleep apnea. N Engl J Med 2002;347(77):498–504.
2. Loube DI, Gay PC, Strohl KP, Pack AI, White DP, Collop NA. Indications for positive airway pressure treatment of adult obstructive sleep apnea patients: a consensus statement. Chest 1999;115(3):863–66.
3. Quan SF, Howard BV, Iber C, et al. The Sleep Heart Health Study: design, rationale, and methods. Sleep 1997;20(12):1077–85.
4. Johns MW. A new method for measuring daytime sleepiness: the Epworth Sleepiness Scale. Sleep 1991;14(6):540–45.
5. Canisius S, Penzel T. Vigilance monitoring – review and practical aspects. Biomed Tech (Berl) 2007;52(1):77–82.
6. Shahar E, Whitney CW, Redline S, et al. Sleep disordered breathing and cardiovascular disease: cross-sectional results of The Sleep Heart Health Study. Am J Respir Crit Care Med 2001;163(1):19–25.
7. He J, Kryger MH, Zorick FJ, Conway W, Roth T. Mortality and apnea index in obstructive sleep apnea. Experience in 385 male patients. Chest 1988;94(1):9–14.
8. Croft CB, Pringle M. Sleep nasendoscopy: a technique of assessment in snoring and obstructive sleep apnoea. Clin Otolaryngol Allied Sci 1991;16(5):504–9.
9. Ahmed MM, Schwab RJ. Upper airway imaging in obstructive sleep apnea. Curr Opin Pulm Med 2006;12(6):397–401.
10. Crookes PF. Surgical treatment of morbid obesity. Annu Rev Med 2006;57:243–64.
11. Kribbs NB, Pack AI, Kline LR, et al. Objective measurement of patterns of nasal CPAP use by patients with obstructive sleep apnea. Am Rev Respir Dis 1993;147(4):887–95.
12. Ferguson KA, Cartwright R, Rogers R, Schmidt-Nowara W. Oral appliances for snoring and obstructive sleep apnea: a review. Sleep 2006;29(2):244–62.
13. Zonato AI, Bittencourt LR, Martinho FL, Gregorio LC, Tufik S. Upper airway surgery: the effect on nasal continuous positive airway pressure titration on obstructive sleep apnea patients. Eur Arch Otorhinolaryngol 2006;263(5):481–86.
14. Kim SH, Eisele DW, Smith PL, Schneider H, Schwartz AR. Evaluation of patients with sleep apnea after tracheotomy. Arch Otolaryngol Head Neck Surg 1998;124:996–1000.

SECTION C — NON-SURGICAL TREATMENT OF OSA/HS

# CHAPTER 8
# Obesity management

*Robert F. Kushner*

## 1 INTRODUCTION

Evaluation and management of obesity is an essential step in the treatment of patients with obstructive sleep apnea (OSA) and snoring based on three important facts. First, 66% of US adults are currently categorized as overweight or obese,[1] placing obesity as one of the most common conditions seen among primary care providers and medical and surgical specialists. Second, obesity is a contributor to poor quality of life and increased morbidity and mortality that involves nine organ systems. Obesity, particularly upper body obesity, is a well-documented risk factor for OSA and is reported to be present in 60% to 90% of OSA patients evaluated in sleep clinics.[2] Additionally, the severity of OSA is directly related to increasing body weight. Population-based studies have consistently shown an increased incidence of sleep disordered breathing with weight gain and obesity.[3–5] Third, weight reduction by dietary and surgical treatment has been shown to improve co-morbid conditions including sleep disordered breathing and sleep quality.[6] For these reasons, a thorough evaluation and treatment plan for OSA should specifically address weight loss for patients who are overweight or obese. This chapter will review current evaluation and treatment guidelines for overweight and obesity with a special focus for the otolaryngologist. For a more comprehensive review, readers are referred to the American Medical Association's *Assessment and Management of Adult Obesity: A Primer for Physicians*.[7]

## 2 EVALUATION OF THE OVERWEIGHT AND OBESE PATIENT

Screening for overweight and obesity should not rely on subjective visual inspection alone. Rather, screening is carried out by performing three simple anthropometric measurements: weight, height and waist circumference. These measurements can be easily obtained by ancillary office personnel. The Body Mass Index (BMI), calculated as weight (kg)/height (m)$^2$, or as weight (pounds)/height (inches)$^2 \times 703$, is used to define classification of weight status and risk of disease (Table 8.1). A BMI table is more conveniently employed for simple reference (Table 8.2). BMI is used since it provides an estimate of body fat and is related to risk of disease.

Excess abdominal fat, assessed by measurement of waist circumference or waist-to-hip ratio, is independently associated with higher risk for metabolic abnormalities, diabetes mellitus, cardiovascular disease and OSA.[8] Although protocols and guidelines differ among investigators, measurement of waist is most commonly performed in the horizontal plane above the iliac crest or at the narrowest point between the costal margin and iliac crest. Cut points that define higher risk are a waist circumference >102 cm (>40 inches) in men and >88 cm (>35 inches) in women when measured superior to the iliac crest.[9] Overweight persons with waist circumferences exceeding these limits should be urged more strongly to pursue weight reduction since it categorically increases disease risk for each BMI class. Measurement of waist circumference should be obtained in those individuals with a BMI ≤35 kg/m$^2$.

Although not specified in the clinical guidelines, it may be useful to measure neck circumference in obese patients presenting with signs and symptoms of OSA. Large neck girth in both men and women who snore is highly predictive

**Table 8.1** Classification of weight status and risk of disease

| | BMI (kg/m$^2$) | Obesity class | Risk of disease |
|---|---|---|---|
| Underweight | <18.5 | | |
| Healthy weight | 18.5–24.9 | | |
| Overweight | 25.0–29.9 | | Increased |
| Obesity | 30.0–34.9 | I | High |
| Obesity | 35.0–39.9 | II | Very high |
| Extreme obesity | ≥BMI 40 | III | Extremely high |

Source (adapted from): National Institutes of Health, National Heart, Lung, and Blood Institute. *Clinical Guidelines on the Identification, Evaluation, and Treatment of Overweight and Obesity in Adults*. US Department of Health and Human Services, Public Health Service; 1998.

### Table 8.2  Body Mass Index (BMI) table

| BMI | 19 | 20 | 21 | 22 | 23 | 24 | 25 | 26 | 27 | 28 | 29 | 30 | 31 | 32 | 33 | 34 | 35 | 36 |
|---|---|---|---|---|---|---|---|---|---|---|---|---|---|---|---|---|---|---|
| Height (inches) | | | | | | | | | Body weight (pounds) | | | | | | | | | |
| 58 | 91 | 96 | 100 | 105 | 110 | 115 | 119 | 124 | 129 | 134 | 138 | 143 | 148 | 153 | 158 | 162 | 167 | 172 |
| 59 | 94 | 99 | 104 | 109 | 114 | 119 | 124 | 128 | 133 | 138 | 143 | 148 | 153 | 158 | 163 | 168 | 173 | 178 |
| 60 | 97 | 102 | 107 | 112 | 118 | 123 | 128 | 133 | 138 | 143 | 148 | 153 | 158 | 163 | 168 | 174 | 179 | 184 |
| 61 | 100 | 106 | 111 | 116 | 122 | 127 | 132 | 137 | 143 | 148 | 153 | 158 | 164 | 169 | 174 | 180 | 185 | 190 |
| 62 | 104 | 109 | 115 | 120 | 126 | 131 | 136 | 142 | 147 | 153 | 158 | 164 | 169 | 175 | 180 | 186 | 191 | 196 |
| 63 | 107 | 113 | 118 | 124 | 130 | 135 | 141 | 146 | 152 | 158 | 163 | 169 | 175 | 180 | 186 | 191 | 197 | 203 |
| 64 | 110 | 116 | 122 | 128 | 134 | 140 | 145 | 151 | 157 | 163 | 169 | 174 | 180 | 186 | 192 | 197 | 204 | 209 |
| 65 | 114 | 120 | 126 | 132 | 138 | 144 | 150 | 156 | 162 | 168 | 174 | 180 | 186 | 192 | 198 | 204 | 210 | 216 |
| 66 | 118 | 124 | 130 | 136 | 142 | 148 | 155 | 161 | 167 | 173 | 179 | 186 | 192 | 198 | 204 | 210 | 216 | 223 |
| 67 | 121 | 127 | 134 | 140 | 146 | 153 | 159 | 166 | 172 | 178 | 185 | 191 | 198 | 204 | 211 | 217 | 223 | 230 |
| 68 | 125 | 131 | 138 | 144 | 151 | 158 | 164 | 171 | 177 | 184 | 190 | 197 | 203 | 210 | 216 | 223 | 230 | 236 |
| 69 | 128 | 135 | 142 | 149 | 155 | 162 | 169 | 176 | 182 | 189 | 196 | 203 | 209 | 216 | 223 | 230 | 236 | 243 |
| 70 | 132 | 139 | 146 | 153 | 160 | 167 | 174 | 181 | 188 | 195 | 202 | 209 | 216 | 222 | 229 | 236 | 243 | 250 |
| 71 | 136 | 143 | 150 | 157 | 165 | 172 | 179 | 186 | 193 | 200 | 208 | 215 | 222 | 229 | 236 | 243 | 250 | 257 |
| 72 | 140 | 147 | 154 | 162 | 169 | 177 | 184 | 191 | 199 | 206 | 213 | 221 | 228 | 235 | 242 | 250 | 258 | 265 |
| 73 | 144 | 151 | 159 | 166 | 174 | 182 | 189 | 197 | 204 | 212 | 219 | 227 | 235 | 242 | 250 | 257 | 265 | 272 |
| 74 | 148 | 155 | 163 | 171 | 179 | 186 | 194 | 202 | 210 | 218 | 225 | 233 | 241 | 249 | 256 | 264 | 272 | 280 |
| 75 | 152 | 160 | 168 | 176 | 184 | 192 | 200 | 208 | 216 | 224 | 232 | 240 | 248 | 256 | 264 | 272 | 279 | 287 |
| 76 | 156 | 164 | 172 | 180 | 189 | 197 | 205 | 213 | 221 | 230 | 238 | 246 | 254 | 263 | 271 | 279 | 287 | 295 |

| BMI | 37 | 38 | 39 | 40 | 41 | 42 | 43 | 44 | 45 | 46 | 47 | 48 | 49 | 50 | 51 | 52 | 53 | 54 |
|---|---|---|---|---|---|---|---|---|---|---|---|---|---|---|---|---|---|---|
| 58 | 177 | 181 | 186 | 191 | 196 | 201 | 205 | 210 | 215 | 220 | 224 | 229 | 234 | 239 | 244 | 248 | 253 | 258 |
| 59 | 183 | 188 | 193 | 198 | 203 | 208 | 212 | 217 | 222 | 227 | 232 | 237 | 242 | 247 | 252 | 257 | 262 | 267 |
| 60 | 189 | 194 | 199 | 204 | 209 | 215 | 220 | 225 | 230 | 235 | 240 | 245 | 250 | 255 | 261 | 266 | 271 | 276 |
| 61 | 195 | 201 | 206 | 211 | 217 | 222 | 227 | 232 | 238 | 243 | 248 | 254 | 259 | 264 | 269 | 275 | 280 | 285 |
| 62 | 202 | 207 | 213 | 218 | 224 | 229 | 235 | 240 | 246 | 251 | 256 | 262 | 267 | 273 | 278 | 284 | 289 | 295 |
| 63 | 208 | 214 | 220 | 225 | 231 | 237 | 242 | 248 | 254 | 259 | 265 | 270 | 278 | 282 | 287 | 293 | 299 | 304 |
| 64 | 215 | 221 | 227 | 232 | 238 | 244 | 250 | 256 | 262 | 267 | 273 | 279 | 285 | 291 | 296 | 302 | 308 | 314 |
| 65 | 222 | 228 | 234 | 240 | 246 | 252 | 258 | 264 | 270 | 276 | 282 | 288 | 294 | 300 | 306 | 312 | 318 | 324 |
| 66 | 229 | 235 | 241 | 247 | 253 | 260 | 266 | 272 | 278 | 284 | 291 | 297 | 303 | 309 | 315 | 322 | 328 | 334 |
| 67 | 236 | 242 | 249 | 255 | 261 | 268 | 274 | 280 | 287 | 293 | 299 | 306 | 312 | 319 | 325 | 331 | 338 | 344 |
| 68 | 243 | 249 | 256 | 262 | 269 | 276 | 282 | 289 | 295 | 302 | 308 | 315 | 322 | 328 | 335 | 341 | 348 | 354 |
| 69 | 250 | 257 | 263 | 270 | 277 | 284 | 291 | 297 | 304 | 311 | 318 | 324 | 331 | 338 | 345 | 351 | 358 | 365 |
| 70 | 257 | 264 | 271 | 278 | 285 | 292 | 299 | 306 | 313 | 320 | 327 | 334 | 341 | 348 | 355 | 362 | 369 | 376 |
| 71 | 265 | 272 | 279 | 286 | 293 | 301 | 308 | 315 | 322 | 329 | 338 | 343 | 351 | 358 | 365 | 372 | 379 | 386 |
| 72 | 272 | 279 | 287 | 294 | 302 | 309 | 316 | 324 | 331 | 338 | 346 | 353 | 361 | 368 | 375 | 383 | 390 | 397 |
| 73 | 280 | 288 | 295 | 302 | 310 | 318 | 325 | 333 | 340 | 348 | 355 | 363 | 371 | 378 | 386 | 393 | 401 | 408 |
| 74 | 287 | 295 | 303 | 311 | 319 | 326 | 334 | 342 | 350 | 358 | 365 | 373 | 381 | 389 | 396 | 404 | 412 | 420 |
| 75 | 295 | 303 | 311 | 319 | 327 | 335 | 343 | 351 | 359 | 367 | 375 | 383 | 391 | 399 | 407 | 415 | 423 | 431 |
| 76 | 304 | 312 | 320 | 328 | 336 | 344 | 353 | 361 | 369 | 377 | 385 | 394 | 402 | 410 | 418 | 426 | 435 | 443 |

To use the table, find the appropriate height in the left-hand column. Move across the row to the given weight. The number at the top of the column is the BMI for that height and weight.

Source: *The Practical Guide: Identification, Evaluation, and Treatment of Overweight and Obesity in Adults*. US Department of Health and Human Services, Public Health Service, National Institutes of Health, National Heart, Lung, and Blood Institute. NIH Publication No. 00-4084, October, 2000.

of sleep apnea.[10] Some studies suggest that neck circumference is a more useful predictor of sleep apnea than BMI[11] or waist circumference.[12] In general, a neck circumference of 17 inches in men or 16 inches in women indicates a higher risk for sleep apnea.

## 3 TAKING AN OBESITY-FOCUSED HISTORY

Once the overweight or obese patient is identified, inclusion of obesity-focused questions in an expanded history will allow the physician to provide tailored treatment recommendations that are more consistent with the needs and goals of the individual patient. Information from the history should address factors that have contributed to the patient's weight gain, how obesity affects the patient's perceived health, the patient's understanding of the relationship between weight and OSA, what the patient's goals and expectations are regarding obesity treatment, whether the patient is ready and motivated to begin a weight management program, and what kind of help the patient needs for treatment.

Although the vast majority of overweight and obesity can be attributed to behavioral changes in diet and physical activity patterns, the patient's history may suggest several less common secondary causes that may warrant further evaluation, such as polycystic ovarian syndrome (PCOS), hypothyroidism, Cushing's syndrome, and hypothalamic tumors or damage to this part of the brain as a consequence of irradiation, infection or trauma. Drug-induced weight gain as well as medications interfering with weight loss also needs to be considered. Common causes include anti-diabetes agents (insulin, sulfonylureas, thiazolidinediones), steroid hormones, psychotropic agents, mood stabilizers (lithium), antidepressants (tricylics, MAOIs, paraxetine, mirtazapine), and antiepileptic drugs (valproate, gabapentin, carbamazepine).

A history of the patient's current diet and physical activity patterns along with existing or potential barriers to change is used to both understand the contributing factors toward the development of obesity as well as target behaviors for treatment. A dietary and physical activity history can be assessed as part of the patient interview.

## 3.1 ASSESSING RISK

The medical history, physical examination and laboratory evaluation should be focused on assessing obesity co-morbid diseases. There is no single laboratory test or diagnostic evaluation that is indicated for all patients with obesity. The specific evaluation performed should be based on presentation of symptoms, risk factors and index of suspicion. However, based on several other screening guideline recommendations, all patients should have a fasting lipid panel (total, LDL and HDL cholesterol and triglyceride levels) and blood glucose measured at presentation along with blood pressure determination. Symptoms and diseases that are directly or indirectly related to obesity are listed in Table 8.3. Although individuals will vary, the number and severity of organ specific co-morbid conditions usually rise with increasing levels of obesity.

An increased waist circumference has been found to be predictive of a constellation of metabolic risk factors termed the metabolic syndrome that includes elevated blood pressure, impaired fasting glucose or glucose intolerance, hypertriglyceridemia, and low HDL cholesterol.[6] Although the components and cutoff values selected to define the metabolic syndrome are useful for clinical practice, the constellation of abnormalities associated with insulin resistance is much broader. These 'non-traditional

**Table 8.3   Obesity-related organ systems review**

| Cardiovascular | Respiratory |
|---|---|
| Hypertension | Dyspnea |
| Congestive heart failure | Obstructive sleep apnea |
| Cor pulmonale | Hypoventilation syndrome |
| Varicose veins | Pickwickian syndrome |
| Pulmonary embolism | Asthma |
| Coronary artery disease | |
| **Endocrine** | **Gastrointestinal** |
| Metabolic syndrome | Gastroesophageal reflux disease (GERD) |
| Type 2 diabetes | Non-alcoholic fatty liver disease (NAFLD) |
| Dyslipidemia | |
| Polycystic ovarian syndrome (PCOS)/angrogenicity | Cholelithiasis |
| Amenorrhea/infertility/menstrual disorders | Hernias |
| | Colon cancer |
| **Musculoskeletal** | **Genitourinary** |
| Hyperuricemia and gout | Urinary stress incontinence |
| Immobility | Obesity-related glomerulopathy |
| Osteoarthritis (knees and hips) | End-stage renal disease |
| Low back pain | Hypogonadism (male) |
| Carpal tunnel syndrome | Breast and uterine cancer |
| | Pregnancy complications |
| **Psychological** | **Neurologic** |
| Depression/low self-esteem | Stroke |
| Body image disturbance | Idiopathic intracranial hypertension |
| Social stigmatization | Meralgia paresthetica |
| | Dementia |
| **Integument** | |
| Striae distensae (stretch marks) | |
| Stasis pigmentation of legs | |
| Lymphedema | |
| Cellulitis | |
| Intertrigo, carbuncles | |
| Acanthosis nigricans | |
| Acrochordon (skin tags) | |
| Hidradenitis suppurativa | |

# SECTION C  NON-SURGICAL TREATMENT OF OSA/HS

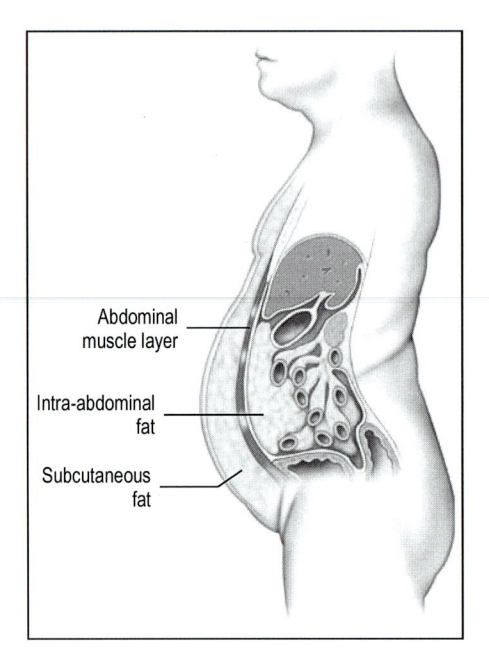

**Fig. 8.1** Waist circumference is an independent prediction of metabolic risk and is a surrogate marker for intra-abdominal or visceral adipose tissue (VAT). VAT is considered an active endocrine organ that is associated with metabolic and inflammatory abnormalities and secretion of adipocyte and adipose connective tissue adipokines. To measure waist, place a measuring tape in a horizontal plane around the abdomen at the level of the iliac crest.

risk factors' include increased biomarkers of chronic inflammation (C-reactive protein, tumor necrosis factor-a, interleukin-6), a prothrombotic state (increased plasma plasminogen activator inhibitor (PAI)-1 and fibrinogen), endothelial dysfunction (decreased endothelium-dependent vasodilatation), hemodynamic changes (increased sympathetic nervous activity and renal sodium retention), hyperuricemia, and non-alcoholic fatty liver disease (NAFLD). OSA often co-exists with these traditional and non-traditional cardiovascular risk factors, leading one author to coin the term 'Syndrome Z'.[13]

Measurement of waist circumference is a surrogate marker for visceral adipose tissue (VAT) which refers to adipose tissue located within the abdominal cavity, below abdominal muscles, and comprising omental and mesenteric adipose tissue, as well as adipose tissue of the retroperitoneal and perinephric regions (Fig. 8.1). Visceral fat accumulation has also been shown to have a significant negative impact on glycemic control in patients with type 2 diabetes. Recent studies have linked the metabolic and inflammatory abnormalities seen in abdominal obesity to the secretion of adipocyte and adipose connective tissue products called adipokines. Secreted factors include leptin, IL-6, TNF-α, angiotensinogen, PAI-1, transforming growth factor (TGF)-β, and adiponectin among many others.[14] Secretion of these products results in altered endocrine, paracrine and autocrine functions. The metabolic dysregulation and systemic inflammation seen in OSA is likely related, in part, to VAT-derived secretory products.[15–17]

## 4 TREATMENT OF THE OVERWEIGHT AND OBESE PATIENT

Guidance for weight loss should be part of the non-surgical treatment for all obese patients with OSA.[18] The evidence that treatment of obesity improves OSA is reasonably well established. Both medical and surgical approaches to weight loss have been associated with a consistent but variable reduction in number of respiratory events, as well as improvement in oxygenation.[10] A critical review of the literature by Strobel and Rosen[6] concluded that obesity treatments have shown varying degrees of improvement in sleep disordered breathing, oxygen hemoglobin saturation, sleep fragmentation, and daytime performance. Dietary weight losses of 9–18% body weight have been associated with reductions in AHI ranging from 30% to 75%. The authors note, however, that it is presently unclear how much weight loss is necessary to achieve significant improvements in sleep disordered breathing and which patients are most likely to benefit from weight loss. In a population-based study, a 10% weight loss was associated with a 26% decrease in the AHI.[5] In general, surgical weight loss interventions have shown greater improvements in the AHI compared to dietary treatments. A recent systematic literature review of bariatric gastric banding surgery noted improvement in OSA in a number of studies.[19] This was consistent with another bariatric surgical meta-analysis that showed striking results with over 85% of patients having complete resolution of the disorder.[20] The authors also report data from a sub-analysis of four studies (92 subjects) that showed a mean decrease of 33.85 apneas or hypopneas per hour after bariatric surgery.

The decision of how aggressively to treat patients and which modalities to use is determined by the patient's risk status, their abilities and desires, and by what resources are available. Table 8.4 provides a guide to selecting adjunctive treatments based on the BMI category. Equally important in choosing a treatment approach is the patient's interest and ability to comply with the regimen and their perceptions of its effectiveness and safety. Therapy for obesity always includes lifestyle management and may include pharmacotherapy or surgery (Fig. 8.2). Since the otolaryngologist is unlikely to manage obesity by him or herself, it is essential to identify resources, e.g. registered dietitian, physician specialist, commercial or internet program, that can provide the needed assistance, monitoring and accountability for successful obesity care. The primary role of the otolaryngologist is to recognize the importance of weight loss, to incorporate weight loss into the treatment plan, and be supportive of the patient's initiatives.

### 4.1 LIFESTYLE MANAGEMENT

Lifestyle management incorporates three essential components of obesity care: dietary therapy, physical activity and

| Table 8.4 | A guide to selecting treatment | | | | |
|---|---|---|---|---|---|
| Treatment | BMI category | | | | |
| | 25–26.9 | 27–29.9 | 30–35 | 35–39.9 | ≥40 |
| Diet, exercise, behavior therapy | With co-morbidities | With co-morbidities | + | + | + |
| Pharmacotherapy | | With co-morbidities | + | + | + |
| Surgery | | | | With co-morbidities | + |
| Source: *The Practical Guide: Identification, Evaluation, and Treatment of Overweight and Obesity in Adults.* US Department of Health and Human Services, Public Health Service, National Institutes of Health, National Heart, Lung, and Blood Institute. NIH Publication No. 00-4084, October 2000. | | | | | |

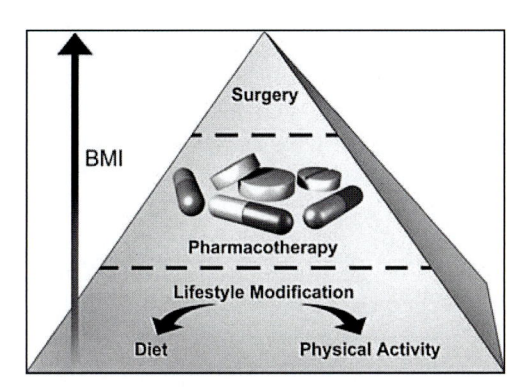

**Fig. 8.2** The clinical approach to obesity can be viewed as a pyramid consisting of several levels of therapeutic options. Lifestyle modification involves diet therapy, physical activity and behavioral modification. Lifestyle modification also should be a component of all other levels of therapy. Pharmacotherapy can be a useful adjunctive measure for properly selected patients. Bariatric surgery is an option for patients with severe obesity, who have not responded to less intensive interventions. The number of obese patients who require a specific level of treatment decreases as one moves up the pyramid.

behavior therapy. Since obesity is fundamentally a disease of energy imbalance, all patients must learn how and when energy is consumed (diet), how and when energy is expended (physical activity) and how to incorporate this information into their daily life (behavior therapy). Lifestyle management has been shown to result in a modest (typically 3–5 kg) weight loss compared to no treatment or usual care.

The primary focus of diet therapy is on reducing overall consumption of calories. The NHLBI guidelines recommend initiating treatment with a diet producing a calorie deficit of 500–1000 kcal/day from the patient's habitual diet with the goal of losing approximately 1–2 lb per week.[21,22] This can be accomplished by suggesting substitutions or alternatives to the diet to achieve the desired calorie deficit. Examples include choosing smaller portion sizes, eating more fruits and vegetables, consuming more whole grain cereals, selecting leaner cuts of meat and skimmed dairy products, reducing fried foods and other added fats and oils, and drinking water instead of caloric beverages. Since portion control is one of the most difficult strategies for patients to manage, use of pre-prepared products, called meal replacements, is a simple and convenient suggestion. Examples include frozen entrees, canned beverages and bars. Use of meal replacements in the diet has been shown to result in a 7–8% weight loss. It is important that the dietary counseling remains patient centered and consistent with his or her cultural preferences.

Although exercise alone is only moderately effective for weight loss, the combination of dietary modification and exercise is the most effective behavioral approach for treatment of obesity. Focusing on simple ways to add physical activity into the normal daily routine through leisure activities, travel and domestic work should be suggested. Examples include walking, using the stairs, doing home and garden work, and engaging in sport activities. Asking the patient to wear a pedometer to monitor total accumulation of steps as part of the activities of daily living, or ADLs, is a useful strategy. Step counts are highly correlated with inactivity (low number of steps) as well as with activity (high number of steps). Studies have demonstrated that lifestyle activities are as effective as structured exercise programs in improving cardiorespiratory fitness and weight loss. The American College of Sports Medicine (ACSM) recommends that overweight and obese individuals progressively increase to a minimum of 150 minutes of moderate-intensity physical activity per week as a first goal.[23] However, for long-term weight loss, higher amounts of exercise (200–300 minutes per week or ≥2000 kcal/week) are needed. The Dietary Guidelines for Americans 2005 found compelling evidence that at least 60–90 minutes of daily moderate-intensity physical activity (420–630 minutes per week) are needed to sustain weight loss.[24] The ACSM also recommends that resistance exercise supplement the endurance exercise program. These recommendations will feel daunting to most patients and need to be implemented gradually. Many patients would benefit from consultation with an exercise physiologist or personal trainer.

When recommending any behavioral lifestyle change, have the patient identify what, when, where and how the behavioral change will be performed, have the patient and yourself keep a record of the anticipated behavioral change, and follow up progress at the next office visit.

## 4.2 PHARMACOTHERAPY

Adjuvant pharmacological treatments should be considered for patients with a BMI of 30 kg/m² or with a BMI of 27 kg/m² who also have concomitant obesity-related risk factors or diseases and for whom dietary and physical activity therapy has not been successful. When prescribing an anti-obesity medication, patients should be actively engaged in a lifestyle program that provides the strategies and skills needed to effectively use the drug since this support increases total weight loss. There are several potential targets of pharmacological therapy for obesity, all based on the concept of producing a sustained negative energy (calorie) balance.[25,26]

## 4.3 CENTRALLY ACTING ANOREXIANT MEDICATIONS

Appetite-suppressing drugs, or anorexiants, affect *satiation* – the processes involved in the termination of a meal, *satiety* – the absence of hunger after eating, and *hunger* – a biological sensation that initiates eating. By increasing satiation and satiety and decreasing hunger, these agents help patients reduce caloric intake while providing a greater sense of control without deprivation. Their biological effect on appetite regulation is produced by variably augmenting the neurotransmission of three monoamines: norepinephrine, serotonin (5-hydroxytryptamine, 5-HT), and, to a lesser degree, dopamine. The classic sympathomimetic adrenergic agents such as phentermine function by either stimulating norepinephrine release or blocking its reuptake. In contrast, sibutramine (Meridia) functions as a serotonin and norepinephrine reuptake inhibitor (SNRI). Sibutramine is not pharmacologically related to amphetamine and has no addictive potential. Sibutramine is the only drug in this class that is approved for long-term use. It produces a dose-dependent weight loss with an average loss of about 5–9% of initial body weight at 12 months. The medication has been demonstrated to be useful in maintenance of weight loss for up to 2 years.

The most commonly reported adverse events of sibutramine are headache, dry mouth, insomnia and constipation. These are generally mild and well tolerated. The principal concern is a dose-related increase in blood pressure and heart rate that may require discontinuation of the medication. A dose of 10–15 mg/day causes an average increase in systolic and diastolic blood pressure of 2–4 mm Hg and an increase in heart rate of 4–6 beats/min. For this reason, all patients should be monitored closely and seen back in the office within 1 month after initiating therapy. The risk of adverse effects on blood pressure is no greater in patients with controlled hypertension than in those who do not have hypertension and the drug does not appear to cause cardiac valve dysfunction. Contraindications to sibutramine use include uncontrolled hypertension, congestive heart failure, symptomatic coronary heart disease, arrhythmias, or history of stroke. Similar to other anti-obesity medications, weight reduction is enhanced when the drug is used along with behavioral therapy.

## 4.4 PERIPHERALLY ACTING MEDICATION

Orlistat (Xenical) is a synthetic hydrogenated derivative of a naturally occurring lipase inhibitor, lipostatin. Orlistat is a potent slowly reversible inhibitor of pancreatic and gastric lipases which are required for the hydrolysis of dietary fat in the gastrointestinal tract. The drug's activity takes place in the lumen of the stomach and small intestine by forming a covalent bond with the active serine residue site of these lipases. Taken at a therapeutic dose of 120 mg tid, orlistat blocks the digestion and absorption of about 30% of dietary fat. On discontinuation of the drug, fecal fat usually returns to normal concentrations within 48–72 hours.

Multiple randomized, 1- to 2-year double-blind, placebo-controlled studies have shown that after 1 year, orlistat produces a weight loss of about 9–10% compared with a 4–6% weight loss in the placebo-treated groups. Since orlistat is minimally (<1%) absorbed from the gastrointestinal tract, it has no systemic side effects. Tolerability to the drug is related to the malabsorption of dietary fat and subsequent passage of fat in the feces. Six gastrointestinal tract adverse effects have been reported to occur in at least 10% of orlistat-treated patients; oily spotting, flatus with discharge, fecal urgency, fatty/oily stool, oily evacuation, and increased defecation. The events are generally experienced early, diminish as patients control their dietary fat intake, and infrequently cause patients to withdraw from clinical trials. Psyllium mucilloid is helpful in controlling the orlistat-induced GI side effects when taken concomitantly with the medication. The manufacturer's package insert for orlistat recommends that patients take a vitamin supplement along with the drug to prevent potential deficiencies. Orlistat was approved for over-the-counter (OTC) use in 2007.

## 4.5 THE ENDOCANNABINOID SYSTEM

Cannabinoid receptors and their endogenous ligands have been implicated in a variety of physiological functions, including feeding, modulation of pain, emotional behavior, and peripheral lipid metabolism.[27] The cannabinoid receptors, the endocannabinoids and the enzymes catalyzing their biosynthesis and degradation constitute the endocannabinoid system or ECS. Cannabis and its main ingredient, $\Delta^9$-tetrahydrocannabinol (THC), is an exogenous cannabinoid compound. Two endocannabinoids have been identified: anandamide and 2-arachidonyl glyceride (2-AG). Two cannabinoid receptors have been cloned termed $CB_1$ (abundant in the brain) and $CB_2$ (present in immune cells). The brain ECS is thought to control food intake through reinforcing motivation to find and consume foods with high incentive value and regulate actions of other mediators of appetite. The first selective cannabinoid $CB_1$ receptor antagonist, called rimonabant, was discovered in 1994. The medication is effective in antagonizing the appetite-stimulating effect of THC and suppressing appetite when given alone in animal models.

Thus far, several large prospective, randomized controlled trials have demonstrated the effectiveness of rimonabant as a weight loss agent.[28] Taken as a 20 mg dose, subjects lost an average of approximately 6.5 kg compared to approximately 1.5 kg for placebo at 1 year. Concomitant improvements were seen in waist circumference and cardiovascular risk factors. The most common reported side effects include depression, anxiety and nausea. Rimonabant is approved for use in Europe and other countries outside the US.

## 4.6 WEIGHT LOSS SURGERY

Bariatric surgery can be considered for patients with severe obesity (BMI = 40 kg/m$^2$) or those with moderate obesity (BMI = 35 kg/m$^2$) associated with a serious medical condition such as OSA.[29] Surgical weight loss functions by reducing caloric intake and, depending on the procedure, macronutrient absorption. The improvement in co-morbid conditions is the result of multiple factors including weight and body fat loss, change in diet, and for the malabsorptive procedures, anatomical changes of the gastrointestinal tract that effect altered responses of several gut hormones involved in glucose regulation and appetite control.

Weight loss surgeries fall into one of two categories: restrictive and restrictive malabsorptive. Restrictive surgeries limit the amount of food the stomach can hold and slow the rate of gastric emptying. The laparoscopic adjustable silicone gastric banding (LASGB) is the most commonly performed restrictive operation. The first banding device, the LAP-BAND, was approved for use in the United States in 2001. In contrast to previous devices, the diameter of this band is adjustable by way of its connection to a reservoir that is implanted under the skin (Fig. 8.3). Injection or removal of saline into the reservoir tightens or loosens the band's internal diameter, respectively, thus changing the size of the gastric opening. Since there is no rerouting of the intestine with LASGB, the risk for developing micronutrient deficiencies is entirely dependent on the patient's diet and eating habits.

The Roux-en-Y gastric bypass (RYGB) is the most commonly performed and accepted of the restrictive-malabsorptive bypass procedures. It involves formation of a 10–30 ml proximal gastric pouch by either surgically separating or stapling the stomach across the fundus (Fig. 8.4). Outflow from the pouch is created by performing a narrow (10 mm) gastrojejunostomy. The distal end of jejunum is then anastomosed 50–150 cm below the gastrojejunostomy.

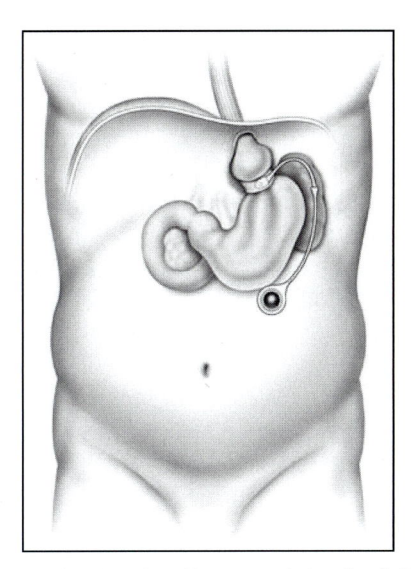

**Fig. 8.3** Laparoscopic adjustable silicone gastric banding (LASGB) is the most commonly performed restrictive operation. The diameter of the band is adjustable by way of its connection to a reservoir that is implanted under the skin. Injection or removal of saline into the reservoir tightens or loosens the band's internal diameter, respectively, thus changing the size of the gastric opening.

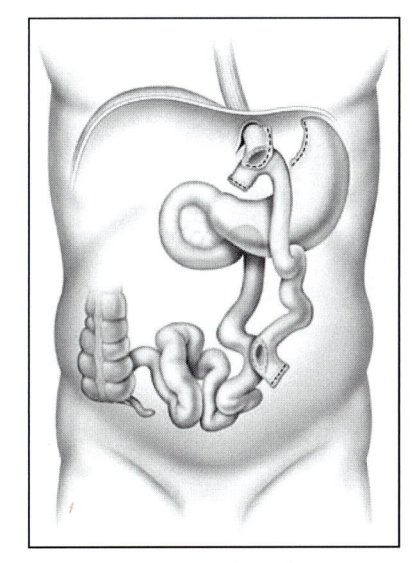

**Fig. 8.4** The Roux-en-Y gastric bypass (RYGB) is the most commonly performed and accepted restrictive-malabsorptive procedure. It involves formation of a 10–30 ml proximal gastric pouch by either surgically separating or stapling the stomach across the fundus. Outflow from the pouch is created by performing a narrow (10 mm) gastrojejunostomy. The distal end of jejunum is then anastomosed 50–150 cm below the gastrojejunostomy.

'Roux-en-Y' refers to the Y-shaped section of small intestine created by the surgery; the Y is created at the point where the pancreo-biliary conduit (afferent limb) and the Roux (efferent) limb are connected. 'Bypass' refers to the exclusion or bypassing of the distal stomach, duodenum and proximal jejunum. RYGB may be performed with an open incision or laparoscopically.

# SECTION C: NON-SURGICAL TREATMENT OF OSA/HS

Although no recent randomized controlled trials compare weight loss after surgical and non-surgical interventions, available data from meta-analyses and large databases primarily obtained from observational studies suggest that bariatric surgery is the most effective weight loss therapy for those with severe obesity. These procedures are generally effective in producing an average weight loss of approximately 30–35% of total body weight that is maintained in nearly 60% of patients at 5 years. In general, mean weight loss is greater after the combined restrictive-malabsorptive procedures compared to the restrictive procedures. An abundance of data supports the positive impact of bariatric surgery on obesity-related morbid conditions including diabetes mellitus, hypertension, OSA, dyslipidemia and non-alcoholic fatty liver disease.

If surgery is considered, the patient should be evaluated by a high patient volume multidisciplinary team that incorporates medical, nutritional and psychological care. Significant and rapid improvement in diabetes control, OSA, gastroesophageal reflux disease and urinary incontinence, among others, is typically seen following surgery. For patients who undergo LASGB, there are no intestinal absorptive abnormalities other than mechanical reduction in gastric size and outflow. Therefore, selective deficiencies occur uncommonly unless eating habits remain restrictive and unbalanced. In contrast, the restrictive-malabsorptive procedures produce a predictable increased risk for micronutrient deficiencies of vitamin $B_{12}$, iron, folate, calcium and vitamin D based on surgical anatomical changes. Patients require lifelong supplementation with these micronutrients.

## 5 CONCLUSIONS

The majority of patients presenting with OSA will be overweight or obese with the distribution of fat located in the central (abdominal) region. The otolaryngologist should routinely use BMI to categorize obesity and evaluate the patient for co-existence of other diseases and disorders that may reduce quality of life and increase morbidity and mortality. Since weight loss has been demonstrated to improve sleep disordered breathing, management of the underlying obesity must be included as one of the most effective non-surgical strategies. Reinforcing behavioral changes in diet and physical activity and use of anti-obesity medications and surgery when indicated have been shown to be useful in obesity treatment. Referral to a physician specialist, registered dietitian, exercise specialist or commercial weight loss program should be included in the long-term treatment plan. The physician can be effective in managing the patient with obesity if he/she takes the initiative and provides targeted supportive strategies and skills.

## REFERENCES

1. Ogden CL, Carroll MD, Curtin LR, et al. Prevalence of overweight and obesity in the United States, 1999–2004. JAMA 2006;295:1549–55.
2. Strohl KP, Redline S. Recognition of obstructive sleep apnea. Am J Crit Care Med 1996;154:279–89.
3. Newman AB, Foster G, Givelber R, et al. Progression and regression of sleep-disordered breathing with changes in weight. The Sleep Heart Health Study. Arch Intern Med 2005;165:2408–13.
4. Young T, Shahar E, Nieto FJ, et al. Predictors of sleep-disordered breathing in community-dwelling adults: the Sleep Heart Health Study. Arch Intern Med 2002;162:893–900.
5. Peppard PE, Young T, Palta M, et al. Longitudinal study of moderate weight change and sleep-disordered breathing. JAMA 2000;284:3015–21.
6. Strobel RJ, Rosen RC. Obesity and weight loss in obstructive sleep apnea: a critical review. Sleep 1996;19:104–15.
7. Kushner RF. Roadmaps for Clinical Practice. Case Studies in Disease Prevention and Health Promotion – Assessment and Management of Adult Obesity. A Primer for Physicians. Chicago, Illinois: American Medical Association; 2003. Available at: www.ama-assn.org/ama/pub/category/10931.html
8. Tishler PV, Larkin EK, Schluchter MD, Redline S. Incidence of sleep-disordered breathing in an urban adult population. The relative importance of risk factors in the development of sleep-disordered breathing. JAMA 2003;289:2230–37.
9. National Institutes of Health. Third Report of the National Cholesterol Education Program Expert Panel on Detection, Evaluation, and Treatment of High Blood Cholesterol in Adults (Adult Treatment Panel III). Bethesda, MD: National Institutes of Health; 2001. NIH Publication No. 01-3670.
10. National Institutes of Health and National Heart, Lung, and Blood Institute. Sleep Apnea: Is Your Patient at risk? NIH Publication No. 95-3803, September 1995.
11. Davies RJO, Ali NJ, Stradling JR. Neck circumference and other clinical features in the diagnosis of the obstructive sleep apnoea syndrome. Thorax 1992;47:101–5.
12. Resta O, Foschino-Barbaro MP, Legari G, et al. Sleep-related breathing disorders, loud snoring and excessive daytime sleepiness in obese subjects. Int J Obesity 2001;25:669–75.
13. Wilcox I, McNamara SG, Collins FL, et al. 'Syndrome Z': the interaction of sleep apnoea, vascular risk factors and heart disease. Thorax 1998;53(Suppl 3):S25–S28.
14. Greenberg AS, Obin MS. Obesity and the role of adipose tissue in inflammation and metabolism. Am J Clin Nutr 2006;83:461S–465S.
15. Brown LK. A waist is a terrible thing to mind. Central obesity, the metabolic syndrome, and sleep apnea hypopnea syndrome. Chest 2002;122:774–78.
16. Coughlin S, Calverley P, Wilding J. Sleep disordered breathing – a new component of syndrome X? Obes Rev 2001;2:267–74.
17. Wolk R, Shamsuzzaman ASM, Somers VK. Obesity, sleep apnea, and hypertension. Hypertension 2003;42:1067–74.
18. Capies SM, Gami AS, Somers VK. Obstructive sleep apnea. Ann Intern Med 2005;142:187–97.
19. Chapman AE, Kiroff G, Game P, et al. Laparoscopic adjustable gastric banding in the treatment of obesity: a systematic literature review. Surgery 2004;135:326–51.
20. Buchwald H, Avidor Y, Braunwald E, et al. Bariatric surgery: a systematic review and meta-analysis. JAMA 2004;292:1724–37.
21. National Heart, Lung, and Blood Institute (NHLBI) Obesity Education Initiative Expert Panel. Identification, Evaluation, and Treatment of Overweight and Obesity in Adults: Evidence Report. NIH Publication NO. 4083, June 1998.
22. National Heart, Lung, and Blood Institute (NHLBI) and North American Association for the Study of Obesity (NAASO). The Practical Guide. Identification, Evaluation, and treatment of Overweight and Obesity in Adults. NIH Publication NO. 00-4084, October 2000.

23. Jakicic JM, Clark. K, Coleman E, et al., for the American College of Sports Medicine Appropriate intervention strategies for weight loss and prevention of Weight Regain for Adults. Med Sci Sports Exerc 2001;33:2145–56.
24. U.S. Department of Health and Human Services and U.S. Department of Agriculture. Dietary Guidelines for Americans 2005, 6th edn. Washington, DC: U.S. Government Printing Office, January 2005. Available at: www.health.gov/dietaryguidelines/dga2005/document/html
25. Yanovski S, Yanovski JA. Obesity. N Engl J Med 2002;346:591–602.
26. Padwal R, Li SK, Lau DCW. Long-term pharmacotherapy for overweight and obesity: a systematic review and meta-analysis of randomized controlled trials. Int J Obesity 2003;27:1437–46.
27. Cota D, Woods SC. The role of the endocannabinoid system in the regulation of energy homeostasis. Curr Opin Endo Diab 2005;12:338–51.
28. Pi-Sunyer FX, Aronne LJ, Heshmati HM, et al. Effect of rimonabant, a cannabinoid-1 receptor blocker, on weight and cardiometabolic risk factors in overweight or obese patients. RIO-North America: a randomized controlled trial. JAMA 2006;295:761–75.
29. Consensus Development Conference Panel. Gastrointestinal surgery for severe obesity. Ann Intern Med 1991;115:956–61.

SECTION C — NON-SURGICAL TREATMENT OF OSA/HS

# CHAPTER 9

# CPAP, APAP and BIPAP

*Terence M. Davidson*

## 1 INTRODUCTION

Positive airway pressure (PAP) therapy, including continuous positive airway pressure (CPAP), adjustable positive airway pressure (APAP), and bi-level positive airway pressure (BI-PAP), is an important, non-invasive treatment for sleep disordered breathing (SDB). PAP therapy as a treatment for obstructive sleep apnea (OSA) was first developed by Colin E. Sullivan and colleagues in 1980 at the University of Sydney, New South Wales, Australia. The effectiveness of CPAP treatment first received public attention in 1981 when Sullivan published his findings, documenting that low pressures of air delivered through the nasal passages had the ability to splint the airway and provide a night of unobstructed, uninterrupted sleep, while reducing daytime somnolence.[1] The recommended and only treatment available for OSA before Sullivan's discovery was the surgical procedure of tracheotomy. Therapy models for PAP treatment have been incorporated into medical practices utilizing a variety of techniques. While surgical procedures are invasive and have variable success for OSA, PAP therapy has proven to be an effective treatment that corrects the obstructed airway, reduces the severity of SDB symptoms and the occurrence of associated co-morbidities, and has no associated risks, although compliance although remains an issue. In any case it is the first-line treatment for OSA. This chapter provides a description of how PAP is administered and a review of its history and efficacies.

## 2 OBJECTIVES OF PAP THERAPY IN AN ENT PRACTICE

Surgeons are understandably interested in surgical therapies for treating OSA. However, to nurture patient referrals, ENT physicians need to incorporate PAP treatments into their practice. Medical colleagues do not always have the resources or interest to examine the upper respiratory tract, diagnose SDB, and recommend appropriate patients for surgical consultations. Unfortunately, the medical community is disenchanted with surgical therapies in treating SDB due to a glaring absence of EBM Level I prospective, controlled studies demonstrating the benefit of surgery.[2] Level II studies are also missing. Furthermore, the sleep physician's anecdotal experience with surgery is not excellent for they rarely see the successes, but all too often see the failures. It is therefore the authors' opinion that if ENT physicians choose to participate in the evaluation and management of SDB, they must offer not only home sleep testing, but also PAP administration as part of their sleep services. Currently, surgeons enjoy patient and primary care physician referrals, but if we are to maintain a position in the sleep market and retain and nurture a steady flow of patients, we must provide comprehensive services. This includes sleep testing and PAP administration in addition to our history, physical examination and surgical procedures. Setting up and managing a polysomnographic operation is time consuming and complex. It is also expensive for patients, insurance companies, and the greater healthcare system.

Shown by numerous validation studies, multi-channel home sleep testing has proven to be highly correlated with polysomnography and equally effective in diagnosing OSA.[3–6] Home sleep testing is easy to perform and fairly reimbursed. PAP therapy is more difficult to perform and is poorly reimbursed. However, if the head and neck surgeon does not provide PAP services, they will not have a comprehensive SDB practice and will ultimately lose their position in the sleep market. There was a time when allergists wished to become the entry point for patients with sinusitis. The head and neck surgery community countered, and today, patients with chronic sinusitis come to our office for evaluation, medical and surgical therapies. The authors propose that the diagnosis and treatment of OSA must follow a similar path in establishing itself within the medical community.

## 3 THERAPEUTIC INDICATIONS

Surgical indications for the treatment of sleep disordered breathing are for the individuals who suffer from severe

## CPAP, APAP and BIPAP

Table 9.1 Medical conditions associated with SDB

| Category | Condition | References |
|---|---|---|
| Cardiac | Hypertension | 35, 36 |
| | Congestive heart failure | 37–41 |
| | Ischemic heart disease | 42–46 |
| | Dysrhythmias | 47–49 |
| Respiratory | Pulmonary hypertension | 50 |
| Neurologic | Stroke | 51–53 |
| | Headache | 54, 55 |
| Metabolic | Insulin resistance | 56–58 |
| | Metabolic syndrome | 59, 60 |
| Gastrointestinal | Gastroesophageal reflux disease | 61–64 |
| Genitourinary | Erectile dysfunction | 65, 66 |
| | Nocturia, enuresis | 67, 68 |

nasal obstruction, most notably nasal polyps, and the patients with four plus tonsils, Friedman Stage 1.[7] Unfortunately, the majority of SDB is obstruction at the tongue base, an area where surgical therapy is not yet uniformly successful. Therefore, a large number of individuals with SDB must be provided PAP therapy, and only if this truly fails, be considered for surgical interventions. The senior author generally advises patients he will only discuss surgical therapies after the SDB patient has learned to use CPAP, and then makes an informed decision to pursue surgical options. Snoring, absent OSA, is still a surgical disease.

The indications for positive airway pressure therapy are individuals with significant SDB. The Center for Medicaid and Medicare Services (CMS) guidelines indicate PAP therapy for individuals with an Apnea Hypopnea Index (AHI) of 15 events per hour or greater or an AHI of five or greater with two or more co-morbidities.[8] Co-morbidities are listed in Table 9.1. There are many individuals with an AHI of five but less than 15, who are diagnosed with mild OSA, for whom PAP therapy should be recommended. This group would include those who are symptomatic, most notably presenting with excessive daytime sleepiness, hypertension and cardiovascular co-morbidities, and those who are not surgical candidates. With the prevalence of obesity increasing, the number of those patients will increase over time.

## 4 ENT PRACTICE MODEL

Positive airway pressure treatment first and foremost requires an individual in the office who is dedicated to this treatment. A trained respiratory therapist or sleep technician is not necessarily needed, but this cannot be an add-on responsibility for an already overworked nurse or medical assistant. Multi-channel home diagnostic devices and PAP machines are evolving technologies that provide automated algorithms within their software and superb technical and educational support from the manufacturers to effectively utilize these products in an office setting.

### 4.1 AUTO-TITRATING PAP

Those who utilize laboratory polysomnography will often initiate PAP therapy from their lab. This is done through a split night titration, where PAP therapy is administered half way through a polysomnography sleep test if the sleep technician believes the patient is positive for SDB. A median pressure is titrated and prescribed for a CPAP machine. Those who conduct multi-channel home sleep testing and provide all their services out of their office can do the same with auto-PAP home titrations. Introduced to the market in 2000, auto-PAP machines have the ability to automatically adjust pressure settings throughout a night's sleep to ensure that the correct pressure is being emitted to splint open the airway.[9] There are several models of auto-adjusting PAP machines available in today's market, and these are used for the initial titration and trial. They can also be used for the PAP treatment. Two recent models are seen in Figures 9.1 and 9.2.

An auto-titrating PAP machine is provided to a SDB patient who typically takes it home and uses it for 3–7 days. They then return the machine to the prescribing physician. If the patient and/or their insurance choose to provide an APAP machine, the prescription is written for the mask and the machine. If the insurance company only covers fixed pressure CPAP, the prescription also includes the 95th percentile pressure for the CPAP machine. This is the pressure that will splint the airway open 95% of the time. Fixed pressure CPAP does well, just not quite as well as APAP. The pros and cons of APAP versus CPAP are an evolving controversy. Typically, a durable medical equipment (DME) provider supplies the equipment. While some patients

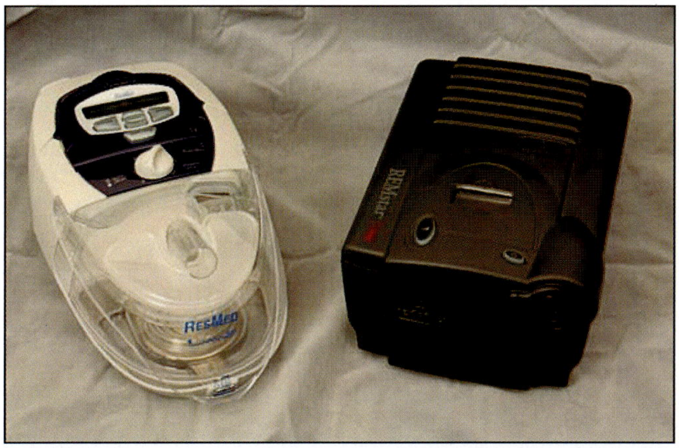

Fig. 9.1

SECTION C  NON-SURGICAL TRETAMENT OF OSA/HS

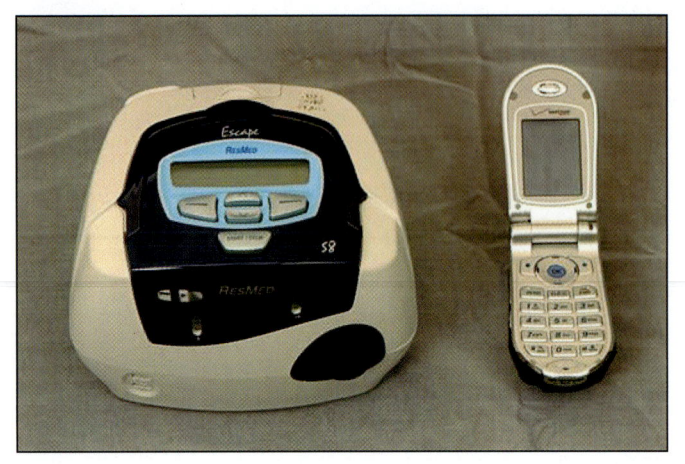

Fig. 9.2

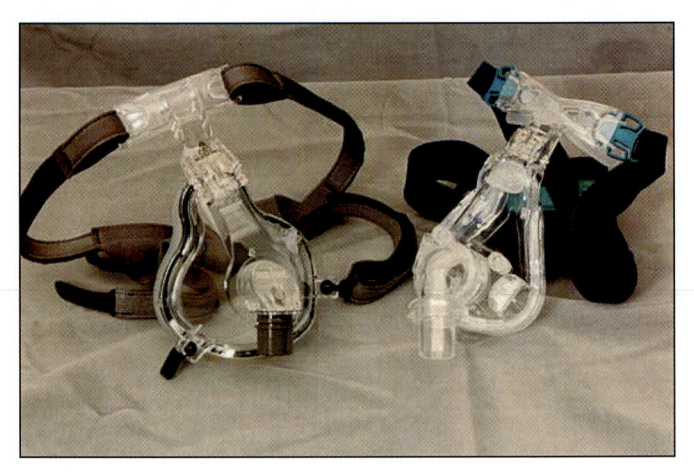

Fig. 9.4

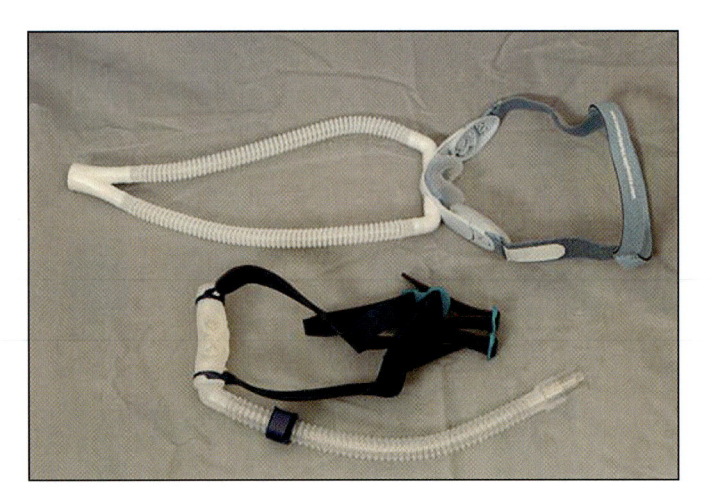

Fig. 9.3

report immediate compliance and benefit, some experience difficulties. These individuals need to be seen in the office, their equipment adjusted, and compliance nurtured.

## 4.2 MASKS

Numerous masks are available, and many believe the mask is the key to PAP therapy. Nasal masks are generally easier to use, as they are less intrusive and certainly less claustrophobic, but individuals who are nighttime mouth breathers will require full face masks. There is no single mask to satisfy everyone, therefore an assortment of nasal masks and full face masks should be maintained. Figures 9.3 and 9.4 show several masks currently on the market. Patients can look at and try these in the office, and select a preference for model and size. The mask is also trialed with the auto-PAP machine for 3–7 days.

## 4.3 THE OFFICE VISIT

After a patient has been informed of their sleep study results and diagnosed with SDB warranting PAP therapy, they are ready to begin their PAP consultation. This visit requires 45 minutes, as informed introduction to the therapy will produce a higher likelihood of compliance. A spouse or bedpartner is strongly encouraged to attend this appointment to address psychosocial sensitivities often associated with PAP therapy, and encourage a support system. This is crucial in achieving compliance. In some areas, the DME can provide this service.

First and foremost, any lingering questions about the patient's sleep study results should be addressed. The diagnosis and the importance of SDB as a health risk should be reiterated. Information in the form of pamphlets and handouts is an excellent supplement. To begin the PAP titration, the patient is asked if they are a mouth breather or a nasal breather to ensure that an appropriate trial mask is chosen. The titration/trial mask is then fitted to the patient and they are asked to practice putting it on their face, preferably in front of a mirror. Once the patient is comfortable handling the mask, it is connected to the titration PAP machine, and the starting procedure is demonstrated. The patient should spend a few minutes with the PAP machine on, to get an idea of how the pressure will feel. At the end of the appointment, logistical information about the PAP titration should be reviewed, and additional questions answered. This is a good time to hand out pamphlets and literature. A list of resourceful websites is generally helpful, as well as contact information, should difficulties arise. A patient should walk out of the PAP consultation with the confidence that the PAP treatment is important to their longevity and that this is a treatment they can do. Figures 9.5 to 9.10 demonstrate an office appointment for PAP fitting.

CHAPTER
CPAP, APAP and BIPAP  9

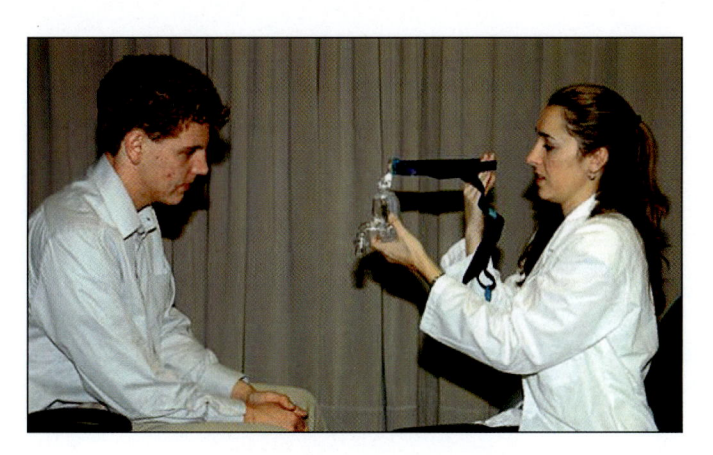

Fig. 9.5

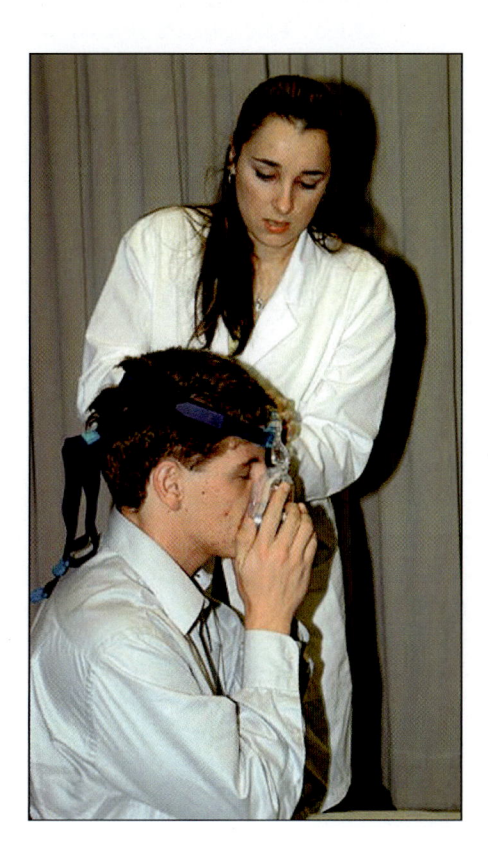

Fig. 9.6

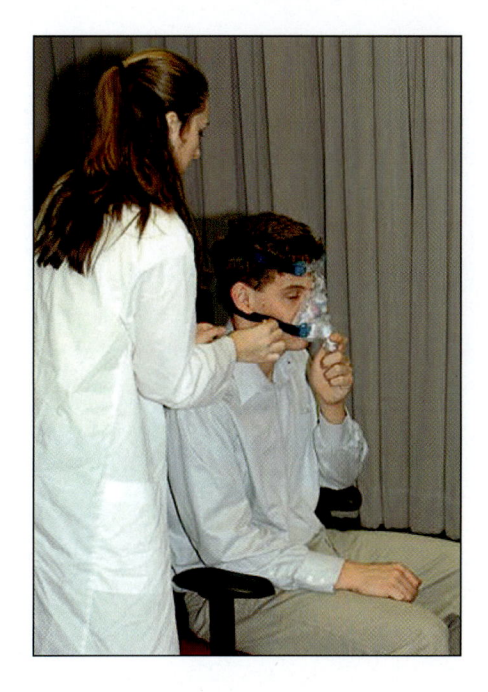

Fig. 9.7

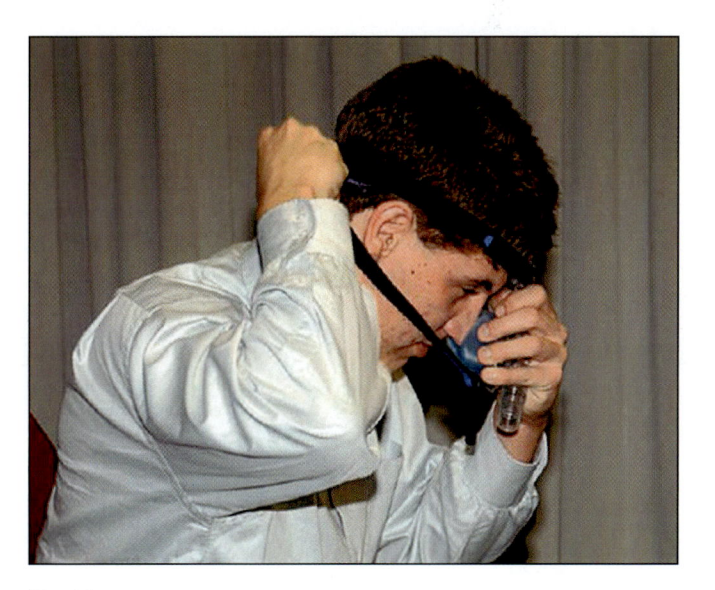

Fig. 9.8

## 4.4 FOLLOW-UP AND COMPLIANCE TECHNIQUES

Many PAP therapy patients take one look at the mask and the machine and announce that they cannot use it. This does not constitute CPAP failure, and the physician and sleep technician must encourage patients to learn to use the PAP machine. Only once patients learn how to use PAP can they make an educated opinion about its long-term use. There are many tricks to nurture PAP use, and each practice needs to develop its own. During the 3–7 day trial, follow-up should be continuously maintained. The first night will be the most difficult for the majority of patients. A follow-up phone call should be made by the sleep technician to inquire about any difficulties the patient may have had with the PAP machine and the mask. At this time, suggestions can be made to nurture compliance. The first seemingly simple aid is to provide the patient with a sleeping pill for the first several nights. Lunesta®, while expensive and often not covered by insurance companies, is probably the preferred sleeping pill, for it is not addictive. Ambien® is an alternative. Tranquilizers and other medications are not ideal, as they will worsen the patient's SDB, and if the patient does not use the PAP treatment, it will place them at risk for SDB difficulties, death included.

| SECTION C | NON-SURGICAL TRETAMENT OF OSA/HS |

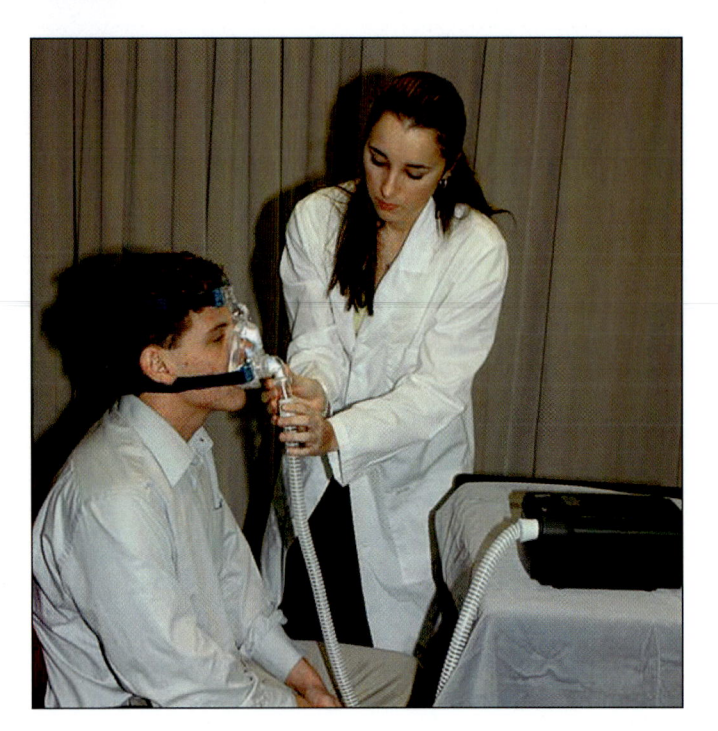

Fig. 9.9

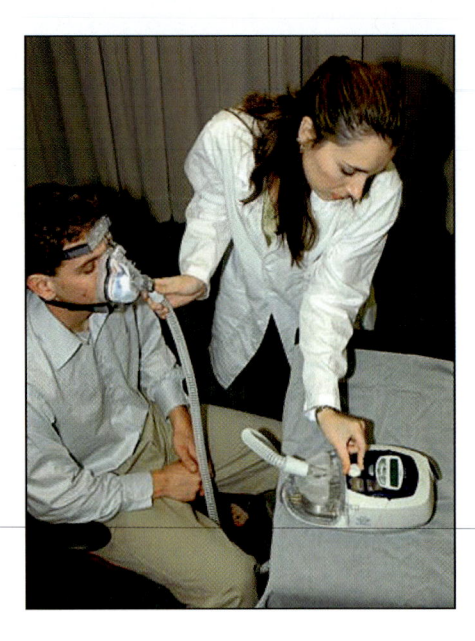

Fig. 9.10

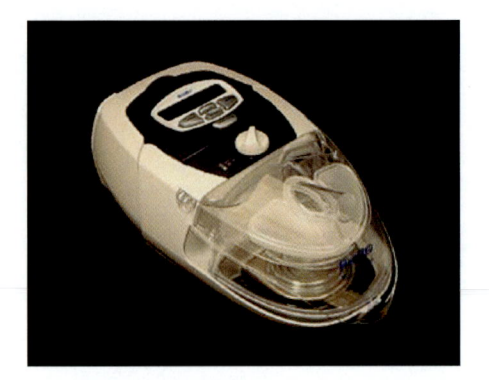

Fig. 9.11

Some patients are claustrophobic and find the mask too frightening to wear. For these patients, a tranquilizer can be considered. Although time consuming, the best approach is probably to develop a program in which the patient slowly gets used to the mask and then the PAP machine. Our paradigm for the 'difficult' patient is to dispense the selected mask from the office and ask the patient to first wear it as an open mask without a hose and the PAP machine, just in the evenings and around their home. As they become used to this, then they can be asked to wear it during sleep. Once they are comfortable with the mask, the hose and PAP machine can be added. This can be started while awake and watching television and only after a few nights should they wear the PAP to bed. A second paradigm is to provide a PAP machine beginning at very low pressures, typically 4–6 cmH$_2$O, increasing the pressure every couple of days until it reaches a therapeutic level. Another paradigm is to dispense an auto-adjusting PAP machine. Theoretically this only provides the required pressure to splint the sleeping airway, and is therefore unobtrusive. If the patient has difficulties, the maximum pressure can be turned down and then increased slowly. For those who experience drying, humidification can be added. In some cases, heated humidification is required. The humidifier seen in Figure 9.11 is typically an external attachment to the PAP machine. Humidification has its complexities, for the equipment and the tubing are prone to mold growth and therefore require a more aggressive daily cleaning program. The experienced PAP sleep technician and the DME can assist the patient in adopting a cleaning regime.

All SDB surgery need not be directed at 'curing' sleep disordered breathing. Surgical procedures can be adopted as a supplement to PAP therapy. There are many individuals for whom selected surgical procedures, most typically of the nose, will allow them to use nasal masks with PAP therapy rather than full face masks, or reduce pressure requirements. When this is the goal, both patient and physician must recognize that a surgical intervention will promote better efficacy of PAP and not a cure for SDB.

## 4.6 THE SURGEON'S ROLE IN PAP COMPLIANCE

While surgery is generally the preferred treatment for palatal snoring in an individual with an AHI of less than 15, without the co-morbidities of sleep disordered breathing, and without the two obvious surgical cures of nasal polyps and four plus tonsils, Friedman Stage I, PAP is considered the primary treatment for SDB. Compliance remains a challenging problem. Surgeons should encourage head and neck surgery evaluation of these patients and explore opportunities to improve CPAP compliance rather than surgical cure.

The evaluation begins with the history of nasal obstruction, most importantly the obligate nighttime mouth breather. A mouth breather requires full face PAP therapy masks. Surgical enlargement of the nasal passage may convert a mouth breather to a nasal breather, but it seems that many are so accustomed to nighttime mouth breathing that even wide enlargement of the nasal passage will not cure the affliction. This does not mean that it should not be attempted, but a high cure rate should not be expected.

The history should also look for inflammatory causes of nasal obstruction, most notably allergic rhinitis, occasionally chronic sinusitis or nasal polyps, and rarely nasal malignancy. The interesting patient is the individual who has nasal obstruction during the day and obstruction that worsens at night. These are cases where head and neck surgery treatment can truly be a benefit. Allergic rhinitis is treated with nasal steroids, environmental control, and leukotriene inhibitors. Skin testing and immunotherapy may be considered.

Chronic sinusitis is documented by a sinus CT scan and is treated with endoscopic sinus surgery. Much of the nasal obstruction occurs in the anterior valve area. For these individuals, sinus cones seen in Figures 9.12 and 9.13 have been found to be useful, particularly for nighttime breathing. For those who have valve problems, septoplasty, spreader grafts, alar battans, and myriad valve plasties may be considered.[10] There is little science to document their benefit in nasal obstruction. There is no science to document their benefit in the treatment of PAP compliance.

Turbinectomy is a widely practiced operation. Limited turbinectomy has minor benefit and little risk. Aggressive turbinectomy has no evidence-based medicine Level I or Level II documented benefit. Aggressive turbinectomy may cause atrophic rhinitis.[11] While many surgeons say it does not, there is an association, called the empty nose association, and a number of rhinological referral nasal practices that say the condition does occur. This is mentioned because those who perform aggressive turbinectomy owe the rest of the head and neck community the dignity of a well-controlled study, at least Level III evidence-based medicine, to show benefit. For the surgeon interested in the nasal surgery of the future, improved valvular surgery is needed. The senior author's prediction is that someone will develop an alloplastic graft that will be placed submucosally, perhaps beneath the upper lateral cartilages, and will hold open the valve. Butterfly grafts also work, but are not aesthetically ideal. This is an area deserving clinical research.

The nasal pharynx should be examined in all patients being evaluated for sleep disordered breathing. An occasional patient will have large adenoids. Assuming that this is not a nasal pharyngeal malignancy or an early warning sign of HIV illness, adenoidectomy can be useful. Oral pharyngeal and tongue base surgeries have not been evaluated in their role for PAP compliance. It would seem that if the surgeon's goals were to improve the pharyngeal airway with the intention of lowering high PAP pressures, there may be indication for surgical intervention.

Lastly, there are numerous patients with sleep disordered breathing who use PAP but would like to be able to travel, camp, or inhabit a mountain cabin without having to cope with the complexities and the embarrassments of PAP machines. For these individuals, snoring surgery can be important; however, this must be done for the expressed purpose of improving snoring, not of curing SDB and not taking on the risks and complications associated with more aggressive SDB surgery.

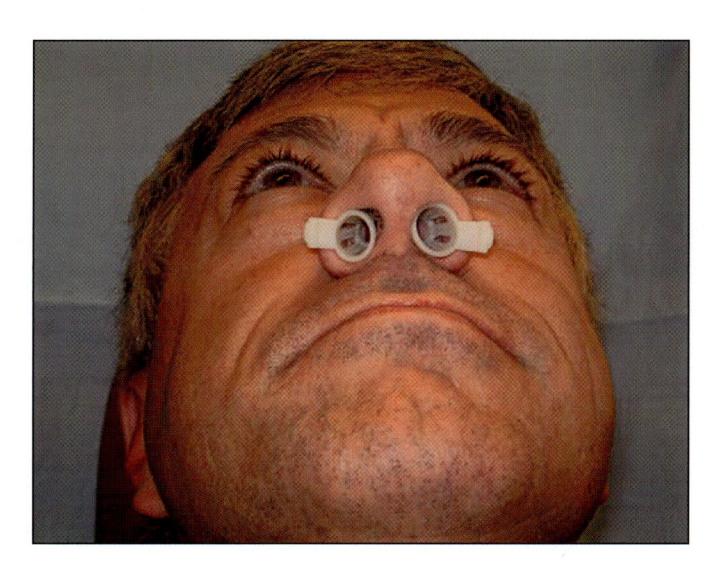

Fig. 9.12

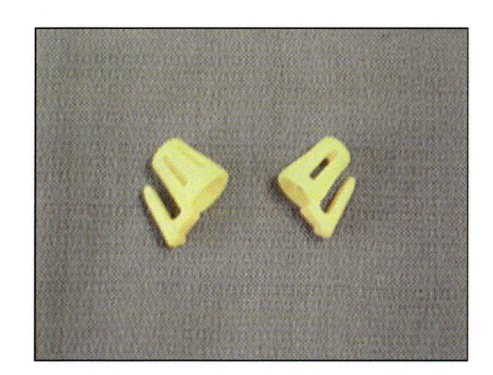

Fig. 9.13

## 4.7 PRESCRIPTIONS

It would be ideal to prescribe an auto-adjusting PAP machine to all patients. Unfortunately, fixed pressure CPAP machines are less expensive so insurance companies will only provide coverage for these. Both the physician and the DME are then challenged to nurture CPAP compliance, and adopt a follow-up procedure for their patients. A drawback to CPAP machines is that the fixed pressure may need adjustment to slightly higher or lower pressures

## 4.8 BI-LEVEL PAP

Bi-level PAP is a machine that delivers one pressure during inspiration and a lower pressure during expiration. These are most commonly needed for individuals who require higher CPAP pressures, typically above 12–14 cmH$_2$O, and have difficulty exhaling against the pressure of the machine. Most bi-level machines require adjustment in the lab; however, evolving products are offering variations of bi-level machines, auto BIPAP included. Recently developed C-Flex technology and expiratory pressure relief (EPR) are touted to work similarly to a bi-level device by offering breath-by-breath exhalation relief and auto-adjusting capabilities during inhalation. BI-PAP is not commonly required but in the rare individual, particularly those with higher CPAP pressures, it may be necessary.

## 4.9 RARE CASES

Occasionally, there are individuals for whom CPAP is difficult. These individuals are typically those with chronic obstructive pulmonary disease (COPD) and those with very high pressures. Cheyne–Stokes breathing requires more complex positive airway pressure paradigms. Cheyne–Stokes breathing is typically seen in Class 3 and Class 4 heart failure and in patients with neurological problems.[12] These rare cases are best referred to a sleep physician with a sleep laboratory for their evaluation and treatment.

## 5 THERAPEUTIC BENEFITS AND RISKS

### 5.1 BENEFITS

PAP therapy offers life-changing benefits for SDB sufferers. Depending on the dedication of the patient to adhere to therapy and frequency of use, results can be seen as early as 1 month. Excessive daytime somnolence can be reduced through long-term use. Depressive symptoms are often reduced and an increase in quality of life has been documented by numerous studies.[13–16] Snoring is eradicated, as PAP keeps the patient's airway open. Often seen in OSA patients, nocturia is also reduced with the use of PAP.[17] Additionally motor vehicle accidents have been shown to decrease among treated OSA sufferers.[18]

Many SDB sufferers often present or are threatened with an increased risk of the aforementioned co-morbidities. Numerous studies have shown that PAP therapy significantly reduces blood pressure levels in systolic and diastolic hypertensive SDB patients, and offers a successful alternative to pharmacological treatments.[19–22] PAP therapy is especially effective in patients with drug-resistant hypertension.[23] Additionally, PAP therapy can benefit SDB patients with type 2 diabetes mellitus, by decreasing insulin sensitivity. Recent studies have shown that elevated glycosylated hemoglobin (HbA1c) levels in type 2 diabetics are reduced through long-term PAP therapy.[24–27]

Cholesterol levels and a decrease in the associated risk for cardiovascular disease have also shown promise from PAP therapy. Studies have shown that clinically significant reductions in cholesterol levels have been demonstrated by PAP therapy use, with results seen as early as 1 month.[28,29] Additionally, poor cardiac indicators such as cardiac contractility, heart rate variability, and hemodynamics at rest can be improved within 1 week of PAP therapy.[30]

Changes in the structure of the upper airway anatomy have also been seen in long-term PAP users. Through continuous splinting of the upper airway, PAP therapy has the ability to permanently morph anatomy that was once causing obstruction. Through the use of magnetic resonance imaging (MRI), studies have shown increase in pharyngeal volume and decrease in tongue volume and upper airway mucosal water in chronic nasal CPAP therapy use.[31]

### 5.2 RISKS

There are risks associated with PAP therapy, none of which is life threatening. Nasal symptoms are often seen with an increased risk of nasal congestion, rhinorrhea, and rare cases of pneumonia.[32,33] These symptoms can be reversed through heated humidification, or nasal steroids. The mask may also elicit claustrophobia in patients.[34] Mold growth in humidifiers that do not have a proper cleaning regime can also cause complex respiratory illnesses. The aforementioned techniques in our practice model can help overcome barriers related to adjustment in wearing the mask. Additionally, the mask may cause skin irritation. The patient should be asked about skin allergies before the prescription is written.

## 6 SUMMARY

The head and neck surgeon who wishes to practice sleep medicine is encouraged to become skilled at the history, upper respiratory tract physical examination, multi-channel home sleep testing and PAP therapies. Not only is this excellent and very satisfying patient care, it also brings substantial surgical opportunities to the practice. Snoring is the premier symptom of sleep disordered breathing, and typically the primary reason that prompts the patient to seek medical care. When a patient's AHI is low and there are no co-morbidities present, snoring surgery can be successful. For those with more complex sleep disordered breathing, PAP therapy is a mandatory, first-line treatment. Those who fail PAP therapy should be considered for surgical therapy, either to make them more compliant or, anatomy permitting, to operate for cure. By incorporating PAP therapy paradigms into an ENT practice, treatment of SDB can achieve high therapeutic and compliance levels.

## REFERENCES

1. Sullivan CE, Issa FG, Berthon-Jones M, Eves L. Reversal of obstructive sleep apnoea by continuous positive airway pressure applied through the nares. Lancet 1981;1(8225):862–65.
2. Sierpina VS, Philips B. Need for scholarly, objective inquiry into alternative therapies. Acad Med 2001;76(9):863–65.
3. Golpe R, Jimenez A, Carpizo R. Home sleep studies in the assessment of sleep apnea/hypopnea syndrome. Chest 2002;122(4):1156–61.
4. Flemons WW, Littner MR, Rowley JA, et al. Home diagnosis of sleep apnea: a systematic review of the literature. An evidence review cosponsored by the American Academy of Sleep Medicine, the American College of Chest Physicians, and the American Thoracic Society. Chest 2003;124(4):1543–79.
5. Reichert JA, Bloch DA, Cundiff E, Votteri BA. Comparison of the NovaSom QSG, a new sleep apnea home-diagnostic system, and polysomnography. Sleep Med 2003;4(3):213–18.
6. ATS/ACCP/AASM Taskforce Steering Committee. Executive summary on the systematic review and practice parameters for portable monitoring in the investigation of suspected sleep apnea in adults. Am J Respir Crit Care Med 2004;169(10):1160–63.
7. Souter MA, Stevenson S, Sparks B, Drennan C. Upper airway surgery benefits patients with obstructive sleep apnoea who cannot tolerate nasal continuous positive airway pressure. J Laryngol Otol 2004;118(4):270–74.
8. Zafar S, Ayappa I, Norman RG, Krieger AC, Walsleben JA, Rapoport DM. Choice of oximeter affects apnea–hypopnea index. Chest 2005;127(1):80–88.
9. d'Ortho MP, Grillier-Lanoir V, Levy P, et al. Constant vs. automatic continuous positive airway pressure therapy: home evaluation. Chest 2000;118(4):1010–17.
10. Egan KK, Kim DW. A novel intranasal stent for functional rhinoplasty and nostril stenosis. Laryngoscope 2005;115(5):903–9.
11. Barbosa Ade A, Caldas N, Morais AX, Campos AJ, Caldas S, Lessa F. Assessment of pre and postoperative symptomatology in patients undergoing inferior turbinectomy. Rev Bras Otorinolaringol (Engl edn) 2005;71(4):468–71.
12. Lorenzi-Filho G, Genta PR, Figueiredo AC, Inoue D. Cheyne–Stokes respiration in patients with congestive heart failure: causes and consequences. Clinics 2005;60(4):333–44.
13. Giles TL, Lasserson TJ, Smith BJ, White J, Wright J, Cates CJ. Continuous positive airways pressure for obstructive sleep apnoea in adults. Cochrane Database Syst Rev 2006;25(1):CD001106.
14. Guilleminault C, Lin CM, Goncalves MA, Ramos E. Related articles. A prospective study of nocturia and the quality of life of elderly patients with obstructive sleep apnea or sleep onset insomnia. J Psychosom Res 2004;56(5):511–15.
15. Haynes PL. The role of behavioral sleep medicine in the assessment and treatment of sleep disordered breathing. Clin Psychol Rev 2005;25(5):673–705.
16. Kawahara S, Akashiba T, Akahoshi T, Horie T. Nasal CPAP improves the quality of life and lessens the depressive symptoms in patients with obstructive sleep apnea syndrome. Intern Med 2005;44(5):422–27.
17. Guilleminault C, Lin CM, Goncalves MA, Ramos E. A prospective study of nocturia and the quality of life of elderly patients with obstructive sleep apnea or sleep onset insomnia. J Psychosom Res 2004;56(5):511–15.
18. George CF. Reduction in motor vehicle collisions following treatment of sleep apnoea with nasal CPAP. Thorax 2001;56(7):508–12.
19. Arias MA, Garcia-Rio F, Alonso-Fernandez A, Martinez I, Villamor J. Pulmonary hypertension in obstructive sleep apnoea: effects of continuous positive airway pressure A randomized, controlled crossover study. Eur Heart J 2006;27(9):1106–13.
20. Dhillon S, Chung SA, Fargher T, et al. Sleep apnea, hypertension, and the effects of continuous positive airway pressure. Am J Hypertens 2005;18(5 Pt 1):594–600.
21. Logan AG, Tkacova R, Perlikowski SM, et al. Refractory hypertension and sleep apnoea: effect of CPAP on blood pressure and baroreflex. Eur Respir J 2003;21(2):241–47.
22. Haas DC, Foster GL, Nieto FJ, et al. Age-dependent associations between sleep-disordered breathing and hypertension: importance of discriminating between systolic/diastolic hypertension and isolated systolic hypertension in the Sleep Heart Health Study. Circulation 2005;111(5):614–21.
23. Poreba R, Derkacz A, Andrzejak R. Sleep apnea syndrome as a cause of secondary hypertension. A case report. Kardiol Pol 2005;63(5):549–51.
24. Hassaballa HA, Tulaimat A, Herdegen JJ, Mokhlesi B. The effect of continuous positive airway pressure on glucose control in diabetic patients with severe obstructive sleep apnea. Sleep Breath 2005;9(4):176–80.
25. Babu AR, Herdegen J, Fogelfeld L, Shott S, Mazzone T. Type 2 diabetes, glycemic control, and continuous positive airway pressure in obstructive sleep apnea. Arch Intern Med 2005;165(4):447–52.
26. Harsch IA, Schahin SP, Bruckner K, et al. The effect of continuous positive airway pressure treatment on insulin sensitivity in patients with obstructive sleep apnoea syndrome and type 2 diabetes. Respiration 2004;71(3):252–59.
27. Harsch IA, Schahin SP, Radespiel-Troger M, et al. Continuous positive airway pressure treatment rapidly improves insulin sensitivity in patients with obstructive sleep apnoea syndrome. Am J Respir Crit Care Med 2004;169(2):156–62.
28. Robinson GV, Pepperell JC, Segal HC, Davies RJ, Stradling JR. Circulating cardiovascular risk factors in obstructive sleep apnoea: data from randomised controlled trials. Thorax 2004;59(9):777–82.
29. Ip MS, Lam KS, Ho C, Tsang KW, Lam W. Serum leptin and vascular risk factors in obstructive sleep apnea. Chest 2000;118(3):580–86.
30. Nelesen RA, Yu H, Ziegler MG, Mills PJ, Clausen JL, Dimsdale JE. Continuous positive airway pressure normalizes cardiac autonomic and hemodynamic responses to a laboratory stressor in apneic patients. Chest 2001;119(4):1092–101.
31. Ryan CF, Lowe AA, Li D, Fleetham JA. Magnetic resonance imaging of the upper airway in obstructive sleep apnea before and after chronic nasal continuous positive airway pressure therapy. Am Rev Respir Dis 1991;144(4):939–44.
32. Kuzniar TJ, Gruber B, Mutlu GM. Cerebrospinal fluid leak and meningitis associated with nasal continuous positive airway pressure therapy. Chest 2005;128(3):1882–84.
33. Hess DR. Noninvasive positive-pressure ventilation and ventilator-associated pneumonia. Respir Care 2005;50(7):924–29. Discussion 929–31.
34. Chasens ER, Pack AI, Maislin G, Dinges DF, Weaver TE. Claustrophobia and adherence to CPAP treatment. West J Nurs Res 2005;27(3):307–21.
35. Nieto FJ, Young TB, Lind BK, et al. Association of sleep-disordered breathing, sleep apnea, and hypertension in a large community-based study. Sleep Heart Health Study. JAMA 2000;283(14):1829–36.
36. Peppard PE, Young T, Palta M, Skatrud J. Prospective study of the association between sleep-disordered breathing and hypertension. N Engl J Med 2000;342(19):1378–84.

37. Lavie P, Herer P, Hoffstein V. Obstructive sleep apnoea syndrome as a risk factor for hypertension: population study. BMJ 2000;320(7233):479–82.
38. Javaheri S, Parker TJ, Liming JD, et al. Sleep apnea in 81 ambulatory male patients with stable heart failure. Types and their prevalences, consequences, and presentations. Circulation 1998;97(21):2154–59.
39. Trupp RJ, Hardesty P, Osborne J, et al. Prevalence of sleep disordered breathing in a heart failure program. Congest Heart Fail 2004;10(5):217–20.
40. Sin DD, Fitzgerald F, Parker JD, Newton G, Floras JS, Bradley TD. Risk factors for central and obstructive sleep apnea in 450 men and women with congestive heart failure. Am J Respir Crit Care Med 1999;160(4):1101–6.
41. Laaban JP, Pascal-Sebaoun S, Bloch E, Orvoen-Frija E, Oppert JM, Huchon G. Left ventricular systolic dysfunction in patients with obstructive sleep apnea syndrome. Chest 2002;122(4):1133–38.
42. Hanly P, Sasson Z, Zuberi N, Lunn K. ST-segment depression during sleep in obstructive sleep apnea. Am J Cardiol 1993;71(15):1341–45.
43. Schafer H, Koehler U, Ploch T, Peter JH. Sleep-related myocardial ischemia and sleep structure in patients with obstructive sleep apnea and coronary heart disease. Chest 1997;111(2):387–93.
44. Mooe T, Franklin KA, Wiklund U, Rabben T, Holmstrom K. Sleep-disordered breathing and myocardial ischemia in patients with coronary artery disease. Chest 2000;117(6):1597–602.
45. Mooe T, Franklin KA, Holmstrom K, Rabben T, Wiklund U. Sleep-disordered breathing and coronary artery disease: long-term prognosis. Am J Respir Crit Care Med 2001;164(10 Pt 1):1910–13.
46. Peker Y, Hedner J, Kraiczi H, Loth S. Respiratory disturbance index: an independent predictor of mortality in coronary artery disease. Am J Respir Crit Care Med 2000;162(1):81–86.
47. Becker H, Brandenburg U, Peter JH, Von Wichert P. Reversal of sinus arrest and atrioventricular conduction block in patients with sleep apnea during nasal continuous positive airway pressure. Am J Respir Crit Care Med 1995;151(1):215–18.
48. Koehler U, Becker HF, Grimm W, Heitmann J, Peter JH, Schafer H. Relations among hypoxemia, sleep stage, and bradyarrhythmia during obstructive sleep apnea. Am Heart J 2000;139(1 Pt 1):142–48.
49. Gami AS, Pressman G, Caples SM, et al. Association of atrial fibrillation and obstructive sleep apnea. Circulation 2004;110(4):364–67.
50. Atwood CW Jr, McCrory D, Garcia JG, Abman SH, Ahearn GS. Pulmonary artery hypertension and sleep-disordered breathing: ACCP evidence-based clinical practice guidelines. Chest 2004;126(1 Suppl):72S–77S.
51. Dyken ME, Somers VK, Yamada T, Ren ZY, Zimmerman MB. Investigating the relationship between stroke and obstructive sleep apnea. Stroke 1996;27(3):401–7.
52. Good DC, Henkle JQ, Gelber D, Welsh J, Verhulst S. Sleep-disordered breathing and poor functional outcome after stroke. Stroke 1996;27(2):252–59.
53. Parra O, Arboix A, Bechich S, et al. Time course of sleep-related breathing disorders in first-ever stroke or transient ischemic attack. Am J Respir Crit Care Med 2000;161(2 Pt 1):375–80.
54. Alberti A, Mazzotta G, Gallinella E, Sarchielli P. Headache characteristics in obstructive sleep apnea syndrome and insomnia. Acta Neurol Scand 2005;111(5):309–16.
55. Goder R, Friege L, Fritzer G, Strenge H, Aldenhoff JB, Hinze-Selch D. Morning headaches in patients with sleep disorders: a systematic polysomnographic study. Sleep Med 2003;4(5):385–91.
56. Ip MS, Lam B, Ng MM, Lam WK, Tsang KW, Lam KS. Obstructive sleep apnea is independently associated with insulin resistance. Am J Respir Crit Care Med 2002;165(5):670–76.
57. Harsch IA, Schahin SP, Radespiel-Troger M, et al. Continuous positive airway pressure treatment rapidly improves insulin sensitivity in patients with obstructive sleep apnea syndrome. Am J Respir Crit Care Med 2004;169(2):156–62.
58. Punjabi NM, Shahar E, Redline S, Gottlieb DJ, Givelber R, Resnick HE. Sleep-disordered breathing, glucose intolerance, and insulin resistance: the Sleep Heart Health Study. Am J Epidemiol 2004;160(6):521–30.
59. Vgontzas AN, Bixler EO, Chrousos GP. Sleep apnea is a manifestation of the metabolic syndrome. Sleep Med Rev 2005;9(3):211–24.
60. Svatikova A, Wolk R, Gami AS, Pohanka M, Somers VK. Interactions between obstructive sleep apnea and the metabolic syndrome. Curr Diab Rep 2005;5(1):53–58.
61. Demeter P, Pap A. The relationship between gastroesophageal reflux disease and obstructive sleep apnea. J Gastroenterol 2004;39(9):815–20.
62. Green BT, Broughton WA, O'Connor JB. Marked improvement in nocturnal gastroesophageal reflux in a large cohort of patients with obstructive sleep apnea treated with continuous positive airway pressure. Arch Intern Med 2003;163(1):41–45.
63. Kerr P, Shoenut JP, Millar T, Buckle P, Kryger MH. Nasal CPAP reduces gastroesophageal reflux in obstructive sleep apnea syndrome. Chest 1992;101(6):1539–44.
64. Berg S, Hoffstein V, Gislason T. Acidification of distal esophagus and sleep-related breathing disturbances. Chest 2004;125(6):2101–6.
65. Margel D, Cohen M, Livne PM, Pillar G. Severe, but not mild, obstructive sleep apnea syndrome is associated with erectile dysfunction. Urology 2004;63(3):545–49.
66. Goncalves MA, Guilleminault C, Ramos E, Palha A, Paiva T. Erectile dysfunction, obstructive sleep apnea syndrome and nasal CPAP treatment. Sleep Med 2005;6(4):333–39.
67. Hajduk IA, Strollo PJ Jr, Jasani RR, Atwood CW Jr, Houck PR, Sanders MH. Prevalence and predictors of nocturia in obstructive sleep apnea–hypopnea syndrome – a retrospective study. Sleep 2003;26(1):61–64.
68. Umlauf MG, Chasens ER. Sleep disordered breathing and nocturnal polyuria: nocturia and enuresis. Sleep Med Rev 2003;7(5):403–11.

SECTION C   NON-SURGICAL TREATMENT OF OSA/HS

CHAPTER 10

# Analysis of NCPAP failures

*Wietske Richard, Jantine Venker, Cindy den Herder, Dennis Kox and Nico de Vries*

## 1 INTRODUCTION

Obstructive sleep apnea syndrome (OSAS) is characterized by intensive snoring and daytime sleepiness, due to repeated obstruction of the upper airway during sleep. OSAS is defined as periods of complete cessation of oronasal airflow for a minimum of 10 seconds (apnea) and periods of more than 30% reduction in oronasal airflow, accompanied by a decrease of more than 4% in ongoing $paO_2$ (hypopnea), with an Apnea/Hypopnea Index (AHI) of more than 5, accompanied by daytime symptoms.[1] The prevalence of obstructive sleep apnea in the middle-aged is 2% of women and 4% of men.[2] It has been estimated that at least 80% of all moderate and severe OSAS in the general population is likely being missed.[3]

OSAS has adverse effects on daytime quality of life such as daytime sleepiness and diminished intellectual performance. OSAS is of growing significance because of its increasingly recognized high incidence and association with neurocognitive symptoms and cardiovascular disease.[4,5] In severe OSAS there is an increased risk of being involved in traffic accidents.[6,7] Therefore OSAS is treated for its symptoms, in the attempt to reduce morbidity and mortality.

In 1981 nasal continuous positive airway pressure (NCPAP), which acts as a pneumatic splint, was introduced as treatment of OSAS and has been considered the gold standard for treatment of severe OSAS since (Fig. 10.1A & B).[8] It is a safe therapeutic option with few contraindications or serious side effects.[9] Unfortunately many patients experience NCPAP therapy as intrusive and the acceptance and (long-term) compliance of NCPAP are at best moderate. A vast body of literature was published in the last decade on the subject of (long-term) compliance of NCPAP, with rates ranging from 46% to 89%.[10–23] Improvements in NCPAP technology, in particular the introduction of automatic adjustments of the NCPAP pressure throughout the night (auto-CPAP), and attempts to enhance acceptance and compliance have been introduced.[24–32] We were interested to see if these actions have led to better acceptance and compliance as compared to earlier reported data.

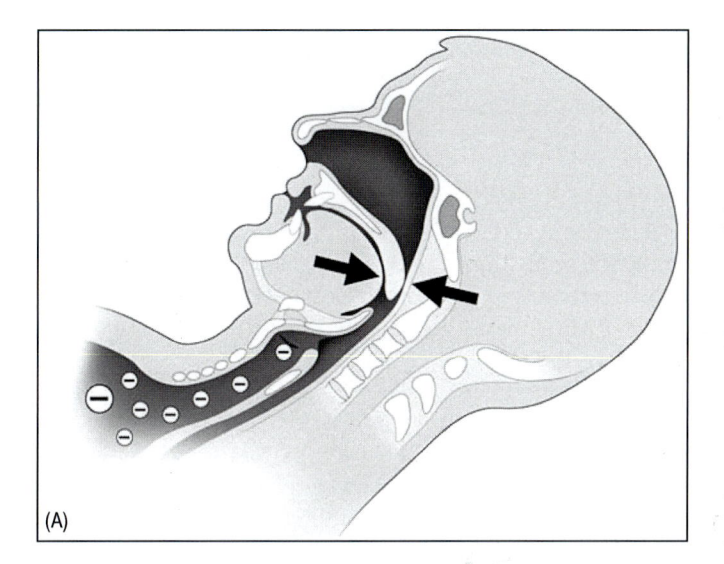

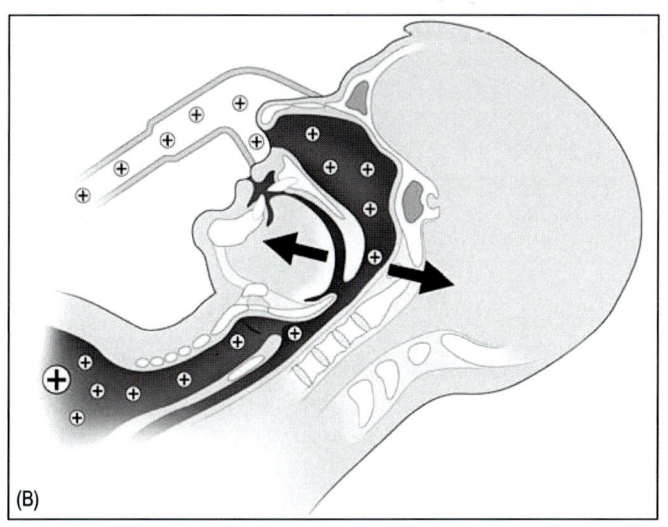

**Fig. 10.1** A, Without NCPAP. Obstruction of the upper airway during sleep, in this case at both retropalatal and retrolingual level. B, With NCPAP. The positive intraluminal pressure keeps the upper airway open.

# SECTION C: NON-SURGICAL TREATMENT OF OSA/HS

## 2 METHODS

We acquired data on (long-term) compliance and therapy failure by sending questionnaires to 256 patients who were offered NCPAP in the past.

### Compliance and failure

- *Compliance* is defined as minimally 4h during five nights per week of CPAP use.
- *Failure* is defined as refusal beforehand, withdrawal directly after use or failure to reduce the AHI.

## 3 RESULTS AND DISCUSSION

OSAS represents a relatively new disease entity, and is currently the most dynamic area in otolaryngology/head and neck surgery, with regard to both diagnostic work-up and therapy.

Treatment of OSAS consists of lifestyle changes (weight reduction, cessation of alcohol misuse, sleep hygiene), and can be subdivided into conservative treatment (oral device or NCPAP), surgery to (minimal invasive to invasive) and combined modalities.

NCPAP has come to be regarded as the gold standard treatment for OSAS in the last decade.[33] In the pioneering phase of management of OSAS this view was understandable as uvulopalatopharyngoplasty (UPPP) was the almost exclusively surgical alternative for OSAS treatment. Metaanalysis by Sher et al. in 1996 showed a success rate of UPPP (in unselected patients) of only 40%.[34]

NCPAP therapy in severe OSAS is successful if it is accepted by the patient. Unfortunately only a limited number of patients are compliant with NCPAP therapy. Many patients refuse its use upfront, or experience problems such as leakage, dry eyes, and blocked nasal passage. Many patients use NCPAP on only a few days per week, and/or only a limited number of hours per night. NCPAP is also troublesome for patients who travel often or sleep on camping grounds. The use of NCPAP therapy does not improve the anatomy of the upper airway, and patients remain dependent on its use lifelong.

Various studies have attempted to analyze compliance. The results vary and do not all apply the same criteria, especially regarding compliance and therapy failure. Furthermore there are no precise recommendations available concerning the necessary duration of daily and weekly use. Twenty-four patients were unavailable for follow-up. Of the remaining 232 patients, 58 (25%) were failures, while 75% were still using NCPAP after 2 months to 8 years of follow-up; 138 (79%) of these 174 patients were considered compliant, as defined above, as compared to 46–89% as reported in earlier series.[10–23] Including the 58 failures, only 59.5% of patients can be seen as compliant.

There were no statistical differences in compliance between the fixed pressure CPAP and auto-CPAP. Although it was to be expected that patients with a higher AHI and higher Epworth Sleepiness Scale (ESS) would be more compliant, we found no difference for AHI and ESS.

Actual use of NCPAP, as reported in the literature, ranged from 3.7 to 7.2h in the years 1992 to 2002.[11,13,14,16–18,20,22,25,26,33,35–42] These data were usually obtained from fixed NCPAP by time counter registration. The average of NCPAP, both fixed and auto-CPAP, in our series is slightly longer (6.4h) as compared to the mean of earlier studies (5.4h) on this subject. The number of hours per night of use in our series was, however, estimated by the patient, and therefore it may be that the actual use is lower.

In conclusion, the long-term compliance with NCPAP therapy has only slightly improved since the introduction of NCPAP 27 years ago, in spite of various efforts to improve it. It seems that a plateau has been reached and that it unrealistic to aim at a substantially higher compliance rate.

At the same time we are witnessing an increasing awareness in the ENT community that an exciting new era in OSAS treatment is dawning. In particular for young patients, the prospect of using NCPAP lifelong is unattractive and with increasing frequency patients ask if surgical alternatives with acceptable success rates are available.

Surgery will not become the first treatment of choice in all patients. However, success rates of UPPP in well-selected patients (obstruction at the retropalatal level only) reach 70–80%.[35,36] In patients with obstruction at the retrolingual level comparable success rates have been reported.[37] In the light of failure rates for NCPAP therapy it is hard to maintain that NCPAP should always be the treatment of first choice. Therefore, a gradual shift can be expected to take place to alternatives to NCPAP, being a combination of surgery,[38,39] and possible positional conditioning,[40,41] in well-selected, well-informed patients, while NCPAP therapy in those patients will still be in reserve in case of surgical failure.

## REFERENCES

1. The Report of an American Academy of Sleep Medicine Task Force. Sleep-related breathing disorders in adults: recommendations for syndrome definition and measurement techniques in clinical research. Sleep 1999;22:667–89.
2. Young T, Palta M, Dempsey J, et al. The occurrence of sleep disordered breathing among middle-aged adults. N Engl J Med 1993;328:1230–5.
3. Young T, Evans L, Finn L, Palta M. Estimation of the clinically diagnosed proportion of sleep apnea syndrome in middle-aged men and women. Sleep 1997;20:705–6.
4. Chesire K, Engleman H, Deary I, et al. Factors impairing daytime performance in patients with sleep apnea/hypopnea syndrome. Arch Intern Med 1992;152:538–41.
5. Shamsuzzaman AS, Gersh BJ, Somers VK. Obstructive sleep apnea, implications for cardiac and vascular disease. JAMA 2003;290:1906–14.

6. Teran-Santos J, Jimenez-Gomez A, Cordero-Guevara J. The association between sleep apnea and the risk of traffic accidents. N Engl J Med 1999;340:847–51.
7. George CF, Smiley A. Sleep apnea and automobile crashes. Sleep 1999;22:790–5.
8. Sullivan CE, Issa FG, Berthon-Jones M, Eves L. Reversal of obstructive sleep apnoea by continuous positive airway pressure applied through the nares. Lancet 1981;1:862–5.
9. Polo O, Berthon-Jones M, Douglas NJ, Sullivan CE. Management of obstructive sleep apnoea/hypopnoea syndrome. Lancet 1994;344:656–60.
10. Sanders MH, Gruendl CA, Rogers RM. Patient compliance with nasal CPAP therapy for sleep apnea. Chest 1986;90:330–3.
11. Rauscher H, Formanek D, Popp W, Zwick H. Self-reported vs measured compliance with nasal CPAP for obstructive sleep apnea. Chest 1993;103:1675–80.
12. Lojander J, Maasilta P, Partinen M, et al. Nasal-CPAP, surgery, and conservative management for treatment of obstructive sleep apnea syndrome. A randomized study. Chest 1996;110:114–9.
13. Hui DS, Choy DK, Li TS, et al. Determinants of continuous positive airway pressure compliance in a group of Chinese patients with obstructive sleep apnea. Chest 2001;120:170–6.
14. Sin DD, Mayers I, Man GC, Pawluk L. Long-term compliance rates to continuous positive airway pressure in obstructive sleep apnea: a population-based study. Chest 2002;121:430–5.
15. Hoffstein V, Viner S, Mateika S, Conway J. Treatment of obstructive sleep apnea with nasal continuous positive airway pressure. Patient compliance, perception of benefits, and side effects. Am Rev Respir Dis 1992;145:841–5.
16. Kribbs NB, Pack AI, Kline LR, et al. Objective measurement of patterns of nasal CPAP use by patients with obstructive sleep apnea. Am Rev Respir Dis 1993;147:887–95.
17. Krieger J. Long-term compliance with nasal continuous positive airway pressure (CPAP) in obstructive sleep apnea patients and nonapneic snorers. Sleep 1992;15:S42–6.
18. Meurice JC, Dore P, Paquereau J, et al. Predictive factors of long-term compliance with nasal continuous positive airway pressure treatment in sleep apnea syndrome. Chest 1994;105:429–33.
19. Nino-Murcia G, McCann CC, Bliwise DL, et al. Compliance and side effects in sleep apnea patients treated with nasal continuous positive airway pressure. West J Med 1989;150:165–9.
20. Pepin JL, Krieger J, Rodenstein D, et al. Effective compliance during the first 3 months of continuous positive airway pressure. A European prospective study of 121 patients. Am J Respir Crit Care Med 1999;160:1124–9.
21. Pieters T, Collard P, Aubert G, et al. Acceptance and long-term compliance with nCPAP in patients with obstructive sleep apnoea syndrome. Eur Respir J 1996;9:939–44.
22. Popescu G, Latham M, Allgar V, Elliott MW. Continuous positive airway pressure for sleep apnoea/hypopnoea syndrome: usefulness of a 2 week trial to identify factors associated with long term use. Thorax 2001;56:727–33.
23. Waldhorn RE, Herrick TW, Nguyen MC, et al. Long-term compliance with nasal continuous positive airway pressure therapy of obstructive sleep apnea. Chest 1990;97:33–8.
24. Fung C, Hudgel DW. A long-term randomized, cross-over comparison of auto-titrating and standard nasal continuous airway pressure. Sleep 2000;23:645–8.
25. Teschler H, Wessendorf TE, Farhat AA, et al. Two months auto-adjusting versus conventional nCPAP for obstructive sleep apnoea syndrome. Eur Resp J 2000;15:990–5.
26. d'Ortho MP, Grillier-Lanoir V, Levy P, et al. Constant vs. automatic continuous positive airway pressure therapy: home evaluation. Chest 2000;118:1010–7.
27. Randerath WJ, Schraeder O, Galetke W, et al. Autoadjusting CPAP therapy based on impedance efficacy, compliance and acceptantance. Am J Respir Crit Care Med 2001;163:652–7.
28. Hukins C. Comparative study of autotitrating and fixed-pressure CPAP in the home: a randomized, single-blind crossover trial. Sleep 2004;27:1512–7.
29. Massie CA, Hart RW, Peralez K, Richards GN. Effects of humidification on nasal symptoms and compliance in sleep apnea patients using positive airway pressure. Chest 1999;116:403–8.
30. Duong M, Jayaram L, Camfferman D, et al. Use of heated humidification during nasal CPAP titration in obstructive sleep apnoea syndrome. Eur Respir J 2005;26:679–85.
31. Mador MJ, Krauza M, Pervez A, et al. Effect of heated humidification on compliance and quality of life in patients with sleep apnea using nasal continuous positive airway pressure. Chest 2005;128:2151–8.
32. Hoy CJ, Vennelle M, Kingshott RN, et al. Can intensive support improve continuous positive airway pressure use in patients with sleep apnea/hypopnea syndrome? Am J Respir Crit Care Med 1999;159:1096–100.
33. Indications and standards for use of nasal continuous positive airway pressure (CAPA) in sleep apnea syndromes. American Thoracic Society. Official statement adopted March 194. Am J Respir Crit Care Med 1994;150:1738–5.
34. Sher AE, Schechtman KB, Piccirillo JF. The efficacy of surgical modifications of the upper airway in adults with obstructive sleep apnea syndrome. Sleep 1996;19:156–77.
35. Friedman M, Ibrahim H, Joseph NJ. Staging of obstructive sleep apnea/hypopnea syndrome: a guide to appropriate treatment. Laryngoscope 2004;114:454–9.
36. Hessel NS, de Vries N. Resutls of uvulopalatopharyngoplasty after diagnostic work-up with polysomnography and sleep endoscopy; a report of 136 snoring patients. Eur Arch Otorhinolaryngol 2003;260:19–25.
37. den Herder C, van Tinteren H, de Vries N. Hyoidthyroidpexia: a surgical treatment for sleep apnea syndrome. Laryngoscope 2005;115:740–5.
38. Verse T, Baisch A, Maurer JT, et al. Multilevel surgery for obstructive sleep apnea: Short-term results. Otolaryngol Head Neck Surg 2006;134:571–7.
39. Richard W, Kox D, den Herder C, et al. One stage multilevel surgery (uvulopalatopharyngoplasty, Hyoid Suspension, Radiofrequent Ablation of the Tongue Base with/without Genioglossus Advancement) in obstructive sleep apnea syndrome. Eur Arch Otorhinolaryngol 2007;264:439–44.
40. Oksenberg A, Silverberg DS, Arons E, Radwan H. Positional versus non-positional obstructive sleep apnea patients. Chest 1997;112:629–39.
41. Richard W, Kox D, den Herder C, et al. The role of sleep position in obstructive sleep apnea syndrome. Eur Arch Otorhinolaryngol 2006;263:946–50.

SECTION C    NON-SURGICAL TREATMENT OF OSA/HS

CHAPTER 11

# Oral appliance and craniofacial problems of obstructive sleep apnea syndrome

*Soichiro Miyazaki and Makoto Kikuchi*

## 1 INTRODUCTION

Pierre Robin (1934) used the monoblock mandible advancement appliance for the purpose of treating patients with obstructive sleep apnea for the first time.[1] Following this, Boraz treated pediatric OSA patients.[2] Cartwright and Samelson (1982)[3] reported the effectiveness of the tongue retaining device (TRD) which retains the tongue in the bulb of the device. Meier-Ewert (1984)[4] used Esmarch–Heiberg manipulation, which opens the airway of a general anesthetized patient, and developed the Esmarch appliance. The tongue retaining appliance represented by the TRD, and the mandible advancing type represented by the Esmarch, are the two main types of oral appliance. Thereafter, other oral appliances were developed such as the adjustable type, which can adjust the amount of mandible advancement. Currently, more than 55 oral appliances (OAs) are on the market.[5]

## 2 PATIENT SELECTION

In 2006, the Standards of Practice Committee of the American Academy of Sleep Medicine published the reports *Oral Appliance for Snoring and Obstructive Sleep Apnea: A Review*[6] and *Practice Parameters for the Treatment of Snoring and Obstructive Sleep Apnea with Oral Appliances: An Update for 2005*.[7] Oral appliances are indicated for use with patients with primary snoring and with mild to moderate OSA, who prefer them to continuous positive airway pressure (CPAP) therapy, or who do not respond to CPAP, are not appropriate candidates for CPAP, or who have failed treatment attempts with CPAP.

## 3 PROCEDURES FOR ORAL APPLIANCE THERAPY

The procedures for oral appliance therapy are as follows.

1. Written referral and diagnostic polysomnographic (PSG) report by the physician or sleep specialist sent to the dentist or dental specialist.
2. Oral examination:
   - number of teeth
   - periodontal evaluation (including dental x-ray and/or panorama x-ray)
   - temporomandibular joints evaluation
   - dental arch and curve of Spee evaluation.
3. Craniofacial skeletal diagnosis:
   - cephalometric radiograph
   - computed tomography
   - magnetic resonance imaging.
4. Taking the impression of both arches.
5. Titration of the mandible position:
   - *George gauge*: This was developed by Peter George of Hawaii to take the bite registration of the upper and lower incisors in the respective notches.[8]
   - *Snoring sound test*: Kazuhisa Esaki developed the snoring sound test to calculate the distance of mandibular advancement that works effectively for oral appliances for OSA. The patient should be placed in the supine position, and while snoring the mandible is gradually moved anteriorly; the site at which the sound of snoring diminishes is then used as the mandible position for the oral appliance.[9]
   - *Initial bite registrations*: These are taken at 70% of maximum protrusion.[10]
6. Appliance determination. This is influenced by the characteristics of the patient, such as number of teeth,

periodontal factors, dental arch, curve of Spee evaluations and craniofacial skeletal diagnosis.
7. Setting the oral appliance for treatment: there should be no pain and a comfortable feeling.
8. Home monitoring to check if the appliance works well.
9. Refer patient back to the physician or sleep specialist for assessment by PSG.

## 4 ORAL APPLIANCE VARIATIONS

With so many different oral appliances available, selection of a specific appliance may appear somewhat difficult, but they are designed around a few major themes. Oral appliances can be classified by mode of action or design variation. Nearly all appliances fall into one of two categories: the tongue retaining type and the mandibular advancing type.

### 4.1 TONGUE RETAINING DEVICE (TRD)

(See Fig. 11.1A&B.)

The TRD functions by holding the tongue in a forward position by means of a suction bulb. When the tongue is in this position, the device keeps the tongue from collapsing during sleep and obstructing the airway in the throat.

### 4.2 MANDIBULAR ADVANCING TYPE

The mandibular advancing type functions by repositioning and maintaining the mandible in a protruded position during sleep. This serves to open the airway by indirectly pulling the tongue forward, keeping the soft palate attached to the tongue (oral seal) by the negative pressure occurring in the mouth and making it more rigid. It also holds the lower jaw and other structures in a stable position to prevent opening of the mouth.

#### 4.2.1 NON-TITRATABLE TYPE

The mandibular advancing and non-titratable type of oral appliance is a custom-made monoblock device connected by two separate arches (maxillary and mandibular) without an advancing mechanism. Several versions are listed below.

1. **Esmarch appliance** (Fig. 11.2A&B). Meier-Ewert developed this mandibular advancing and non-titratable type of oral appliance, using the Esmarch–Heiberg manipulation method, which opens the airway of the general anesthetized patient.
2. **Nocturnal airway patency appliance (NAPA)** (Fig. 11.3A &B). With this appliance, the mandible is in a protruded position during sleep. This serves to open the airway by indirectly pulling the tongue forward and keeping the soft palate attached to the tongue. This device has a hole in the front extended portion, to enable inhaling from the mouth.

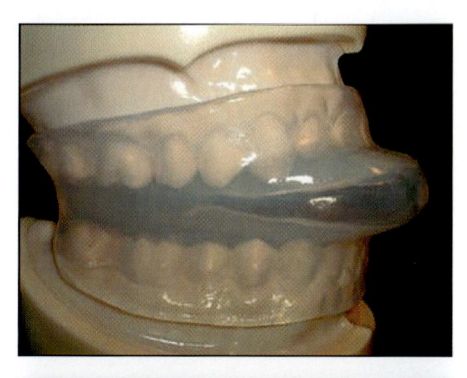

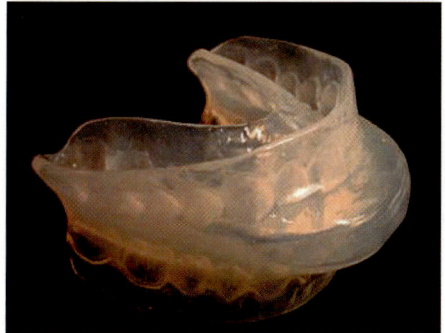

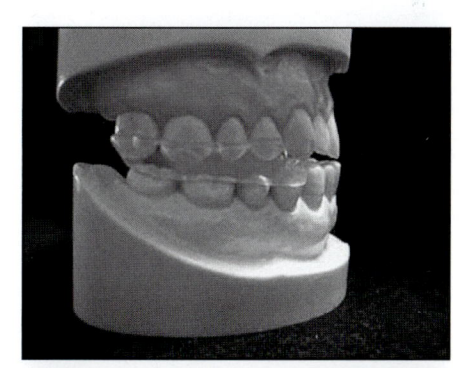

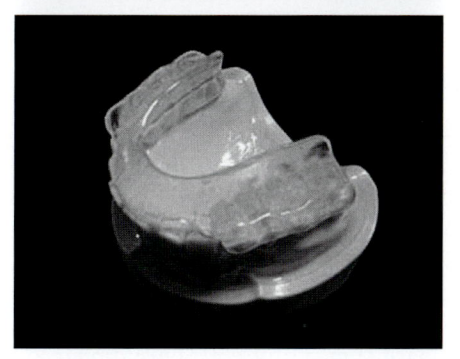

Fig. 11.1

Fig. 11.2

SECTION C — NON-SURGICAL TREATMENT OF OSA/HS

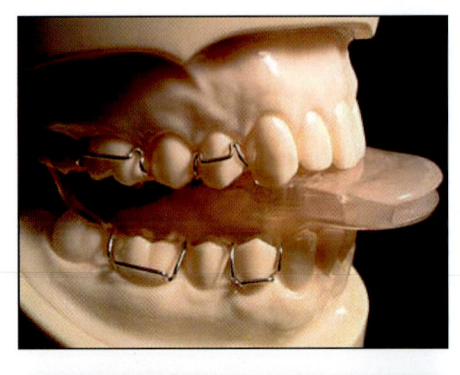

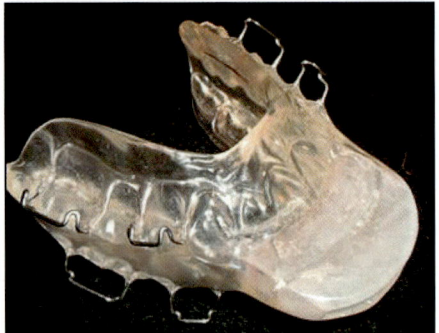

Fig. 11.3

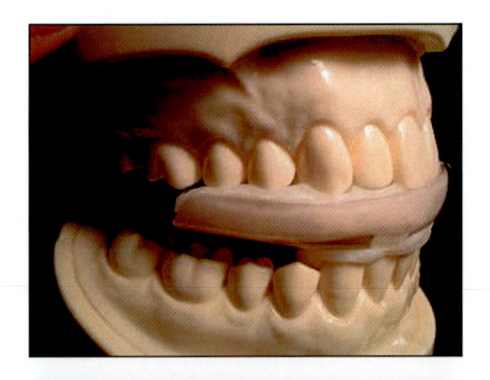

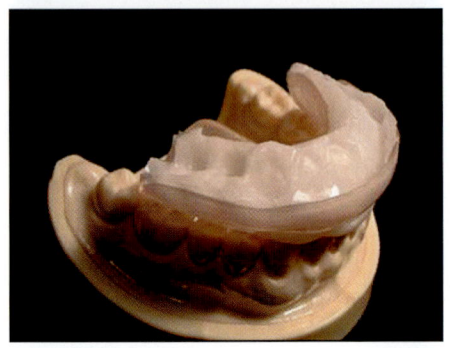

Fig. 11.5

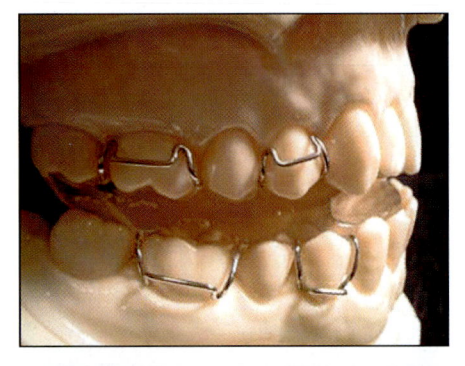

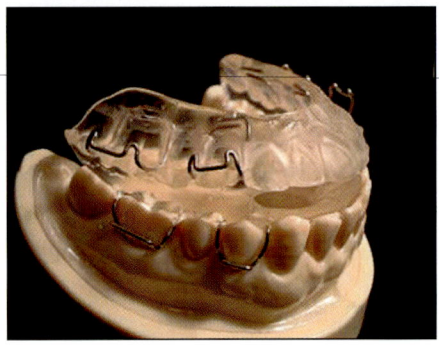

Fig. 11.4

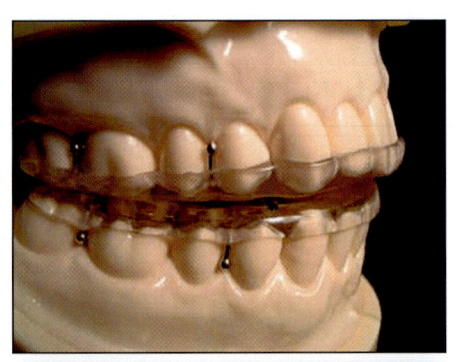

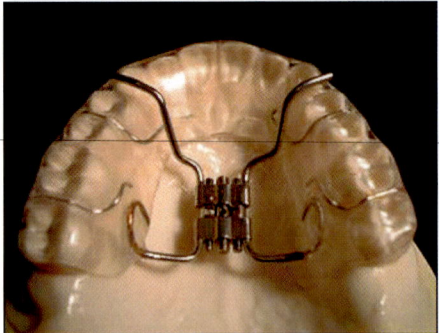

Fig. 11.6

3. **Mandibular repositioner** (Fig. 11.4A&B). This appliance also has a hole in the front to enable inhaling from the mouth.
4. **Snore guard** (Fig. 11.5A&B). This appliance is made of heat-activated resin.

## 4.2.2 TITRATABLE TYPE

The mandibular advancing and titratable type of oral appliance is a custom-made two-piece appliance composed of two separate arches (maxillary and mandibular) containing an advancing mechanism. Examples are listed below.

1. **Klearway** (Fig. 11.6A&B). This custom-made two-piece appliance is composed of two separate arches (maxillary and mandibular) to advance the mandible with a screw (0.25 mm/1 turn) to determine the ideal forward position of the mandible required to adequately open the airway. A total of 44 forward positions are available in increments of 0.25 mm, which covers a full 11.0 mm range of anterior–posterior movement.
2. **Thornton adjustable positioner (TAP)** (Fig. 11.7A&B). This appliance is composed of two separate arches (maxillary and mandibular) containing an advancing mechanism and a base and hook assembly with an internal adjustment mechanism.
3. **Herbst** (Fig. 11.8A&B). This device contains an advancing mechanism which has two sets of pistons and tubes to keep the mandible in the forward position required to adequately open the airway.

Oral appliances may be used alone or in combination with other means of treating OSA, including weight control, surgery, or CPAP.

Recently, oral appliance therapy was performed along with CPAP therapy to reduce the pressure flow of the CPAP machine; however, there will be a growing number of combination treatments developed in the near future. We currently have no data available concerning the percentage of patients treated with both the oral appliance and CPAP therapy. However, we have a number of patients using the CPAP on a daily basis who prefer to use an oral appliance for traveling, even though the CPAP machines are getting smaller.

## 5 POSTOPERATIVE MANAGEMENT AND SIDE EFFECTS OF ORAL APPLIANCE

Follow-up dental appointments at least every 6 months to monitor subjective effectiveness, comfort, and temporomandibular joint and dental status are needed.

### 5.1 CHANGING THE OCCLUSION

Patients have to use oral appliances for long periods of time to maintain the airway patency every night. Consequently, the vigorous force applied to the teeth changes the occlusion. The occlusal change of the patient during oral appliance therapy conducted for 12 years can be seen in Figures 11.9 and 11.10. Sometimes teeth and/or prosthetic crowns can be broken by this force (Fig. 11.11). We should not only take care of the teeth, but also the occlusion and temporomandibular joint.

### 5.2 EFFICACY OF ORAL APPLIANCES

The Standards of Practice Committee of the American Academy of Sleep Medicine reported that the efficacy of OAs was established for controlling OSA in some but not all patients with success (defined as no more than 10 apneas or hypopneas per hour of sleep) achieved in an average of 52% of treated patients.[6]

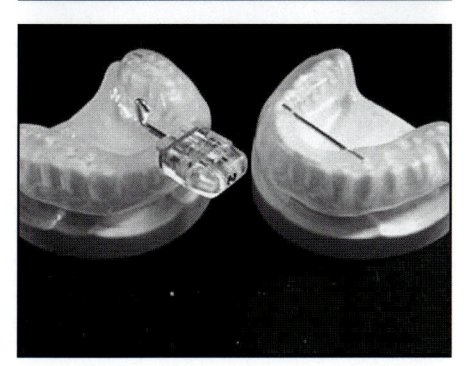

Fig. 11.7

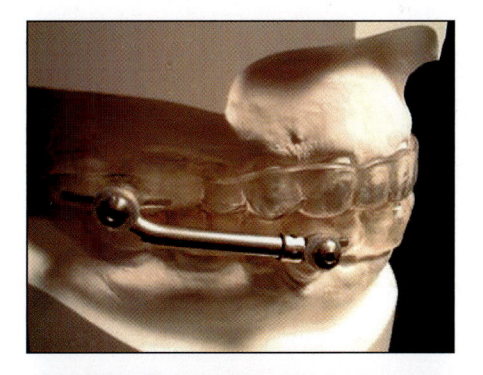

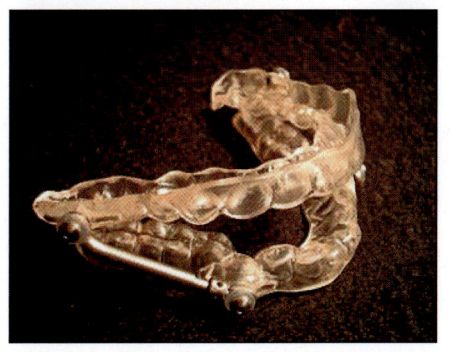

Fig. 11.8

SECTION C  NON-SURGICAL TREATMENT OF OSA/HS

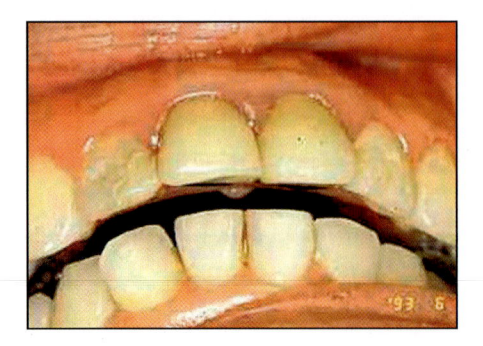

Fig. 11.9

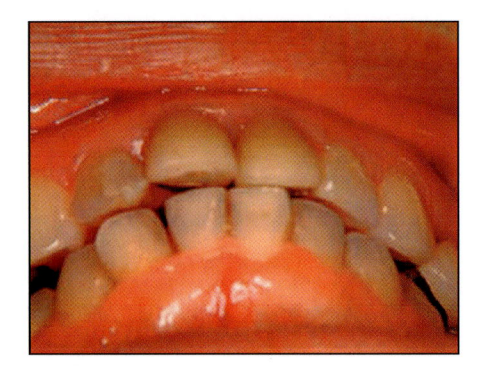

Fig. 11.10

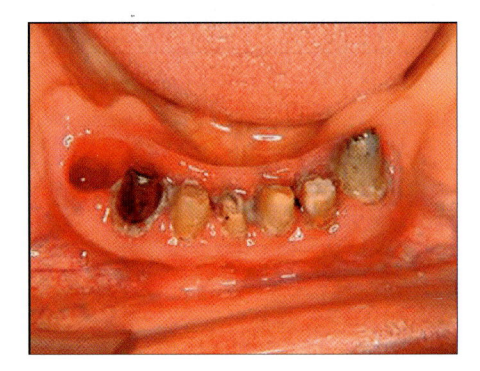

Fig. 11.11

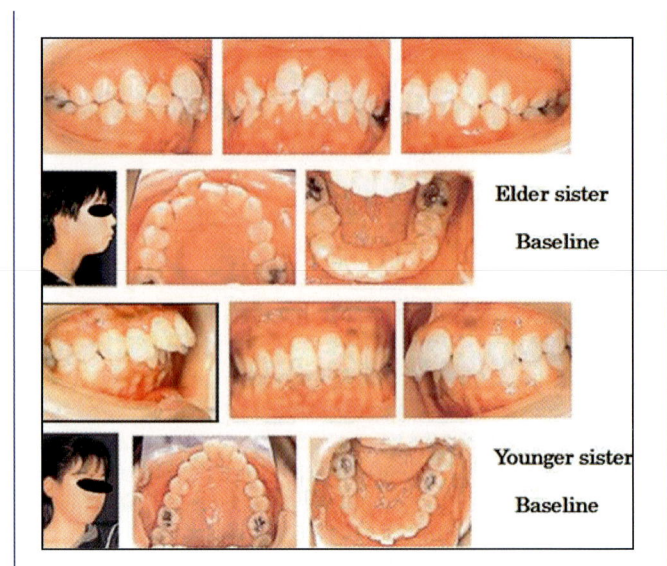

Fig. 11.12

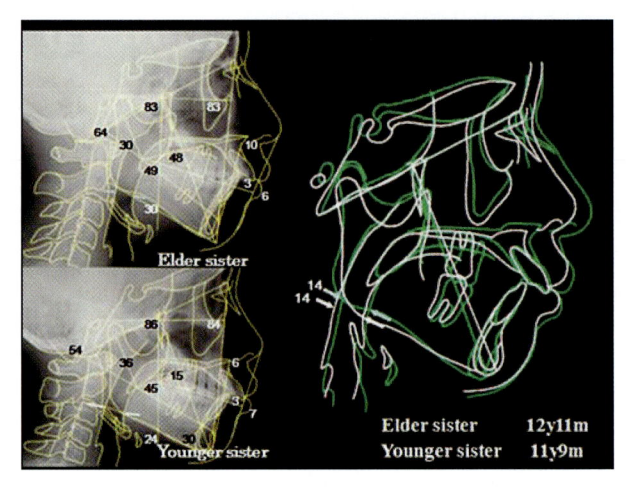

Fig. 11.13

## 5.3 ORTHODONTIC TREATMENT AND AIRWAY

Orthodontic treatment can influence the size and the function of the airway.

### Cases 1 & 2

These patients were sisters aged 12 years 11 months and 11 years 9 months, so they were still growing. They complained about their maxillary protrusion. The elder sister was treated by the extraction of five teeth because she had one congenitally missing tooth and one root resorbed tooth. The younger sister, however, was treated by non-extraction with the Herbst appliance. The treatment term was 3 years 11 months for the elder sister and 3 years 2 months for the younger sister. Both sisters had a typical muscle strain on the chin when they closed the lips together (Fig. 11.12).

When we superimposed the cephalograms at the baseline of these sisters, there were a few differences between the sisters before treatment; for instance, the nose of the elder sister was bigger than that of the younger sister. However, the superimposition of the cephalograms of both cases revealed these sisters were almost identical. Their lower pharynx was the same width at the baseline (Fig. 11.13).

In both cases, the muscle strain on the chin disappeared after orthodontic treatment. Both sisters recovered with better facial appearance, and had a satisfactory result. There was little difference between the appearance of the sisters (Fig. 11.14).

When we superimposed the cephalograms of the baseline and the result of the elder sister, only her nose grew; the other part did not grow at all and the width of the lower pharynx was reduced from 12 mm to 10 mm. Conversely, the mandible of the younger sister grew a lot. As a consequence, the width of the lower pharynx was increased from 12 mm to 17 mm. The lower pharynxes of the sisters were the same, 12 mm before the treatment; however, the lower pharynx of elder sister reduced to 10 mm and that of younger sister increased to 17 mm. Thus, there was a total difference of 7 mm after the treatment (Fig. 11.15).

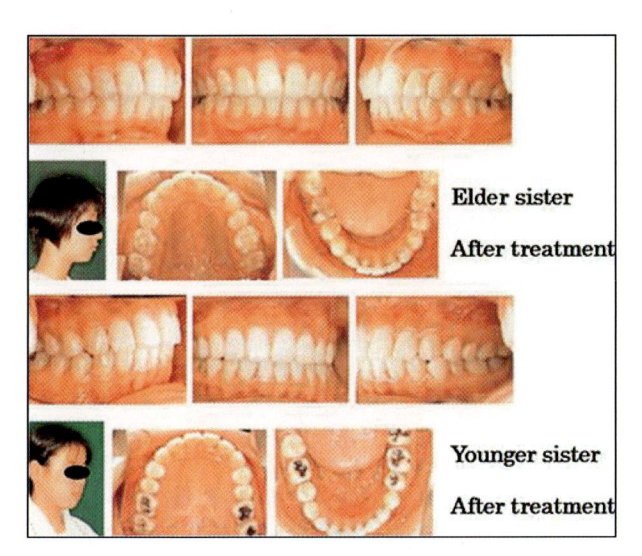

**Fig. 11.14**

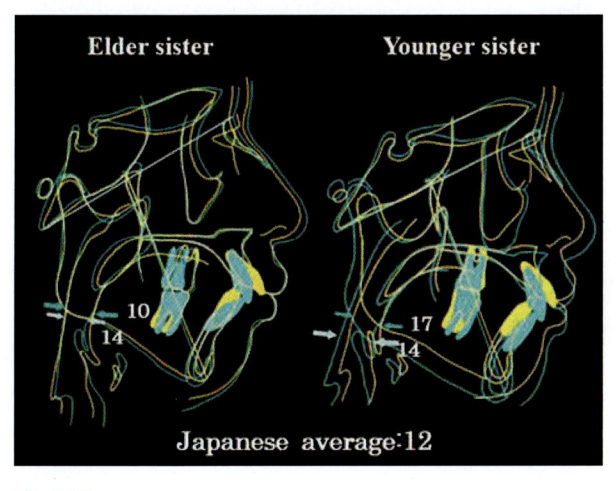

**Fig. 11.15**

The result of the treatment looks almost the same from the outward appearance; there were, however, significant differences between the sisters inside the face involving the size of the airway. It may be that orthodontic treatment influences the size of the airway; evidence for this is still being investigated.

## 6 CRANIOFACIAL PATTERN OF OSA

The craniofacial characteristics of obstructive sleep apnea patients have been reported as follows.

1. Short anterior cranial base.[11,12]
2. Less obtuse cranial base flexure angle.[13]

| Table 11.1 | Cephalometric variables | | |
|---|---|---|---|
| | Control (adult) (n = 26) | Patient (child) (n = 29) | OSAS (adult) (n = 31) |
| FX (°) | 84.3 ± 4.8 | 81.8 ± 3.1 | 79.8 ± 4.7 |
| FD (°) | 87.3 ± 3.4 | 84.8 ± 3.2 | 86.4 ± 4.3 |
| MP (°) | 27.6 ± 5.7 | 31.9 ± 5.6 | 29.4 ± 7.0 |
| LFH (°) | 50.8 ± 4.7 | 54.6 ± 5.3 | 55.7 ± 5.4 |
| MA (°) | 27.7 ± 5.1 | 21.2 ± 4.8 | 24.3 ± 5.8 |
| TFH (°) | 64.8 ± 5.2 | 68.4 ± 4.5 | 69.8 ± 6.3 |

The cephalometric measurements were (i) facial axis angle (FX): BA-CC-GN; (ii) facial depth angle (FD): crossing of facial plane to FH; (iii) mandibular plane angle (MP): crossing of mandibular plane to FH; (iv) lower facial height angle (LFH): ANS-XI-PM; (v) mandibular arc angle (MA): crossing of condylar axis to corpus axis; (vi) total facial height angle (TFH): crossing of corpus axis to cranial base plane.
Adapted from Kikuchi M.[15,18]

3. Retroposition of the mandible.[11,14]
4. Small mandible.[12]
5. Small maxilla.[12,16]
6. Steep mandibular plane.[14]
7. Long soft palate.[11,13,15]
8. Decreased airway space.[11,13–15]
9. Lowered position of hyoid bone.[13,15–17]
10. Increased anterior facial height.[11,14–17]

We reported that craniofacial patterns of OSA patients were: the dolichofacial pattern (increased anterior facial height) by cephalometric analysis of Ricketts' and OSA patients having their mandible retropositioned; a long soft palate; decreased airway space; and a lowered position of the hyoid bone.[15]

### 6.1 CRANIOFACIAL PATTERN OF CHILD OSA

We also reported that the craniofacial pattern of child OSA was intermediate between adult OSA and adult control (Table 11.1).[15,18] All the data showed intermediate values from the adult control to adult OSA. This may mean that the continuation of OSA makes the craniofacial pattern worsen year by year.

## 7 IMPORTANCE OF THE ORAL SEAL TO BREATHING

Frankel[19] noted that the impact of the 'space problem' in the physiology of the orofacial complex has been emphasized by Moss.[20–22] He maintains that the proper functioning of the digestive and respiratory systems depends on a functionally adequate patency of the oral and the

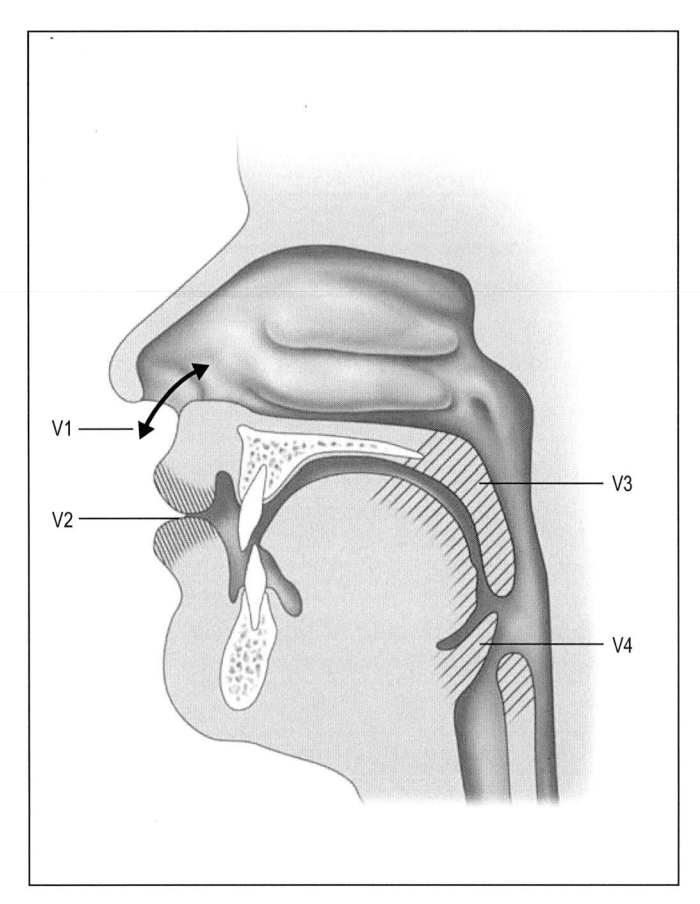

**Fig. 11.16**

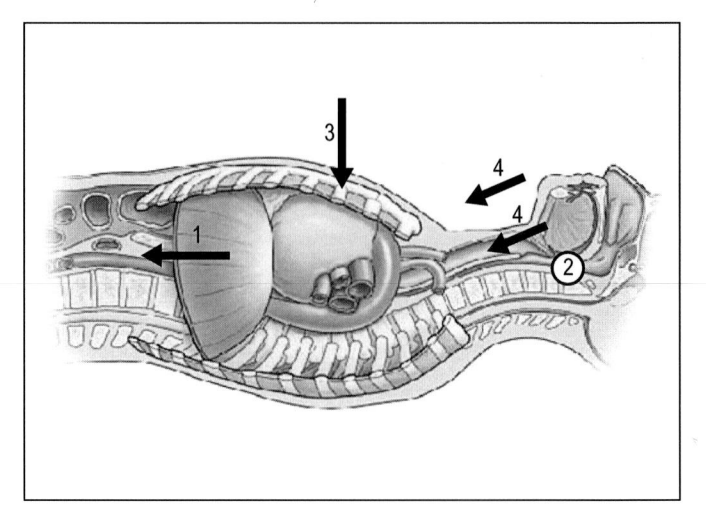

**Fig. 11.17**

nasopharyngeal passageways. This assumption receives significant support from the work of Bosma[23] who emphasized the impact of adequate space conditions in the physiology of the orofacial complex, with particular emphasis on airway maintenance. The life-sustaining functions of breathing as well as intake and transport of food are dependent on the adequate patency of these spaces and the proper functioning of the various valves as seen in Figure 11.16.

Frankel emphasized that there are four valves in the dentofacial skeleton: the V1 nasal valve, the V2 lip valve (the so-called lip seal), the V3 tongue and soft palate valve (the so-called oral seal) and the V4 epiglottis valve, and that we could maintain physiological atmospheric pressure in the oral and nasopharyngeal spaces in the presence of a competent oral seal.

Bosma[23] emphasized that the posterior soft tissue barrier formed by the soft palate and the tongue is an important factor for airway maintenance. The positional stabilization of the pharyngeal airway is the initial manifestation of the distinctive coordination of posture. The physiological relevance of the infantile performance of the stabilization of the airway is identified by its impairment in Pierre Robin syndrome. When these afflicted children are lying on their backs, the apposition of the tongue to the palate cannot take place because of the hypoplasia of the dorsal portion of the palate mostly associated with the cleft. The infantile mechanism of pharyngeal airway maintenance fails to operate, and the tongue falls downward and backward, occluding the pharynx. In a prone position, the tongue approximates the palate by the force of gravity, permitting nasal portal respiration. Bosma[23] noted that mandibular retrusion in Pierre Robin syndrome may be interpreted as an appropriate component of a regional failure of a positional function which emphasizes the physiological relevance of the muscular barrier separating the oral cavity from the pharyngeal space.

*Hypothesis: Negative pressure produced in the chest inhibits growth of the mandible.*[24]

We propose the hypothesis that the mechanism of thoracic negative pressure inhibits the backward and downward growth of the mandible. When the obstruction occurs in the pharyngeal area, the patient wants to move down the diaphragm to take in air; accordingly, pressure is produced in the chest. The negative pressure produced in the chest (of the obstructive sleep apnea patient) is detected by intraesophageal pressure monitoring. The deformity of the chest appears when the patient inhales, which is the opposite of that which occurs in breathing. The mechanism of negative pressure inhibits the growth of the mandible as follows (Fig. 11.17).

1. Diaphragm moves downward to inhale.
2. Obstruction at the pharyngeal region.
3. Negative pressure produced in the chest (esophagus).
4. This negative pressure pulls the tongue and mandible downward and backward.

If we stand by this hypothesis and the functional matrix hypothesis, it is easier to interpret why OSA patients tend to have the dolichofacial pattern (long face) and lower positioned hyoid bone, longer soft palate and narrow airway. These may be the result of negative pressure in the

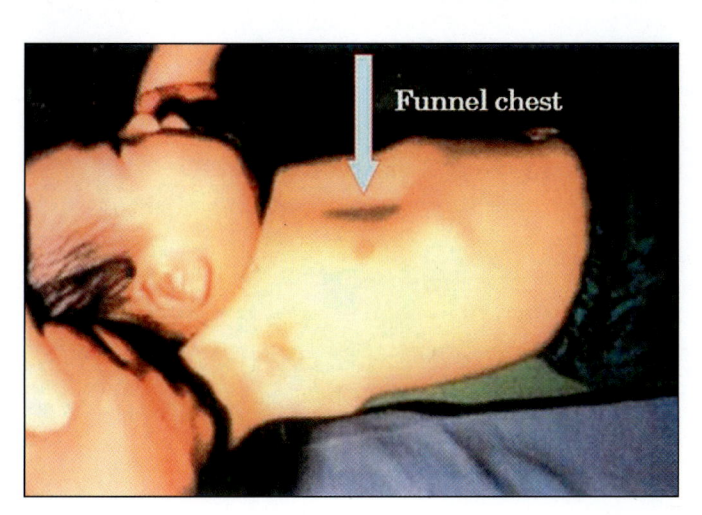

**Fig. 11.18**

chest. This negative pressure may cause funnel chest (Fig. 11.18). Castiglione[25] reported that 82% of 23 children affected by chronic upper airway obstruction showed pectus excavatum and 82% showed enlarged tonsils and adenoids. If this negative pressure disappears as a result of the removal of the tonsils or adenoids, or by orthodontic treatment to improve patency of the airway, the mandible may grow normally, and we could prevent or reduce sleep apnea in the future.

## REFERENCES

1. Robin P. Glossoptsis due to atresia and hypotrophy of the mandible. Am J Dis Child 1934;48:541–47.
2. Boraz R, Martin H, Michel J. Sleep apnea syndrome: report of case. J Dent Child 1979;46:50–52.
3. Cartwright R, Samelson C. The effects of a nonsurgical treatment for obstructive sleep apnea – the tongue retaining device. JAMA 1982;248:705–9.
4. Meir-Ewert K, Schafer H, Kloe W. Treatment of sleep apnea by a mandibular protracting device. Berichtsband 7th European Congress on Sleep Research. Munich, Germany: 1984;217.
5. Lowe A. Oral appliance for sleep breathing disorders. In: Principles and Practice of Sleep Medicine, 3rd edn. Kryger M, Roth T, Dement W, eds. Philadelphia: WB Saunders; 2000, pp. 929–39.
6. Kushida C, Morgenthaler T, Littner M. Oral appliance for snoring and obstructive sleep apnea: a review. Sleep 2006;29(2):244–62.
7. Kushida C, Morgenthaler T, Littner M. Practice parameters for the treatment of snoring and obstructive sleep apnea with oral appliances: an update for 2005. Sleep 2006;29(2):240–43.
8. George PT. A new instrument for functional appliance bite registration. J Clin Orthodont 1992;26:721–3.
9. Esaki K, Kanegae H, Uchida T, et al. Treatment of sleep apnea with a new separated type of dental appliance (mandibular advancing positioner). Kurume Med J 1997;44:315–19.
10. Tsuiki S, Hiyama S, Ono T, et al. Effects of a titratable oral appliance on supine airway size in awake non-apneic individuals. Sleep 2001;24(5):554–60.
11. Bacon WH, Turlot JC, Krieger J, et al. Cephalometric evaluation of pharyngeal obstructive factors in patients with sleep apneas syndrome. Angle Orthod 1990;60(2):115–22.
12. Andersson L, Brattstrom V. Cephalometric analysis of permanently snoring patients with and without obstructive sleep apnea syndrome. Int J Oral Maxillofac Surg 1991;20(3):159–62.
13. Jamieson A, Guilleminault C, Partinen M, et al. Obstructive sleep apneic patients have craniomandibular abnormalities. Sleep 1986;9(4):469–77.
14. Lowe AA, Santamaria JD, Fleetham JA, et al. Facial morphology and obstructive sleep apnea. Am J Orthod Dentofacial Orthop 1986;90(6):484–91.
15. Kikuchi M, Higurashi N, Miyazaki S, et al. Facial patterns of obstructive sleep apnea patients using Ricketts' method. Psychiatr Clin Neurosci 2000;54(3):336–7.
16. Tangugsorn V, Skatvedt O, Krogstad O, et al. Obstructive sleep apnoea: a cephalometric study. Part I. Cervico-craniofacial skeletal morphology. Eur J Orthod 1995;17(1):45–56.
17. Lyberg T, Krogstad O, Djupesland G. Cephalometric analysis in patients with obstructive sleep apnoea syndrome. I. Skeletal morphology. J Laryngol Otol 1989;103(3):287–92.
18. Kikuchi M, Higurashi N, Miyazaki S, et al. Facial pattern categories of sleep breathing disordered children using Ricketts analysis. Psychiatr Clin Neurosci 2002;56(3):329–30.
19. Frankel R, Frankel C. Orofacial Orthopedics with the Function Regulator. Basel: Karger; 1989. pp. 19–21
20. Moss ML. Differential roles of the periosteal and capsular matrices in orofacial growth. Trans Eur Orthod Soc 1969;45:193–206.
21. Moss ML, Rankow R. The role of the functional matrix in mandibular growth. Angle Orthod 1968;38:95–103.
22. Moss ML, Salentijn L. The capsular matrix. Am J Orthod 1969;55:566–77.
23. Bosma JF. Form and function in the mouth and pharynx of the human infant. In: Control Mechanism in Craniofacial Growth. Monograph 3: Craniofacial Growth Series, Center for Human Growth and Development. McNamara JA Jr., ed. Ann Arbor, MI: University of Michigan; 1975.
24. Kikuchi M. Orthodontic treatment in children to prevent sleep-disordered breathing in adulthood. Sleep Breath 2005;9:146–58.
25. Castiglione N, Eterno C, Sciuto C, et al. The diagnostic approach to and clinical study of 23 children with an obstructive sleep apnea syndrome. Pediatr Med Chir 1992;14(5):501–6.

# SECTION D — SURGICAL TREATMENT OF OSA/HS

## CHAPTER 12

# Rationale and indications for surgical treatment

*Donald M. Sesso, Robert W. Riley and Nelson B. Powell*

## 1 INTRODUCTION

Obstructive sleep apnea syndrome (OSAS), upper airway resistance syndrome (UARS) and snoring are collectively referred to as sleep-related breathing disorders (SRBD). Although the specific etiology is unknown, SRBD involves repeated partial or complete obstructions of the upper airway during sleep. The obstructions can be due to anatomical or central neural abnormalities. Loss of airway patency may cause sleep fragmentation and subsequent neurocognitive derangements, such as excessive daytime sleepiness.[1] The objective of surgical treatment is to alleviate this obstruction and the associated cardiovascular and neurobehavioral sequelae by increasing airway patency.

Tracheotomy was the first therapeutic modality employed to treat OSAS. Although effective, tracheotomy is not readily accepted by most patients due to its morbidity. Sullivan et al. reported the application of nasal continuous positive airway pressure (CPAP) to maintain upper airway patency as an alternative to tracheotomy.[2] Because of its efficacy, CPAP is usually the first-line treatment for OSAS.[3] Yet, a subset of patients struggle to accept or comply with CPAP therapy.[4] Thus, those patients who cannot tolerate medical therapy may be candidates for surgery.

Recognizing that multiple levels of airway obstruction exist in OSAS is essential to achieve a cure. Consequently, the surgical armamentarium has evolved to create techniques which address the specific anatomical sites of obstruction. The surgeon must be willing to treat all levels of obstruction in an organized and safe manner. Therefore, we developed a two-phase surgical protocol (Powell–Riley protocol) to target the specific anatomical sites of obstruction (nasal cavity/nasopharynx, oropharynx and hypopharynx). This protocol was created to minimize surgical interventions and avoid unnecessary surgery, while alleviating SRBD.[5,6]

Prior to any intervention, the surgeon must be familiar with the rationale and indications for each surgery. A systematic review of the patient will aid in identification of regions of obstruction and minimize risk and potential complications. Hence, this chapter will summarize our approach to the surgical treatment of OSAS.

## 2 RATIONALE FOR SURGICAL TREATMENT

The rationale for surgical treatment of the upper airway is to eliminate or minimize the neurocognitive and pathophysiologic derangements associated with OSAS. These neurocognitive derangements are the result of sleep fragmentation and hypoxemia. Patients with excessive daytime sleepiness (EDS) may experience emotional, social and economic problems.[7] Furthermore, uncontrollable fatigue may predispose a patient to automobile or occupational accidents.[8] Morbidity is seen from the associated sequelae of these pathophysiologic derangements such as hypertension, congestive heart failure, myocardial infarction, cardiac arrhythmias and cerebrovascular disease.[9,10] Thus, reducing the Apnea/Hypopnea Index (AHI) by 50% is no longer deemed acceptable. Rather, the goal is to treat to cure (elimination of hypoxemia and normalization of respiratory events). Ultimately, the surgeon's objective is to achieve outcomes that are equivalent to those of CPAP management. Ideally, surgical intervention seeks to improve the quality of life, enhance longevity and reduce the risk of medical morbidity.

## 3 SURGICAL INDICATIONS

The indications for surgery are listed in Table 12.1. For patients whose AHI is less than 20, surgical treatments may still be an option. Surgery is considered appropriate if these patients have associated EDS which results in impaired cognition or comorbidities as recognized by the Center for Medicare and Medicaid Services (including hypertension, stroke and ischemic heart disease). Consideration may be given to obtaining a multiple sleep latency test (MSLT) or the maintenance of wakefulness test (MWT) to determine

| Table 12.1 Surgical indications |
|---|
| • Apnea/Hypopnea Index (AHI) ⩾ 20* events/per hour of sleep<br>• Oxygen desaturation nadir < 90%<br>• Esophageal pressure (PES) more negative than −10 cm H$_2$O<br>• Cardiovascular derangements (arrhythmia, hypertension)<br>• Neurobehavioral symptoms (excessive daytime sleepiness [EDS])<br>• Failure of medical management<br>• Anatomical sites of obstruction (nose, palate, tongue base) |
| *Surgery may be indicated with an AHI < 20 if accompanied by excessive daytime fatigue.<br>From Powell NB, Riley RW, Guilleminault C. Surgical management of sleep-disordered breathing. In: Kryger MH, Roth T, Dement WC, eds. Principles and Practices of Sleep Medicine, 4th edn. Philadelphia: Elsevier Saunders; 2005, pp. 1081–97. |

| Table 12.2 Contraindications for surgery |
|---|
| • Severe pulmonary disease<br>• Unstable cardiovascular disease<br>• Morbid obesity<br>• Alcohol or drug abuse<br>• Psychiatric instability<br>• Unrealistic expectations |
| From Powell NB, Riley RW, Guilleminault C. Surgical management of sleep-disordered breathing. In: Kryger MH, Roth T, Dement WC, eds. Principles and Practices of Sleep Medicine, 4th edn. Philadelphia: Elsevier Saunders; 2005, pp. 1081–97. |

other etiologies of EDS for those patients whose symptoms are not obviated with CPAP therapy or for those whose symptoms of fatigue seem out of proportion to the severity of their apnea. In this subgroup of patients, surgery is unlikely to be beneficial. Other factors exist which could predict poor surgical outcomes and consequently render a patient to be an unsuitable candidate for surgery.[11] These factors are detailed in Table 12.2.

## 4 PATIENT SELECTION

Proper screening and selection of patients for surgery is vital to achieve successful outcomes and to minimize postoperative complications. Because daytime fatigue has numerous etiologies, such as periodic limb movement disorder and narcolepsy, a complete sleep history must be obtained. Furthermore, the preoperative evaluation requires a comprehensive medical history, head and neck examination, polysomnography (PSG), fiberoptic nasopharyngolaryngoscopy and lateral cephalometric analysis. A thorough review of these data will identify probable sites of obstruction and direct a safe, organized surgical protocol.[11]

A complete physical exam with vital signs, weight and neck circumference should be performed on every patient.

Specific attention is focused in the regions of the head and neck that have been well described as potential sites of upper airway obstruction, such as the nose, palate and base of tongue. Nasal obstruction, which can occur as a result of septal deviation, turbinate hypertrophy, alar collapse or sinonasal masses, can be identified on anterior rhinoscopy. The oral cavity should be examined for periodontal disease and dental occlusion. Examination of the oropharyngeal and hypopharyngeal regions includes a description of the palate, lateral pharyngeal walls, tonsils and tongue base. Mallampati and Friedman have proposed standardized grading systems to describe the degree of obstruction caused by these structures.[12,13]

Fiberoptic examination is used to identify obstruction of the nasopharynx, oropharynx and hypopharynx, as well as any laryngeal abnormalities. The airway is examined at rest and during provocative maneuvers. One such technique, Mueller's maneuver, exposes the upper airway to negative intraluminal pressure in an attempt to identify anatomical regions of obstruction. Fiberoptic examination is not only important to evaluate the upper airway for obstruction, but aids in determining ease of intubation. Furthermore, photodocumentation of the airway findings may be a useful tool in patient education.

The lateral cephalogram allows measurement of the length of the soft palate, posterior airway space, hyoid position and skeletal proportions. It is the most cost-effective radiographic study of the bony facial skeleton and soft tissues of the upper airway. Studies have shown the cephalogram to be valid in assessing obstruction, and in fact, it compares favorably to three-dimensional volumetric computed tomographic scans of the upper airway.[14] Since the cephalogram is not performed while the patient is sleeping, the degree of obstruction may be underestimated. Therefore, the results of this imaging test should be correlated with the fiberoptic examination.

The polysomnogram (PSG) is critical in the evaluation of a patient with OSAS. No patient should undergo airway surgery without this study. An attended, full-night PSG is considered the gold standard. Surgeons should pay particular attention to the AHI and the oxygen desaturation nadir. These data will guide appropriate surgical treatment, as well as preoperative and postoperative management. Patients must be counseled about the need for a postoperative PSG to assess their response to surgery. A patient may be inadequately treated if this study in not obtained.

Proper patient selection requires the surgeon to determine if a patient is medically stable for surgery. We recommend obtaining a comprehensive metabolic panel, complete blood count, thyroid stimulating hormone, electrocardiogram and chest x-ray on all patients. Additional testing or consultation with the appropriate medical specialist should be sought in patients with comorbid medical conditions.

Preoperative CPAP can alleviate the issues associated with sleep deprivation and may reduce the risk of postobstructive pulmonary edema. Consequently, all patients who

# SECTION D: SURGICAL TREATMENT OF OSA/HS

### Table 12.3 Powell–Riley protocol surgical procedures

*Phase I*

Nasal surgery (septoplasty, turbinate reduction, nasal valve grafting)
Tonsillectomy
Uvulopalatopharyngoplasty (UPPP) or uvulopalatal flap (UPF)
Mandibular osteotomy with genioglossus advancement
Hyoid myotomy and suspension
Temperature-controlled radiofrequency (TCRF)*-turbinates, palate, tongue base

*Phase II*

Maxillomandibular advancement osteotomy (MMO)
Temperature-controlled radiofrequency (TCRF)*-tongue base

*TCRF is typically used as an adjunctive treatment. Select patients may choose TCRF as primary treatment. From Powell NB, Riley RW, Guilleminault C. Surgical management of sleep-disordered breathing. In: Kryger MH, Roth T, Dement WC, eds. Principles and Practices of Sleep Medicine, 4th edn. Philadelphia: Elsevier Saunders; 2005, pp. 1081–97.

### Table 12.4 Rationales for Powell–Riley surgical protocol

- Provides a systematic and thorough evaluation of each patient
- Surgery is directed to the specific sites of anatomical obstruction
- Reduces risk of over-operating
- Limits pain and recovery time
- Better accepted by most patients
- Improves cure rates of phase II surgery

From Powell NB, Riley RW, Guilleminault C. Surgical management of sleep-disordered breathing. In: Kryger MH, Roth T, Dement WC, eds. Principles and Practices of Sleep Medicine, 4th edn. Philadelphia: Elsevier Saunders; 2005, pp. 1081–97.

### Table 12.5 Definition of surgical responders

- Apnea/Hypopnea Index (AHI) <20 events/per hour of sleep*
- Oxygen desaturation nadir ≥90%
- Excessive daytime fatigue (EDS) alleviated
- Normalization of sleep architecture
- Response equivalent to CPAP on full-night titration

*A reduction of the AHI by 50% or more is considered a cure if the preoperative AHI is less than 20.
From Powell NB, Riley RW, Guilleminault C. Surgical management of sleep-disordered breathing. In: Kryger MH, Roth T, Dement WC, eds. Principles and Practices of Sleep Medicine, 4th edn. Philadelphia: Elsevier Saunders; 2005, pp. 1081–97.

are tolerant of CPAP are encouraged to use this modality for at least 2 weeks prior to surgery. In 1988, Powell et al. recommended the use of preoperative CPAP for all patients who have a Respiratory Disturbance Index (RDI) greater than 40 and an oxygen desaturation of 80% or less. According to this protocol, the surgeon must consider insertion of a temporary tracheotomy for those patients with a RDI greater than 60 and/or a $SaO_2$ less than 70% who are intolerant of CPAP therapy.[15]

Prior to surgical intervention, all medical and surgical options should be reviewed with the patient. A discussion regarding the potential risks, benefits and likelihood of success should occur. Only after the patient fully comprehends the process and has consented to surgery can the treatment plan proceed.

## 5 POWELL–RILEY TWO-PHASE SURGICAL PROTOCOL

This protocol has two distinct phases which direct treatment towards the specific sites of obstruction during sleep. The procedures included in each phase are listed in Table 12.3. The rationale for the protocol is to limit unnecessary surgery (Table 12.4). This approach limits postoperative complications, pain and hospital stay. Furthermore, the surgeon's main objective is to treat to cure. Since it is difficult to predict outcomes, all patients are counseled on the possibility of needing both phases of surgery in order to achieve a cure (Table 12.5). Conservative surgery (phase I) is recommended initially with the plan to re-evaluate the patient with a postoperative PSG in three to four months. Patients have a reasonable expectation to be cured by phase I surgery alone. If incompletely treated, those patients are prepared for phase II surgery. However, there are instances when phase II surgery may be the appropriate initial procedure. A non-obese patient with marked mandibular deficiency and a normal palate may be most appropriately treated with phase II surgery.[6]

Essentially, phase I surgery is directed towards the soft tissues of the upper airway. The nose, palate and tongue base can be simultaneously treated. Neither dental occlusion nor the facial skeleton is altered.

Phase II surgery or maxillomandibular advancement osteotomy (MMO) enlarges the hypopharyngeal and pharyngeal airway by expanding the skeletal framework. MMO is the only surgery which creates more space for the tongue to be advanced anteriorly.

## 6 RATIONALE FOR SURGICAL PROCEDURES

### 6.1 NASAL RECONSTRUCTION

Nasal obstruction is often encountered in the form of septal deviation, turbinate hypertrophy or nasal valve incompetence. The rationale of surgery is to maintain nasal airway patency and minimize mouth breathing. Mouth opening causes a posterior displacement of the tongue into the hypopharyngeal airway with narrowing of the airway. Surgery may consist of septoplasty, turbinate reduction or alar grafting. While nasal reconstruction is unlikely to cure OSAS, it can improve quality of life and potentially reduce the severity of this syndrome. Furthermore, treating the nasal airway may improve a patient's tolerance of nasal CPAP.

## 6.2 UVULOPALATOPHARYNGOPLASTY (UPPP)/ UVULOPALATAL FLAP (UPF)

The rationale of UPPP is to reposition the redundant soft tissues of the palate and lateral pharyngeal walls. Collapse of the oropharyngeal airway is well documented in patients with SRBD. UPPP is an excellent technique to treat isolated retropalatal obstruction. However, there is often a stigma associated with this procedure due to its intense postoperative pain and variable success rates. Sher et al. documented that UPPP had a cure rate of 39%.[16] Unrecognized hypopharyngeal obstruction is thought to be the primary reason for such a high failure rate. If UPPP is performed on patients with obstruction localized to the palate or combined with procedures directed towards other sites of obstruction, the results can be much more gratifying.

The indications and rationale for the UPF are the same as UPPP. The technique was developed to reduce the risk of velopharyngeal insufficiency by using a potentially reversible flap that could be 'taken down' if complications arose. Additionally, the UPF is associated with less postoperative pain, as compared to UPPP. The UPF is contraindicated in patients with long and thick palates. In these patients, the flap will be too bulky and could result in a negative outcome.[17]

## 6.3 MANDIBULAR OSTEOTOMY WITH GENIOGLOSSUS ADVANCEMENT

The rationale of genioglossus advancement (GA) is to limit the posterior displacement of the tongue into the hypopharyngeal airway during sleep. The genial tubercle, genioglossus muscle and tongue base are advanced anteriorly by creating a rectangular osteotomy in the mandible as described by Riley et al.[18] GA is a conservative technique that does not change dental occlusion or jaw position. However, a limitation of this surgery is that no additional room is created for the tongue, in contrast to maxillomandibular advancement.

## 6.4 HYOID MYOTOMY WITH SUSPENSION

The genioglossus, geniohyoid and middle pharyngeal constrictor muscles insert on the hyoid bone. These muscles are vital to maintain the integrity of the hypopharyngeal airway. Thus, the rationale of hyoid suspension is to alleviate hypopharyngeal obstruction by advancing the hyoid complex in an anterior direction. Hyoid suspension may be performed as an isolated procedure or in combination with GA to treat tongue base obstruction.[19]

## 6.5 MAXILLOMANDIBULAR ADVANCEMENT OSTEOTOMY (MMO)

MMO is considered phase II treatment and is the only surgery which creates more space for the tongue in the oral cavity. The rationale for MMO is to ameliorate refractory hypopharyngeal obstruction by expanding the skeletal facial framework of the maxilla and mandible. This surgical technique combines a Le Fort I osteotomy and a mandibular sagittal split osteotomy. While the efficacy of MMO has been clearly demonstrated, we typically reserve this surgery for patients who are incompletely treated with phase I surgery to prevent unnecessary procedures. Furthermore, the success rate of MMO appears to increase when phase I procedures are included in the treatment plan.[20,21]

## 7 POSTOPERATIVE MANAGEMENT AND COMPLICATIONS

The postoperative management of OSA patients can be challenging. Proper planning and foresight can reduce the incidence of complications. Our two-phase protocol includes a risk management strategy to ensure patient safety.[22] Maintaining the integrity of the airway remains the overriding principle of this protocol.

ICU admission is recommended for patients with comorbid medical conditions, moderate to severe OSA, multi-level surgery or MMO for the first day. Intravenous analgesics and antihypertensives can be safely administered in this setting. Continuous pulse oximetry and hemodynamic monitoring is required. Morphine sulfate 1 to 5 milligrams is administered every 3 hours. The staff must be educated to avoid over-sedation. Patient-controlled analgesia (PCA) is contraindicated. Medications which have the potential to depress respiration or cause sedation should be avoided. An emergent airway kit should be readily available at the bedside.

Although airway edema is expected in the postoperative period, every effort must be made to limit swelling. This can be achieved intraoperatively by judicious fluid replacement and meticulous hemostasis. Antihypertensives are administered to maintain a mean arterial pressure (MAP) between 80 and 100 mm Hg. All patients receive 24 hours of intravenous corticosteroid treatment unless medically contraindicated. Furthermore, we strongly encourage patients to use their CPAP immediately after surgery to reduce airway edema.[15] When stable, the patients are transferred to the ward.

Antibiotics are administered for 7 days. Fiberoptic evaluation is performed on all patients prior to discharge to ensure a patent airway. Pain is managed at home with hydrocodone and acetaminophen elixir. Requirements for discharge include reasonable pain control, adequate oral intake and a patent airway.[22]

# 8 SUCCESS RATE

Clinical response to phase I surgery ranges from 42% to 75%.[20,23,24] Our data demonstrate that approximately 60% of all patients are cured with phase I surgery.[20] Factors that predict a less successful outcome include a mean RDI greater than 60, oxygen desaturation below 70%, mandibular deficiency (sella nasion point B <75°) and morbid obesity (body mass index [BMI] >33 kg/m$^2$).

However, it is imprudent to forego phase I surgery in these patients, since a reasonable percentage may not need more aggressive surgery.[20]

Patients who are incompletely treated by phase I surgery have persistent hypopharyngeal obstruction. Phase II surgery (MMO) would then be offered to those patients. Maxillomandibular advancement osteotomy has documented success rates >90%.[20]

## REFERENCES

1. Schwab RJ, Kuna ST, Remmers JE. Anatomy and physiology of upper airway obstruction. In: Principles and Practices of Sleep Medicine, 4th edn. Kryger MH, Roth T, Dement WC, eds. Philadelphia: Elsevier Saunders; 2005, pp. 983–1000.
2. Sullivan CE, Issa FG, Berthon-Jones M, et al. Reversal of obstructive sleep apnoea by continuous positive airway pressure applied through the nares. Lancet 1981;1:862–65.
3. Ballestar E, Badia JR, Hernandez L, et al. Evidence of the effectiveness of CPAP in the treatment of sleep apnea/hypopnea syndrome. Am J Respir Crit Care Med 1999;159(5 Pt 1):495–501.
4. Sin DD, Mayers I, Man GC, et al. Long-term compliance rates of CPAP in obstructive sleep apnea: a population-based study. Chest 2002;121:430–35.
5. Riley R, Powell N, Guilleminault C, et al. Obstructive sleep apnea syndrome: a surgical protocol for dynamic upper airway reconstruction. J Oral Maxillofac Surg 1993;51:742–47.
6. Powell NB, Riley RW. A surgical protocol for sleep disordered breathing. Oral Maxillofac Surg Clin North Ann 1995;7:345–56.
7. Bonnet MH. The effect of sleep disruption on performance, sleep and mood. Sleep 1985;8:11–19.
8. Powell NB, Schechtman KB, Riley RW, et al. Sleepy driving: accidents and injury. Otolaryngol Head Neck Surg 2002;126:217–27.
9. Shahar E, Whitney CW, Redline S, et al. SDB and cardiovascular disease: cross-sectional results of the sleep heart health study. Am J Respir Crit Care Med 2001;163:19–25.
10. Yaggi HK, Concato J, Kernan WN, et al. Obstructive sleep apnea as a risk factor for stroke and death. N Engl J Med 2005;353:2034–41.
11. Powell NB, Riley RW, Guilleminault C. Surgical management of sleep-disordered breathing. In: Principles and Practices of Sleep Medicine, 4th edn. Kryger MH, Roth T, Dement WC, eds. Philadelphia: Elsevier Saunders; 2005, pp. 1081–97.
12. Mallampati SR, Gatt SP, Gugino LD, et al. A clinical sign to predict difficult tracheal intubation: a prospective study. Can Anaesth Soc J 1985;32:429–34.
13. Friedman M, Ibrahim H, Joseph NJ. Staging of obstructive sleep apnea/hypopnea syndrome: a guide to appropriate treatment. Laryngoscope 2004;114:454–59.
14. Riley R, Powell N, Guilleminault C. Cephalometric roentgenograms and computerized tomographic scans in obstructive sleep apnea. Sleep 1986;9:514–15.
15. Powell N, Riley R, Guilleminault C, et al. Obstructive sleep apnea, continuous positive airway pressure, and surgery. Otolaryngol Head Neck Surg 1988;99:362–69.
16. Sher AE, Schechtman KB, Piccirillo JF. The efficacy of surgical modifications of the upper airway in adults with obstructive sleep apnea syndrome. Sleep 1996;19:156–77.
17. Powell NB, Riley RW, Guilleminault C, et al. A reversible uvulopalatal flap for snoring and obstructive sleep. Sleep 1996;19:593–99.
18. Riley R, Powell N, Guilleminault C. Inferior sagittal osteotomy of the mandible with hyoid myotomy-suspension: a new procedure for obstructive sleep apnea. Otolaryngol Head Neck Surg 1986;94:589–93.
19. Riley R, Powell N, Guilleminault C. Obstructive sleep apnea and the hyoid: a revised surgical procedure. Otolaryngol Head Neck Surg 1994;111:717–21.
20. Riley R, Powell N, Guilleminault C. Obstructive sleep apnea syndrome: a review of 306 consecutively treated surgical patients. Otolaryngol Head Neck Surg 1993;108:117–25.
21. Hochban W, Brandenburg U, Hermann PJ. Surgical treatment of obstructive sleep apnea by maxillomandibular advancement. Sleep 1994;17:624–29.
22. Riley RW, Powell NB, Guilleminault C, et al. Obstructive sleep apnea surgery: risk management and complications. Otolaryngol Head Neck Surg 1997;117:648–52.
23. Johnson NT, Chinn J. Uvulopalatopharyngoplasty and inferior sagittal mandibular osteotomy with genioglossus advancement for treatment of obstructive sleep apnea. Chest 1994;105:278–83.
24. Lee N, Givens C, Wilson J, et al. Staged surgical treatment of obstructive sleep apnea syndrome: a review of 35 patients. J Oral Maxillofac Surg 1999;57:382–85.

# SECTION D  SURGICAL TREATMENT OF OSA/HS

## CHAPTER 13

# The impact of surgical treatment of OSA on cardiac risk factors

*Darius Bliznikas and Ho-Sheng Lin*

Evidence supporting the association between OSA and cardiovascular diseases is compelling. In a retrospective analysis of 182 men without history of cardiovascular disease at baseline, Peker et al. found that incompletely treated OSA was an independent predictor for cardiovascular disease in this group of patients at 7 years of follow-up.[1] Several case–control studies in patients with myocardial infarction also support an increased risk of cardiovascular morbidity in patients with OSA, with odds ratios in the range of 4.1 to 4.5 over control population.[2] Partinen et al. followed 198 patients with OSA for 5 to 7 years and showed that patients who were treated conservatively had more than twice the risk of developing new cardiovascular disease and nearly five times the risk of cardiovascular or stroke-related death when compared to those patients treated by tracheotomy.[3]

A number of possible mechanisms by which OSA might affect cardiovascular function have been hypothesized. Repetitive hypoxemia and hypercapnia throughout the night may be responsible for vascular injury and acceleration of atherosclerosis,[4] chronic sympathetic hyperactivity,[5] elevation of fibrinogen,[6] pulmonary hypertension, right heart hypertrophy[7] and failure,[8] and increased risk of plaque ruptures and subsequent cardiovascular event.[9]

In recent years, several serum markers have been investigated as potential surrogate biomarkers for monitoring and predicting cardiovascular events. These serum biomarkers include leptin, matrix metalloperoxidase, proteins involved in the angiotensin–aldosterone axis, nitric oxide, plasma cytokines, tumor necrotizing factor a (TNF-a), interleukin-1 (IL-1), IL-6, IL-8, IL-10, IL-18, and inflammation markers such as fibrinogen, high-sensitivity C-reactive protein (hs-CRP), and serum amyloid A (SAA). The important role that inflammation played in the process of atherosclerosis has become well established over the past decade.[10] Inflammatory cells and cytokines are involved in virtually every step in atherogenesis.[11]

The inflammatory cascade can be activated by noxious stimuli such as the repetitive hypoxemia associated with untreated or poorly treated OSA. Activation of the inflammatory cascade leads to secretion of proinflammatory cytokines, such as TNF-a and IL-1. IL-1 then activates IL-6 which upregulates the production of CRP in the liver. CRP is a pro-oxidant that induces expression of adhesion molecules, such as ICAM-1 and VCAM-1, and production of monocyte chemoattractant protein-1[12] (Fig. 13.1). These factors facilitate the attachment and migration of monocytes into the subintimal spaces of the blood vessels. The monocytes are then transformed into macrophages and take up cholesterol lipoproteins which lead to fatty deposits in the subintimal space. Further injurious stimuli propagate the attraction and accumulation of macrophages, mass cells, and activated T cells, with resultant formation and growth of atherosclerotic plaque. Secretions of

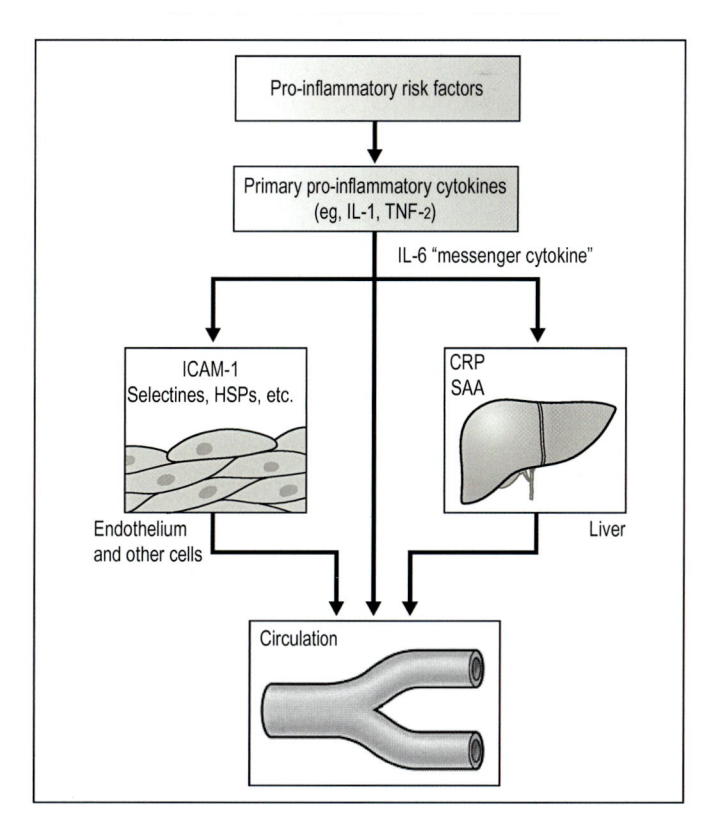

**Fig. 13.1** The inflammatory cascades.

metalloproteinases and other connective tissue enzymes by activated macrophages may cause breakdown of collagen and make these plaques more prone to rupture. Disruption of the atherosclerotic plaque exposes the atheronecrotic core to arterial blood and leads to thrombosis.[13]

Evidence suggesting an association between OSA and inflammatory factors includes the findings of increased plasma IL-6, CRP, and fibrinogen in patients under hypoxic conditions at high altitude,[14] as well as increased daytime plasma levels of IL-6 in patients after sleep deprivation and patients with excessive daytime sleepiness.[15] A study by Shamsuzzaman et al. indicated a strong association of OSA and elevated CRP levels.[16] In their study, 22 patients with newly diagnosed OSA showed significantly higher CRP levels compared to the control group (0.81 ± 0.15 mg/dl vs. 0.28 ± 0.12 mg/dl). Minoguchi et al. measured carotid intima-media thickness (IMT) and serum CRP, IL-6, and IL-18 levels in patients with OSA ($n = 36$) and compared these measurements to an obese control group ($n = 16$). They found that carotid IMT and serum levels of CRP, IL-6 and IL-18 were significantly higher in patients with OSA than in the obese control group. In addition, carotid IMT was significantly correlated with levels of CRP, IL-6, and IL-18, duration of OSA-related hypoxia and severity of OSA. Moreover, the duration of hypoxia during total sleep time was the strongest independent predictor of carotid IMT in patients with OSA and obese control subjects.[17]

Although there are numerous commercial kits available for assessment of cardiovascular risk, the majority of these tests suffer from lack of standardization, consistency, and rigorous scientific evidence to support their use. At a recent workshop on inflammatory markers and cardiovascular disease sponsored by CDC and AHA in Atlanta, it was concluded that the current use of assays for assessment of cardiovascular risk should be limited to measurement of hs-CRP.[18] The hs-CRP should be measured twice, either fasting or non-fasting, with the average expressed in mg/l, in metabolically stable patients. Relative risk categories of low, average and high correspond to hs-CRP values of less than 1, between 1 to 3, and greater than 3 mg/l, respectively.

Interventions targeted to correct sleep disordered breathing should result in improvement in sleep architecture, sleep quality and nocturnal oxygenation. This in turn should lead to reduction in the level of bioactive proteins in the serum and thus reduction of cardiovascular risk in patients with OSA. Yokoe et al. reported significant decrease in levels of CRP after 1 month of CPAP treatment in patients with moderate to severe OSA.[19] Similarly, Minoguchi et al. found that treatment with CPAP significantly improved sleep quality and decreased serum levels of TNF-a. On multiple regression analysis, the strongest predictor of spontaneous production of TNF-a by monocytes was the percentage of time with $SaO_2$ <90%.[20]

Although CPAP devices are highly successful, their use is limited by poor patient compliance. Patients often turn to surgical treatment when non-surgical treatment fails. Although the treatment of OSA using CPAP is different from surgical treatment (overcoming upper airway obstruction via positive pressure versus removal of the obstruction site), both treatment modalities are focused on reduction of apnea events, reduction in sleep fragmentation, increase in total sleep time, and reduction of nocturnal hypoxia. Thus, surgical treatment may be as successful as CPAP in reduction of cardiovascular risks. A study presented by Friedman et al.[21] showed statistically significant mean CRP level reduction from 0.33 mg/dl preoperatively to 0.16 mg/dl postoperatively (Fig. 13.2). This study involved 23 patients with moderate-to-severe OSA who underwent a variety of procedures including uvulopalatopharyngoplasty ($n = 15$), palatal stiffening procedure with pillar implants ($n = 8$), and thyrohoid suspension procedure ($n = 1$). Interestingly, they found that there is a statistically significant reduction in CRP levels in patients who were surgical responders based on polysomnogram (PSG) criteria as well as patients who were surgical failures. The CRP levels dropped from 0.33 to 0.17 in patients who were surgical responders and from 0.32 to 0.16 in patients who were non-responders (Figs 13.3 and 13.4). Sleep parameters such as Apnea Index (AI), Apnea/Hypopnea Index (AHI) and lowest oxygen saturation (LSAT) may impact synthesis of CRP. (Classically, surgical 'success' is arbitrarily defined as a 50% reduction in preoperational AHI with a posttreatment AHI of <20.)

Statistically significant difference of preoperative and postoperative PSG results was found in both surgical responders and non-responders. Even though some patients do not achieve 'success' in surgical treatment, positive changes in AI, AHI and LSAT were accompanied by significant reduction of serum CRP levels.[21] Based on this study, we suggest that the benefits of surgical treatment may be greater than indicated by 'cure' rates based on classic PSG criteria. However, further study with a control

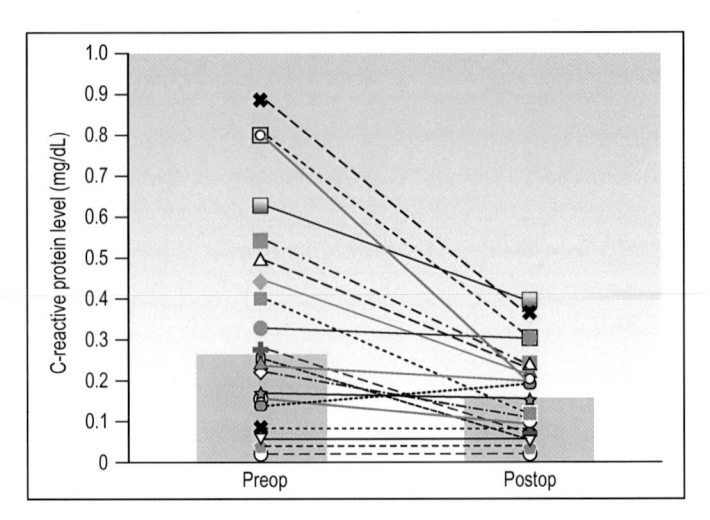

**Fig. 13.2** Effect of surgical treatment on serum levels of CRP in patients with preoperatively elevated CRP ($n = 23$).

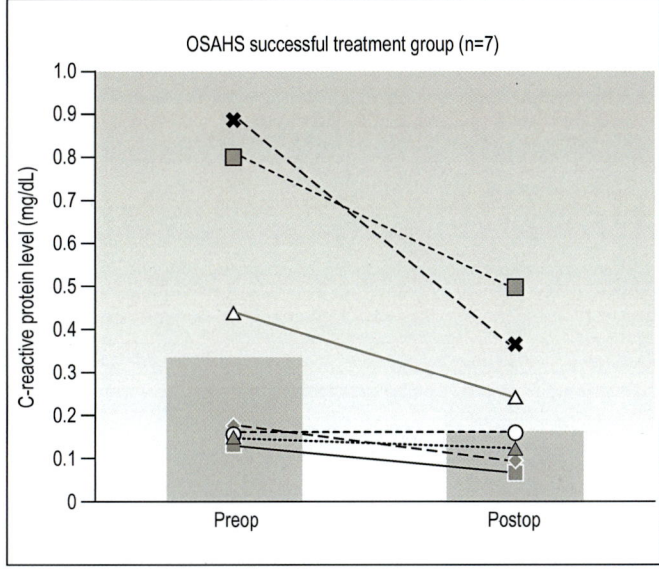

**Fig. 13.3** Effect of surgical treatment on CRP levels in surgical 'cure' or responder group ($n = 7$).

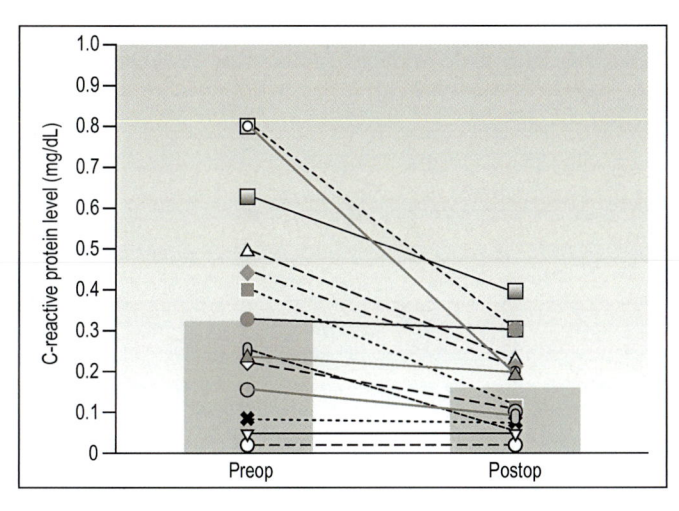

**Fig. 13.4** Effect of surgical treatment on CRP levels in surgical 'failure' or non-responder group ($n = 16$).

group and adjustment for potentially confounding variables is needed to validate this hypothesis.

## REFERENCES

1. Peker Y, Hender J, Norum J, et al. Increased incidence of cardiovascular disease in middle-aged men with obstructive sleep apnea: a 7-year follow-up. Am J Respir Crit Care Med 2002;166:159–65.
2. D'Alessandro R, Magelli C, Gamberini G, et al. Snoring every night as a risk factor of myocardial infarction: a case–control study. BMJ 1990;300:1557–58.
3. Mooe T, Rabben T, Wiklund U, et al. Sleep-disordered breathing in men with coronary artery disease. Chest 1996;109:659–63.
4. Gainer JL. Hypoxia and atherosclerosis: re-evaluation of an old hypothesis. Atherosclerosis 1987;68:263–66.
5. Carlson JT, Hedner J, Elam M, et al. Augmented resting sympathetic activity in awake patients with obstructive sleep apnea. Chest 1993;103:1763–68.
6. Wessendorf TE, Thilmann AF, Wang YM, et al. Fibrinogen levels and obstructive sleep apnea in ischemic stroke. Am J Respir Crit Care Med 2000;162:2039–42.
7. Lavie P, Hoffstein V. Sleep apnea syndrome: a possible contributing factor to resistant hypertension. Sleep 2001;24:721–25.
8. Bradley TD. Right and left ventricular functional impairment and sleep apnea. Clin Chest Med 1992;13:459–79.
9. Hedner JA, Wilcox I, Sullivan CE. Speculations on the interaction between vascular disease and obstructive sleep apnea. In: Sleep and Breathing, 2nd edn. Sauders NA, Sullivan CE, eds. New York: Marcel Dekker; 1994, pp. 823–46.
10. Tracy RP. Inflammation in cardiovascular disease. Circulation 1998;97:2000–2.
11. Plutzky J. Inflammatory pathways in atherosclerosis and acute coronary syndromes. Am J Cardiol 2001;88:10K–15K.
12. Libby P, Ridker PM. Novel inflammatory markers of coronary risk. Circulation 1999;100:1148–50.
13. Pearson TA, Mensah GA, Alexander WR, et al. Markers of inflammation and cardiovascular disease. Application to clinical and public health practice. A statement for healthcare professionals from the Centers for Disease Control and Prevention and the American Heart Association. Circulation 2003;107:499–511.
14. Hartmann G, Tschop M, Fisher R, et al. High altitude increases circulating interleukin-6, interleukin-1 antagonist and C-reactive protein. Cytokine 2000;12:246–52.
15. Vgontzas AN, Papanicolaou DA, Bixter EO, et al. Circadian interleukin-6 secretion and quantity and depth of sleep. J Clin Endocrinol Metab 1999;84:2603–7.
16. Shamsuzzaman ASM, Winnicki M, Lanfranchi P, et al. Elevated C-reactive protein in patients with obstructive sleep apnea. Circulation 2002;105:2462–64.
17. Minoguchi K, Yokoe T, Tazaki T, et al. Increased carotid intima-media thickness and serum inflammatory markers in obstructive sleep apnea. Am J Respir Crit Care Med 2005;172:625–30.
18. Pearson TA, Mensah GA, Hong Y, Smith SC. CDC/AHA workshop on markers of inflammation and cardiovascular disease. Application to clinical and public health practice overview. Circulation 2004;110:e543–e544.
19. Yokoe T, Minoguchi K, Matsuo H, et al. Elevated levels of C-reactive protein and interleukin-6 in patients with obstructive sleep apnea syndrome are decreased by nasal continuous positive airway pressure. Circulation 2003;107:1129–34.
20. Minoguchi K, Tazaki T, Yokoe T, et al. Elevated production of tumor necrosis factor-a by monocytes in patients with obstructive sleep apnea syndrome. Chest 2004;126:1473–79.
21. Friedman M, Bliznikas D, Vidyasagar R, Woodson TB. Reduction of cardiovascular risks with surgical treatment of obstructive sleep apnea hypopnea syndrome. Presented at the Academy of Otolaryngology – Head and Neck Surgery Annual Meeting, New York, NY, September 2004.

SECTION E  ANESTHESIA FOR OSA/HS

# CHAPTER 14
# Perioperative monitoring in obstructive sleep apnea hypopnea syndrome

*Samuel A. Mickelson*

## 1 INTRODUCTION

Obstructive sleep apnea hypopnea syndrome (OSAHS) is a prevalent condition resulting from a decrease in upper airway size and patency during sleep. Apneas, hypopneas and episodes of airflow limitation occur during sleep resulting in physiological changes including reductions in oxygen saturation and arousals from sleep. Arousals lead to cessation of the respiratory event, only to be followed by repetitive airflow obstructions and arousals. The arousals cause sleep fragmentation, and secondary daytime symptoms including non-restorative sleep, excessive daytime somnolence, memory loss and other psychometric changes. Arousals also lead to a rise in sympathetic tone, with secondary changes in blood pressure, pulse and cardiac output. In addition to the nocturnal and daytime symptoms, obstructive sleep apnea may contribute to significant complications including hypertension, cardiac arrhythmias, myocardial infarction, and stroke.

Safe perioperative management of patients with obstructive sleep apnea requires special attention to preoperative, intraoperative and postoperative care. These patients are more likely to have hypertension, esophageal and laryngopharyngeal reflux disease, coronary artery disease and obesity. Operative treatment of these patients requires special care due to these co-morbidities.

In addition, anatomical features (retrognathia, micrognathia, macroglossia, tonsil and uvula hypertrophy, nasal obstruction, abnormal epiglottis position, anterior positioning of the larynx, elongation of the airway) and alterations in arousal responses may lead to difficulty with ventilation and intubation. Airway narrowing may predispose to increased risk of complications including intraoperative airway obstruction, postoperative airway obstruction, myocardial infarction, stroke and cardiac arrhythmia. These patients are also prone to complications associated with reducing their arousal response. Anesthetic agents, narcotic analgesics, and sedative hypnotics reduce arousals responses and may lengthen respiratory events, hypoxemia and hypercarbia during sleep thus leading to postoperative airway obstruction, myocardial infarction, stroke, cardiac arrhythmia and sudden death. Obesity may also contribute to deep vein thrombosis and pulmonary emboli. There is growing evidence that sleep apnea is a risk factor for anesthetic morbidity and mortality. These risks are present when undergoing upper airway surgery or any surgical procedure. The care of these patients requires vigilance before, during and after surgery in order to minimize risks associated with their underlying diseases. This chapter discusses these potential complications along with avoidance strategies.

## 2 PREOPERATIVE MANAGEMENT

### 2.1 SELECTION OF A SURGICAL FACILITY

The surgeon must select an operating room with personnel and equipment adequate for an elective and controlled management of the patient's airway. Preoperative preparation is intended to improve a patient's medical status and reduce the risk of complications. The literature is insufficient to offer guidance regarding which patients can be safely managed as an outpatient as opposed to an inpatient basis or the appropriate time for discharge from the surgical facility.[1]

Upper airway surgery in sleep apnea patients can temporarily worsen the sleep apnea and lead to serious and potentially fatal complications, including acute upper airway obstruction, hypoxemia, hypercarbia, myocardial infarction, cardiac arrhythmias, stroke and death. Prevention of these complications requires early detection of pending airway problems. Postoperative monitoring is performed in order to detect and prevent potential complications. While there are insufficient published data, it is assumed that patients with more severe sleep apnea are at greater risk for perioperative complications.

The determination to perform surgery as an outpatient, in an outpatient surgery center with ambulance transfer to a hospital facility, admit for a short extended recovery room stay, admit to a 23-hour unit, regular hospital room or an intensive care unit should be made with consideration of associated co-morbidities, severity of apnea, sites of airway narrowing, type of anesthesia, length of time for anesthesia, need for postoperative narcotic agents, and type of surgery being performed. This determination should be made preoperatively.[1] Confusing the matter is the use of the term 'outpatient' by some organizations to refer to all surgical stays less than 24 hours and by other organizations to label any stay after midnight as 'inpatient.' In a recent report of the American Society of Anesthesiologists,[1] consultants were surveyed using a non-validated scoring system about opinions regarding outpatient surgery in patients with OSAS. This survey suggested that a patient with mild sleep apnea undergoing uvulopalatopharyngoplasty (UPPP) or nasal surgery was not at increased risk, while a patient with moderate sleep apnea undergoing UPPP was at increased risk of complications.[1]

Care should be taken in selecting patients for outpatient procedures. It is my opinion that most patients with mild or moderate sleep apnea undergoing nasal surgery only may safely be treated as an outpatient, while those with severe sleep apnea may require some observation before discharge. Similarly, most patients with mild OSAHS undergoing UPPP or other pharyngeal airway surgeries should at least be observed for several hours prior to discharge, while those with moderate or severe OSAHS should stay as an inpatient or for a longer observation period. The importance of the postoperative observation period is to document the presence or absence of sleep apnea and oxygen desaturation in the patient while sleeping without supplemental oxygen. The need for postoperative monitoring depends upon the procedure performed and associated co-morbid conditions. The quality of the hospital nursing care and skill of the anesthesiologist also have an impact on the level and type of postoperative monitoring. Some facilities can perform continuous pulse oximetry in the extended recovery unit or regular nursing unit, while others require an intensive care unit to administer this same level of care.

## 2.2 CHOICE OF ANESTHESIA TECHNIQUE (LOCAL, GENERAL OR MONITORED ANESTHESIA CARE)

The literature is insufficient to evaluate the effects of different anesthetic techniques on surgical outcomes after surgery for OSAS. Since airway reconstructive surgery for sleep apnea causes blood to enter the airway, it would be safest to perform these surgeries under general anesthesia, in order to control and protect the airway. When a patient with OSAS is undergoing non-airway related surgery, then a local anesthesia, or monitored anesthesia care (MAC) would be preferred. If the patient is to undergo any sedation during a non-airway surgery, then oximetry and $CO_2$ monitoring should be used. General anesthesia with a secure airway is preferred if the patient is going to require moderate or deep sedation.

## 2.3 USE OF CONTINUOUS POSITIVE AIRWAY PRESSURE (CPAP)

There is an alteration of sleep architecture and frequently sleep deprivation prior to and after surgery, including sleep deprivation due to anxiety about the surgery.[2,3] Once surgery is done and these factors are gone, however, the patient is more likely to enter deeper levels of sleep and may be predisposed to more severe sleep apnea.[4] It would therefore seem to be beneficial to improve sleep quality as much as possible before and after surgery. When possible, a patient should be asked to use CPAP for several weeks prior to and after surgery and to bring their machine into the hospital for perioperative use. While the majority of patients are undergoing surgery because they cannot tolerate CPAP, even moderate use of CPAP preoperatively may be beneficial.

## 2.4 USE OF NARCOTICS AND SEDATIVE AGENTS

Use of narcotics, sedative hypnotics and anxiolytic agents should be avoided prior to surgery in a patient with OSAS. These agents have been reported to lead to sudden death, even in the preoperative holding area.[5] These drugs suppress respiration, blunt the arousal response and may lead to life-threatening hypoxemia. Benzodiazepine agonists affect upper airway muscle tone and worsen sleep apnea.[6] Flurazepam has been shown to increase the Apnea Index[7] and triazolam increased the arousal threshold to airway obstruction, apnea and hypopnea duration and oxygen desaturation.[8] If a sleep apnea patient requires sedation or an anxiolytic, this necessitates require continuous pulse oximetry, and possibly supplemental oxygen.

## 2.5 REFLUX/ASPIRATION PRECAUTIONS

Obesity is common in patients with sleep disordered breathing, leading to an increased risk of gastroesophageal reflux[9,10] which is caused by increased intra-abdominal fat, intra-abdominal pressure and higher incidence of hiatal hernia. Ninety percent of obese patients have greater than 25 ml of gastric fluid prior to surgery, a pH under 2.5 and will be at increased risk of aspiration during induction of anesthesia[11] or upon extubation. In order to reduce these risks, obese patients should receive an $H_2$ blocker, proton pump inhibitor or esophageal motility stimulant prior to surgery.[12]

## 2.6 MEDICAL/ANESTHESIA/CARDIOLOGY CLEARANCE

A consultation with the primary physician, cardiologist, anesthesiologist or other specialist should be considered in patients with complicated co-morbid conditions, or in patients with multiple co-morbidities. For example, a patient with hypertension requiring three antihypertensive agents may require a consultation for medical clearance. A patient with poorly controlled diabetes may benefit from a preoperative clearance. The selection of an internist, cardiologist or anesthesiologist may be based on availability or expertise of the consultant. The purpose of the preoperative clearance is to optimize control of the co-morbidities prior to surgery and to reduce the risk of surgical complications.

Patients with OSAS are at increased risk of hypertension due to an increased sympathetic drive.[13,14] Undiagnosed hypertension is common in the sleep apnea patient. Blood pressure screening should be done at the time of initial evaluation or after initial diagnoses of OSAS. If blood pressure is elevated, these patients should be referred for treatment. Blood pressure should again be checked at a preoperative visit to be sure that hypertension is well controlled.

## 2.7 COMMUNICATION WITH ANESTHESIA TEAM

As the head of the surgical team, it is the responsibility of the surgeon to advise the anesthesia team about any potential difficulty with the airway. While it should be assumed that all OSAS patients may be more difficult to ventilate or intubate, there will be some with macroglossia, retrognathia or micrognathia who are going to be particularly challenging. In these patients, the surgeon may wish to have difficult airway instruments in the operating room, a tracheostomy set available or to be ready to assist with a fiberoptic intubation. I have found that patients are typically more difficult to intubate or ventilate if they have Friedman palate/tongue position IV or if the larynx is not visible with a mirror on indirect laryngoscopy.

## 3 INTRAOPERATIVE MANAGEMENT

### 3.1 PREPARATION FOR INTUBATION (VENTILATION)

Prior to surgery, an anti-reflux agent and anti-sialogogue should be administered to reduce the risk of aspiration and reduce saliva production.[12] It is important to maintain continuous control of the airway by the anesthesiologist. In order to ventilate the patient, the anesthetized patient

**Table 14.1** Available methods for difficult ventilation

| |
|---|
| Oral airway |
| Long nasopharyngeal airways |
| Laryngeal mask airway |
| Esophageal–tracheal combitube |
| Rigid ventilating bronchoscope |
| Intratracheal jet stylet |
| Transtracheal jet ventilation |

will require positive pressure breathing by mask, head and neck extension, jaw protrusion, and insertion of a properly sized oral airway or long nasal airway in order to keep the tongue from falling posteriorly. A two-person ventilation approach may be needed, one for jaw positioning and mask seal and the other for ventilation.[15] A 3–5 minute period of ventilation is used to increase oxyhemoglobin saturation and reduce the rate of desaturation, prior to intubation.

A variety of methods are available to maintain ventilation in a difficult airway (Table 14.1). The simplest approach is to insert a long nasopharyngeal airway that extends inferior to the base of tongue. A laryngeal mask airway (LMA) is another excellent way to stabilize the airway and allow ventilation.[16,17] The LMA is inserted blindly, and keeps the base of tongue and epiglottis from collapsing posteriorly. Other options require additional equipment and expertise such as use of a rigid ventilating bronchoscope, an esophageal–tracheal combitube, or the placement of a 14 gauge angiocath into the cricothyroid membrane followed by transtracheal jet ventilation.

### 3.2 INTUBATION TECHNIQUES

The sleep apnea patient can be a challenge to intubate due to the combination of skeletal deficiency, a long airway, excessive oropharyngeal and hypopharyngeal soft tissue, and a relatively anterior larynx. If easily ventilated, then short-acting paralyzing agents such as succinylcholine may be used. Oral intubation may not be feasible if the larynx cannot be visualized. Alternative methods (Table 14.2) are available for difficult intubations. The safest approach is an awake oral or nasal intubation as the patient continues breathing. A more comfortable approach for the patient is a planned awake transnasal fiberoptic intubation performed with the patient in a sitting or semi-sitting position. Another simple option is the use of a light wand (lighted stilet) inserted into the endotracheal tube, with transcutaneous guidance into the trachea, in a darkened room. If the patient is ventilated through an LMA, then the easiest intubation approach is through the LMA. One of the newest approaches is the use of a video laryngoscope, which has a small video camera on the end, allowing the anesthesiologist to visualize the larynx on a screen. As a result, the

| Table 14.2 Available methods for difficult intubation |
|---|
| Awake intubation |
| Light wand |
| Fiberoptic intubation |
| Video laryngoscopes |
| Intubation through laryngeal mask airway (LMA) |
| Retrograde intubation |
| Blind nasal intubation |

endotracheal tube can be guided through the vocal cords, by visualizing the video screen.

A patient may also require a planned temporary or skinned lined tracheostomy. Planned tracheostomy should be considered in those with severe sleep apnea and failure of CPAP, those with life-threatening cardiac arrhythmias or severe oxygen desaturation,[18] or in those with a failed intubation at a prior surgery. Temporary tracheostomy should also be considered if significant postoperative edema is expected. An emergency tracheostomy or cricothyrotomy may be needed if a patient cannot be ventilated or intubated.

## 3.3 EXTUBATION

Extubation is another critical time due to potential airway obstruction. Full reversal of neuromuscular block should be verified prior to extubation. The patient should have purposeful movement, recovery of neuromuscular activity, sustainable head lift for at least 5 seconds, and an adequate voluntary tidal volume. Whenever possible, the patient should be in the semi-upright or lateral position. In addition, it is generally accepted that patients should be extubated awake.[1,19] Most anesthesiologists prefer not to extubate 'deep' as the airway may obstruct. However, if extubated light or awake, the patient may cough or buck on the tube and cause bleeding into the airway. As a result, there are certainly medical and surgical contraindications to awake extubation. In children, postobstructive pulmonary edema may occur with deep extubation due to negative pressure breathing against a closed airway. In general, if the patient was easy to ventilate with induction, there should be no difficulty ventilating after extubation. The patient should only be extubated with appropriate personnel and equipment present so as to be able to replace the tube if necessary.

It is unclear whether adjunctive local anesthetic agents improve operative safety. Use of long-acting local anesthetics at the conclusion of surgery may reduce the need for narcotic analgesics but may worsen apnea due to blockage of airway mechanoreceptors that contribute to the arousal stimulus and apnea termination.[20] Narcotic agents should be minimized during surgery, as their effect may persist postoperatively and lead to postoperative complications.

## 3.4 SURGEON AVAILABILITY

The surgeon and anesthesiologist should both be in the operating room at time of induction, intubation, and extubation for all sleep apnea patients.

## 4 POSTOPERATIVE MANAGEMENT

Several studies have shown that apnea severity is unchanged or worse one to two nights following UPPP.[21,22] Following surgery, multiple approaches are required to reduce those factors which may exacerbate sleep apnea and to closely monitor patients in order to give early warning of potential serious or fatal airway complications such as airway obstruction, hypoxemia, myocardial infarction, cardiac arrhythmias, stroke and death.

## 4.1 PATIENT POSITIONING

Sleep apnea severity and hypoxemia tend to improve when adult OSAS patients are tested in the sleep laboratory in the lateral, prone, or sitting positions rather than supine. Elevation of the head of the bed after surgery reduces soft tissue edema and turbinate engorgement, and improves the nasal airway. Since there are no valves in the veins of the head and neck, lying flat increases venous pressure and increases tissue edema. While the literature is insufficient to provide guidance for the postoperative period, most physicians agree that after airway surgery, the head of the bed should be elevated and the supine position should be avoided.[1]

## 4.2 PATIENT ANALGESIA

Reconstructive surgery for sleep apnea is often painful, requiring narcotic agents for adequate pain control.[23] All opiate agents including morphine, meperedine, hydromorphone and fentanyl cause dose-dependent reduction of respiratory drive, respiratory rate, and tidal volume and can lead to hypoventilation, hypoxemia and hypercarbia.[24,25] The literature is insufficient to evaluate the effects of different analgesic techniques and there is no agreement about the safety of nurse-administered versus patient-controlled analgesia with systemic opioids.[1]

In general, narcotic agents should be titrated for pain severity and used only as needed. Stronger narcotic agents should be used only when weaker analgesic agents are not adequate. Mild to moderate pain should be treated with oral opioid agents such as codeine, hydrocodone, oxycodone and propoxyphene, as these agents have only mild respiratory suppressing effects. Non-narcotic options include centrally acting agents such as tramadol hydrochloride and acetaminophen, which is often used in combination with opioid agents. Non-steroidal anti-inflammatory agents (ibuprofen, naproxen, ketorolac, tromethamine) may also be helpful but should be used with caution due to the potential for increased bleeding. Newer COX-2 non-steroidal antiinflammatory agents (celocoxib) probably have minimal bleeding risk. Topical anesthetics such as benzocaine may also be helpful for pain control.

## 4.3 OXYGENATION

Maintaining adequate oxygenation is mandatory following surgery. Supplemental oxygen should be continued in order to maintain the oxygen saturation above 90%. Supplemental oxygen may be discontinued when the patient is able to maintain their baseline oxygen saturation while breathing room air. CPAP can be safely used after most upper airway surgeries to prevent desaturation during sleep[26] and should be used as soon as feasible after surgery in patients who were using it prior to surgery. Following surgery, CPAP may also reduce the risk of gastroesophageal reflux.[27] Patients should be instructed to bring their own PAP machine to the surgery facility for postoperative use during sleep at the preset pressure. The CPAP pressure may be changed if needed: higher due to tissue edema or muscle relaxation; lower due to enlargement of the airway. CPAP should be avoided after maxillary advancement due to the risk of subcutaneous emphysema. After nasal surgery, CPAP can be used with a full face mask instead of a nasal mask or nasal pillows.

## 4.4 REDUCING AIRWAY EDEMA

Despite surgical correction of the upper airway, edema caused by surgical trauma or difficult intubation may cause airway compromise, especially in those with severe apnea, multiple sites of airway compromise, and multiple airway surgeries. Tissue edema occurs even after laser and radiofrequency (RF) procedures.[28,29] Systemic steroids can reduce edema in the upper airway.[30] Dexamethasone (10–15 mg/dose in adults) is the preferred corticosteroid agent due to the limited effect on sodium retention. I administer steroids prior to surgery and several doses postoperatively.

Soft tissue edema may be reduced by tissue cooling. Tissue precooling reduces edema in thermal wounds from lasers[30] or cautery units. Application of external ice packs or sucking on ice chips may also reduce swelling. Topical or systemic antibiotic prophylaxis may also reduce edema by reducing bacterial contamination of the surgical wound.

Perioperative use of a broad-spectrum antibiotic agent with anaerobic coverage is recommended with oral or nasal surgery and topical chlorhexidine oral rinse has been shown to reduce bacterial counts in the oral cavity.

Nasal obstruction may cause or worsen sleep apnea[31] while improving the nasal airway can improve sleep apnea.[32] Nasal packing should be avoided in patients undergoing nasal surgery. Alternatives to packing include use of quilting septal sutures, septal splints, nasal tubes such as Doyle splints, or nasopharyngeal airways sewn into place. Use of a decongestant nasal spray (oxymetazoline) or a systemic decongestant postoperatively is also helpful following nasal surgery or nasal intubation.

## 4.5 POSTOPERATIVE MONITORING

The first 24 hours after surgery are probably the most critical time for complications, though deaths from complications have also occurred later, potentially from the accumulated effects of sleep deprivation, narcotic agents and REM rebound.[33,34] Unfortunately, the literature is insufficient to offer guidance regarding the impact of telemetry monitoring, ICU or stepdown units versus routine hospital ward settings, or the appropriate duration of monitoring.[1]

Postoperative monitoring is performed in order to detect and prevent potential complications. Continuous pulse oximetry is the easiest and most reliable method for early detection of postoperative hypoventilation as it can alert the nursing staff and physician to a pending airway complication, and should be used for all OSAS patients following upper airway surgery. Intermittent spot checking of oxygen saturation typically has no benefit since the patent will usually be awakened by putting on the oximetry probe. Some surgical facilities can perform continuous pulse oximetry in the extended recovery unit or hospital ward setting while others require an intensive care unit to administer continuous monitoring. While there is no consensus about whether cardiac monitoring affords any protection to the patient after sleep apnea surgery, it should be used in patients with a history of significant cardiac disease or cardiac arrhythmias.

Monitoring in the ICU has been recommended as a measure to decrease the risk of complications after OSAS surgery.[35,36] Some older publications have recommended ICU monitoring to monitor oxygen saturation and cardiac arrhythmias[21,22] while others have advocated ICU monitoring due to the high incidence of serious airway complications (13–25%) in patients undergoing UPPP.[36,37] Newer publications have noted a much lower complication rate, likely due to more aggressive perioperative precautions to avoid tissue edema and excessive sedation.[38,39] Other authors[40] used the precautions listed in this chapter and reported an overall complication rate of 4% (1.4% airway issues, 1.4% bleeding) in 347 consecutive patients.

## 4.6 USE OF SEDATIVES POSTOPERATIVELY

Sedative hypnotics are frequently administered after surgery for complaints of insomnia. As discussed earlier in this chapter, sedative hypnotics and anxiolytics should be avoided due to the adverse effects on arousal thresholds, as well as apnea duration and severity. For patients with OSAS, short-acting non-benzodiazapine hypnotic agents may be safer than benzodiazepine hypnotics. Zaleplon (half-life 1 hour) and zolpidem tartrate (half-life 2.5 hours) have no significant effect on the Apnea/Hypopnea Index compared to placebo in mild to moderate sleep apnea patients.[41] However, while zaleplon had no effect on the oxygen saturation, zolpidem reduced the lowest oxygen saturation compared to placebo as well as the total time with $SaO_2 < 90\%$ and 80%, compared to the placebo group.

## 4.7 DVT PROPHYLAXIS

Obesity, advanced age, long surgical procedures and prolonged bed-rest can predispose to deep vein thrombosis (DVT) and pulmonary emboli. Methods to reduce the risk of this complication include application of sequential compression stockings, elastic stockings and subcutaneous heparin. DVT prophylaxis is indicated for the majority of patients undergoing surgery for sleep apnea.

## 4.8 BLOOD PRESSURE CONTROL

Patients with OSAS have a higher prevalence of hypertension and are at increased risk of postoperative hypertension due to an increased sympathetic tone.[13,14] To maintain a postoperative systolic blood pressure below 160 mm Hg and diastolic below 90 mm Hg, over half of the patients undergoing upper airway surgery for OSAS will require an antihypertensive agent in the recovery room (unpublished observations, S. Mickelson MD). Blood pressure control during and after surgery is imperative in order to reduce the risk of postoperative bleeding and tissue edema. Blood pressure control is most important after osseous surgeries, since postoperative bleeding from bone is blood pressure dependent.

## 4.9 GENERIC PATIENT CARE PROTOCOLS

Physician and hospital patient care protocols for preoperative instructions and postoperative orders are often utilized for surgery.[42] Institution protocols should be examined to be sure that routine recovery room, surgical ward, or extended recovery unit orders are appropriate for the sleep apnea patient (see Tables 14.3 and 14.4). Nursing checks should be more frequent than for the non-OSAS patient, in order to visually check the patient's breathing status and be sure there is no labored breathing.

**Table 14.3 Standard preop orders for sleep apnea surgery**

1. Pepcid ____ mg PO 30–60 minutes prior to surgery
2. Reglan ____ mg PO 30–60 minutes prior to surgery
3. Robinol ____ mg IM 30–60 minutes prior to surgery
4. Ancef ____ mg IVPB 30–60 minutes prior to surgery
5. Dexametasone ____ mg IV 30–60 minutes prior to surgery
6. Oxymetazoline nasal spray, ____ sprays each nostril, to be given 10–20 minutes preop if patient is to undergo nasal surgery or nasal intubation
7. No narcotic or sedative agents to be given prior to surgery

**Table 14.4 Standard postop orders after sleep apnea surgery**

1. Recovery room orders: No IV or IM narcotics 30 minutes prior to transfer to room.
2. Wean oxygen to room air but maintain $O_2$ saturation above 90%.
3. Vitals: per recovery room, then routine.
4. Check patient's breathing effort and record results at least every 2 hours.
5. Continuous pulse oximetry.
6. Elevate head of bed 30–45 degrees.
7. Ice collar to neck prn.
8. Sequential compression stockings to be on while in bed.
9. Clear liquid diet. Advance as tolerated. Encourage PO intake. Monitor oral intake.
10. IV D5 LR at ____ ml per hour.
11. Cefazolin sodium ____ mg IVPB q 8 hours.
12. Pt is to wear his/her own CPAP/BIPAP machine, whenever sleeping, beginning in recovery room. If patient underwent nasal surgery, use a CPAP full face mask.
13. For pain:
    Chloroseptic spray to oral cavity prn, keep at bedside.
    *Mild:* Hydrocodone and acetaminophen elixir 2.5/166 mg/5 ml: ____ mL PO q 6 hours prn.
    *Moderate:* Oxycodone and acetaminophen elixir 5/325 mg/5 ml: ____ mL PO q6 hours prn.
    *Severe:* Nalbuphine hydrochloride ____ mg IM or slow IV q 3–6 hours prn.
14. Dexametasone sodium phosphate ____ mg IVPB at ____ pm today and ____ am tomorrow.
15. Oxymetazoline nasal spray: ____ sprays to each nostril q 8hours.
16. For blood pressure elevation: systolic > 160 or diastolic > 90 give:
    Apresoline ____ mg IV, may repeat q 15 minutes up to 4 doses total or
    Labatolol ____ mg IV, may repeat q 15 minutes up to 4 doses total.
17. Call physician for:
    Active bleeding from nose or mouth.
    Any evidence of respiratory distress.
    Oxygen saturation below 90% or inability to wean off supplemental oxygen.
    Temperature above 101° (oral).
18. Systolic BP > 160; Diastolic > 90, not controlled with prescribed medication.

# SECTION E: ANESTHESIA FOR OSA/HS

## 4.10 CRITERIA FOR DISCHARGE

The patient should not be discharged home until swallowing is adequate to maintain hydration and adequate nutrition at home. The patient should not be discharged until there is adequate pain control with oral analgesics. The literature is insufficient to offer guidance about the appropriate time for discharge of these patients. Consultants to the ASA agreed that the room air oxygen saturation should return to its preoperative baseline, that patients should not be hypoxemic or develop airway obstruction when left undisturbed, and that these patients should be monitored for 7 hours after the last episode of airway obstruction or hypoxemia while breathing room air in a non-stimulating environment.[1]

## 5 CONCLUSIONS

Obstructive sleep apnea increases the risk for anesthetic and postoperative complications, including postoperative airway obstruction, myocardial infarction, stroke and cardiac arrhythmia. The sleep apnea patient poses a challenge for the surgeon, anesthesiologist and surgical facility in order to administer safe perioperative care. To reduce this risk, precautions are required before, during and after surgery. The important concepts for safe perioperative management are constant control of the airway during surgery, judicious use of sedating medications and proper monitoring following surgery. While the literature is lacking for specific measures, the recommendations presented here are based on a combination of 25 years of experience supported by the peer-reviewed medical literature available.

## REFERENCES

1. American Society of Anesthesiologists. Practice guidelines for the perioperative management of patients with Obstructive Sleep Apnea. A report by the ASA Task Force on Perioperative Management of Patients with Obstructive Sleep Apnea. Anesthesiology 2006;104:1081–93.
2. Aurell J, Elmqvist D. Sleep in the surgical intensive care unit: continuous polygraphic recording of nine patients receiving postoperative care. BMJ Clin Res Ed 1985;290:1029–32.
3. Rosenberg J, Rosenberg-Adamsen S, Kehlet H. Post-operative sleep disturbances: causes, factors and effects on outcome. Eur J Anaesthesiol 1995;10(Suppl):28–30.
4. Cullen DJ. Obstructive sleep apnea and postoperative analgesia – a potentially dangerous combination. J Clin Anesth 2001;13:83–5.
5. Fairbanks DNF. Uvulopalatopharyngoplasty complications and avoidance strategies. Otolaryngol Head Neck Surg 1990;102:239–45.
6. Bonara M, St John WM, Bledsoe TA. Differential elevation by protriptyline and depression by diazepam of upper airway motor activity. Am Rev Respir Dis 1985;131:41–5.
7. Guilleminault C, Silvestri R, Mondini S, Coburn S. Aging and sleep apnea: action of benzodiazipine, acetozolamide, alcohol and sleep deprivation in a healthy elderly group. J Gerontol 1984;39:655–66.
8. Berry RB, Kouchi K, Bower J, Prosise G, Light RW. Triazolam in patients with obstructive sleep apnea. Am J Respir Crit Care Med 1995;151:450–54.
9. DeMeester TR, Johnson LF, Joseph GJ, Toscano MS, Hall AW, Skinner DB. Patterns of gastroesophageal reflux in health and disease. Ann Surg 1976;184:459–70.
10. Mercer CD, Wren SF, DaCosta LR, Beck IT. Lower esophageal sphincter pressure and gastroesophageal pressure gradients in excessively obese patients. J Med 1987;18:135–46.
11. Vaughan RW, Bauer S, Wise L. Volume and pH of gastric juice in obese patients. Anesthesiology 1975;43:686–9.
12. Warwick JP, Mason DG. Obstructive sleep apnoea in children. Anaesthesia 1998;53:571–9.
13. Worsnop CJ, Pierce RJ, Naughton M. Systemic hypertension and obstructive sleep apnea. Sleep 1993;16:S148–9.
14. Bonsignore MR, Marrone O, Insalaco G, Bonsignore G. The cardiovascular effects of obstructive sleep apnoeas: analysis of pathogenic mechanisms. Eur Respir J 1994;7:786–805.
15. Benumof JL. Management of the difficult airway. Anesthesiology 1991;75:1087–110.
16. Practice Guidelines for Management of the Difficult Airway. Anesthesiology 1993;78:597–602.
17. Benumof JL. Laryngeal mask airway and the ASA difficult airway algorithm. Anesthesiology 1996;84:686–99.
18. Mickelson SA. Upper airway bypass surgery for obstructive sleep apnea syndrome. Otolaryngol Clin North Am 1996;31:1013–23.
19. Meoli AL, Rosen CL, Kristo D, et al. Report of the AASM clinical practice review committee. Upper airway management of the adult patient with obstructive sleep apnea in the perioperative period – avoiding complications. Sleep 2003;26:1060–65.
20. Berry RB, Kouchi KG, Bower JL, et al. Effect of upper airway anesthesia on obstructive sleep apnea. Am J Respir Crit Care Med 1995;151:1857–61.
21. Sanders MH, Johnson JT, Keller FA, Seger L. The acute effects of uvulopalatopharyngoplasty on breathing during sleep in sleep apnea patients. Sleep 1988;11:75–89.
22. Johnson JT, Sanders MH. Breathing during sleep immediately after uvulopalatopharyngoplasty. Laryngoscope 1986;96:1236–8.
23. Troell RJ, Powell NB, Riley TW, et al. Comparison of postoperative pain between laser assisted uvulopalatoplasty, uvulopalatopharyngoplasty, and radiofrequency volumetric tissue reduction of the palate. Otolaryngol Head Neck Surg 2000;122:402–9.
24. Bailey PL, Egan TD, Stanley TH. Intravenous opioid anesthetics. In: Anesthesia, 5th edn. Miller RD, ed. Philadelphia: Churchill Livingstone; 2000, pp. 273–376.
25. Mickelson SA. Perioperative and anesthesia management. In: Obstructive Sleep Apnea Surgery. Fairbanks DNF, Mickelson SA, Woodson BT, eds. Philadelphia: Lippincott Williams & Wilkins; 2003, pp. 223–32.
26. Powell NB, Riley RW, Guilleminault C, Murcia GN. Obstructive sleep apnea, continuous positive airway pressure, and surgery. Otolaryngol Head Neck Surg 1988;99:362–69.
27. Kerr P, Shoenut JP, Millar J, Buckle P, Kryger MH. Nasal CPAP reduces gastroesophageal reflux in obstructive sleep apnea syndrome. Chest 1992;101:1539–44.
28. Terris DJ, Clerk AA, Norbash AM, Troell RJ. Characterization of postoperative edema following laser-assisted uvulopalatoplasty using MRI and polysomnography: implications for the outpatient treatment of obstructive sleep apnea syndrome. Laryngoscope 1996;106:124–28.
29. Powell NB, Riley RW, Troell RJ, Blumen MB, Guillemenault C. Radiofrequency volumetric reduction of the tongue. A porcine pilot study for the treatment of obstructive sleep apnea syndrome. Chest 1997;111:1348–55.
30. Sheppard LM, Werkhaven JA, Mickelson SA. The effect of steroids or tissue pre-cooling on edema and tissue thermal coagulation after $CO_2$ laser impact. Lasers Surg Med 1992;12:137–46.
31. Olsen KD. The nose and its impact on snoring and obstructive sleep apnea. In: Snoring and Obstructive Sleep Apnea. Fairbanks DNF, ed. New York: Raven Press; 1987, pp. 199–226.
32. Dayall VS, Phillipson EA. Nasal surgery in the management of sleep apnea. Ann Otol Rhinol Laryngol 1985;94:550–54.
33. Rosenberg J, Rasmussen GI, Wojdemann KR, et al. Ventilatory pattern and associated episodic hypoxaemia in the late postoperative period in the general surgical ward. Anaesthesia 1999;54:323–28.

34. Knill RL, Moote CA, Skinner MI, Rose EA. Anesthesia with abdominal surgery leads to intense REM sleep during the first postoperative week. Anesthesiology 1990;73:52–61.
35. Macaluso RA, Reams C, Vrabec DP, Gibson WS, Matragrano A. Uvulopalatopharyngoplasty: post-operative management and evaluation of results. Ann Otol Rhinol Laryngol 1989;98:502–7.
36. Esclamado RM, Gleen MG, McCulloch TM, Cummings CW. Perioperative complications and risk factors in the surgical treatment of obstructive sleep apnea syndrome. Laryngoscope 1989;99:1125–29.
37. Haavisto L, Suonpaa J. Complications of uvulopalatopharyngoplasty. Clin Otolaryngol 1994;9:243–47.
38. Hathaway B, Johnson JT. Safety of uvulopalatopharyngoplasty as outpatient surgery. Otolaryngol Head Neck Surg 2006;134:542–44.
39. Kezirian EJ, Weaver EM, Yuen B, et al. Incidence of serious complications after uvulopalatopharyngoplasty. Laryngoscope 2004;114:450–53.
40. Mickelson SA, Hakim I. Is post operative intensive care monitoring necessary after uvulopalatopharyngoplasty? Otolaryngol Head Neck Surg 1998;119:352–56.
41. George CFP. Perspectives on the management of insomnia in patients with chronic respiratory disorders. Sleep 2000;23(Suppl 1):S31–35.
42. Mickelson SA. Avoidance of complications in sleep apnea patients. In: Surgical Management of Sleep Apnea and Snoring. Terris DJ, Goode RL, eds. Boca Raton: Taylor & Francis; 2005, pp. 453–64.

# SECTION E — ANESTHESIA FOR OSA/HS

## CHAPTER 15
# Perioperative and anesthesia management

*Arthur J. Klowden, Usharani Nimmagadda and Benjamin Salter*

> **Keys to anesthetic management of obstructive sleep apnea/hypopnea syndrome**
> - Anticipate co-morbid conditions
> - Be prepared for difficult intubation
> - Avoid long-acting sedatives/narcotics
> - Expect violent/combative emergence
> - Do not extubate when patient is combative
> - Extubate only when patient can follow commands
> - Use nasopharyngeal airway after extubation

## 1 INTRODUCTION

As the population in the United States becomes more obese every year, the incidence of obstructive sleep apnea/hypopnea syndrome (OSAHS) is also increasing. In the general population, the incidence of OSAHS is 2% in women and 4% in men.[1] An increase in the body mass index (BMI) of one standard deviation increases the likelihood of co-existing OSAHS by a factor of 4.[1] In the morbidly obese population, the incidence of OSA is 3% to 25% in women and 40% to 77% in men.[2] Conversely, 90% of OSAHS subjects have a BMI greater than $28\,kg/m^2$. Some subjects have severe (BMI = 35 to $39\,kg/m^2$) and even morbid (BMI = $40\,kg/m^2$) obesity.

The airway obstruction in OSAHS patients is due to a decrease in the upper airway muscle tone during sleep and airway narrowing due to the deposition of adipose tissue in pharyngeal structures. The structures that may increase in size due to deposition of fat are the uvula, tonsils, tonsillar pillars, tongue, aryepiglottic folds and the lateral pharyngeal walls (Fig. 15.1). The deposition of fat in the lateral pharyngeal walls not only narrows the airway, but also changes the shape of the pharynx. The normal shape of the pharynx with a long transverse (lateral) and a short anterior–posterior axis changes into an ellipsoid with a short transverse and a long anterior–posterior axis. This change in shape makes the action of the anterior pharyngeal dilator airway muscles (tensor palitini, genioglossus, and hyoid) less efficient (Fig. 15.2).[3]

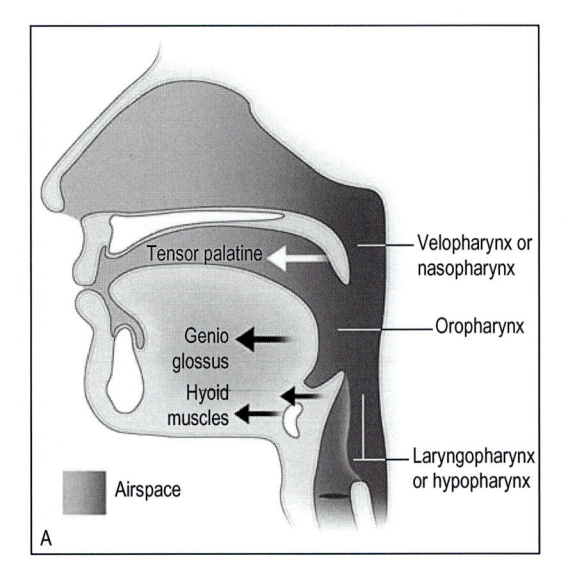

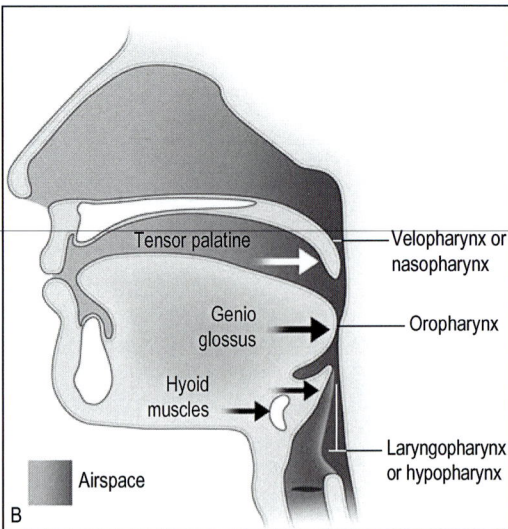

**Fig. 15.1** A, The action of the most important dilator muscles of the upper airway. The tensor palatine, genioglossus, and hyoid muscles enlarge the nasopharynx, oropharynx, and the laryngopharynx, respectively. B, Collapse of the nasopharynx at the palatal level, the oropharynx at the glottic level, and the laryngopharynx at the epiglottic level. Modified from Benumof JL. Obstructive sleep apnea in the adult obese patient: implications for airway management. J Clin Anesth 2001;13(2):144–56, with permission.

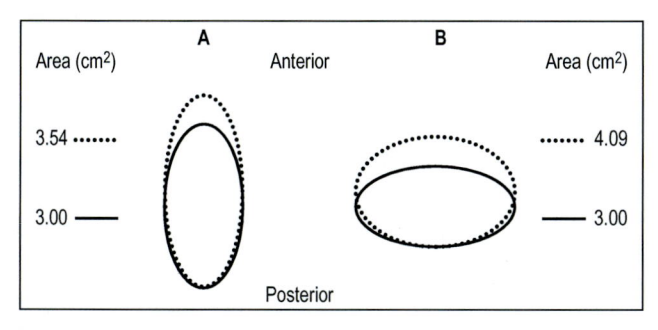

**Fig. 15.2** The effects of a 5 mm change in the anteroposterior (AP) diameter of the airway on airway cross-sectional area is shown for two equally elliptical airways with different lateral/AP ratios. A, The lateral/AP ratio = 0.5. B, The lateral/AP ratio = 2. The lateral dimension of each ellipse was held constant. The solid line represents the starting area (3 cm² in both ellipses), and the dotted line represents the area after a 5 mm increase in the AP diameter. The area change is greater in the ellipse with a more lateral orientation B, From Leiter JC. Upper airway shape. Is it important in the pathogenesis of obstructive sleep apnea? Am J Respir Crit Care Med 1996;153:894–8, with permission.

Respiratory outcomes during the perioperative management of patients with OSAHS are a major concern for anesthesiologists. The inability to tracheally intubate the patient, respiratory obstruction soon after tracheal extubation at the end of the procedure, and severe respiratory depression and respiratory arrest after the administration of sedatives and narcotics are the biggest concerns.[4]

Recently, the American Society of Anesthesiologists (ASA) developed practice guidelines for the perioperative management of patients with OSAHS.[5] These guidelines proposed a scoring system, which can be used to estimate whether a patient is at increased risk for perioperative complications from OSAHS (Table 15.1). The scoring system depends upon three factors: (1) the severity of OSAHS disease; (2) the invasiveness of the surgery and anesthesia; and (3) the requirement for postoperative opioids. The estimation of perioperative risk is based on the overall score; patients with an overall score of 5 or greater have an increased risk of perioperative complications.

## 2 PREOPERATIVE ASSESSMENT OF THE PATIENT

Ideally, evaluation of the patient should take place in a preoperative clinic, several days before surgery. Unfortunately, many patients will not be seen by the anesthesiologist until the day of surgery. The evaluation should include a review of the current and previous medical records, an interview of the patient, and a physical examination.

A careful review of all medical records is very important. The preoperative diagnosis, exact surgical procedure being performed and proper consent for anesthesia and surgery should be noted. Reviewing old medical records can be particularly useful with regard to previous anesthetic history, which may reveal airway difficulties, an unusual response to anesthetic agents and the postoperative course. All co-existing medical conditions and treatments should be noted. In addition to the routine laboratory values, any work-up that has been done specific to OSAHS (such as polysomnographic testing, cephalometric measurements, cardiac or pulmonary function studies) should be checked. All consultations should be reviewed and if a specific question arises, the consultant in question should be contacted. A detailed history from the patient (and bedpartner if possible) should identify patients with undiagnosed OSAHS.

A thorough physical examination of the patient is essential. Many OSAHS patients have several co-existing diseases due to hypoxic episodes and obesity. Careful examination of the cardiovascular system should be done. Bradycardia occurs during apneic spells due to hypoxia and reverts to baseline during and after arousal. In about half of the patients, long sinus pauses, second-degree heart block and ventricular arrhythmias occur. When arterial oxygen saturation ($SaO_2$) decreases below 60%, the severity of the bradycardia and the onset of arrhythmias markedly increase.[6]

---

**Table 15.1 Scoring system for calculation of perioperative risk in patients with OSAHS‡**

A. Severity of sleep apnea based on sleep study (or clinical indicators if sleep study not available). Point score _____ (0–3).*†
   0. None (AHI = 0–5)
   1. Mild (AHI = 6–20)
   2. Moderate (AHI = 21–40)
   3. Severe (AHI > 40)
B. Invasiveness of the surgery and anesthesia. Point score _____ (0–3).
   0. Superficial surgery under local or peripheral nerve block without sedation
   1. Superficial surgery with moderate sedation or general anesthesia or peripheral surgery with spinal or epidural anesthesia
   2. Peripheral surgery with general anesthesia or airway surgery with moderate sedation
   3. Major surgery or airway surgery with general anesthesia
C. Requirement of postoperative opioids. Point score _____ (0–3).
   0. None
   1. Low-dose oral opioids
   2. High-dose oral, parenteral or neuroaxial opioids

Estimation of perioperative risk is calculated as follows: Overall score = the score for A plus the greater of the score for either B or C.
*One point may be subtracted if a patient has been on CPAP or NIPPV before surgery and will be using his or her appliance consistently during the postoperative period.
†One point should be added if a patient with mild or moderate OSAHS also has a resting $PaCO_2$ greater than 50 mm Hg.
‡Patients with a score of 5 or 6 may be at significantly increased perioperative risk from OSAHS. Modified from Gross JB, Bachenberg KL, Benumof JL, et al. American Society of Anesthesiologists Task Force on Perioperative Management. Practice guidelines for the perioperative management of patients with obstructive sleep apnea: a report by the American Society of Anesthesiologists Task Force on perioperative management of patients with obstructive sleep apnea. Anesthesiology 2006;104(5):1081–93, with permission.

---

Patients with diagnosed OSAHS may come to surgery for either OSAHS corrective surgery or for some other procedure. In addition, many patients coming for surgeries other than OSAHS correction may have undiagnosed OSAHS.

# SECTION E: ANESTHESIA FOR OSA/HS

**Table 15.2 Components of the preoperative airway physical examination**

| Airway examination component | Non-reassuring findings |
|---|---|
| Length of upper incisors | Relatively long |
| Relation of maxillary and mandibular incisors during normal jaw closure | Prominent 'overbite' (maxillary incisors anterior to mandibular incisors) |
| Relation of maxillary and mandibular incisors during voluntary protrusion of mandible | Patient cannot bring mandibular incisors anterior to (mandible in front of) maxillary incisors |
| Interincisor distance | Less than 3 cm |
| Visibility of uvula | Not visible when tongue is protruded with patient in sitting position (e.g. Mallampati class greater than II) |
| Shape of palate | Highly arched or very narrow |
| Compliance of mandibular space | Stiff, indurated, occupied by mass, or non-resilient |
| Thyromental distance | Less than three ordinary finger breadths |
| Length of neck | Short |
| Thickness of neck | Thick |
| Range of motion of head and neck | Patient cannot touch tip of chin to chest or cannot extend neck |

This table displays some findings of the airway physical examination that may suggest the presence of a difficult intubation. The decision to examine some or all of the airway components shown in this table depends on the clinical context and judgment of the practitioner. The table is not intended as a mandatory or exhaustive list of the components of an airway examination. The order of presentation in this table follows the 'line of sight' that occurs during conventional oral laryngoscopy.

Many patients develop both systemic and pulmonary hypertension. Systemic hypertension is present in half the patients due to repetitive increases in sympathetic tone during each hypoxic/hypercapnic arousal event.[7] Pulmonary hypertension has several possible etiologies.

Special attention must be paid to the airway of the patient. In general, obese patients are more difficult to tracheally intubate.[10] Since many OSAHS patients are obese, the same principles should be applied when securing the airway of an OSAHS patient. These patients have a large tongue and a thick neck. The probability of difficult tracheal intubation is 5% when the neck circumference is 40 cm whereas the probability increases to 35% when the neck circumference is 60 cm.[11] The fact that the excess pharyngeal tissue that is deposited in the lateral walls of the pharynx may not be visible on routine examination is another cause for an unanticipated difficult tracheal intubation. During laryngoscopy, the commonly seen excessive adipose tissue in the interscapular region ('buffalo hump') causes malalignment of the oral, pharyngeal and tracheal axes. In addition, since these patients are more prone to aspiration of gastric contents, the Sellick maneuver (cricoid pressure) used during induction of anesthesia before tracheal intubation may also misalign the axes.[12] These misalignments can interfere with the 'line of sight' and make visualization of the larynx more difficult.

Whether tracheal intubation should be performed with the patient awake or under general anesthesia must be individualized on the basis of a methodical, complete airway examination (Table 15.2). Thus, a multivariate airway risk index should be performed.[13] This index identifies several criteria including:

1. Mouth opening including temporomandibular joint function.
2. Modified Mallampati classification of the airway.[14,15]
3. Atlanto-occipital joint mobility.
4. Ability to prognath.
5. Thyromental distance.
6. History of previous difficult tracheal intubation.
7. Weight of the patient.

Using rigid laryngoscopy, the multivariate risk index predicts the difficulty of laryngeal visualization better than a single criterion such as the Mallampati classification of the oropharyngeal view.

## 2.1 PREMEDICATION

Sedatives and narcotics have a propensity to exacerbate the sleep-related apneic episodes and may impair life-saving arousal in patients with OSAHS. Benzodiazepines and barbiturates preferentially decrease neural input to the upper airway dilating muscles, leading to airway obstruction.[16] Even small doses of narcotics given intravenously or epidurally can cause severe airway obstruction and apnea.[17,18] Administration of a combination of sedatives and narcotics can be disastrous. Anxiolytic drugs such as midazolam should only be administered when close monitoring of the patient by appropriate personnel is possible. This means that the drug should not be given until the patient is about to enter the operating room for surgery. Because of the increased incidence of aspiration of gastric contents, an antacid and/or metoclopramide should be given to decrease the gastric acidity and volume. Glycopyrrolate to reduce oral secretions and dexametasone to reduce airway edema and nausea and vomiting are generally administered.

## 2.2 MONITORING

In addition to the standard monitors (electrocardiogram, non-invasive blood pressure, pulse oximetry, end-tidal carbon dioxide), some patients may require an indwelling arterial catheter. In obese patients, the blood pressure cuff may not fit the upper arm properly, and thus may not read correctly. In addition, tongue advancement and mandibular osteotomy procedures may require hypotensive anesthesia where accurate blood pressure readings are essential. An indwelling arterial catheter also allows easy access to blood for arterial blood gases and other laboratory testing, intraoperatively and postoperatively. Very rarely, patients with advanced cardiac or pulmonary dysfunction may need a pulmonary artery catheter. If the procedure is very long and necessitates administration of large quantities of fluids, a Foley catheter should be considered. A depth of anesthesia monitor, when available, may facilitate rapid awakening of the patient at the end of the procedure. For all long procedures, some form of temperature monitor should be used.

## 2.3 POSITIONING OF THE PATIENT FOR SURGERY

Accommodating these large patients appropriately on the narrow operating tables is a common problem. If a wide operating table is not used, the arms may have to be placed on arm boards and positioned in such a way that the surgeon will have proper access to the surgical site, and at the same time the patient is protected from neurological damage.

Obese patients have increased oxygen consumption ($VO_2$) and decreased lung volumes. Functional residual capacity (FRC) and expiratory reserve volume (ERV) are small and patients become desaturated faster during apnea.[19] The supine position is the most common position for OSAHS surgery. In this position the abdominal contents and the diaphragm are pushed into the chest cavity, further decreasing the lung volumes and exaggerating the problem of desaturation.[20] A 'ramped' position (Fig. 15.3), in which the upper body, neck and head are elevated to a point where an imaginary horizontal line can be drawn from the sternal notch to the external ear, not only improves the comfort of the patient but also improves the laryngeal view during intubation when compared to the 'sniffing' position.[21] Once the endotracheal tube (ETT) is safely secured, some of the blankets can be removed before surgery commences.

## 2.4 PREOXYGENATION OF THE PATIENT

Maximally preoxygenating obese, OSAHS patients is absolutely essential for many reasons, including a higher incidence of difficulty in securing the airway, not ventilating the patient during a rapid sequence induction before securing the airway, decreased lung volumes, and increased $VO_2$, which lead to faster desaturation during apnea. In addition, these patients may be difficult to ventilate after induction agents are given since they can become obstructed very easily due to redundant soft tissue. Although the original ASA difficult airway algorithm made no mention of preoxygenation, an updated task force report includes facemask preoxygenation before initiating management of the difficult airway.[22] The same ramped position (Fig. 15.3) that was mentioned earlier can also improve the preoxygenation.[23] In obese patients with a large head, selecting the proper size facemask and maintaining a tight seal around the mask are very important to achieve a maximal inspired oxygen concentration. In normal patients, a minimum of 3 minutes of tidal volume breathing or eight deep breaths in 1 minute is necessary to sufficiently increase oxygen stores. In the obese OSAHS patient, a longer duration of preoxygenation (at least 5 minutes of tidal volume breathing) is necessary to increase the oxygen stores in the body. Oxygen insufflation into the pharynx via a small naso- or oropharyngeal catheter during laryngoscopy may further delay the onset of desaturation.[24]

## 3 INTRAOPERATIVE CARE

In the operating room, the anesthetic management ranges from essentially 'routine' to treacherous. As previously indicated, these cases require communication and discussion between the surgeon and the anesthesiologist, creating a team approach. Extra thought, extra planning, and extra care are indicated. There is a level of unpredictability associated with all phases of the perioperative period, particularly with (OSAHS) patients. Can the patient be mask ventilated? Should we even try? Can the patient's trachea be intubated easily? Can the patient's trachea be intubated with a laryngoscope? Experience shows that not all Mallampati Grade 1 airways[14] are easily intubated, but also, not all Mallampati 3 or 4 airways require an awake or fiberoptic intubation.

At least two people should be present for the tracheal intubation of severe OSAHS patients, and at least one of them should be an experienced anesthesiologist. Familiarity with the ASA practice guidelines for management of the difficult airway,[22] the difficult airway algorithm and the new

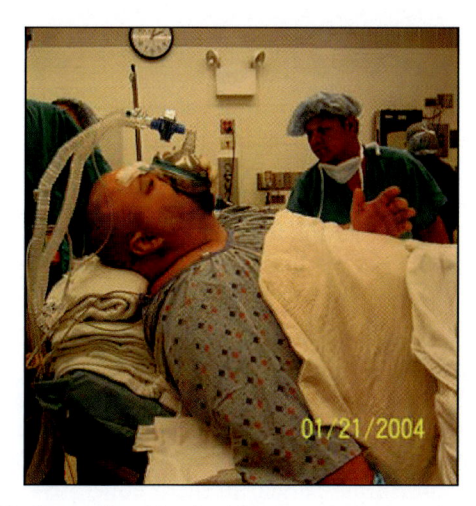

**Fig. 15.3** The 'ramped' position, in which the upper body, neck and head are elevated to a point where an imaginary horizontal line can be drawn from the sternal notch to the external ear, not only improves the comfort of the patient but also improves the laryngeal view during intubation. Once the endotracheal tube (ETT) is safely secured, some of the blankets can be removed before surgery commences.

practice guidelines for the management of patients with obstructive sleep apnea[4] seem mandatory.

The importance of positioning, and in particular the 'ramped' position,[21] has already been mentioned. Taking time to optimize the view is vital. Many anesthesiologists start the process in the prep-and-hold area, although others do it only in the operating room. The 'sniffing' position was the standard for many years, with up to 35 degrees flexion of the neck on the chest, up to 15 degrees extension of the facial plane and up to 85 degrees extension of the neck at the atlanto-occipital joint.[26] Elevating the head even further, the 'head-elevated' laryngoscopy position, has been claimed[27] to further improve the success rate of intubation. Many anesthesiologists, however, now believe that the 'ramped' position with blankets or other padding placed under the shoulders, head and neck is optimal. In some patients, however, no amount of position change improves 'the view'.

Although succinylcholine seems to be the relaxant of choice for most patients with severe OSAHS, in some cases, where there is easy, comfortable mask ventilation after intravenous induction, some anesthesiologists may elect to give a nondepolarizing relaxant, usually rocuronium, for intubation. If the virtue of succinylcholine is its rapid onset and relatively rapid recovery, what is the virtue of rocuronium? Its slower onset necessitates longer mask ventilation with an inhalational anesthetic (sevoflurane). This can be advantageous in augmenting the relaxation, helping to guarantee amnesia, and raising the arterial oxygen tension ($PaO_2$) even further. This, of course, assumes that the easy mask ventilation continues. A second benefit to the use of rocuronium is the prolonged relaxant effect, avoiding the problem of succinylcholine wearing off quickly, leading to less than optimal relaxation and failed intubation. The anesthesiologist must, of course, realize the 'commitment' he/she is making by using rocuronium, and having committed, not underdose. Relaxation with rocuronium also allows time for the use of the intubating LMA (LMA Fastrach™, LMA-North America, San Diego, CA) or for fiberoptic intubation, if necessary.

It is reasonable to have multiple laryngoscopes available. If possible, a Macintosh 3, Macintosh 4, and Miller and/or Phillips blades should be ready, each on its own handle to speed up the laryngoscopic process. The ETT should be styletted, with the stylet pushed down to the Murphy eye of the ETT, and the tip bent in a curve similar to a hockey stick. An Eschmann tube exchanger, sometimes called a gum elastic bougie, or a newer variation of this must also be within reach. An appropriately sized LMA or intubating LMA may also prove useful. Attempts at laryngoscopy must be done expeditiously and in a planned, orderly manner. The first attempt can be a longer and a more 'exploratory' look around. It is usually the anesthesiologist's best attempt. If it fails, adjustments are made quickly. These adjustments may include changing the depth of anesthesia, the dose of muscle relaxant, the head and neck position, the type of laryngoscope blade, the lighting and the assistant. The anesthesiologist may attempt to optimize laryngeal view with external manipulations of the larynx and neck. Maneuvers such as BURP (backwards, upwards, rightward pressure) or OLM (optimal laryngeal manipulation) may make the larynx more visible.[12] If necessary, the anesthesiologist should call for help from a colleague before a crisis arises. Once the airway is established, maintenance of anesthesia is routine.

## 3.1 EMERGENCE

Emergence after sleep apnea surgery is perhaps the most critical time for both the anesthesiologist and the patient. These patients, in particular, require extra vigilance because of their increased susceptibility to airway compromise and the deleterious effects of anesthetic medications given throughout the procedure.

Preparation for emergence from anesthesia and tracheal extubation begins when the surgeon approximates a time when the procedure will be completed. Usually, the volatile anesthetic is removed from the patient's breathing circuit as the surgery comes to an end and the patient is kept anesthetized with nitrous oxide or intravenous propofol. There are several precautions the anesthesiologist should take before emergence from anesthesia and tracheal extubation. Some sleep apnea surgeries require manipulation of the ETT, so it is important to re-secure it after the surgery is completed. An oral airway should always be used to prevent obstruction by the tongue, which may or may not have been operated on. Some surgeons insert nasal trumpets that maintain a patent nasopharynx and may further assist with preventing airway obstruction. Although airway control is always of paramount importance to the anesthesiologist, OSAHS patients have an especially dynamic airway that requires extra support. Additional measures include insuring adequate reversal of all muscle relaxants, and adequate support staff to help control what is frequently a slow to awaken, agitated and aggressive postoperative patient. Tracheal extubation should never be rushed in OSAHS patients. When a patient tells you that it took six people to hold him down the last time he had surgery, believe him. One anesthesiologist and one nurse should not be expected to awaken a 130 kg patient who feels that he cannot breathe and must sit up or roll over.

The goal should be to awaken the patient with adequate spontaneous ventilation as soon as possible. The patient with OSAHS requires a cautious evaluation prior to tracheal extubation, including the demonstration of deliberate and appropriate responses to multiple commands. It is helpful to inform the patient in the preoperative area what they will be asked to do, and to confirm the name that they prefer to be called upon awakening. There are a number of ways to assess a postoperative patient and it is important to include several of these when considering extubation in OSAHS patients. The anesthesiologist's goal is to determine the patient's ability to protect their airway. More common methods include neck flexion or fist clenching for greater than 5 seconds, sustained tongue protrusion, and eye opening. Regardless of the technique used, the anesthesiologist looks for the ability of the patient to follow verbal commands repetitively; often the patient may raise his or her head for a very short time, but then falls back to sleep very quickly. 'Do not interpret mindless reaching for the ETT as purposeful movement.'[30] The more difficult the tracheal intubation, the more patience is needed waiting for the tracheal extubation. The patient should be asked to nod if awake, nod if they want the ETT removed, attempt to head raise, etc. The return of rhythmic, spontaneous ventilation of good tidal volume is also sought. If there is any doubt, the anesthesiologist should leave the ETT in place.

Once the patient seems ready for extubation, the anesthesiologist should run through another last moment checklist. Check that the IV is running and has sufficient intravenous solution left in the bag. If not, flush it or re-establish it before proceeding or hang another bag. Make sure that succinylcholine is ready if needed, that the suction is still working, and that adequate help is present should trouble arise. Available airway devices on hand should include a nasopharyngeal airway, a new styletted ETT, and a tube exchanging device. The worst patients probably should have their tracheas extubated over either an Eschmann tube exchange catheter (rigid but solid) or a ventilating catheter (longer and hollow) (Cook Airway Exchange Catheter, Cook Medical Inc., Bloomington, IN) (Fig. 15.4). Both catheters, once placed into the trachea, are usually well tolerated provided that they are not pushed in too far. Each serves as an introducer to facilitate the potential re-insertion of an ETT, although neither can absolutely guarantee the success of that re-insertion attempt. The Cook catheter has the added advantage of being hollow, and having a 15 mm adaptor to allow for ventilation or oxygen insufflation of the lungs, should that be necessary. The amount of positive pressure that can be achieved, however, is limited due to the relatively small inner diameter of the Cook catheter.

When the patient is considered ready, the extubation procedure begins by moving the patient into a semi-upright position (approximately 45 degrees) to help move the tongue forward and the abdominal contents down and away from the diaphragm. After the throat is suctioned thoroughly, positive pressure is administered. The ETT is removed and 100% oxygen is given immediately via facemask, along with a jaw thrust. If a Cook catheter has been placed, the majority of patients are observed in the operating room for about 10 minutes and then extubated there. The worst cases may be transported to the PACU with the catheter in place and extubated later when they are fully awake. Some anesthesiologists believe that there is a role for doxapram (0.5–1.0 mg/kg) during emergence to stimulate ventilation and to help speed up awakening. The first minutes after tracheal extubation are crucial, as direct access to the airway has been lost, and postoperative edema and airway closure may ensue. Previously placed nasopharyngeal airway devices bypass the surgical site and decrease the patient's work of breathing significantly. An oropharyngeal airway is not as well tolerated as a nasal, but may be used if needed. In addition, elevation of the head of the bed after surgery reduces soft tissue edema at the surgical sites and turbinate engorgement, thus improving the nasal airway diameter and airflow.

Two other immediate concerns after sleep apnea surgery (and tracheal extubation) are laryngospasm and obstruction secondary to local analgesic use and the presence of blood and other secretions. Although preoperative glycopyrrolate and judicious postoperative suctioning minimize the risk, laryngospasm may still occur. Treatment should include head extension, anterior displacement of the mandible, and positive airway pressure. If these maneuvers fail to stabilize the airway, direct laryngoscopy with tracheal reintubation is necessary; cricothyrotomy may be performed on rare occasions. Local anesthetics like bupivacaine and lidocaine are frequently used in sleep apnea surgeries and may exhibit unwanted side effects. For example, tongue ablation procedures require the injection of local anesthetic into the tongue base to diminish postoperative pain. However, when the operation is over, patients can experience difficulty with tongue proprioception, leading to feelings of obstruction and possible airway impediment. Minimizing the dose of local anesthetics, postoperative patient reassurance, and meticulous postoperative airway management are important.

## 4 POSTOPERATIVE CARE

The anesthesiologist's primary concerns for the postoperative period center on the patency of the airway and the adequacy of ventilation and oxygenation. Potential edema, bleeding, or opioid-induced airway obstruction/hypoventilation are the factors that have led to a tendency to monitor these patients in the intensive care unit (ICU), but recent studies indicate ICU admissions may not be necessary for all patients. Significant complications generally emerge within the immediate postoperative period. Accordingly, a patient's status should be evaluated frequently in the postanesthesia care unit and the level of postoperative care should be decided upon then. If in doubt, the conservative approach is to admit the patient to a surgical intensive care unit.

Airway edema is a major concern for patients undergoing surgical repair for OSAHS. Small airways compounded with surgical trauma or a difficult intubation put OSAHS patients at a higher risk for airway compromise. It is of paramount importance for both the anesthesiologist and the surgeon to make all attempts at reducing airway edema in patients undergoing OSAHS surgery. Preoperative and postoperative intravenous steroids have routinely been shown to be effective in the reduction of airway edema. Dexametasone

# SECTION E: ANESTHESIA FOR OSA/HS

**Difficult airway algorithm**

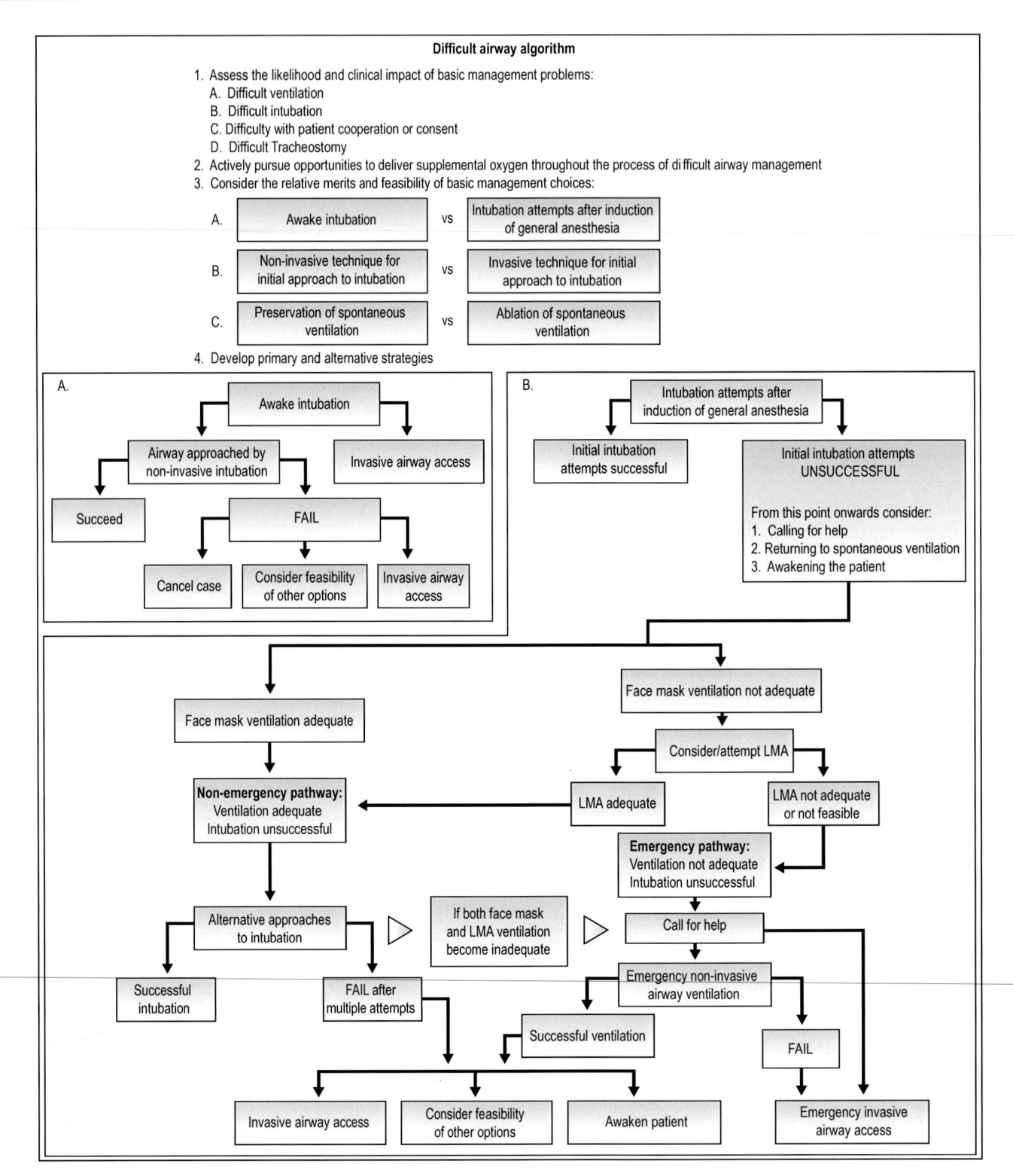

1. Assess the likelihood and clinical impact of basic management problems:
   A. Difficult ventilation
   B. Difficult intubation
   C. Difficulty with patient cooperation or consent
   D. Difficult Tracheostomy
2. Actively pursue opportunities to deliver supplemental oxygen throughout the process of difficult airway management
3. Consider the relative merits and feasibility of basic management choices:

   A. Awake intubation **vs** Intubation attempts after induction of general anesthesia
   B. Non-invasive technique for initial approach to intubation **vs** Invasive technique for initial approach to intubation
   C. Preservation of spontaneous ventilation **vs** Ablation of spontaneous ventilation

4. Develop primary and alternative strategies

**A. Awake intubation**
- Airway approached by non-invasive intubation → Succeed / FAIL → Cancel case / Consider feasibility of other options / Invasive airway access
- Invasive airway access

**B. Intubation attempts after induction of general anesthesia**
- Initial intubation attempts successful
- Initial intubation attempts UNSUCCESSFUL
  From this point onwards consider:
  1. Calling for help
  2. Returning to spontaneous ventilation
  3. Awakening the patient

Face mask ventilation adequate → **Non-emergency pathway:** Ventilation adequate, Intubation unsuccessful → Alternative approaches to intubation → Successful intubation / FAIL after multiple attempts

Face mask ventilation not adequate → Consider/attempt LMA → LMA adequate / LMA not adequate or not feasible

**Emergency pathway:** Ventilation not adequate, Intubation unsuccessful → Call for help → Emergency non-invasive airway ventilation → Successful ventilation / FAIL → Emergency invasive airway access

If both face mask and LMA ventilation become inadequate

Invasive airway access / Consider feasibility of other options / Awaken patient

**Fig. 15.4** The difficult airway algorithm. From the American Society of Anesthesiologists Task Force on Management of the Difficult Airway. Practice guidelines for management of the difficult airway: an updated report by the American Society of Anesthesiologists Task Force on Management of the Difficult Airway. Anesthesiology 2003;98(5):1269–77, with permission.

(8–12 mg), which is administered just prior to surgery, should be repeated every 8 hours postoperatively (8 mg).

Adequate blood pressure control is very important in the management of a postoperative OSAHS patient. Hypertension is more commonly seen in OSAHS patients secondary to their heightened sympathetic drive. Consequently, elevated blood pressure leads to more bleeding and increased tissue swelling. Although induced hypotension is not currently used for OSA surgeries, the patient's blood pressure should be managed prior to the procedure and controlled throughout the perioperative period. Another aspect of postoperative edema control is hemostasis. Current options for managing intraoperative bleeding are electrocautery, vessel ligature, thrombin on absorbable gelatin sponge (Gelfoam®, Pharmacia & Upjohn Co., Kalamazoo, MI), or a topical gelatin hemostatic matrix (Floseal, Baxter Bioscience, Fremont, CA). Finally, other means of controlling postoperative edema include elevating the head of the bed to improve venous return and tissue cooling with ice packs and ice chips.

Postoperative pain management for OSAHS patient is another topic with a debated and well-studied history. Ideally, the selected analgesic should have minimal effect on respiratory drive and airway muscle tone while supplying strong, adequate pain control. In addition, it is important to remember the sedatives and narcotics used throughout the case, because of their lingering analgesic and depressant effects on the patient. Unfortunately, the spectrum of pharmaceutical options for analgesia ranges from minimal pain relief with a low incidence of side effects, to good pain relief with a higher incidence of side effects. Non-steroidal anti-inflammatory drugs (NSAIDs) are usually inadequate for postoperative pain control, and standard narcotic dosing or patient-controlled analgesic infusions (PCAs) put the patient at increased risk of obstructive complications. One regimen found to be effective involves lower dosed intravenous narcotics for immediate pain control and oral hydrocodone or acetaminophen with codeine once the patient resumes eating.

## REFERENCES

1. Young T, Palta M, Dempsey J, Skatrud J, Weber S, Badr S. The occurrence of sleep-disordered breathing among middle-aged adults. N Engl J Med 1993;328(17):1230–35.
2. van Boxem TJ, de Groot GH. Prevalence and severity of sleep disordered breathing in a group of morbidly obese patients. Neth J Med 1999;54(5):202–6.
3. Leiter JC. Upper airway shape: is it important in the pathogenesis of obstructive sleep apnea? Am J Respir Crit Care Med 1996;153(3):894–98.
4. Benumof JL. Obstructive sleep apnea in the adult obese patient: implications for airway management. J Clin Anesth 2001;13(2):144–56.
5. Gross JB, Bachenberg KL, Benumof JL, et al. American Society of Anesthesiologists Task Force on Perioperative Management. Practice guidelines for the perioperative management of patients with obstructive sleep apnea: a report by the American Society of Anesthesiologists Task Force on perioperative management of patients with obstructive sleep apnea. Anesthesiology 2006;104(5):1081–93. quiz 1117–8.
6. Orr WC. Sleep apnea, hypoxemia, and cardiac arrhythmias [Editorial]. Chest 1986;89(1):1–2.
7. Fletcher EC. The relationship between systemic hypertension and obstructive sleep apnea: facts and theory. Am J Med 1995;98(2):118–28.
8. Schafer H, Hasper E, Ewig S, et al. Pulmonary haemodynamics in obstructive sleep apnoea: time course and associated factors. Eur Respir J 1998;12(3):679–84.
9. Berman EJ, DiBenedetto RJ, Causey DE, et al. Right ventricular hypertrophy detected by echocardiography in patients with newly diagnosed obstructive sleep apnea. Chest 1991;100(2):347–50.
10. Wilson ME, Spiegelhalter D, Robertson JA, Lesser P. Predicting difficult intubation. Br J Anaesth 1988;61(2):211–16.
11. Brodsky JB, Lemmens HJ, Brock-Utne JG, Vierra M, Saidman LJ. Morbid obesity and tracheal intubation. Anesth Analg 2002;94(3):732–36.
12. Vanner RG, Clarke P, Moore WJ, Raftery S. The effect of cricoid pressure and neck support on the view at laryngoscopy. Anaesthesia 1997;52(9):896–900.
13. el-Ganzouri AR, McCarthy RJ, Tuman KJ, Tanck EN, Ivankovich AD. Preoperative airway assessment: predictive value of a multivariate risk index. Anesth Analg 1996;82(6):1197–204.
14. Mallampati SR, Gatt SP, Gugino LD, et al. A clinical sign to predict difficult tracheal intubation: a prospective study. 1985;32(4):429–34.
15. Samsoon GL, Young JR. Difficult tracheal intubation: a retrospective study. Anaesthesia 1987;42(5):487–90.
16. Bonora M, St John WM, Bledsoe TA. Differential elevation by protriptyline and depression by diazepam of upper airway respiratory motor activity. Am Rev Respir Dis 1985;131(1):41–45.
17. VanDercar DH, Martinez AP, De Lisser EA. Sleep apnea syndromes: a potential contraindication for patient-controlled analgesia. Anesthesiology 1991;74(3):623–24.
18. Lamarche Y, Martin R, Reiher J, Blaise G. The sleep apnoea syndrome and epidural morphine. Can Anaesth Soc J 1986;33(2):231–33.
19. Jense HG, Dubin SA, Silverstein PI, O'Leary-Escolas U. Effect of obesity on safe duration of apnea in anesthetized humans. Anesth Analg 1991;72(1):89–93.
20. Ferretti A, Giampiccolo P, Cavalli A, Milic-Emili J, Tantucci C. Expiratory flow limitation and orthopnea in massively obese subjects. Chest 2001;119(5):1401–408.
21. Collins JS, Lemmens HJ, Brodsky JB, Brock-Utne JG, Levitan RM. Laryngoscopy and morbid obesity: a comparison of the 'sniff' and 'ramped' positions. Obes Surg 2004;14(9):1171–75.
22. American Society of Anesthesiologists Task Force on Management of the Difficult Airway. Practice guidelines for management of the difficult airway: an updated report by the American Society of Anesthesiologists Task Force on Management of the Difficult Airway. Anesthesiology 2003;98(5):1269–77.
23. Dixon BJ, Dixon JB, Carden JR, et al. Preoxygenation is more effective in the 25 degrees head-up position than in the supine position in severely obese patients: a randomized controlled study. Anesthesiology 2005;102(6):1110–15. discussion 5A.
24. Teller LE, Alexander CM, Frumin MJ, Gross JB. Pharyngeal insufflation of oxygen prevents arterial desaturation during apnea. Anesthesiology 1988;69(6):980–82.
25. Cormack RS, Lehane J. Difficult tracheal intubation in obstetrics. Anaesthesia 1984;39(11):1105–111.
26. Benumof JL. Difficult laryngoscopy: obtaining the best view. Can J Anaesth 1994;41(5 Pt 1):361–65.
27. Levitan RM, Mechem CC, Ochroch EA, Shofer FS, Hollander JE. Head-elevated laryngoscopy position: improving laryngeal exposure during laryngoscopy by increasing head elevation. Ann Emerg Med 2003;41(3):322–30.
28. Benyamin RM, Wafai Y, Salem MR, Joseph NJ. Two-handed mask ventilation of the difficult airway by a single individual. Anesthesiology 1998;88(4):1134.
29. El-Orbany MI, Joseph NJ, Salem MR. Tracheal intubating conditions and apnoea time after small-dose succinylcholine are not modified by the choice of induction agent. Br J Anaesth 2005;95(5):710–14.
30. Benumof JL. Obesity, sleep apnea, the airway and anesthesia. Abstracted summary of Audio-Digest Anesthesiol 2004;46(247):221.

# SECTION F   TREATMENT SELECTION

# CHAPTER 16

# Friedman tongue position and the staging of obstructive sleep apnea/hypopnea syndrome

*Michael Friedman*

## 1 INTRODUCTION

Obstructive sleep apnea/hypopnea syndrome (OSAHS) is often the result of obstruction at multiple anatomic sites. Nasal, palatal and hypopharyngeal obstruction, acting alone or in concert, are frequently identified as the cause of snoring and OSAHS. Even in cases where a single site is primarily involved, the increase in negative pressure may induce further obstruction in other areas. When surgical management of OSAHS is considered, a clear understanding of the complex relationship between the sites of obstruction is essential to surgical success.

The importance of determining the sites of obstruction has led to the development of numerous methods that attempt to predict the location of the upper airway obstruction. These include snoring sound analysis, physical examination, computed tomography, magnetic resonance imaging, cephalometric studies and fluoroscopy, among others. Although these methods have demonstrated value, the number of methods described is evidence of the lack of agreement that any single method is perfect. The most commonly used method is the Mueller maneuver (MM). Borowiecki and Sassin first described this maneuver for the preoperative assessment of sleep-disordered breathing (SDB).[1] The MM consists of having the patient perform a forced inspiratory effort against an obstructed airway with fiberoptic endoscopic visualization of the upper airway. The test is widely used and simple to perform. Despite this, its use is controversial and certainly no studies have been able to associate the maneuver as a tool for patient selection. It is within this context that the Friedman tongue positions (FTP) emerged.

Initially presented by Friedman et al. in 1999,[2] FTP (previously identified as the Mallampati palate position and subsequently as the Friedman palate position) has been found to be a simple method to approximate obstruction at the hypopharyngeal level. This classification is based on observations by Mallampati, who published a paper on palate position as an indicator of the ease or difficulty of endotracheal intubation by standard anesthesiologist techniques.[3] The Mallampati stages had only been studied in the context of difficult intubations; therefore two major modifications were incorporated into FTP for its use in sleep medicine. First, the anesthesiologist assessment is based on the patient sticking out their tongue and the observer then noting the relationship of the soft palate to the tongue. FTP is based on evaluating the tongue in a neutral, natural position inside the mouth. Second, the Mallampati system had only three grades. Initially, FTP included four distinct positions, but we now believe that five positions are necessary to best describe the anatomy (Table 16.1). Due to these modifications and because this system describes the position of the tongue relative to the tonsils/pillar, uvula, soft palate, and hard palate, we have identified it as the Friedman tongue position (FTP). FTP has been studied extensively as it relates to OSAHS. As there are no studies that have been done on the 'Mallampati position' in sleep medicine, the use of the term is inaccurate in the context of OSAHS.

The procedure for identifying FTP involves asking the patient to open their mouth widely without protruding the tongue. The procedure is repeated five times so that the observer can assign the most consistent position as the FTP. FTP I allows the observer to visualize the entire uvula and tonsils or pillars (Fig. 16.1). FTP IIa allows visualization of the uvula but only parts of the tonsils are seen. FTP IIb allows visualization of the complete soft palate down to the base of the uvula, but the uvula and the tonsils are not seen. FTP III allows visualization of some of the soft palate but the distal soft palate is eclipsed. FTP IV allows visualization of the hard palate only (Fig. 16.1).

Earlier publications have described only four FTPs. In our experience with the system over the years, we have found that the previous staging system a majority of patients were classified as FTP III. With such a large number of subjects categorized into this one position we believe that it is clinically relevant to further stratify this group in terms of characteristics and response to surgical outcomes. We have found that expanding FTP II into two groups, FTP IIa and FTP IIb, provides the means for achieving this stratification. Patients with FTP IIb, although they may have been formerly classified as FTP III

Table 16.1 Comparison of the original and the new FTP

| Original | | | New | | |
|---|---|---|---|---|---|
| FTP | Anatomical structures visualized | Anatomical structures not visualized | FTP | Anatomical structures visualized | Anatomical structures not visualized |
| I | Tonsils and pillars Entire uvula | | I | Tonsils and pillars Entire uvula | |
| II | Uvula | Tonsils and pillars | II a | Uvula | Tonsils and pillars |
| III | Most of the soft palate Base of the uvula | Uvula Tonsils and pillars | II b | Most of the soft palate Base of the uvula | Uvula Tonsils and pillars |
| IV | Only the hard palate | Tonsils and pillars Uvula | III | Some of soft palate | Tonsils and pillars Distal soft palate Base of the uvula |
| | | | IV | Only the hard palate | Tonsils and pillars Uvula |

in the earlier staging system, share surgical response rates more characteristic of FTP II.

Once FTP is determined, the information can be incorporated into two distinct algorithms which can provide insights on the diagnosis and management of OSAHS. First, the use of FTP enables the clinician to predict the presence of OSAHS. A thorough history is most often the only screening for OSAHS. Unfortunately, many patients who are in denial about their symptoms cannot be identified by history alone, and therefore go undiagnosed. Routine use of FTP can be utilized as a cost-effective, non-invasive screening tool that will allow ready identification of patients that may suffer from OSAHS. Second, since FTP estimates the presence hypopharyngeal obstruction, determining FTP prior to surgical intervention can be instrumental in guiding the surgical management of OSAHS. Previous studies have demonstrated its ability to separate patients that will likely benefit from uvulopharyngopalatoplasty (UPPP) as a single modal treatment from those that will require multilevel surgical intervention.[4,5]

## 2 THE OSAHS SCORE

The estimated prevalence of OSAHS is 2% in women and 4% in men.[6] There is also clear evidence that associates OSAHS with hypertension, insulin resistance, coronary heart disease, myocardial infarction and stroke, as well as compromised quality of life and significant social and emotional problems;[7] yet it estimated that approximately 80% of cases remain undiagnosed.[8] The primary screening for OSAHS is by a thorough history. Patients who complain of snoring, excessive daytime sleepiness or observed apnea are usually the only ones who are further tested for OSAHS. The major inaccuracy of such a screening system is that history, in the context of OSAHS, has a low sensitivity.

The obstacles in eliciting history in sleep apnea patients are two-fold. First, because the patient is asleep when the pathology occurs, they are largely unaware of the problem and often deny symptoms. In such cases, only a history elicited from a bedpartner can offer sufficient insight into symptomology. Second, symptoms of OSAHS often overlap with other pathologies physical findings can help direct further testing. For example, a patient complaining of excessive sleepiness and fatigue may very likely receive a full work-up for depression and not OSAHS.

History is always the starting point for the screening and diagnosis of any medical condition. This is generally followed by a physical examination that can confirm the history or can bring to attention new concerns not identified in the history. The known physical findings that are associated with OSAHS include BMI, neck circumference, and tonsil size, are routinely assessed and are well defined. Descriptions of hypopharyngeal obstruction, however, have not been standardized. Often times the similar physical findings are reported with many arbitrary terms such as 'crowded oropharynx', 'macroglossia', 'retrognathia', etc. This causes much confusion in both patient care and in reporting data. The routine use of FTP in the context of OSAHS can help standardize the description of hypopharyngeal obstruction.

FTP can be employed in an algorithm that can help identify patients with OSAHS. This system is based on three readily identifiable and reproducible physical exam findings and can provide a simple means for screening patients. The system relies on calculating the patient's Body Mass Index (BMI), along with the assessment of the patient's tonsil size and FTP. FTP position is assessed according to the system stated in the previous section. Tonsil size and BMI are assessed as follows. Tonsil size is graded from 0 to 4. Tonsil size 1 implies tonsils hidden within the pillars. Tonsil size 2 implies the tonsil extending to the pillars. Size 3 tonsils are beyond the pillars but not to the midline. Tonsil size 4 implies tonsils that extend to the midline (Fig. 16.2).

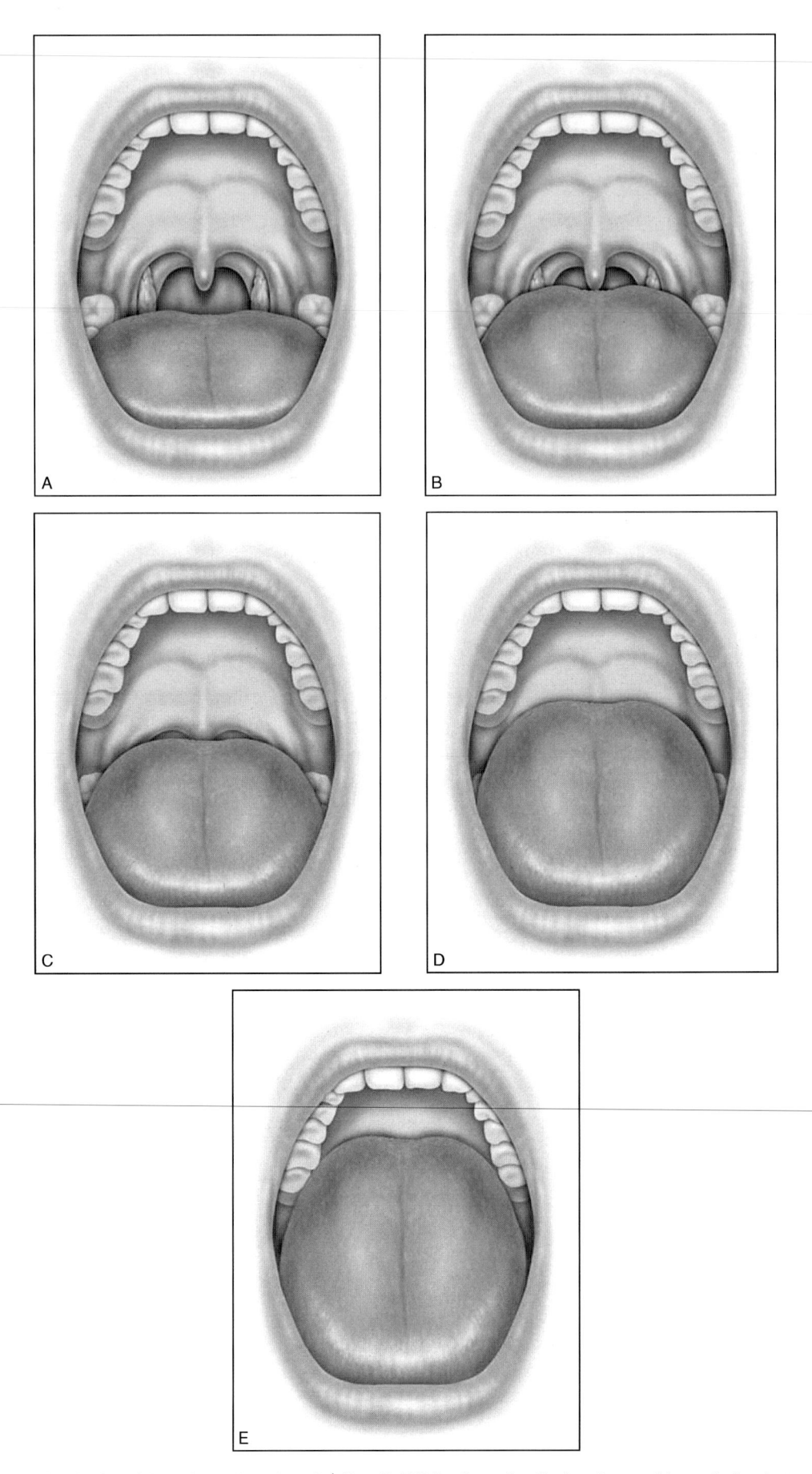

**Fig. 16.1** A, FTP I allows visualization of the entire uvula and tonsils/pillars. B, FTP IIa allows visualization of most of the uvula, but the tonsils/pillars are absent. C, FTP IIb allows visualization of the entire soft plate to the base of the uvula. D, In FTP III some of the soft palate is visualized but the distal structures are absent. E, FTP IV allows visualization of the hard palate only.

A BMI is derived from the height and weight of the patient and is calculated using the formula BMI = weight (kg)/height$^2$ (m$^2$). The BMI is graded as grade 0 (<20 kg/m$^2$), grade 1 (20–25 kg/m$^2$) grade 2 (25–30 kg/m$^2$), grade 3 (30–40 kg/m$^2$), and grade 4 (>40 kg/m$^2$) according to previously published standards for obesity. Neck circumference has been shown to correlate well as a clinical predictor, but BMI is an alternative measure that was used.

Once known, these three findings can be combined to calculate an OSAHS score. The OSAHS score can help identify patients that may have OSAHS via physical exam alone and does not rely on history. To calculate the OSAHS score the numerical values of these findings are summed:

$$\text{OSAHS score} = \text{FTP (0–IV)} + \text{tonsil size (0–4)} + \text{BMI value (0–4)}$$

Any value above an 8 is considered as a positive OSAHS score, whereas any value below 4 is considered a negative OSAHS score. A positive score has a positive predictive value of moderate OSAHS (defined as Apnea/Hypopnea Index (AHI) > 20) of 90%, and was 74% effective in predicting severe OSAHS (defined as AHI > 45). A negative score was 67% effective in predicting an AHI of <20.

With the use of FTP and the OSAHS score, the number of undiagnosed cases may also fall. In cases where history is unclear, this algorithm may help identify patients that may have otherwise gone unnoticed. In other cases, this algorithm may provide the impetus for eliciting a more detailed history and performing further tests to confirm suspicion of OSAHS.

## 3 SURGICAL STAGING OF OSAHS

Uvulopalatopharyngoplasty (UPPP) is the most common surgical procedure performed by otolaryngologists for the treatment of OSAHS. Unfortunately, a meta-analysis of unselected patients treated with UPPP revealed that only 40.79% of patients had a 'successful' surgery defined by an AHI reduction of 50% and a postoperative AHI < 20 or an Apnea Index (AI) reduced by 50% and a postoperative AI < 10.[9] Surgery with a 40% success rate is certainly less than ideal and our ultimate goal, of course, is to develop a treatment with a much higher success rate. But in the absence of such a treatment, our goal would be to identify those patients who are likely to benefit from UPPP, which is a valuable procedure for those patients who can be cured with it. The ideal system would identify those patients with a high likelihood of successful UPPP and separate them from those with a high likelihood of failure, thus guiding patient selection and improving outcomes.

Currently, the most common method used to identify patients for surgery is based on the misconception that patients with mild/moderate disease are better candidates for UPPP than those patients with severe disease. Therefore, the procedure is often recommended for patients with mild/moderate OSAHS. Severity of disease as determined by clinical symptoms, polysomnography results, or tools such as the Epworth Sleepiness Scale has been shown not to correlate with surgical success. Studies have shown that patients with mild SDB based on clinical and polysomnographic data have no better chance of successful treatment with UPPP than patients with severe disease.[5] In fact, one study demonstrated that UPPP performed on unselected patients with mild OSAHS (AHI < 15) not only does not cure disease in 60% of cases but often makes it worse.[10] Using severity of disease for the identification of UPPP candidates is tenuous at best, and at times results in negative outcomes.

The failure of UPPP to cure OSAHS has been clearly associated with sites of obstruction in the upper airway not corrected by the procedure. It is well known that OSAHS involves obstruction of the airway at multiple levels. Although palatal obstruction accounts for a large portion of the obstruction, hypopharyngeal obstruction can also play a significant role. UPPP alleviates obstruction at the level of the soft palate and tonsils, but does not address obstruction at the level of the hypopharynx. This is clearly a significant cause of the failure of UPPP. Therefore when devising a system that is intended to predict UPPP outcomes, the anatomical considerations must be incorporated.

FTP, used as an estimation of hypopharyngeal obstruction, can be integrated into an anatomical staging system that can reliably predict surgical outcomes. This system relies on BMI, tonsil size and FTP and can separate patients who will benefit from UPPP alone from those that will require multilevel surgical intervention. In this system stage I disease is defined as those patients with FTP I, IIa or IIb, tonsil size 3 or 4, and BMI < 40. Stage II disease is defined as FTP I, IIa or IIb and tonsil size 0, 1, or 2, or FTP III and IV with tonsil size 3 or 4, and BMI < 40. Stage III disease is defined as FTP III or IV and tonsil size 0, 1, or 2. Although somewhat controversial, most surgeons have found that patients with BMI > 40 have a poor prognosis for corrective UPPP and therefore these patients are automatically assigned to stage IV (Table 16.2). In addition, all patients with skeletal deformities such as micrognathia or mid-face hypoplasia are considered stage IV.

The rationale for such a staging system is that the success of UPPP is highly dependent on the anatomical relationship between palatal and hypopharyngeal obstruction. Stage I patients are those with favorable tongue position (I, IIa, IIb) indicating minimal hypoglossal obstruction and large tonsils. They are most likely to benefit from UPPP with tonsillectomy as hypopharyngeal obstruction does not represent a significant component of their disease. Stage

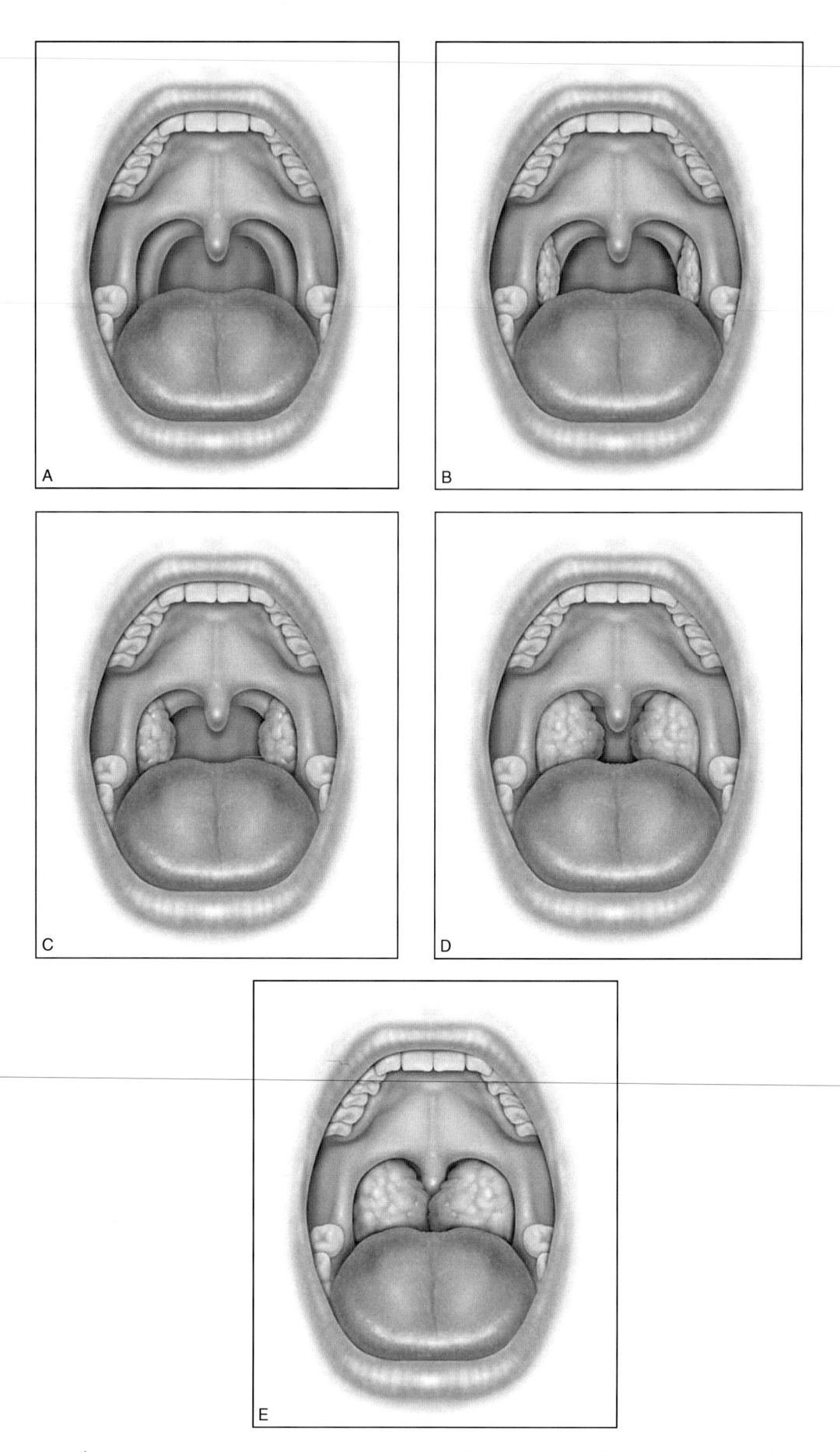

**Fig. 16.2** A, Tonsils, size 0, s/p tonsillectomy. B, Tonsils, size 1, within the pillars. C. Tonsils, size 2, extend to the pillars. D. Tonsils, size 3, extend past the pillars. E, Tonsils, size 4, extend to the midline.

| Table 16.2 | Staging system | | |
|---|---|---|---|
| Stage | FTP | Tonsil size | BMI |
| I | I, IIa, IIb | 3 or 4 | <40 |
| II | I, IIa, IIb | 0, 1 or 2 | <40 |
|  | III or IV | 3 or 4 | <40 |
| III | III or IV | 0, 1 or 2 | <40 |

Table 16.3 Success rate of uvulopalatopharyngoplasty in the treatment of SDB

| Stage | Unsuccessful | Successful | Total |
|---|---|---|---|
| I | 6 (19.4%) | 25 (80.6%) | 31 (100%) |
| II | 18 (62.1%) | 11 (37.9%) | 29 (100%) |
| III | 68 (91.9%) | 6 (8.1%) | 74 (100%) |

III patients are on the opposite extreme of the spectrum with small or no tonsils and unfavorable tongue position (III or IV) indicating significant hypopharyngeal obstruction. They are least likely to benefit from UPPP as UPPP will not address their hypopharyngeal obstruction. Stage II patients are those with either large tonsils and unfavorable tongue position or small tonsils and a favorable tongue position.

Table 16.3 demonstrates the evidence of success and failure rates of UPPP for the treatment of OSAHS according to aforementioned stages. Chi-square analysis demonstrates a highly significant relationship between stage and success of surgery. The Pearson chi-square = 54.2, with two degrees of freedom, and a two-sided $P < 0.0001$. Successful treatment of SDB with UPPP was most likely achieved in stage I patients (80.6%) and least likely in stage III patients (8.1%).

To further explore the relationship between the stages of disease and the efficacy of surgical treatment with UPPP, a stepwise multivariate discriminant analysis was performed. The preoperative criteria used to stratify patients into stages (BMI, tonsil, size and FTP) were the only indices introduced into the stepwise analysis. The success or failure of treatment with UPPP was used as the categorical end point. Using F values of 3.84 for entry and 2.71 for removal, stepwise analysis eliminated BMI, keeping tonsil size and FTP as the best combination of indices for differentiating between success and failure. The classification coefficients calculated for tonsil size and FTP were used to construct Fisher's linear classification functional equations. Fisher's linear classification equation for each group takes the form:

$$CF = \text{tonsils (Coef tonsils)} + \text{FTP (Coef FTP)} + \text{Constant}$$

where CF is group classification function; tonsils is tonsil size; Coef tonsils is group classification coefficient for tonsil size; FTP is FTP classification; Coef FTP is group classification coefficient for FTP; Constant is group constant.

A separate equation is constructed for each result, unsuccessful and successful.

In the present case:

$$\text{Unsuccessful result} = ((\text{tonsils})\,0.870) + ((\text{FTP})\,5.319) + (-10.563)$$

$$\text{Successful result} = ((\text{tonsils})\,2.284) + ((\text{FTP})\,2.333) + (-6.001)$$

To predict the success of UPPP in patients with OSAHS, enter the patient's tonsil size and FTP into each of the above formulas and calculate. The equation totaling the numerical highest value is the predicted result. In the validation study, the above formulas were applied casewise to the 134 patients and correctly predicted 95% of the cases by result.

While results of surgical treatment are never completely predictable for any disorder, clinical staging of the disorder offers several important benefits. Staging systems are created to identify those clinical features of the disease process that can predict whether any particular treatment option will be valuable. The use of the anatomic staging system in OSAHS offers a cost-effective, non-invasive, reproducible method to stratify patients based on anatomic variations. The use of this system in addition to detailed clinical examination, cephalometrics and Mueller maneuver can help improve surgical outcomes in OSAHS. Patients with stage I disease have better than an 80% chance of success with UPPP and should therefore undergo the procedure when non-surgical treatment has failed. Even patients with severe SDB had an 80% success rate if they had stage I disease based on this staging system. Patients with stage III disease should never undergo UPPP alone as a surgical cure for SDB. With an 8.1% success rate, the surgery is destined to fail. They should be treated with a combination of procedures that address both the palate and the hypopharynx. In our study, 78.3% of patients can be stratified into stage I or III. Patients with stage II disease do not fall into either extreme but probably can be treated similar to stage III patients.

## 4 CONCLUSIONS

Friedman tongue position (FTP) is a physical finding that can help with the diagnosis and surgical management of OSAHS. FTP describes the position of the tongue relative to the tonsils/pillar, uvula, soft palate, and hard palate and is easily assessed by physical examination of the oropharynx.

When combined with tonsil size and BMI, FTP can be used to calculate an OSAHS score, which can help screen for OSAHS in patients. FTP can also be integrated into an anatomical staging system that can help predict the likelihood of surgical success with UPPP. Stage I patients would most likely benefit from UPPP alone whereas stage II and stage III patients will likely need additional treatment to the hypopharynx.

## REFERENCES

1. Borowiecki BD, Sassin JF. Surgical treatment of sleep apnea. Arch Otolaryngol 1983;109:508–12.
2. Friedman M, Tanyeri H, La Rosa M, et al. Clinical predictors of obstructive sleep apnea. Laryngoscope 1999;109:1901–7.
3. Mallampati SR, Gatt SP, Gugino LD, et al. A clinical sign to predict difficult tracheal intubation: a prospective study. Can Anaesth Soc J 1985;32:429–34.
4. Friedman M, Ibrahim H, Joseph NJ. Staging of obstructive sleep apnea/hypopnea syndrome: a guide to appropriate treatment. Laryngoscope 2004;114:454–59.
5. Friedman M, Ibrahim H, Lee G, et al. Combined uvulopalatopharyngoplasty and radiofrequency tongue base reduction for treatment of obstructive sleep apnea/hypopnea syndrome. Otolaryngol Head Neck Surg 2003;129:611–21.
6. Young T, Palta M, Dempsey J, et al. The occurrence of sleep-disordered breathing among middle-aged adults. New Engl J Med 1993;328:1230–35.
7. Shahar E, Whitney CW, Redline S, et al. Sleep-disordered breathing and cardiovascular disease: cross-sectional results of the Sleep Heart Health Study. Am J Respir Crit Care Med 2001;163:19–25.
8. Young T, Evans L, Finn L, et al. Estimation of the clinically diagnosed proportion of sleep apnea syndrome in middle-aged men and women. Sleep 1997;20:705–6.
9. Sher AE, Schechtman KB, Piccirillo JF. The efficacy of surgical modifications of the upper airway in adults with obstructive sleep apnea syndrome. Sleep 1996;19:156–77.
10. Senior BA, Rosenthal L, Lumley A, et al. Efficacy of uvulopalatopharyngoplasty in unselected patients with mild obstructive sleep apnea. Otolaryngol Head Neck Surg 2000;123:179–82.

# SECTION F  TREATMENT SELECTION

## CHAPTER 17

# Multilevel surgery for obstructive sleep apnea/hypopnea syndrome

*Michael Friedman, Hsin-Ching Lin, T.K. Venkatesan and Berk Gurpinar*

Effective surgical treatment for obstructive sleep apnea/hypopnea syndrome (OSAHS) must be designed to eliminate collapsible soft tissue in the upper airway without interfering with normal function. Creation of a non-collapsible airspace and reduction of airway resistance enables maintenance of adequate airflow with normal inspiratory effort. This translates into elimination or reduction of apneic/hypopneic episodes during sleep, control of symptoms and further minimizes ongoing multi-system damage in OSAHS patients. OSAHS is often caused by multiple levels of obstruction and therefore requires multilevel treatment. In the last decade, several surgical advances have been made in the management of OSAHS.

In this chapter, we review the concept, techniques, evidence-based review of the literature and clinical highlights with respect to multilevel surgery for OSAHS.

## 1 CONCEPT OF MULTILEVEL TREATMENT – ESTABLISHING THE BASIS

### 1.1 INCIDENCE OF MULTILEVEL OBSTRUCTIONS IN OSAHS PATIENTS

The true incidence of multilevel obstruction is a subject of much debate. Fujita[1] first described different anatomic levels of obstruction in OSAHS. He recognized that half of the patients who underwent uvulopalatopharyngoplasty (UPPP) were non-responders. Most of the non-responders were identified as having multilevel obstruction. Combined oropharyngeal and hypopharyngeal obstruction was noted in 54.5% (36/66) of patients in his study. Thus, it is clear that Fujita himself never intended to suggest that UPPP will cure most patients with OSAHS. In 1993, Riley et al.[2] reported their surgical experience, outlining a multilevel concept. Each patient was classified as having single level obstruction involving oropharynx only – type 1 – or the hypopharynx only – type 3. Multilevel obstruction was identified as type 2 and implied a combination of oropharyngeal and hypopharyngeal obstruction. Of the 239 patients, 93.3% (223 patients) were identified as having multilevel obstruction, type 2. Only 16 patients (6.7%) had single level obstruction. Of these, 10 patients had type 1 obstruction and six patients had type 3 obstruction.

This early classification by Fujita and Riley was based on physical examination of the patients with vague guidelines. Specific criteria for identifying unilevel versus multilevel obstruction were not reported. Subsequent development of the Friedman tongue position (FTP) allowed for a simplified method of staging the levels of obstruction.[3,4] The early data based on FTP indicated that approximately 25% of patients presenting with OSAHS had unilevel obstruction, while 75% had multilevel obstruction.

To more precisely identify the anatomic sites of obstruction during sleep, sleep endoscopy was proposed as a preferred method. den Herder et al.[5] reported an unusually high number of single level obstructions. In their study of 127 patients, 63% had single level obstruction while only 37% had multilevel disease. The study, however, may have misidentified the level of obstruction; tongue base obstruction pushing the palate backward causing secondary palatal obstruction may have been classified as primary palatal obstruction.[6] Another study by Abdullah van Hasselt confirmed the high incidence of multilevel disease and 87% of their 893 patient populations had multilevel obstruction.[7]

Many other techniques to identify levels of obstruction have been reported. The most popular are the Mueller maneuver and cephalometry. Both of these are used to identify the levels of obstruction. Other diagnostic aids such as sleep MRI have also been reported. The other techniques are reviewed in other chapters.

### 1.2 SINGLE LEVEL SURGERY CANNOT BE THE ONLY TREATMENT FOR MOST OSAHS PATIENTS

UPPP was designed to enlarge the oropharyngeal airway[8] and remains the most common surgical intervention for OSAHS. Review of the literature indicates the success rate (a 50% reduction in Apnea/Hypopnea Index (AHI) and a postoperative AHI of less than 20) for UPPP as an isolated procedure ranges from 25% to 80%. However, Sher et al.[9] reported success rates for UPPP around 41% based on a meta-analysis of unselected cases. Although there are many reasons UPPP may fail, uncorrected retrolingual obstruction has been clearly identified as a major cause. This seems to support the concept that multiple levels of obstruction exist and explains why UPPP alone frequently results in failure.

## 1.3 MULTILEVEL SURGERY IS NOT LIMITED TO SEVERE DISEASE

Many otolaryngologists presume that although UPPP may not cure the patients with severe OSAHS, it is likely to be effective for patients with mild disease. There are however many studies indicating that the severity of disease is not a predictor of success with single level surgery.[3,4,10] Senior et al.[11] studied a group of patients with mild OSAHS (AHI less than 15). These patients underwent UPPP and the success rate was only 40%. Friedman further studied a series of patients with mild disease and showed an overall success rate of approximately 40% as well.[3,4] If indeed most patients have multilevel disease, the success for the surgical treatment of mild OSAHS is not better than those for treating severe disease. In fact, the basis of the Friedman staging system is that anatomic findings are the most significant factors, rather than severity of disease. Multilevel surgery should not be reserved exclusively for the treatment of severe disease. It is therefore reasonable that multilevel treatment should be considered for most patients with mild disease as well as most patients with severe disease. Since the majority of patients suffering from OSAHS do have multilevel disease and directing the therapy to a single anatomic level has a high potential for failure, the need for multilevel therapy is evident.

## 2 HISTORY OF MULTILEVEL TREATMENT

Historically, surgical treatment for OSAHS was often based on trial and error. Patients would invariably undergo UPPP as a first stage. If the disease was not eliminated, they would go on to have hypopharyngeal surgery. Planned multilevel surgery at a single phase however has now become standard in many centers.

Published data on multilevel treatment can be divided into four groups.

1. The most commonly performed multilevel approach includes a UPPP as a basic technique with a second procedure designed to improve the hypopharyngeal airway. Most commonly this includes genioglossus advancement, thyrohyoid advancement, radiofrequency tissue volume reduction of the tongue base, and in some cases tongue base suspension.[12–15] The success rate for these procedures has been reported to be between 20% and 100% and was based on retrospective studies on small groups of patients. The largest series reported by a single group was by Riley et al.[2] who studied 239 patients who underwent what they describe as phase I surgery. In their study, 223 patients (93.3%) underwent multilevel surgery (UPPP + GAHM) in the initial phase. Their success rate based on single stage multilevel treatment for patients with mild, moderate and severe OSAHS was 60%.
2. The second group of patients studied who have undergone multilevel treatment include those who have had more invasive and more radical hypopharyngeal surgery such as open tongue base resection. Because of the aggressive nature of these procedures, most of these patients had a temporary tracheotomy and required significant hospitalization. There was significant postoperative morbidity as well. The success rate in this group varied between 44% and 100%.[2,15–18]
3. The third group of multilevel surgery for OSAHS included those patients undergoing bimaxillary advancement as part of the multilevel treatment program. Most of these patients had undergone a staged surgery often, with UPPP and genioglossus advancement as their primary procedure. This group was not included in the overall discussion and recommendation for treatment in this chapter.
4. 'Multilevel minimally invasive treatment for mild/moderate OSAHS' will be discussed in the next section. This section also lists minimally invasive as well as invasive procedures to address obstruction at the level of the nose, oropharynx and hypopharynx.

## 3 MULTILEVEL MINIMALLY INVASIVE TREATMENT FOR MILD/MODERATE OSAHS

The ideal procedure for OSAHS patients would have low morbidity, allow reasonable success, have low risk of alteration of the original upper aerodigestive tract function, and could be performed in a single stage. In our experience, patients with severe disease and obvious daytime sleepiness often have strong motivation for multilevel surgery with invasive procedures to address the obstructed sites. However, patients with mild or moderate obstructive sleep apnea are less likely to be willing to undergo aggressive surgical procedures.

Many options are available for minimally invasive treatment of palatal obstruction. Minimally invasive treatment options for retrolingual obstruction are limited, but have been in clinical use. There have been a few studies that looked at multilevel minimally invasive treatment. Steward[19] studied 22 patients who underwent combined radiofrequency reduction of the palate and the base of tongue and reported a success rate of 59%. None of the patients had concomitant nasal surgery. Fischer et al. presented a similar study about multilevel minimally invasive surgery with radiofrequency on the palate, tonsil and tongue base for 15 OSAHS patients.[20] The results showed that the AHI changed from 32.6 ± 17.4 preoperatively to 22 ± 15 for a success rate of 33%. Whereas the majority of Fischer's patients had moderate disease, Steward's patients had mild-to-moderate disease.

In 2004, Stuck et al.[21] published their surgical results with radiofrequency on the palate and base of the tongue for 18 OSAHS patients with mild/moderate disease. They reported their success rate as 33.3% (by their definition of success, a postoperative AHI reduction of at least 50% and below a value of 15).

In 2007, we presented our experience on minimally invasive single-stage multilevel surgery (MISSMLS) for patients with mild/moderate OSAHS.[22] Our patients underwent three-level treatment that included nasal surgery, palatal stiffening by pillar implant technique and radiofrequency volume reduction of the tongue base with a minimum follow-up of 6 months. The results in a retrospective review of a prospective dataset showed that both subjective and objective outcomes improved significantly, and treatment morbidity was minimal and only temporary. Mean bedpartner's snoring visual analog scale (VAS) decreased from 9.4 ± 0.9 preoperatively to 3.2 ± 2.4 postoperatively. Epworth Sleepiness Scale (ESS) decreased from 9.7 ± 3.9 preoperatively to 6.9 ± 3.3 postoperatively. Mean AHI was reduced from 23.2 ± 7.6 to 14.5 ± 10.2. Classic success was achieved in 54 of 122 patients (47.5%).

Although there was a significant failure rate, patients that failed were candidates for additional procedures. The first stage procedures that were performed including pillar palatal implantation and radiofrequency tongue base tissue volume reduction in no way negatively affected their ability to undergo secondary UPPP or additional tongue base procedures. Thus, many of the patients in our study who failed went on to undergo classic UPPP combined with additional hypopharyngeal procedures. Presence of pillar implants in the palate did not affect the UPPP in any way that could be determined by the surgeons. Patients who underwent previous radiofrequency tongue base reduction were still candidates for additional radiofrequency treatment or other hypopharyngeal procedures. This MISSMLS approach resulted in a fairly high patient satisfaction rate even though many patients required secondary procedures.

MISSMLS offers reasonable improvement of both subjective symptoms and objective PSG findings in patients with mild/moderate OSAHS. Polysomnographic respiratory parameters, ESS and snoring VAS show statistically significant improvement in patients with mild/moderate OSAHS treated with MISSMLS.

The success rate of any protocol has to be weighed against associated morbidity and risks. The relatively low morbidity combined with reasonable success makes multilevel minimally invasive surgery for OSAHS worthwhile. It should be offered to patients when multilevel obstruction is identified in the context of mild/moderate disease and other non-surgical options have been excluded.

## 4 SYSTEMATIC REVIEW OF LITERATURE ON MULTILEVEL TREATMENT FOR OSAHS PATIENTS

There has been a significant increase in publications on the multilevel approach for OSAHS patients within the last 5 years. The procedures include modification of previously invasive procedures, combination of minimally invasive techniques and classic surgery, and even minimally invasive single-stage multilevel surgery.

We recently reported on a systematic review of all English language literature on multilevel surgery for OSAHS patients as of 31 March 2007.[23] Article titles and abstracts were reviewed to determine article eligibility. We also identified relevant publications from the lists of references in this subset of articles. The study design and its corresponding level of evidence were clarified as follows: (1) Level 1 – randomized controlled trials or a systematic review; (2) Level 2 – prospective cohort study; (3) Level 3 – case–control study; (4) Level 4 – case series; and (5) Level 5 – expert opinion.

There were 49 papers (58 groups) selected for final inclusion after detailed review (Table 17.1). There were 1978 subjects included in the study with a pooled mean age of 46.2 years. The mean minimal time period from multilevel surgery to postoperative PSG was 7.3 months (range, 1–100 months).

The originally reported success rate in the included literature was 64.5%. However, the definition of success used by the authors of the various papers reviewed was not consistent. Therefore, a meta-analysis was performed to redefine the success rate to be consistent with the commonly agreed upon criteria – namely 'a reduction in AHI of 50% or more and an AHI of less than 20'. The recalculated success rate was 66.4%.

An improvement in lowest saturation of oxygen (LSAT) was reported in 18 out of 33 groups (54.5%) and the weighted average percentage change showed a 10.8% improvement after multilevel surgery. Bedpartner's snoring VAS revealed an improvement in eight out of nine groups (88.9%) and the weighted average percentage change demonstrated a 65.1% decrease postoperatively. ESS showed an improvement in 23 of 26 groups (88.4%) and the weighted average percentage change improved by 43.0% postoperatively.

Multilevel surgery for OSAHS is obviously associated with improved outcomes, although this benefit is supported largely by level 4 evidence. Future research should conduct larger, higher level and longer-term studies to further validate the results.

# SECTION F: TREATMENT SELECTION

**Table 17.1** Peer reviewed studies on multilevel surgery for OSAHS

| Author, year | N | Approach levels | Severity of OSAHS | F/U (month) | Original success (%) | Original def. for success | Redefining success (%) | EBM level |
|---|---|---|---|---|---|---|---|---|
| Waite,[24] 1989 | 23 | 3 | All | 1.5 | 65.2 | 6 | 69.6 | 4 |
| Riley[25]-phase 1, 1989 | 55 | 2 | Mo-Se | 6 | 67.3 | 1 | 67.3 | 4 |
| Riley,[26] 1990 | 40 | 2 | Se | 6 | 97.5 | 1 | 97.5 | 4 |
| Djupesland,[27] 1992 | 20 | 2 | mi-Se | 3.5 | 50 | 5 | NA | 4 |
| Riley[2]-phase 1, 1993 | 239 | 2, 3 | mi-Se | 6 | 60 | 1 | 60 | 4 |
| Johnson,[28] 1994 | 9 | 2 | Mo-Se | 3 | 77.8 | 5 | 77.8 | 4 |
| Ramirez,[29] 1996 | 12 | 2, 3 | Se | 6 | 41.7 | 1 | 41.7 | 4 |
| Mickelson,[30] 1997 | 12 | 2 | Mo-Se | 2 | 25 | 5 | 25 | 4 |
| Hochban,[31] 1997 | 38 | 2 | Mo-Se | 2 | 97.4 | 6 | 97.4 | 4 |
| Elasfour,[18] 1998 | 18 | 2 | Se | 3 | 61.1 | 5 | 44.4 | 4 |
| Chabolle,[17] 1999 | 10 | 2, 3 | Se | 3 | 80 | 1 | 80 | 4 |
| Li,[32] 1999 | 175 | 2, 3 | Se | 6 | 94.9 | 1 | 94.9 | 4 |
| Lee,[33] 1999 | 35 | 2 | mi-Se | 4 | 68.6 | 4 | 68.6 | 4 |
| Andsberg,[34] 2000 | 16 | 2 | mi-Se | 100 | 56.3 | 3 | NA | 4 |
| Battega[35]-group 1, 2000 | 44 | 2, 3 | Mo-Se | 6 | 22.7 | 2 | NA | 4 |
| Riley,[36] 2000 | 40 | 2 | Se | 12 | 90 | 1 | 90 | 4 |
| Li,[37] 2000 | 19 | 2 | Se | 6 | 94.7 | 1 | 94.7 | 4 |
| Hendler,[38] 2001 | 33 | 2 | mi-Se | 6 | 48.5 | 5 | 45.5 | 4 |
| Nelson[39]-group 1, 2001 | 7 | 2 | mi-Se | 2 | 57.1 | 1 | 57.1 | 4 |
| Nelson[39]-group 2, 2001 | 10 | 3 | mi-Se | 2 | 50 | 1 | 50 | 4 |
| Hsu,[40] 2001 | 13 | 2 | Mo-Se | NA | 76.9 | 1 | 76.9 | 4 |
| Terris,[41] 2002 | 12 | 2 | Mo-Se | 3 | 66.7 | 1 or 3 | NA | 4 |
| Miller,[42] 2002 | 15 | 2 | Mo-Se | 3 | 20 | 1 | 20 | 4 |
| Kao,[43] 2003 | 42 | 2, 3 | mi-Se | NA | 83.3 | 1 | 83.3 | 4 |
| Woodson,[44] 2003 | 26 | 2 | mi-Mo | 6 | NA | NA | NA | 1 |
| Friedman,[45] 2003 | 143 | 2 | mi-Se | 6 | 40.9 | 1 | 40.9 | 4 |
| Thomas[46]-group 1, 2003 | 8 | 2 | Mo-Se | 4 | 50 | 2 | NA | 3 |
| Thomas[46]-group 2, 2003 | 9 | 2 | Mo-Se | 4 | 57.1 | 2 | NA | 3 |
| Fischer,[20] 2003 | 15 | 2 | mi-Mo | 3 | 33.3 | 1 | 33.3 | 4 |
| Neruntarat,[47] 2003 | 31 | 2 | Mo-Se | 3 | 70.1 | 1 | 70.1 | 4 |
| Neruntarat,[48] 2003 | 46 | 2 | Se | 37 | 65.2 | 1 | 65.2 | 4 |
| Neruntarat,[49] 2003 | 32 | 2 | Mo-Se | 5 | 78.1 | 1 | 78.1 | 4 |
| Stuck,[21] 2004 | 18 | 2 | mi-Mo | 3 | 33.3 | 2 | 44.4 | 4 |
| Li[16]-group 1, 2004 | 6 | 2 | Se | NA | 83.3 | 1 | 83.3 | 4 |
| Li[16]-group 2, 2004 | 6 | 2 | Se | NA | 0 | 1 | 0 | 4 |
| Steward,[19] 2004 | 22 | 2 | mi-Mo | NA | 59.1 | 1 | 59.1 | 4 |
| Miller,[13] 2004 | 24 | 2 | Mo-Se | 3 | 66.7 | 1 | 66.7 | 4 |
| Dattilo[50]-phase 1, 2004 | 42 | 2 | mi-Se | 2 | 78.6 | 7 | 71.4 | 4 |
| Dattilo[50]-phase 2, 2004 | 15 | 2 | Mo-Se | 2 | 93.3 | 2 | 93.3 | 4 |
| Omur,[51] 2005 | 22 | 2 | Mo-Se | 6 | 81.8 | 1 | 81.8 | 4 |
| Pang[52]-group 1, 2005 | 12 | 3 | Mo-Se | NA | 75 | 1 | 75 | 4 |
| Li[53]-group 1, 2005 | 55 | 2 | Mo-Se | 6 | 81.8 | 1 | 81.8 | 4 |
| Li[53]-group 2, 2005 | 30 | 2 | Mo-Se | 6 | 73.3 | 1 | 73.3 | 4 |
| Steward,[54] 2005 | 29 | 2 | mi-Mo | 12 | NA | NA | NA | 4 |
| Bowden,[55] 2005 | 29 | 2, 3 | mi-Se | 4 | 17.2 | 1 | 17.2 | 4 |
| Liu,[56] 2005 | 44 | 2 | Se | 3 | 52.3 | 1 | 52.3 | 4 |
| Smatt,[57] 2005 | 18 | 2 | Se | 6 | 83.3 | 2 | NA | 4 |
| Sorrenti,[15] 2006 | 10 | 2 | Se | 6 | 100 | 1 | 100 | 4 |
| Jacobowitz,[58] 2006 | 37 | 2 | Mo-Se | 3 | 75.7 | 1 | 75.7 | 4 |
| Verse[12]-group 1, 2006 | 45 | 2 | Mo-Se | 2 | 51.1 | 2 | NA | 3 |
| Verse[12]-group 2, 2006 | 15 | 2 | Mo-Se | 2 | 40 | 2 | NA | 3 |
| Vicente,[14] 2006 | 55 | 2, 3 | Se | 36 | 76.4 | 1 | 76.4 | 4 |
| Friedman[59]-group 2a, 2006 | 22 | 2 | Mi | 4 | 36.4 | 1 | 36.4 | 4 |
| Friedman[59]-group 2b, 2006 | 15 | 2 | Mo | 4 | 46.7 | 1 | 46.7 | 4 |
| Friedman[59]-group 3, 2006 | 55 | 2 | mi-Se | 4 | 38.2 | 1 | 38.2 | 4 |

*(Continued)*

| Table 17.1 (Continued) | | | | | | | | | |
|---|---|---|---|---|---|---|---|---|---|
| Author, year | N | Approach levels | Severity of OSAHS | F/U (month) | Original success (%) | Original def. for success | Redefining success (%) | EBM level |
| Baisch[60]-group 1, 2006 | 67 | 3 | mi-Se | 1 | 59.7 | 2 | NA | 4 |
| Baisch[60]-group 2, 2006 | 16 | 3 | mi-Se | 1 | NA | 2 | NA | 4 |
| Richard,[61] 2007 | 22 | 2 | Mo-Se | 2 | 45 | 1 | 45 | 4 |

**Abbreviations:** OSAHS, Obstructive sleep apnea/hypopnea syndrome; Def., definition; EBM, evidence-based medicine; mi, mild OSAHS; Mo, moderate OSAHS; Se, severe OSAHS; F/U: follow up; NA: not available.

**Original definition for success:**

1. Definition of success: 50% reduction in AHI *and* an AHI < 20 events per hour.
2. Definition of success: a postoperative AHI reduction of at least 50% *and* below a value of 15.
3. Definition of success: a reduction of greater than 50% *and* an AHI of less than 10 events per hour.
4. Definition of success: an AHI <20 events per hour, with normal $O_2$ saturation ($\geq$95%).
5. Definition of success: 50% reduction in preoperative AHI.
6. Definition of success: an AHI <10 events per hour.
7. Definition of success: a postoperative AHI reduction of at least 50% *or* below an AHI value of 15.

## 4.1 SHORT-TERM VERSUS LONG-TERM RESULTS OF MULTILEVEL TREATMENT

Most of the literature on multilevel treatment of OSAHS reported short-term surgical results at 6 months or less after surgery. The success rate varied from 0% to 100%. Vicente[14] studied the long-term efficacy of UPPP and tongue base suspension with the Repose system for severe OSASHS and reported a 78% success rate at 3 years after surgery. Neruntarat[48] performed uvulopalatal flap in conjunction with GAHM in 46 patients and followed the short-term (6 months after surgery) and long-term (at least 37 months postoperatively) outcome. The short-term and long-term success rates were 78.3% and 65.2%, respectively. Six (16.7%) patients with short-term success failed over the long term and these patients had significant increase in BMI.

The longest follow-up result in multilevel treatment was reported by Andsberg et al.[34] using a 50% reduction in the Apnea Index as the definition for success. They reported on 16 patients at 1 year and 8.4 years after surgery. Their success rates were 56% and 56%, respectively. The weights of the patients remained stable during the follow-up period. Although there is a perception that the long-term results are poorer than the short-term results for surgical treatment of OSAHS, the studies showed the reduction in surgical success was only moderate and that the majority of patients at 6 months maintain long-term successful outcomes.

## 4.2 SINGLE STAGE OR MULTI-STAGED SURGERY IN MULTILEVEL TREATMENT

Multilevel treatment can be performed in a single stage or in multiple stages. The major concern about single stage multilevel surgery for OSAHS involves its safety. Staging multiple procedures may be inconvenient for patients, but by doing so one can reduce the surgical morbidity per session. Single stage versus multi-stage treatment remains an area of controversy. Proponents of each approach have valid evidence that either approach is reasonable and safe. If the procedures are staged, the order in which sites are corrected is also controversial.

Olsen[62] stated that when nasal obstruction is identified, it is usually addressed with a multi-staged procedure after the palate and hypopharyngeal areas are treated. Hsu[40] also stated that the timing of nasal surgery in patients undergoing other procedures for OSAHS remains controversial. He feels that performing multi-staged procedures is a safer option in the surgical management of patients with moderate to severe OSAHS. The presence of blood, secretion or edema may add to the severity of obstruction in an already narrow and obstructed upper airway in patients with moderate to severe OSAHS. The addition of nasal packing may further compromise the airway.

However, most studies revealed that single stage surgery at multiple levels did not increase postoperative complications.[52,53,63] Single stage multilevel surgery can lower total hospitalization expenses when compared to multi-staged surgery.[53] Kieff and Busaba[64] studied the safety of same-day or overnight discharge and concluded that same-day discharge for patients who have undergone combined nasal and palatal surgery for OSAHS is relatively safe in selected cases when significant comorbid diseases are not present.

Most of the above literature preferred single stage surgery primarily focusing on nasal and palatal surgery; however, there was no additional hypopharyngeal procedure included. Experience with multilevel surgery with a hypopharyngeal procedure has shown the postoperative morbidity (the highest complication rate) of single stage and multi-staged surgeries to be 40.9% and 39.1%, respectively.[19,48] All of the complications were temporary.

Thus, on the issue of single or multiple stage surgery, our opinion is that it is safe and efficacious to perform multilevel surgery in one surgical session using minimally invasive techniques and with adequate postoperative monitoring for patients with mild/moderate OSAHS. When multilevel invasive procedures are necessary, the authors prefer to limit the number of levels to one or two per stage. Three-level invasive surgery is never performed in a single stage.

## 4.3 ROLE OF NASAL SURGERY IN MULTILEVEL TREATMENT

Multilevel treatment generally includes the palate and tonsil, as well as the hypopharynx. Often, a nasal corrective procedure is included as well. The importance of nasal breathing during sleep has been documented.[65] Nasal obstruction also plays a role in the pathogenesis of OSAHS.[66] According to the Bernouilli principle (Venturi effect), intraluminal pressure in the compromised airspace suddenly drops if the inspired airway accelerates to keep ventilatory volume constant. The effect further narrows the airspace (hypnogenic stenosis). When inspiratory negative pressure reaches a certain critical point in the effort to overcome increased upper airway resistance, a combination of redundant soft tissues and loss of pharyngeal muscle tone and decreased tongue muscle tone causes complete upper airway collapse on inspiration.

It is well known that nasal cross-sectional area reduced by septal deviation or other pathology causes increased nasal resistance and predisposes the OSAHS patients to downstream inspiratory collapse of the oropharynx, hypopharynx or both.[67,68] Correction of the nasal airway, however, does not always improve OSAHS. In fact it may result in an unexpectedly worse AHI postoperatively. Friedman[69] conducted a prospective study of 50 consecutive patients with nasal airway obstruction and OSAHS to compare the effect of an improved nasal airway on OSAHS by use of subjective and objective measures. The results demonstrated that although 98% of patients had subjective improvement in nasal breathing, 66% of patients did not notice any significant change in their snoring. Review of the polysomnographic data demonstrated that the group overall did not have significant changes in AHI or LSAT. The subgroup of patients with mild OSAHS showed the most significant worsening in their AHI. CPAP levels, however, required to correct OSAHS decreased significantly after nasal surgery. Verse et al.[70] also reported a similar study with 26 adult patients who underwent nasal surgery as single level treatment of their sleep-related breathing disorders. They concluded that nasal surgery alone had a limited efficacy in the treatment of adult patients with OSAHS. Nevertheless, nasal surgery significantly improves sleep quality and daytime sleepiness independent of the severity of OSAHS.

Thus, nasal surgery alone does not consistently improve OSAHS when measured objectively. Depending on the severity of OSA, nasal airway reconstruction as an isolated procedure may contribute to decrease in CPAP pressures and improve CPAP compliance. The most important value, however, of nasal surgery is as one stage in the multilevel treatment plan for OSAHS. The role of nasal surgery in OSAHS is discussed in detail in another chapter.

## 5 SUGGESTED TECHNIQUES FOR MULTILEVEL TREATMENT

When making a decision to select a treatment plan for the OSAHS patient, the balance between morbidity of treatment and severity of disease needs to be considered. We present an algorithm (Tables 17.2 to 17.5) used in our practice to plan treatment on the nose, palate, tonsil and hypopharynx. The entire surgical plan should be outlined prior to onset of treatment rather than embarking on a series of trial and error procedures. It is also important to emphasize that the severity of disease and ease or difficulty of correction in OSAHS do not always correlate with the severity of anatomical obstruction.[10] Thus, an algorithm for successful surgical treatment of

**Table 17.2** Surgical techniques for OSAHS patients with multilevel treatment at the *nasal* level

| Anatomical deformity | N0 | N1 | N2 |
|---|---|---|---|
|  | No intervention | Minimally invasive technique | Invasive technique |
| Nasal septum | – | Endoscopic septoplasty (No packing) | Septoplasty (+/– packing) |
| Nasal valve | – | Valve suspension | Open valve repair |
| Inferior turbinate | – | RF, laser or microdebrider inferior turbinoplasty | Submucosal resection of turbinate |

**Table 17.3** Surgical techniques for OSAHS patients with multilevel treatment at the *palatal* level

| Anatomical deformity | P0 | P1 | P2 |
|---|---|---|---|
|  | No intervention | Minimally invasive technique | Invasive technique |
| Palate and uvula | – | RF soft palate, pillar implants, CAPSO, laser-assisted uvuloplasty, uvulectomy, uvulopalatal flap | UPPP, Z-PP, lateral pharyngopalatoplasty, transpalatal advancement pharyngoplasty |

**Table 17.4** Surgical techniques for OSAHS patients with multilevel treatment at the *tonsils*

| Anatomical deformity | T0 | T1 | T2 |
|---|---|---|---|
| | No Intervention | Minimally invasive technique | Invasive technique |
| Tonsil | – | RF tonsillar reduction, coblation tonsillectomy | Tonsillectomy |

**Table 17.5** Techniques for OSAHS patients with multilevel treatment at the *hypopharyngeal* level

| Anatomical deformity | H0 | H1 | H2 |
|---|---|---|---|
| | No intervention | Minimally invasive technique | Invasive technique |
| Tongue base | – | RFBOT, BOT coblation, tongue base suspension (soft tissue-to-bone anchor system), oral appliance | Midline glossectomy, genioglossal advancement, thyrohyoid suspension, maxillomandibular advancement |

OSAHS should be based on the combination of the anatomic abnormality and severity of disease (the symptoms of snoring alone vs. snoring and excessive daytime sleepiness, and PSG data). The anatomic sites, nose, palate, tonsil and hypopharynx, are identified by N, P, T and H. The level of treatment is described by a number between 0 and 2 (0: no abnormality and therefore no intervention; 1: mild abnormality requiring minimally invasive intervention; 2: severe abnormality/disease requiring invasive correction). Each patient is identified as NxPxTxHx for treatment plan, where x represents a number from 0–2.

## 5.1 SUGGESTED TECHNIQUES FOR MULTILEVEL TREATMENT ON OSAHS PATIENTS

If BMIs of the OSAHS patients are greater than 40, being automatically assigned to Friedman's stage IV, they will not be candidates for the following suggested techniques and will suggest the treatment of CPAP, bariatric surgery or tracheostomy.

If BMI is less than 40 and the Friedman's stage is I, II or III, the patient will be offered surgical modalities on nose, palate, tonsil and hypopharynx from minimal invasive techniques to invasive correction.

## 6 RISK MANAGEMENT AND COMPLICATIONS OF MULTILEVEL TREATMENT

The complication rate for multilevel treatment is the sum of the complications for each of the individual procedures. In our systematic review[23] of multilevel surgery for OSAHS patients, the overall complication rate is 14.6%. The complication rates developed in mild/moderate disease and severe disease were 16% and 14.2%, respectively.

Preoperative assessment for OSAHS patients should be performed by the anesthesiologist and discussed with the sleep surgeon. Eschmann catheter, rigid bronchoscopy and flexible intubation equipment should be available. Extubation is preferably carried out in the operating room when the patients understand and follow commands and should not be done when they are combative. Airway compromise usually occurs in the immediate postextubation phase. In the perioperative period, use of the nasopharyngeal airway may help stent the compromised upper airway and can often be life saving. Details of anesthetic management are discussed in another chapter.

## 7 CONCLUSION

CPAP remains the initial treatment for OSAHS. However, there is a significant percentage of OSAHS patients who either fail or are unwilling to pursue CPAP therapy. For these patients, surgery offers a viable alternative chance to control OSAHS. The subjective and objective severity of OSAHS integrated with the degree of anatomic abnormality dictates the choice of surgical procedure(s). These vary from single to multilevel therapy using either minimally invasive or classic invasive techniques in various combinations. Multilevel treatment should be dictated by the presence of multilevel obstruction. Most patients with OSAHS have multilevel obstruction and should be considered for MISSMLS. It should not be reserved only for patients with severe OSAHS.

Although surgery for the treatment of OSAHS remains a relatively young medical discipline, more evidence-based data could help direct optimal surgical intervention for each patient and ultimately reverse or at least halt the multi-system damage caused by OSAHS.

## REFERENCES

1. Fujita S. UPPP for sleep apnea and snoring. Ear Nose Throat J 1984;63:227–35.
2. Riley RW, Powell NB, Guilleminault C. Obstructive sleep apnea syndrome: a review of 306 consecutively treated surgical patients. Otolaryngol Head Neck Surgery 1993;108:117–25.
3. Friedman M, Tanyeri H, La Rosa M, Landsberg R, Vaidyanathan K, Pieri S, Caldarelli D. Clinical predictors of obstructive sleep apnea. Laryngoscope 1999;109:1901–1907.
4. Friedman M, Ibrahim H, Bass L. Clinical staging for sleep-disordered breathing. Otolaryngol Head Neck Surg 2002;127:13–27.

5. den Herder C, van Tinteren H, de Vries. Sleep endoscopy versus modified Mallampati score in sleep apnea and snoring. Laryngoscope 2005;115:735–39.
6. Friedman M. Letter to the editor. Comment in Sleep endoscopy versus modified Mallampati score in sleep apnea and snoring. Laryngoscope 2005; 115: 2072–2073
7. Abdullah VJ, van Hasselt CA. Video sleep nasendoscopy. In: Surgical Management of Sleep Apnea and Snoring. Terris DJ, Goode RL, eds. Boca Raton, FL: Taylor & Francis; 2005, pp. 143–54.
8. Fujita S, Conway W, Zorick F, Roth T. Surgical correction of anatomic abnormalities in obstructive sleep apnea syndrome: uvulopalatopharyngoplasty. Otolaryngol Head Neck Surg 1981;89:923–34.
9. Sher AE, Schechtman KB, Piccirillo JF. The efficacy of surgical modifications of the upper airway in adults with obstructive sleep apnea syndrome. Sleep 1996;19:156–77.
10. Friedman M, Vidyasagar R, Bliznikas D, Joseph N. Does severity of obstructive of sleep apnea/hypopnea syndrome predict uvulopalatopharyngoplasty outcome?. Laryngoscope 2005;115:2109–13.
11. Senior BA, Rosenthal L, Lumley A, Gerhardstein R, Day R. Efficacy of uvulopalatopharyngoplasty in unselected patients with mild obstructive sleep apnea. Otolaryngol Head Neck Surg 2000;123:179–82.
12. Verse T, Baisch A, Maurer JT, Stuck BA, Hormann K. Multilevel surgery for obstructive sleep apnea: short-term results. Otolaryngol Head Neck Surg 2006;134:571–77.
13. Miller FR, Watson D, Boseley M. The role of the genial bone advancement trephine system in conjunction with uvulopalatopharyngoplasty in the multilevel management of obstructive sleep apnea. Otolaryngol Head Neck Surg 2004;130:73–79.
14. Vicente E, Marin JM, Carrizo S, Naya MJ. Tongue-base suspension in conjunction with uvulopalatopharyngoplasty for treatment of severe obstructive sleep apnea: long-term follow-up results. Laryngoscope 2006;116:1223–27.
15. Sorrenti G, Piccin O, Mondini S, Ceroni AR. One-phase management of severe obstructive sleep apnea: tongue base reduction with hyoepiglottoplasty plus uvulopalatopharyngoplasty. Otolaryngol Head Neck Surg 2006;135:906–10.
16. Li HY, Wang PC, Hsu CY, Chen NH, Lee LA, Fang TJ. Same-stage palatopharyngeal and hypopharyngeal surgery for severe obstructive sleep apnea. Acta Otolaryngol 2004;124:820–26.
17. Chabolle F, Wagner I, Blumen MB, Sequert C, Fleury B, De Dieuleveult T. Tongue base reduction with hyoepiglottoplasty: a treatment for severe obstructive sleep apnea. Laryngoscope 1999;109:1273–80.
18. Elasfour A, Miyazaki S, Itasaka Y, Yamakawa K, Ishikawa K, Togawa K. Evaluation of uvulopalatopharyngoplasty in treatment of obstructive sleep apnea syndrome. Acta Otolaryngol Suppl 1998;537:52–56.
19. Steward D. Effectiveness of multilevel (tongue and palate) radiofrequency tissue ablation for patients with obstructive sleep apnea syndrome. Laryngoscope 2004;114:2073–84.
20. Fischer Y, Khan M, Mann WJ. Multilevel temperature-controlled radiofrequency therapy of soft palate, base of tongue, and tonsils in adults with obstructive sleep apnea. Laryngoscope 2003;113:1786–91.
21. Stuck BA, Starzak K, Hein G, Verse T, Hormann K, Maurer JT. Combined radiofrequency surgery of the tongue base and soft palate in obstructive sleep apnoea. Acta Otolaryngol 2004;124:827–32.
22. Friedman M, Lin HC, Gurpinar B, Joseph NJ. Minimally invasive single-stage multilevel treatment for obstructive sleep apnea/hypopnea syndrome. Laryngoscope 2007;117:1859–63.
23. Lin HC, Friedman M, Chang HW, Gurpinar B. The efficacy of multilevel surgery of the upper airway in adults with obstructive sleep apnea/hypopnea syndrome, Lanyngoscope 2008;18:902–8.
24. Waite PD, Wooten V, Lachner J, Guyette RF. Maxillomandibular advancement surgery in 23 patients with obstructive sleep apnea syndrome. J Oral Maxillofac Surg 1989;47:1256–60.
25. Riley RW, Powell NB, Guilleminault C. Maxillofacial surgery and obstructive sleep apnea: a review of 80 patients. Otolaryngol Head Neck Surg 1989;101:353–61.
26. Riley RW, Powell NB, Guilleminault C. Maxillary, mandibular, and hyoid advancement for treatment of obstructive sleep apnea: a review of 40 patients. J Oral Maxillofac Surg 1990;48:20–26.
27. Djupesland G, Schrader H, Lyberg T, Refsum H, Lilleas F, Godtlbsen OB. Palatopharyngoglossoplasty in the treatment of patients with obstructive sleep apnea syndrome. Acta Otolaryngol Suppl 1992;492:50–54.
28. Johnson NT, Chinn J. Uvulopalatopharyngoplasty and inferior sagittal mandibular osteotomy with genioglossus advancement for treatment of obstructive sleep apnea. Chest 1994;105:278–83.
29. Ramirez SG, Loube DI. Inferior sagittal osteotomy with hyoid bone suspension for obese patients with sleep apnea. Arch Otolaryngol Head Neck Surg 1996;122:953–57.
30. Mickelson SA, Rosenthal L. Midline glossectomy and epiglottidectomy for obstructive sleep apnea syndrome. Laryngoscope 1997;107:614–19.
31. Hochban W, Conradt R, Brandenburg U, Heitmann J, Peter JH. Surgical maxillofacial treatment of obstructive sleep apnea. Plast Reconstr Surg 1997;99:619–26.
32. Li KK, Riley RW, Powell NB, Troell R, Guilleminault C. Overview of phase II surgery for obstructive sleep apnea syndrome. Ear Nose Throat J 1999;78:851, 854–7.
33. Lee NR, Givens CD, Wilson J, Robins RB. Staged surgical treatment of obstructive sleep apnea syndrome: a review of 35 patients. J Oral Maxillofac Surg 1999;57:382–85.
34. Andsberg U, Jessen M. Eight years of follow-up – uvulopalatopharyngoplasty combined with midline glossectomy as a treatment for obstructive sleep apnoea syndrome. Acta Otolaryngol Suppl 2000;543:175–78.
35. Bettega G, Pépin JL, Veale D, Deschaux C, Raphaël B, Lévy P. Obstructive sleep apnea syndrome. Fifty-one consecutive patients treated by maxillofacial surgery. Am J Respir Crit Care Med 2000;162:641–49.
36. Riley RW, Powell NB, Li KK, Troell RJ, Guilleminault C. Surgery and obstructive sleep apnea: long-term clinical outcomes. Otolaryngol Head Neck Surg 2000;122:415–21.
37. Li KK, Riley RW, Powell NB, Guilleminault C. Maxillomandibular advancement for persistent obstructive sleep apnea after phase I surgery in patients without maxillomandibular deficiency. Laryngoscope 2000;110:1684–88.
38. Hendler BH, Costello BJ, Silverstein K, Yen D, Goldberg A. A protocol for uvulopalatopharyngoplasty, mortised genioplasty, and maxillomandibular advancement in patients with obstructive sleep apnea: an analysis of 40 cases. J Oral Maxillofac Surg 2001;59:892–97.
39. Nelson LM. Combined temperature-controlled radiofrequency tongue reduction and UPPP in apnea surgery. Ear Nose Throat J 2001;80:640–44.
40. Hsu PP, Brett RH. Multiple level pharyngeal surgery for obstructive sleep apnoea. Singapore Med J 2001;42:160–64.
41. Terris DJ, Kunda LD, Gonella MC. Minimally invasive tongue base surgery for obstructive sleep apnoea. J Laryngol Otol 2002;116:716–21.
42. Miller FR, Watson D, Malis D. Role of the tongue base suspension suture with The Repose System bone screw in the multilevel surgical management of obstructive sleep apnea. Otolaryngol Head Neck Surg 2002;126:392–98.
43. Kao YH, Shnayder Y, Lee KC. The efficacy of anatomically based multilevel surgery for obstructive sleep apnea. Otolaryngol Head Neck Surg 2003;129:327–35.
44. Woodson BT, Steward DL, Weaver EM, Javaheri S. A randomized trial of temperature-controlled radiofrequency, continuous positive airway pressure, and placebo for obstructive sleep apnea syndrome. Otolaryngol Head Neck Surg 2003;128:848–61.
45. Friedman M, Ibrahim H, Lee G, Joseph NJ. Combined uvulopalatopharyngoplasty and radiofrequency tongue base reduction for treatment of obstructive sleep apnea/hypopnea syndrome. Otolaryngol Head Neck Surg 2003;129:611–21.
46. Thomas AJ, Chavoya M, Terris DJ. Preliminary findings from a prospective, randomized trial of two tongue-base surgeries for sleep-disordered breathing. Otolaryngol Head Neck Surg 2003;129:539–46.
47. Neruntarat C. Genioglossus advancement and hyoid myotomy under local anesthesia. Otolaryngol Head Neck Surg 2003;129:85–91.
48. Neruntarat C. Genioglossus advancement and hyoid myotomy: short-term and long-term results. J Laryngol Otol 2003;117:482–86.
49. Neruntarat C. Hyoid myotomy with suspension under local anesthesia for obstructive sleep apnea syndrome. Eur Arch Otorhinolaryngol 2003;260:286–90.

50. Dattilo DJ, Drooger SA. Outcome assessment of patients undergoing maxillofacial procedures for the treatment of sleep apnea: comparison of subjective and objective results. J Oral Maxillofac Surg 2004;62:164–68.
51. Omur M, Ozturan D, Elez F, Unver C, Derman S. Tongue base suspension combined with UPPP in severe OSA patients. Otolaryngol Head Neck Surg 2005;133:218–23.
52. Pang KP. One-stage nasal and multi-level pharyngeal surgery for obstructive sleep apnoea: safety and efficacy. J Laryngol Otol 2005;119:272–76.
53. Li HY, Wang PC, Hsu CY, Lee SW, Chen NH, Liu SA. Combined nasal-palatopharyngeal surgery for obstructive sleep apnea: simultaneous or staged?. Acta Otolaryngol 2005;125:298–303.
54. Steward DL, Weaver EM, Woodson BT. Multilevel temperature-controlled radiofrequency for obstructive sleep apnea: extended follow-up. Otolaryngol Head Neck Surg 2005;132:630–35.
55. Bowden MT, Kezirian EJ, Utley D, Goode RL. Outcomes of hyoid suspension for the treatment of obstructive sleep apnea. Arch Otolaryngol Head Neck Surg 2005;131:440–45.
56. Liu SA, Li HY, Tsai WC, Chang KM. Associated factors to predict outcomes of uvulopharyngopalatoplasty plus genioglossal advancement for obstructive sleep apnea. Laryngoscope 2005;15:2046–50.
57. Smatt Y, Ferri J. Retrospective study of 18 patients treated by maxillomandibular advancement with adjunctive procedures for obstructive sleep apnea syndrome. J Craniofac Surg 2005;16:770–77.
58. Jacobowitz O. Palatal and tongue base surgery for surgical treatment of obstructive sleep apnea: a prospective study. Otolaryngol Head Neck Surg 2006;135:258–64.
59. Friedman M, Vidyasagar R, Bliznikas D, Joseph NJ. Patient selection and efficacy of pillar implant technique for treatment of snoring and obstructive sleep apnea/hypopnea syndrome. Otolaryngol Head Neck Surg 2006;134:187–96.
60. Baisch A, Maurer JT, Hörmann K. The effect of hyoid suspension in a multilevel surgery concept for obstructive sleep apnea. Otolaryngol Head Neck Surg 2006;134:856–61.
61. Richard W, Kox D, den Herder C, van Tinteren H, de Vries N. One stage multilevel surgery (uvulopalatopharyngoplasty, hyoid suspension, radiofrequent ablation of the tongue base with/without genioglossus advancement), in obstructive sleep apnea syndrome. Eur Arch Otorhinolaryngol 2007;264:439–44.
62. Olsen KD. The role of nasal surgery in treatment of OSA. Op Tech in Otolaryngol Head Neck Surg 1991;2:63–68.
63. Busaba NY. Same-stage nasal and palatopharyngeal surgery for obstructive sleep apnea: is it safe? Otolaryngol Head Neck Surg 2002;126:399–403.
64. Kieff DA, Busaba NY. Same-day discharge for selected patients undergoing combined nasal and palatal surgery for obstructive sleep apnea. Ann Otol Rhinol Laryngol 2004;113:128–31.
65. Lavie P. Rediscovering the importance of nasal breathing in sleep or, shut your mouth and save your sleep. J Laryngol Otol 1987;101:558–63.
66. Busaba NY. The nose in snoring and obstructive sleep apnea. Curr Opin Otolaryngol Head Neck Surg 1999;7:11–13.
67. Olsen KD, Kern EB, Westbrook PR. Sleep and breathing disturbance secondary to nasal obstruction. Otolaryngol Head Neck Surg 1981;89:804–10.
68. Cole P, Haight JS. Mechanisms of nasal obstruction in sleep. Laryngoscope 1984;94:1557–79.
69. Friedman M, Tanyeri H, Lim JW, Landsberg R, Vaidyanathan K, Caldarelli D. Effect of improved nasal breathing on obstructive sleep apnea. Otolaryngol Head Neck Surg 2000;122:71–74.
70. Verse T, Maurer JT, Pirsig W. Effect of nasal surgery on sleep-related breathing disorders. Laryngoscope 2002;112:64–68.

# SECTION G — NASAL SURGERY FOR TREATMENT OF OSA/HS

## CHAPTER 18

# Nasal obstruction and sleep-disordered breathing

*Kristin K. Egan, David Kim and Eric J. Kezirian,*

## 1 FUNCTIONAL VALVULAR ANATOMY

Anatomic models (Figs 18.1 and 18.2) in combination with objective measurements have shown that nasal airflow follows a parabolic curve directed superiorly through the nostril, upwards through the nasal cavity past the turbinates, and posteriorly to the nasopharynx during inspiration.[1,2]

The internal nasal valve area is the narrowest part of the nasal passage and is the major source of nasal resistance in normal patients. Four structures compose the internal nasal valve: the upper lateral cartilage superiorly, nasal septum medially, pyriform aperture inferiorly, and the head of the inferior turbinate posteriorly.[3] The narrowest portion of the internal nasal valve area is the region between the septum and the caudal border of the upper lateral cartilage. This structure is approximately 10–15° in Caucasian subjects and can be wider in subjects of African and Asian descent. Patients with internal nasal valve angles of <10° are more prone to internal nasal valve collapse on inspiration.

The external nasal valve is composed of the nares and the nasal vestibule. The nasal vestibule lies just inside the external naris and is located caudal to the internal nasal valve area. The septum is located medially along with the columella, and the alar sidewalls are lateral to the vestibule. Vibrissae are located within the vestibule under the lateral crus and function as a filter for the inspired air. They also serve to direct the air posteriorly into the nasal cavity and to slow the inspired air.[4] The nares are composed of the alar margin, the soft tissue triangle, the columella and the nasal sill. The position of the medial crural footplates, the nasal spine and the caudal septum may all change the location and shape of the columella, thereby influencing the nares.

The internal and external nasal valves function together to deliver a smooth air current to the nasal cavities for humidification. The nasal valves can have a greater influence during deep inspiration when the nostrils flare and the diameter of the external nasal valve is increased. The Bernoulli principle is responsible for this effect in that the intraluminal pressure in the internal valve area decreases when the airflow is increased through it. The cartilaginous

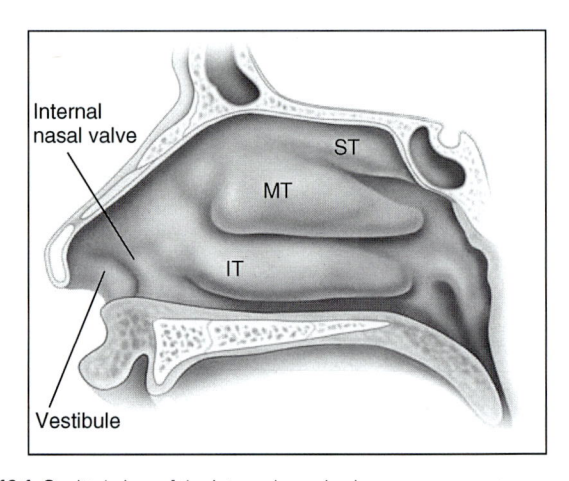

Fig. 18.1 Sagittal view of the internal nasal valve.

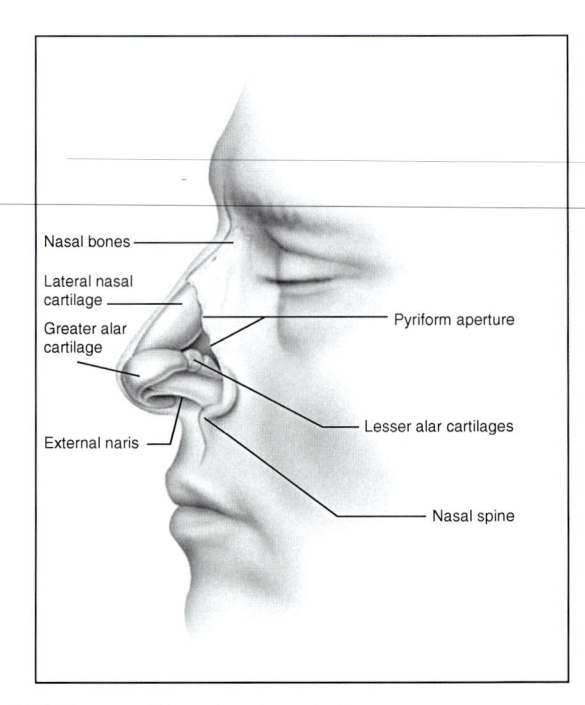

Fig. 18.2 Diagram of the external nasal valve.

structure of the nose serves as a counterbalance to this tendency toward internal nasal valve collapse. The investing nasal musculature consists of elevator muscles, including the procerus, levator labii superioris alaeque nasi and anomalous nasi. The depressor muscles include the alar nasalis and the depressor septi nasi while the compressor muscles include the transverse nasalis and the compressor narium minor. There are also minor dilator muscles. The alar muscles contract and dilate the internal nasal valve area in order to keep the lumen open. Throughout normal nasal function, the internal nasal valve area should remain unchanged,[5] although collapse demonstrable only during forced inspiration does not require intervention.[6]

Subjects with certain nasal anatomical characteristics may be predisposed to nasal obstruction; for example, those individuals with a narrow upper cartilaginous vault have a narrower internal nasal valve and may exhibit collapse in the resting state. The impact of a relatively small decrease in cross-sectional area of the internal nasal valve can be substantial due to Poiseuille's law, which indicates that the rate of airflow is proportional to the fourth power of the radius of the conduit. Those subjects who possess weak upper lateral cartilages and/or lateral nasal walls may be more predisposed to collapse of the internal nasal valve during inspiration.

The otolaryngologist should be aware of those characteristics that contribute to nasal obstruction. Those patients who have pre-existing or traumatic septal deviation can suffer nasal obstruction. Insufficient support of the alar rim and alar lobule may lead to external valve collapse on inspiration. Short nasal bones and a long upper cartilaginous vault; narrow, projecting nose; slit-like nostrils; exaggerated supra-alar creases; visible pinching of the lateral wall with inspiration; thin cartilages and skin; and cephalically positioned lateral crura which provide minimal support to the alar margins are all attributes that the surgeon should consider when planning surgical correction.[7]

## 2 NASAL OBSTRUCTION AND SDB

Case reports and case series as early as the 1890s showed an association between the nasal valve and sleep-disordered breathing (SDB). Today, we are all familiar with the fact that nasal obstruction and SDB often co-exist. Among patients referred to sleep clinics, studies have shown that subjective or objective nasal obstruction is a risk factor for SDB.[2-4] Approximately 15% of patients with SDB also have nasal obstruction,[8] but there is no correlation between the severity of obstructive sleep apnea and an objective measure of nasal resistance – acoustic rhinometry.[9] Lofaso analyzed cephalometrics, body mass index and posterior rhinometry and showed that daytime nasal obstruction is an independent risk factor for obstructive sleep apnea.[10] Others have explored the relationship between nasal obstruction and SDB showing that there is no association between SDB severity and the severity of the nasal obstruction.[11-15]

Beyond a simple association, however, nasal obstruction often plays a major role in SDB and its treatment. Nasal obstruction itself may contribute substantially to SDB by being an independent source of airway obstruction. The evidence supporting the role of nasal obstruction in SDB comes from a variety of sources. Normal patients have been shown to experience sleep disturbances – including sleep stage disruption as well as new-onset snoring and even mild obstructive sleep apnea – after acute, complete bilateral nasal obstruction such as abrupt occlusion of their nose.[16] One study demonstrated that SDB was related to nasal cross-sectional area objectively assessed using acoustic rhinometry and both titrated nasal continuous positive airway pressure (CPAP) and the Respiratory Disturbance Index (RDI); however, these associations were only present in patients with normal Body Mass Index (BMI).[17]

Besides the simple effect of nasal obstruction on breathing patterns during sleep, the nose is a major conduit for treatment of obstructive sleep apnea with positive airway pressure therapy. Nasal obstruction can therefore interfere with treatment. Lafond and Series showed that nasal obstruction can increase the required continuous positive airway pressure in obstructive sleep apnea patients.[18] They induced an increased nasal resistance with histamine and demonstrated that this increased flow limitation in two commonly used CPAP devices. Zozula and Rosen also showed that nasal obstruction can affect positive airway pressure therapy tolerance and adherence in their study examining and classifying reasons for CPAP non-compliance.[19]

Three different theories have been proposed to explain the relationship between nasal obstruction and SDB. These will be considered separately.

## 2.1 INCREASED AIRWAY RESISTANCE

In 1912, Knowlton and Starling described a new model to explain flow through blood vessels. Previously, simpler models of fluid mechanics had suggested that fluid, in this case blood, flows in a tube with higher pressure at one end and lower pressure at the other. Their contribution in describing flow through a *collapsible* tube was to incorporate the extraluminal pressure of this collapsible segment. By considering the collapsibility of this tube, they showed that if the extraluminal pressure was greater than the pressure of the downstream segment, flow was related not to pressure differential across the whole tube, but rather to inflow pressure minus the extraluminal pressure.

Applying the Starling model to the pharynx (Fig. 18.3), maximal airflow is based on three factors: upstream pressure, resistance in the upstream segment, and the extraluminal pressure. Increased nasal resistance is an increase in resistance of the upstream segment and therefore reduces

# SECTION G: NASAL SURGERY FOR TREATMENT OF OSA/HS

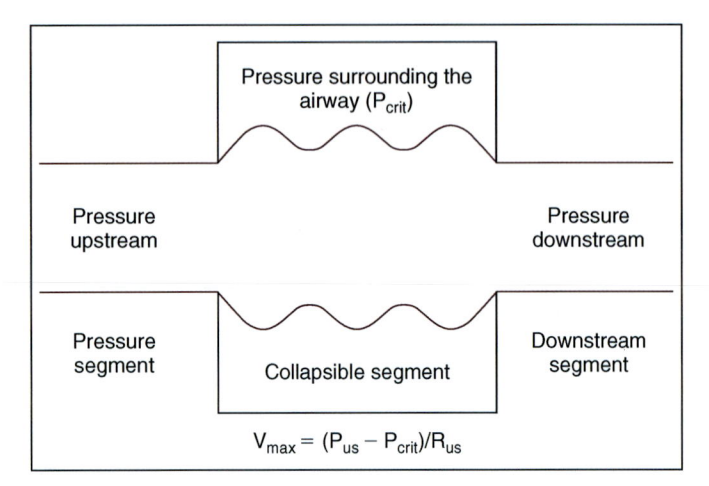

**Fig. 18.3** Starling resistor. The maximal velocity of air through the nose is proportional to the pressure surrounding the tube ($P_{crit}$) subtracted from the upstream pressure ($P_{us}$) and is inversely proportional to the resistance of the upstream segment ($R_{us}$).

flow through the collapsible tube, the pharynx. The maximal velocity of air through the nose is proportional to the pressure surrounding the tube ($P_{crit}$) subtracted from the upstream pressure ($P_{us}$) and is inversely proportional to the resistance of the upstream segment ($R_{us}$).

From a teleological standpoint, nasal resistance functions as an upstream resistor of nasal airflow. In this capacity, nasal resistance matches the impedance of upper and lower airways to prolong inspiration and expiration. On expiration, this prolongation has the beneficial effect of improving pulmonary compliance and increasing gas exchange. On inspiration, however, as suggested by the Starling model, nasal resistance can augment pharyngeal resistance to promote upper airway collapse. The decline in tidal volume and minute ventilation has been shown in several studies.[20,21]

## 2.2 UNSTABLE ORAL BREATHING

The second theory describing nasal obstruction and its connection to SDB is based on the instability of oral breathing compared with nasal breathing. With nasal obstruction, patients open their mouth. This reflexive compensation contributes to SDB by narrowing the pharyngeal lumen in two ways. First, the chin and rest of the mandible move posteriorly and inferiorly with mouth opening to displace the tongue in that direction. This directly narrows the pharyngeal airway. Second, this maneuver decreases the length and tension of the muscles surrounding the airway, and the compliance of the pharynx increases.[22] It has been shown that opening of the mouth to provide a 1.5 cm separation between incisors moves the angle of the mandible posteriorly 1 cm, a substantial change.[23] In fact, two studies have demonstrated that oral breathing is associated with increased airway resistance during sleep compared to nasal breathing.[24,25]

## 2.3 IMPAIRED NASAL REFLEXES

The third mechanism focuses on important nasal reflexes. Nasal breathing stimulates ventilation, and the best evidence of this in normal patients comes from a study showing that not only is minute ventilation higher with nasal compared to oral breathing, but also that augmented nasal airflow increases minute ventilation.[26] Furthermore, the evidence that this response is due to neural regulation in humans comes from studies which show that application of topical anesthesia in the nose and nasopharynx specifically increases nasal and pharyngeal resistance,[27] and that topical nasal anesthesia actually leads to increased SDB – whether this is measured as the number of apneas, apnea duration, or a decrease in genioglossus muscle activity.[28]

## 3 EFFECTS OF TREATMENT

Treatment of nasal obstruction has three potential goals. It can reduce nasal obstruction, reduce the severity of – possibly even eliminating – SDB, or it can facilitate SDB treatment by allowing the nose to be used more easily as a conduit for positive airway pressure therapy. Because there are multiple causes of nasal obstruction, the combination of history, physical exam, and accurate diagnosis is critical to selecting from the long list of medical and surgical treatments. A wide variety of treatments have demonstrated benefits in improving nasal obstruction, but the discussion of this evidence is beyond the scope of this chapter.

In contrast, isolated treatment of nasal obstruction does not successfully treat obstructive sleep apnea for most patients. Verse and Pirsig performed a literature review that showed that medical treatment produced resolution of obstructive sleep apnea in 9% of patients and surgical treatment in 18%.[29] Nasal corticosteroids can produce small changes in snoring and the Apnea/Hypopnea Index, but the degree of improvement varies widely.[30] A few studies specifically looking at surgical treatment showed that there was minimal to no change in Apnea/Hypopnea Index, but some patients experienced improvements in sleep quality and symptoms of daytime somnolence.[31]

Because the improvement in SDB associated with isolated treatment of nasal obstruction varies among patients, Series et al. examined 14 patients with nasal obstruction and SDB (Apnea/Hypopnea Index > 5) who were treated for nasal obstruction alone. Of the seven patients who had a normal Apnea/Hypopnea Index postoperatively, six out of seven of the patients with good outcomes had mild SDB (Apnea/Hypopnea Index 5–15) at the beginning of the study and had normal cephalometric imaging. This was among the first studies to identify factors that may be associated with better outcomes after nasal surgery designed to treat SDB.[32]

Finally, there is evidence showing that nasal treatments can facilitate the treatment of SDB by decreasing the magnitude of the positive airway pressure necessary to treat SDB. Friedman showed a reasonable improvement (9.3–6.7 cm water) for septoplasty with or without inferior turbinate reduction,[7] and a smaller effect (8.6–8.0 cm water) was seen with an external nasal valve dilator device.[33] Two additional studies have shown that nasal surgery can increase the adherence to continuous positive airway pressure devices.[34,35]

## 4 CONCLUSIONS

Overall, the patient population in whom SDB presents will commonly also show concurrent nasal obstruction. Selecting the potential medical and surgical treatment options requires an understanding of nasal anatomy and physiology and the combination of history, physical examination, and accurate diagnosis. There are three potential mechanisms for the association between nasal obstruction and SDB: an increase in airway resistance; the transition to unstable oral breathing; and the impairment of nasal reflexes. Treatment can effectively reduce nasal obstruction, although the effects are more variable in the reduction of SDB severity (when treating nasal obstruction alone) and the facilitation of SDB treatment.

## REFERENCES

1. Tarabichi M, Fanous N. Finite element analysis of airflow in the nasal valve. Arch Otolaryngol Head Neck Surg 1993;119(6):638–42.
2. Proctor DF. The upper airways. I. Nasal physiology and defense of the lungs. Am Rev Respir Dis 1977;115:97–129.
3. Kasperbauer JL, Kern EB. Nasal valve physiology. Implications in nasal surgery. Otolaryngol Clin North Am 1987;20:699–719.
4. Cottle MH. Structures and function of the nasal vestibule. Arch Otolaryngol Head Neck Surg 1955;62:173.
5. Cole P. The four components of the nasal valve. Am J Rhinol 2003;17:107–10.
6. Goode RL. Surgery of the incompetent nasal valve. Laryngoscope 1985;95:546–55.
7. Constantian MB. Four common anatomic variants that predispose to unfavorable rhinoplasty results: a study based on 150 consecutive secondary rhinoplasties. Plast Reconstr Surg 2000;105:316–31.
8. Mayer-Brix J, Muller-Marschhausen U, Becker H, Peter JH. How frequent are pathologic ENT findings in patients with obstructive sleep apnea syndrome? HNO 1989;37(12):511–16.
9. Young T, Finn L, Kim H. Nasal obstruction as a risk factor for sleep disordered breathing. J Allergy Clin Immunol 1997;99:S757–S762.
10. Lofaso F, Coste A, d'Ortho M, et al. Nasal obstruction as a risk factor for sleep apnea syndrome. Eur Respir J 2000;16:639–43.
11. Blakley BW, Mahowald M. Nasal resistance and sleep apnea. Laryngoscope 1987;97:752–54.
12. Miljeteig H, Hoffstein V, Cole P. The effect of unilateral and bilateral nasal obstruction on snoring and sleep apnea. Laryngoscope 1992;102:1150–52.
13. Atkins M, Taskar V, Clayton N, Stone P, Woodcock A. Nasal resistance in obstructive sleep apnea. Chest 1994;105:1133–35.
14. Riechelmann H, Furst G. Medical ENT diagnosis and therapy of sleep-associated respiratory disorders with obstruction of the upper airways. Pneumologie 1995;49:523–27.
15. Liistro G, Rombaux P, Belge C, Dury M, Aubert G, Rodenstein DO. High Mallampati score and nasal obstruction are associated risk factors for obstructive sleep apnea. Eur Respir J 2003;21:248–52.
16. Olsen KD, Kern EB, Westbrook PR. Sleep and breathing disturbance secondary to nasal obstruction. Otolaryngol Head Neck Surg 1981;89:804–10.
17. Morris LG, Burschtin O, Lebowitz RA, Jacobs JB, Lee KC. Nasal obstruction and sleep-disordered breathing: a study using acoustic rhinometry. Am J Rhinol 2005;19(1):33–39.
18. Lafond C, Series F. Influence of nasal obstruction on auto-CPAP behaviour during sleep in sleep apnoea/hypopnea syndrome. Thorax 1998;53:780–83.
19. Zozula R, Rosen R. Compliance with continuous positive airway pressure therapy: assessing and improving treatment outcomes. Curr Opin Pulm Med 2001;7(6):391–98.
20. Iber C, Berssenbrugge A, Skatrud JB, Dempsey JA. Ventilatory adaptations to resistive loading during wakefulness and non-REM sleep. J Appl Physiol 1982;52(3):607–14.
21. Henke KG, Sullivan CE. Effects of high-frequency pressure waves applied to upper airway on respiration in central apnea. J Appl Physiol 1992;73(3):1141–45.
22. Basner RC, Simon PM, Schwartzstein RM, et al. Breathing route influences upper airway muscle activity in awake normal adults. J Appl Physiol 1989;66:1766–71.
23. Kuna ST, Remmers JE. Neural and anatomic factors related to upper airway occlusion during sleep. Med Clin North Am 1985;69(6):1221–42.
24. Olsen KD, Suh KW, Staats BA. Sleep and breathing disturbance secondary to nasal obstruction. Otolaryngol Head Neck Surg 1981;89(5):804–10.
25. Meurice JC, Marc I, Carrier G, Series F. Effects of mouth opening on upper airway collapsibility in normal sleeping subjects. Am J Respir Crit Care Med 1996;153(1):255–59.
26. McNicholas WT, Coffey M, Boyle T. Effects of nasal airflow on breathing during sleep in normal humans. Am Rev Respir Dis 1993;147(3):620–23.
27. White D, Cadieux R, Lomard R, et al. The effects of nasal anesthesia on breathing during sleep. Am Rev Respir Dis 1985;132:972–75.
28. Garpestad E, Basner RC, Ringler J, et al. Phenylephrine-induced hypertension acutely decreases genioglossus EMG activity in awake humans. J Appl Physiol 1992;72:110–15.
29. Verse T, Pirsig W. Impact of impaired nasal breathing on sleep-disordered breathing. Sleep Breath 2003;7(2):63–76.
30. Kiely JL, Nolan P, McNicholas WT. Intranasal corticosteroid therapy for obstructive sleep apnoea in patients with co-existing rhinitis. Thorax 2004;59(1):50–55.
31. Friedman M, Tanyeri H, Lim JW, Landsberg R, Vaidyanathan K, Caldarelli D. Effect of improved nasal breathing on obstructive sleep apnea. Otolaryngol Head Neck Surg 2000;122(1):71–74.
32. Series F, St Pierre S, Carrier G. Surgical correction of nasal obstruction in the treatment of mild sleep apnoea: importance of cephalometry in predicting outcome. Thorax 1993;48(4):360–63.
33. Schonhofer B, Kerl J, Suchi S, Kohler D, Franklin KA. Effect of nasal valve dilation on effective CPAP level in obstructive sleep apnea. Respir Med 2003;97(9):1001–5.
34. Powell NB, Riley RW, Guilleminault C, Murcia GN. Obstructive sleep apnea, continuous positive airway pressure, and surgery. Otolaryngol Head Neck Surg 1988;99(4):362–69.
35. Series F, St Pierre S, Carrier G. Effects of surgical correction of nasal obstruction in the treatment of obstructive sleep apnea. Am Rev Respir Dis 1992;146(5 Pt 1):1261–65.

# SECTION G  NASAL SURGERY FOR TREATMENT OF OSA/HS

# CHAPTER 19

# Effects of nasal surgery on snoring and sleep apnea

*Michael Friedman and Paul Schalch*

## 1 INTRODUCTION: NASAL SURGERY AND OBSTRUCTIVE SLEEP APNEA

The location of obstruction in the obstructive sleep apnea/hypopnea syndrome (OSAHS) is variable and can often be localized to several levels in the upper airway. In fact, the level of obstruction can vary in the same patient among consecutive episodes of apnea.[1] In normal circumstances, the normal nose contributes to 50% of upper airway resistance, adding to the resistance provided by both oropharyngeal tissues and the tongue.[2] In fact, resistance at the level of the nose is more constant in both sleep and awake states, due to the more rigid frame provided by the septum and the lower and upper lateral cartilages. If, however, the upper or lower lateral cartilages are weak, damaged, resected, or otherwise structurally affected, this stability is lost. Patients in such cases are subject to an increased tendency towards collapse during sleep, even with a normal nasal airway in the awake state. The association between nasal obstruction and sleep disturbances was probably what first led to the description of sleep-related breathing disorders,[3] or sleep-disordered breathing (SDB), the group of disorders that includes snoring, the upper airway resistance syndrome, and OSAHS. It is currently recognized that nasal obstruction interferes with pressure titration in nasal continuous positive airway pressure (nCPAP) for the management of OSAHS, and that treatment of such obstruction improves patient compliance with nCPAP.[4,5] The cause–effect relationship of nasal obstruction and OSAHS, however, remains unclear. While surgical correction of obstructed nasal airways is, without a doubt, an important component of the surgical management of OSAHS,[6-8] the expectations of improvement after performing nasal procedures alone are still, at best, unclear. Another important factor in the relationship between nasal obstruction and SDB is the tendency that patients with obstructed nasal airways have to mouth breathe, which decreases the hypopharyngeal space by moving the mandible posteriorly and, most importantly, by pushing the base of the tongue backwards.

The primary sites of nasal obstruction are the nasal vestibule, the nasal valves, and the turbinates.[9] The nasal septum, when deviated, also has a significant impact on these areas of obstruction. Of these three sites, the nasal valve is the site of major resistance.[2] Many authors have shown that, in fact, nasal valve incompetence may equal, or even exceed, septal deviation or turbinate hypertrophy as the prime cause of nasal airway obstruction.[10] The *internal* nasal valve is defined as the area between the caudal end of the upper lateral cartilages and the cartilaginous septum, and the entire nasal valve complex is bounded superiorly by the reflection between the upper lateral cartilages and the septum, posteriorly by the head of the inferior turbinate, inferiorly by the floor of the nose, and laterally by the bony piriform aperture.[11] During inspiration, particularly during the forced inspiration that occurs during an apneic episode, the negative nasopharyngeal and intranasal pressures increase to generate more flow, creating a transmural pressure gradient, which, when a critical value is reached, causes collapse of the upper lateral cartilages.[12] Thus, the flow-limiting segment constituted by the nasal site of obstruction acts as a Starling resistor, not only at the level of the nose (in the case of inspiratory nasal valve collapse), but also for further 'downstream' structures like the soft palate and the oro- and hypopharynx.[7,13] Nasal obstruction leads to mouth opening and transition to oral breathing, which contributes to airway flow limitation and collapse, mainly due to inferior movement of the mandible,[14] a backward fall of the base of the tongue, resulting in a reduction of the posterior pharyngeal space and diameter[15] and an increased respiratory effort that causes collapse of the pharyngeal tissues due to greater negative pressures.

## 2 CAUSES OF NASAL OBSTRUCTION

The causes for nasal obstruction can be broadly divided into structural, mucosal, or neuromuscular.[14] Structural causes may include septal deviation, hypertrophy of the inferior or middle turbinates and fixed and inspiratory nasal valve collapse, which may or may not be secondary to prior nasal surgery or trauma. Of these causes, nasal valve dysfunction may contribute to symptoms in as many as 13% of adults that report chronic nasal obstruction.[11] Although no data are available, it is likely that the increased respiratory efforts by OSAHS patients during episodes of apnea caused by palatal or tongue base obstruction make these patients more prone to nasal valve collapse. In children, in addition to developmental abnormalities like choanal atresia and craniofacial syndromes (e.g. Pierre Robin sequence), adenoidal and – to a lesser degree – tonsillar hypertrophy also constitute an important cause for nasal obstruction,[16] both of which have an important correlation with OSAHS in this patient population. Chronic mouth breathing in these patients actually leads to acquired craniofacial abnormalities (e.g. the 'adenoid face'), which further compromise the stability of the upper airway.[17] The consequences of these alterations in cephalometric measurements that may originate during infancy may actually constitute the origin of the relationship between SDB and nasal obstruction. Earlier studies by Series[4] established that sleep apneic patients with septal deviation that had subjective symptoms of nasal obstruction and subjectively disturbed sleep (mostly in the form of arousals) were more likely to improve both subjectively and objectively after correction of nasal obstruction if their cephalometric measurements were within normal ranges.

Nasal symptoms, findings, and even anatomical abnormalities (e.g. nasal septal deviation) are common in patients with sleep apnea,[18] and data suggest that increased nasal resistance is more prevalent in patients who snore.[19]

Alterations in the nasal mucosa lead to nasal congestion, which involves the cavernous tissues of the turbinates. Common causes of nasal congestion include allergic rhinitis, vasomotor rhinitis, chronic sinusitis, and upper respiratory tract viral infections.[20] These conditions are often associated with structural abnormalities, like septal deviation, which may also cause alterations in the nasal cycle. Chronic inflammation, as well as conditions like asthma, aspirin sensitivity or cystic fibrosis, lead to the development of nasal or nasopharyngeal polyps, which cause obstruction.[20] Medical management of these conditions is an essential component in addressing nasal obstruction. Intranasal corticosteroid therapy for rhinitis showed improvement of OSAHS, but not snoring, in a randomized, placebo-controlled, crossover trial involving a group of 24 patients with mild to moderate sleep apnea, as reported by Kiely et al.[21]

Facial muscular weakness and impaired nasal reflexes (especially the ones involved in dilating the nose prior to inspiration), which occur secondary to neuropathy and facial palsy, are also important neuromuscular causes of nasal obstruction.[2,11,12]

## 3 DIAGNOSTIC EVALUATION OF NASAL OBSTRUCTION

The evaluation of nasal obstruction in the context of sleep-disordered breathing is based on nasal airway assessment while the patient is awake and asleep. Elements that should be included in the history include whether the obstruction is uni- or bilateral, intermittent or persistent, seasonal or perennial, and whether it is worse while in the supine position, particularly at night. A detailed medication history is essential, in order to document the effects of medications, particularly decongestants and topical steroids. History of previous surgery is also an important aspect that guides the therapeutic decision making. There is no simple way to assess the patient's nasal airway during sleep. A therapeutic trial of topical decongestants and systemic steroids may be useful in assessing the effect on snoring and overall quality of sleep in OSAHS patients.

### 3.1 NASAL AIRWAY STRUCTURE

The physical exam must include an examination of the internal and external nasal valves and the septum by means of anterior rhinoscopy. The nasal valves are common sites of obstruction in sleep apneic patients (see also Chapter 20), even more than deviated septa.[10] The Cottle maneuver still remains an essential trial in the diagnosis of nasal valve obstruction. Fiberoptic endoscopy enables the surgeon to rule out the presence of any obstructing masses such as nasal polyps or nasopharyngeal tumors. Radiologic evaluation with CT scans may also have a confirmatory or strategic role for the preoperative evaluation in select cases, but is not essential.

### 3.2 THERAPEUTIC TRIALS

Therapeutic trials help confirm the causes and sites of nasal obstruction, and also help in determining the potential success of both medical and surgical interventions.

Medication trials include the administration of topical nasal steroids, sympathomimetic agents, and antihistamines, as well as allergic management in the form or desensitization. Patients that show significant improvement may choose not to undergo surgery. However, an underlying anatomical cause for obstruction needs to be addressed if a patient is unwilling to take medications permanently. The impact of decongestants such as oxymetazoline during nighttime sleep is valuable in assessing the impact of nasal obstruction in symptoms like snoring and overall in sleep-disordered breathing. The role of nasal valve collapse in nasal obstruction can also be confirmed with a trial of Breathe Right™ nasal strips (CNS Inc., Whippany, NJ), which help maintain the valves open through external dilatation, and prevent collapse during deep inspiration. Patients that have an adequate response in the form of reduced snoring and improved breathing are likely to benefit from nasal valve suspension procedures. Sleep partners may report decrease in snoring levels and observe how the patient is able to breathe through the nose alone, without opening the mouth.

## 3.3 NASAL AIRFLOW EVALUATION

Even a thorough clinical evaluation can oftentimes be unreliable and even contradictory. Patients are often not completely aware of the magnitude of nasal obstruction they might be experiencing, particularly during sleep. In the awake state, patients with atrophic rhinitis secondary to extensive turbinate resection have a persistent feeling of obstruction in spite of objective evidence of patency, whereas patients with deviated septa or nasal polyposis report no obstruction symptoms, despite evidence against a patent nasal airway.[9] The objective evaluation of the nose can be divided into static or dynamic, depending on whether the structure of the nose or the airflow as a measure of the nasal function is being evaluated. In general, the evaluation of nasal airflow is a key element in the evaluation of improvement after surgical intervention. Measurements are performed at baseline and after procedures, in order to compare values and confirm improvement. Nasal airflow tests show a wide variety of normal values, which limits their use as stand-alone diagnostic tests.[22]

## 3.4 RHINOMANOMETRY AND ACOUSTIC RHINOMETRY

Nasal resistance can be calculated on the basis of the pressure gradients formed in the nose during inspiration. Rhinomanometry (RM) measures nasal airway resistance and airflow. It has two phases, passive and active, and it can be divided into anterior and posterior. Active RM requires the patient to generate airflow through inspiration. Passive RM utilizes external generation of airflow through the nose at a constant pressure. Anterior RM may reflect the status of the nares, nasal valves, and nasal cycling, and utilizes a device inserted into the nares. Posterior RM, in turn, utilizes a sensor inserted into the mouth which measures the nasopharynx, hence requiring substantial patient co-operation. These tests are also usually performed before and after the administration of nasal decongestants.[23]

Acoustic rhinometry evaluates nasal obstruction by analyzing reflected sound waves introduced through the nares. It is not invasive, is easily reproducible and it does not require patient co-operation. The results are expressed as cross-sectional dimensions of the nasal cavity, which closely approximate the smallest cross-sectional area and volume.[24]

The cross-sectional area (CSA) is measured at different points from the nares to the closest area of narrowing, which corresponds to the nasal valve area. Since a 'normal' CSA varies so much from patient to patient, an absolute value is not very useful for diagnosis or for confirmation of nasal valve area obstruction. Previously published work by the authors, however, has demonstrated that the ratio of the CSA during inspiration to the CSA at rest is highly diagnostic of nasal valve collapse.[25] Normally, deep inspiration should not decrease the CSA. If it does, it is a sign of nasal valve collapse.

## 4 IMPACT OF NASAL SURGERY ON SNORING AND OSAHS

The most direct way to study the impact of an obstructed nasal airway is to examine the effect surgical correction of obstruction has on patients with SDB. A number of studies have been published that studied the effects on subjective (daytime somnolence, snoring) and objective parameters (Polysomnography) by addressing obstruction caused by the nasal valve, the septum, and the turbinates. A small study showed improvement in both subjective and objective parameters,[26] but it only involved a total of six patients, without controls. A bigger, non-controlled study by Fairbanks[27] showed improvement in snoring in 47 out of 113 enrolled subjects. Perhaps the only study to show consistent improvement of the Apnea/Hypopnea Index (AHI) was the study performed by Series et al.[17] In this study, patients with mild OSAHS underwent lateral radiographs, from which cephalometric measurements were taken. Patients that showed an improvement on the AHI were those that had normal cephalometric measurements preoperatively (specifically mandibular plane to hyoid, decreased posterior airspace, or length of the soft palate). Patients with abnormal measurements did not improve with nasal surgery alone.

Contradicting these earlier findings, more recent reports show that less than 20% of patients achieve a 50% reduction in AHI with nasal surgery alone.[28] A recent report by Virkkula et al. also failed to show improvement in snoring intensity or daytime sleepiness symptoms in a group of 40 patients after nasal surgery for an obstructed nasal airway, in spite of decreased nasal resistance as measured by rhinomanometry.[29] Data on patients undergoing nasal surgery alone for the treatment of OSAHS[30] showed that, despite subjective improvement in patients undergoing submucous resection (SMR) of the septum with or without SMR of the inferior turbinates, an overall improvement in OSAHS on the basis of polysomnographic data could not be demonstrated in most patients. In fact, when pre- and postnasal surgery AHI have been compared in mild, moderate, and severe OSAHS patients, a tendency towards worsening of this parameter has been observed, although statistical significance for the postoperative increase in AHI was only observed in mild OSAHS cases[26] (Table 19.1). This paradoxical effect has been previously described,[4] and the numerous hypotheses that have been proposed for this phenomenon are based on the increased comfort that

| Table 19.1 Respiratory Disturbance Index and OSAHS procedure | | |
|---|---|---|
| OSAHS classification/type of procedure | Mean RDI | |
| | Pre-op | Post-op |
| Mild/nasal | 8.69 | 18.7 |
| Mild/nasal + PIT | 12.9 | 9.3 |
| Moderate/nasal | 19.4 | 28.9 |
| Moderate/nasal + PIT | 30.3 | 26.2 |
| Severe | 55.8 | 56 |

patients experience by being able to breathe through the nose. Better subjective sleep quality due to a patent nasal airway is achieved, which leads to deeper and more comfortable sleep, resulting in increased apneic episodes due to increased collapsibility of the upper airway. Sleep fragmentation results, particularly in moderate to severe sleep apnea patients. The experimental and clinical evidence of less sleep fragmentation and disturbance, thus, applies only to non-OSAHS patients in whom nasal breathing is improved after surgery.[7,31] Another possible explanation for worsening of the AHI from the first to the second night of study might occur because the patients experience what is also known as the 'first night effect',[29] where they become adapted to the test environment after the second or third night of study, and thus are able to sleep better.

Finally, the increased airflow in a patient's nasal airway creates more turbulence by the Bernoulli effect, thus promoting the collapse of the airway at the site of greatest pressure, which corresponds to the narrowest point.

Intervention at other levels of obstruction, without a doubt, increase the impact that relieving nasal obstruction has on the overall picture of OSAHS, and even on nasal obstruction by itself. Correction of nasal airway obstruction has been shown to have a significant impact on OSAHS when performed as a part of a multilevel approach to treat patients with OSAHS. Friedman et al. have shown that patients with nasal obstruction and OSAHS achieved significantly better objective and subjective success rates when soft palate implant insertion for the treatment of snoring and mild to moderate OSAHS was performed together with nasal surgery[32] (Table 19.1). A more rigid palate is probably less prone to collapsing (requiring an increased pharyngeal closing pressure) and thus the increased flow of air through the operated nose, which actually counteracts a normal effect of increased nasal resistance in the recumbent position,[33] does not have the negative effect on the patient's OSAHS.

## 5 IMPACT OF NASAL SURGERY ON BLOOD OXYGEN SATURATION

Olsen and Kern, in an excellent review of nasal influences on OSAHS,[34] documented the importance of the nasal cycle and the nasopulmonary reflex in maintaining adequate blood oxygenation. The lowest oxygen saturation levels ($LSaO_2$) are directly affected by the patency of the nasal airway, with or without persistent OSAHS. While the increase in $LSaO_2$ might be discrete, nasal interventions might at least maintain adequate blood oxygenation levels.[30] This supports the necessity of correcting an obstructed nasal airway as part of the overall strategy of surgical intervention for OSAHS.

## 6 IMPACT OF NASAL SURGERY ON NASAL CONTINUOUS AIRWAY PRESSURE (NCPAP) THERAPY

Continuous positive airway pressure (CPAP) is currently the mainstay for the management of OSAHS. Poor compliance (sometimes less than 50%) with this management strategy[35] – particularly of nCPAP – has been attributed to the discomfort of the high-pressure air being delivered through partially obstructed nasal airways. Surgical correction of nasal obstruction can have a significant Impact on the nCPAP pressure needed to decrease the Respiratory Disturbance Index as much as possible without disrupting the patient's sleep. This makes it more tolerable, which results in an increase in compliance in some patients.[36] Friedman et al. confirmed a significant decrease in CPAP titration levels after nasal surgery alone[30] (Table 19.2), after Series et al. initially described this finding in a small series of patients.[4] Powell showed that patients actually report a subjective improvement in nasal obstruction, which seemed to be in direct relationship with the degree of adherence to CPAP therapy.[5] In fact, it has been proposed that CPAP in itself might promote the development of nasal inflammation, and in some patients even vasomotor rhinitis, particularly when using CPAP machines that do not control the temperature of the delivered air nor humidify it. It is likely that this effect might be even more pronounced in patients with an underlying cause for nasal obstruction.

## 7 CONCLUSION

Although nasal obstruction may be a major contributing factor of OSAHS in some patients, this is certainly not the case in the majority. Selected patients who respond to a diagnostic trial of artificial nasal airway improvement with topical and systemic decongestants and steroids, along with external nasal dilators (e.g. Breathe Right™ strips), may also benefit from definitive correction of the nasal airway, with elimination of snoring and improvement in OSAHS. The majority of patients with nasal obstruction and OSAHS will likely benefit from a multilevel surgical approach. If nasal surgery is undertaken alone, it is important

# SECTION G: NASAL SURGERY FOR TREATMENT OF OSA/HS

**Table 19.2** CPAP titration levels before and after nasal surgery for OSA

| OSAHS patients | Mean CPAP (cm H$_2$O) Pre-op | Mean CPAP (cm H$_2$O) Post-op |
|---|---|---|
| Total (n = 22) | 9.3 | 6.7 |
| Severe (n = 13) | 10.07 | 7.42 |
| Moderate (n = 4) | 9.5 | 6.5 |
| Mild (n = 5) | 7.2 | 5 |

to inform patients that it may not only fail to cure, but may even aggravate snoring and OSAHS in certain cases. Nasal surgery also has a significant impact in improving patients' subjective symptoms, like daytime sleepiness and quality of sleep. It also constitutes a valuable intervention in patients that need nCPAP management for their OSAHS.

## REFERENCES

1. Boudewyns AN, Heyning PHVD, Backer WAD. Site of upper airway obstruction in obstructive sleep apnea and influence on sleep stage. Eur Respir J 1997;10:2566–72.
2. Mirza N, Lanza DC. The nasal airway and obstructed breathing during sleep. Otolaryngol Clin North Am 1999;32:243–62.
3. Carpenter JE. Mental aberration and attending hypertrophic rhinitis with subacute otitis media. JAMA 1892;19:539–42.
4. Series F, St Pierre S, Carrier G. Effects of surgical correction of nasal obstruction in the treatment of obstructive sleep apnea. Am Rev Respir Dis 1992;146:1261–65.
5. Powell N. Radiofrequency treatment of turbinate hypertrophy in subjects using CPAP: a randomized, double-blind, placebo-controlled trial. Laryngoscope 2001;111:1783–90.
6. Vijay SD, Phillipson EA. Nasal surgery in the management of sleep apnea. Ann Otol Rhinol Laryngol 1985;94:550–54.
7. Olsen KD, Kern EB, Westbrook PR. Sleep and breathing disturbance secondary to nasal obstruction. Otolaryngol Head Neck Surg 1981;89:804–10.
8. Papsidero MJ. The role of nasal obstruction in obstructive sleep apnea syndrome. Ear Nose Throat J 1993;72:82–4.
9. Rappai M, Collop N, Kemp S, deShazo R. The nose and sleep-disordered breathing: what we know and what we do not know. Chest 2003;124:2309–23.
10. Constantian MB, Clardy RB. The relative importance of septal and nasal valvular surgery in correcting airway obstruction in primary and secondary rhinoplasty. Plast Reconstr Surg 1996;98:38–54.
11. Schlosser RJ, Park SS. Functional nasal surgery. Otolaryngol Clin North Am 1999;32:37–51.
12. Tarabichi M, Fanous N. Finite element analysis of airflow in the nasal valve. Arch Otolaryngol Head Neck Surg 1993;119:638–42.
13. Cole P, Haight JS. Mechanisms of nasal obstruction in sleep. Laryngoscope 1984;94:1557–59.
14. Chen W, Kushida CA. Nasal obstruction in sleep-disordered breathing. Otolaryngol Clin North Am 2003;36:437–60.
15. De Vito A, Berrettini S, Carabelli A, et al. The importance of nasal resistance in obstructive sleep apnea syndrome: a study with positional rhinomanometry. Sleep Breath 2001;5:3–11.
16. Rizzi M, Onorato J, Andreoli A, et al. Nasal resistances are useful in identifying children with severe obstructive sleep apnea before polysomnography. Int J Pediatr Otorhinolaryngol 2002;65:7–13.
17. Series F, Pierre SS, Carrier G. Surgical correction of nasal obstruction in the treatment of obstructive sleep apnea: importance of cephalometry in predicting outcome. Thorax 1993;48:360–63.
18. Ancoli-Israel S, Kripke DF, Mason W, Messin S. Sleep apnea and nocturnal myoclonus in a senior population. Sleep 1981;4:349–58.
19. Young T, Finn L, Kim H. Nasal obstruction as a risk factor for sleep-disordered breathing. J Allergy Clin Immunol 1997;99:S757–S762.
20. Corey JP, Houser SM, Ng BA. Nasal congestion: a review of its etiology, evaluation, and treatment. Ear Nose Throat J 2000;79:690–693, 696, 698.
21. Kiely JL, Nolan P, McNicholas WT. Intranasal corticosteroid therapy for obstructive sleep apnea in patients with co-existing rhinitis. Thorax 2004;59:50–55.
22. Corey JP, Gungor A, Nelson R, Liu X, Fredberg J. Normative standards for nasal cross-sectional areas by race as measured by acoustic rhinometry. Otolaryngol Head Neck Surg 1998;119:389–93.
23. Grymer LF, Hilberg O, Pedersen OF, Rasmussen TR. Acoustic rhinometry: values from adults with subjective normal nasal patency. Rhinology 1991;29:35–47.
24. Fisher EW, Daly NJ, Morris DP, Lund VJ. Experimental studies of the resolution of acoustic rhinometry in vivo. Acta Otolaryngol 1994;114:647–50.
25. Vidyasagar R, Friedman M, Ibrahim H, Bliznikas D, Joseph NJ. Inspiratory and fixed nasal valve collapse: clinical and rhinomanometric assessment. Am J Rhinol 2005;19:370–74.
26. Dayal VS, Phillipson EA. Nasal surgery in the management of sleep apnea. Ann Otol Rhinol Laryngol 1985;94:550–54.
27. Fairbanks D. Effect of nasal surgery on snoring. South Med J 1985;78:268–70.
28. Verse T, Maurer JT, Pirsig W. Effect of nasal surgery on sleep-related breathing disorders. Laryngoscope 2002;112:64–8.
29. Virkkula P, Bachour A, Hytonen M, Salmi T, Malmberg H, Hurmerinta K, Maasita P. Snoring is not relieved by nasal surgery despite improvement in nasal resistance. Chest 2006;129:81–7.
30. Friedman M, Tanyeri H, Lim JW, Landsberg R, Vaidyanathan K, Caldarelli D. Effect of improved nasal breathing on obstructive sleep apnea. Otolaryngol Head Neck Surg 2000;122:71–4.
31. Zwillich CW, Pickett J, Hanson FN, Weil JV. Disturbed sleep and prolonged apnea during nasal obstruction in normal men. Am Rev Respir Dis 1981;124:158–60.
32. Friedman M, Vidyasagar R, Bliznikas D, Joseph NJ. Patient selection and efficacy of pillar implant technique for the treatment of snoring and obstructive sleep apnea/hypopnea syndrome. Otolaryngol Head Neck Surg 2006;134:187–96.
33. Tvinnereim M, Cole P, Haight JS, Mateika S, Hoffstein V. Sleep and posture. Laryngoscope 1994;104:846–49.
34. Olsen KD, Kern EB. Nasal influences on snoring and obstructive sleep apnea. Mayo Clin Proc 1990;65:1095–105.
35. Practice parameters for the treatment of obstructive sleep apnea in adults: the efficacy of surgical modifications of the upper airway. An American Sleep Disorders Association Report. Sleep 1996;19:152–55.
36. Pirsig W, Verse T. Long-term results in the treatment of obstructive sleep apnea. Eur Arch Otolaryngol 2000;257:570–77.

# SECTION G — NASAL SURGERY FOR TREATMENT OF OSA/HS

## CHAPTER 20

# Nasal valve repair

*Michael Friedman and Paul Schalch*

## 1 INTRODUCTION

The nasal valve is defined as the flow-limiting segment of the nasal airway, located at the triangular aperture between the upper lateral cartilage and the septum. The angle formed by these two structures ranges from 10° to 15°, and is maintained by the relationships between the nasal septum, the lower lateral cartilage, and the attachments of the facial muscles.[1]

Nasal valve collapse is a common cause of nasal airway obstruction. In fact, nasal valvular incompetence may equal or even exceed septal deviation as the prime cause of nasal airway obstruction.[2] The valve area may be obstructed secondary to surgical procedures (such as rhinoplasty), trauma, or even aging. The complexity of nasal valve repair techniques and its variable results, coupled with the difficulty of treating previously operated patients or even the fact that advanced-age patients often do not seek medical attention for this problem, make nasal valve collapse an issue that oftentimes remains unresolved. In many cases, nasal valve collapse is not diagnosed until surgical treatment, in the form septoplasty or turbinate reduction, fails to relieve symptoms of nasal obstruction, in which case further causes are investigated. It is often impossible to know if the correction of the obstruction caused by a deviated septum and the turbinates actually unmasked an underlying valve collapse problem, or whether the ensuing increased airflow actually makes the valve collapse. Classically, obstruction of the valve area has been attributed to insufficient support of the upper or lower lateral cartilages. This represents true valve collapse. Fixed valve obstruction, however, may be secondary to a persistently deviated caudal septum after septoplasty. In these cases, lateral displacement of the valve area can overcome this obstruction.

Various techniques aimed at correcting nasal valve collapse have been described.[3] Techniques designed to lateralize the superior segment of the upper lateral cartilage, involving cartilage and spreader grafts, are effective when this portion has been medially displaced.[4,5] Nasal valve obstruction may be secondary to the position of the septum (e.g. after septoplasty), and in selected cases, also amenable for repair using a nasal valve suspension technique.

The original description of a technique for repair of the nasal valve by means of a suspension of the valve to the orbital rim was described by Paniello.[6] Significant modifications to this original technique which simplified this technique, and made it safer and equally effective were later introduced by Friedman et al.[7] In this chapter, we describe the patient selection criteria and the simplified technique for nasal valve suspension for patients with nasal valve collapse and obstruction. The effect of improved nasal breathing in patients with OSAHS is discussed in detail in Chapter 19.

## 2 PATIENT SELECTION

In general, four categories of nasal valve obstruction can be identified, based on the involved valve (external or internal), and whether it is always present (fixed), or present during inspiration only (inspiratory, also referred to as nasal valve collapse). It should be noted that both types of obstruction can be present at the same time. While examining the nasal valve, both the external and the internal valves should be visualized, in order to determine the presence of obstruction. The internal valve is located at the level of the border of the upper lateral cartilage and the piriform aperture. Not only can this area be easily distorted during anterior rhinoscopy, it can also be completely overlooked with nasal endoscopy; hence, it should actually be examined prior to the introduction of the speculum or endoscope into the nose. As part of the routine evaluation, patients should be asked to take a deep breath while observing the nasal valve. A normally functioning nasal valve widens together with the nasal alae external dilator muscles, whereas in patients with inspiratory obstruction, the nasal valve collapses during inspiration. Nasal strips (Breathe Right™, CNS Inc., Whippany, NJ) are usually effective in improving airflow by widening the nasal valve area in these patients, and may serve as a kind of confirmatory test to identify potential candidates for nasal valve suspension.

Patients may have nasal valve obstruction secondary to a deviated caudal septal position, which may nevertheless be correctable by valve suspension in selected situations. The decision to correct the valve or the septum is based on the response to the Cottle maneuver, the position of the entire septum, and whether the patient has had previous septal surgery. The Cottle maneuver consists of superolateral traction being applied to the nasofacial groove, and is considered positive when it causes improvement of the nasal airway, as perceived by the patient. A positive Cottle maneuver is an adequate predictor of a successful outcome of nasal valve suspension for the treatment of nasal airway obstruction.[8] The area of obstruction can then be identified by intranasal examination at the valve region. Direct superolateral displacement (with a cotton-tip applicator) should significantly improve the patients' nasal airway. Patients with associated rhinitis or other causes of nasal airway obstruction should be treated appropriately prior to surgery.

## 3 SURGICAL TECHNIQUE (OUTLINE OF PROCEDURE)

Several key points simplify the procedure and deserve special mention before describing the technique for nasal valve suspension in detail. The necessary equipment, which includes the bone anchoring device (Mitek Soft Tissue Anchor system™, DePuy Mitek Inc., Raynham, Mass.) and needle (Fig. 20.1), has been carefully tested and chosen based on trial and error, and has proven to be crucial to the simplicity and effectiveness of the technique. The drill bit is included with the disposable bone anchor set, and it fits into the specific drill used for the procedure. The needle is perfectly sized and its contour allows for easy placement of the suture from the orbital rim to the valve area. Equipment or instrument substitutions are likely to complicate these important steps.

The procedure can be performed under local or general anesthesia. The nasal valve area is examined to identify the area of collapse prior to injection of local anesthesia, in order to avoid tissue distortion. Two points representing the caudal and cephalad margins of the collapsed area are marked, and an incision is made through the mucosa, connecting both points (Fig. 20.2). This mucosal incision is an important modification from a previously reported technique.[7] It ensures that the suture, once it is looped at the level of the nasal valve and back into the orbital rim, is buried underneath the healing mucosa, instead of remaining exposed, which used to promote the development of granulation along the valve area in patients who had a reaction to the suture material. A natural skin crease along the orbital rim is also marked (Fig. 20.3), where the incision for the infraorbital approach will be performed. Alternatively, a transconjunctival approach that provides access to the infraorbital rim can be performed on patients who refuse facial incisions (Fig. 20.4). No significant scarring results from the facial incision, however, and since this approach is significantly more direct and simple than the transconjunctival approach, we prefer and recommend the infraorbital approach. Local anesthesia with epinephrine is then injected into the valve area, along the maxilla, near the infraorbital nerve, and along the orbital rim. A 3 mm incision is made in the medial aspect of the orbital rim. The skin incision is carried down through the subcutaneous tissue. The orbicularis

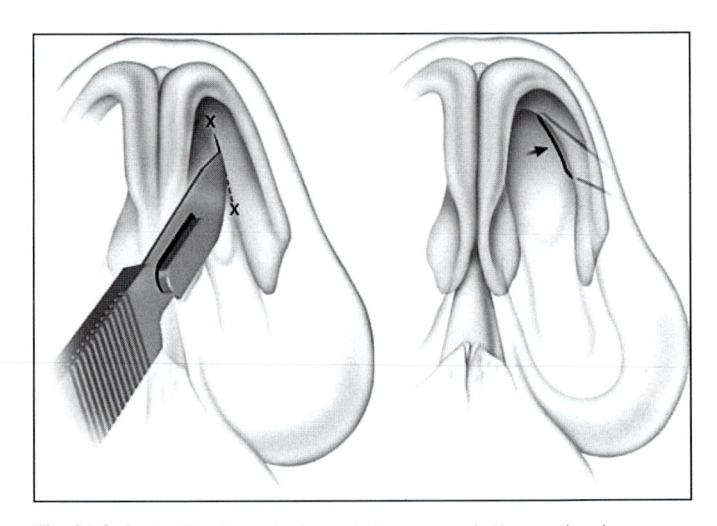

**Fig. 20.2** An incision is made through the mucosa in the previously identified area of internal valve collapse.

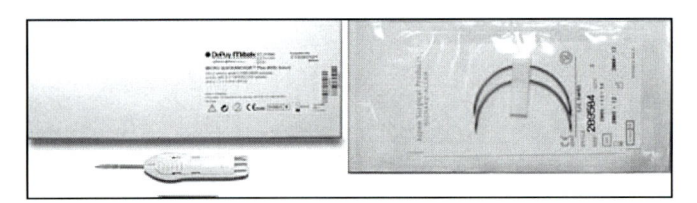

**Fig. 20.1** The bone anchoring device (Mitek Soft Tissue Anchor system™, DePuy Mitek Inc., Raynham, Mass.) and needle.

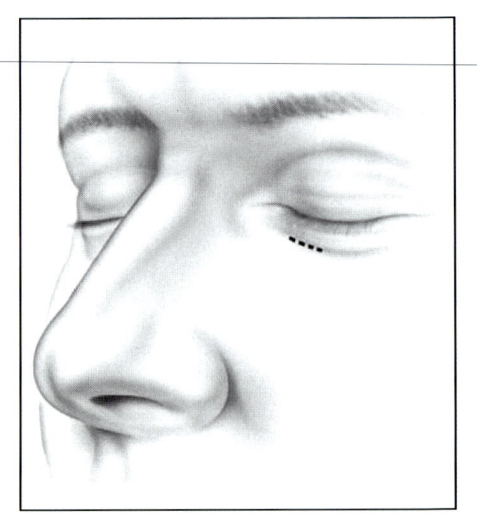

**Fig. 20.3** A natural skin crease along the orbital rim serves as the site for incision for the infraorbital approach.

oculi muscle fibers are then separated with blunt dissection using a Dunning elevator. The orbital periosteum is exposed, incised, and elevated. Bleeding is rarely encountered, and can be easily controlled with bipolar cautery. The periosteum is elevated away from the orbital rim with two Dunning elevators, in order to expose a 3 × 3 mm area. The bone anchor system is used to anchor the suture to this exposed area in the orbital rim. The drill bit included with the bone anchor system is compatible with the battery-operated Stryker™ (Kalamazoo, MI) drill. A small drill hole is made into the bone, with or without a guide, and the anchor is easily inserted into the bone (Fig. 20.5). Should the drill hole enter the maxillary sinus, the anchor should not be placed, since the thin bone will not provide adequate support. It is crucial for the anchor to be placed at the orbital rim, where the bone is thick enough to engage the anchor. The anchor is designed to be placed beneath the bone surface, thus eliminating the possibility of protruding above the surface and causing symptoms. The longer end of the suture (3-0 Ethibond™, Ethicon, Sommerville, NJ) is then passed with a curved, tapered needle (Fig. 20.6) into the nasal valve area and passed through the incised mucosa (Fig. 20.7). After identifying the site of collapse and the intended site of suspension, the needle is then rethreaded and passed through the opening in the mucosa and toward the anchor (Fig. 20.8). Another important technical point is for the needle and suture to 'hug' the periosteum of the maxilla, so that the suture is along the surface of the bone and not running through the subcutaneous tissue. Subcutaneous placement can cause pain or discomfort. The suture is then tightened and tied with the amount of tension necessary to ensure support of the valve, but avoiding significant distortion of the external valve area. The suture is buried underneath the incised mucosa, which avoids the

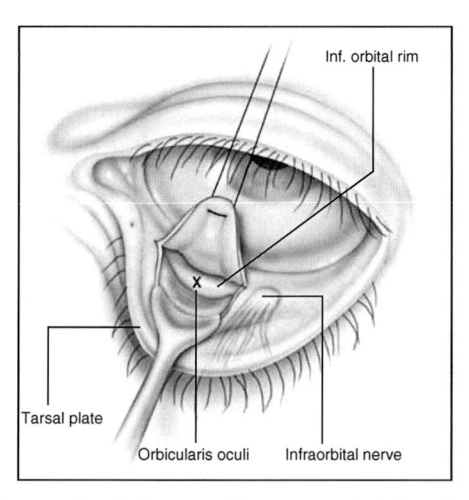

**Fig. 20.4** Transconjunctival approach for access to the infraorbital rim without facial incisions.

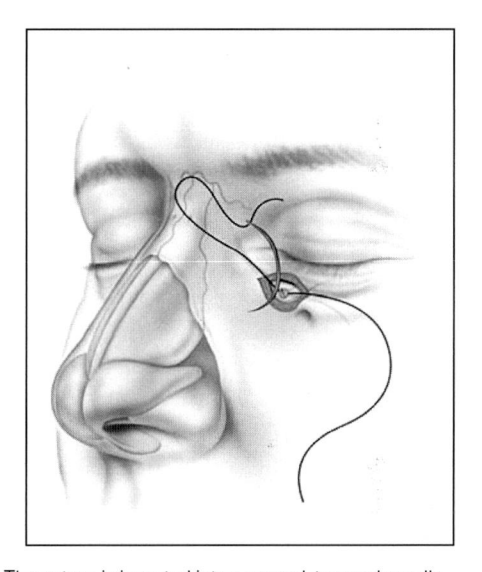

**Fig. 20.6** The suture is inserted into a curved, tapered needle.

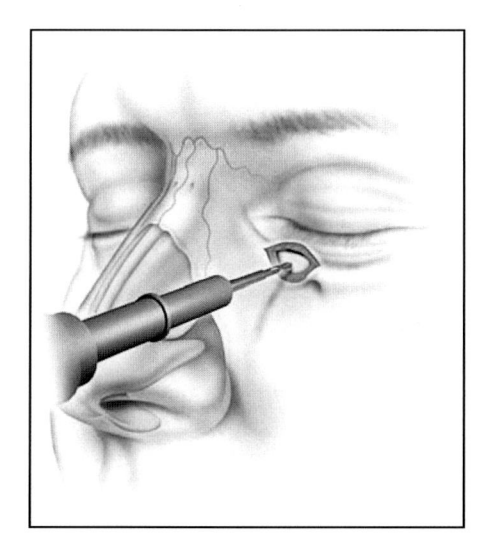

**Fig. 20.5** A small drill hole is made into the bone, in preparation for insertion of the anchoring system and suture.

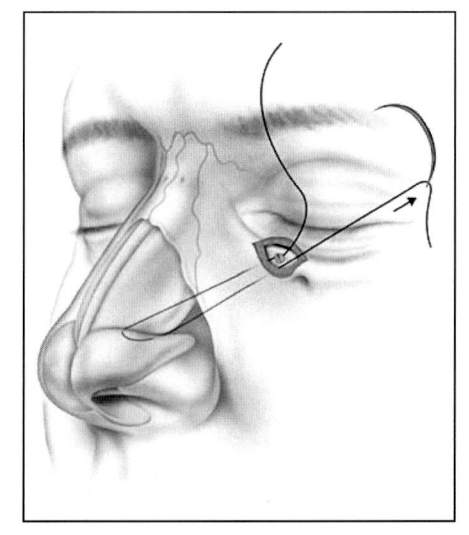

**Fig. 20.7** The suture is then passed into the nasal valve area, through the incised mucosa.

# SECTION G
## NASAL SURGERY FOR TREATMENT OF OSA/HS

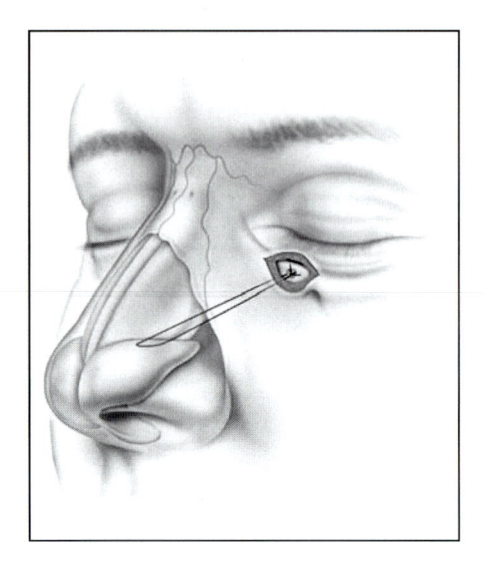

**Fig. 20.8** The needle is then rethreaded and passed through the opening in the mucosa and toward the anchor.

development of granulation tissue. The orbital rim incision is closed with Steri-strips (3M, St Paul, MN). Although usually only one bone anchor and suture are needed on each affected side, some patients may require additional suspension with two anchors and their corresponding sutures on a single side. The orbicularis oculi fibers are not sutured to avoid ectropion. Patients are told to expect some fullness in the nasofacial groove. The vast majority of patients find this tolerable, and patients reluctant to tolerate this side effect of the procedure should be counseled against undergoing nasal valve suspension.

## 4 POSTOPERATIVE MANAGEMENT AND COMPLICATIONS

Due to the simplicity of this procedure, patients can be discharged on the same day, with a 1-week postoperative follow-up appointment. Patients usually receive a prescription for postoperative antibiotics for 5–7 days, and are instructed to take over-the-counter analgesics in case of significant postoperative pain. No additional postoperative instructions are necessary. Nasal valve suspension does not require postoperative packing, which not only makes the postoperative course much more comfortable for the patient, but it also eliminates an important source of morbidity when combined with other procedures, like uvulopalatopharyngoplasty, in patients who undergo combined procedures for OSAHS.[9] For this same reason, nasal valve suspension allows for the resumption of nasal continuous positive airway pressure during the immediate postoperative period, if necessary.

The fact that the patient will experience fullness in the nasofacial groove after this procedure is reiterated to the patient upon discharge. This is an important point to make before the procedure, in order to ensure realistic expectations on behalf of the patient.

In general, no major complications have been identified. Minor complications include, but are not limited to, persistent pain at the orbital suspension site, which may require removal of the suture. This pain might be due to the close proximity to the infraorbital nerve, which may be confirmed by means of a computed tomography (CT) scan. This is a rare complication, since the placement of the anchor is usually 2.5 cm medial to the infraorbital nerve. The pain intensity may range from vague discomfort or a sensation of fullness to significant pain, and should be addressed appropriately. The more likely cause of persistent pain is the subcutaneous placement of the suture, which pulls on the tissues. This symptom usually resolves after removal of the suture. Implant removal is more difficult and almost never required. Infection and abscess formation is a rare complication. Should they present, incision and drainage of the abscess, together with suture removal, will appropriately resolve these complications. In most cases, a change in the external appearance of the nose is considered inconsequential by patients. Scars at the infraorbital level are, likewise, not considered significant. The overall rate of complications, requiring suture removal, is about 3%, as described by Friedman et al.[8] It is also important to note that this procedure is completely reversible, and that the common complications can be addressed in an outpatient setting. Removal of the suture is more difficult than placement of the suture, but can be performed with local anesthesia. Suture removal will almost always resolve uncontrolled infection, pain, or deformity. It is rarely necessary to remove the bone anchor, which could require drilling of the surrounding bone.

## 5 SUCCESS RATE OF THE PROCEDURE

Over 90% of patients who experience relief of nasal airway obstruction by using breathing strips report subjective improvement after nasal valve suspension, based on short- and long-term studies (6-month follow-up). As measured by standardized symptom and quality-of-life questionnaires specifically designed to assess nasal obstruction symptoms,[10] significant improvement has also been shown in over 80% of patients who underwent bilateral nasal valve suspension, even considering the fact that some of the most popular instruments used, like the Sino-nasal Outcome Test (SNOT-20), do not specifically explore symptoms relative to nasal stuffiness or obstruction. Objective improvement, as shown by comparing pre- and postoperative nasal cross-sectional area (CSA) with acoustic rhinometry (AR) for the left and right nasal cavities, also has shown consistent and significant improvement. AR is probably not valuable as an isolated diagnostic test in evaluating nasal valve obstruction due to its wide range of normal values.[11,12] It does, however, provide a good objective value for comparison, and to establish improvement. Improvement of CSA correlates with subjective improvement in relief of nasal obstruction. Nasal valve suspension can also be combined with other airway procedures, when performed for the surgical treatment of OSAHS, and this significantly impacts the effectiveness of nasal obstruction relief in the treatment of such patients (see Chapter 19). A significant number of patients will undergo nasal valve suspension after having previously undergone procedures like rhino- or septoplasty, or even endonasal repair attempts with alar cartilage or spreader grafts for persistent nasal obstruction. These patients also show significant improvement after nasal valve suspension, and find this surgical alternative more acceptable than additional endonasal surgery, mostly because of the possibility of undergoing the procedure with local anesthesia only, not requiring postoperative packing or splinting, and not having the potential for donor site morbidity, as is the case for cartilage-grafting techniques. Long-term controlled studies have not been done, and the success rate of the procedure would likely drop after longer follow-up.

## 5.1 WHAT TO DO IF THE PROCEDURE FAILS

While the procedure described in this chapter is not a substitute for the standard reconstructive techniques, it can serve as an option for patients who do not want to accept the morbidity of open nasal surgery or cartilage-grafting procedures. It is also an option for patients who have failed previous attempts at correction surgery for valve collapse. Lack of improvement is presumably due to failure to suspend the nasal valve because of insufficient tension of the suture. Other potential causes may be tearing of the suture, inadequate positioning of the suture or the bone anchor, or weakening of the tissues. If nasal valve obstruction is not resolved or if it recurs, a second suspension can easily be performed, which constitutes a distinct advantage of this procedure. Persistent obstruction after nasal valve suspension probably requires more aggressive reconstructive techniques, like septorhinoplasty and alar cartilage or spreader raft reconstruction, after appropriately analyzing the potential structural cause for failure.

## 6 CONCLUSION

The bone anchor technique for nasal valve suspension is a simple, minimally invasive alternative to address nasal obstruction secondary to fixed or inspiratory nasal valve collapse. The procedure can be done under local anesthesia and has minimal postoperative morbidity. It is reversible and it has been shown to be effective in over 90% of patients in relieving subjective symptoms of nasal obstruction. Nasal valve suspension is an alternative for patients who have already undergone rhino- or septoplasty or endonasal procedures to relieve nasal obstruction, and are reluctant to undergo additional endonasal surgery. It also constitutes a valuable component of a multilevel surgical approach for the treatment of OSAHS.

## REFERENCES

1. Bridger G. Physiology of the nasal valve. Arch Otolaryngol 1970;92:543–53.
2. Constantian M, Clardy R. The relative importance of septal and nasal valvular surgery in correcting airway obstruction in primary and secondary rhinoplasty. Plast Reconstr Surg 1996;98:38–54. discussion 55–8.
3. Goode R. Surgery of the incompetent nasal valve. Laryngoscope 1985;95:546–55.
4. Lee D, Glasgold A. Correction of nasal valve stenosis with lateral suture suspension. Arch Facial Plast Surg 2001;3:237–40.
5. Sheen J. Spreader graft: a method of reconstructing the roof of the middle nasal vault following rhinoplasty. Plast Reconstr Surg 1984;73:230–39.
6. Paniello R. Nasal valve suspension. An effective treatment for nasal valve collapse. Arch Otolaryngol Head Neck Surg 1996;122:1342–46.
7. Friedman M, Ibrahim H, Syed Z. Nasal valve suspension: an improved, simplified technique for nasal valve collapse. Laryngoscope 2003;113:381–85.
8. Friedman M, Ibrahim H, Lee G, et al. A simplified technique for airway correction at the nasal valve area. Otolaryngol Head Neck Surg 2004;131:519–24.
9. Dorn M, Pirsig W, Verse T. [Postoperative management following rhinosurgery interventions in severe obstructive sleep apnea. A pilot study]. HNO 2001;49:642–45.
10. Piccirillo J, Merritt MJ, Richards M. Psychometric and clinimetric validity of the 20-Item Sino-Nasal Outcome Test (SNOT-20). Otolaryngol Head Neck Surg 2002;126:41–7.
11. Corey J, Gungor A, Nelson R, et al. A comparison of the nasal cross-sectional areas and volumes obtained with acoustic rhinometry and magnetic resonance imaging. Otolaryngol Head Neck Surg 1997;117:349–54.
12. Hamilton J, McRae R, Phillips D, et al. The accuracy of acoustic rhinometry using a pulse train signal. Clin Otolaryngol Allied Sci 1995;20:279–82.

SECTION G    NASAL SURGERY FOR TREATMENT OF OSA/HS

CHAPTER
21

# Correction of nasal obstruction due to nasal valve collapse

*Maria T. Messina-Doucet*

## 1 INTRODUCTION

Airway obstruction or difficulty breathing through the nose is one of the most frequent complaints presented to an otolaryngologist. Nasal septal deviation and turbinate hypertrophy are easily identified as areas of anatomic obstruction. One area that can be overlooked as an etiology for obstruction is an incompetent nasal valve. Nasal valve obstruction can markedly reduce airflow through the anterior nostril. This reduction in flow can contribute to snoring. A patient who complains of snoring is indicating that something more serious may be occurring. Snoring can present as a symptom of obstructive sleep apnea. Many people who snore also admit to excessive daytime sleepiness and fatigue.[1]

Incompetence of the nasal valve, either internal or external, may arise from several factors. Congenital weakness of the nasal sidewalls may allow for easier collapse. As age progresses nasal ptosis and sagging of the sidewalls can occur. This can contribute to nasal obstruction. An anatomically narrow nasal valve may contribute to nasal valve collapse, which can be congenital or present years after cosmetic rhinoplasty surgery.

Anything that increases the resistance of nasal airflow can be markedly perceived as obstruction by the patient. During rhinoplasty, specifically hump reduction, the internal nasal valve can be interrupted. Interruption of the attachment of the septum to the upper lateral cartilages allows for collapse of the weakened cartilage. The interrupted support for the upper lateral cartilage can cause it to fall towards the dorsal septal edge, narrowing the internal nasal valve. The external nasal valve can be weakened by overzealous resection of the lower lateral cartilage. Scar tissue formation can also contribute to weakening of the remaining alar cartilage. A weakened alar sidewall with less support can easily collapse and obstruct the anterior nostril.

The internal valve is the area in which the septum articulates with the lower border of the upper lateral cartilage (Fig. 21.1A). The angle of this area is normally 10° to 15°. Minimal reduction in this angle can substantially restrict nasal airflow. The external nasal valve is an area composed of the alar or lower lateral cartilage with its associated cutaneous support as a mobile alar wall (Fig. 21.1B). It is bordered superiorly by the caudal edge of the upper lateral cartilages, inferiorly by the nasal floor, and posteriorly by the inferior turbinate. Laterally it is supported by the pyriform aperture of the maxilla and fibrofatty tissue of the ala.[2]

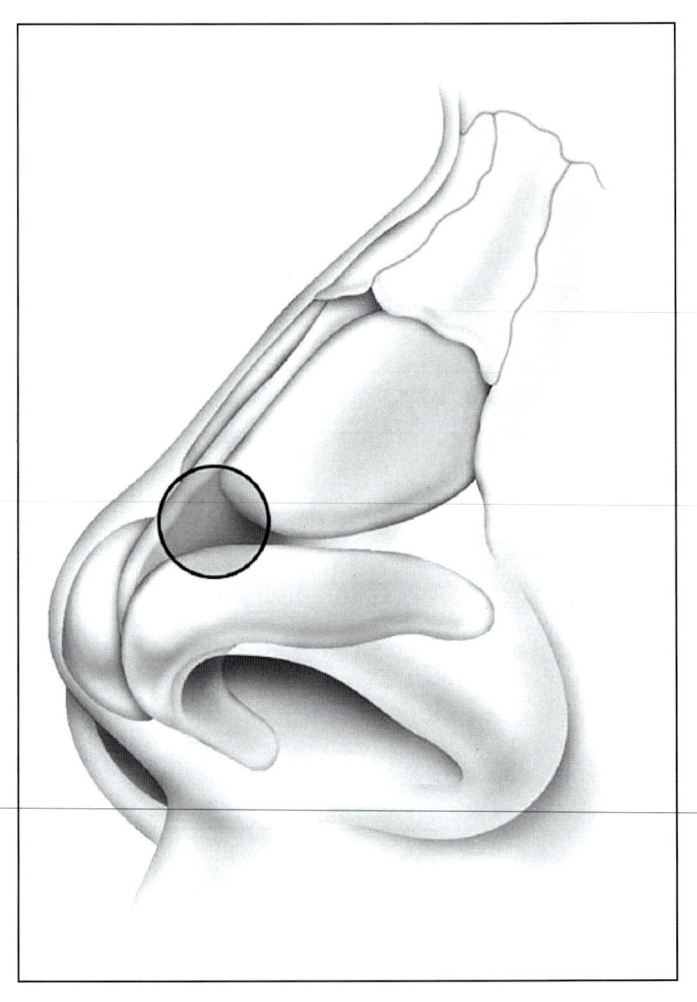

**Fig. 21.1** A, Internal nasal valve.

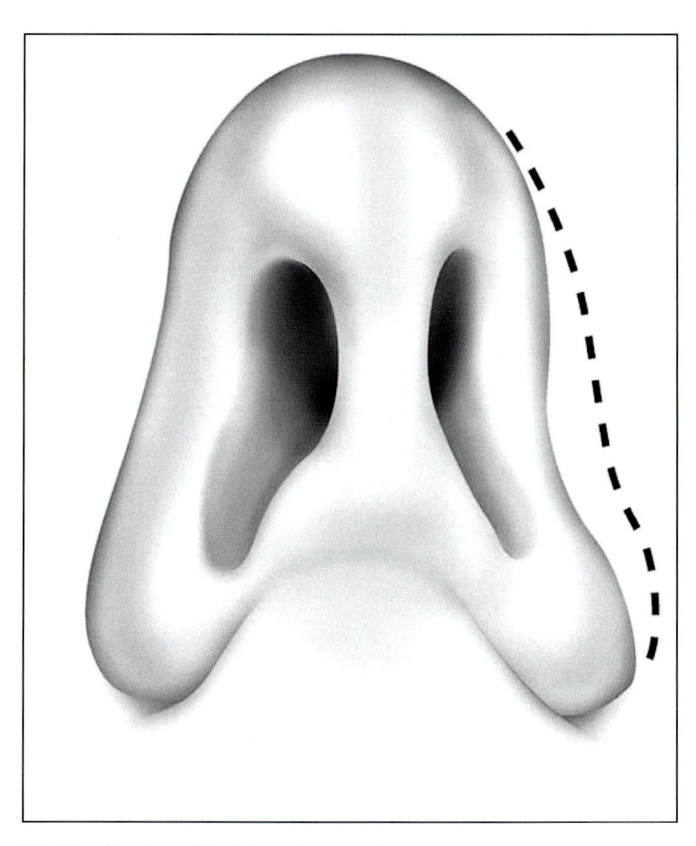

**Fig. 21.1** (Continued) B, External nasal valve.

In consideration of surgical approaches to correct nasal obstruction, all possible causes must be entertained. Correction of septal deviation alone may not alleviate obstruction. Valvular effects may equal or surpass a deviation of the septum as the cause of airflow obstruction. In an excellent study by Constantain it was shown that septoplasty in addition to internal and external valve reconstruction offered the best relief in nasal obstruction. This combined approach offered significantly improved airflow in comparison to septoplasty alone.[3]

## 2 EXAMINATION

Examination before and after the application of topical vasoconstrictors can allow the effects of turbinate hyperplasia to be evaluated. The use of a standard nasal speculum spreads the valve open and can allow a narrowed valve to go undetected. An otoscope is a useful tool to evaluate internal valve collapse as it dose not splay open the area of concern. Some advocate the use of a Q-tip or cerumen spoon to elevate the sidewall of the nose 1–2 mm. If the patient reports improved breathing with this conservative maneuver, valve restriction is contributing to the patient's obstruction.[4] It is important to evaluate the competence of both the internal and the external nasal valves as concurrent correction is often required in order to alleviate the symptoms of nasal obstruction.

## 3 SURGICAL APPROACHES

This is by no means a complete review of all of the techniques that are available to surgically address incompetent valves. However, it will serve as a guideline of the most commonly accepted techniques.

### 3.1 INTERNAL NASAL VALVE

The spreader graft as described by Sheen in 1984[5] has been the most common approach to correct internal nasal valve collapse. Several adaptations to this technique have been reported in the literature.[6-9] Each offers a varying twist of the standard that may accommodate specific circumstances pertaining to individual patients. An open approach is preferable as it allows superior visualization of anatomy.

#### 3.1.1 TECHNIQUES FOR INTERNAL VALVE REPAIR

**Spreader graft**

1. For an open approach: an 11 blade is used to make an inverted V transcolumellar incision. Marginal incisions are made in the nasal vestibule of each nostril. Soft tissue is elevated off the medial crus of the lower lateral cartilages with care taken not to disrupt this delicate cartilage. A converse scissors is used to create a subperiosteal plane that allows for a clean dissection. Tissue is elevated following each lower lateral cartilage laterally. By exposing the cartilages in this way, multiple problem areas can be corrected through the same approach.
2. Dissection then follows at the septal edge and mucoperiosteal flaps are elevated from both sides of the septum. If septal cartilage is available this is the graft material of choice as it is in the same operative field. Otherwise, auricular cartilage can be harvested. Leaving a 1 cm strut to both the caudal septal edge as well as to the dorsal aspect of the septum, septal cartilage is harvested. The cartilage is then carved with either a 15 blade or a 64 beaver blade into two grafts 15 mm in length and 2–3 mm in thickness.
3. The grafts are placed on either side of the septum as high as possible. Try to place the grafts at the same height as the septum so that they sit flush at the nasal dorsum. The use of a 25-gauge 1 inch straight needle helps to hold the grafts in place on each side of the septum while preparing to place sutures. At the caudal edge of the graft, a 5.0 absorbable suture (Vicryl) is placed through the spreader

SECTION G  NASAL SURGERY FOR TREATMENT OF OSA/HS

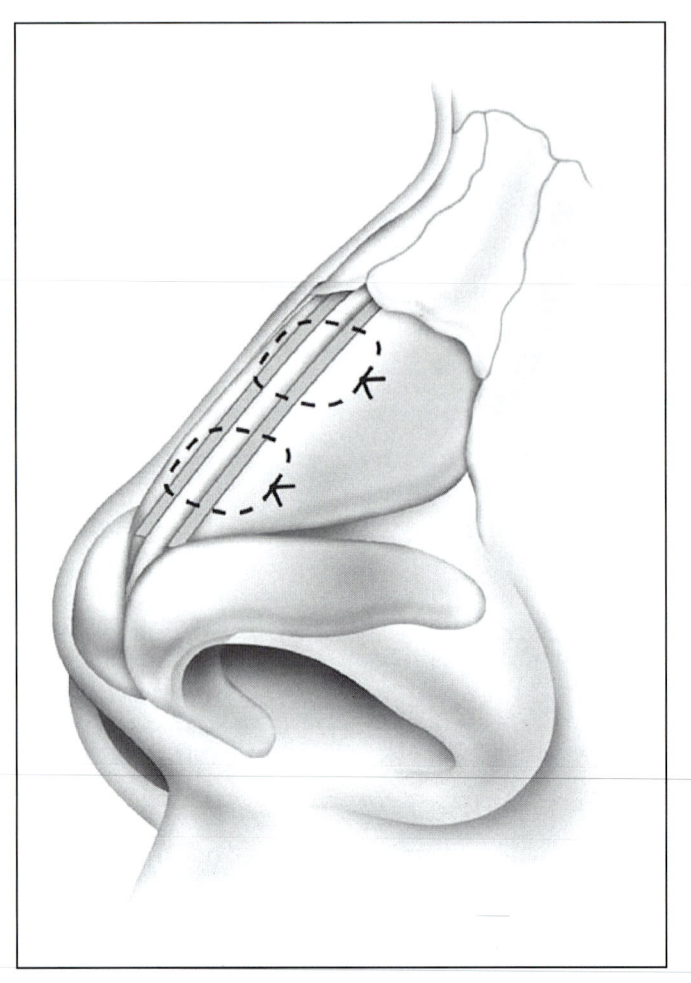

**Fig. 21.2** Spreader graft.

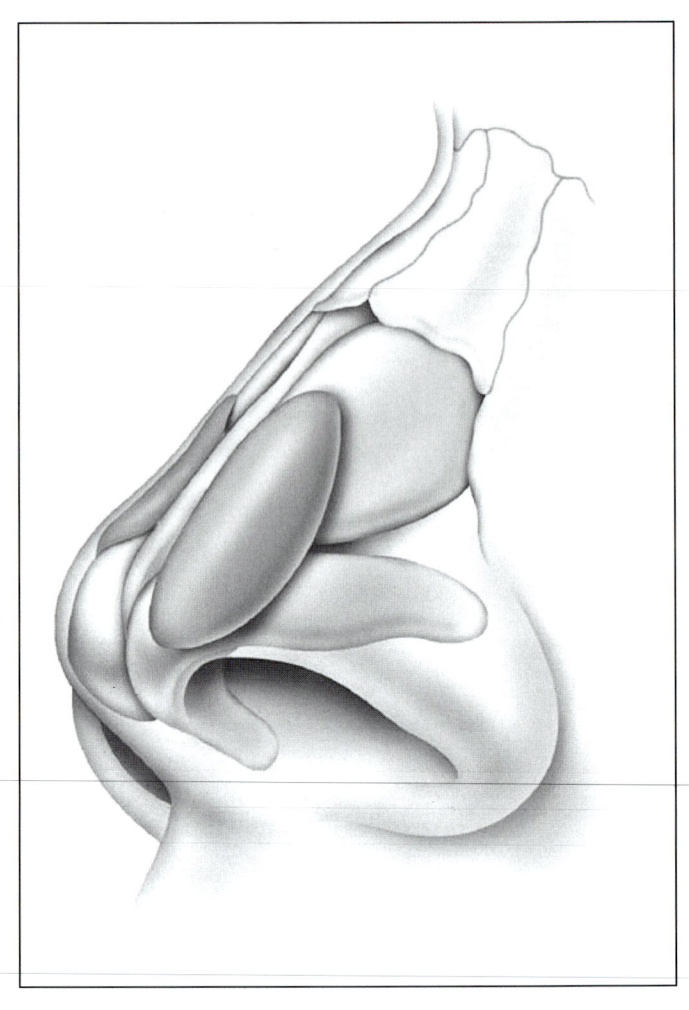

**Fig. 21.3** Cartilage spanning graft.

graft, the septum, and the other spreader graft in a mattress fashion (Fig. 21.2). Approximately 1 cm posterior another suture is placed from the upper lateral cartilage, through the spreader graft, septum spreader graft, and upper lateral cartilage in a mattress fashion (Fig. 21.2).

The advantage of this technique is that it causes little nasal deformity. It can widen the dorsum but this trade-off is usually acceptable as the function of the nose is improved as the obstruction may be alleviated.

### Cartilage spanning graft

Occasionally, spreader grafts alone are not sufficient especially in a patient with weak septal cartilages. Even if auricular cartilage is used for spreader grafts sometimes the septum is very thin and another option must be considered. Cartilage placed over the area of internal valve collapse can provide structural support and prevent collapse of the internal nasal valve.

*Technique*
1. Prior to anesthesia, the area on the external nose that corresponds to the internal nasal valve is observed. A Q-tip is used to view the internal valve area and a surgical marking pen is used to mark the surface of the skin on the lateral nose that sits above this weak area.
2. An open approach, as described above, is then used to expose the area of the septum and the upper lateral cartilage. Cartilage is harvested and a 64 beaver blade is used to configure a graft that is circular in fashion and large enough to cover the defect as determined by preoperative markings. Tapering the edges improves cosmetic camouflage and makes the graft less visible postoperatively.
3. The graft is placed spanning the upper lateral cartilage and the lower lateral cartilage, lateral to the septum (Fig. 21.3). The graft is sutured percutaneously with a 4.0 PDS in order to coapt tissues, prevent graft migration, and prevent the accumulation of fluid between the graft and the skin (Fig. 21.3). The PDS is removed in 7 days.

This technique is advantageous in elderly patients with thin septal cartilages. It can also be used in patients with thick skin. The disadvantage of this method is that the tip

CHAPTER 21
Correction of nasal obstruction due to nasal valve collapse

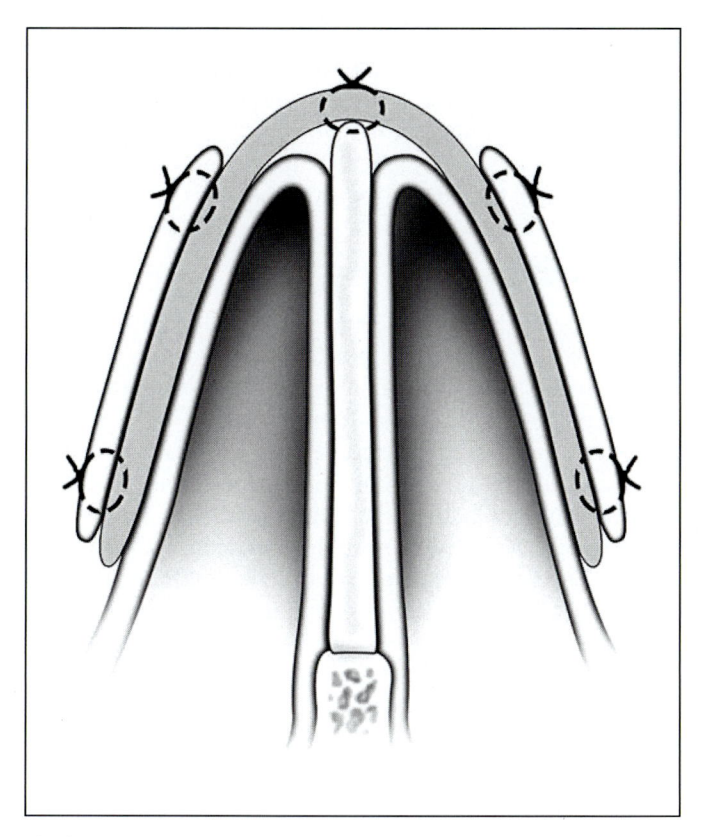

**Fig. 21.4** Splay conchal graft.

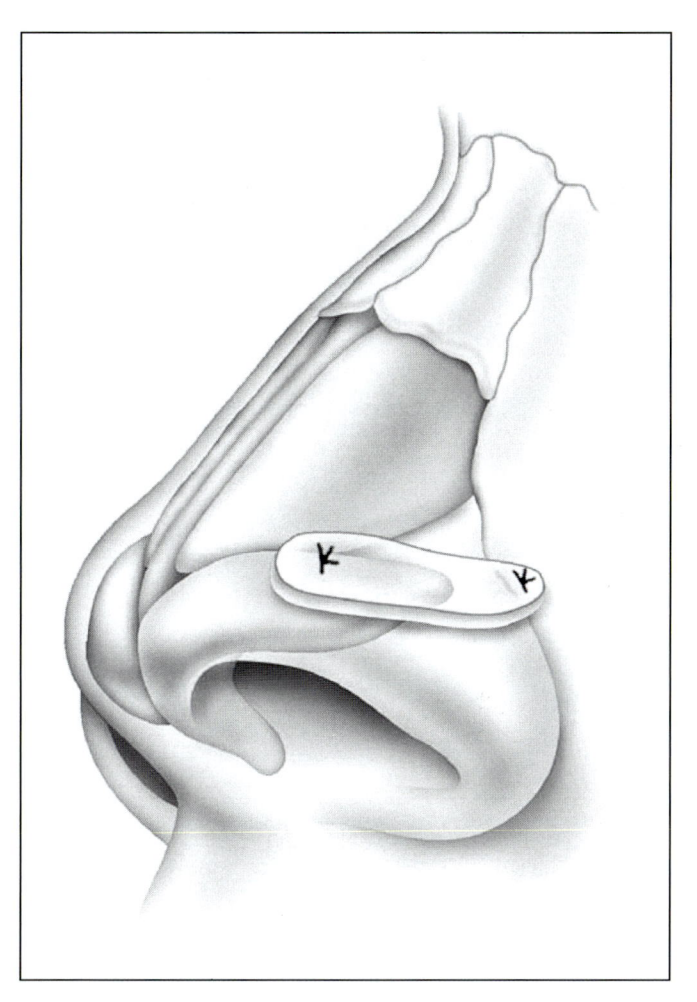

**Fig. 21.5** Alar batten graft.

is made to appear wider, and may not be acceptable to a cosmetic rhinoplasty patient or patients with thin skin.

### Splay conchal graft[1,10,11]
1. The open technique is initiated as described above.
2. Conchal cartilage is harvested by making a postauricular incision. The perichondrium is left intact on the posterior surface. The entire concha is harvested.
3. A 15 blade is used to sculpt the graft to fit over the anatomic deformity that extends laterally to cover both internal nasal valve areas. The area of deformity usually sits between the septum and upper lateral cartilage on both sides, and cephalic to the lower lateral cartilage. The size of the graft ranges from 0.9 to 1.2 cm in length, by 2.2 to 2.5 cm in width.[1] The edges of the concealed graft are beveled.
4. The graft is placed on the nasal dorsum, over the upper lateral cartilages, with the concave side facing down and the periosteal covered side facing up. A 5.0 Vicryl is used to attach the graft to both upper lateral cartilages in a single interrupted fashion (Fig. 21.4).
5. The skin flap is then replaced and percutaneous suture is placed in a mattress fashion to coapt the skin and endonasal lining to the graft using a 5.0 PDS suture. The suture is removed in 5 days.

This is a very simple technique especially in a patient with weak septal cartilage or in a patient in whom septal cartilage is unavailable for graft harvest. It can widen the nasal dorsum but if sculpted properly this widening is not perceived as a problem to the patient. It is most applicable for use on a patient with thick skin.

### 3.1.2 TECHNIQUES TO RECONSTRUCT THE EXTERNAL NASAL VALVE

### Alar batten graft[2,12,13]
1. Prior to anesthesia, a surgical marking pen is used to mark the area of the lateral nasal sidewall corresponding to external valve or sidewall collapse. As the patient inhales, the area of maximum flaccidity is marked.
2. An open rhinoplasty approach is recommended. Septal cartilage or auricular cartilage is harvested. The graft is fashioned to meet the required length per preoperative markings. Effective graft size is approximately 14 mm in length and 8 mm in width. The width of the graft should be 4–5 mm wider than the existing alar cartilage (Fig. 21.5).
3. The graft is placed anterior to the pyriform aperture and extends 2 mm superior to the rim. Using 5.0 Vicryl, the graft is sutured medially, centrally and laterally.

## SECTION G  NASAL SURGERY FOR TREATMENT OF OSA/HS

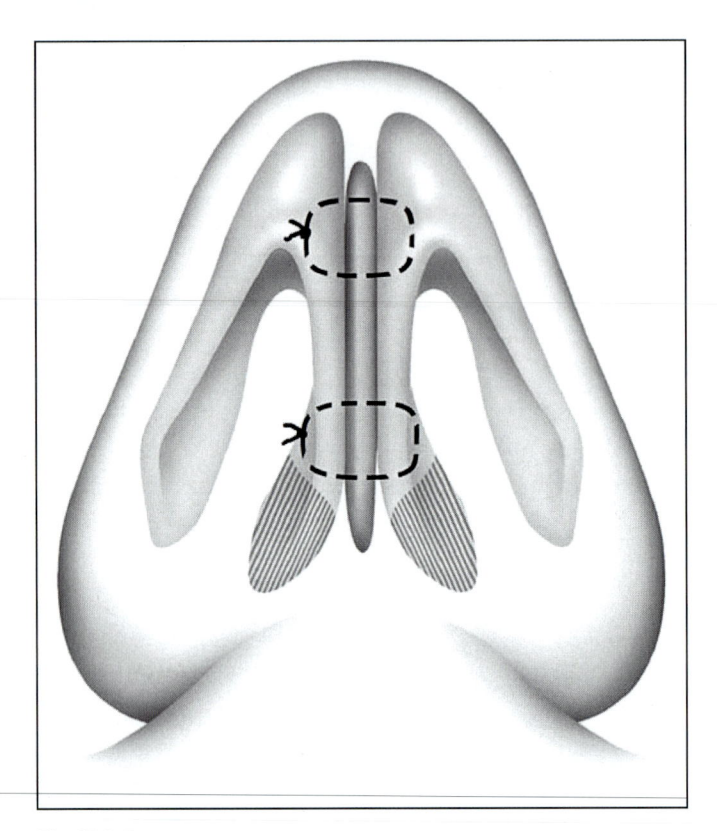

**Fig. 21.6** Columelloplasty.

### Columelloplasty

The width of the columella often plays an important role in narrowing the nostril. Strengthening the columella and narrowing the footplates can improve nasal airflow.[14]

1. Using an open approach, the columellar footplates are exposed. Soft tissue is dissected from the caudal edges of the medial alar crura.
2. The basal third of the medial crural footplate is exposed and a 15 blade is used to transect the cartilage.
3. A strut graft is then fashioned from septal cartilage and placed between the footplates. The graft and footplates are then sutured together using a 5.0 Vicryl (Fig. 21.6).

This procedure is not indicated on all patients. It is useful to narrow the columella and widen the nostril sill. Sometimes the bony nasal spine and pyriform crest contribute to narrowing and need to be trimmed as well. This procedure can also correct abnormalities at the base of the nostril due to wide or asymmetric columellar footplates.

### NASAL VALVE SUSPENSION TECHNIQUE

This technique is a simple approach, providing an internal suspension suture to elevate the nasal valve. It is most beneficial for the treatment of internal nasal valve collapse but I have seen improvement in external valve collapse also. The technique involves anchoring sutures into the inferior orbital rim and guiding sutures to suspend the nasal valve. Cartilage harvesting is not involved. The technique was originally described by Paniello[15] and advancements in this technique have been described over the years.[16]

### TECHNIQUE

1. The area of nasal collapse is marked preoperatively. Specifically, the caudal and cephalad margins that represent the area of maximal collapse are marked. These two points should be about 5 mm apart.
2. Under general anesthesia, orbital shields are placed. Access to the infraorbital rim can be through a standard transconjunctival incision medially or a subciliary incision. The incision should be medial to the infraorbital nerve and lateral to the lacrimal punctae. In patients with thick skin or rhytids, a natural crease can be used.
3. An 11 blade is used to make a small 3 mm incision down to the periosteum. A periosteal elevator facilitates clearing a 3 × 3 mm area on the orbital rim. A Mitek Soft tissue anchor system is optimal for anchoring sutures to the orbital rim (1.3 mm Micro quick anchor; Ethicon). A drill is used to make a small hole in the orbital rim. The anchor is then placed into the hole and the sutures released. The bone anchor must sit flush with the bone in order to prevent a palpable foreign body sensation postoperatively.
4. The end of one suture is threaded through a large curved needle. The needle is then advanced through the incision toward the endonasal mucosa. The plane of advancement is deep to the facial muscles and superficial to the maxillary periosteum. The needle should exit at the cephalad point of nasal valve collapse first. The needle is then retrieved intranasally and passed from the internal nasal mucosa back toward the orbital rim incision (Fig. 21.7).
5. The suture is then tied. Once the sutures are tightened, observe the area of collapse and adjust the tightness of the suture accordingly. Slight overcorrection may be necessary. If there is any skin dimpling, this indicates that the needle tract passed too superficially and will need to be redirected in a deeper plane.
6. The skin incision is closed with a 6.0 chromic.

The advantage of this technique is that it is simple and effective. It does not require cartilage harvesting. In my experience the results have not caused widening of the nasal tip or dorsum. This is a good procedure to consider in cosmetic surgical patients.

In summary, no one procedure will be applicable to all patients. Knowledge of a variety of techniques is essential in order to customize your approach to correct the patient's specific defect.

## REFERENCES

1. Akcam T, Freidman O, Cook T. The effect on snoring of structural nasal valve dilation with a butterfly graft. Arch Oto Head Neck Surg 2004;130:1313–18.
2. Kosh M, Jen A, Honrado C, Pearlman S. Nasal valve reconstruction. Arch Facial Plastic Surg 2004;6:167–71.
3. Constantain M, Clardy R. The relative importance of septal and nasal valvular surgery in correcting airway obstruction in primary and secondary rhinoplasty. Plastic Reconst Surg 1996;98(1):38–58.
4. Becker D, Becker S. Treatment of nasal obstruction from nasal valve collapse with alar batten grafts. J Long-Term Effects Med Implants 2003;13(3):259–69.
5. Sheen JH. Spreader graft: a method of reconstructing the roof of the middle nasal vault following rhinoplasty. Plast Reconstr Surg 1984;73:230–39.
6. Ozturan O. Techniques for improvement of the internal nasal valve in functional-cosmetic nasal surgery. Acta Otolaryngol 2000;120:312–15.
7. Andre R, Paun S, Vuyk H. Endonasal spreader graft placement as treatment for internal nasal valve insufficiency. Arch Facial Plast Surg 2004;6:36–40.
8. Gupta A, Brooks D, Stager S, Lindsey W. Surgical access to the internal nasal valve. Arch Facial Plast Surg 2003;5:155–8.
9. Boccieri A. Mini spreader grafts: a new technique associated with reshaping of the nasal tip. Plastic Reconst Surg 2005;116(5):1525–34.
10. Deylamipour M, Azarhoshandh A, Karimi H. Reconstruction of the internal nasal valve with a splay conceal graft. Plastic Reconst Surg 2005;116(3):712–22.
11. Stucker F, Lian T, Karen M. Management of the keel nose and associated valve collapse. Arch Otolaryngol Head Neck Surg 2002;128:842–6.
12. Kalan A, Kenyon G, Seemungal T. Treatment of external nasal valve (alar rim) collapse with an alar strut. J Laryngol Otol 2001;115:788–91.
13. Romo III T, Sclafani A, Sabini P. Use of porous high density polyethylene in revision rhinoplasty and in the plattyrrhine nose. Aesth Plast Surg 1998;22:211–21.
14. Ghidini A, Dallari S, Marchioni D. Surgery of the nasal columella in external valve collapse. Ann Otol Rhinol Laryngol 2002;11:701–3.
15. Paniello R. Nasal valve suspension. Arch Otolaryngol Head Neck Surg 1996;122:1342–6.
16. Friedman M, Ibrahim H, Syed Z. Nasal valve suspension: an improved, simplified technique for nasal valve collapse. Laryngoscope 2003;113:381–5.

SECTION G  NASAL SURGERY FOR TREATMENT OF OSA/HS

CHAPTER 22

# Radiofrequency volumetric reduction for hypertrophic turbinate

*Kasey K. Li*

**Summary**

Inferior turbinate hypertrophy is a frequent cause of nasal obstruction. It is well accepted that turbinate reduction by radiofrequency energy achieves excellent result in improving nasal breathing. The need for medical therapy such as topical corticosteroid sprays or antihistamines after treatment is usually reduced or eliminated. This chapters describes the technique of radiofrequency turbinate reduction.

## 1 INTRODUCTION

Inferior turbinate hypertrophy can be caused by generalized nasal mucosal diseases in allergic and vasomotor rhinitis, as well as compensatory enlargement due to a long-standing septal deviation.[1-3] Medical treatments such as topical corticosteroid sprays, antihistamines and allergic desensitization are usually the first-line therapy. However, these treatment modalities may be inadequate in achieving significant resolution of nasal obstruction. Surgical reduction of the hypertrophic inferior turbinate has been advocated after failure of medical therapy. The surgical techniques usually involve resection in the form of partial or total turbinectomy with electrocautery, scissors, or laser.[4-8] Although successful outcomes following these procedures are often reported, the associated complications including pain, bleeding, crusting, dryness, infection, adhesion, foul odor and the need for nasal packing are also well known. Furthermore, most of these techniques result in mucosal injury, thus potentially affecting the nasal physiology.

Radiofrequency (RF) volumetric reduction uses RF energy to create submucosal tissue injury leading to the reduction of tissue volume. Li et al.[9] first reported the use of RF for the treatment of hypertrophic inferior turbinate. This article describes the author's technique of RF reduction for turbinate hypertrophy.

## 2 TECHNIQUE

| | |
|---|---|
| **Candidates:** | Any patient with hypertrophic inferior turbinates resulting in nasal obstruction. |
| **Diagnosis:** | Anterior rhinoscopy and possibly nasal endoscopy. |
| **Facility:** | Outpatient-office setting. |
| **Anesthesia:** | Cotton ball (saturated with 2% lidocaine without epinephrine) applied to the anterior aspect of the inferior turbinate for 1 minute followed by a local anesthetic injection (2–3 milliliters of 2% lidocaine without epinephrine). |
| **Temperature:** | 85°C. |
| **Energy:** | 300–600 joules per lesion. |
| **Tx site:** | Anterior one-third to one-half of the inferior turbinate. |
| **Tx number:** | 1–2 lesions per turbinate. |
| **Post tx:** | Cotton ball applied to the puncture site for 2 minutes. |
| **Post op:** | No restriction, over-the-counter analgesics as needed. |
| **Recovery:** | Increased nasal obstruction for 2–5 days. |
| **Improvement:** | 10–14 days following treatment. |

### 2.1 DESCRIPTION OF TECHNIQUE

The procedure is routinely performed in an office setting. Treatment begins with topical anesthetic (cotton swab saturated with 2% lidocaine without epinephrine) applied to the anterior aspect of the inferior turbinate for 1 minute followed by a local anesthetic injection (3 milliliters of 2% lidocaine without epinephrine). The RF needle electrode (Gyrus

CHAPTER 22 Radiofrequency volumetric reduction for hypertrophic turbinate

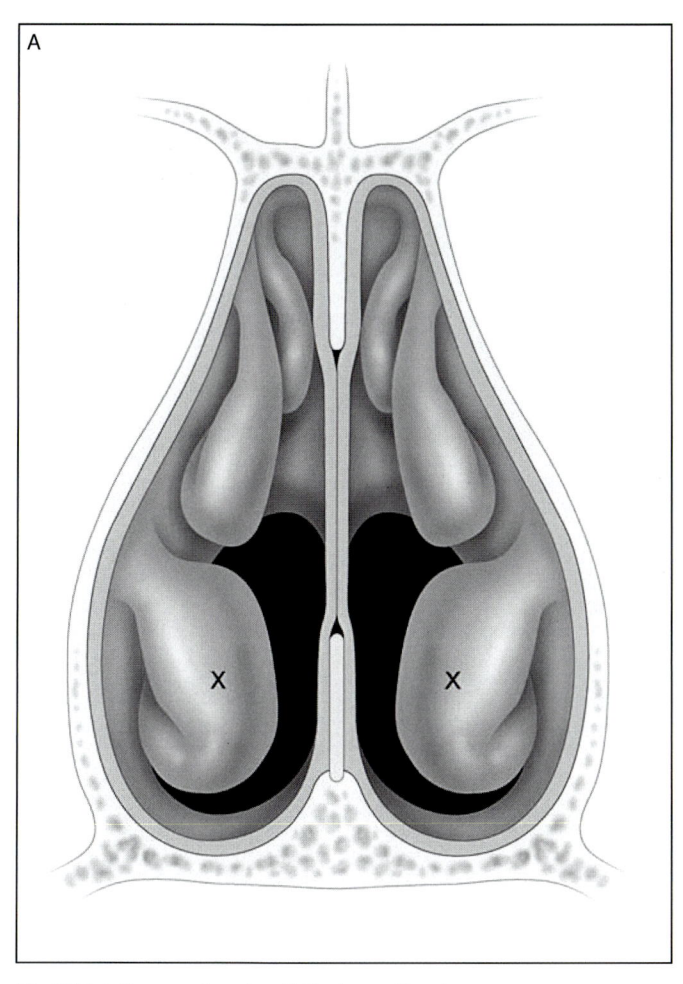

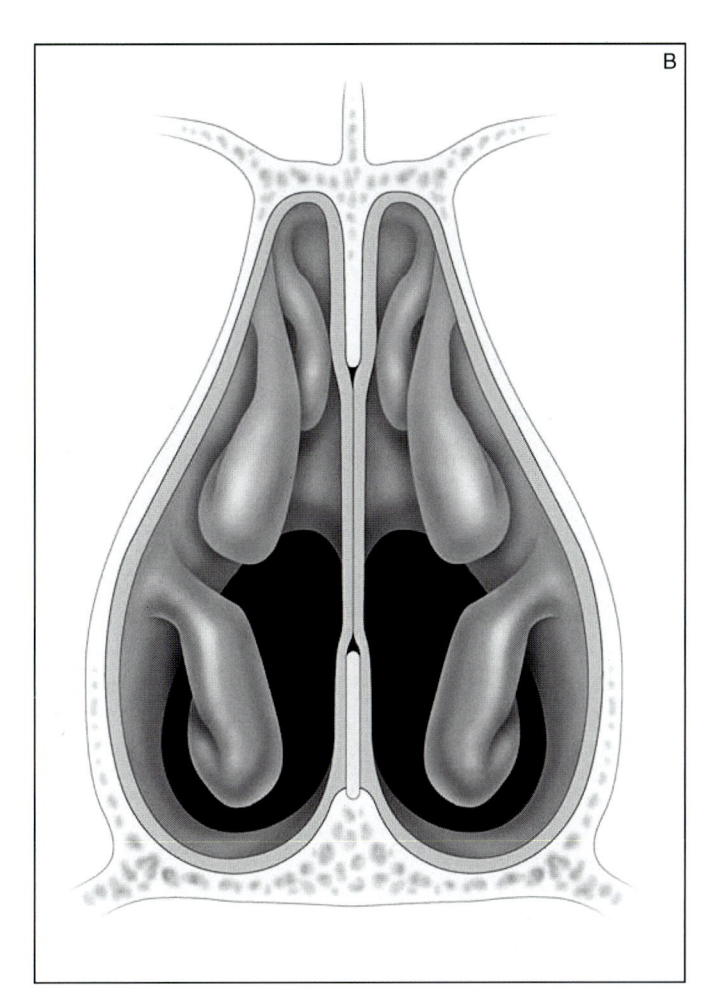

**Fig. 22.1** A, Preoperative view. B, Postoperative view.

Medical, Minneapolis, MN) containing a 10 mm active length is inserted 12 mm submucosally into the anterior head of the inferior turbinate (Fig. 22.1). Care should be taken not to breach the mucosa posterior to the puncture site. The settings on the RF generator include energy delivery (range 400–700 joules) and temperature (85°C). In general, only one treatment is required per turbinate and 300–600 joules are delivered. Obviously, the amount of energy delivered is related to the size of the turbinate. Occasionally, if the turbinate is extremely large, two treatments per turbinate can be given. Immediately following the procedure, a cotton ball is applied over the puncture site for 2 minutes, and the patient is discharged without restrictions on normal daily activities. No nasal packing, topical ointment, steroids or nasal spray are required. Occasionally, patients may complain of burning sensation at the treated area. This is well managed with any over-the-counter analgesics.

## 3 DISCUSSION

RF turbinate reduction has been extensively published. The most widely used RF generator is by Gyrus Medical, which has the most literature support. Turbinate reduction while avoiding mucosal disruption is not a new concept. Submucosal diathermy has been the most commonly used technique. However, submucosal diathermy lacks well-established parameters for the energy requirement, thus could lead to unpredictable results and risks excessive tissue injury with complicatons.[10,11] RF volumetric reduction of hypertrophic turbinate results in predictable tissue injury and minimizes potential complications due to the biophysics of RF energy. The controlled submucosal heating by the small turbinate probe reliably avoids mucosal injury, thus minimizing complications while reducing turbinate size.

The anterior third to half of the inferior turbinate was selected as the treatment site because this is the location of the nasal valve. Engorgement of the erectile turbinate tissue in this location significantly increases nasal resistance leading to nasal airway obstruction.[12] Although greater improvement may be possible if treatment is extended toward the posterior, the diminished visibility and increased energy delivery could increase mucosal injury. RF turbinate reduction reduces nasal obstruction and the postoperative discomfort and adverse effects are minimal.[13–16] The improvement of nasal breathing appears to last on long-term follow-up.[17,18]

Furthermore, multiple studies have demonstrated that nasal physiology is unaltered after treatment.[19]

## REFERENCES

1. Mabry RL. Surgery of the inferior turbinates: how much and when? Otolaryngol Head Neck Surg 1984;92:571–76.
2. Lai VWS, Corey JP. The objective assessment of nasal patency. Ear Nose Throat J 1993;72:395–400.
3. Wood RP, Jafek BW, Eberhard R. Nasal obstruction. In: Head and Neck Surgery – Otolaryngology. Bailey BJ, ed. London: J.B. Lippincott; 1993, pp. 303–28.
4. Ophir D, Shapira A, Marshak G. Total inferior turbinectomy for nasal airway obstruction. Arch Otolaryngol Head Neck Surg 1985;111:93–5.
5. Rejali SD, Upile T, McLellan D, Bingham BJ. Inferior turbinate reduction in children using Holmium YAG laser – a clinical and histological study. Laser Surg Med 2004;34:310–14.
6. Wexler D, Braverman I. Partial inferior turbinectomy using the microdebrider. J Otolaryngol 2005;34:189–93.
7. Elwany S, Harrison R. Inferior turbinectomy: comparison of four techniques. J Laryngol Otol 1990;104:206–9.
8. Gupta A, Mercurio E, Bielamowicz S. Endoscopic inferior turbinate reduction: an outcomes analysis. Laryngoscope 2001;111:1957–9.
9. Li KK, Powell NB, Riley RW, Troell RJ, Guilleminault C. Radiofrequency volumetric tissue reduction for treatment of turbinate hypertrophy – a pilot study. Otolaryngol Head Neck Surg 1998;119:569–73.
10. Woodhead CJ, Wickham MH, Smelt GJC, MacDonald AW. Some observations on submucous diathermy. J Laryngol Otol 1989;103:1047–9.
11. Williams HOL, Fisher EW, Holding-Wood DG. 'Two-stage turbinectomy': sequestration of the inferior turbinate following submucosal diathermy. J Laryngol Otol 1991;105:14–16.
12. Haight SJ, Cole PH. The site and function of the nasal valve. Laryngoscope 1983;93:49–55.
13. Utley DS, Goode RL, Hakim I. Radiofrequency energy tissue ablation for the treatment of nasal obstruction secondary to turbinate hypertrophy. Laryngoscope 1999;109:683–6.
14. Smith TL, Correa AJ, Kuo T, Reinisch L. Radiofrequency tissue ablation of the inferior turbinates using a thermocouple feedback electrode. Laryngoscope 1999;109:1760–65.
15. Fischer Y, Gosepath J, Amedee RG, Mann WJ. Radiofrequency volumetric tissue reduction (RFVTR) of inferior turbinates: a new method in the treatment of chronic nasal obstruction. Am J Rhinol 2000;14:355–60.
16. Lin HC, Lin PW, Su CY, Chang HW. Radiofrequency for the treatment of allergic rhinitis refractory to medical therapy. Laryngoscope 2003;113:673–8.
17. Sapci T, Sahin B, Karavus A, Akbulut UG. Comparison of the effects of radiofrequency tissue ablation, $CO_2$ laser ablation, and partial turbinectomy applications on nasal mucociliary functions. Laryngoscope 2003;113:514–19.
18. Rhee CS, Kim DY, Won TB, et al. Changes of nasal function after temperature-controlled radiofrequency tissue volume reduction for the turbinate. Laryngoscope 2001;111:153–8.
19. Porter MW, Hales NW, Nease CJ, Krempl GA. Long-term results of inferior turbinate hypertrophy with radiofrequency treatment: a new standard of care? Laryngoscope 2006;116:554–7.

SECTION G  NASAL SURGERY FOR TREATMENT OF OSA/HS

CHAPTER 23

# Bipolar radiofrequency cold ablation turbinate reduction for obstructive inferior turbinate hypertrophy

*Neil Bhattacharyya*

## 1 INTRODUCTION

Nasal obstruction secondary to inferior turbinate hypertrophy is a common compounding problem for many patients with obstructive sleep apnea and/or snoring (OSA/S).

As such, medical or surgical treatment of inferior turbinate hypertrophy may improve symptoms associated with OSA and/or snoring in many ways. Enhancement of nasal airflow may allow for increased nasal versus mouth breathing or improved tolerance of continuous positive airway pressure (CPAP). Given the association between allergic rhinitis alone and reduced sleep quality, improvement of nasal obstruction may also independently improve sleep quality.

When pharmacologic management of nasal obstruction secondary to inferior turbinate hypertrophy fails, surgical therapy should be considered. Many treatment modalities for inferior turbinate hypertrophy have been prescribed including partial turbinectomy (bone and soft tissue) and turbinate reduction by various modalities including electrocautery, radiofrequency ablation, laser ablation, radiofrequency cold ablation (coblation) and submucous resection. Since most of these methods have demonstrated good clinical effectiveness, those procedures that are minimally invasive with limited side effects have been recently favored including office-based radiofrequency techniques. This chapter details patient selection procedural details, perioperative management and outcomes with coblation inferior turbinate reduction.

## 2 PATIENT SELECTION

As with any surgical procedure, patient selection has a tremendous impact on postsurgical outcomes. Although many patients with OSA and/or snoring complain of nasal obstruction or nasal congestion, the etiologies for these symptoms may be multiple and multifactorial. Conversely, a number of patients with OSA/S may complain little about symptomatic nasal obstruction but upon examination are found to have several anatomic factors that may contribute to nasal obstruction. Therefore, independent of reported symptoms, all patients with OSA/S require a detailed nasal examination, typically including fiberoptic transnasal endoscopy. The examiner must note the presence or absence of inferior turbinate hypertrophy, nasal septal deviation, sinonasal polyposis and adenoid hypertrophy. Other factors that may also contribute to nasal obstruction (i.e. making one or more of the above more symptomatic) but may be less anatomically evident include nasal valve collapse and the relative size of the piriform aperture.

With respect to inferior turbinate hypertrophy, the relative size of the inferior turbinate along its full length must be assessed. It is not uncommon to find patients with relatively normal-appearing anterior inferior turbinates, but with very pronounced posterior (tail) cobblestoned turbinate hypertrophy. The relationship of the inferior turbinate hypertrophy to nasal septal deviation in particular should be assessed. Some patients with septal deviation may yet still be candidates for inferior turbinate reduction alone if the turbinate component is felt to contribute substantially more to the nasal obstruction. Unfortunately, no clear-cut testing modality will define the individual contributions to nasal obstruction for these anatomic factors. However, we and others have found that a topical nasal decongestant test with neosynephrine or oxymetazoline may help identify patients more likely to benefit from inferior turbinate reduction. Patients must be cautioned that this pharmacologic turbinate reduction is supraphysiological and may exaggerate what is achievable with mechanical inferior turbinate reduction. Those patients who demonstrate an improvement in their subjective sense of nasal breathing and/or objectively demonstrate improvement in their nasal patency (as measured by acoustic rhinometry or nasal endoscopy) are more likely to achieve benefit with inferior turbinate reduction alone. We avoid mixing topical lidocaine in conjunction with topical decongestants because it may confound the patient's subjective assessment of their nasal breathing. A small fraction of patients will have

# SECTION G: NASAL SURGERY FOR TREATMENT OF OSA/HS

limited improvement with topical decongestion, still demonstrating large inferior turbinates. These patients often have a large bony (concha) inferior turbinate and may be better candidates for submucous resection techniques. Patients with significant nasal septal deviation (especially in the anterior or mid-nasal cavity), sinonasal polyposis or adenoid hypertrophy are often not good candidates for inferior turbinate reduction alone.

Part of patient selection is appropriate patient counseling and ensuring the patient's understanding of the goals of the procedure as well as treatment outcomes. Patients should be informed and understand that coblation inferior to reduction may be only component in addressing nasal obstruction with further therapy being required. Further therapy may include repeated coblation inferior turbinate reduction sessions to address middle or posterior turbinate hypertrophy or further sessions to achieve the desired volume of turbinate reduction.

## 3 OUTLINE OF PROCEDURE

Patients are typically apprised of the procedure and given perioperative instructions prior to the procedure. Informed consent is obtained for all patients and includes a discussion of the risks and benefits of procedure, including the rare risk of smell disturbance as well as the infrequent risks of postoperative crusting, bleeding and/or pain.

The coblation inferior turbinate reduction procedure is most commonly performed in the outpatient setting. In patients who have isolated turbinate hypertrophy as a cause of their nasal obstruction (or minimally impacting nasal septal deviation) we prefer to perform this procedure in the outpatient setting prior to any adjunctive sleep apnea procedures. This allows patients to maintain a patent nasal airway in the immediate postoperative period after other surgical procedures for OSA. However, the procedure can be performed simultaneously with nasal septoplasty and/or other adjunctive surgical procedures for OSA in the operating room setting provided the plasma field generator is available.

Patients are positioned upright in the procedure chair in the clinical examination room. Visualization of the anterior aspect of the nasal cavity is readily provided by a nasal speculum and headlight illumination as seen in Figure 23.1. The inferior turbinate dimensions both in terms of cross-sectional area occupied and anterior–posterior length of hypertrophy are determined. Infrequently, preoperative sedation or preoperative pre-emptive pain medication may be provided for anxious individuals. The procedure for anesthesia of the nasal cavity is a very important component of outpatient coblation inferior turbinate reduction and actually takes up much of the operative time. The nasal cavity is sequentially anesthetized, first with spray application of a lidocaine/phenylephrine mixture. After a few minutes,

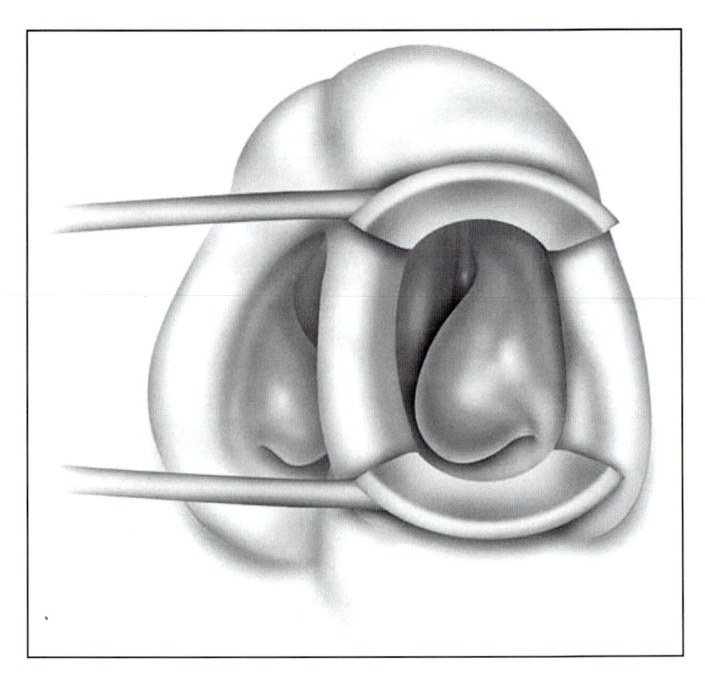

**Fig. 23.1** Anterior rhinoscopy demonstrating inferior turbinate hypertrophy and exposure for anesthesia and subsequent coblation of the inferior turbinate.

this is then followed by a direct contact anesthesia applied in the form of a cottonoid pledget soaked in cetaccaine phenylephrine which is placed in the anterior one half of the nasal cavity, maximizing contact with the inferior turbinate. After an additional few minutes have elapsed, these pledgets are removed, an additional 2–3 ml up 2% lidocaine has infiltrated in each anterior inferior turbinate head, extending from the mucosal surface to the periosteum of the inferior concha. Additionally, we have found that further anesthetic injections just lateral to the piriform aperture, slightly anterior to the anterior head of the inferior turbinate, provide additional anesthesia to the infraorbital nerve branches to the inferior turbinate, increasing patient comfort and tolerance for the procedure. Occasionally, even after these steps with anesthesia, patients still may have some pain with the coblation procedure, especially as the middle to posterior aspects of the inferior turbinate are treated. In these patients, it is helpful to provide a sphenopalatine nerve block with a slightly bent spinal needle as indicated in Figure 23.2. For a sphenopalatine nerve block, 1–2 ml of 1% lidocaine with epinephrine are instilled just posterior and slightly inferior to the posterior attachment of the middle turbinate. This is best done with a 3 ml injection syringe coupled to a slightly bent 22-gauge spinal needle (Fig. 23.3). On occasion, endoscopic guidance may facilitate this posterior nerve block. Alternatively, a transoral, greater palatine foramen approach to the sphenopalatine ganglion for this additional nerve block may be employed.

For typical inferior turbinate reduction procedures, the coblation radiofrequency controller (ENTec/Arthrocare Corp., Sunnyvale, CA) is set to a power level of 6. We prefer

CHAPTER 23
Bipolar radiofrequency cold ablation turbinate reduction

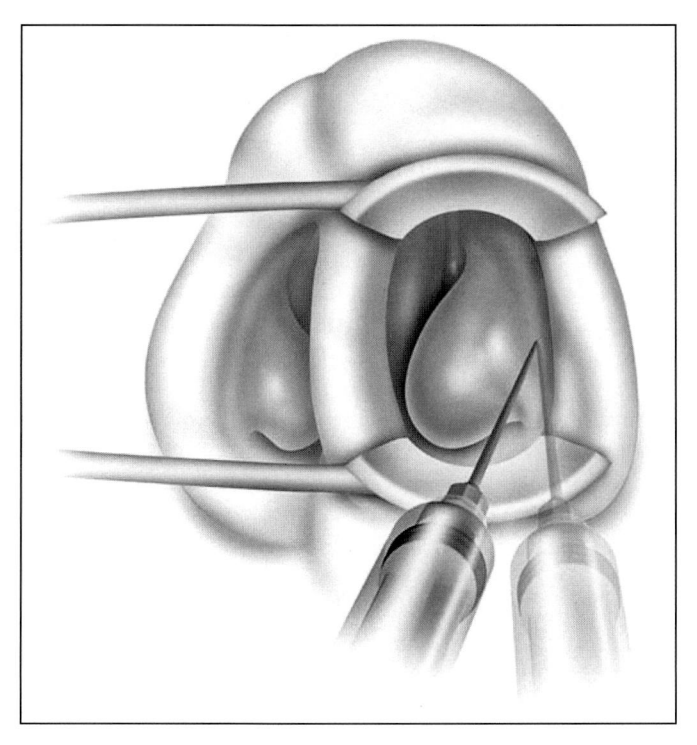

**Fig. 23.2** Lateral piriform aperture and periosteal anesthesia of the inferior turbinate for coblation inferior turbinate reduction.

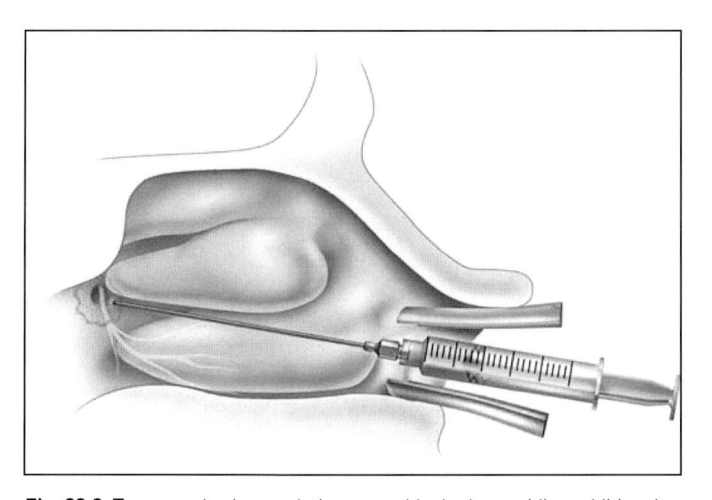

**Fig. 23.3** Transnasal sphenopalatine nerve blockade providing additional anesthesia for inferior turbinate reduction.

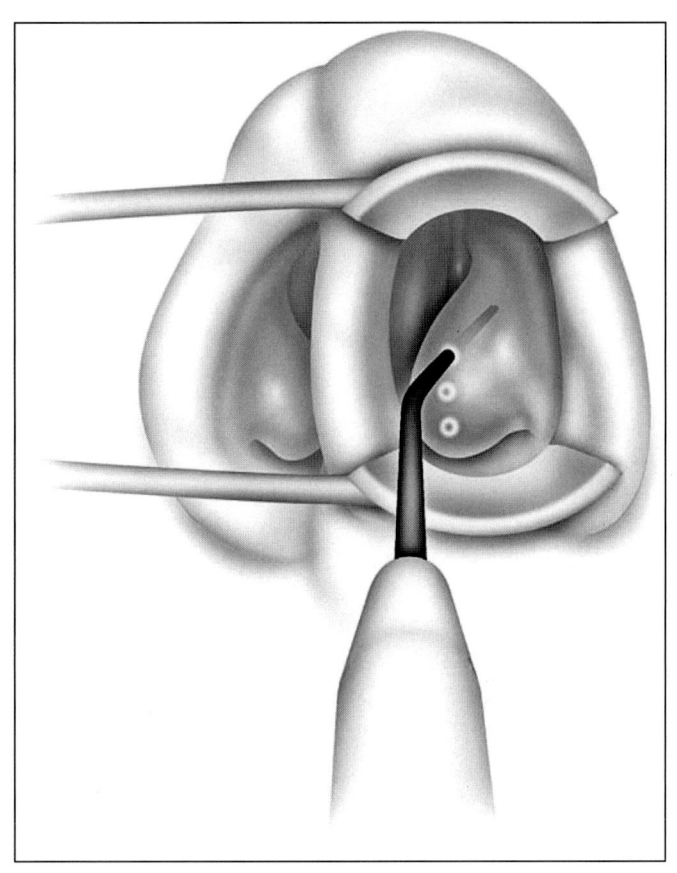

**Fig. 23.4** Anterior rhinoscopy view of left inferior turbinate reduction with the coblation technique. Here, the wand is placed with three passes in a submucosal plane midway between the mucosal surface of the inferior turbinate and the inferior turbinate concha.

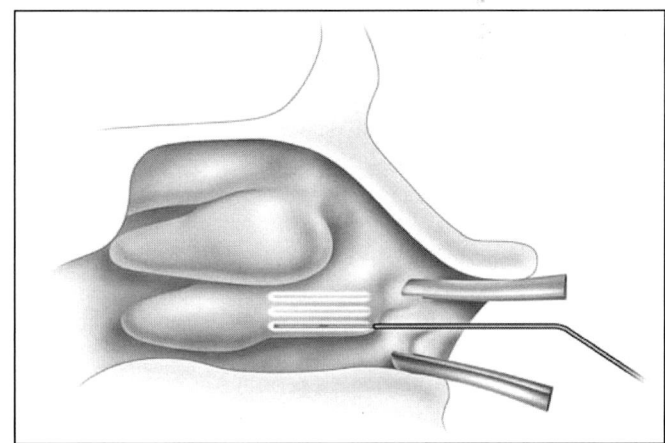

**Fig. 23.5** Sagittal view of multiple passes of the coblation wand in the inferior turbinate for inferior turbinate reduction. Multiple passes may be made as required depending on the depth and volume of turbinate reduction required.

to use this turbinate setting and conduct multiple passes rather than increasing power level for larger turbinates. Next, a small amount of nasal saline gel is placed on the tip of the coblation wand. This nasal saline gel as a conductive medium is essential to provide smooth entry into the surface of the inferior turbinate without thermally related damage. Using a small nasal speculum to dilate and protect the limen nasi, the coblation wand is placed against the anterior aspect of the inferior turbinate. The wand is activated by the foot pedal, and the probe is carefully passed into the inferior turbinate in a submucosal plane (Figs 23.4 and 23.5). Depending on the degree of turbinate hypertrophy and the desired volume of tissue reduction, anything from one to six passes may be made. The coblation wand is maintained in the active state as the wand is

145

# SECTION G: NASAL SURGERY FOR TREATMENT OF OSA/HS

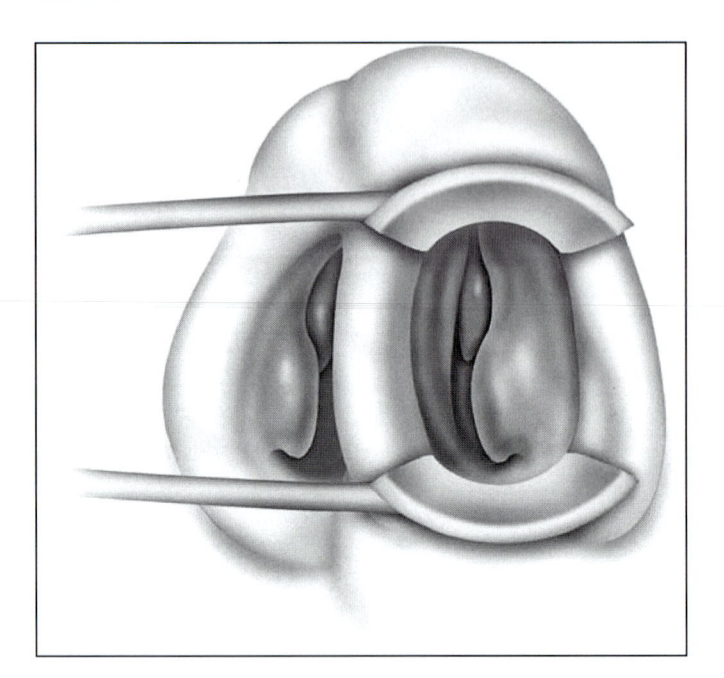

**Fig. 23.6** Optimal appearance of the left inferior turbinate after left inferior turbinate coblation reduction. Typically a visible reduction in the turbinate size is almost immediately evident after coblation treatment.

removed from the turbinate, thereby providing additional exit point hemostasis. For each pass, approximately 10–15 seconds are required. The same procedure is repeated for the contralateral turbinate. Again, the desired volume of tissue reduction may be achieved by adjusting the number of passes and depth of entry into the inferior turbinate. Commonly, though not always, there is a visual reduction in turbinate size immediately during the procedure (Fig. 23.6). Any minor oozing after the procedure is handled by replacement of the cottonoid pledget into the nasal cavity. We commonly leave a cottonoid pledget in the nasal cavity to be removed by the patient approximately 4–6 hours later, depending on the degree of minor mucosal oozing.

As noted, the coblation inferior turbinate reduction procedure may be performed as a stand-alone procedure (i.e. in the office-based setting) or it may be conducted in concert with other obstructive sleep apnea surgical procedures, more typically done concurrently in the operating room. There is no contraindication to simultaneous performance of nasal septoplasty, nasal polypectomy, adenoidectomy with coblation inferior turbinate reduction. Furthermore, we commonly combine inferior turbinate reduction with palatal implant placement (i.e. the pillar procedure) for the treatment of obstructive sleep apnea and/or snoring (approximately 20% of cases). Patients tolerate simultaneous procedures quite well and prefer a single sitting for their procedures rather than separate office visits. Coblation inferior turbinate reduction also serves a useful purpose in addressing recurrent or persistent inferior turbinate virtually after nasal septoplasty in the office-based setting.

## 4 POSTOPERATIVE MANAGEMENT AND COMPLICATIONS

For patients undergoing office-based coblation inferior turbinate reduction, postoperative morbidity and management requirements are minimal. For most patients, postoperative analgesia is provided by acetaminophen or acetaminophen with codeine. Usually by the third postoperative day, pain scores are quite minimal. Patients are instructed not to blow their nose for the first 24–48 hours to prevent hemorrhage. Minor venous oozing after the coblation procedure is typically handled with over-the-counter application of oxymetazoline or phenylephrine spray during the first 3 days.

Patients should be warned to expect approximately 7–10 days of increasing nasal congestion due to intranasal new coastal swelling. Many patients do not experience this, but patients should plan for some increased congestion and possibly adverse effects on sleep in the first week after procedure. Oxymetazoline spray may be used sparingly for nighttime nasal obstruction within the first postoperative week.

Complications after coblation inferior turbinate reduction are quite rare. Approximately 2–4% of patients will have some venous bleeding typically handled with self-application of nasal decongestant sprays. Rarely, temporary packing with a dissolvable material such as Gelfoam is required. Because of the risk of postoperative bleeding, patients should refrain from strenuous exercise or lifting for approximately 7 days after the procedure. We have not seen any significant cases of postoperative nasal crusting requiring substantial débridement after the coblation inferior turbinate reduction procedure.

As with any procedure, the amount of inferior turbinate reduction must be judged carefully. Excessively superficial passes in a submucosal plane will result in loss of nasal mucosa and thereby promote crusting and bleeding in the early postoperative phase. In addition, unusually deep passes close to the periosteum or bone of the inferior concha run the risk of turbinate necrosis and excessive perioperative and/or postoperative pain. It is generally better to treat (reduce) somewhat conservatively and have the patient return for a second round of inferior turbinate reduction rather than attempting to produce all of the benefit in a single sitting.

## 5 SUCCESS RATE OF PROCEDURE AND WHAT TO DO IF THE PROCEDURE FAILS

Success of inferior turbinate reduction may be measured on many scales including degree of relief in terms of structuring, time spent with nasal obstruction, nasal stuffiness, mucus production, postnasal discharge, snoring and overall symptoms. With follow-up ranging from 6 months and beyond, the vast majority of patients perceive significant

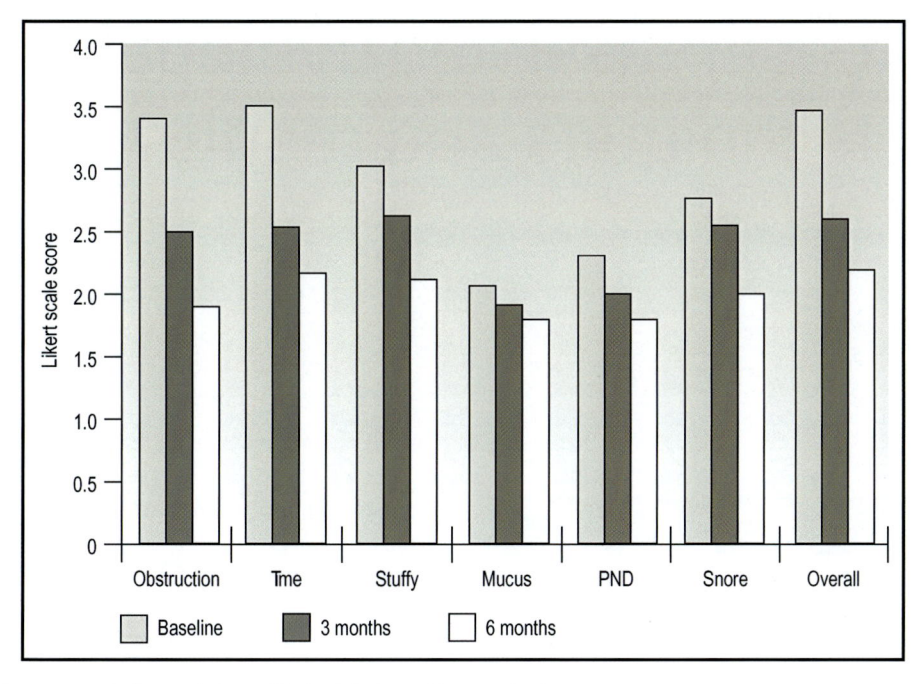

**Fig. 23.7** Individual nasal symptoms before and after coblation inferior turbinate reduction.

benefit from coblation inferior turbinate reduction with statistically and clinically significant decreases in most nasal symptoms. For example, nasal obstruction, the amount of time spent with nasal obstruction and nasal stuffiness decreased by 43%, 35% and 27% after a single treatment with coblation inferior turbinate reduction. Overall nasal symptoms decreased by 34% at 6 months follow-up. Overall, seven out of 10 patients can expect overall perceived clinical success with one treatment, and an additional two patients out of 10 will obtain substantial clinical improvement after a second treatment (Fig. 23.7).

In cases of failure, patients may be treated with additional coblation treatments. Most commonly, this involves treatment of more distal posterior turbinate hypertrophy. In select cases, the size of the bony concha may be a substantial portion of the problem. These patients are best served with a submucous resection of a portion of the bony inferior turbinate. As the nasal mucosa is dynamic and changes over time, the inferior turbinate is no exception. Patients sometimes require a secondary or supplementary procedure at a 1 year interval or beyond. Thus far, in cases of subsequent turbinate hypertrophy after initial treatment, the coblation procedure has been repeatable with very similar subjective patient benefit without a higher rate of supplementary treatment side effects or complications.

## FURTHER READING

Atef A, Mosleh M, El Bosraty H, et al. Bipolar radiofrequency volumetric tissue reduction of inferior turbinate: does the number of treatment sessions influence the final outcome? Am J Rhinol 2006;20:25–31.

Berger G, Gass S, Ophir D. The histopathology of the hypertrophic inferior turbinate. Arch Otolaryngol Head Neck Surg 2006;132:588–94.

Bhattacharyya N, Kepnes LJ. Bipolar radiofrequency cold coblation turbinate reduction for obstructive inferior turbinate hypertrophy. Operat Tech Otolaryngol Head Neck Surg 2002;13:170–74.

Bhattacharyya N, Kepnes LJ. Clinical effectiveness of coblation inferior turbinate reduction. Otolaryngol Head Neck Surg 2003;129:365–71.

Cavaliere M, Mottola G, Iemma M. Comparison of the effectiveness and safety of radiofrequency turbinoplasty and traditional surgical technique in treatment of inferior turbinate hypertrophy. Otolaryngol Head Neck Surg 2005;133:972–78.

Farmer SE, Eccles R. Understanding submucosal electrosurgery for the treatment of nasal turbinate enlargement. J Laryngol Otol 2006; 28:1–8.

Grutzenmacher S, Lang C, Mlynski G. The combination of acoustic rhinometry, rhinoresistometry and flow simulation in noses before and after turbinate surgery: a model study. ORL J Otorhinolaryngol Relat Spec 2003;65:341–47.

Zonato AI, Bittencourt LR, Martinho FL, et al. Upper airway surgery: the effect on nasal continuous positive airway pressure titration on obstructive sleep apnea patients. Eur Arch Otorhinolaryngol 2006;263:481–6.

SECTION H — MINIMALLY INVASIVE PALATAL PROCEDURES

# CHAPTER 24

# Laser-assisted uvulopalatoplasty: techniques and results

*Andrew N. Goldberg and Amol M. Bhatki*

## 1 INTRODUCTION

Laser-assisted uvulopalatoplasty (LAUP) is a surgical procedure for the treatment of snoring and mild obstructive sleep apnea hypopnea syndrome (OSAHS) that involves a sequential reduction and reshaping of the tissues of the uvula and soft palate. Initially described by Dr Yves-Victor Kamami in 1986, LAUP has been widely performed in the United States since 1993 to remove excessive vibratory tissue of the velopharynx.[1] This procedure can often be performed in the office setting under local anesthesia in one to four stages that are typically 6 weeks apart.

## 2 PATIENT SELECTION

As with many surgical procedures, a systematic preoperative assessment and appropriate patient selection are critical elements in maximizing success and meeting patient expectations.

A thorough preoperative evaluation is necessary prior to considering patient selection for LAUP. The medical history is best taken with the patient and the bedpartner present. The sleep history should include discussion of sleep habits, daytime symptoms of fatigue, and observations of the bedpartner. A detailed inventory of alcohol and caffeine consumption, as well as prescription and nonprescription medications is also necessary. Validated questionnaires (e.g. Epworth Sleepiness Scale) may be used as an adjunctive objective measure of symptoms.

A complete head and neck physical examination should include calculation of a Body Mass Index (BMI), measurement of the neck circumference, and flexible laryngoscopy. During an exam for all sleep disordered breathing patients, the surgeon must attempt to identify the site or sites of potential obstruction. All patients considering LAUP should also undergo some formal objective sleep assessment. The Standards of Practice Committee of the American Academy of Sleep Medicine recommends a preoperative polysomnogram or cardiorespiratory study prior to LAUP.[2]

There are several key features that can help a practitioner identify the ideal patient for LAUP. First, polysomnography should reveal the patient to either be a non-apneic snorer or have mild obstructive sleep apnea. Although some studies have shown benefit in patients with moderate and severe OSAS, the long-term outcomes in the improvement of objective indices are controversial. Although the American Academy of Otolaryngology – Head and Neck Surgery declared that LAUP is considered a part of the comprehensive management of adults with OSAHS in 1997, the American Academy of Sleep Medicine did not recommend LAUP for the treatment of sleep-related breathing disorders in 2000.[3]

Second, the patient's physical exam should indicate obstruction at the level of the velum. Patients with Friedman Tongue Position (FTP) I or II are ideal candidates. Patients with FTP III or IV would need additional treatment to address retrolingual obstruction. Stigmata include an elongated or thick uvula, webbing of the posterior pillars/soft palate, and a long and thickened soft palate. Caution should be exercised in patients with a narrow framework to the oropharyngeal inlet as they may be at increased risk for stenosis after LAUP. Clearly obstruction from septal deviation, hypertrophied tonsils or adenoids, base of tongue prolapse, or hypopharyngeal collapse will not be relieved by reduction of the uvula and soft palate; obstruction in these areas will limit the success of LAUP.

A third important selection factor is the patient's BMI. Rollheim and colleagues were able to demonstrate a statistically significant difference in snoring outcomes 3 months after surgery in patients with a BMI less than 28 kg/m$^2$ as compared to those with a BMI greater than or equal to 28 kg/m$^2$.[4] This disparity is most likely related to a greater incidence of obstruction at levels other than the soft palate in patients with a higher BMI, and thus persistent snoring.

There are also several more subtle patient factors to consider in patient selection. Patient co-operation is essential to success if the procedure is to be performed in an outpatient setting. A nervous patient or one with an uncontrollable gag reflex may not be able to tolerate one, or even several, procedures. A small mouth opening or trismus may limit the surgeon's access to the oropharynx. Lastly, any medical condition, such as a hemostatic disorder, that may decrease the safety of the procedure should be considered a relative contraindication. In the above circumstances, the procedure alternatively may be conducted in the operating room under general anesthesia.

## 3 PROCEDURE

When initially described by Kamami, the LAUP procedure consisted of two paramedian vertical incisions extending superiorly from the free edge of the soft palate.[5] The uvula was largely resected in order to reshape a new, shorter one. This French method was later modified by Woolford and Farrington.[6] Their British technique involved vaporization of a strip of mucosa from the uvula to the hard palate. This area is left bare to contract and scar, resulting in increased rigidity of the velum soft tissues. The authors prefer to utilize both modifications, often in a sequential, staged fashion. The following procedure is described with a $CO_2$ laser, but other lasers and cutting/coagulating instruments can also be used, such as electrocautery.

The procedure is performed in an outpatient setting under local anesthesia without conscious sedation. Patients should limit their oral intake prior to the procedure to reduce the incidence of nausea and vomiting. The patient is given an appropriate antibiotic (e.g. amoxicillin) to take the day of the procedure; this is especially important if that patient has a heart murmur or valvular disease. Also, if the patient desires, a dose of an oral benzodiazepine (e.g. Valium) to reduce anxiety, but not enough to induce somnolence, can also be administered prior to the procedure.

With the patient in the upright, sitting position, a topical anesthetic spray (benzocaine) is generously applied to the oropharynx (Fig. 24.1). Next, lidocaine 1% with epinephrine (1:100,000) is infiltrated into the base of the uvula, posterior soft palate, and the superior aspect of the tonsillar pillars (Fig. 24.2). The injected volume is small (approximately 3 ml) since soft tissue distortion and added water content may compromise the surgeon's ability to precisely shape the palate. To minimize the painful burning associated with infiltration, the lidocaine may be mixed with bicarbonate solution (9:1 ratio) prior to injection. Further anesthetic may be readministered to alleviate any discomfort during the procedure.

The authors use a $CO_2$ laser to perform the surgery (Lumenis 30-C $CO_2$ Laser, Lumenis, Inc, New York, New York). Lasers of other wavelengths can be used as well. The hand piece has a 'backstop' that protects the posterior pharyngeal mucosa from inadvertent injury. A typical laser setting is 20 watts with a focused beam in a continuous

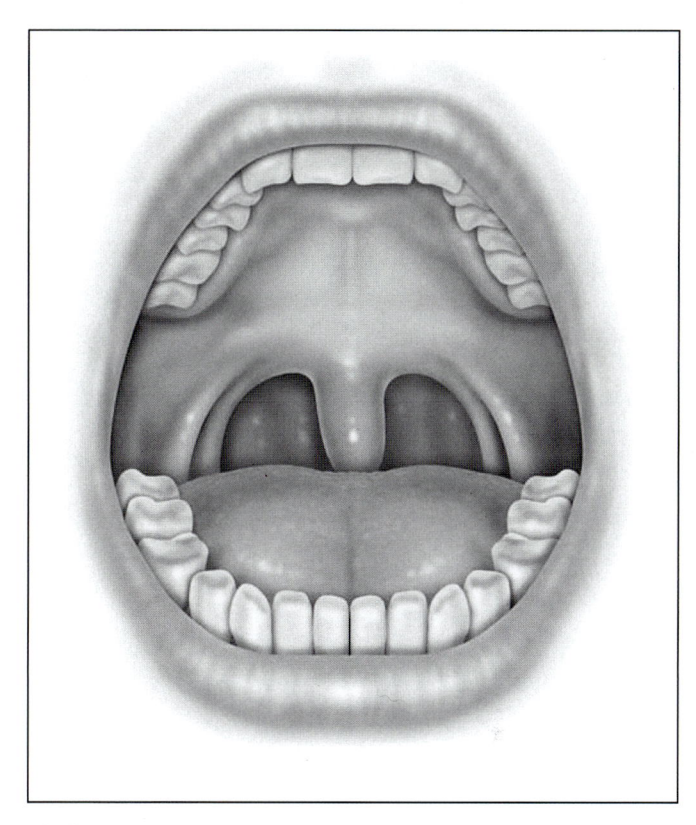

**Fig. 24.1** Oropharyngeal exam. Note the elongated and thick uvula and webbing of the posterior pillars. (Courtesy of Dr. Andrew N. Goldberg.)

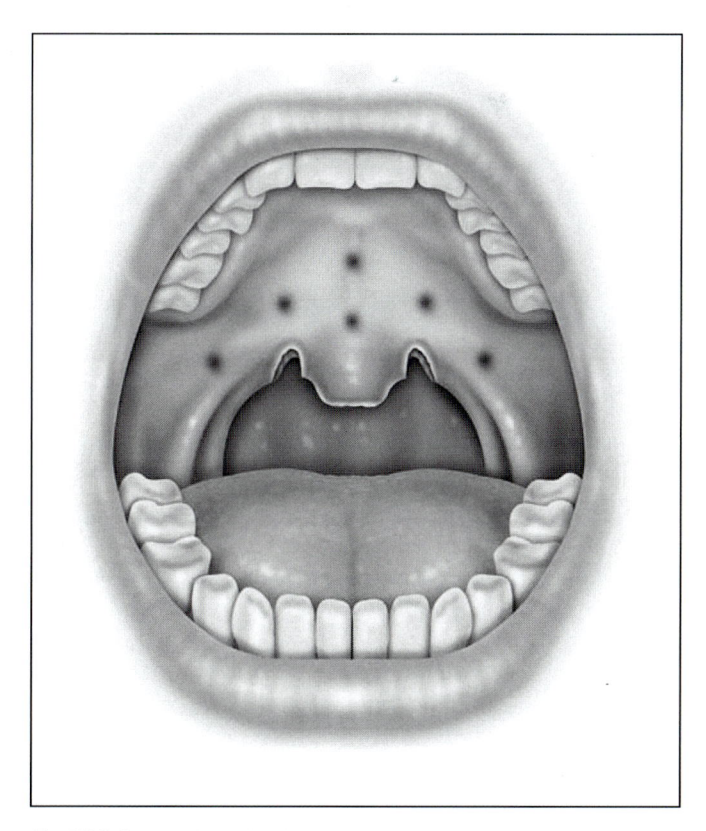

**Fig. 24.2** Six injection points in the uvular base and soft palate are present. Parauvular incision as well as uvular reduction has been performed.

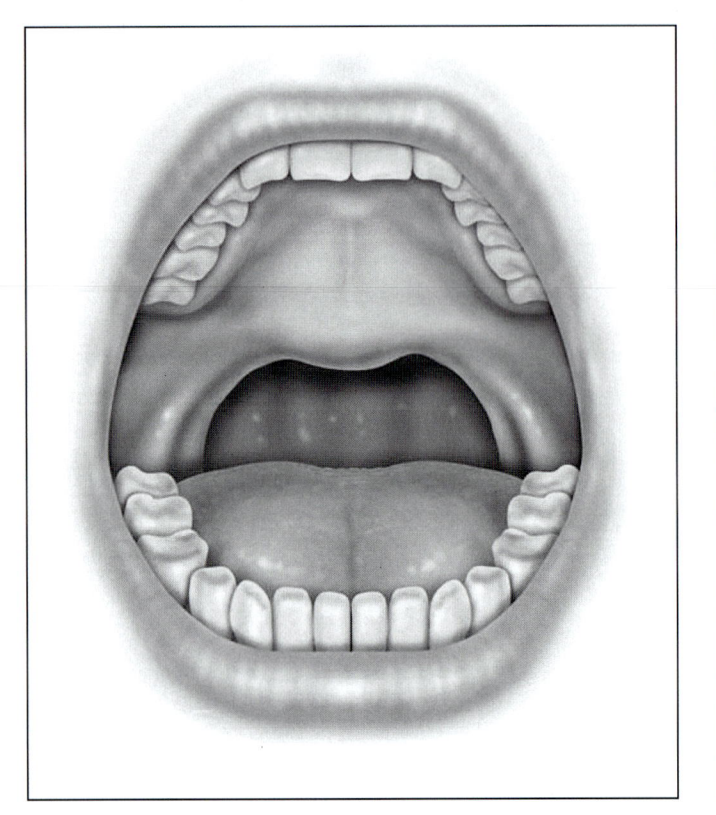

| SECTION H | MINIMALLY INVASIVE PALATAL PROCEDURES |

**Fig. 24.3** Typical reduction in uvular size and shortening of the soft palate after first treatment.

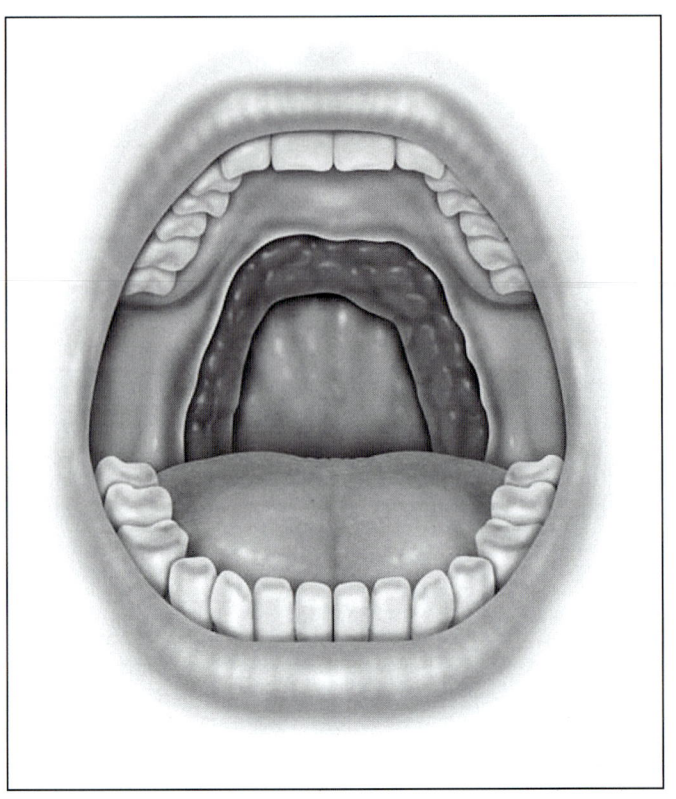

**Fig. 24.4** Extensive mucosal obliteration and circumferential soft tissue injury may result in poor outcomes and pharyngeal stenosis.

mode. The patient and all members of the surgical team must wear eye protection prior to laser deployment.

Initially, the laser is used to create vertical trenches in the soft palate on either side of the root of the uvula. From inferior to superior, a through-and-through incision cutting the oral and nasal mucosa of the soft palate and the intervening soft tissue is made (Fig. 24.2). The length of the trench should be guided by the patient's anatomy. Typically, the palatal musculature is not exposed. The tip of the uvula is obliterated and made to take on the desired contour (a scanning beam is helpful but not essential for this).

Next, the thickness of the uvula and free edge of soft palate is reduced by excision of the submucosal tissue and part of the uvularis muscle. The anterior uvular mucosa is grasped and rotated superiorly so that the tissue between the oral and nasal mucosa can be reduced with a scanning laser beam. By 'fish mouthing' the uvula, the anterior and posterior mucosa are left intact and will heal with minimal granulation at the free edge. These tissues then subsequently scar and contract over the subsequent weeks (Fig. 24.3).

The laser is a useful tool for this procedure mainly because controlled tissue incision and obliteration can be performed with great accuracy. Especially with the protective backstop, collateral tissue damage is quite minimal. It is clear, moreover, that the surgical result and patient outcomes are technique sensitive; precision in tissue reduction and contouring is essential. Specific caution should be exercised to avoid a circumferential wound or continuous raw surface that will predispose to pharyngeal contraction and stenosis (Fig. 24.4). Extensive and imprecise mucosal obliteration will not only lead to failure of symptomatic improvement, but also increase the chance of complications.

For subsequent stages, the vertical trenches can be serially recreated and extended to obtain the desired contour and symptomatic improvement (Fig. 24.5). The uvula, in general, should be conservatively addressed after the initial stage. Furthermore, the British method of soft palate mucosal vaporization can be used as an adjunct in second or third stages. The scanning beam of the laser is used with a power setting of 20W. Approximately 2cm of mucosa and submucosa on the oral side of the soft palate and uvular base is vaporized (Fig. 24.6). The underlying median raphe and palatal musculature should, however, be carefully preserved. Subsequent scarring of this bare area may result in increased rigidity of the velum so that it may resist collapse and vibration during inspiration.

## 4 POSTOPERATIVE MANAGEMENT

Prior to discharge, an examination of the pharynx confirms hemostasis. A mild narcotic with acetaminophen (e.g. hydrocodone) is used for pain management and the patient maintains 5 days of oral antibiotics. The patient

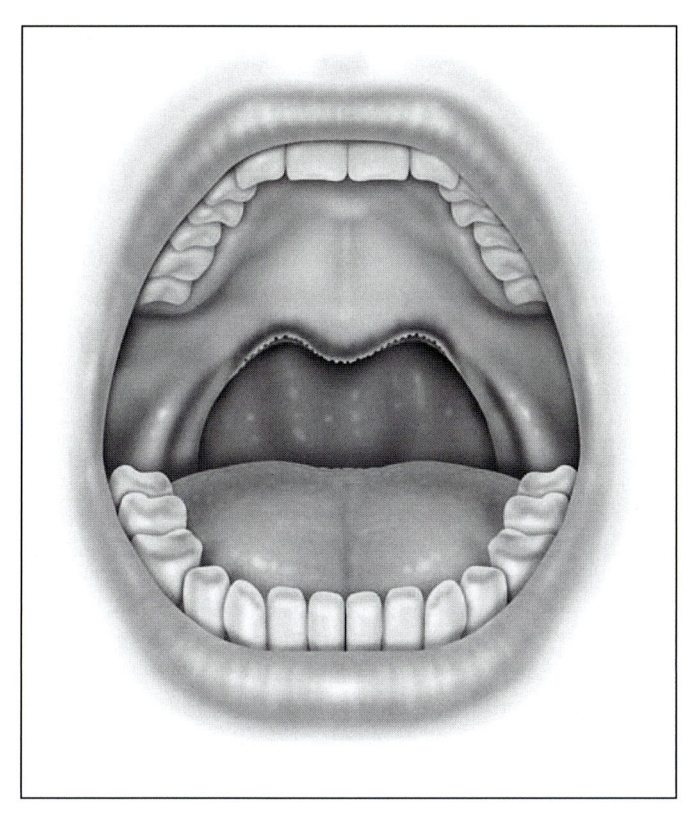

**Fig. 24.5** Conservative contouring of the soft palate and uvula may be performed in subsequent stages.

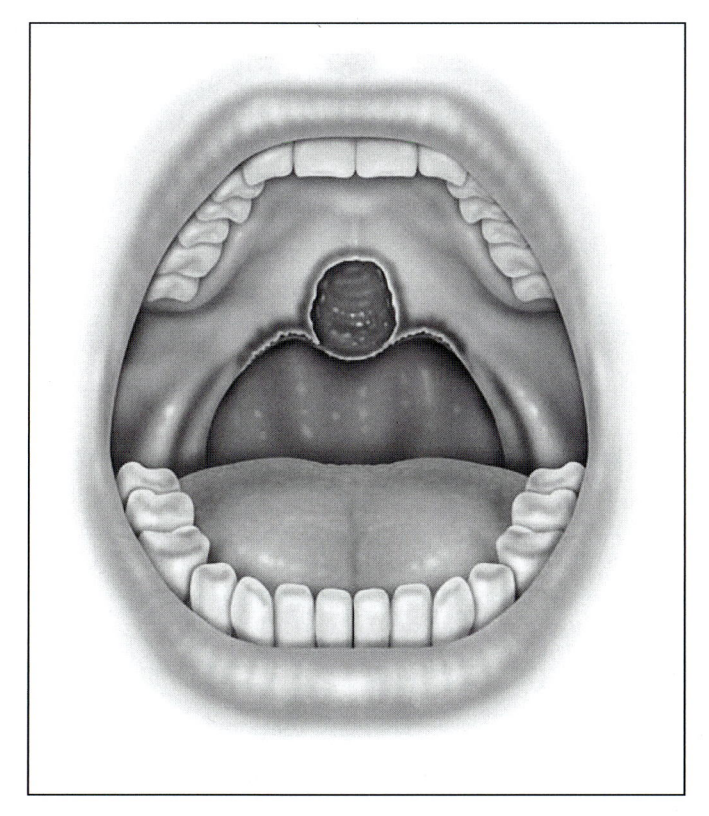

**Fig. 24.6** The British method of anterior uvular and soft palate mucosal vaporization can be used as an adjunct in the subsequent stages. Tissue injury does not extend to the palatal musculature.

is instructed to avoid aspirin and other non-steroidal anti-inflammatory drugs (NSAIDs). Furthermore, a viscous lidocaine (2%) solution may be used every 2 hours as a mouth rinse to reduce the pain.

In general, this procedure produces a significant amount of postoperative pain and discomfort. Although this improves with convalescence, several days of throat pain necessitating narcotics are common. Although LAUP may be perceived as less painful than uvulopalatopharyngoplasty (UPPP), pain from both procedures is approximately equivalent in both severity and duration to UPPP.[7] The patient should, therefore, be appropriately counseled preoperatively and treated with appropriate narcotics postoperatively.

Oral sucralfate, a drug used for peptic ulcer disease, has been recently shown to reduce pain after LAUP. Sucralfate adheres to proteins at the ulcer site and forms a viscous adhesive barrier on the surface of injured mucosa, resulting in a cytoprotective effect. When 5 ml of sucralfate (1 g/5mL) was gargled for 5 minutes every 6 hours, there was a statistically significant improvement in throat pain, oral analgesic requirement, and return to normal diet in a randomized controlled trial.[8]

Patients are typically seen in follow-up 6 weeks after each stage of the procedure. The patient's snoring or sleep apnea symptoms are reassessed and the palate is re-examined. Most patients require two to four stages to achieve optimal outcomes. For snoring patients, this includes reduction of snoring volume and snoring time. However, for sleep apnea, goals include alleviation of daytime somnolence and overall improvement in alertness. If being performed for obstructive sleep apnea, the patient should undergo a polysomnogram 3 months after the final LAUP stage.

## 5 COMPLICATIONS

Although laser-assisted uvulopalatoplasty is considered a relatively safe procedure, complications including persistent foreign body sensation, pharyngeal dryness, postoperative hemorrhage, infection, palatal incompetence, taste alteration, nasopharyngeal stenosis, and even airway compromise or death can occur. The overall complication rate for the procedure is 3.5%;[9] since a patient undergoes several serial procedures, the complication rate for a given individual may be slightly higher.

Because of the inherent vascularity of the soft palate, hemorrhage is the most common complication after LAUP and occurs in 2–3% of patients. In a study of 754 LAUP procedures by Walker and Gopalsami, 16 patients (2.1%) developed postoperative hemorrhage.[9] All of these patients bled within 48 hours of a procedure, with the vast majority occurring within 24 hours. None of the cases necessitated blood transfusion and the site of bleeding was always the apex of the parauvular vertical trench. Approximately

# SECTION H: MINIMALLY INVASIVE PALATAL PROCEDURES

half of the patients required no medical intervention as the bleeding ceased spontaneously. The remainder were controlled with silver nitrate cautery or suture ligation.

To minimize bleeding complications, patients are restricted from aspirin, non-steroidal anti-inflammatory drugs (NSAIDs), and other anticoagulation medication for 2 weeks before surgery. As with all surgery, the surgeon should question the patient for a history of liver disease, bleeding after previous surgery, or a family history of blood dyscrasias and bleeding disorders.

Postoperative infection is rarely seen and occurs in less than 1% of cases. Both bacterial and fungal infections may occur. Prophylactic perioperative oral antibiotics covering oral flora are administered prior to each procedure and continued for 5 days to minimize the risk of wound infection. Fungal infections, usually candidiasis, can easily be treated with topical antifungal medications should they occur.

Velopharyngeal insufficiency is also an infrequent complication of LAUP, occurring in less than 1% of cases. The vast majority of patients will have only temporary palatal insufficiency and will often lack the stereotypical hypernasal speech. Velopharyngeal stenosis may also occur in rare cases. Care must be taken to avoid circumferential scarring of the velopharynx to prevent this complication.

Few studies have analyzed the long-term effectiveness of LAUP. The problem with such longitudinal assessments is the presence of other confounding variables. The patient's body habitus, for example, may change with time or new-onset nasal obstruction may develop. Furthermore, a bed-partner's retrospective recall of snoring severity may become unreliable over time. Mickelson and Ahuja reported an initial total to near-total improvement in snoring in 90% of their patients at 6 to 12 weeks.[13] However, when these patients were re-evaluated after 2 years, the effectiveness was reduced to 62%. In a Thai study, Neruntarat analyzed long-term outcomes in 340 non-apneic snorers that underwent LAUP.[14] Although a small portion of his cohort underwent adjunctive procedures (e.g. tonsillectomy, turbinate reduction), 75% of patients had at least a 50% improvement in their snoring after 3 years. More prospective study with standardized techniques and grading criteria is definitely necessary to reliably establish long-term effectiveness.

Patient selection is an integral element in achieving good outcomes and patient satisfaction. As mentioned earlier, careful preoperative assessment localizing the velum as the primary level of upper airway obstruction will improve success. In a similar vein, patients with a BMI under 28 kg/m$^2$ will also have more statistically significant snoring improvement than those above 28 kg/m$^2$.[4] It is likely that patients with a higher BMI will have secondary levels of obstruction other than the soft palate, resulting in LAUP failure.

## 6 RESULTS

### 6.1 SNORING

The LAUP procedure has been conventionally used in the treatment of snoring without obstructive sleep apnea. The initial report on LAUP by Kamami[5] revealed that 77% of non-apneic snorers had complete or near-complete resolution of snoring. A follow-up study by Walker and colleagues[10] echoed these results. In their series, 60% of 105 snorers had total or near-total elimination of snoring, with an additional 29% who reported partial improvement. Other studies show patient satisfaction ranging from 60% to 84%.[1] However, the surgical techniques, timing of serial sessions, and criteria for 'cure' differed among these studies and may limit extrapolation of this information.

Quality of life data from several studies also indicate an improvement corresponding to decreased snoring. Armstrong and colleagues demonstrated a statistically significant improvement in quality of life for the patient and bedpartner for non-apneic snorers who underwent LAUP.[11] Another study revealed that 72% of bedpartners were satisfied with the procedure, and close to two-thirds no longer slept in separate rooms.[12] As most patients often seek medical attention for the sake of their bedpartner, these data realize the main outcome for which they seek care.

### 6.2 OBSTRUCTIVE SLEEP APNEA

LAUP may be a reasonable treatment option for carefully selected patients with obstructive sleep apnea. Mickelson and Ahuja[13] studied a cohort of 36 patients who underwent LAUP for obstructive sleep apnea. In postoperative sleep studies, the Apnea Index decreased from 14.4 to 5.8 and the Respiratory Disturbance Index (RDI) decreased from 28.1 to 17.9, both of which were statistically significant. The RDI decreased by at least 50% in 39% of patients overall and 44% of patients dropped to less than 10 events per hour. Another study by Walker and associates[15] confirmed these findings. Their study of 38 patients revealed that surgical response rates, as defined by 50% decrease in RDI and postoperative RDI less than 20, were seen in 47% of mild apneics, 42% of moderate apneics, and 46% of severe apneics.

There are other studies, however, that temper the enthusiasm for LAUP as a standard treatment in the sleep apnea algorithm. When evaluating 44 consecutive patients with mild to moderate OSA, Ryan and Love found that only 27% of patients had a good response to LAUP in postoperative sleep studies performed at least 3 months after intervention.[16] Subjective improvements in quality of life and daytime somnolence were present, but the snoring index did not show statistically significant improvement. Moreover, 30% of their patients were worse and had an AHI twice that of their preoperative sleep study. This unusual finding also occurred in a study by Finkelstein and colleagues.[17] In their study of 26 patients, 31% actually had a worsening of the post-procedure RDI. They surmised that velopharyngeal narrowing from progressive palatal fibrosis might actually aggravate obstruction in some individuals and, thereby, worsen their sleep apnea. Indeed, a review of illustrations confirms that assumption and highlights the need to avoid circumferential scarring. Long-term satisfaction after LAUP appears to be dependent on technique and patient selection, the two most crucial aspects to successful outcomes.

## 7 CONCLUSION

LAUP is a technique that has demonstrated effectiveness in the treatment of snoring and sleep apnea. Appropriate patient selection and execution of the technique are critical to success and the prevention of stenosis. Pain from the procedure, the possible need for serial procedures, and return of snoring and symptoms are limitations of the technique.

## REFERENCES

1. Remacle M, Betsch C, Lawson G, et al. A new technique for laser-assisted uvulopalatoplasty: decision-tree analysis and results. Laryngoscope 1999;109:763–8.
2. Littner M, Kushida CA, Hartse K, et al. Practice parameters for the use of laser-assisted uvulopalatoplasty: an update for 2000. Sleep 2001;24:603–19.
3. Walker RP. Laser assisted uvulopalatoplasty. In: Snoring and Obstructive Sleep Apnea, 3rd edn. Fairbanks D, Mickelson SA, Woodson BT, eds. Philadelphia: Lippincott Williams and Wilkins; 2003: 144–50.
4. Rollheim J, Miljeteig H, Osnes T. Body mass index less than 28 kg/m$^2$ is a predictor of subjective improvement after laser-assisted uvulopalatoplasty for snoring. Laryngoscope 1999;109:411–14.
5. Kamami Y. Laser $CO_2$ for snoring, preliminary results. Acta Otorhinolaryngol Belg 1990;44:45–56.
6. Woolford T, Farrington T. Laser-assisted uvulopalatoplasty – the British method. Oper Tech Otolaryngol Head Neck Surg 1994;5:292–93.
7. Troell RJ, Powell NB, Riley RW, et al. Comparison of postoperative pain between laser-assisted uvulopalatoplasty, uvulopalatopharyngoplasty, and radiofrequency volumetric tissue reduction of the palate. Otolaryngol Head Neck Surg 2000;122:402–9.
8. Kyrmizakis DE, Papadakis CE, Bizakis JG, et al. Sucralfate alleviating post-laser-assisted uvulopalatoplasty pain. Am J Otolaryngol 2001;22:55–58.
9. Walker RP, Gopalsami C. Laser-assisted uvulopalatoplasty: postoperative complications. Laryngoscope 1996;106:834–8.
10. Walker RP, Grigg-Damberger MM, Gopalsami C, et al. Laser-assisted uvuloplasty for snoring and obstructive sleep apnea: results in 170 patients. Laryngoscope 1995;105:938–43.
11. Armstrong MW, Wallace CL, Marais J. The effect of surgery upon the quality of life in snoring patients and their partners: a between-subjects case-controlled trial. Clin Otolaryngol Allied Sci 1999;24:510–22.
12. Prasad KR, Premraj K, Kent SE, Reddy KT. Surgery for snoring: are partners satisfied in the long run? Clin Otolaryngol Allied Sci 2003;28:497–502.
13. Mickelson SA, Ahuja A. Short-term objective and long-term subjective results of laser-assisted uvulopalatoplasty for obstructive sleep apnea. Laryngoscope 1999;109:362–7.
14. Neruntarat C. Laser-assisted uvulopalatoplasty: short-term and long-term results. Otolaryngol Head Neck Surg 2001;124:90–93.
15. Walker RP, Garrity T, Gopalsami C. Early polysomnographic findings and long-term subjective results in sleep apnea patients treated with laser-assisted uvulopalatoplasty. Laryngoscope 1999;109:1438–41.
16. Ryan CF, Love LL. Unpredictable results of laser assisted uvulopalatoplasty in the treatment of obstructive sleep apnoea. Thorax 2000;55:399–404.
17. Finkelstein Y, Stein G, Ophir D, et al. Laser-assisted uvulopalatoplasty for the management of obstructive sleep apnea. Arch Otolaryngol Head Neck Surg 2002;128:429–34.

# SECTION H — MINIMALLY INVASIVE PALATAL PROCEDURES

## CHAPTER 25

# Snare uvulectomy for upper airway resistance

*James Newman*

## 1 INTRODUCTION

The upper airway resistance syndrome (UARS) defines a group of patients with clinical signs and symptoms of excessive daytime somnolence in absence of obstructive sleep apnea. Often these patients complain of snoring. These patients have increased upper airway resistance which is characterized by partial collapse of the airway resulting in increased resistance to airflow. Physical findings often include excessive palatal tissue and narrowing of the oropharynx and hypopharynx. The increased respiratory effort required results in multiple sleep fragmentations as measured by very short alpha EEG arousals.[1] In some cases, snoring may not be a feature of UARS. The resistance to airflow is typically subtle and does not result in apneic or hypopneic events; therefore a normal respiratory index is recorded. However, it does result in increasingly negative intrathoracic pressure during inspiration, which can be measured using an esophageal manometer as an adjunct to a polysomnogram. Therefore, diagnosis rests on symptoms of excessive daytime somnolence coupled with polysomnographic documentation of >10 EEG arousals per hour of sleep. These EEG arousals are correlated with episodes of reduced intrathoracic pressure, as noted on esophageal manometry. The esophageal pressure monitoring is an indirect measurement of upper airway collapse and when the esophageal pressure readings exceed −10 cm of water the work of breathing is increased and polysomnogram with electroencephalogram monitoring will pick up these alpha arousals.[2] The frequency of alpha arousals during sleep is thought to be the major contributing factor for daytime somnolence.

## 2 PATIENT SELECTION

Patients with symptoms of UARS and normal respiratory disturbance indices should be considered for snare uvulectomy if the palate has already been treated or excluded as part of the pathology of sleep disordered breathing.[2] Patients with an elongated uvula which touches the base of the tongue or those with an edematous mucosal uvula are considered to have uvular hypertrophy and will have the most significant tissue volume reduction. The uvula is targeted in other minimally invasive surgery to treat UARS which has included laser-assisted uvulopalatoplasty, bovie uvulectomy, injection snoreplasty, and radiofrequency submucosal needle therapy. The purpose of this chapter will be to describe the current technique of palatal volume reduction through the means of uvulectomy with a hot snare. It has the advantage of limiting thermal mucosal injury because the precision of the wire and the central squeeze makes for a clean amputation. It should be noted that the procedure itself is not a new one; indeed it dates back to Greek physicians in the Byzantium era.[3] The modern form of the procedure is performed strictly in a clinical setting with local anesthesia. In cases where both palatal and/or uvulectomy do not improve the UARS, procedures related to the tongue base or medical treatment with CPAP are alternatives.

## 3 OUTLINE OF THE PROCEDURE

Equipment needed includes a headlight, tongue depressor, bayonet forceps with Brown–Adson tissue grasping tips, and a standard cautery source for attachment to a standard hand-controlled snare. Several manufacturers supply cautery snares for otolaryngology including Karl Strorz Instruments (Culver City, California) and Ellman International Inc. (Hewlitt, New York).

The anesthetic technique is similar to that of preparation for laser uvulopalatoplasty. The oropharynx is sprayed with 20% benzocaine (Hurricane Spray, Beutlich, Waukegan, IL) followed by injection with 1.5 ml of equal mixture of 1% lidocaine with 1:100,000 epinephrine (Abbott, North Chicago, IL) and 0.25% bupivacaine through a one and a quarter inch 27-gauge needle attached to a 3 ml syringe (Figs 25.1 and 25.2).

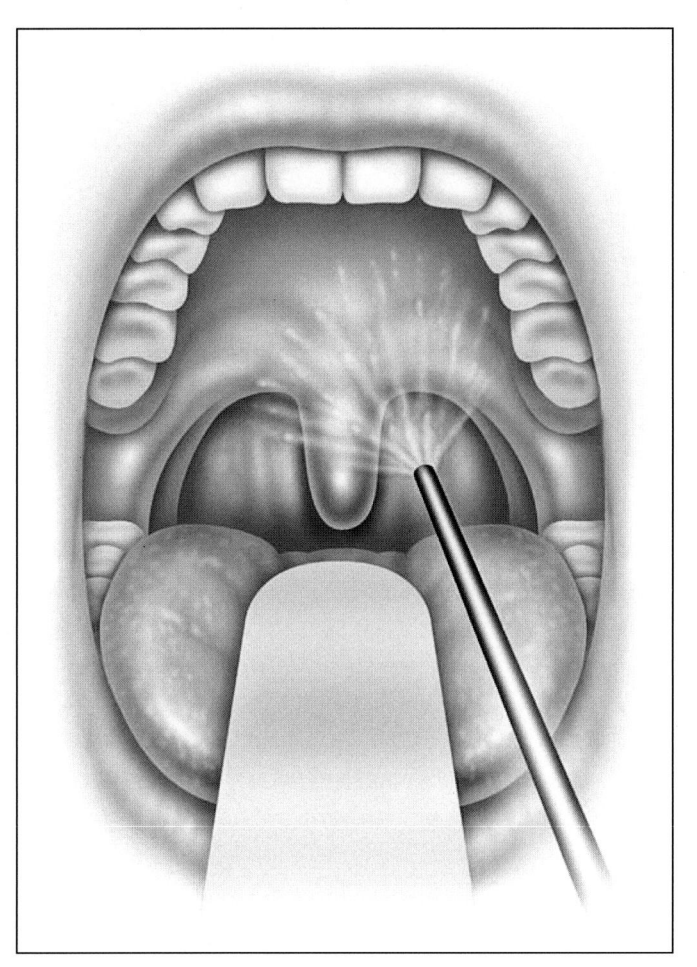

# Snare uvulectomy for upper airway resistance

**CHAPTER 25**

**Fig. 25.1** Application of topical anesthesia into the oral cavity and oropharynx.

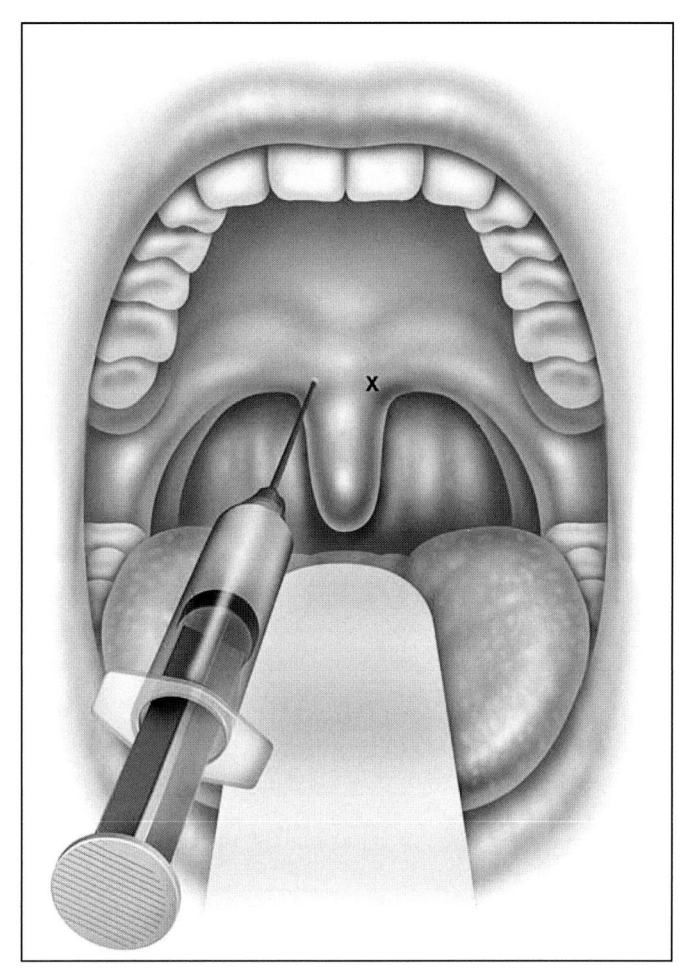

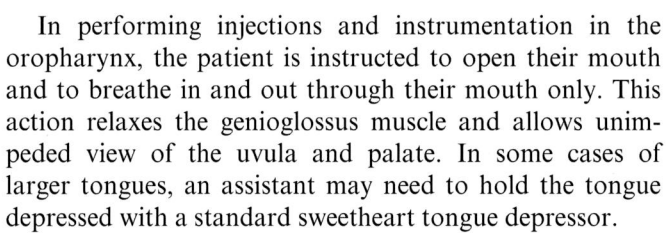

**Fig. 25.2** Injection of local anesthetic at the neck of the uvula. Injection is within the muscle layer.

In performing injections and instrumentation in the oropharynx, the patient is instructed to open their mouth and to breathe in and out through their mouth only. This action relaxes the genioglossus muscle and allows unimpeded view of the uvula and palate. In some cases of larger tongues, an assistant may need to hold the tongue depressed with a standard sweetheart tongue depressor.

During the preoperative examination, the patient is asked to elevate the palate for general muscle tone and the palate is palpated to assess for any submucous cleft of the hard palate. The thickness of the palate and uvula base is also assessed to help determine the duration of cauterization and speed of snare tightening. The snare is always tested prior to introduction and then relaxed so that the initial diameter of the loop opening is the size of a quarter. A 'dry run' placement of the snare is performed so the operator can anticipate movements of the palate and to determine the position of the uvula amputation. Sometimes a cautery mark is scored with the tip of the snare to mark the level of amputation and to confirm adequate anesthesia.

After pretreatment, preparations are checked and to ensure proper grounding an assistant stands to the right of the patient with a hand-held suction and tongue depressor. The patient is given a 500 ml emesis basin to hold. The physician with a headlight, Brown–Adson bayonet forceps in the left hand and the control snare in the right hand, is ready to begin the procedure. With the mouth open, the procedure is initiated by engaging the uvula and snugging the snare at the indicated level for amputation (Figs 25.3 and 25.4). The cautery settings depend on the source to be used. In my experience, three different cautery sources have been utilized with equally satisfactory results in hemostasis. The Cameron Miller radiofrequency source is typically set between 3 and 4. The Ellman radiotron box is set on 4–5 with a partially rectified current. The Valley Lab Force 2 electrosurgical generator is set in the cut mode with a blend of 2 and power setting of 3. Regardless of the generator used, one should be familiar with the current device, and practice the procedure on a template from an uncooked piece of chicken breast.

The procedure is then begun with depression of the footswitch and closing of the snare loop. During the procedure, there is an absence of smoke plume because no tissue is being vaporized as in laser or free hand cautery techniques. This is an important advantage, as there is no risk of visual

155

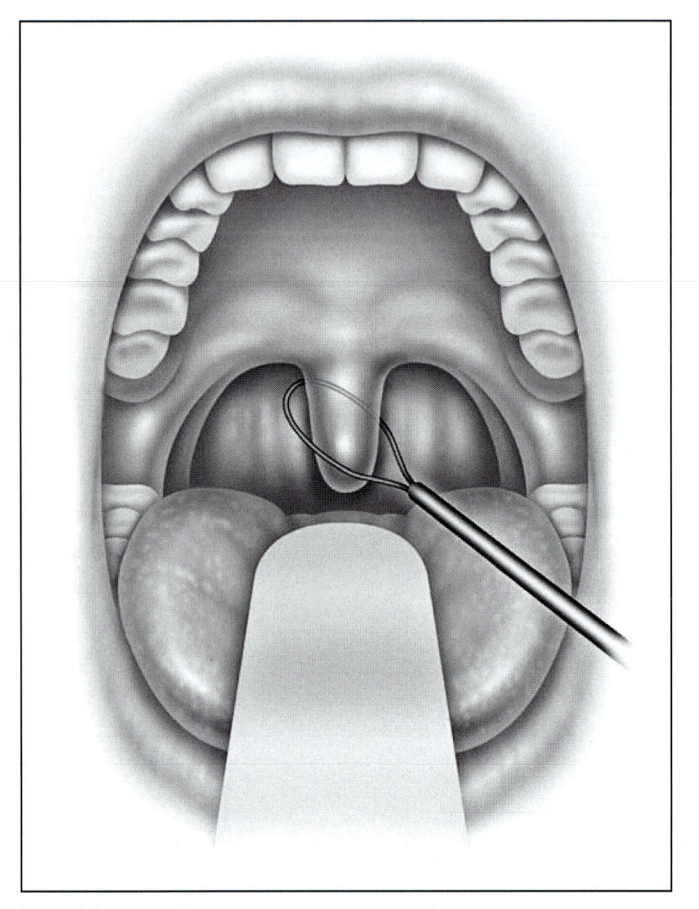

# SECTION H  MINIMALLY INVASIVE PALATAL PROCEDURES

**Fig. 25.3** Depressing the tongue and securing the snare around the uvula.

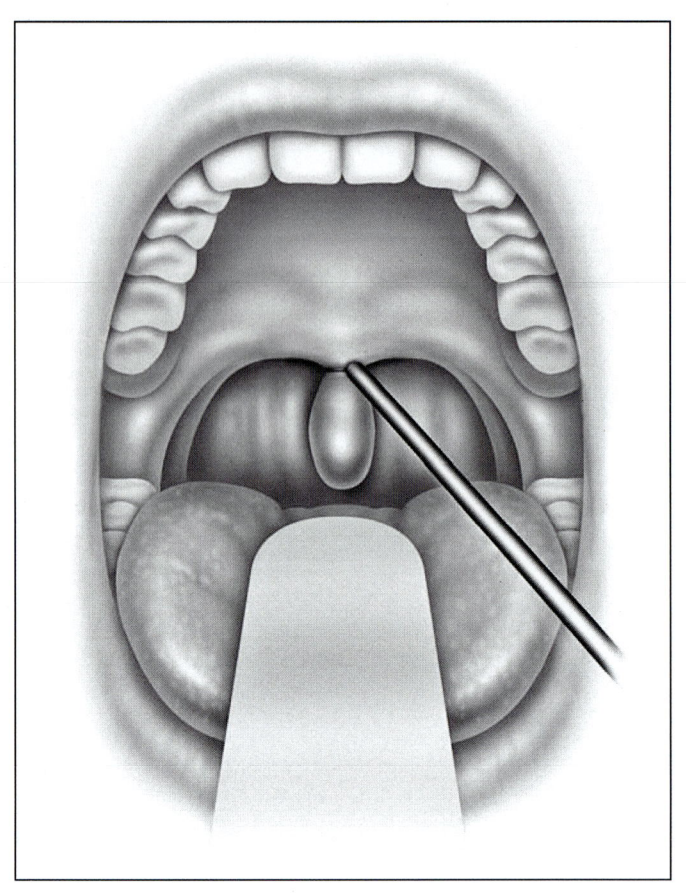

**Fig. 25.4** Snare is tightened around the base of the uvula and heat cauterization is initiated.

obstruction by an assistant's hand or suction tip device trying to evacuate a plume. The procedure culminates in the forceful closure of the snare, resulting in amputation of the uvula which is then removed from the mouth with the bayonet forceps (Fig. 25.5). After the specimen is removed, the stump is observed for any potential sites of bleeding (Fig. 25.6). If any red spots are seen, they can be point cauterized with the partially drawn closed free snare which makes the end into a narrow wire cautery tip.

Choosing the location of amputation is the most variable portion of the procedure as a low, mid, or high amputation can be performed:

- low amputation is defined as a site of tissue cut inferior to the midway length of the uvula;
- mid amputation is defined as the site of tissue cut exactly at the midline length of the uvula;
- high amputation is defined as a site of tissue cut above the midway length of the uvula.

The length of the uvula is observed beginning at the muscular base and extending to the free tip of the uvula. Treatments for simple snoring can also be performed in similar locations. More risk of bleeding is possible with high amputations performed due to the larger size diameter vessels which include arterioles in this location.

## 4 POSTOPERATIVE MANAGEMENT AND COMPLICATIONS

The patients are usually impressed with the brief nature of the procedure and lack of discomfort. Patients are observed for 15 minutes and then allowed to go home with a prescription for 3 days of penicillin and a week's supply of liquid codeine with acetaminophen or liquid hydrocodone with acetaminophen. Patients are instructed to return to the office in 3 weeks. If there is bleeding or increased pain after the first 3 days, they are encouraged to come in for an office visit prior to their routine 3-week visit. Their return visit at 3 weeks usually shows a well-healed mucosa and normal palate contraction.

Possible complications include vasovagal responses from patients during local anesthetic administration, bleeding, and excessive scarring; all these have been reported with this procedure.[4] Excessive pain, infection and dysphagia

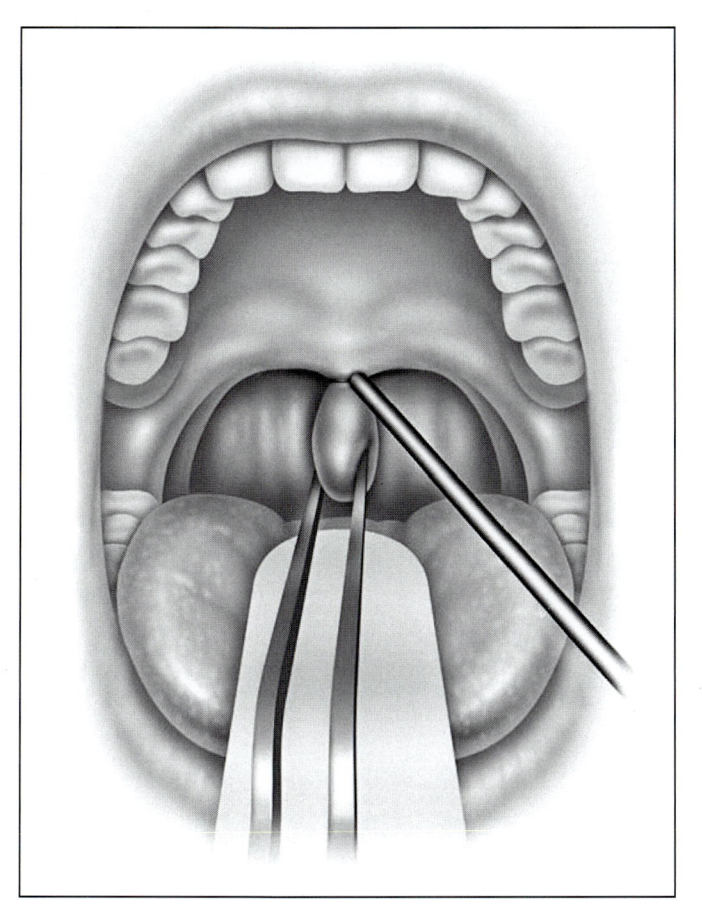

**Fig. 25.5** Grasping of the uvula from the oral cavity after its transection by closing the snare across the base of the uvula.

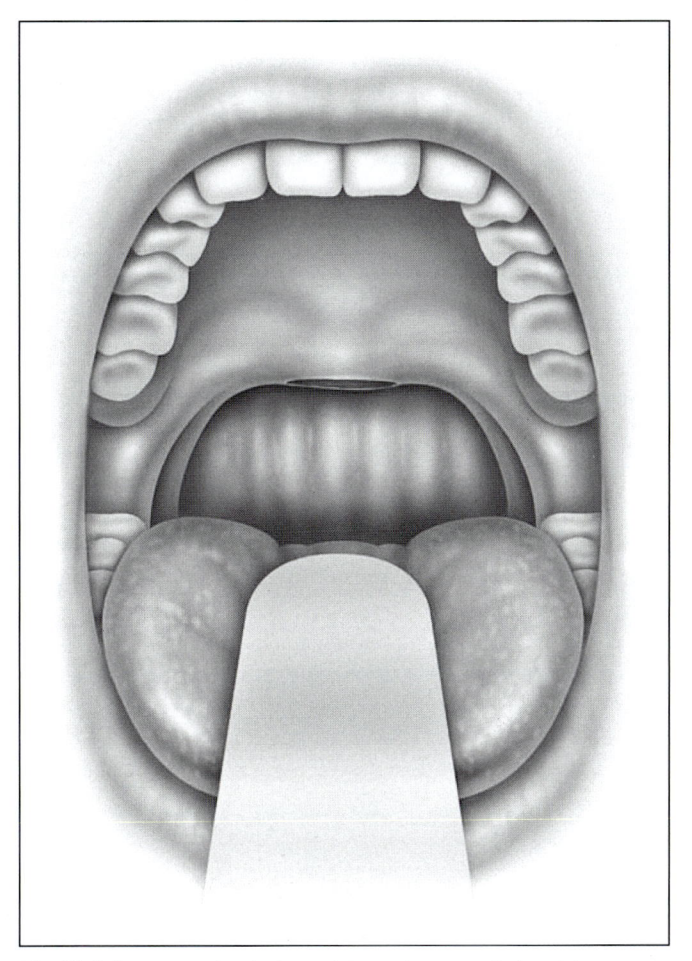

**Fig. 25.6** Open wound at the base of the uvula at completion of the procedure.

## 5 RESULTS AND DISCUSSION

There have been no cases of bleeding with the first 70 cases performed to date. Patients have reported pain lasting from 3 days to 20 days. No cases of stenosis, voice disturbance, infection, or excessive scarring have been noted. Most patients report that their symptoms of excessive daytime somnolence and snoring when present have been eliminated or significantly reduced. We have been unsuccessful in our attempts to universally obtain post-treatment polysomnograms with esophageal monitoring to confirm the abatement of signs associated with UARS. It is important to stress that some sort of clinical follow-up or testing is recommended during the following 2 years to check for continued success. In cases where the symptoms of excessive daytime somnolence have not improved, CPAP or surgery to address tongue base collapse should be discussed.

are also possibilities, but have not been reported. The author is not aware of any other complications associated with this procedure and continues to offer it for cases of UARS and simple snoring.

This particular procedure seems to offer several advantages when compared to similar treatments for UARS or even snoring. It is a single procedure with minimal risks and does not require the expenditure of a unique piece of equipment for the sole purpose of snare uvulectomy. The anatomic configuration of the uvula makes it an ideal candidate for amputation with a snare. The ability to produce circumferential cauterization and cutting makes for excellent hemostasis as well as limiting collateral thermal damage. Loop tip cauteries have limited collateral damage when used in pure cutting modes. Performance of the procedure requires an appreciation of the anatomy and a feel for the amount of manual squeeze over the course of the procedure. The main risks of other uvulectomy procedures have included bleeding and excessive scarring resulting in stenosis of the oropharynx inlet. Compared to the laser, there is less chance of pass pointing or posterior wall injury. Compared to free hand bovie tip cautery amputation, there is less chance of collateral heat damage and less smoke and a more stable target is present as the single instrument both grasps and cuts. The lack of smoke plume makes for better visualization when compared to other techniques and the limited lateral thermal damage to the palate makes for quick recovery and diminished discomfort when compared to laser uvulectomy or laser palatoplasty.

The author is not aware of any other complications associated with this procedure and continues to offer it for cases of UARS and simple snoring.

## REFERENCES

1. Guilleminault C, Stoohs R. The upper airway resistance syndrome. Sleep Res 1991;20:250.
2. Newman JP, Moore M, Utley D, Terris DJ, Clerk A. Recognition and surgical management of the upper airway resistance syndrome. Laryngoscope 1996;106:1089–93.
3. Lascaratos J. Surgery on the larynx and pharynx and Byzantium AD (324–1453): early scientific descriptions of these operations. Otolaryngol Head Neck Surg 2000;122:579–83.
4. Coleman J, Rathfoot C. Oropharyngeal surgery in the management of upper airway obstruction during sleep. Otolaryngol Clin North Am 1999;32:263–76.

SECTION H  MINIMALLY INVASIVE PALATAL PROCEDURES

CHAPTER 26

# Cautery-assisted palatal stiffening operation

*Kenny P. Pang and David J. Terris*

## 1 INTRODUCTION

Snoring is caused by the vibration of the structures in the oral cavity and oropharynx – namely the soft palate, uvula, tonsils, base of tongue, epiglottis and pharyngeal walls. Most authorities would concur that over 80% of snoring is due to palatal flutter, caused by vibration of the uvula and the soft palate. Hence, it would be conceivable that techniques to stiffen the palate would be beneficial in reducing snoring. Different techniques using various instruments (e.g. the laser, cautery and coblator) have been used to achieve the same outcome. The palatal stiffening operation was first introduced by Ellis in 1994[1] and improvised by Mair in 2000.[2] Both authors utilized cautery to stiffen the palate. The original cautery-assisted palatal stiffening operation (CAPSO) procedure was based on stripping a 'diamond' shaped area of mucosa off the soft palate and uvula, with the aid of cautery under local anesthesia (Figs 26.1 to 26.4). Although good results were reported, the procedure produced a stellate puckered scar on the soft palate that resulted in tenting of the lateral pharyngeal walls and therefore narrowing of the lateral distance between the tonsillar pillars (Fig. 26.5). These anatomic manifestations may explain why some patients did not have any clear benefit from the procedure.

Several of the newer methods involve the use of expensive implants or sophisticated equipment. The ideal technique would be an office-based procedure which would require no special equipment or implants, and which achieves effective results in a reliable and predictable fashion. We describe a modified palatal stiffening technique designed to create the palatal scar and fibrosis that is anatomically sounder and which results in retraction of the palate superiorly, avoiding the puckered scar and stenosis of the lateral pharyngeal walls.

## 2 PATIENT SELECTION

This modified CAPSO (Fig. 26.6) procedure is performed for patients with mild obstructive sleep apnea (OSA) (Apnea/Hypopnea Index (AHI) < 15) or patients who are primary snorers (AHI < 5). The inclusion criteria include patients above 18 years of age, Body Mass Index (BMI) < 33, tonsil size grade 1 and 2, elongated uvula, all Mallampati grades, minimal base of tongue collapse (<25%) as seen on Mueller's maneuver.

All patients undergo a thorough physical examination, nasoendoscopy, and a level I overnight attended polysomnography (PSG). Patients also complete the Epworth Sleepiness Scale (ESS) and a visual analogue scale (VAS) for snoring before surgery and 7, 14, 30, 60 and 90 days after

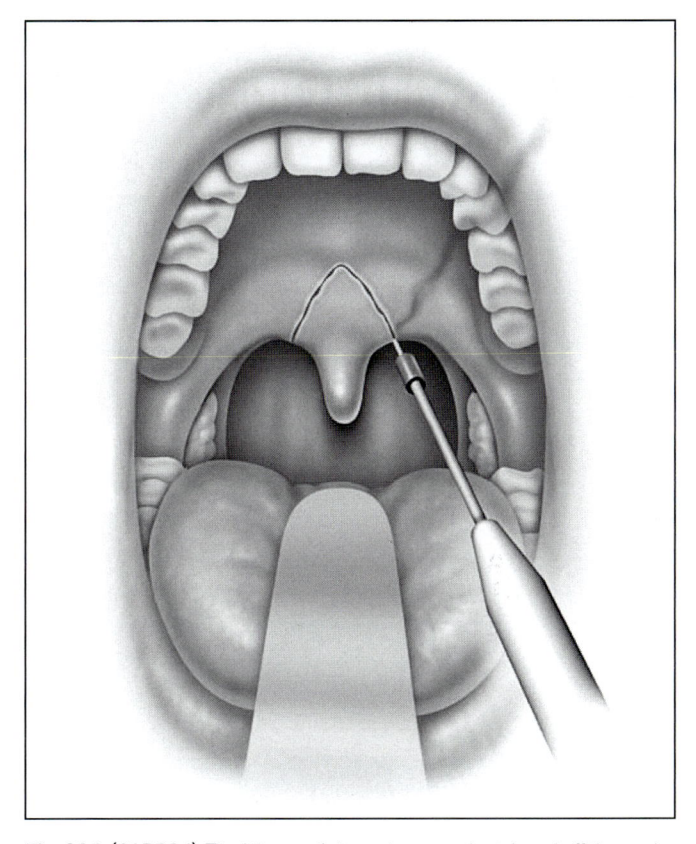

**Fig. 26.1** (CAPSO 1). The 'diamond' shaped mucosa is stripped off the uvula and the soft palate.

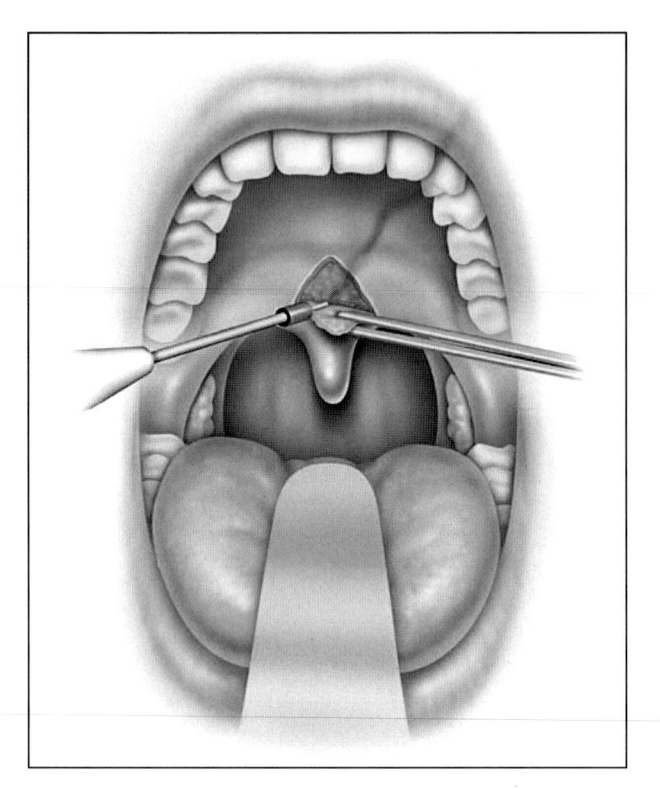

# SECTION H  MINIMALLY INVASIVE PALATAL PROCEDURES

**Fig. 26.2** (CAPSO 2). With the aid of an artery forceps and cautery, the mucosa is removed.

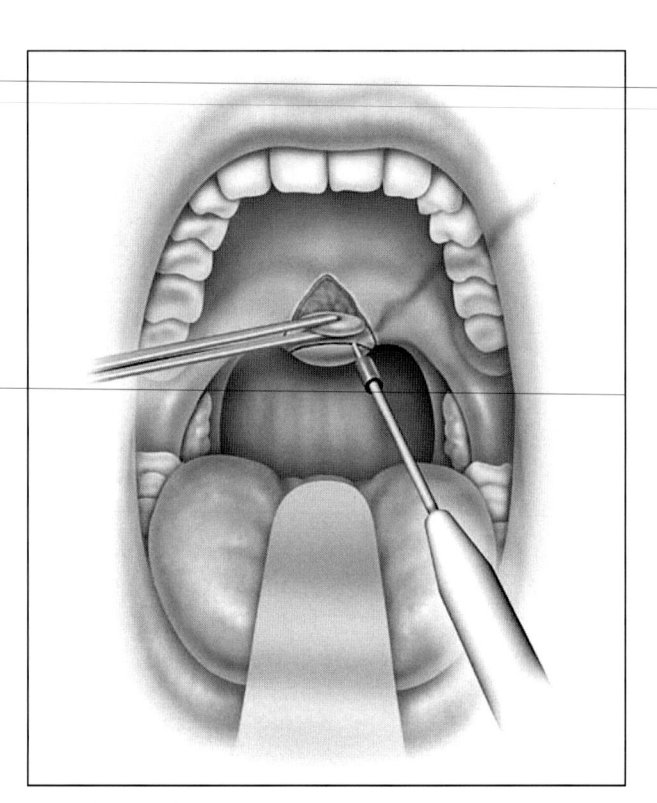

**Fig. 26.3** (CAPSO 3). The uvulectomy is also performed with cautery.

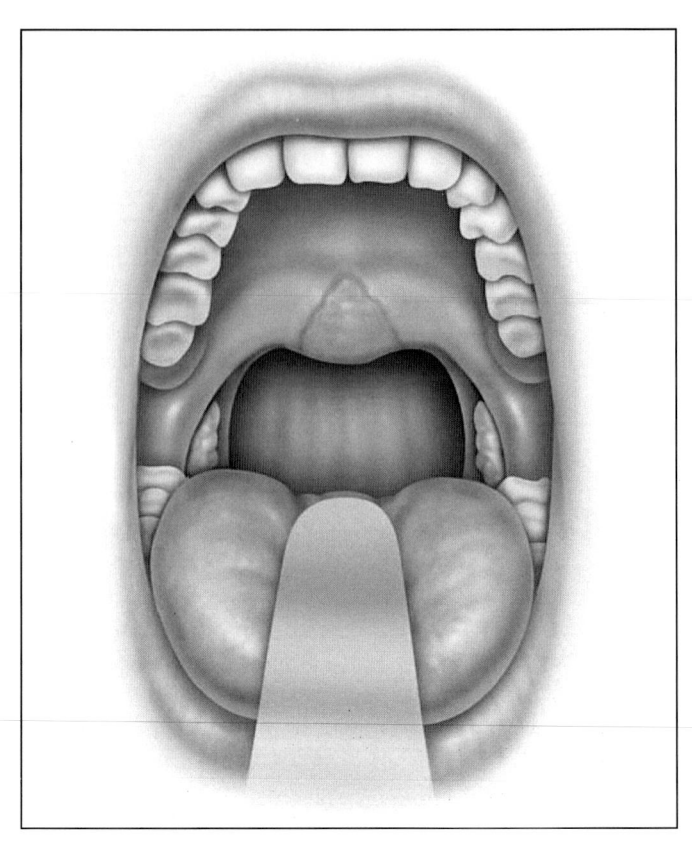

**Fig. 26.4** (CAPSO 4). The fibrotic scar starts to form as healing takes place.

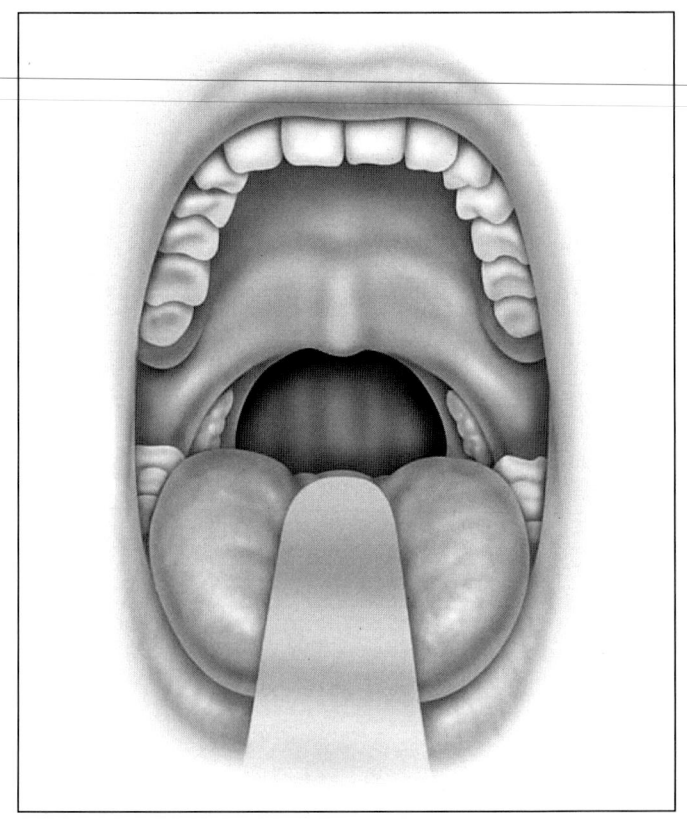

**Fig. 26.5** (CAPSO 5). A puckered stellate scar results that causes narrowing of the lateral pharyngeal pillars and tonsillar pillars medially, hence narrowing the oropharyngeal space.

Cautery-assisted palatal stiffening operation **CHAPTER 26**

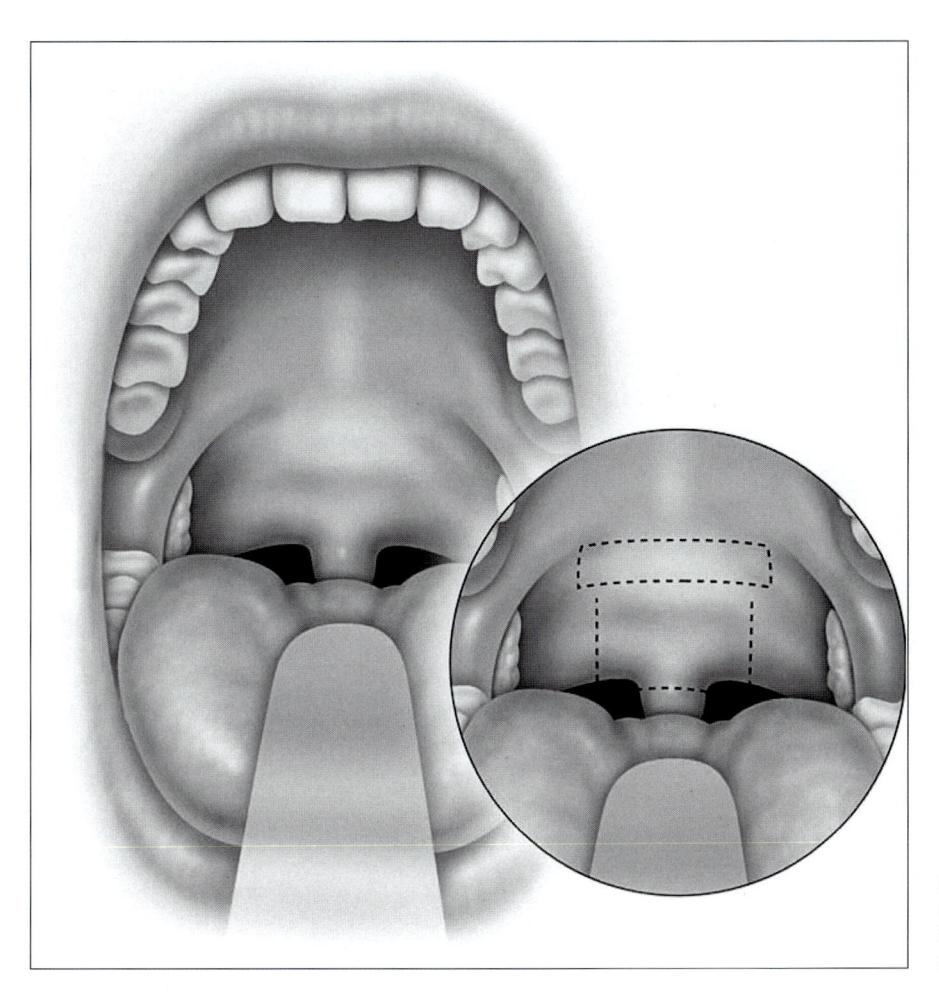

**Fig. 26.6** (1 Oral cavity insert). Showing the uvulectomy, and bilateral vertical trenches. The horizontal strip of mucosa is removed down to muscle.

surgery. The sleep partner also completes a similar scale for snoring. Patients also complete a VAS for pain on postoperative days 1, 3, 7 and 14. Examination includes height, weight, neck circumference, BMI, and assessment of the nasal cavity, posterior nasal space, oropharyngeal area, soft palatal redundancy, uvula size and thickness, tonsillar size and Mallampati grade. Flexible nasoendoscopy is performed for all patients, and collapse during a Mueller's maneuver is graded for the soft palate, lateral pharyngeal walls and base of tongue on a five-point scale.[3]

Outcome measures include subjective improvement in snoring based on the VAS and improvement in sleepiness as indicated by the Epworth scale. Objective changes are judged by the polysomnographic findings. The success criterion is a reduction of at least 50% of the pre-procedure AHI and post-procedure AHI below 15.

## 3 SURGICAL TECHNIQUE

The procedure is done under local anesthesia in the office as an outpatient. The patient is seated in an examination chair with the mouth open. Topical benzocaine (14%) is used to anesthetize the palatal region. A total of 3 ml of 1:100,000 adrenaline and 2% xylocaine is injected into three sites of the soft palate. An uvulectomy is performed (Fig. 26.7), followed by vertical cuts on either side of the uvula (Fig. 26.8), through both soft palatal arches. A horizontal rectangular strip of mucosa is removed from the soft palate (50 mm in length by 7 mm in width), down to the muscle layer (Fig. 26.9). Hemostasis is achieved with electrocautery. All patients are prescribed with anesthetic gargles (Difflam) and lozenges (Difflam), non-steroidal anti-inflammatory agents (Naproxen sodium), narcotics (like codeine), and cyclo-oxygenase-2 inhibitors. The co-blator technique may also be used as an instrument for this technique.

With the healing process, as the palatal tissue heals, a fiberoptic palate results and retracts superiorly, with the oropharyngeal airway widened superiorly (Fig. 26.10).

## 4 POSTOPERATIVE MANAGEMENT AND COMPLICATIONS

All patients are monitored in the recovery room for a further 30 minutes, with monitoring of their blood pressure, pulse rate and oxygen saturation. They are given adequate

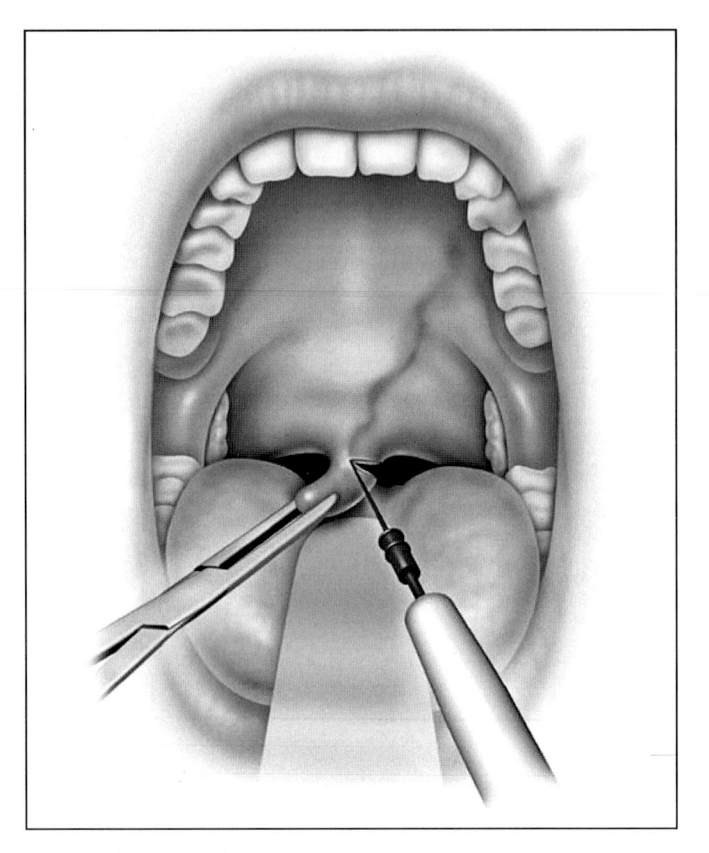

SECTION H — MINIMALLY INVASIVE PALATAL PROCEDURES

**Fig. 26.7** (2 Oral cavity). Uvulectomy is performed.

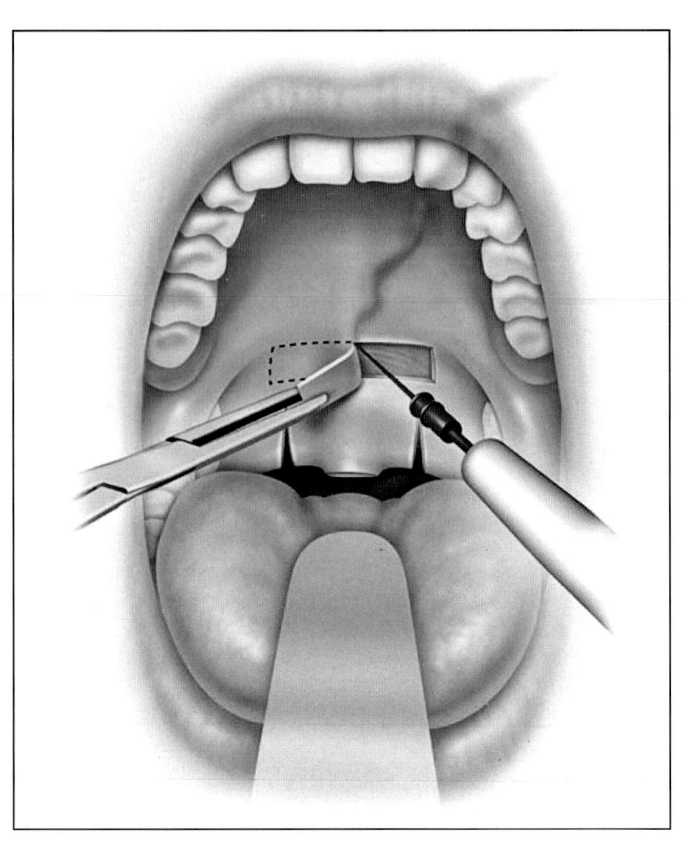

**Fig. 26.9** (4 Oral cavity). Horizontal strip of mucosa is removed down to muscle. The edges may be apposed with absorbable Vicryl 3/0 suture.

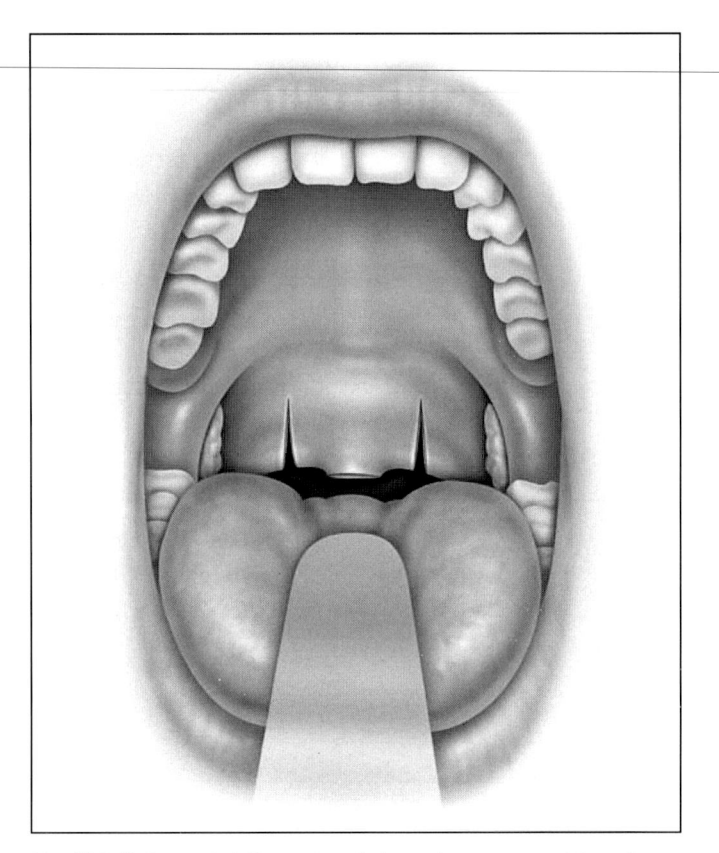

**Fig. 26.8** (3 Oral cavity). Bilateral vertical trenches are created through-and-through mucosa and muscle.

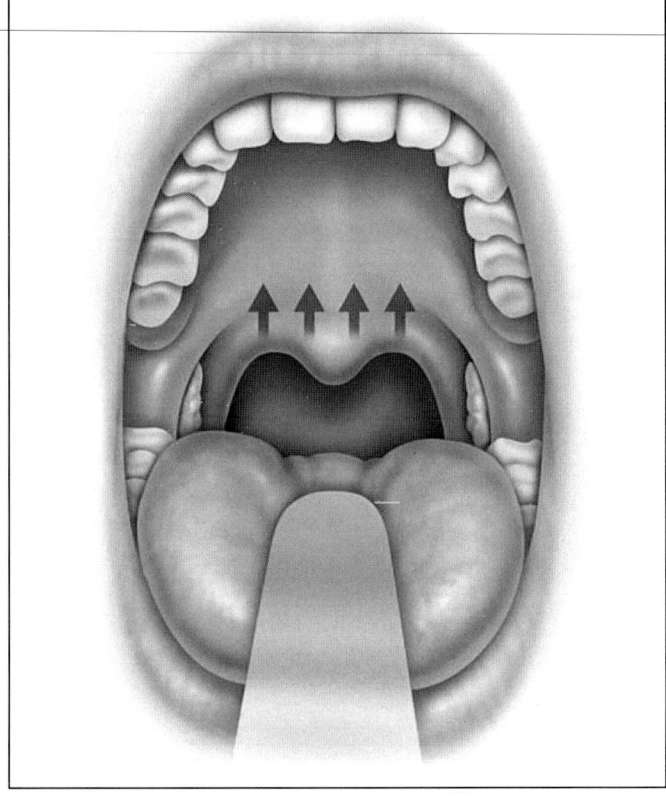

**Fig. 26.10** (5 Oral cavity). Final result showing superior retraction and fibrosis of the soft palate resulting in a larger oropharyngeal airway.

analgesia in the form of anesthetic gargles (Difflam) and lozenges (Difflam), non-steroidal anti-inflammatory agents (Naproxen sodium), narcotics (like codeine), and cyclo-oxygenase-2 inhibitors. All patients are advised to take adequate oral fluid hydration and soft blended diet in the first postoperative week.

Complications from this procedure are rare. However, primary or secondary hemorrhage is possible. Other potential complications that are very rare include velopharyngeal incompetence, fistula of the soft palate and nasopharyngeal stenosis.

## 4.1 SUCCESS RATE OF PROCEDURE

In this series, there were 13 patients who underwent this procedure for management of their snoring or mild OSA. All 13 patients were males, with a mean age of 35.7 years old (range of 24 to 47 years old). The mean BMI was 28.4 (range of 21.6 to 31.2). All patients were classified as Friedman stage II and III,[4] with tonsil size 0, 1 or 2. The mean preoperative AHI was 11.6 (range of 3.5 to 14.8), with a mean preoperative Apnea Index (AI) of 5.6 (range 0.5 to 9.1). The mean preoperative lowest oxygen saturation (LSAT) was 91.4% (range of 88% to 94%). All patients had a 3-month postoperative polysomnogram done. There were five patients who were simple snorers (mean AHI of 3.9) and eight patients who had mild OSA (mean AHI of 12.3).

The mean operative time was 15.6 minutes (range 12 minutes to 25 minutes). There were no complications of velopharyngeal incompetence, fistula, primary or secondary hemorrhage.

All patients (13/13) had reduction in their snoring intensity. The patients and their sleep partners were satisfied with the result at 3 months postoperatively. The VAS showed gradual reduction in the snoring intensity with time, ranging from a preoperative level of 8.3 (range 7.5 to 9.1) to a low of 3.3 (range 2.5 to 4.6) at 90 days postoperative.

Improvements were also noted in the Epworth Sleepiness Scale which decreased from 12.2 (range 8 to 15) to 8.9 (range 5 to 13) at 90 days postoperatively, although two patients (25.4%) did not subjectively improve. Subjectively, most patients felt that they experienced more dreams during their sleep, and much less choking sensation at night. Pain was the most common complaint. The VAS revealed significant pain, which reached a maximum on day 2 (mean of 8.6, range 7.3 to 9.1). The pain score reduced to a mean of 2.2 (range 1.8 to 3.6) at day 14.

Objective polysomnographic improvements were noted in six out of the eight patients (75%) with mild OSA. The mean preoperative AHI improved from 12.3 to 5.2 postoperatively ($P < 0.05$). The lowest oxygen saturation improved from 88.3% to 92.5% ($P < 0.05$). There were, however, no improvements in the proportion of slow wave sleep (SWS) or rapid-eye movement (REM) sleep. None of the patients suffered worsening of their AHI.

Mair and Day[2] reported a 77% success rate for reduction of snoring in 206 patients, at 1 year, who underwent the cautery-assisted palatal stiffening operation (CAPSO). Ellis[1] similarly revealed excellent results with this procedure. Kamami first described the laser-assisted uvulopalatoplasty (LAUP)[5] for patients with snoring. Kamami studied 417 snorers who underwent LAUP and found a reduction of snoring in 95% of the patients, after 1 year. Most authors report modest improvement after LAUP for patients with mild OSA, although a success rate as high as 75% was described by Walker et al.[6]

By combining the use of cautery with the principles of the laser palatoplasty technique and the creation of a horizontal denuded mucosal strip on the soft palate, in order to create a superior scar tissue. In this small cohort of simple snorers and patients with mild OSA, there were improvements in the VAS for snoring and the Epworth Sleepiness Scale. Most of the sleep partners were also happy with the reduction in snoring intensity at 90 days post-procedure. Subjectively, many patients reported improvements in daytime sleepiness and felt that they were no longer tired during the day. The frequency of choking sensation and gasping at night had also reduced and patients reported more dreams during their sleep. All patients had improvements in their AHI and LSAT; however, there was no significant increase in the SWS and REM sleep. The results reflect the scarring and fibrosis of the soft palate and the 'pull' of the scar superiorly that shortens and stiffens the soft palate. The effect is also enhanced by the shortening of the soft palate which increases the anteroposterior distance of the velopharynx.

The advantages of this procedure are that:

1. it produces a superior scar that pulls the entire soft palate upwards, in order to expand the oropharyngeal airway;
2. it is done as an office-based procedure on an out-patients basis;
3. it is low-cost and requires no special equipment nor implants; and
4. the results are excellent.

Patient selection is prudent: patients who are simple snorers and patients with mild obstructive sleep apnea, with primarily retropalatal flutter and/or obstruction, with small tonsils and BMI < 33, will benefit from the modified CAPSO technique.

## REFERENCES

1. Ellis PD. Laser palatoplasty for snoring due to palatal flutter: a further report. Clin Otolaryngol Allied Sci 1994;19(4):350–1.
2. Mair EA, Day RH. Cautery-assisted palatal stiffening operation. Otolaryngol Head Neck Surg 2000;122(4):547–56.

3. Terris DJ, Hanasono MM, Liu YC. Reliability of the Muller maneuver and its association with sleep-disordered breathing. Laryngoscope 2000;110:1819–23.
4. Friedman M. Clinical staging. Uvulopalatopharyngoplasty. In: Snoring and Obstructive Sleep Apnea, 3rd edn, Chapter 9, Section 9.2. Fairbanks DNF et al., eds. Lippincott Williams & Wilkins; 2003:120–27.
5. Kamami YV. Outpatient treatment of sleep apnea syndrome with $CO_2$ laser, LAUP: laser-assisted UPPP results on 46 patients. J Clin Laser Med Surg 1994;12(4):215–9.
6. Walker RP, Grigg-Damberger MM, Gopalsami C. Laser-assisted uvulopalatoplasty for the treatment of mild, moderate, and severe obstructive sleep apnea. Laryngoscope 1999;109(1):79–85.

SECTION H — MINIMALLY INVASIVE PALATAL PROCEDURES

CHAPTER 27

# Injection snoreplasty*

*Scott E. Brietzke and Eric A. Mair*

## 1 INTRODUCTION

There is a vast array of choices available to the otolaryngologist to treat simple snoring. The majority of these procedures function via the principle of palatal stiffening in which the vibrating floppy soft palate of the snoring patient is stiffened by creating scar tissue in or on the palate. Injection snoreplasty (IS) was originally developed as a modification of a solitary, indistinct case series published in the 1940s in which fish oil was injected into the pharynx of three patients to 'alter the "flutter ratio" of these tissues as to reduce or eliminate snoring.'[1] IS serves well as an alternative to the currently available snoring treatments that are either painful and/or expensive.[2] IS is highly effective in the majority of patients, is easily performed in the office with inexpensive materials, and typically results in mild pain only that does not prevent the patient from returning to the majority of their daily activities.

## 2 PATIENT SELECTION

IS is most effective in patients who suffer from socially bothersome palatal flutter snoring. IS has not been found to be effective in managing obstructive sleep apnea syndrome (OSAS) (author's unpublished data) and therefore, it is strongly recommended that OSAS be objectively excluded prior to snoring treatment. This is best accomplished with polysomnography as the history and physical exam are limited in their accuracy in diagnosing and excluding OSAS.[3]

IS (and most currently available snoring treatments) targets only the soft palate for snoring treatment. Fortunately, it appears the majority (estimated to be approximately 85%) of snoring patients suffer from palatal flutter snoring.[4] Ascertaining that the patient does indeed suffer from palatal flutter snoring, as opposed to other sites of snoring noise production, can translate to increased success with IS and other palatal snoring procedures.[5] Commercially available 'take-home' polysomnographic technology does exist that appears to reliably identify palatal flutter snoring that translates into improved treatment success rates. However, one must be careful in relying on objective snoring analysis to the point where the ultimate goal of improving the patient's subjective, social problem of snoring is overlooked.

As with any palatal procedure, patients should be screened carefully for any systemic conditions which may adversely affect wound healing. Examples include vascular disease, poorly controlled diabetes, and chronic steroid use. Additionally, patients with a strong gag reflex that is not abated with topical anesthesia may be very difficult to treat with IS or any office-based snoring procedure. Lastly, any pre-existing allergies to the injected agents should be excluded.

## 3 DESCRIPTION OF THE PROCEDURE

IS can be easily accomplished in a typical 20-minute office visit.[2] Informed consent is first obtained in all cases. Topical anesthesia is obtained with a thorough application of benzocaine spray or gel. This will also help the majority of patients with a problematic gag reflex. Local injected anesthesia (1% or 2% lidocaine without epinephrine) can be used to further anesthetize the soft palate, but is not necessary as the procedure can be quickly accomplished with a brief, mildly uncomfortable single injection that would be analogous to a local anesthetic injection.

IS has been successfully performed with three different sclerosing agents. The authors have reported the safe and effective use of two different agents in large numbers of patients. Three percent sodium tetradecyl sulfate (STS) (30 mg/ml Sotradecol™, Bioniche Pharma, Lake Forest, Illinois, USA, http://www.sotradecolusa.com/) was used in

---

*The opinions or assertions of the authors contained herein are the private views of the authors and are not to be construed as official or as reflecting the views of the Department of the Army, the Department of the Air Force, or the Department of Defense.

# SECTION H: MINIMALLY INVASIVE PALATAL PROCEDURES

the original developmental animal model and in the initial IS human use studies.[6] Three percent STS has been used for over five decades for varicose vein therapy and has an excellent safety record. It is inexpensive (less than $30 per treatment at the time of writing), easily obtained, and requires no dilution or mixing. It is highly effective and is the agent of choice for us. It is important to note that STS has NOT been FDA approved for palatal sclerotherapy and its use as such entails 'off label' use. It is unlikely that an FDA approval trial will ever be performed due to the fact that STS is no longer under patent protection.

IS has also been extensively performed by the authors with a 50–50 combination of 2% lidocaine (no epinephrine) and 98% dehydrated ethanol (sterile for injection). The safety and efficacy of dehydrated alcohol were demonstrated in an animal and human use study.[7] Ethanol was chosen as an alternative to STS given its equally excellent long-term safety record, its widespread availability, and its low cost (less than $20 per at the time of writing). There does not appear to be any significant difference in the effectiveness and discomfort level in STS and ethanol.[7] Again it is noted that ethanol is also not FDA approved for palatal sclerotherapy and will likely never undergo an approval trial for the same reasons as STS.

IS has also been successfully performed by published report using a lesser known sclerosing agent called Aethoxysklerol (AES).[8] The authors have not used this agent and refer the interested reader to the original article for more information.

After topical anesthesia is obtained and the sclerosing agent is selected, the procedure is simply accomplished with a single midline soft palate injection. Typically a 2 ml syringe and a 27-gauge inch and a half needle are used and 1.5–2.0 ml of sclerosing agent is injected. The location of the injection is important to the success of the procedure and in minimizing patient discomfort (Fig. 27.1). The injection is best placed in the midline soft palate approximately 1 cm proximal to the edge of the soft palate near the hard palate junction. It should NOT be placed into the uvula as this will produce significant uvular swelling that is often distressing to the patient. The injection is placed submucosally and NOT deep to the palatal muscle. The goal of the injection is to create a superficial sloughing of the soft palate mucosa that will be replaced by scar tissue, thereby stiffening the palate and reducing the patient's snoring.

After completion of the injection, the patient is observed for 10 minutes for development of possible hypersensitivity to the injected agent and then released with a follow-up scheduled in approximately 6 weeks.

In rare cases, the initial injection will not be completely successful. In this case, a second injection can be performed. This is typically placed in two separate sites in the lateral edges of the previous injection to produce more widespread palatal stiffening (Fig. 27.2). The injection is again placed submucosally with approximately 1.0 ml placed in each site.

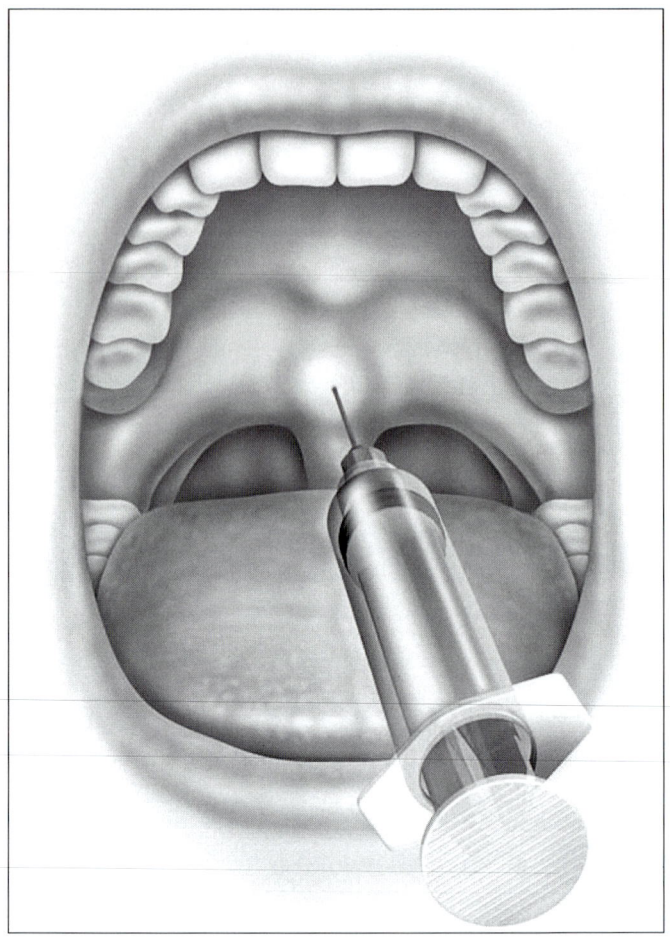

**Fig. 27.1** The injection snoreplasty procedure. Approximately 1.5 ml of the selected sclerotherapy agent is injected submucosally into the central soft palate with a 27-gauge needle creating an easily visible bulla. Care is taken not to allow the injected agent to spread into the uvula to avoid bothersome uvular swelling.

## 4 POSTOPERATIVE MANAGEMENT AND COMPLICATIONS

Pain is typically reported by IS patients to be mild. Pain is usually well controlled with ibuprofen and/or acetaminophen and over-the-counter throat lozenges. Pain typically is reported to last 3–5 days. No dietary restrictions are imposed. Most patients will note a swelling sensation in the roof of their mouth immediately after the procedure that typically abates over several hours. No significant airway obstruction has ever been noted to result from the procedure in the author's experience. Patients should be carefully counseled that snoring will typically worsen during the next 1–2 weeks after the procedure until scarring/stiffening begins. Maximal treatment effect is expected to occur at about 6–8 weeks after injection.

All patients should be cautioned that palatal ulceration and sloughing will likely occur after IS. This should not be considered a complication as this tissue injury and the

Injection snoreplasty | CHAPTER 27

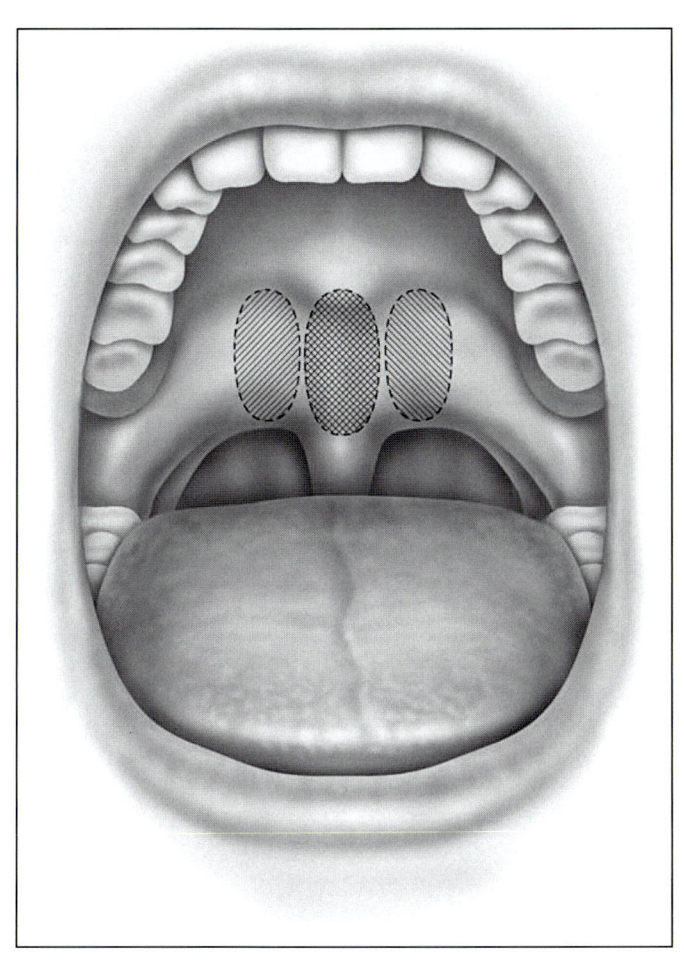

**Fig. 27.2** In unusual cases where the first injection is only partially successful, more scar tissue can be created in the soft palate with a second set of injections. These second injections are best placed in the lateral areas of the soft palate (diagonal lined areas) as opposed to the original central injection zone (cross-hatched area). Re-injection into the previously injected central injection zone may be difficult due to previously created submucosal scar tissue.

procedure) have a high probability of being non-palatal flutter snorers. If a patient reports no benefit from the procedure and scar tissue is visible and/or palpable on the soft palate after the procedure, then no further treatment is recommended. If no visible/palpable scar tissue is present (rare) then further treatment with IS or another palatal stiffening procedure can be attempted until scar tissue is produced and snoring is reassessed. If scar tissue is observed yet there has been a less than complete response to the treatment, a second injection can be performed (see Fig. 27.2). This is unusual in our experience.

It is known that all snoring treatments (with the possible exception of palatal implants for which there are limited long-term data) have reduced effectiveness over time. This is likely the result of the softening and/or remodeling of scar tissue within the soft palate that occurs over time. Fortunately, it has been demonstrated that repeating IS after a relapse of snoring can be effective.[9] In fact, if it turns out that snoring treatment must be maintained with serial treatments as opposed to being cured with a single treatment, then IS lends itself well to this concept as it is simple, only mildly painful, and very inexpensive.

## 6 CONCLUSION

IS is a simple, safe, well-tolerated palatal stiffening procedure that is easily performed in the office setting. It provides an effective but inexpensive alternative to currently popular 'high tech' procedures that pass on high costs to patients.

resulting replacement with scar tissue is the directed goal of the procedure. However, we have observed in rare cases (less than 1%) that a complete palatal fistula can occur.[9] These case have all been managed conservatively with antibiotics and observation. All observed fistulae have closed spontaneously and no lasting velopharyngeal insufficiency (VPI) has ever been observed.

## 5 SUCCESS/FAILURE RATES

IS has been found to be successful short term in approximately 76.7% to 92% of patients.[2,5,7,8,9] This result is most likely due to the fact that palatal snoring is the predominant form of snoring in approximately 85–90% of snorers.[4] Therefore, it can be deduced that those patients who report no benefit from IS (or likely any other palatal snoring

## REFERENCES

1. Straus JF. A new approach to the treatment of snoring. Arch Otolaryngol 1943;38:225–29.
2. Brietzke SE, Mair EA. Injection snoreplasty: how to treat snoring without all the pain and expense. Otolaryngol Head Neck Surg 2001;124(5):503–10.
3. Ross SD, Sheinhait IA, Harrison KJ, et al. Systematic review and meta-analysis of the literature regarding the diagnosis of sleep apnea. Sleep 2000;23(4):519–32.
4. Miyazaki S, Itasaka Y, Ishikawa K, et al. Acoustic analysis of snoring and the site of airway obstruction in sleep related respiratory disorders. Acta Otolaryngol Supp 1998;537:47–51.
5. Brietzke SE, Mair EA. The acoustical analysis of snoring: can the probability of success be predicted? Otolaryngol Head Neck Surg 2006;135(3):417–20.
6. LaFrentz JR, Brietzke SE, Mair EA. Evaluation of palatal snoring surgery in an animal model. Otolaryngol Head Neck Surg 2003;129(4):343–52.
7. Brietzke SE, Mair EA. Injection snoreplasty: investigation of alternative sclerotherapy agents. Otolaryngol Head Neck Surg 2004;130(1):47–57.
8. Iseri M, Balcioglu O. Radiofrequency versus injection snoreplasty in simple snoring. Otolaryngol Head Neck Surg 2005;133(2):224–8.

167

# SECTION H: MINIMALLY INVASIVE PALATAL PROCEDURES

9. Brietzke SE, Mair EA. Injection snoreplasty: extended follow-up and new objective data. Otolaryngol Head Neck Surg 2003;128(5):605–15.

## FURTHER READING

Brietzke SE, Mair EA. Injection snoreplasty: how to treat snoring without all the pain and expense. Otolaryngol Head Neck Surg 2001;124(5):503–10.

Brietzke SE, Mair EA. Injection snoreplasty: extended follow-up and new objective data. Otolaryngol Head Neck Surg 2003;128(5):605–15.

Brietzke SE, Mair EA. Injection snoreplasty: investigation of alternative sclerotherapy agents. Otolaryngol Head Neck Surg 2004;130(1):47–57.

SECTION H — MINIMALLY INVASIVE PALATAL PROCEDURES

# CHAPTER 28
# Palatal implants for primary snoring: short- and long-term results of a new minimally invasive surgical technique

*Joachim T. Maurer*

## 1 INTRODUCTION

Snoring is a widespread symptom affecting about 50% of the adult population. Primary snoring without sleep disordered breathing is not harmful in itself. However, as snoring often causes social embarrassment and marital disharmony, affected patients apply to their physicians for treatment.

The primary therapeutic aim of all available therapies is a reduction in the duration and intensity of snoring to a tolerable degree without harming the patient. Apart from conservative treatments that require patient compliance to be successful, various kinds of surgical procedures exist, with techniques for the soft palate being the most widespread. All these procedures intend to reduce palatal flutter, the major cause of non-apneic snoring. Uvulopalatopharyngoplasty (UPPP) and laser-assisted uvulopalatoplasty (LAUP) are well known, but associated with a significant morbidity. Furthermore, these treatments are invasive, destructive, painful, and irreversible to a certain extent. UPPP even requires general anesthesia.

Therefore, both patients and physicians prefer a minimally invasive and less painful procedure as a primary option for the treatment of snoring. Since its invention in 1998 interstitial radiofrequency treatment of the soft palate has gained increasing interest among the public because it was the first minimally invasive surgical treatment bearing a low morbidity as well as a remarkable success rate.[1] However, it is not a single-step procedure and treating the palate excessively may still impair the various functions of the soft palate in very few cases. Furthermore, a considerable relapse of snoring 1 to 1½ years after the last radiofrequency treatment has to be considered.[2] Due to this relapse of snoring, alternative therapies with minimal morbidity and long-term efficacy are desired. Therefore, a new procedure was developed in 2001 where woven cylindrical implants are placed within the soft palate in order to stiffen the soft palate and thus reduce snoring. These implants are made of polyethylene terephtalate, a material which has been used in heart valve surgery for the last decades.

In this chapter, the patient selection criteria for the insertion of palatal implants in the treatment of snoring and its success rate as well as its morbidity are described according to the literature and to our own experience. The procedure is described in detail. It is performed identically in snorers as well as sleep apnea patients. During the last few years the delivery tool has been modified three times. It became smaller and contains more safety precautions against unwanted or incorrect implant deployment (Fig. 28.1).

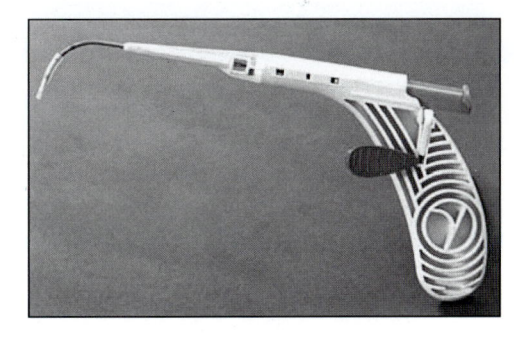

Fig. 28.1

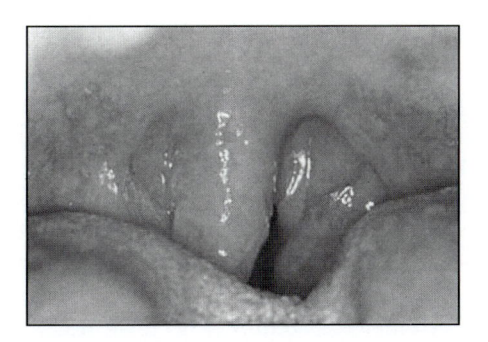

Fig. 28.2

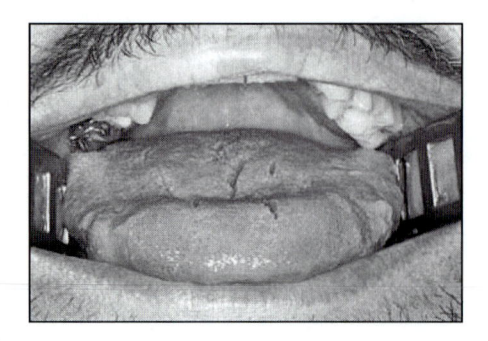

# SECTION H  MINIMALLY INVASIVE PALATAL PROCEDURES

Fig. 28.3

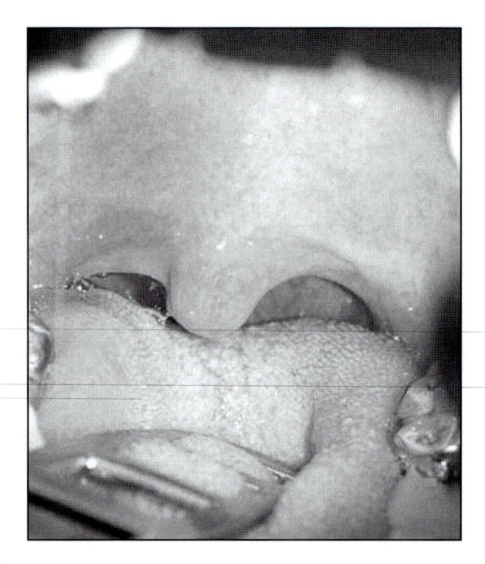

Fig. 28.4

## 2 PATIENT SELECTION

The Pillar® procedure consists of inserting implants into the junction of hard and soft palate in order to extend the hard palate, thus reducing the vibrating parts of the palate. The nature of the procedure where there is no resection or ablation of palatal tissue makes the patient selection criteria for this operation comprehensible. Patients with the following findings at the upper pharyngeal level should not receive palatal implants as a *solitary* intervention: nasal obstruction for whatever reason, distance between both tonsils less than 2 cm, excessive palatal and pharyngeal mucosa, and an uvula longer than 1 cm (Fig. 28.2). Patients with signs of tongue base snoring or obstruction in the clinical examination such as Friedman Tongue Position 3 or 4 (Fig. 28.3), tongue base hypertrophy, retrognathia, and floppy epiglottis are also not suitable candidates for this procedure. Obesity with a BMI above 32 kg/m² is known to impair any surgical intervention at the upper pharyngeal level and therefore is considered to be an exclusion criterion. In brief, patients without any obvious morphological anomaly in their nose and pharynx except a sufficiently long soft palate are suitable candidates for a solitary Pillar® procedure (Fig. 28.4). It has to be kept in mind that in all publications concerning the efficacy of palatal implants themselves, only those patients who fulfilled the above-mentioned inclusion criteria were treated.

The impact of nasal obstruction on snoring can be easily detected by applying a nasal decongestant and/or a nasal dilator before bedtime for a period of 7 days. If the improvement of nasal breathing during the night does not lead to a decrease of snoring, a combined versus a stepwise operation of the nose and the Pillar® procedure may be discussed with the patient. Of course, an adjunct conservative treatment with a mandibular advancement device, positional therapy, and/or weight reduction is possible at any time and vice versa. It is well documented in sleep apnea patients that palatal implants can be inserted synchronously to or as a second step after other soft palate procedures like UPPP.[3] It is also possible in the case of a recurrence of symptoms after such operations.[4] Future studies have to show whether this is also true for primary snorers. Radiofrequency of the soft palate, injection snoreplasty, and cautery-assisted palatal stiffening operations are not recommended as additional surgeries by us, because the tissue necrosis they induce is likely to increase the risk of implant extrusion and infection (see Complications below). There are no data concerning the combination with tongue base procedures (i.e. radiofrequency, laser resection of the lingual tonsil, genioglossus advancement, hyoid suspension), but obviously there is no surgical contraindication as different anatomical sites are addressed. However, tongue base procedures are rarely used in primary snoring anyway.

If palatal implants are used as additional surgery, one will lose the minimally invasive character of the intervention in most cases. Therefore, it has to be investigated whether the indication for an isolated Pillar® procedure may generally be extended to patients considered less suitable up to now, in order to offer this minimally invasive procedure as a real alternative to more aggressive operations as mentioned above. Furthermore, it is not yet clear whether additional methods for the assessment of the site of snoring sound generation can improve the selection process towards a better outcome. Regarding this issue, sound analysis using the SNAP® system did not increase the success rate.[5] Multi-channel pressure recordings during natural sleep and videoendoscopy during wakefulness as well as under sedation are still under investigation.

So far, there are no data concerning the treatment of children with palatal implants. As children mainly have shorter palates than adults, the size of the implants would probably not fit for most children.

## 3 OUTLINE OF PROCEDURE

The implant is a braided segment of polyester filaments intended for permanent implantation. The implant is 18 mm in length and has an outer diameter of 1.5 mm. The delivery tool (See Fig. 28.1) consists of a handle and 14-gauge needle, with the implant preloaded. The implant is deployed by pushing the thumb switch. Three implants are placed near the midline into the soft palate near the junction of hard and soft palate as if the hard palate was extended by the implants. The curved needle has three markings: a full insertion marking, a halfway depth marking, and a needle tip marking. Care must be taken to remove the transport lock and the plastic sleeve covering the tip of the needle, before attempting insertion of the implants. Each delivery tool contains one implant. The delivery tools are not reusable, and should be appropriately disposed of in a sharps container after the procedure.

The Pillar® Implant Technique can be performed in the office under local anesthesia or as part of a combination of procedures in patients under general anesthesia in the operating room.

After mucosal disinfection with hexetidine 0.1% and topical anesthesia with lidocaine gel 2%, the total length of the soft palate is infiltrated in the midline and approximately 5 mm laterally with a total of approximately 3 ml of prilocaine 2% with epinephrine 1:200000. Meanwhile 2 g cefazoline are administered intravenously and antibiotic prophylaxis is continued for 5 days with cefuroxime $2 \times 500$ mg per day. Midazolam is used for sedation if desired by the patient.

The exact location of the insertion sites is determined by palpating the junction of the soft and hard palate and may be marked by the surgeon. The needle is inserted in the midline first while the neck is slightly extended, thus giving more space between chest and delivery tool and making it easier to follow the angle and curvature of the soft palate. The needle is then advanced towards the free margin of the soft palate to the full insertion marking which still has to remain visible. Care must be taken to always stay in the muscle layer (Fig. 28.5). Correct positioning of the needle can be checked either by palpation or, more easily, by making the soft palate move anteriorly and posteriorly with the needle.

At this point the device is unlocked by pressing the lock located beneath the slider downwards. The slider is pushed halfway, until a click is heard. The needle is then withdrawn until the halfway depth marker, and the slider is pushed all the way in, thus deploying the implant into the channel which has been created in the soft palate by the needle. The position of the slider can be determined by looking at the windows on the side of the delivery tool. The needle is then withdrawn following the curvature of the needle, by moving the delivery tool in an arching fashion. If resistance is felt while delivering the implant, it usually means that the implant is pushing against the end of the previously created tunnel. Withdrawing the needle as the slider is pushed all the way in will usually result in adequate placement of the implant. The two lateral implants are inserted in the same fashion, as close as possible to the midline implant, about 2 mm apart (Fig. 28.6). A good way of estimating this distance is by using the diameter of the needle (approx. 2 mm).

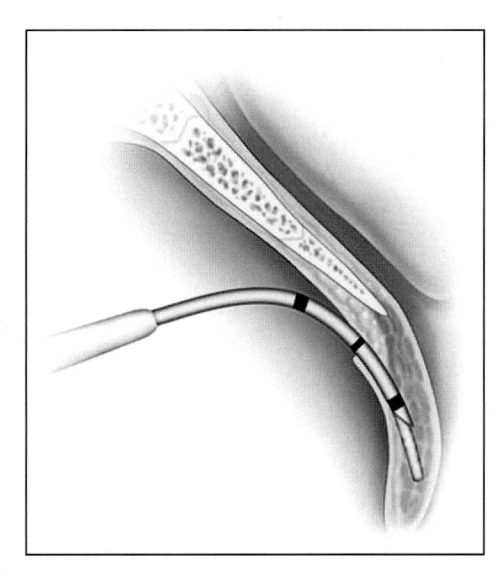

Fig. 28.5

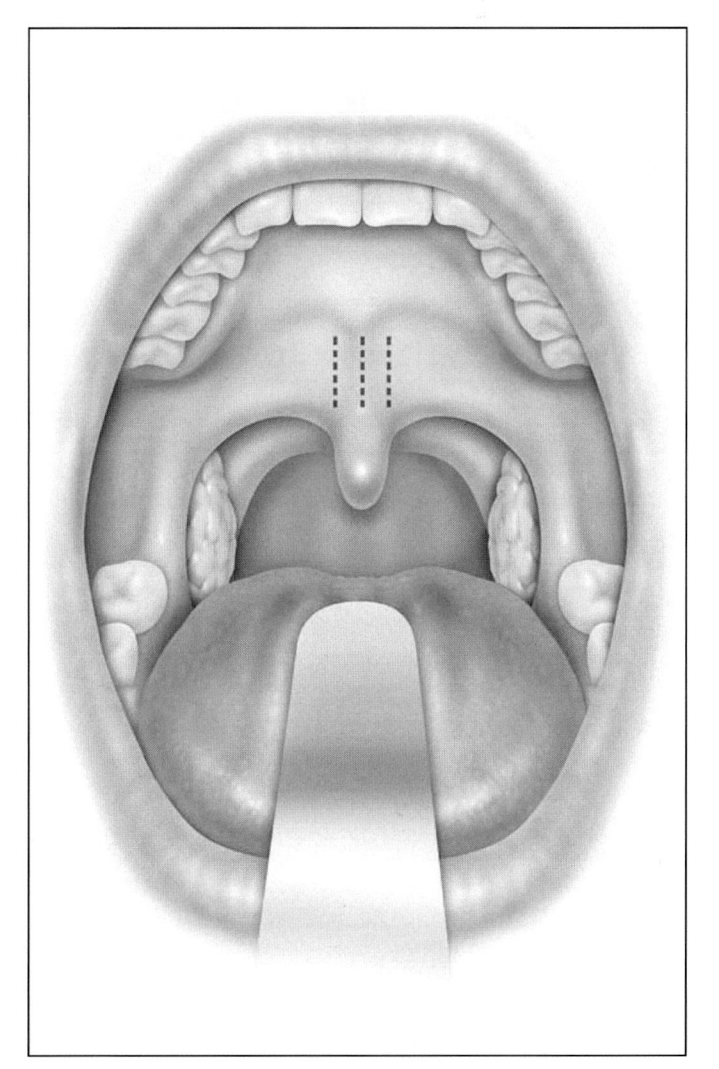

Fig. 28.6A

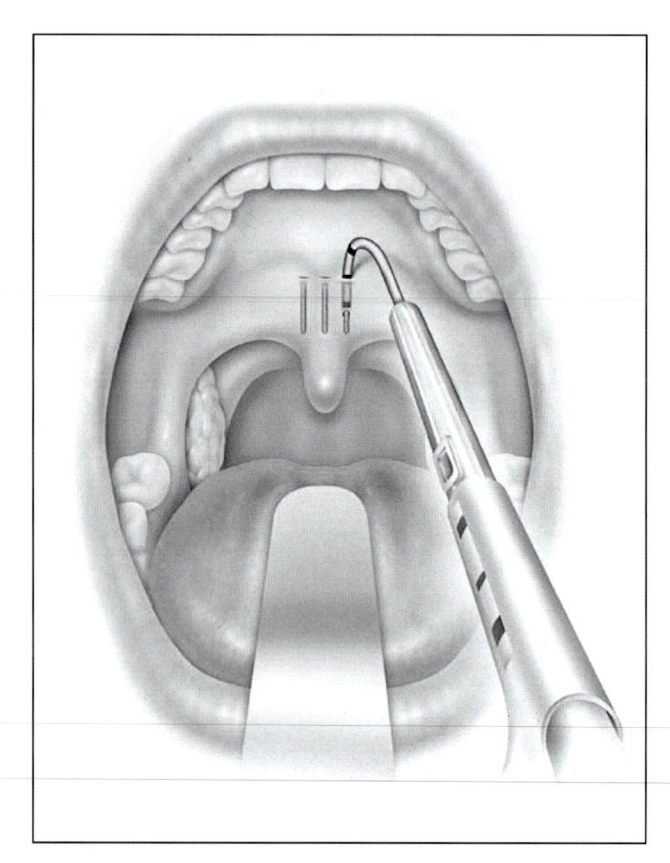

# SECTION H  MINIMALLY INVASIVE PALATAL PROCEDURES

**Fig. 28.6B** (Continued)

The correct positioning of all three implants is finally verified by palpation and transnasal pharyngoscopy.

## 4 POSTOPERATIVE MANAGEMENT AND COMPLICATIONS

Our own data and the literature demonstrate that palatal implants can be easily implanted under local anesthesia. Sedation is usually not necessary. If – due to a sudden gagging of the patient – an implant is pushed through the mucosa at either side of the soft palate, it can be pulled out easily at once with tweezers or a forceps. A new implant can be implanted at minimal distance of the extracted implant during the same operation. Apart from that there are no relevant perioperative complications. The mean postoperative pain levels and use of analgesics are comparable to the data obtained after radiofrequency treatment (RF) of the soft palate and considerably lower than after UPPP or LAUP.[6] There were no mucosal ulcerations, palatal sloughing, or fistulas detected which have been described after RF procedures[7] and injection snoreplasty.[8] Swallowing and speech were not subjectively affected. On the other hand, partial extrusions of one or more implants were noted during the first postoperative year in 25% of our first group of 40 snorers.[9] In one patient all three implants extruded. The

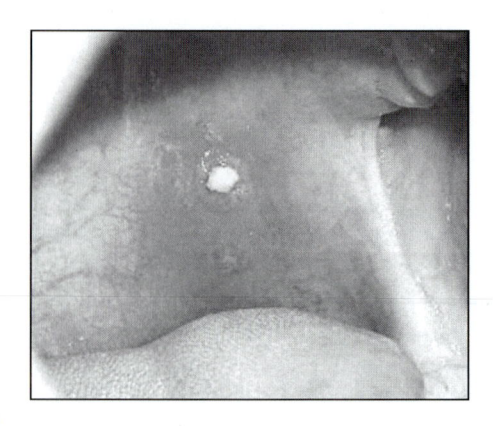

**Fig. 28.7**

implants never extruded completely, making an aspiration impossible. However, we saw an ongoing extrusion of up to one-third of an implant over 2 weeks in one patient. Patients experience this partial implant extrusion either like a mild sore throat due to the concomitant or responsible infection, a foreign body, or they do not feel anything particular but discover a white spot at the oral surface of the soft palate accidentally (Fig. 28.7). If the implant is extruded through the posterior palatal surface, patients always feel a foreign body sensation or a sore throat. Therefore, a fibroscopic control of the nasopharynx is always necessary if any suspicion about implant extrusion arises. Ho et al.[10] reported about 8.8% partial extrusions in 16.7% of the patients after 3 months; Nordgard[11] and co-workers mentioned only two partial extrusions in 35 patients (2% of the implants) and one additional removal due to foreign body sensation during the first 90 days after the procedure. Our partial extrusion rate after 3 months is comparable. However, almost half of the partial extrusions occurred later than 90 days after implantation. There were more extrusions in the first half of the study population. Using more rigid implants increased the number of partial extrusions (five partial extrusions in 10 patients) whereas efficacy decreased compared to regular implants.[12] In our own last 20 patients we did not see any extrusions during the first year after the implantation. The data available are summarized in Table 28.1.

All this indicates that there is a certain learning curve. In the beginning the surgeon may tend to place the implants too superficially in order to avoid penetrating the soft palate to the nasopharynx. Second, it is rather difficult to penetrate the mucosa near the junction of the hard and soft palate as recommended. In the beginning the surgeon may thus place the implants too close to the edge of the soft palate, where it becomes rather thin. Both factors increase the risk of partial implant extrusion.

The removal of partially extruded implants is always simple if extruded to the oral surface. In some cases it can even be done without any local anesthesia. Implants extruding to the nasopharynx may eventually require general anesthesia to be removed. If desired by the patient and if there are no signs of infection (Fig. 28.8) the surgeon may substitute the removed implants during the same session. It

### Table 28.1 Extrusions of implants

| Author (Reference) | Number | Follow-up (days) | Extrusion rates (per implant) | (per patient) | Site (median/lateral) |
|---|---|---|---|---|---|
| Friedman (3) | 125 | 300 | 10 (2.7%) | 10 (8%) | n.a. |
| Friedman (4) | 23 | 180 | 0 (0%) | 0 (0%) | n.a. |
| Maurer (9) | 40 | 365 | 13 (11%) | 10 (25%) | 5/8 |
| Ho (10) | 11 | 90 | 3 (8.8%) | 2 (16.7) | n.a. |
| Nordgard (11) | 35 | 365 | 9 (8.6%) | 6 (17.1%) | 0/9 |
| Skjostad (12) | 10 | 180 | 0 (0%) | 0 (0%) | n.a. |
| Romanow (13) | 25 | 90 | 2 (2.7%) | 1 (4%) | n.a. |
| Nordgard (14) | 26 | 365 | 3 (3.8%) | 3 (11.5%) | 2/1 |
| Goessler (15) | 16 | 90 | 0 (0%) | 0 (0%) | n.a. |
| **All** | **311** | **273** | **40 (4.3%)** | **32 (10.3%)** | |

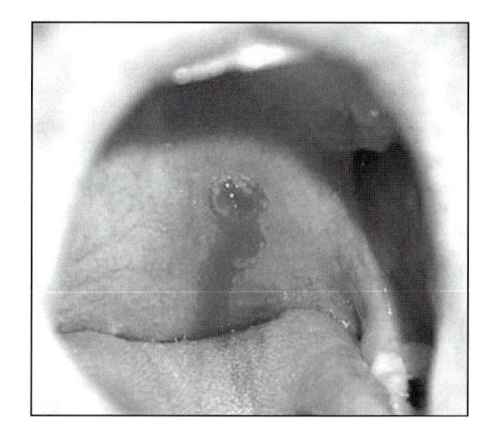

Fig. 28.8

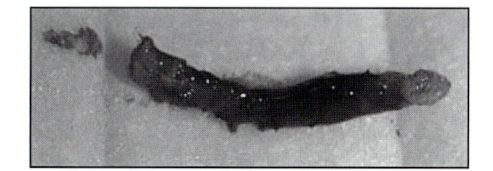

Fig. 28.9

is also possible to remove non-irritating implants if desired by the patient for any reason. However, this may be more difficult and destructive and may require general anesthesia as the implants are intact (Fig. 28.9) and thoroughly anchored in scar tissue. Therefore, we suggest not removing ineffective implants which do not cause any problems.

A worsening of snoring was only reported if two implants were removed but snoring could be improved by replacing them. There seems to be some additional anti-snoring effect due to scarring, explaining the ongoing efficacy after partial extrusion of one implant. However, this effect seems insufficient if only one implant is left. Our patients with a partial extrusion were neither snoring more nor were less satisfied with the procedure than patients without partial extrusions.

Thus we consider a partial extrusion to be of rather minor importance, but the patient must be well informed about that risk. When taking into consideration the different aspects of morbidity, the Pillar® palatal implant system is a safe procedure with only minor complications.

## 5 SUCCESS RATE OF THE PROCEDURE

In the majority of primary snorers the soft palate is the main source of sound generation. Therefore, the first studies using palatal implants were performed on primary snorers. All patients had palatal implants as a solitary intervention and fulfilled the inclusion and exclusion criteria mentioned above. All patients received three implants. Snoring was mainly assessed using visual analogue scales which were filled in by the bedpartner. In some studies, the SNAP® recording system was additionally used in order to obtain some objective data. However, there was no relationship between subjective and objective outcome.[5,9,11,16] On average, snoring could be reduced significantly from 7.7 to 4.0 on the VAS after 3 months and from 7.1 to 4.8 after 1 year (Fig. 28.10). The available data concerning 3-month and 1-year results are summarized in Tables 28.2 and 28.3. These raw results are similar to radiofrequency treatment of the soft palate. In the light of the limited data available the recurrence of snoring after an initial success seems lower with Pillar® compared to radiofrequency treatment of the soft palate. Long-term data over several years are being collected currently. More than 90% of patients and bedpartners would recommend the procedure to others, although only a few bedpartners reported a complete elimination of snoring (Fig. 28.11). Mostly snoring decreased but could still be heard. A reason for the surprisingly good patient acceptance might be the low morbidity of the procedure combined with a recognizable reduction of snoring sound intensity. However, placebo-controlled randomized trials as published for RF of the palate[18] are necessary to assess the impact of Pillar® implants on simple snoring.

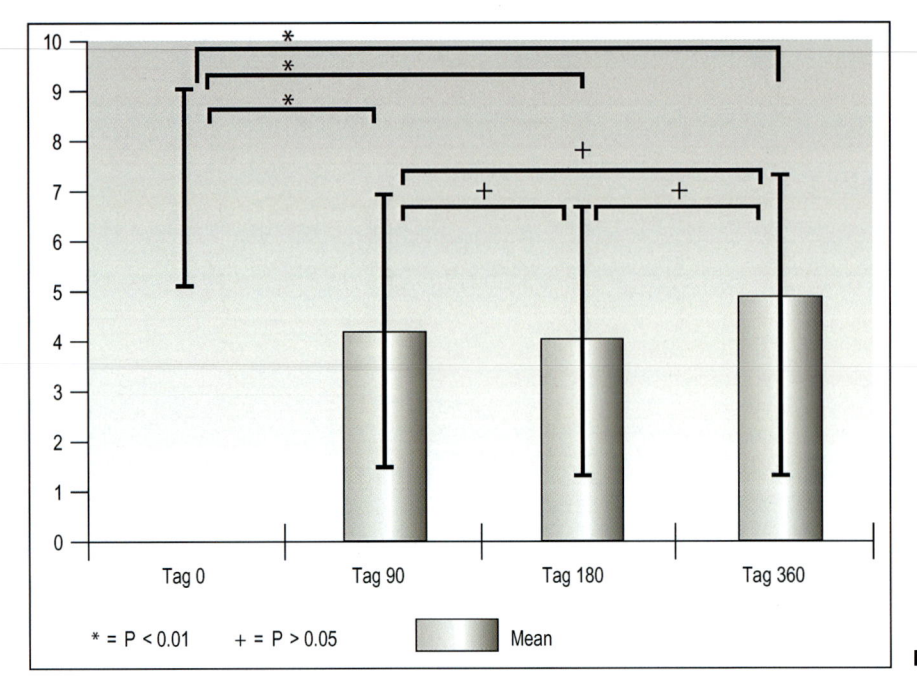

Fig. 28.10

* = P < 0.01    + = P > 0.05    Mean

Table 28.2 Impact of palatal implants on snoring intensity in primary snorers, measured by visual analogue scale (VAS, 0–10 cm) after 3 months

| Author (Reference) | Number | VAS before | VAS day 90 |
|---|---|---|---|
| Maurer (5) | 15 | 7.3 | 2.5 |
| Ho (10) | 9 | 7.9 | 4.8 |
| Skjostad (12) | 10 | 7.7 | 4.7 |
| Romanow (13) | 25 | 8.5 | 4.4 |
| Nordgard (16) | 35 | 7.3 | 3.6 |
| Kühnel (17) | 95 | 7.7 | 3.7 |
| **All** | **189** | **7.7** | **4.0** |

Table 28.3 Impact of palatal implants on snoring intensity in primary snorers, measured by visual analogue scale (VAS, 0–10 cm) after 1 year

| Author (Reference) | Number | VAS before | VAS day 360 |
|---|---|---|---|
| Maurer (9) | 32 | 7.1 | 4.8 |
| Nordgard (11) | 34 | 7.1 | 4.8 |
| **All** | **66** | **7.1** | **4.8** |

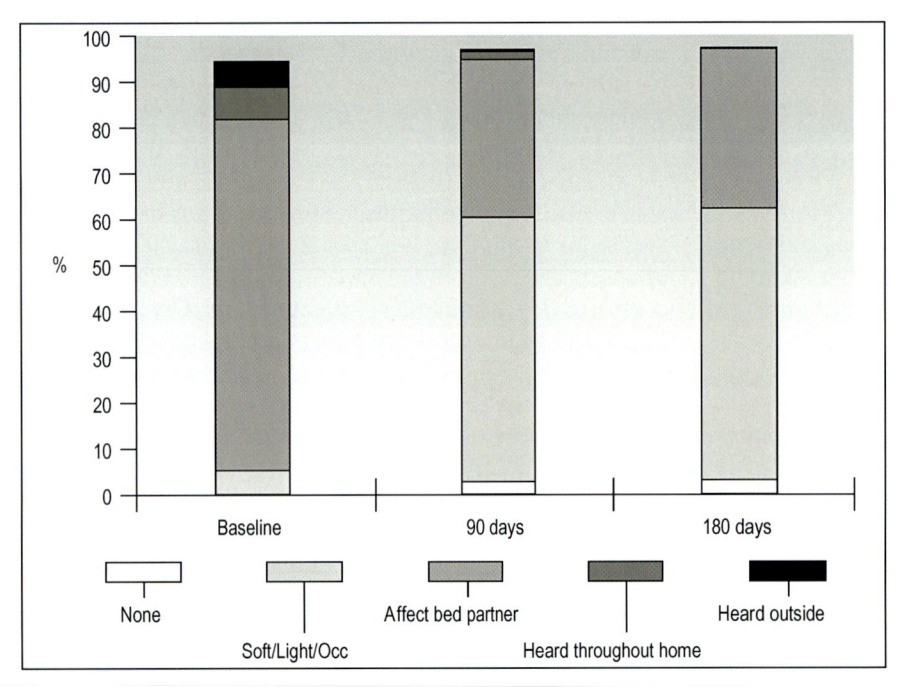

Fig. 28.11

## 5.1 WHAT TO DO IF THE PROCEDURE FAILS

If there are extrusions causing a recurrence of socially disturbing snoring, palatal implants can be reinserted easily in most cases with an anew snoring reduction. If patients are not satisfied by the snoring reduction 3 months after the procedure, two additional implants – one at each side – can be placed laterally in the same way as during the initial treatment. On the other hand, if the upper airway examination or the control polygraphy reveals a clear pathology that may need correction one should address this factor first. Useful treatments in such cases may be: nasal surgery, LAUP, mandibular advancement or positional devices. It is not recommended to reduce the soft palate with radiofrequency if implants have been placed, because of the risk of implant extrusion, and soft palate perforation is likely to increase. Tongue base procedures should be regarded with caution as the main snoring sound generation is due to soft palate flutter even after residual snoring. More aggressive procedures such as UPPP, multilevel or maxillomandibular surgery are not recommended as primary snoring does not bear any health risk.

## 6 CONCLUSION

The Pillar® implant technique is a non-destructive treatment option for palatal snorers due to its low morbidity in combination with an acceptable success rate. It has to be investigated whether additional implants during the initial operation or as a second step after initial failure can improve the success rate.

## REFERENCES

1. Powell NB, Riley RW, Troell RJ, et al. Radiofrequency volumetric tissue reduction of the palate in subjects with sleep-disordered breathing. Chest 1998;113:1163–74.
2. Li KK, Powell NB, Riley RW, et al. Radiofrequency volumetric reduction of the palate: an extended follow-up study. Otolaryngol Head Neck Surg 2000;122:410–14.
3. Friedman M, Vidyasagar R, Bliznikas D, Joseph NJ. Patient selection and efficacy of Pillar implant technique for the treatment of snoring and obstructive sleep apnea/hypopnea syndrome. Otolaryngol Head Neck Surg 2006;134:187–96.
4. Friedman M, Schalch P, Joseph NJ. Palatal stiffening after failed uvulopalatopharyngoplasty with the Pillar Implant System. Laryngoscope 2006;116:1956–61.
5. Maurer JT, Verse T, Stuck BA, Hormann K, Hein G. Palatal implants for primary snoring: short-term results of a new minimally invasive surgical technique. Otolaryngol Head Neck Surg 2005;132:125–31.
6. Troell RJ, Powell NB, Riley RW, et al. Comparison of postoperative pain between laser-assisted uvulopalatoplasty, uvulopalatopharyngoplasty, and radiofrequency volumetric tissue reduction of the palate. Otolaryngol Head Neck Surg 2000;122:402–9.
7. Stuck BA, Starzak K, Verse T, et al. Complications of temperature-controlled radiofrequency volumetric tissue reduction for sleep-disordered breathing. Acta Otolaryngol 2003;123:532–5.
8. Brietzke SE, Mair EA. Injection snoreplasty: extended follow-up and new objective data. Otolaryngol Head Neck Surg 2003;128:605–15.
9. Maurer JT, Hein G, Verse T, et al. Long-term results of palatal implants for primary snoring. Otolaryngol Head Neck Surg 2005;133:573–78.
10. Ho WK, Wei WI, Chung KF. Managing disturbing snoring with palatal implants: a pilot study. Arch Otolaryngol Head Neck Surg 2004;130:753–8.
11. Nordgard S, Stene BK, Skjostad KW, et al. Palatal implants for the treatment of snoring: long-term results. Otolaryngol Head Neck Surg 2006;134:558–64.
12. Skjostad KW, Stene BK, Norgard S. Consequences of increased rigidity in palatal implants for snoring: a randomized controlled study. Otolaryngol Head Neck Surg 2006;134:63–6.
13. Romanow JH, Catalano PJ. Initial U.S. pilot study: palatal implants for the treatment of snoring. Otolaryngol Head Neck Surg 2006;134:551–7.
14. Nordgard S, Hein G, Stene BK, et al. One-year results: palatal implants for the treatment of obstructive sleep apnea. Otolaryngol Head Neck Surg 2007;136:818–22.
15. Goessler UR, Hein G, Verse T, et al. Soft palate implants as a minimally invasive treatment for mild to moderate obstructive sleep apnea. Acta Otolaryngol 2007;127:527–31.
16. Nordgard S, Wormdal K, Bugten V, et al. Palatal implants: a new method for the treatment of snoring. Acta Otolaryngol 2004;124:970–5.
17. Kuhnel TS, Hein G, Hohenhorst W, Maurer JT. Soft palate implants: a new option for treating habitual snoring. Eur Arch Otorhinolaryngol 2005;262:277–80.
18. Stuck BA, Sauter A, Hormann K, et al. Radiofrequency surgery of the soft palate in the treatment of snoring. A placebo-controlled trial. Sleep 2005;28:847–50.

# SECTION I  PALATAL SURGERY

## CHAPTER 29
# Uvulopalatopharyngoplasty

*George P. Katsantonis*

## 1 INTRODUCTION

Although the surgical armamentarium for snoring and obstructive sleep apnea (OSA) has, in the last several years, expanded significantly to include many procedures, uvulopalatopharyngoplasty (UPPP) still remains the most widely performed operation for these conditions. The procedure was first introduced by Fujita in 1981 and is designed to enlarge the airway lumen at the level of the velopharynx and decrease the collapsibility of the pharyngeal walls.

A large number of UPPP procedures were performed in the 1980s, because with the exception of tracheostomy, UPPP was the only available treatment for OSA during that period. This provided adequate material for an accurate assessment of the efficacy of the operation in both selected and unselected patients. Although UPPP enjoyed success in reducing snoring, it had unpredictable results in curing apnea. The success rate of the procedure in unselected OSA patients was only 20–25%. Uvulopalatopharyngoplasty results continued to be unpredictable even after careful selection of candidates, although its success rate increased to 50–60% in groups of selected patients. Further investigation of the upper airway mechanics of obstruction revealed that the pharynx of OSA patients collapses in more than one site. This realization offered some understanding of the limitations of the isolated UPPP procedure in curing OSA and the concept of multilevel airway surgery was born. Uvulopalatopharyngoplasty nowadays is frequently performed in conjunction with other airway procedures in multi- or single-stage fashion. The original technique has also undergone many modifications in order to comply with anatomical variations of the velopharynx and minimize morbidity.

## 2 PATIENT SELECTION

Theoretically patients who have airway collapse at the level of the velopharynx should respond well to UPPP. However, so far, identification of the site of collapse has proven to be a difficult task. Furthermore, even patients whose site of collapse is documented to be in the velopharynx may have poor response to the UPPP. Fiberoptic and manometric studies have shown that many patients who failed UPPP continue to have obstruction at the level of the velopharynx, although it is speculated that increased resistance due to narrowing (without obstruction) at the base of tongue level causes the more collapsible velopharynx to obstruct. There is a plethora of methods to evaluate the airway in OSA patients, but the efficacy of most of them in predicting UPPP success is limited. It would be beyond the scope of this chapter to elaborate on methods of airway evaluation. From a practical view point, information obtained by physical examination (PE), awake fiberoptic endoscopy and cephalometric analysis is quite valuable and these three methods are utilized by majority of otolaryngologists for preoperative airway evaluation.

Physical examination factors important in airway evaluation are:

- size of tonsils;
- length of uvula;
- Friedman tongue position;
- presence of palatal and pillar webbing;
- presence of posterior pharyngeal folds and mandibular position.

Endoscopic factors are:

- retropalatal and retrolingual airway cross-section;
- lateral pharyngeal wall position (bulge);
- airway orientation (circular, sagittal);
- presence of lingual tonsil;
- shape and position of epiglottis and presence of retrodisplacement of the tongue.

Cephalometric indices are:

- length of soft palate–uvula (posterior nasal spine to tip of uvula distance);
- posterior airway space (PAS);
- mandibular plane to hyoid distance (MP–H);
- the presence of retrognathia.

# CHAPTER 29 Uvulopalatopharyngoplasty

| Table 29.1 Indications for UPPP | |
|---|---|
| Posterior nasal spine to uvula tip distance | >38 mm |
| Tonsil size | +++ – ++++ |
| Posterior airway space | >10 mm |
| Mandibular plane to hyoid distance | <27 mm |
| Friedman tongue position | I or II |
| Absence of retrognathia | |
| Absence of retroglossia | |
| Absence of hypopharyngeal narrowing | |
| Absence of lateral pharyngeal wall bulging | |
| Absence of morbid obesity | BMI > 40 |
| Absence of sagittal orientation of airway | |

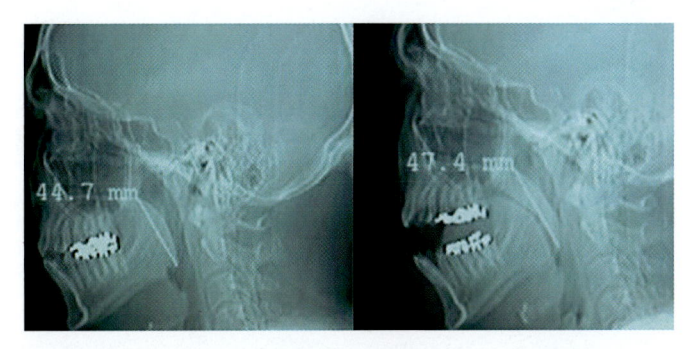

**Fig. 29.2** CT topogram of the airway showing long uvula (44.7–47.4 cm with open mouth), short MP–H distance (22.5 cm) and adequate PAS (11.6 cm). This patient is a reasonably good candidate for UPPP.

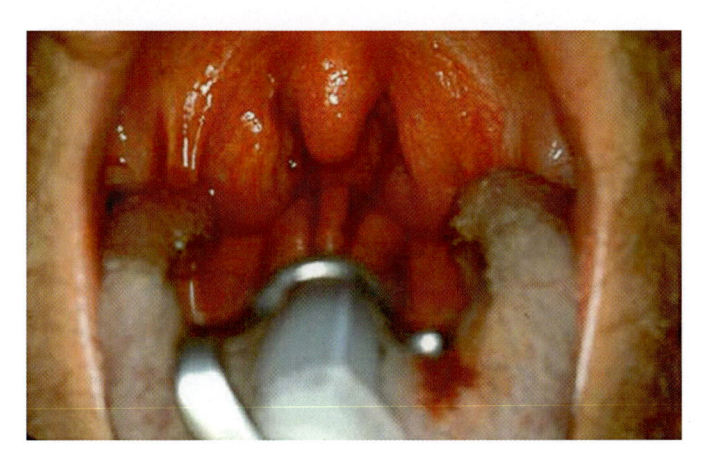

**Fig. 29.1** OSA patient with marked tonsillar and uvular hyperplasia. Physical examination suggests that he is a reasonably good UPPP candidate.

There are no widely accepted standardized methods or algorithms and frequently surgeons utilize their own judgment in interpreting such indices for patient selection. General points by which UPPP candidates can be identified are seen in Table 29.1. It should be pointed out that when UPPP is performed as part of a multilevel approach, most of these criteria are not relevant.

Obviously there is only a small fraction of OSA patients that can satisfy all the aforementioned selection criteria. Friedman et al., using a standardized method of airway evaluation based on assessment of palatal position and tonsillar size, found that only 23.5% of OSA patients were considered acceptable UPPP candidates. This fact emphasizes the concept that if surgical correction of OSA is deemed necessary, the vast majority of patients will require a multilevel approach to their airway. It would be incorrect for one to utilize rigid criteria and a 'cook book' approach for patient selection. Instead the process should be individualized and the surgeon should implement her/his judgment keeping always in mind that additional surgery may be necessary.

In general patients with large tonsils, elongated uvula and palatal redundancy position who do not have hypopharyngeal narrowing or tongue enlargement and are not extremely obese will be advised to have UPPP (Figs 29.1 and 29.2).

Because of its relative simplicity and low morbidity UPPP is usually performed as part of a multilevel approach in many patients, even if there is no overt evidence of velopharyngeal pathology.

## 3 TECHNIQUE

Uvulopalatopharyngoplasty is an evolving procedure and has undergone many modifications since its introduction primarily in order to comply with the variability of the pharyngeal anatomy and physiology and to reduce morbidity. Generally emphasis is placed on maximal tissue removal from the lateral pharyngeal walls and conservative resection of the palate and uvula. In a technique called palatal advancement with pharyngoplasty proposed by Woodson, the soft palate is elevated by advancing it towards the hard palate in order to totally preserve its functionality. The Z-palatoplasty technique has been designed for individuals without tonsillar hypertrophy and elongated palate. Another modification proposed by Pirsig describes complete preservation of the palatoglossus, palatopharyngeus and uvularis muscles thus leaving all velar muscles intact. I have used the technique described here in the last few years for the majority of patients undergoing the operation. Some of the reported modifications are utilized on an individual basis.

The procedure is performed under general anesthesia. The anesthesiology staff should be alerted about the diagnosis and the likelihood of difficult intubation. If deemed necessary fiberoptically aided awake intubation is carried out. Administration of narcotics should be kept to a minimum because of the likelihood of airway obstruction and depressed respiratory drive post extubation. Dexametasone and a broad-spectrum antibiotic are administered IV preoperatively.

### Step 1
Following orotracheal intubation and deep muscle relaxation, the mouth gag is positioned. This routinely provides

# SECTION I  PALATAL SURGERY

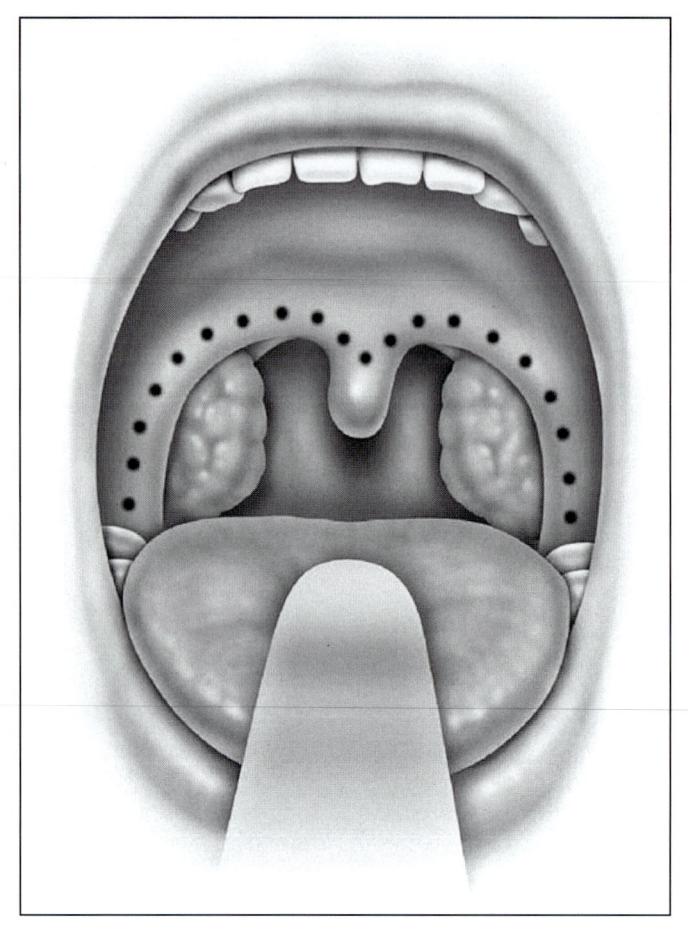

**Fig. 29.3** The incision is marked on the anterior pillars and ventral surface of the palate with electrical cautery.

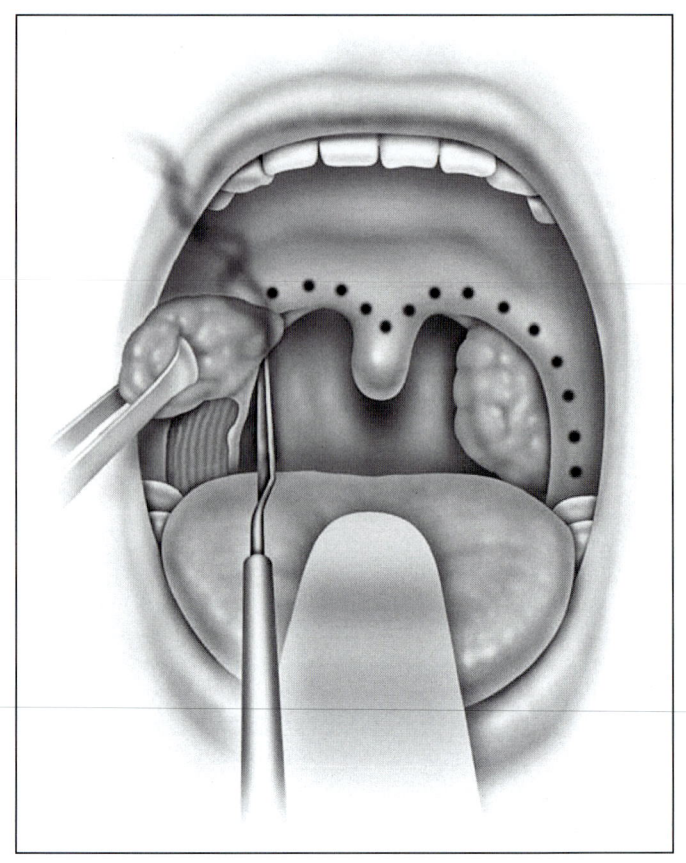

**Fig. 29.4** Dissection begins at the right inferior tonsillar pole.

adequate visualization and exposure. Local infiltration with epinephrine solution is not performed. In the past the amount of palate to be resected was determined by gently pushing the palate to the posterior pharyngeal wall and marking on its ventral surface the point where the palate met the posterior pharyngeal wall. Currently soft palate resection is conservative and is determined by gently curving the anterior pillar incision towards the base of the uvula, leaving only 5–10 mm of soft palate to be resected. The incision is marked with electrical cautery on the most lateral aspect of the anterior pillar in order to maximally resect this structure and the underlying palatoglossus muscle. The incision is then gently curved towards the base of the uvula and is continued in an identical fashion onto the opposite side (Fig. 29.3).

## Step 2
The incision is then completed with a #15 scalpel by simply 'connecting the dots'. Dissection commences by mobilizing and delivering the inferior tonsillar pole. The tonsil along with the anterior pillar and portion of the palatoglossus muscle is resected in a retrograde fashion. Most of the posterior pillar and glossopharyngeus muscle is preserved to be used for resurfacing the lateral pharynx (Fig. 29.4).

If the tonsils have been previously removed the tonsillar fossa mucosa and scar tissue is resected. Dissection then continues on the soft palate, leaving a slightly longer posterior (dorsal) mucosa flap. When the uvula is reached the ventral incision is carried close to its base. The uvular muscle is now transected and partially removed, preserving a longer dorsal uvular flap. The dissection is now carried to the opposite side in identical fashion. The entire dissection is performed with electrical cautery.

## Step 3
The ventral mucosal flap is retracted using forceps and an oblique incision is made, measuring 1–2 cm at the junction of the posterior tonsillar pillar and soft palate bilaterally (Fig. 29.5).

## Step 4
Closure begins at the oblique incisions at the posterior palatal/pillar flap. The corners of the flaps are retracted anteriorly and laterally and sutured onto the superior aspect of the anterior pillar and lateral aspect of the palate respectively (Fig. 29.6). Sutures are then placed at the region of the tonsillar fossae. Substantial bites are taken through mucosa and musculature for a sturdier lateral closure because of the susceptibility of this portion of the incision to dehiscence. Satisfactory stretching and elimination of the posterior pharyngeal mucosa redundancy must be

CHAPTER 29 — Uvulopalatopharyngoplasty

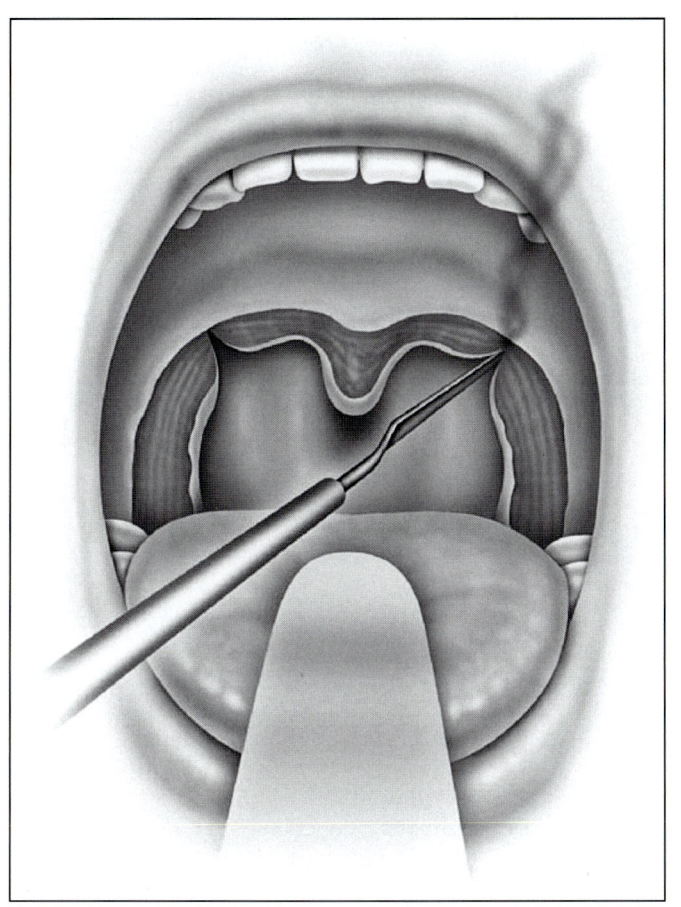

**Fig. 29.5** Incisions are made at the junction between the dorsal palatal and posterior pillar flaps.

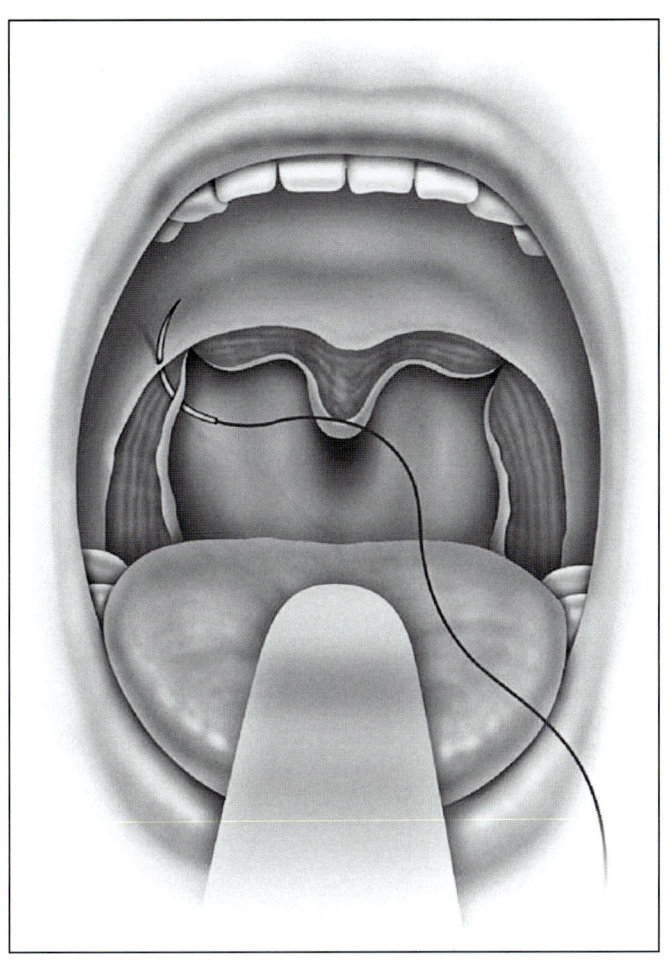

**Fig. 29.6** The upper part of the posterior pillar flap is approximated to the ventral palatal mucosa.

achieved. If the posterior pillars are redundant, further excision of mucosa and palatopharyngeus muscle is performed. If, on the other hand, approximation of the mucosal edges produces extreme wound tension or a ridge on the posterior pharyngeal wall, then the mucosal edges are sutured to the tonsillar fossa musculature instead. Undermining of the posterior pharyngeal mucosa is not recommended because of the risk of devascularization, which may result in scarring and pharyngeal stenosis. Finally suturing continues on to the palate and uvula, meticulously approximating the mucosal edges. Sutures are placed 1 to 1½ cm apart (Fig. 29.7). The preferred suture material is 2-0 chromic cat-gut on an atraumatic needle. Polyglycolic sutures do not prevent dehiscence and remain in the tissues for several weeks, thus prolonging the patient's discomfort.

## 4 POSTOPERATIVE MANAGEMENT AND COMPLICATIONS

The majority of patients undergoing UPPP are hospitalized at least for the first night after surgery. If UPPP is part of a multilevel approach and particularly if hypopharyngeal or base of tongue surgery is performed, longer hospitalization may be necessary until the patient gains satisfactory oral intake and pain is adequately controlled with oral medications. Only relatively healthy patients with mild OSA may have UPPP on an outpatient basis. Intensive care monitoring is not required unless patients have severe OSA, significant co-existing medical conditions, or are undergoing multiple procedures.

Patients with severe OSA and patients using nasal CPAP are placed on CPAP postoperatively. After discharge from the recovery room, analgesia is usually managed with hydrocodone elixir. Intravenous or intramuscular narcotics-analgesics are avoided. All staff caring for patients with OSA should be educated about the mechanism of sleep apnea and the risk of using narcotics. Oral hydrocodone and antibiotic suspension (cefalexin or erythromycin) is used after discharge.

Regardless of the surgical procedure performed, OSA patients are predisposed to specific complications because of anatomical abnormalities of their airway and the underlying disease. Complications related to the OSA are usually perioperative (Table 29.2). The majority of them (75%) are related to airway loss, a potentially disastrous complication which is associated with high mortality

# SECTION I PALATAL SURGERY

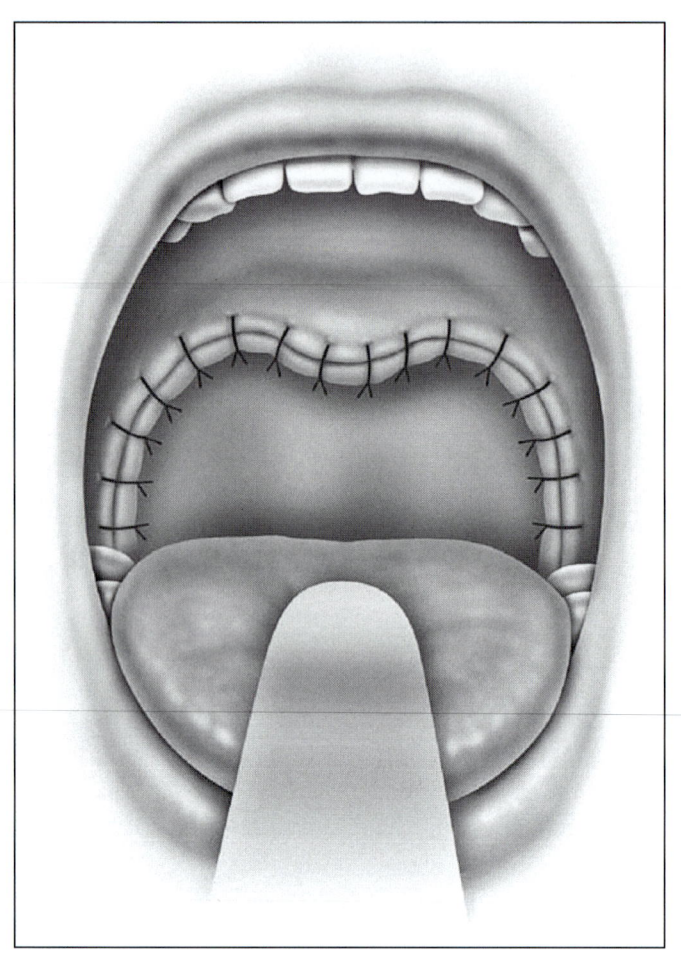

**Fig. 29.7** The mucosa suturing has been completed.

**Table 29.3 Causes of perioperative airway loss**

Use of perioperative narcotics
Failed intubation
Postoperative edema
Postoperative hemorrhage

**Table 29.4 Postoperative UPPP complications**

| Early | Late |
| --- | --- |
| Transient velopharyngeal insufficiency | Pharyngeal symptoms: 'tightness' 'dryness' 'drainage' 'food caught in throat' |
| Wound dehiscence<br>Bleeding | Prolonged pain<br>Taste disturbance<br>Voice disturbance<br>Velopharyngeal insufficiency<br>Nasopharyngeal stenosis<br>Deterioration of OSA |

**Table 29.2 Perioperative complications of UPPP**

Airway obstruction
Accentuation of OSA
Cardiopulmonary sequelae:
- hypertension
- arrhythmia
- congestive heart failure

Hemorrhage

rates. Causes of perioperative airway obstruction are seen in Table 29.3. Perioperative use of narcotics is the most common cause of airway obstruction. Utilization of nasal CPAP in the immediate postoperative period makes the use of parenteral narcotics safer. Cardiopulmonary complications are primarily related to hypertension. The majority of OSA patients undergoing UPPP require postoperative or intraoperative antihypertensive medications. Even patients without history of hypertension are at significant risk of developing hypertension intraoperatively or immediately.

Complications directly related to UPPP can be classified into early postoperative and late postoperative (Table 29.4). Transient velopharyngeal insufficiency is usually manifested with nasal regurgitation and less commonly with detectable hypernasal speech. In the vast majority of cases symptoms are mild. The patients usually complain of regurgitation of liquids when bending down to drink (on a water faucet) or when they attempt to swallow large amount of liquids in a single gulp. In the majority of patients these symptoms disappear once the postoperative pain and edema subside. A small number of patients may continue to display slight regurgitation indefinitely but self-training may control the problem and it rarely requires correction. It is not clear whether dehiscence of the lateral pharyngeal incisions should be considered as a complication. It is yet undetermined if healing of these wounds by secondary intention has any implications on the postoperative results. Some surgeons leave the lateral wall mucosa unsutured, while most advocate the use of polyglycolic (semipermanent) sutures. We believe that dehiscence is a common occurrence because of continuous pharyngeal wall motion during swallowing and tension of the mucosal flaps. Meticulous suturing with reasonable tension and with substantial 'bites' through both mucosal flaps and musculature may decrease the incidence of dehiscence postoperatively. The incidence of postoperative bleeding is approximately 2%. It usually occurs 4–8 days after surgery, but in some cases bleeding has occurred as late as 12–15 days postoperatively.

A significant percentage of patients (30–40%) have prolonged complaints related to the pharynx. These are usually expressed as 'throat dryness', 'throat drainage', 'throat tightness', 'food caught in the throat'. These complaints are thought to be related to wound healing, scarring and contracture. However, the absence of the uvula may also be responsible. This structure possesses an abundance of seromucinous salivary glands, supporting the notion that

CHAPTER 29 Uvulopalatopharyngoplasty

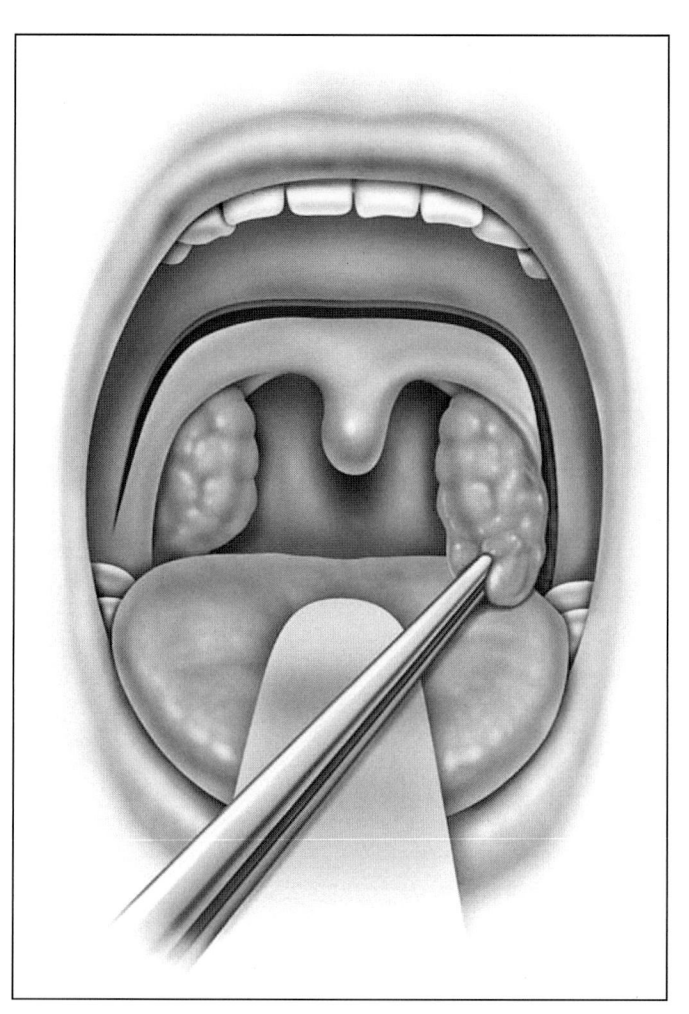

**Fig. 29.8** Old UPPP technique. The incision is carried out with electrical cautery.

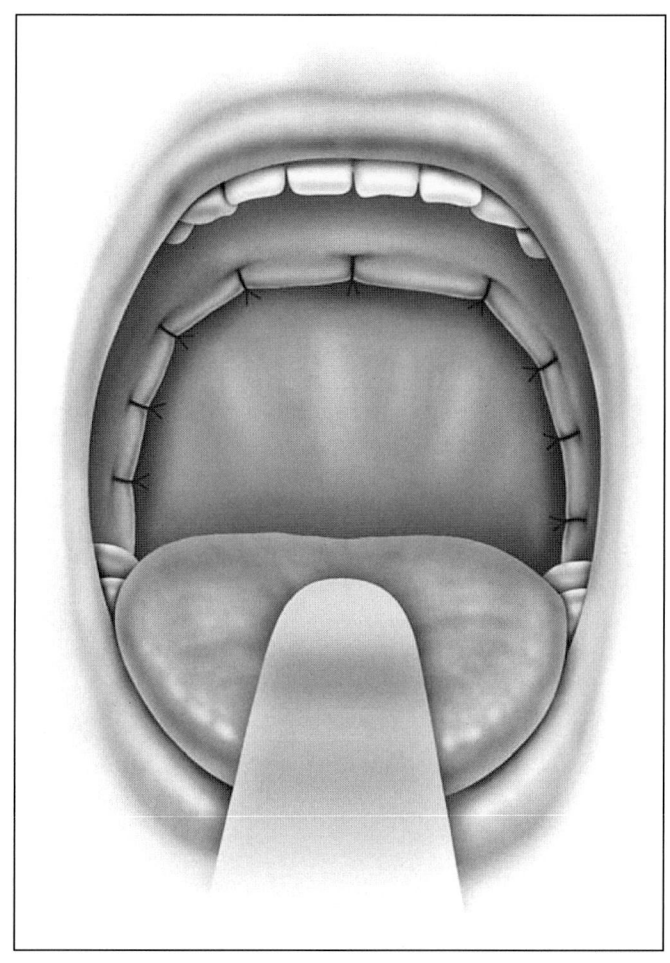

**Fig. 29.9** Old UPPP technique. Note that significant amount of palate has been removed.

the uvula is a lubricating organ useful in both speech and deglutition. Uvulopalatopharyngoplasty causes mild albeit permanent changes in voice and speech characteristics. There is a rise of the fundamental speech frequency up to 10 Hz. In addition there is lowering of the second formant in some of the vowels. These changes may be significant to singers and those relying on their voice for professional reasons and should be mentioned to them preoperatively. The uvula is the primary structure responsible for the vocal trill, a sound used in some languages (Dutch, French, German, Arabic, Hebrew, Greek, Russian, Spanish, Persian and Turkish). The loss of this sound may be extremely bothersome to individuals speaking these languages. Professional wind instrument players seeking UPPP should be advised against the procedure because it will render the velum incapable of resisting the high pressures generated in the oral cavity of these individuals during performances.

Occasionally patients complain of distortion of taste and/or numbness of the tongue. A possible explanation is the prolonged pressure by the blade of mouth gag. Taste disturbance could also be related to glossopharyngeal nerve injury at the inferior aspect of the tonsillar fossa.

The incidence of permanent velopharyngeal insufficiency (VPI), severe enough to warrant intervention, was approximately 2% when older UPPP techniques were used (Figs 29.8 and 29.9). If surgical correction of VPI is deemed necessary, the severity of OSA should be considered because OSA will most likely deteriorate following correction. For this reason the author advocates against palate push-back procedures or palatal flaps. Teflon paste injection in the submucosal layer of the posterior pharyngeal wall is an effective method of treating VPI. Furthermore, its effects can be easily reversed. The procedure is relatively simple and well tolerated and can be performed in an office setting.

Nasopharyngeal stenosis is a dreadful post-UPPP complication because it results in significant disability and it is extremely difficult to correct. Prevention of this complication cannot be overemphasized. One should be aware of surgical pitfalls and predisposing factors. Possible causes of nasopharyngeal stenosis following UPPP are listed in Table 29.5. Stenosis usually develops 6–8 weeks after UPPP and can present with various grades of severity. Mild forms of nasopharyngeal stenosis present with adherence of the lateral aspects of the palate to the posterior pharyngeal

| Table 29.5 Risk factors in post-UPPP nasopharyngeal stenosis |
|---|
| Aggressive posterior pillar resection |
| Aggressive undermining of posterior pharyngeal wall mucosa |
| Excessive mucosa destruction |
| Infection |
| Necrosis |
| Excessive electrocautery |
| Adenoidectomy? |
| Wound dehiscence? |

| Table 29.6 UPPP results ($n = 46$) | | |
|---|---|---|
| | Preop | Postop |
| BMI | 34.5 ± 9.8 | 33.0 ± 11.5 |
| RDI | 48.6 ± 21.2 | 24.7 ± 14.5 |
| ESS | 14 | 8 |

RDI, Respiratory Disturbance Index; ESS, Epworth Sleepiness Scale

| Table 29.7 UPPP response rate ($n = 46$) | | |
|---|---|---|
| | No | % |
| Good responders | 27 | 58.6 |
| Poor responders | 19 | 41.4 |

walls and they are usually asymptomatic. More severe forms range from excessive scarring of the velum with a cicatricial band on the posterior pharyngeal wall, with a small opening remaining to complete fusion of the palate to the pharynx. In many of these cases in addition to partial nasal obstruction, symptoms of VPI can also be present.

Surgical correction of nasopharyngeal stenosis is a formidable task as indicated by the numerous techniques utilized so far. These include pharyngeal, palatal and combination flaps, Z-plasty, skin grafting and stenting. I have experienced satisfactory results with superiorly based palatopharyngeal flaps that are rotated and sutured to the dorsal surface of the palate. The velopharynx is stented postoperatively with a custom-made obturator which is anchored on a maxillary dental plate, worn intermittently for a period of 4–6 months. We feel that stenting is necessary regardless of the surgical technique used, because of the inexorable tendency of the nasopaharyngeal wound for circumferential scarring and constriction. Application of mitomycin may play a role in preventing restenosis after repair.

## 5 SUCCESS RATE OF UPPP

It is generally accepted that successful surgical treatment of OSA is considered at least 50% reduction of the Respiratory Disturbance Index (RDI) and a postoperative RDI of less than 20. In carefully selected patients UPPP can be successful in 55% to 85% of patients, while there is a 60% to 80% failure rate in groups of unselected patients. From 1982 until 1988 I performed UPPP on all patients who desired to be treated for their apnea, because, with the exception of tracheostomy, UPPP was the only available method of treatment during that period. Many of these patients had severe OSA and were extremely obese. In these series of such patients (unselected) the UPPP success rate was 52% as documented by polysomnography performed approximately 3 months postoperatively. Later in a series of patients selected for UPPP by fiberoptic pharyngoscopy with Mueller maneuver, the success rate improved to 58%. Currently patients are selected for UPPP primarily according to the Friedman staging system. In addition, cephalometric data are taken into consideration in many of these patients. Our most recent series includes stage I and II patients. In stage II patients hypopharyngeal surgery is also recommended, but many decline it or prefer to have it in a staged fashion. The UPPP success rates in these series are seen in Table 29.6 and Table 29.7.

There is little debate that the beneficial effects of UPPP decline with time. The rate of apnea and snoring relapse ranges from 15% to 40% 3–5 years after surgery. An explanation is that surgical modifications of soft tissue structures such as the tongue, palate and pharyngeal walls may not have a lasting effect because of progressive laxity and volume increase of these structures. Patients undergoing UPPP should be warned about the possibility of relapse of OSA and that long-term follow-up is necessary.

## FURTHER READING

Brosch S, Matthes C, Pirsig W, et al. Uvulopalatopharyngoplasty changes in the fundamental frequency of the voice: A prospective study. J Laryngol Otol 2000;114(2):113–8.

Cahali MB. Lateral pharyngoplasty: a new treatment for obstructive sleep apnea hypopnea syndrome. Laryngoscope 2003;113(11):1961–8.

Fairbanks DN, Fujita S. Snoring and Obstructive Sleep Apnea, 2nd edn. New York: Raven Press; 1994.

Farmer WC, Giudici SC. Site of airway collapse in obstructive sleep apnea after uvulopalatopharyngoplasty. Ann Otol Rhinol Laryngol 2000;109(6):581–4.

Finkelstein Y, Talmi YP, Raveh E, et al. Can obstructive sleep apnea be a complication of uvulopalatopharyngoplasty? J Laryngol Otol 1995;109(3):212–7.

Friedman MA, Ibrahim HA, Lee Bass A. Clinical staging for sleep-disordered breathing. Otolaryngol Head Neck Surg 2002;127(1):13–21.

Friedman M, Ibrahim HZ, Vidyasagar R, et al. Z-palatoplasty (Z-PP): a technique for patients without tonsils. Otolaryngol Head Neck Surg 2004;131(1):89–100.

Isono S, Shimada A, Tanaka A, et al. Effects of uvulopalatopharyngoplasty on collapsibility of the retropalatal airway in patients with obstructive sleep apnea. Laryngoscope 2003;113(2):362–7.

Katsantonis GP. Uvulopalatopharyngoplasty for obstructive sleep apnea and snoring. Operat Tech Otolaryngol Head Neck Surg 1991;2(2):100–103.

Katsantonis GP. Complications of surgical treatment for obstructive sleep apnea. Operat Tech Otolaryngol Head Neck Surg 1991;2(2):143–7.

Katsantonis GP, Friedman WH, Rosenblum BN, et al. The surgical treatment of snoring: a patient's perspective. Laryngoscope 1990;100(2):138–40.

Kim JA, Lee JJ, Jung HH. Predictive factors of immediate postoperative complications after uvulopalatopharyngoplasty. Laryngoscope 2005;115(10):1837–40.

Riley RW, Powell NB, Guilleminault C, et al. Obstructive sleep apnea surgery: risk management and complications. Otolaryngol Head Neck Surg 1997;117(6):648–52.

Senior BA, Rosenthal L, Lumley A. Efficacy of uvulopalatopharyngoplasty in unselected patients with mild obstructive sleep apnea. Otolaryngol Head Neck Surg 2000;123(3):179–82.

Sher AE, Schechtman KB, Piccirillo JF. The efficacy of surgical modifications of the upper airway in adults with obstructive sleep apnea syndrome. Sleep 1996;19(2):156–77.

Woodson BT. Acute effects of palatopharyngoplasty on airway collapsibility. Otolaryngol Head Neck Surg 1999;121(1):82–6.

Woodson BT, Marvin MR. Manometric and endoscopic localization of airway obstruction after uvulopalatopharyngoplasty. Otolaryngol Head Neck Surg 1994;111(1):38–43.

# SECTION I  PALATAL SURGERY

# CHAPTER 30
# Uvulopalatopharyngoplasty – effects on the airway

*Aaron E. Sher*

## 1 HISTORY OF UVULOPALATOPHARYNGOPLASTY

Uvulopalatopharyngoplasty (UPPP) was first described by Fujita in 1981. It represented the first surgical procedure specifically designed to treat obstructive sleep apnea (OSA).[1] Fujita modified an earlier procedure applied by Ikematsu as a treatment for snoring.

UPPP enlarges the retropalatal airway by excision of the tonsils (if not previously extirpated), trimming and reorienting the posterior and anterior tonsillar pillars, and excising the uvula and posterior portion of the soft palate (Fig. 30.1). A number of modifications of Fujita's procedure were described shortly after his publication, but none has clearly improved outcome, nor become the predominant technique.[2] However, more recent modifications seem promising: UPPP with creation of a uvulopalatal flap in lieu of extirpation of the uvula and posterior soft palate;[3] tonsil reduction by coblation (rather than tonsillectomy) combined with a palatal flap technique.[4] Different surgical tools can be applied to achieve UPPP, such as electrocautery vs. scalpel.[5] UPPP can include tonsillectomy, but can also be performed in a patient previously tonsillectomized.[6] A procedure described as lateral pharyngoplasty focuses on splinting the lateral pharyngeal walls through microdissection of the superior pharyngeal constrictor muscles within the tonsillar fossa, sectioning this muscle, and suturing the laterally based flap consisting of that muscle to the same side palatoglossus muscle. A palatopharyngeal Z-plasty is performed to prevent retropalatal collapse.[7,8] Laser-assisted uvulopalatoplasty (LAUP) is performed with laser, under topical and local anesthesia, without tonsillectomy. Though it may (in some cases) be applied in treatment for OSA, particularly in previously tonsillectomized patients, LAUP is not generally included among the surgical armamentaria for OSA, but rather for snoring.[9]

## 2 UPPP: THE PROCEDURE

See Figure 30.1.

1. Tonsillectomy is performed or (if patient was previously tonsillectomized) the mucosa of the tonsillar fossa is excised.
2. An incision is made in the soft palate, several millimeters lateral to the medial margin of the glossopalatal arch, extending from the inferior pole of the tonsillar fossa to the root of the uvula, then to its tip, then up the pharyngeal side of the uvula, continuing along the pharyngopalatal arch to the inferior pole of the tonsillar fossa (see Fig. 30.1A–H).
3. Alternatively, tonsillectomy is performed with electrocautery, and dissection is performed horizontally across the soft palate, extirpating the uvula and posterior margin of the soft palate (at the level of the superior pole of the tonsillar fossa or the 'palatal dimple') en bloc with the tonsils.

## 3 WHY DOES UPPP WORK?

Structurally, the dorsum of the tongue is anterior to the soft palate. The dorsum of the tongue may push the anterior wall of the soft palate posteriorly during obstructive events (maintaining closure of the retropalatal airway). Depending upon specifics of pharyngeal anatomy, there is dynamic interaction between the tongue and soft palate during obstructive apnea, reflecting an abnormally highly collapsible airway at the retropalatal level.[10] A model of the upper airway in OSA syndrome (OSAS) likens it to a simple collapsible tube. The tendency of the upper airway to collapse can be expressed quantitatively in terms of a critical pressure ($P_{crit}$), defined as the pressure surrounding the focus of collapse. If atmospheric pressure

CHAPTER 30
Uvulopalatopharyngoplasty – effects on the airway

is designated zero, then airway collapse will occur whenever $P_{crit}$ is a positive number (indicating that it is higher than atmospheric pressure). $P_{crit}$ levels are higher during sleep than during wakefulness in both normal individuals and OSAS patients. In normals, $P_{crit}$ rises from awake values that are more negative than $-41\,cm\,H_2O$ to values in sleep of $-13\,cm\,H_2O$.[11–13] This means that, in normals, atmospheric pressure is greater than $P_{crit}$ even during sleep and the pharynx will not collapse. In OSAS patients, the spectrum of awake values of $P_{crit}$ is $-40\,cm\,H_2O$ to $-17\,cm\,H_2O$ and $P_{crit}$ during sleep is $+2.5\,cm\,H_2O$.[11,12,14,15] Although the pharyngeal airway of awake OSAS patients tends to be more collapsible than that of awake normals, $P_{crit}$ does not cross the critical line of zero (i.e. atmospheric pressure) except when the individual with OSAS has sleep onset, at which time an obstructive event results.[11] Patients who have varying degrees of partial pharyngeal collapse have intermediate, but negative, levels of $P_{crit}$ during sleep: $-6.5\,cm\,H_2O$ for asymptomatic snorers and $-1.6\,cm\,H_2O$ for patients with hypopneas but no apneas.[11,15] In general, $P_{crit}$ must be below

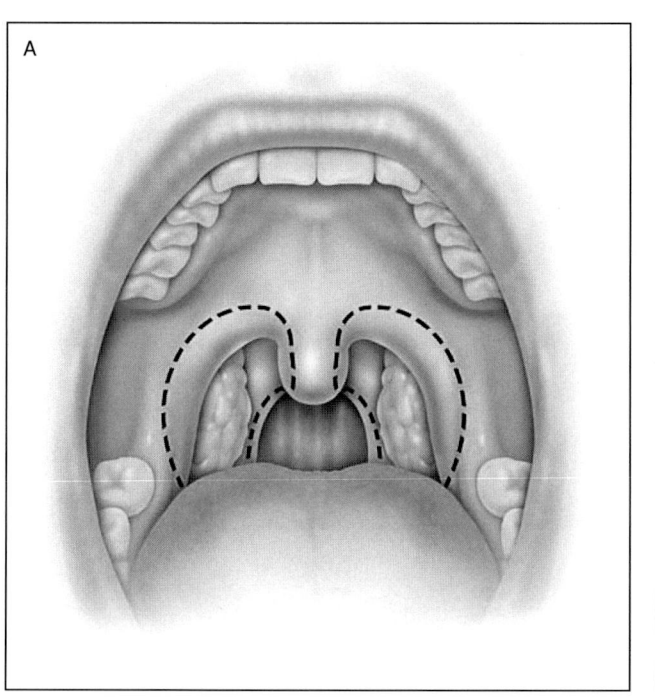

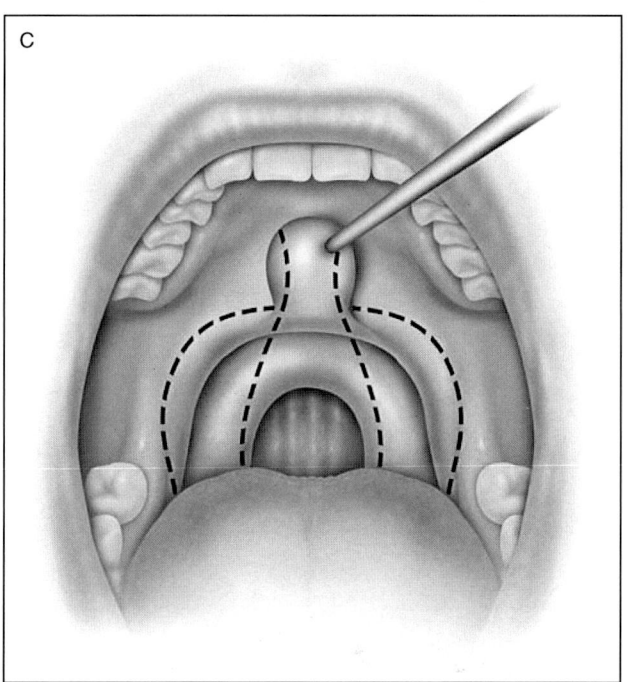

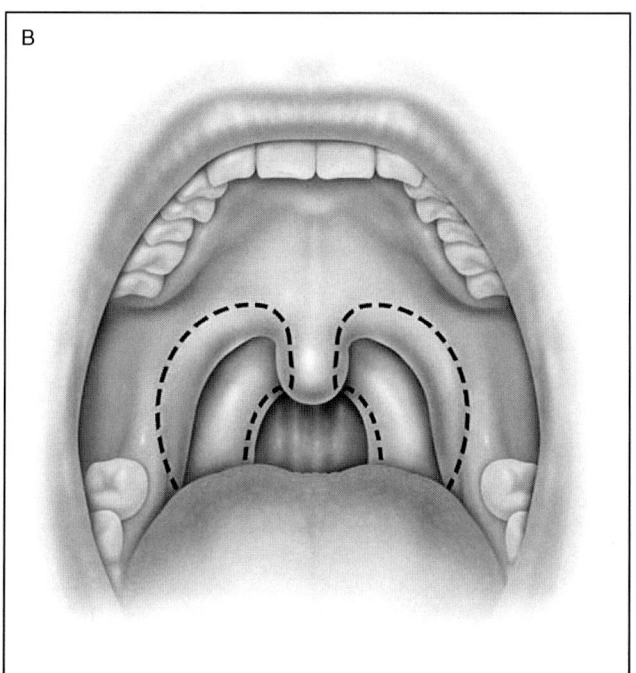

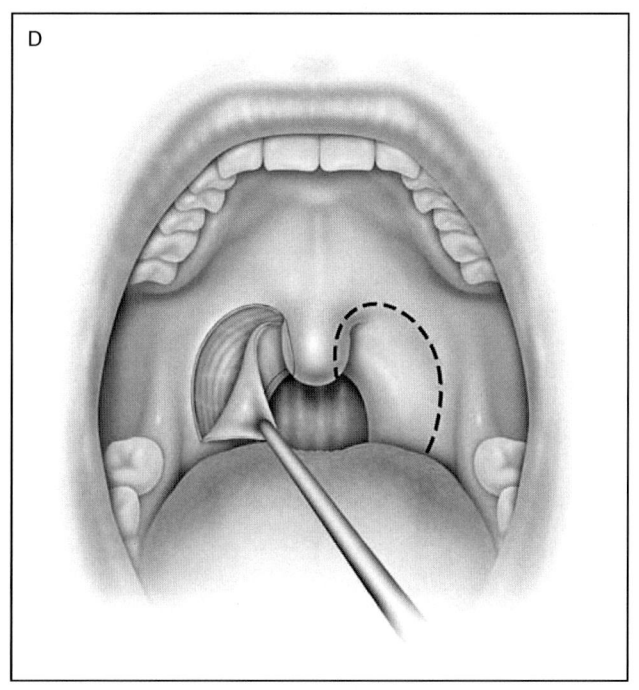

**Fig. 30.1** A, UPPP incision in patient who has not had prior tonsillectomy. B, UPPP incision in patient who has had prior tonsillectomy. C, Incision demonstrated on the posterior (nasopharyngeal) surface of the uvula. D, Mucosa is stripped off in a patient with previous tonsillectomy.

# SECTION I PALATAL SURGERY

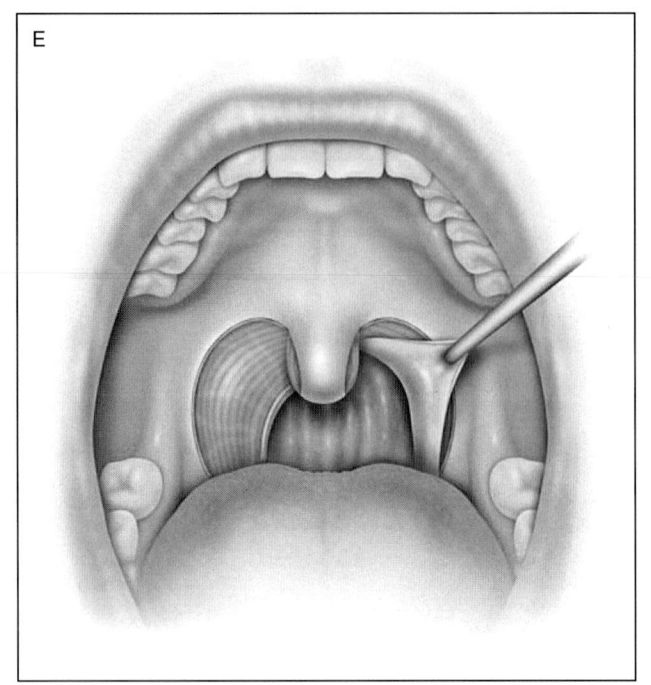

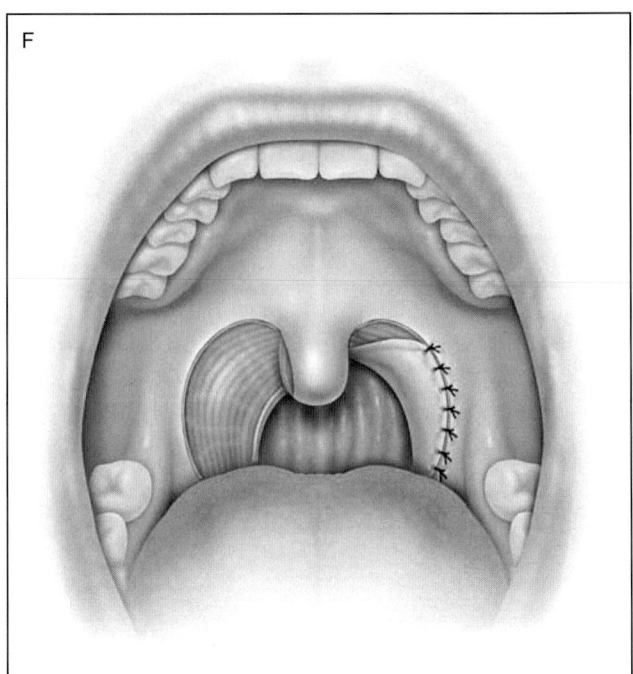

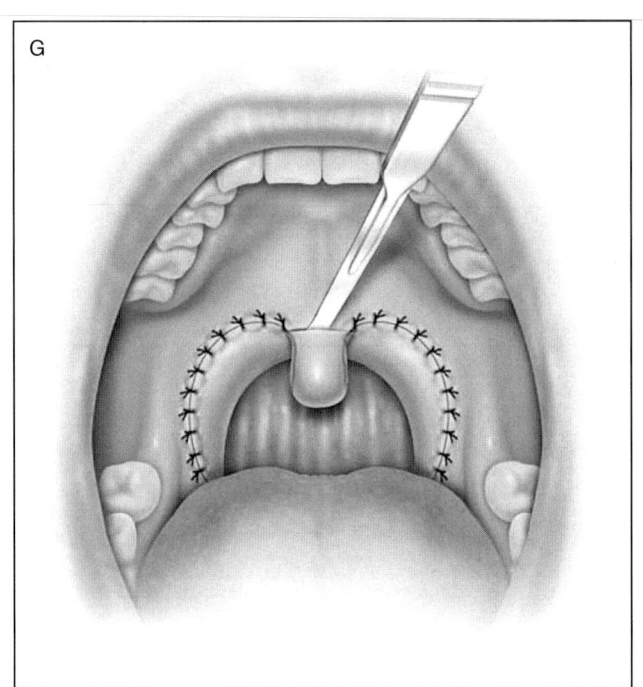

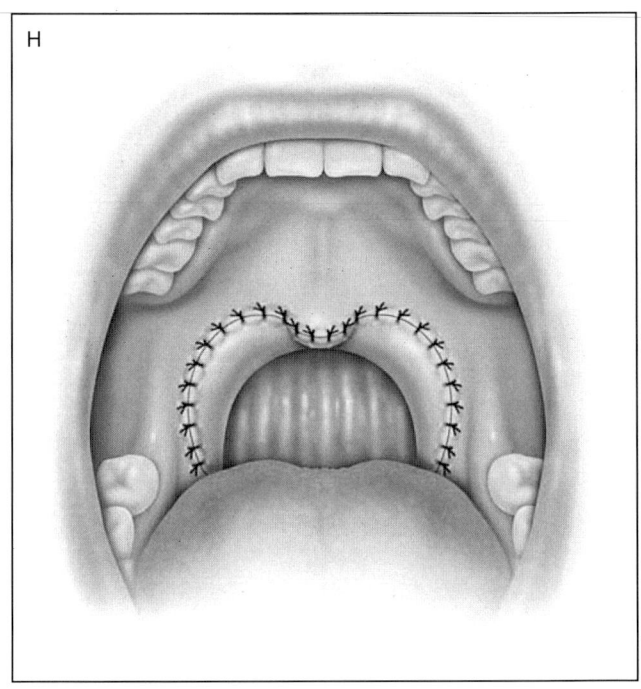

**Fig. 30.1** (Continued). E, Posterior pillar remnant brought forward for closure. F, Single layer closure. G, Excess tissue of anterior uvula removed. H, Uvula remnant closed.

−5 cm $H_2O$ to eliminate obstructive sleep disordered breathing.[11] $P_{crit}$ for an OSAS patient can, alternatively, be defined as the lowest level of nasal continuous positive airway pressure (CPAP) at which airflow is maintained.[16] Examples of the decrement in $P_{crit}$ that can be achieved by non-surgical interventions are −6 cm $H_2O$ through loss of 15% of body weight; −3 to −4 cm $H_2O$ through protriptyline treatment; and −4 to −5 cm $H_2O$ through the avoidance of sleeping in the supine position.[11] $P_{crit}$ decrement resulting from upper airway surgery has been documented for UPPP. When 13 patients undergo UPPP, $P_{crit}$ decreases from a level of 0 to a level of −3 cm $H_2O$ ($P = 0.016$). In those patients who have greater than 50% decrease in Respiratory Disturbance Index (RDI) in non-REM sleep, $P_{crit}$ decreases from −1 to −7 cm $H_2O$ ($P = 0.01$). The degree of improvement in sleep disordered breathing is correlated significantly with the change of $P_{crit}$ ($P = 0.001$), and the decrease in RDI is determined by the magnitude of the drop in $P_{crit}$ rather than by the initial level of $P_{crit}$. No significant change in $P_{crit}$ is detected in non-responders.[16,17] In a study performed under anesthesia and induced paralysis, 18 patients were analyzed for retropalatal pharyngeal closing pressure before and 3 months and 1 year after UPPP. UPPP decreased retropalatal airway closing pressure by 3.5 cm H₂O. A direct correlation existed between the severity of OSA and retropalatal airway closing pressure. Patients who failed at UPPP had postoperative retropalatal airway closing pressure greater than zero. Reduced retropalatal airway collapsibility was maintained up to 1 year after UPPP.[10,18]

## 4 WHY DOES UPPP FAIL TO CORRECT OSAS, AND WHY DO SALVAGE PROCEDURES WORK?

The likely explanation is that upper airway collapsibility has been inadequately addressed. The degree of improvement in severity of OSAS is correlated significantly with the change in $P_{crit}$ ($P = 0.001$). The decrease in RDI is determined by the magnitude of the fall in $P_{crit}$. No significant change in $P_{crit}$ is detected in non-responders. UPPP failures reveal retropalatal airway closing pressure greater than zero.[10,16–18] Alternative (not mutually exclusive) explanations for UPPP failure are: (1) UPPP does not address all sites of narrowing or collapse; or (2) UPPP addresses sites of narrowing or collapse in an inadequate manner. Evidence for these explanations has been documented through application of upper airway manometry, measurement of pharyngeal cross-sectional area, videoendoscopy, and cephalometry.[19–22] Further evidence comes from clinical experience. Surgical modification of the upper airway at sites other than those addressed by UPPP may salvage UPPP failures. Thus, procedures believed to diminish collapsibility of the retrolingual airway (unlike UPPP which addresses primarily the retropalatal airway) may achieve surgical salvage after UPPP failure. These procedures include: mandibular advancement, laser midline glossectomy, lingualplasty, radiofrequency tongue base ablation, genioglossal advancement and hyoid myotomy and suspension. Maxillomandibular advancement enlarges the retropalatal and retrolingual airway and may achieve surgical salvage after failure of various combinations of UPPP and the other procedures outlined above.[16,23] On the other hand, additional surgical modification of the palate (addressing the retropalatal airway, as does UPPP) also salvages UPPP failures. Transpalatal advancement pharyngoplasty (TPAP) increases the retropalatal airway size by excising posterior hard palate and advancing the soft palate. Sequential performance of TPAP after UPPP results in incremental decrease in $P_{crit}$ to a level below that resulting from UPPP alone. When four patients underwent TPAP after previous UPPP, mean post-UPPP $P_{crit}$ of 5 was decreased to –4 after TPAP ($P < 0.01$). TPAP increased the post-UPPP retropalatal airway cross-sectional area from 30 to 95 cm² ($P < 0.01$).[24] Other studies have demonstrated that the degree of improvement in OSAS is correlated significantly with the change of $P_{crit}$ ($P = 0.001$), and the decrease in RDI is determined by the magnitude of the fall in $P_{crit}$.[13] It is likely that each surgical procedure successfully decreasing OSAS severity results in decreased $P_{crit}$, and that procedures performed concomitantly or in sequence (at a single or at multiple sites of airway narrowing/collapse) result in incremental decreases in $P_{crit}$. Further data are needed for confirmation.[11]

## 5 WHAT ARE LONG-TERM POLYSOMNOGRAPHY OUTCOMES OF UPPP?

Efficacy of UPPP may diminish over time: 60% success (defined as RDI diminished by 50%) at mean of 6 months postoperatively declined to 50% at mean of 46 months postoperatively. Success of 64% (defined as RDI diminished by 50% and postoperative RDI < 10 apneas and hypopneas per hour) at mean of 6 months postoperatively declined to 48% at mean 48–96 months postoperatively. Success of 67% (defined as RDI diminished by 50%) at 3–6 months postoperatively declined to 33% at mean of 88 months postoperatively. Weight gain was implicated as an explanation for long-term recurrence in some, but not all cases.[25–27]

## 6 CAN PATIENT SELECTION IMPACT UPPP OUTCOME?

Lateral cephalometry and fiberoptic endoscopy have been widely applied for preoperative characterization of the pharyngeal airway (as Type 1, 2, or 3) and, hence, as a method of patient selection. The assumption was that Type 1 patients were favorable for UPPP, whereas Types 2 and 3 were not. The original goal of patient characterization was to permit selection of a candidate pool for UPPP who would exceed the 50% success rate (PSG criteria) reported in the literature. Neither of these approaches has been clearly documented to be an effective screening tool. Indeed, different investigators have widely different degrees of success predicting UPPP success through application of fiberoptic endoscopy and lateral cephalometry.[23,28–38]

Weaknesses of each technique are readily apparent. Both are applied in the awake patient, while OSAS occurs only in the asleep patient. Both are generally applied in a sitting position, while the sleeping patient is generally not in this position. Lateral cephalometry is adynamic and assesses the airway in only two dimensions, while airway collapse in OSAS is dynamic and occurs in three dimensions. Endoscopic data are highly subjective and dependent on observer interpretation, while the quality of cephalometric films can be variable and dependent on attention to detail in shooting. Nonetheless, pharyngeal classification into Types 1–3 by techniques including fiberoptic endoscopy and lateral cephalometry permitted identification of two subgroups with markedly different UPPP success rates: 52% success for Type 1 and 5% for types 2 and 3.[23] It also provided the basis for development of new surgical procedures designed to salvage UPPP failures.

Several reports document OSAS cure rates (by PSG criteria) close to 100%, achieved by complex upper airway modification utilizing these procedures. Depending upon the complexity of anatomical compromise, one or multiple procedures may be required.[39–42] However, the pharyngeal classification system does not explain failure of UPPP in 48% of patients classified as Type 1. It is likely that nuances of pharyngeal anatomy and function are not discriminated by these techniques of evaluation. Alternatively, lack of consistency in interpretation of endoscopic data may be a consequence of its subjective nature, and interpretation of cephalometric views may be compromised by lack of attention to detail in execution and interpretation of cephalometric analysis. Studies comparing fiberoptic endoscopy with pharyngeal manometry (awake and asleep) demonstrate disagreement between these techniques in identifying pharyngeal dynamics as well as discrepancies in observation with the same technique applied in wakefulness and in sleep.[19,37,38] An alternative approach to prognostic classification of patients being considered for UPPP was introduced. A total of 134 patients were retrospectively classified by means of a staging system which included: (a) palate position in relationship to tongue (b) tonsil size, and Body Mass Index (BMI). This staging system did correlate success of UPPP based on postoperative PSG results with palate position and tonsil size (Table 30.1). Success rate for Stage I was 81%, for Stage II was 37%, and for Stage III was 8%. Success was defined as reduction of the RDI by at least 50% to an RDI less than 20 apneas and hypopneas per hour. Statistical analysis demonstrated a highly significant relationship between Friedman stage and success of surgery ($P < 0.0001$).

Friedman further explored the relationship between stage and the efficacy of UPPP, applying stepwise multivariate discriminant analysis. Preoperative criteria used to stratify patients into stages (BMI, tonsil size and palate position) were the only indices introduced into the stepwise analysis. Success or failure of surgical treatment with UPPP was used as the categorical endpoint. Friedman derived equations with representation of tonsil size and palate position which permitted correct outcome in 95% of 134 patients.[43] It was subsequently demonstrated that preoperative application of a modified version of this staging paradigm permitted improvement of surgical outcomes through application of UPPP with additional surgical intervention aimed at the retrolingual area in patients having an unfavorable prognostic prediction for UPPP as a sole procedure.[44]

**Table 30.1** Postoperative PSG results with palate position and tonsil size

| | | | |
|---|---|---|---|
| I | I, IIa, IIb | 3 or 4 | <40 |
| II | I, IIa, IIb | 0, 1 or 2 | <40 |
| | III or IV | 3 or 4 | <40 |
| III | III or IV | 0, 1 or 2 | <40 |
| IV | Any | Any | >40 |

## REFERENCES

1. Fujita S, Conway W, Zorick F, et al. Surgical correction of anatomic abnormalities in obstructive sleep apnea syndrome: uvulopalatopharyngoplasty. Otolaryngol Head Neck Surg 1981;89:923–34.
2. Ikematsu T, Fujita S, Simmons BF, et al. Uvulopalatopharyngoplasty: variations. In: Snoring and Obstructive Sleep Apnea, 2nd edn. Fairbanks DNF, Fujita S, eds. New York: Raven Press; 1994.
3. Powell N, Riley R, Guilleminault C, et al. A reversible uvulopalatal flap for snoring and sleep apnea syndrome. Sleep 1996;19:593–9.
4. Friedman M, Ibrahim H, Lowenthal S, et al. Uvulopalatoplasty (UP2): a modified technique for selected patients. Laryngoscope 2004;114:441–9.
5. Altman JS, Senior B, Ransom E. The effect of electrocautery vs. cold scalpel technique on the incidence of early postoperative tonsillar pillar dehiscence after uvulopalatopharyngoplasty with tonsillectomy. Laryngoscope 2004;114:294–6.
6. McGuirt WF Jr, Johnson JT, Sanders MH. Previous tonsillectomy as prognostic indicator for success of uvulopalatopharyngoplasty. Laryngoscope 1995;105:1253–5.
7. Cahali MB. Lateral pharyngoplasty: a new treatment for obstructive sleep apnea hypopnea syndrome. Laryngoscope 2003;113:1961–8.
8. Cahali MB, Formigoni GG, Gebrim EM, et al. Lateral pharyngoplasty versus uvulopalatopharyngoplasty: a clinical, polysomnographic and computed tomography measurement comparison. Sleep 2004;27:942–50.
9. Littner M, Kushida CA, Hartse K, et al. Practice parameters for the use of laser-assisted uvulopalatoplasty: an update for 2000. Sleep 2000;24:603–19.
10. Isono S, Shimada A, Tanaka A, et al. Effects of uvulopalatopharyngoplasty on collapsibility of the retropalatal airway in patients with obstructive sleep apnea. Laryngoscope 2003;113:362–7.
11. Winokur SJ, Smith PL, Schwartz AR. Pathophysiology and risk factors for obstructive sleep apnea. Semin Resp Crit Care Med 1998;19:999–1112.
12. Suratt PM, Wilhoit SC, Cooper K. Induction of airway collapse with subatmospheric pressure in awake patients with sleep apnea. J Appl Physiol 1984;57:140–6.
13. Schwartz AR, Smith PL, Wise RA, et al. Induction of upper airway occlusion in sleeping individuals with subatmospheric pressure in awake patients with sleep apnea. J Appl Physiol 1988;64:535–42.
14. Horner RL, Mohiaddin RH, Lowell DG, et al. Sites and sizes of fat deposits around the pharynx in obese patients with obstructive sleep apnoea and weight matched controls. Eur Resp J 1989;2:6113–22.
15. Gleadhilll IC, Schwartz AR, Schubert OI, et al. Upper airway collapsibility in snorers and in patients with obstructive hypopnea and apnoea. Am Rev Respir Dis 1991;143:1300–3.
16. Sher AE. Upper airway surgery for obstructive sleep apnea. Sleep Med Rev 2002;6:195–212.
17. Schwartz AR, Schiebert N, Rothman W, et al. Effect of uvulopalatopharyngoplasty on airway collapsibility in obstructive sleep apnea. Am Rev Respir Dis 1992;145:522–32.
18. Isono S, Tanaka A, Nishino T. Dynamic interaction between the tongue and soft palate during obstructive apnea in anesthetized patients with sleep disordered breathing. J Appl Physiol 2003;95:2257–64.
19. Sher AE. Soft tissue surgery for obstructive sleep apnea syndrome. Semin Resp Crit Care Med 1998;19:165–73.
20. He J, Kryger M, Zorick F, et al. Mortality and apnea index in obstructive sleep apnea. Experience in 385 male patients. Chest 1988;94:9–14.
21. Guilleminault C, Stoohs R, Clerk A, et al. A cause of excessive daytime sleepiness: the upper airway resistance syndrome. Chest 1993;104:7810–17.
22. Osnes T, Rollheim J, Hartmann E. Effect of UPPP with respect to site of pharyngeal obstruction in sleep apnoea: follow-up at 18 months by overnight recording of airway pressure and flow. Clin Otolaryngol Allied Sci 2002;27:38–43.

23. Sher AE, Schechtman KB, Piccirrillo JF. The efficacy of surgical modifications of the upper airway in adults with obstructive sleep apnea syndrome. Sleep 1996;19:156–77.
24. Woodson BT. Retropalatal airway characteristics in uvulopalatopharyngoplasty compared with tranpalatal advancement pharyngoplasty. Laryngoscope 1997;107:735–40.
25. Larsson LH, Carlsson-Nordlander B, Svanborg E. Four-year follow-up after uvulopalatopharyngoplasty in 50 unselected patients with obstructive sleep apnea syndrome. Laryngoscope 1994;104:1362–8.
26. Janson C, Gislason T, Bengtsson H, et al. Long term follow-up of patients with obstructive sleep apnea treated with uvulopalatopharyngoplasty. Arch Otolaryngol Head Neck Surg 1997;123:257–62.
27. Lee S-J, Chong S-Y, Shiao G-M. Comparison between short-term and long-term post-operative evaluation of sleep apnoea after uvulopalatopharyngoplasty. J Laryngol Otol 1995;109:308–12.
28. Hessel NS, de Vries N. Results of uvulopalatopharyngoplasty after diagnostic workup with polysomnography and sleep endoscopy: a report of 136 snoring patients. Eur Arch Otorhinolaryngol 2002;260:91–5.
29. Millman RP, Carlisle CC, Rosenberg C, et al. Simple predictors of uvulopalatopharyngoplasty outcome in the treatment of obstructive sleep apnea. Chest 2000;118:1025–30.
30. Boot H, Poublon RM, Van Wegen R, et al. Uvulopalatopharyngoplasty for the obstructive sleep apnea syndrome: value of polysomnography, Mueller manoeuvre and cephalometry in predicting surgical outcome. Clin Otolaryngol Allied Sci 1997;22:504–10.
31. Woodson BT, Conley SF. Prediction of uvulopalatopharyngoplasty response using cephalometric radiographs. Am J Otolaryngol 1997;18:179–84.
32. Woodson BT, Conley SF, Dohse A, et al. Posterior cephalometric radiographic analysis in obstructive sleep apnea. Ann Otol Rhinol Laryngol 1997;106:310–13.
33. Aboussouan LS, Golish JA, Wood BG, et al. Dynamic pharyngoscopy in predicting outcome of uvulopalatopharyngoplasty for moderate and severe obstructive sleep apnea. Chest 1995;107:946–51.
34. Doghramji K, Jabourian AH, Pilla M, et al. Predictors of outcome for uvulopalatopharyngoplasty. Laryngoscope 1995;105:311–14.
35. Petri N, Suadicani P, Wildschiodtz G, et al. Predictive value of Muller maneuver, cephalometry, and clinical features for the outcome of uvulopalatopharyngoplasty. Acta Otolaryngol (Stockh) 1994;114:565–75.
36. Sher AE, Thorpy MJ, Shprintzen RJ, et al. Predictive value of Muller maneuver in selection of patients for uvulopalatopharyngoplasty. Laryngoscope 1985;95:1483–7.
37. Woodson BT, Wooten MR. Comparison of upper airway evaluation during wakefulness and sleep. Laryngoscope 1994;104:821–8.
38. Skatvedt O. Localization of site of obstruction in snorers and patients with obstructive sleep apnea syndrome: a comparison of fiberoptic nasopharyngoscopy and pressure measurements. Acta Otolaryngol (Stockh) 1993;113:206–9.
39. Chabolle F, Wagner I, Blumen M, et al. Tongue base reduction with hyoepiglottoplasty: a treatment for severe obstructive apnea. Laryngoscope 1999;109:1273–80.
40. Riley RW, Powell NB, Guilleminault C, et al. Obstructive sleep apnea syndrome: a review of 306 consecutively treated surgical patients. Otolaryngol Head Neck Surg 1993;108:117–25.
41. Troell RJ, Powell JB, Riley RW. Hypopharyngeal airway surgery for obstructive sleep apnea syndrome. Semin Resp Crit Care Med 1998;19:175–83.
42. Prinsell JR. Maxillomandibular advancement surgery in a site-specific treatment approach for obstructive sleep apnea in 50 consecutive patients. Chest 1999;116:1519–29.
43. Friedman M, Ibrahim H, Bass C. Clinical staging for sleep disordered breathing. Otolaryngol Head Neck Surg 2002;127:13–21.
44. Friedman M, Ibrahim H, Joseph N. Staging of obstructive sleep apnea/hypopnea syndrome: a guide to appropriate treatment. Laryngoscope 2004;114:454–9.

## FURTHER READING

American Academy of Sleep Medicine Task Force on Sleep Related Breathing Disorders in Adults. Recommendations for syndrome definition and measurement techniques in clinical research. Sleep 1999;5:667–89.
Boudewyns A, DeCock W, Willemen M, et al. Influence of UPPP on alpha-EEG arousals in nonapnoeic snorers. Eur Respir J 1997;10:129–32.
Esclamado RM, Glenn MG, McCulloch TM, et al. Perioperative complications and risk factors in the surgical treatment of obstructive sleep apnea syndrome. Laryngoscope 1989;99:1125–9.
Farmer WC, Giudici SC. Site of airway collapse in obstructive sleep apnea after uvulopalatopharyngoplasty. Ann Otol Rhinol Laryngol 2000;109:581–4.
Haavisto L, Suonpaa J. Complications of uvulopalatopharyngoplasty. Clin Otolaryngol 1994;19:243–7.
Haraldsson P.-O, Carenfelt C, Lysdahl M, et al. Does uvulopalatopharyngoplasty inhibit automobile accidents? Laryngoscope 1995;105:657–661.
Keenan SP, Heather B, Ryan CF, et al. Long-term survival of patients with obstructive sleep apnea treated by uvulopalatopharyngoplasty or nasal CPAP. Chest 1994;105:155–9.
Kezirian EJ, Weaver EM, Yuch B, et al. Risk factors for serious complication after uvulopalatopharyngoplasty. Arch Otolaryngol Head Neck Surg 2006;132:1091–8.
Langin T, Pepin JL, Pendlebury S, et al. Upper airway changes in snorers and mild sleep apnea sufferers after uvulopalatopharyngoplasty (UPPP). Chest 1998;113:1595–603.
Li HY, Lee LA, Wang PC, et al. Taste disturbance after uvulopalatopharyngoplasty for obstructive sleep apnea. Otolaryngol Head Neck Surg 2006;134:985–90.
Lysdahl M, Haraldsson P-O. Long-term survival after UPPP in non-obese heavy snorers. Arch Otolaryngol Head Neck Surg 2000;126:1136–40.
Marti S, Sampol G, Munoz X, et al. Mortality in severe sleep apnoea hypopnea syndrome patients: impact of treatment. Eur Respir J 2002;20:1511–8.
Mickelson SA, Hakim I. Is postoperative intensive care monitoring necessary after uvulopalatopharyngoplasty? Otolaryngol Head Neck Surg 1998;119:352–6.
Milljetieg H, Mateika S, Haight JS, et al. Subjective and objective assessment of uvulopalatopharyngoplasty for treatment of snoring and obstructive sleep apnea. Am J Respir Crit Care Med 1994;150:1286–90.
Mortimer IL, Bradley PA, Murray JA, et al. Uvulopalatopharyngoplasty may compromise nasal CPAP therapy in sleep apnea syndrome. Am J Respir Crit Care Med 1996;154:1759–62.
Peker Y, Hedner J, Norum J, et al. Increased incidence of cardiovascular disease in middle-aged men with obstructive sleep apnea: a 7-year follow-up. Am J Respir Crit Care Med 2002;166:159–65.
The International Classification of Sleep Disorders: Diagnostic and Coding Manual, 2nd edn. Westchester, IL: AASM; 2005:51–3.
Weaver EM, Maynard C, Yueh B. Survival of veterans with sleep apnea: continuous positive airway pressure vs. surgery. Otolaryngol Head Neck Surg 2004;130:659–65.
Weaver EM, Sher AE, in preparation.
Weaver EM, Woodson BT, Steward DL. Polysomnography indexes are discordant with quality of life, symptoms, and reaction times in sleep apnea patients. Otolaryngol Head Neck Surg 2005;132:255–62.
Woodson BT, Wooten MR. Manometric and endoscopic localization of airway obstruction after uvulopalatopharyngoplasty. Otolaryngol Head Neck Surg 1994;111:38–43.
Zohar Y, Finkelstein Y, Talmi YP, et al. Uvulopalatopharyngoplasty: evaluation of complications, sequelae, and results. Laryngoscope 1991;101:775–9.
Zorick F, Roehrs T, Conway W, et al. Effects of uvulopalatopharyngoplasty on the daytime sleepiness associated with sleep apnea syndrome. Bull Europ Physiopath Resp 1983;19:600–3.

# SECTION I  PALATAL SURGERY

# CHAPTER 31

# Uvulopalatopharyngoplasty – the Fairbanks technique

*David N.F. Fairbanks*

## 1 INTRODUCTION

Uvulopalatopharyngoplasty (UPPP) is generally both safe and effective as a surgical treatment for non-obese patients who suffer with mild to moderate sleep apnea and severe snoring. This refinement in surgical technique[1] employs strategies for avoidance of complications and improvement of efficacy. Palatal dysfunction is avoided by minimization of soft palate shortening in the midline (uvula) area. Nasopharyngeal stenosis is avoided by minimization of posterior pillar resection and avoidance of pharyngeal undermining. Effectiveness of surgery is improved when emphasis is placed on opening the nasopharynx widely in the lateral port areas. Also, tissue removal deep in the inferior tonsillar poles (and hypopharynx) with mucosal advancement and suturing is emphasized.

### 1.1 PATIENT SELECTION

UPPP can generally be recommended for treatment of young to middle-aged non-obese (or mildly obese) offensive snorers in whom correctable anatomical abnormalities in the oropharyngeal and palatal areas are identifiable. Often, such patients who also suffer with mild to moderate obstructive sleep apnea are likewise good candidates, especially when they are resistant to (or intolerant of) use of positive pressure breathing devices, such as continuous positive airway pressure (CPAP). Some such patients who even have moderate to severe obstructive sleep apnea may also be good candidates for UPPP, but for them success is less predictable, obesity, hyperglossia, retrognathia and neuromuscular disorders being limiting factors.

### 1.2 OBJECTIVES

The technique described here resembles the original descriptions of Ikematsu[2] and Fujita.[3] However, it is modified to achieve the following desirable objectives.

1. Maximize the lateralization of the posterior pharyngeal pillars, including submucosal musculature, which will increase the lateral dimension of the oropharyngeal airway.
2. Interrupt some of the sphincteric action of the palatonasopharyngeal musculature, which will increase the patency of the nasopharyngeal airway.
3. Maximize shortening of the soft palate in the lateral ports while sparing midline musculature (resulting in a 'squared off' soft palate appearance), which will prevent palatal tethering and nasopharyngeal stenosis, yet will preserve mobility and function of the palate for purposeful closure.

## 2 SURGICAL PROCEDURE AND TECHNIQUE

Prophylactic antimicrobials (with anaerobic activity) are initiated 1 hour before surgery, with intravenous ampicillin/sulbactam (Unasyn 3 g) or clindamycin (900 mg). A preoperative corticosteroid intravenous injection is also given (Solu-Medrol 125 mg or dexametasone 10–15 mg). Preoperative sedatives are avoided because obstructive sleep apnea patients are often over-reactive to them and airway crisis may occur. Likewise, an anesthesiologist should be selected who is well aware of the compromised status of the airway in such patients. The orally intubated and anesthetized patient is placed in the head-extended supine position with the Crowe–Davis tonsillectomy mouth gag and the Ring tongue blade in place.

The areas to be surgically excised are injected with small amounts of epinephrine 1:100,000 solution (usually provided in 1% lidocaine). This is to promote hemostasis and is done by prior agreement with the anesthesiologist, who selects an appropriate inhalation agent.

The mucosa on either side of the uvula is clamped with hemostats and then incised in an oblique direction as in Figure 31.1. This severs the drooping mucosal web between the uvula and the posterior pillar, increases the mobility of the pillar, prevents soft palatal scar contraction (with 'tethering'), and incises some of the lowermost fibers of the nasopharyngeal sphincter. Typically, the low-hanging soft palate of an apnea patient contains few muscular fibers of the nasopharyngeal sphincter.

# Uvulopalatopharyngoplasty – the Fairbanks technique

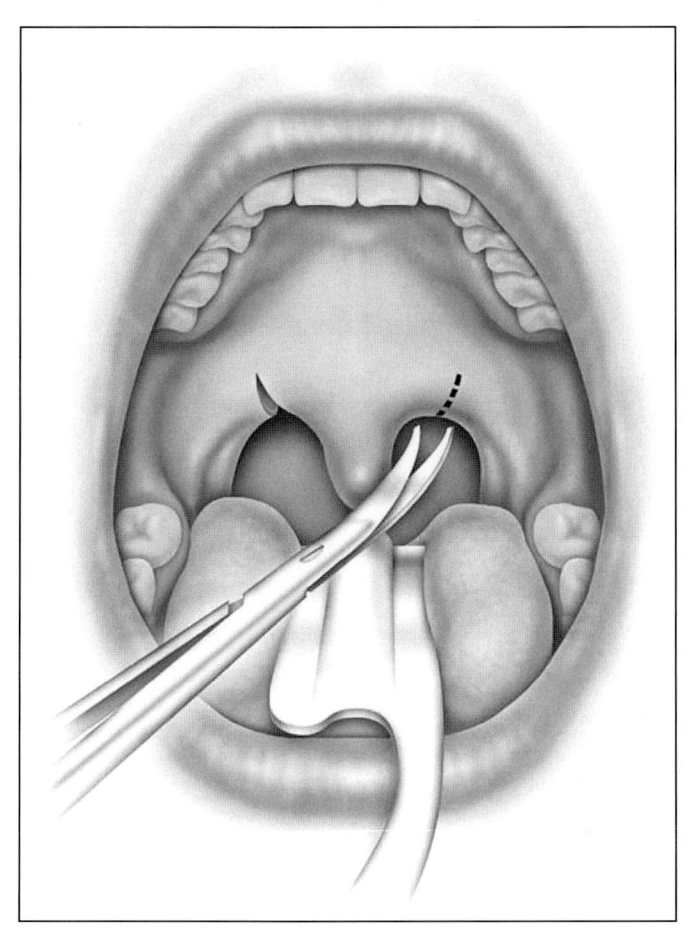

**CHAPTER 31**

**Fig. 31.1** Pharyngeal view of apnea patient with absent tonsils, redundant mucosa, and drooping soft palate with webbing between uvula and tonsillar pillars. Begin by severing the uvulopalatal webs. This mobilizes the posterior pillars, releases the contracture, and prevents palatal tethering.

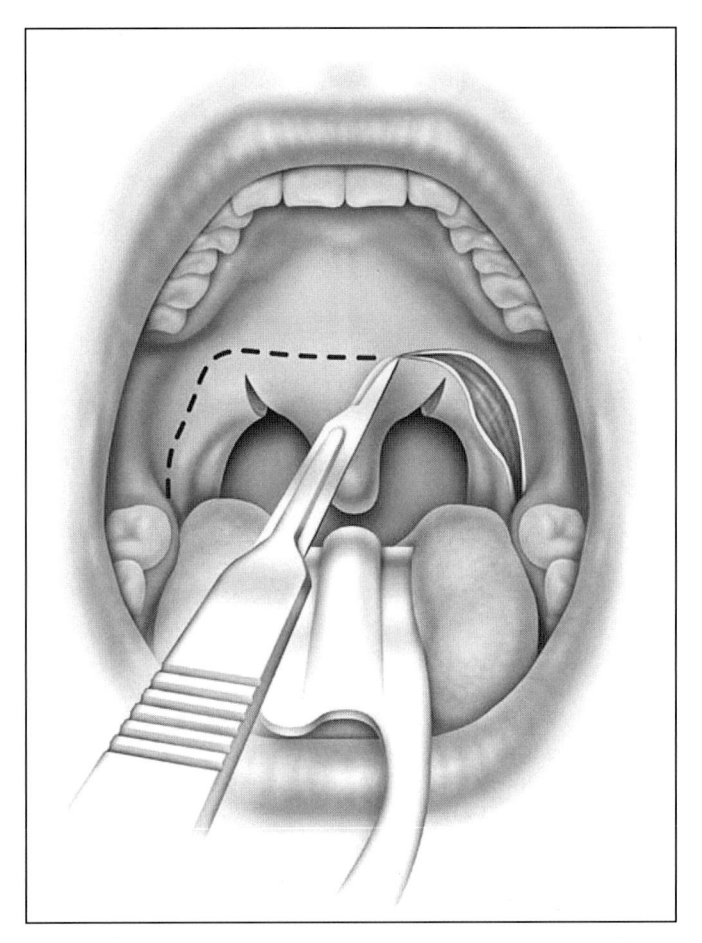

**Fig. 31.2** Box-shaped mucosal incision begins at tongue base, ascends in sulcus between anterior pillar and mandible, and then turns medially to cross soft palate about midway between trailing edges of soft and hard palates.

The palatopharyngeal incision is designed as three sides of a rectangle, as in Figure 31.2. It begins at the base of the tongue lateral to the inferior tonsillar pole and extends cephalad in the sulcus or angle formed between the internal surface of the mandible and the anterior tonsillar pillar. At about 1 cm above the level of the trailing edge of the soft palate, the incision makes a 90° angle, transverses the soft palate horizontally, then angles 90° downward again symmetrical to the opposite side. The ideal level for the horizontal palatal incision is at the location of the palatal 'dimple' as described by Dickson.[4]

The soft palatal mucosa and submucosa (with glands and fat) are then stripped away from the muscular layers, beginning at the horizontal palatal incision and moving caudally toward the trailing edge of the soft palate and uvula. One or two brisk bleeders will often be encountered near the corners of the incision, and they must be suture-ligated with O plain catgut. (Cautery is inadequate and tissue-destructive, and it encourages stenosis.[5]) The uvula is amputated at the level of the trailing (caudal) edge of the soft palatal muscle fibers (Fig. 31.3). A tiny bleeder on each side of the uvula responds to a brief touch of electrocautery.

Traction on the uvula during its amputation should be avoided because that results in excessive shortening of the uvula with interruption of the insertions of the levator palati muscles into the musculus uvulae. Loss of palatal sphincteric action (required for closure during speech and swallowing) has been attributed to excessive excision of the uvula and midline palatal tissue.

Tonsils (present in one-third of snoring and apnea patients) are excised, and other soft tissues between the posterior tonsillar pillars and the lateral incisions are all stripped out, down to the muscular layers. The plane of dissection is readily apparent when a tonsillectomy is performed. However, if a previous tonsillectomy was done, dense fibrous scar tissue will be encountered that will inhibit mobilization of the posterior pillars. This fibrous scar should be carefully stripped away from the underlying muscle fibers of the tonsillar fossa (superior pharyngeal constrictors); the dissection should avoid damage (and cautery) to the musculature so as to avoid penetration through the muscle into the underlying structures of the carotid sheath.[5]

Bleeders are clamped and suture-ligated (which is less traumatic to the musculature and carotid sheath than is

191

# SECTION I  PALATAL SURGERY

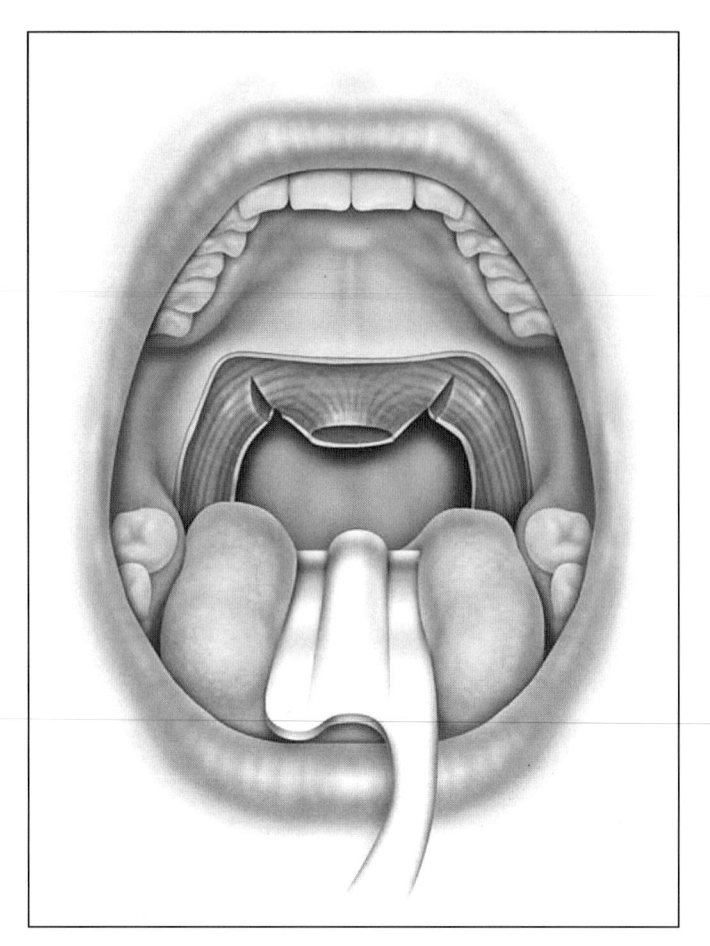

**Fig. 31.3** Mucosa, glands, fat, and fibrous tissue removed down to but not through muscular layers. Uvula amputated at trailing edge of soft palatal muscle fibers.

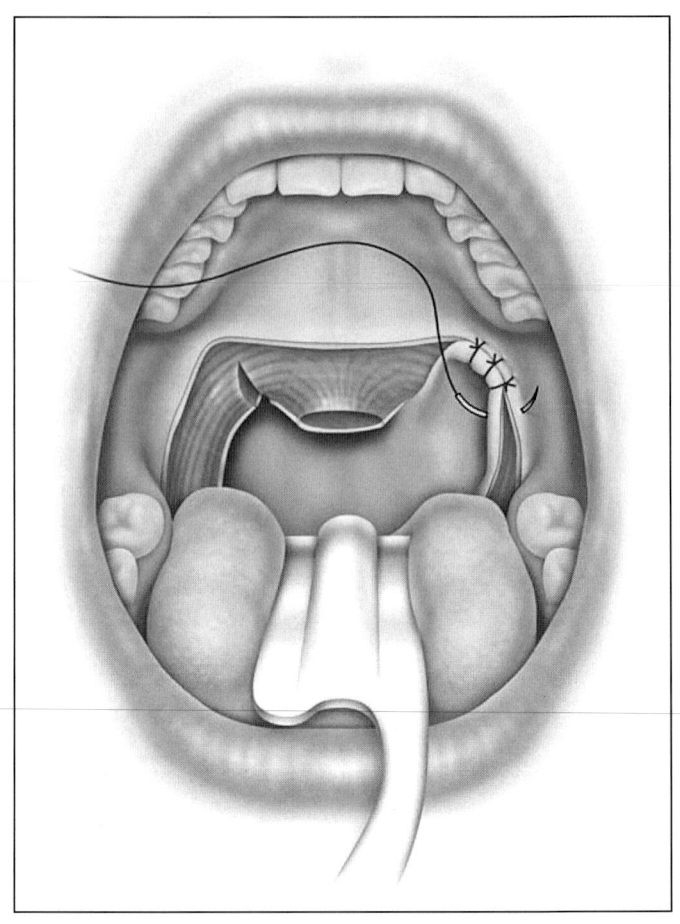

**Fig. 31.4** Posterior pillar is advanced in cephalad-lateral direction to increase lateral dimension of oropharyngeal airway. Pharyngeal redundancy is reduced.

heavy electrocoagulation); good hemostasis is essential. Dissection below (caudal to) the lower pole of the tonsil is carried as far as visibility and safety allow, at which point lymphoid aggregations there and on the base of the tongue (lingual tonsils) may be reduced with gentle electrocoagulation.

The posterior tonsillar pillar is then advanced in a lateral-cephalad direction toward the corner of the original palatopharyngeal incision (Fig. 31.4). Contiguous submucosal muscle fibers should be incorporated in this advancement because such a maneuver will increase the lateralizing effect and will expand the lateral dimension of the pharyngeal airway. This should also smooth and flatten out the redundancy and vertical folds of the posterior pharyngeal mucosa.[3]

Note that the best results are obtained from resection of the anterior pillar rather than the posterior pillar. This is because, when the intact posterior pillar is pulled forward (to cover the tonsillar fossa and to meet the incision of the resected anterior pillar), the soft palate will move along with it in a forward direction, thus *enlarging* the anterior posterior dimension of the nasopharynx. Conversely (and adversely), if the posterior pillar were to be resected, the closure would pull the anterior pillar and soft palate posteriorly, thus *narrowing* the nasopharynx.[1]

The pillar is advanced and fixated into its new, lateralized position with multiple sutures of 3–0 polyglycolic acid (Dexon-'S') or polyglactin 910 (Vicryl). The sutures should pass through the mucosa into superficial muscular layers so as to lateralize the muscular as well as the mucosal elements of the pillars (see Fig. 31.5). Furthermore, such closure eliminates 'dead space' where hematomas might accumulate. I prefer to put in the second stitch before I tie the first knot so that the positioning is more visible. Suturing then progresses downward (caudally) toward the tongue base, where a small opening is left unsutured to allow for spontaneous drainage.

The dissection and closure on the opposite side are identical (see Fig. 31.5).

Then the palatal closure is accomplished as the nasopharyngeal (posterior) surface of the soft palate mucosa is advanced over onto the oral (anterior) surface (Fig. 31.6). Redundant or flabby mucosa is trimmed, and the sutures are put into place, including a small amount of muscle fiber in the closure. Notice that the incisional/suture lines face forward (anteriorly), away from the nasopharynx and

# Uvulopalatopharyngoplasty – the Fairbanks technique

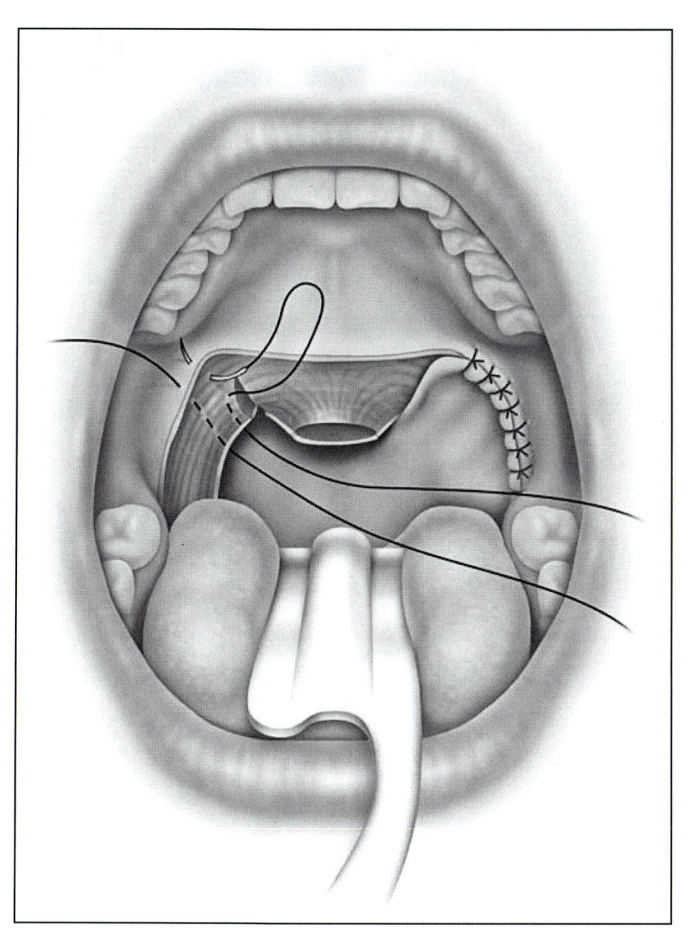

**CHAPTER 31**

**Fig. 31.5** Sutures pass through mucosal edges and also through superficial muscular layers to maximize lateralization of posterior pillar, to prevent hematoma formation, and to provide mucosal coverage of surgical defect.

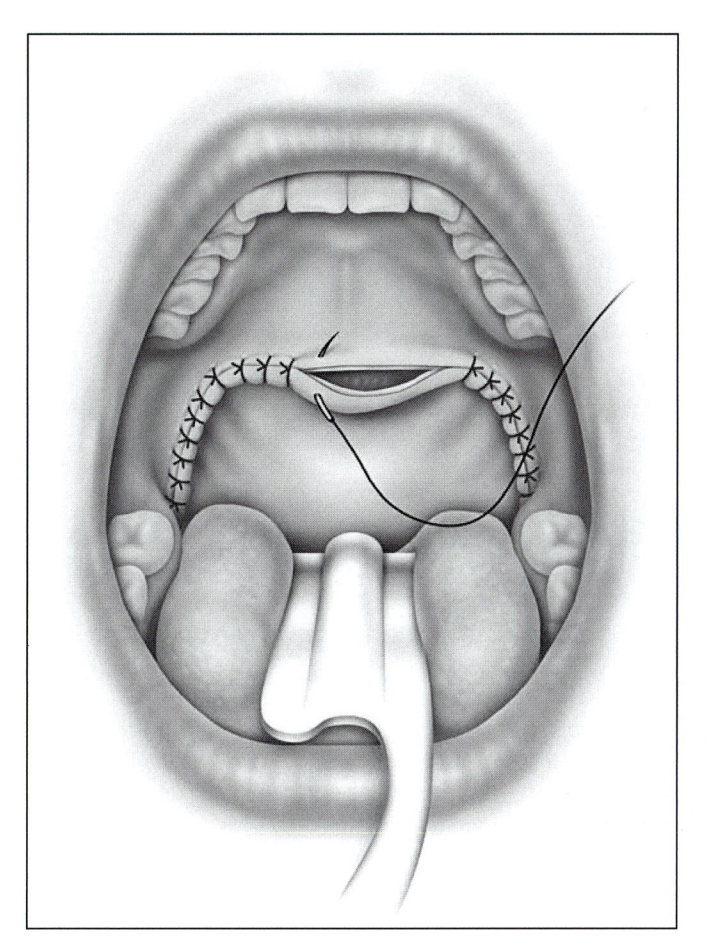

**Fig. 31.6** Nasopharyngeal surface of soft palate is advanced forward to meet the incision on the oral surface and to cover the surgical defect on the oral surface. Forward-facing suture line minimizes risk of stenosis. It also expands the anterior–posterior dimension of the nasopharyngeal airway. Note rectangular appearance designed to minimize nasopharyngeal regurgitation.

away from the caudal margin of the soft palate. This gives added protection against nasopharyngeal stenosis.

## 3 POSTOPERATIVE MANAGEMENT

Intravenous antimicrobial prophylaxis is maintained for 48 hours (Unasyn or clindamycin). During surgery a single dose of a corticosteroid is given (e.g. dexametasone 10–15 mg intravenously) and if swelling/edema or excess pain begins to be apparent early in the postoperative period, a short course of corticosteroids is given (up to every 4 hours for four doses, then every 8 hours for four doses). Many apneic patients are already hypertensive before surgery or are hypertensive immediately afterwards. Salt overloading with intravenous fluids contributes to this problem, and anti-hypertensive therapy is often required.

Any patient with significant obstructive sleep apnea before surgery will need vigilant postoperative monitoring of respirations. The intensive care unit is frequently the ideal place for the first 24 hours after surgery.[6]

Postoperative care for simple-snoring patients is the same as that for adult tonsillectomy patients. However, for obstructive sleep apnea patients, pain medication is given more cautiously (i.e. low-dose parenteral morphine or oral elixir of acetaminophen with added codeine, 30 mg/5 ml), with the recognition that apnea is aggravated by narcotics, and that life-threatening loss of airway can be precipitated, especially in the postanesthetic period or the period of postoperative edema of the airway.[1,5,6]

Similarly, anti-emetics, sleeping medications, and sedating tranquilizers can precipitate an apneic crisis; therefore, my nurses are instructed never to accept a telephone order for any of those medications by a physician who is not personally acquainted with my particular patient and his or her disease.

The criteria for discharge include a secure airway, adequate intake of fluids, and pain control with oral medications. The patient is sent home with instructions to avoid foods or drinks that are salty, scratchy, or sour. Liquid acetaminophen with codeine suffices for pain relief. Superficial wound contamination with oral microbial flora creates the equivalent of aphthous stomatitis at the surgical site. Recovery proceeds more rapidly if the patient uses the following 'canker-sore' mixture and procedure[7]:

diphenhydramine (Benadryl) liquid – 100 mg
dexametasone 0.5 mg/5 ml elixir – 20 ml
nystatin suspension – 60 ml
tetracycline (from disassembled capsules) – 1500 mg.

Sig.: One teaspoonful six times daily, after and between each meal, and at bedtime. Swish in mouth, gargle, swallow.

Sutures that have not disappeared within 2 weeks may be removed in the office setting to improve the patient's comfort.

## 4 RESULTS

Many – but not all – patients who undergo UPPP achieve remarkable relief of their snoring and excessive daytime sleepiness. Patient testimonials abound about lives having been dramatically changed. Furthermore, some studies suggest that the surgery, if successful, reduces to normal the exaggerated cardiovascular death rates seen in untreated obstructive sleep apneic patients.[8]

Unfortunately, UPPP does not always yield favorable results, and sometimes patients who enjoyed initial improvements will regress within 6–12 months later, especially if they regain body weight (against the physician's strenuous advice). Furthermore, other sites of airway compromise may need to be addressed, such as nasal airway obstruction, hyperglossia, or skeletal deformities such as retrognathia.

## ACKNOWLEDGMENT

Figures 31.1–31.6 are reprinted from Snoring and Obstructive Sleep Apnea, 3rd edn. Fairbanks DNF, Mickelson SA, Woodson BT, eds. Philadelphia: Lippincott Williams & Wilkins; 2003, with permission.

## REFERENCES

1. Fairbanks DNF. Uvulopalatopharyngoplasty techniques, pitfalls, and risk management. In: Fairbanks DNF, Mickelson SA, Woodson BT, eds. Snoring and Obstructive Sleep Apnea, 3rd edn. Philadelphia: Lippincott Williams & Wilkins; 2003, pp. 107–20.
2. Ikematsu T. Study of snoring, 4th report: therapy. J Jpn Otol Rhinol Larynogol 1964;64:434–5.
3. Fujita S, Conway W, Zorick F, et al. Surgical corrections of anatomic abnormalities in obstructive sleep apnea syndrome: uvulopalatopharyngoplasty. Otolaryngol Head Neck Surg 1981;89:923–34.
4. Dickson R, Blokmanis A. Treatment of obstructive sleep apnea by uvulopalatopharyngoplasty. Laryngoscope 1987;97:1054–8.
5. Fairbanks DNF. Uvulopalatopharyngoplasty complications and avoidance strategies. Otolaryngol Head Neck Surg 1990;102:239–45.
6. Mickelson SA, Hakim I. Is postoperative intensive care monitoring necessary after uvulopalatopharyngoplasty?. Otolaryngol Head Neck Surg 1998;119:352–6.
7. Fairbanks DNF. Pocket Guide to Antimicrobial Therapy in Otolaryngology Head and Neck Surgery, 12th edn. Alexandria, VA: American Academy of Otolaryngology Head and Neck Surgery Fdn; 2005, p. 38.
8. Lysdahl M, Haraldsson PO. Long-term survival after uvulopalatopharyngoplasty in non-obese heavy snorers. Arch Otolaryngol Head Neck Surg 2000;119:352–6.

SECTION I   PALATAL SURGERY

CHAPTER 32

# Submucosal uvulopalatopharyngoplasty

*Michael Friedman and Paul Schalch*

## 1 INTRODUCTION

Uvulopalatopharyngoplasty (UPPP) is a widely accepted surgical procedure for the treatment of obstructive sleep apnea/hypopnea syndrome (OSAHS)[1] and the only one recommended by the American Sleep Disorders Association. Due to the inaccuracy of current diagnostic methods for preoperatively determining the level of upper airway obstruction in OSAHS patients, as well as the inherent technical limitations of UPPP in dealing the relevant anatomical factors, success rates in attaining objective cure of about 40% after a long-term follow-up are far from desirable.[2] Recent studies, however, have established a staging system that can result in success rates as high as 80% in select patients[3] (see Chapter 16: Friedman Tongue Position and the Staging of Obstructive Sleep Apnea/Hypopnea Syndrome). In addition, UPPP is often part of a multilevel treatment strategy, which significantly improves success rates (see Chapter 17: Multilevel Surgery for Obstructive Sleep Apnea/Hypopnea). In addition to a considerable failure rate, complications of UPPP include nasopharyngeal stenosis, velopharyngeal insufficiency, pharyngeal dryness, hemorrhage, wound dehiscence, excessive palatal scarring, persistent dysphagia, and severe postoperative pain, not to mention rare but serious complications such as airway obstruction due to postoperative edema, leading to emergency reintubation or tracheotomy.[4–7]

Traditionally, UPPP is designed to eliminate palatal and pharyngeal redundancy by resection of excess loose palatal and pharyngeal mucosal and submucosal tissue, in addition to tonsillectomy. The initial procedure, described by Fujita,[8] as well as many other modifications, recommends excision of redundant mucosa, with a single-layer closure under tension. A widely accepted surgical principle is that epithelial surfaces should never be closed under tension. Repositioning of tissues should be accomplished at a muscular or subepithelial level, so that epithelium can be closed with minimal or no tension. The tense mucosal closure in traditional UPPP has resulted in two common sequelae.

1. Dehiscence of the suture line.
2. Severe postoperative pain, lasting as long as 2 weeks in some cases.

Likewise, epithelial tension may also be responsible for common complications that contribute to failure of the procedure and require surgical correction.[9]

Since its description by Fujita in 1981,[8] many authors writing about UPPP have actually re-described the original procedure, with important technical modifications. Submucosal UPPP focuses on the importance of epithelial preservation, and tension-free closure of the epithelium; and on the preservation of the majority of the mucosa of the soft palate and the anterior and posterior pillars. Elimination of palatal and pharyngeal tissue redundancy (the palatoplasty and the pharyngoplasty components, respectively) is accomplished by subepithelial and muscular stretching and closure. Epithelial closure is accomplished without tension.

In this chapter, we describe the patient selection criteria, surgical technique, and postoperative complications for submucosal UPPP.

## 2 PATIENT SELECTION

Candidates for surgical intervention must experience significant symptoms of snoring and/or daytime somnolence, documented failure of a continuous positive airway pressure (CPAP) trial, and documented failure of conservative measures such as dental appliances, changes in sleeping position, and sleep hygiene in general. Apparent obstruction at the level of the soft palate must be determined by fiberoptic nasopharyngolaryngoscopy and Mueller maneuver or sleep endoscopy. Adequate medical clearance and a

# SECTION I PALATAL SURGERY

thorough review of the procedure with the patient, as well as its implications, potential outcomes, and complications are essential components of the preoperative work-up.

Patient selection criteria for UPPP have been previously described by Friedman et al.[3] (see Chapter 16: Friedman Tongue Position and the Staging of Obstructive Sleep Apnea/Hypopnea). Specific criteria for submucosal UPPP are the same as for classic UPPP, and include patients classified as Friedman Tongue Position (FTP) I or II with tonsil sizes 1–4. Patients with FTP III and IV are less than ideal candidates for UPPP, and should therefore undergo a combined procedure that addresses both the palate and the hypopharynx (e.g. radiofrequency base of the tongue reduction).[10] An alternative technique, the Z-palatoplasty[11] (see Chapter 33: Zetapalatopharyngoplasty), was developed as a more aggressive technique for patients with stage II and III disease. This includes all patients who have had previous tonsillectomy, as well as patients with small tonsils and those with unfavorable tongue positions.

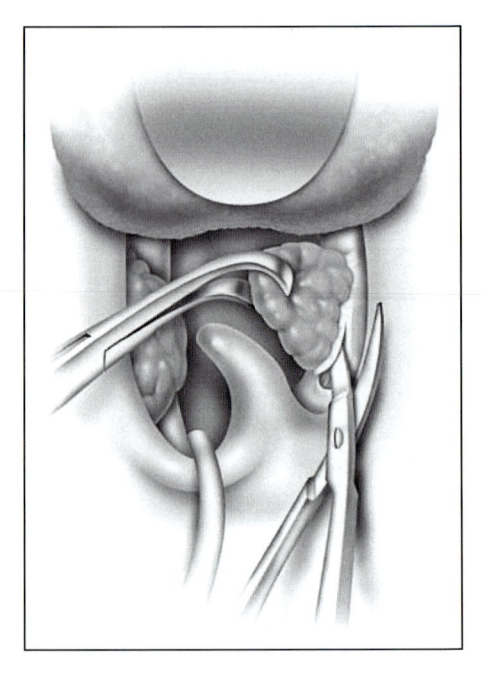

**Fig. 32.1** The tonsil is grasped with curved Allis forceps and pushed laterally to help identify the capsule. The authors prefer the cold steel technique in order to minimize trauma to the anterior and posterior pillars.

## 3 SURGICAL TECHNIQUE

Prior to the procedure, good communication with the anesthesiologist is of great importance, considering the distinct anatomic characteristics that cause OSAHS patients to have an increased risk for complications with general anesthesia. After oral intubation, the patient is placed in the head-extended position with the Crowe–Davis tonsillectomy mouth gag in place. Intravenous antibiotics and dexametasone are administered before incision. The surgeon should be comfortably positioned at the patient's head, with headlight illumination.

### 3.1 TONSILLECTOMY

The tonsils, if present, can be excised using any technique, but the authors prefer the cold steel technique to minimize trauma to the anterior and posterior pillars. The tonsil is grasped with curved Allis forceps and pushed laterally to help identify the capsule. This allows for assessment of the lateral extent of the tonsil, and exposes the proper plane of dissection (Fig. 32.1). An incision through the anterior pillar and the posterior pillar is made, preserving as much tissue as possible. If necessary, excess anterior pillar can be trimmed at closure. Posterior pillar resection results in posterior pull of the palate, which decreases the retropalatal space. The dissection is carried out using Metzenbaum scissors or a Herd dissector, dividing the tonsil capsule from the superior constrictor muscle. Constant traction of the tonsil is maintained, allowing the tissue to separate as it is dissected. The removal of the tonsil proceeds within its anatomic boundaries, and the musculature of the tonsil fossa is left intact. Dissection is carried out inferiorly, towards the base of the tongue, and a snare is applied to complete the dissection. If done carefully, at the end of tonsillectomy, the tonsillar fossa is dry and the muscle fibers are still covered by fascia.

### 3.2 SUBMUCOSAL UVULOPALATOPHARYNGOPLASTY

After removal of both tonsils, the palate is addressed. The uvula is grasped with Allis forceps and retracted anteriorly for optimal approach to the posterior surface of the soft palate. A curvilinear horizontal incision is made on the mucosa at the base of the uvula posteriorly, preserving almost the entire posterior soft palate mucosa (Fig. 32.2). Using a cold knife, the mucosa is separated from the muscle, releasing the posterior soft palatal mucosa. A trapezoid incision is outlined at the anterior mucosa of the soft palate (Fig. 32.3). This level is identified preoperatively in the awake patient, just below the 'dimpled' area. The incision is carried bilaterally and horizontally across the soft palate, until the anterior pillar starts sloping downward (Fig. 32.4). The uvula and the submucosal tissue of the lower edge of the soft palate are excised (Fig. 32.5). Based on Fairbanks' technique, an incision dividing the superior third from the inferior two-thirds of the posterior pillar is performed. The posterior pillar is then advanced anterolaterally, towards the corner of the palatal-pharyngeal junction

CHAPTER 32
Submucosal uvulopalatopharyngoplasty

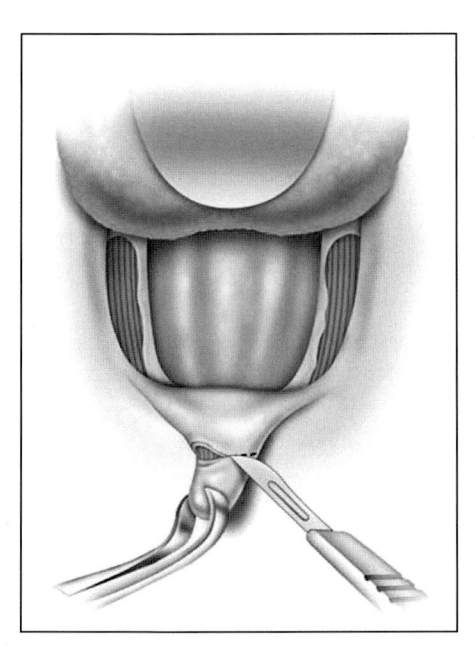

**Fig. 32.2** The uvula is grasped with Allis forceps and retracted anteriorly. A curvilinear horizontal incision is made on the mucosa at the base of the uvula posteriorly, preserving almost the entire posterior soft palate mucosa.

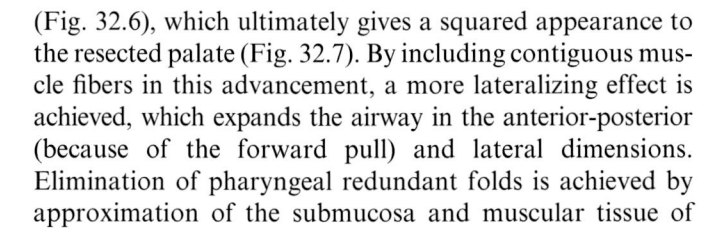

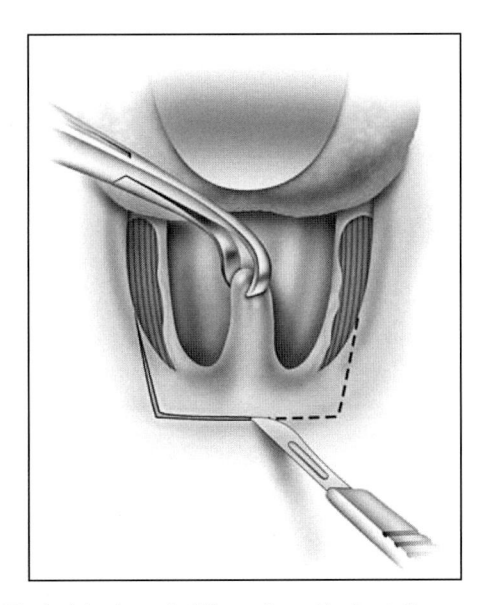

**Fig. 32.4** The incision is carried bilaterally and horizontally across the soft palate, until the anterior pillar starts sloping downward.

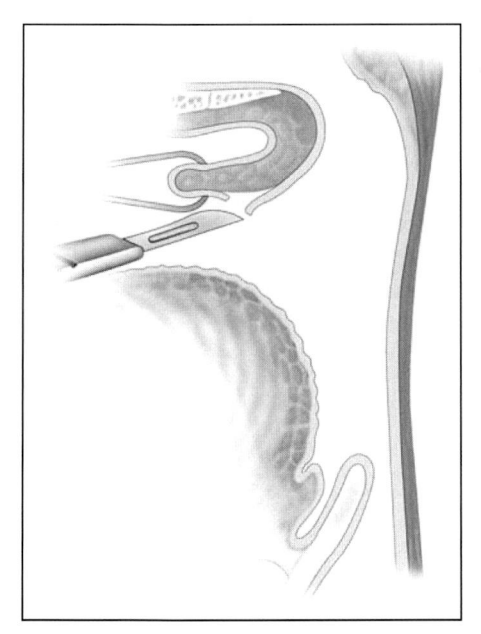

**Fig. 32.3** A trapezoid incision is outlined at the anterior mucosa of the soft palate.

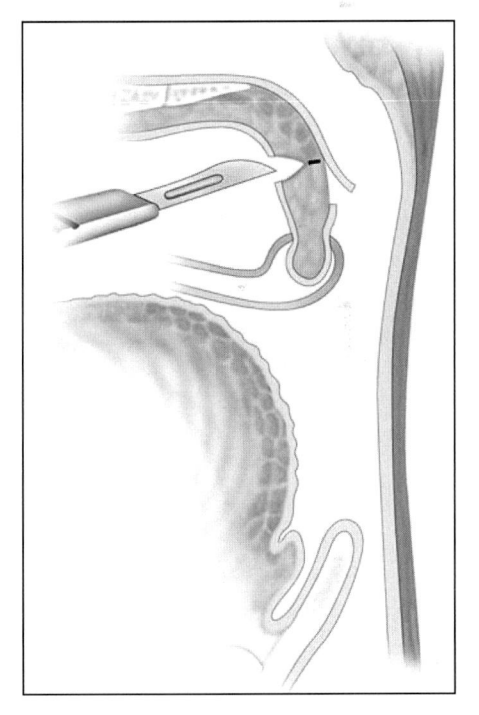

**Fig. 32.5** The uvula and the submucosal tissue of the lower edge of the soft palate are excised.

(Fig. 32.6), which ultimately gives a squared appearance to the resected palate (Fig. 32.7). By including contiguous muscle fibers in this advancement, a more lateralizing effect is achieved, which expands the airway in the anterior-posterior (because of the forward pull) and lateral dimensions. Elimination of pharyngeal redundant folds is achieved by approximation of the submucosa and muscular tissue of the tonsillar fossa and the soft palate, using interrupted 2-0 Vicryl™ (Ethicon, Inc., Sommerville, NJ) sutures through the exposed pharyngeal musculature (Fig. 32.8). These sutures also prevent the formation of a dead space, where a seroma or hematoma might develop. The mucosal flap edges are then loosely approximated, taking care not to undermine, using 3-0 chromic sutures (Fig. 32.9).

# SECTION I
## PALATAL SURGERY

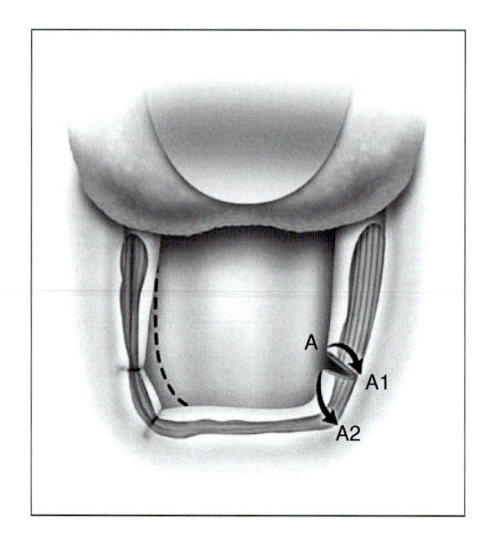

**Fig. 32.6** After making a small incision which creates two corners at the edge of the posterior pillar, the corners are then advanced anterolaterally, towards the palatal–pharyngeal junction, which eventually creates a squared appearance once both edges are sutured together.

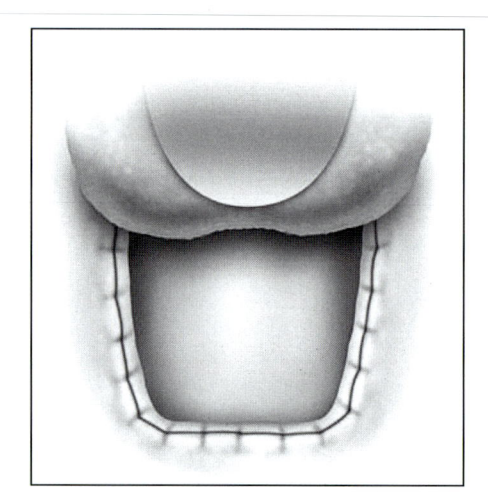

**Fig. 32.7** Squared appearance to the resected palate, after suturing.

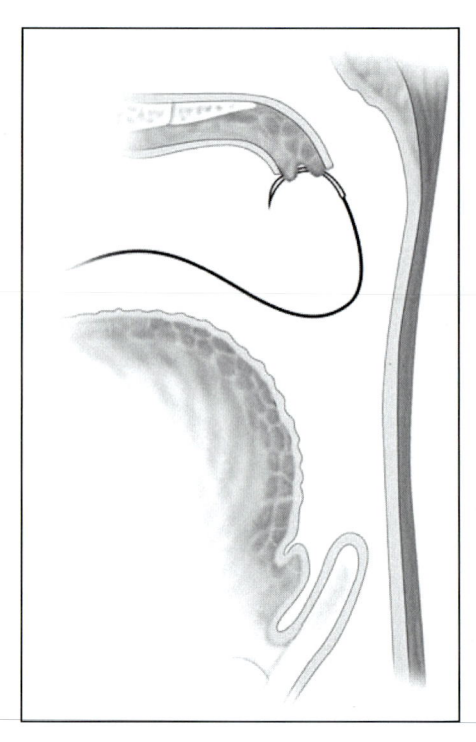

**Fig. 32.8** The submucosa and muscular tissue of the tonsillar fossa and the soft palate are then approximated, which eliminates the creation of redundant folds.

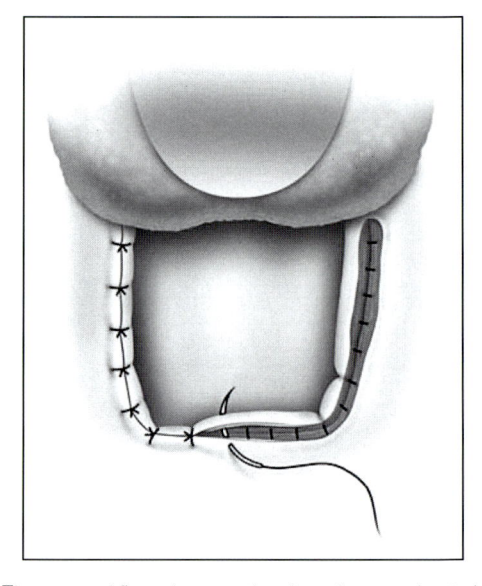

**Fig. 32.9** The mucosal flap edges are then loosely approximated, taking care not to undermine.

### 3.3 ADJUNCTIVE SURGICAL PROCEDURES

All patients with anatomical Stage II or greater also undergo serial tongue base reductions. This adjunctive technique is performed in all patients by administering 3000 joules (rapid lesion technique, Gyrus ENT, Memphis, TN), which are distributed to ten points along the midline of the tongue behind the circumvallated papillae. This initial treatment is followed by monthly sessions, as needed, with radiofrequency. In most cases, patients discontinue treatment when they achieve subjective improvement (in snoring levels and daytime sleepiness symptoms), which usually precedes normalization of objective parameters on polysomnography (PSG).

### 4 POSTOPERATIVE MANAGEMENT AND COMPLICATIONS

Significant morbidity is observed during the first 24–72 hours postoperatively, in the form of significant pain and

Table 32.1 Comparison of narcotic medication use, return to normal diet, and morbidity in a series of patients undergoing uvulopalatoplasty and uvulopalatopharyngoplasty

|  | UPP (n = 30) | UPPP (n = 33) |
|---|---|---|
| Postoperative narcotic use (in days) | 5.1±1.8 | 7.6±3.7 |
| Return to normal diet (in days) | 4.6±2.0 | 8.7±3.3 |
| Postoperative hemorrhage | 0% | 9.1% |
| Dysphagia | 10% | 18.2% |
| Foreign body sensation | 23.3% | 57.6% |
| Velopharyngeal insufficiency | 0% | 9.1% |

UPP, uvulopalatoplasty; UPPP, uvulopalatopharyngoplasty. Modified from Friedman et al.[13]

dysphagia. However, patients who undergo UPPP with tension-free closure show significantly less postoperative pain, when compared with patients post conventional UPPP.[12] Clearly, a dehiscent suture line produces far more pain. The ability of the patient to tolerate at least a liquid diet, oral pain medications, antibiotics and steroids determines the need to keep the patient hospitalized. In general, patients diagnosed with moderate and severe OSAHS preoperatively are admitted to the intensive care unit for overnight monitoring. Most patients will need one or two days of intravenous fluids and medications before they can start taking an oral diet. Prior to discharge, patients are prescribed acetaminophen with codeine elixir as needed for pain. Pain medication requirements average 7–10 days. Postoperative antibiotics and steroids are also recommended, for a total of 7 days.

A summary of complications and the comparative incidence thereof between submucosal UPPP and UPP is listed in Table 32.1. Bleeding is always a potential complication and the risk is significant. Mild velopharyngeal insufficiency (VPI) may manifest when drinking quickly, and may persist for up to 3 months. After 3 months, patients have normal deglutition. Severity of VPI symptoms diminish with time and it is expected to progressively resolve. Permanent VPI is a potential complication that must be considered in every patient. Additional morbidity of the procedure is usually related to throat discomfort symptoms, including globus sensation, mild dysphagia, dry throat, and inability to clear the throat. These symptoms are almost universal after any form of palatopharyngoplasty. Nasopharyngeal stenosis of varying degrees may occur, which may be caused by many factors, including the patient's original anatomy.[9] Fortunately, this is not a frequent complication after submucosal UPPP.[12]

The submucosal tension-free technique does appear to allow for faster wound healing, and all the significant complications appear to occur less frequently than with traditional UPPP.

## 5 SUCCESS RATE OF THE PROCEDURE

### 5.1 SUBJECTIVE AND OBJECTIVE SYMPTOM ELIMINATION

Subjective success is based on the assessment of patients and their bedpartners regarding symptom improvement, mainly snoring level and daytime sleepiness symptoms, by comparing these symptoms before and after treatment. Patients who underwent submucosal UPPP and the modified UPP technique achieved subjective improvement of symptoms in 97% and 87% of cases, respectively,[13] which compares favorably to traditional UPPP. Significant improvement is achieved in quality-of-life parameters as well, as determined by the SF-36v2™ Quality of Life Survey. A greater degree of improvement is observed in several parameters, mostly bodily pain and psychological distress/well-being, which may relate specifically to less short- and long-term morbidity, particularly in the case of UPP, where by virtue of modification of the pharyngoplasty component of the technique, the major source of morbidity is eliminated.

When focusing on objective success, there were no significant differences between UPPP and UPP in achieving a subjective cure in a series of 63 patients. The overall surgical success for both techniques is 55% and 70%, which compares favorably to previously described success rates of classic UPPP.

### 5.2 WHAT TO DO IF THE PROCEDURE FAILS

This procedure, like any other, may fail. Failure can be defined as a persistence of symptoms, which would demand additional treatment. Failure can also occur when symptoms of snoring and daytime sleepiness are eliminated, but PSG scores indicate persistent disease. Typically, patients who fail after UPPP will show a pattern of elimination of apneas, but persistent hypopneas. Failure in achieving satisfactory results always requires the patient to restart or continue CPAP. When CPAP is not accepted by the patient, further evaluation and treatment are essential.

Uvulopalatopharyngoplasty failure is multi-faceted, as is OSAHS itself, which only stresses the importance of appropriate patient selection before performing any surgical intervention. Pan-airway obstruction, which may be present before surgery or may become manifest or more pronounced after UPPP, may be the source of failure. However, in up to 75% of patients, persistent retropalatal obstruction is usually the cause for initial failure or recurrence of symptoms and deterioration in PSG parameters after UPPP.[14] The first step should be a thorough investigation, in order to identify the site of failure. Sleep endoscopy evaluation may be a valuable test at this point. If the level of obstruction is confirmed to be retropalatal, a revision uvulopalatoplasty by Z-palatoplasty (ZPP) is one option for revision, with a success rate of about 68%[15] (see Chapter 62: Revision Uvulopalatoplasty by Z-Palatoplasty [ZPP]). Transpalatal advancement pharyngoplasty can also be considered as an alternative.[16] In order to address the persistence of obstruction at the tongue base or hypopharyngeal level, genioglossus advancement alone or in combination with thyrohyoid suspension could be an option. Bimaxillary advancement should be kept in mind as a second-line procedure, if the above interventions fail. This procedure will correct failures at both the retropalatal and retrolingual levels.[17]

## 6 CONCLUSION

The key element in prevention of wound dehiscence is submucosal pharyngeal and palatal closure, followed by a tension-free epithelial closure. Submucosal uvulopalatopharyngoplasty is a successful procedure for the treatment of OSAHS, from both the objective and subjective perspectives, in appropriately selected patients. Postoperative pain is comparatively less than in patients who undergo classic UPPP, which has a significant impact on quality of life. Wound healing is faster and suture line dehiscence is rare. Postoperative complications (such as hemorrhage, nasopharyngeal stenosis and permanent VPI) are rare, which makes this procedure a good first-line option in patients with snoring and moderate to severe OSAHS, either alone or in combination with radiofrequency base of the tongue reduction.

## REFERENCES

1. Littner M, Kushida C, Hartse K, et al. Practice parameters for the use of laser-assisted uvulopalatoplasty: an update for 2000. Sleep 2001;24:603–19.
2. Sher AE, Schechtman KB, Piccirillo JF. The efficacy of surgical modifications of the upper airway in adults with obstructive sleep apnea syndrome. Sleep 1996;19:156–77.
3. Friedman M, Ibrahim H, Joseph N. Staging of obstructive sleep apnea/hypopnea syndrome: a guide to appropriate treatment. Laryngoscope 2004;114:454–9.
4. Fairbanks D. Uvulopalatopharyngoplasty complications and avoidance strategies. Otolaryngol Head Neck Surg 1990;102:239–45.
5. Katsantonis G, Friedman W, Krebs F, et al. Nasopharyngeal complications following uvulopalatopharyngoplasty. Laryngoscope 1987;97:309–14.
6. Haavisto L, Suonpää J. Complications of uvulopalatopharyngoplasty. Clin Otolaryngol Allied Sci 1994;19:243–7.
7. Kezirian E, Weaver E, Yueh B, et al. Incidence of serious complications after uvulopalatopharyngoplasty. Laryngoscope 2004;114:450–3.
8. Fujita S, Conway W, Zorick F, et al. Surgical correction of anatomic abnormalities in obstructive sleep apnea syndrome: uvulopalatopharyngoplasty. Otolaryngol Head Neck Surg 1981;89:923–34.
9. Krespi Y, Kacker A. Management of nasopharyngeal stenosis after uvulopalatoplasty. Otolaryngol Head Neck Surg 2000;123:692–5.
10. Friedman M, Ibrahim H, Lee G, et al. Combined uvulopalatopharyngoplasty and radiofrequency tongue base reduction for treatment of obstructive sleep apnea/hypopnea syndrome. Otolaryngol Head Neck Surg 2003;129:611–21.
11. Friedman M, Ibrahim H, Vidyasagar R, et al. Z-palatoplasty (ZPP): a technique for patients without tonsils. Otolaryngol Head Neck Surg 2004;131:89–100.
12. Friedman M, Landsberg R, Tanyeri H. Submucosal uvulopalatopharyngoplasty. Oper Tech Otolaryngol Head Neck Surg 2000;11:26–29.
13. Friedman M, Ibrahim H, Lowenthal S, et al. Uvulopalatoplasty (UP2): a modified technique for selected patients. Laryngoscope 2004;114:441–9.
14. Woodson B, Wooten M. Manometric and endoscopic localization of airway obstruction after uvulopalatopharyngoplasty. Otolaryngol Head Neck Surg 1994;111:38–43.
15. Friedman M, Duggal P, Joseph N. Revision uvulopalatoplasty by Z-palatoplasty. Otolaryngol Head Neck Surg 2007;136:638–43.
16. Woodson B, Toohill R. Transpalatal advancement pharyngoplasty for obstructive sleep apnea. Laryngoscope 1993;103:269–76.
17. Li K, Riley R, Powell N, et al. Maxillomandibular advancement for persistent obstructive sleep apnea after phase I surgery in patients without maxillomandibular deficiency. Laryngoscope 2000;110:1684–88.

# SECTION I  PALATAL SURGERY

# CHAPTER 33

# Zetapalatopharyngoplasty (ZPP)

*Michael Friedman and Paul Schalch*

## 1 INTRODUCTION

Due to its limited success in curing obstructive sleep apnea/hypopnea syndrome (OSAHS),[1] many adjunctive procedures and modifications were proposed after the introduction of the classic uvulopalatopharyngoplasty (UPPP) by Fujita et al. in 1981.[2] Its role as part of a comprehensive treatment plan remains, however, solidly accepted in most situations in which the palate, with or without the tonsils, is contributing to airway turbulence and obstruction. The goal of UPPP is to widen the airspace in three areas:

1. the retropalatal space;
2. the space between tongue base and palate;
3. the lateral dimensions.

This is accomplished through two components: (a) the palatoplasty component, which involves palatal shortening with closure of mucosal incisions; and (b) the pharyngoplasty component, which is composed of a classic tonsillectomy with pharyngeal closure. These goals, however, are not always achieved with classic UPPP and, in spite of our best efforts, patients may end up with an extremely narrow palatal arch in which the diameter of the oropharyngeal inlet is decreased due to a forward approximation of the posterior palatal mucosa. The resulting new shape of the free edge of the palate is triangular, rather than square. Further contraction of the wound occurs due to scarring secondary to the resection of the posterior tonsillar pillars, and additional narrowing is caused, which further affects long-term results (Fig. 33.1)[3] (see also Chapter 32: Submucosal Uvulopalatopharyngoplasty). Additionally, patients who previously underwent tonsillectomy are particularly poor candidates for classic UPPP due to scarring or absence of the posterior pillar from the previous tonsillectomy. These patients have an already narrowed space between the soft palate and the posterior pharyngeal wall and often do not have any redundant pharyngeal folds. Important modifications of the classic UPPP proposed by Fairbanks, in which the posterior pillar is advanced lateral cephalad in order to widen the retropalatal space,[4] are, hence, not possible. It is well known

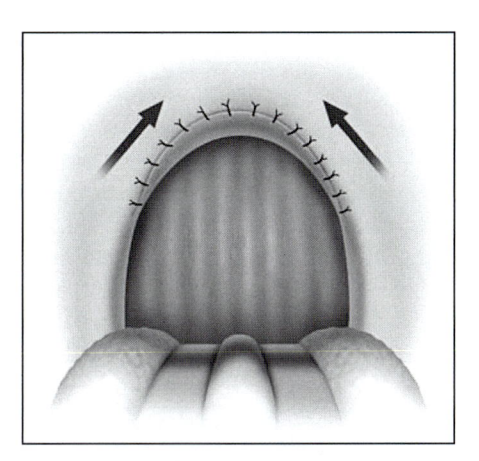

**Fig. 33.1** After traditional UPPP, an anteriomedially directed pull eventually causes narrowing of the pharyngeal airway at the midline.

that when UPPP fails, the severity of obstruction may actually worsen.[5]

It became apparent that appropriate selection criteria needed to be implemented in order to identify the patients with a higher likelihood of cure after UPPP. A staging system introduced by Friedman et al.[6] identified that patients with anatomic stage I disease (Friedman Tongue Position (FTP) I and II) with large tonsils have a better than 80% chance of success, whereas patients with stage II and III disease (FTP III and IV) are less than ideal candidates and should therefore undergo a combined procedure that addresses both the palate and the hypopharynx. The zetapalatopharyngoplasty (ZPP) technique was developed as a more aggressive technique for patients with stage II and III disease. This includes all patients who have had previous tonsillectomy, as well as patients with small tonsils and those with unfavorable tongue positions. A modification, useful for revision UPPP, is presented in Chapter 62.

The goal of ZPP is to widen the space between the palate and the posterior pharyngeal wall, between the palate and the tongue base and to either maintain or even widen the lateral dimensions of the pharynx. This is accomplished by changing the scar contracture tension line to an anterolateral vector and by widening the anteroposterior and

# SECTION I PALATAL SURGERY

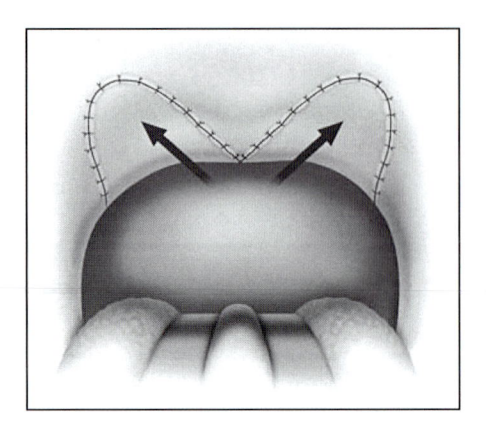

**Fig. 33.2** After ZPP, the anterolateral direction of pull on the soft palate widens the retropharyngeal space.

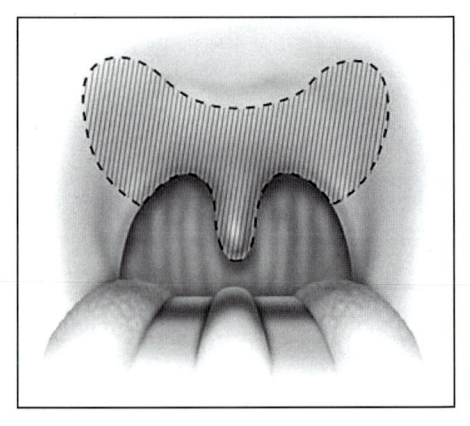

**Fig. 33.3** Outline of the palatal flaps, marked before incision.

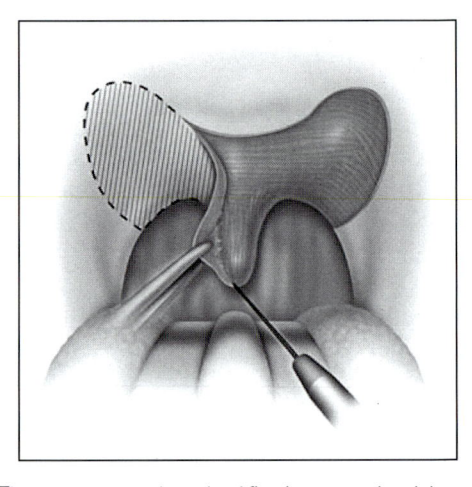

**Fig. 33.4** The mucosa over the palatal flap is removed and the palatal musculature is exposed.

lateral oropharyngeal air spaces at the level of the palate. By splitting the soft palate and retracting it anterolaterally, an effective anterolateral pull is created, which actually continues to widen the airway as healing and contracture occur (Fig. 33.2). None of the palatal musculature is resected, in spite of the aggressive palatal shortening, thereby addressing and minimizing the risk for permanent velopharyngeal insufficiency (VPI). This procedure is performed with adjunctive tongue base reduction by radiofrequency (TBRF), which addresses the hypopharyngeal airway.

## 2 PATIENT SELECTION

General guidelines for surgical intervention include significant symptoms of snoring and daytime somnolence, documented failure of a continuous positive airway pressure (CPAP) trial, documented failure of conservative measures such as dental appliances, changes in sleeping position and sleep hygiene in general. Apparent obstruction at the level of the soft palate must be determined by fiberoptic nasopharyngolaryngoscopy and Mueller maneuver, or sleep endoscopy. Adequate medical clearance and a thorough review of the procedure, its implications, potential outcomes and complications with the patient are essential components of the preoperative work-up.

Specific criteria for ZPP include patients classified as stage II and III according to Friedman's Anatomic Staging System[7] (see also Chapter 16). Because ZPP produces a significant widening of the retropalatal space, it is an aggressive procedure, with significant temporary VPI and the risk for permanent VPI. It should be reserved for patients with moderate to severe OSAHS with moderate to severe symptoms. It is not a surgical option for snoring only.

## 3 SURGICAL TECHNIQUE

Candidates eligible to undergo a modified uvulopalatopharyngoplasty technique can be divided into patients with intact tonsils and patients status post tonsillectomy. The revision UPPP technique is outlined in Chapter 62.

The key main goals of ZPP are the removal of the anterior mucosa only and the splitting of the soft palate in the midline. The key features are the cutting of the palatoglossus muscle, and the sewing of the posterior palatal mucosa to the anterior resection margin, which retracts the midline anterolaterally and widens the retropharyngeal area.

The surgical technique for the modified ZPP is illustrated in Figures 33.3 to 33.10.

Two adjacent flaps are outlined in the palate (Fig. 33.3). The anterior midline margin of the flap is halfway between the hard palate and the free edge of the soft palate, and the distal margin corresponds to the free edge of the palate and uvula. The lateral extent is posterior to the midline, and extends to the lateral extent of the palate. The mucosa from only the anterior aspect of the two flaps is subsequently removed (Fig. 33.4). Figure 33.5 illustrates how the preoperative uvula and palate hang close to the posterior pharyngeal wall, narrowing the retropharyngeal space. The two flaps are then separated from each other by splitting the palatal segment down the midline (Fig. 33.6), extending them

# Zetapalatopharyngoplasty (ZPP)
## CHAPTER 33

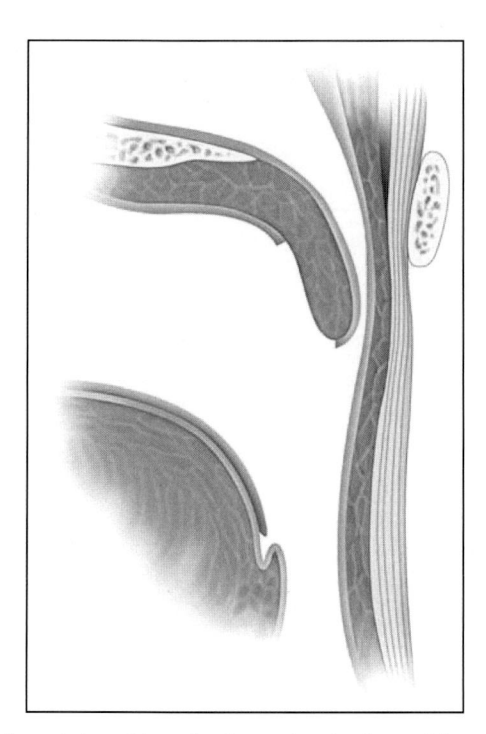

**Fig. 33.5** Lateral view of the soft palate and uvula after excision of the anterior mucosa. The uvula and palate hang close to the posterior pharyngeal wall, narrowing the retropharyngeal space.

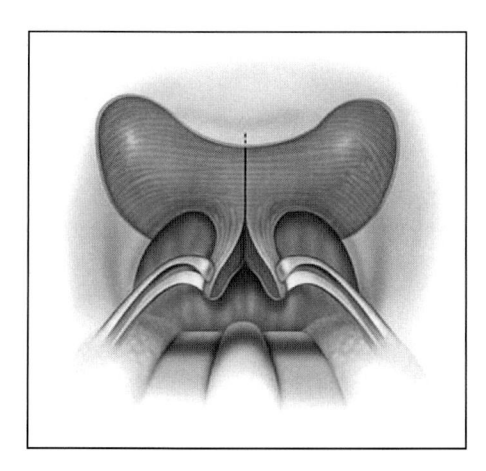

**Fig. 33.6** The uvula and palate are split in the midline with a cold knife.

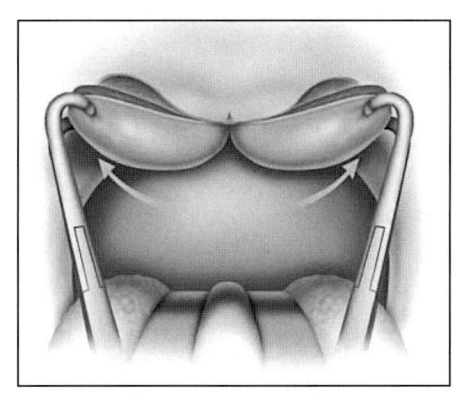

**Fig. 33.7** The uvular flaps along with the soft palate are reflected back and laterally, over the soft palate.

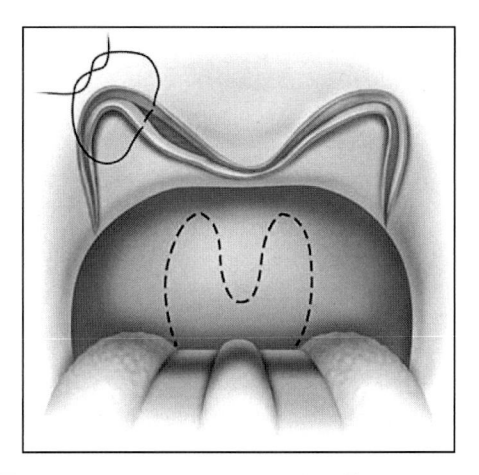

**Fig. 33.8** Two-layered closure of the palatal flaps. The submucosal layer is approximated first with 2-0 Vicryl™ (Ethicon, Inc., Somerville, NJ).

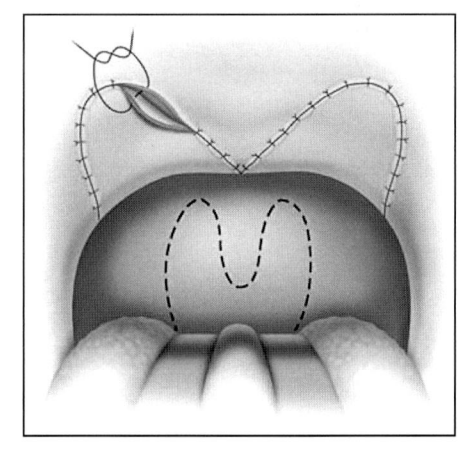

**Fig. 33.9** Two-layered closure of the palatal flaps with 3-0 chromic suture.

laterally, in a butterfly fashion (Fig. 33.7), and dividing the palatoglossus muscle. A two-layer closure is then done, which brings the midline all the way to the anterolateral margin of the palate (Figs 33.8 and 33.9). The primary closure is done at the submucosal level, which then enables a tension-free closure of the mucosa. A distance of at least 3–4 cm between the posterior pharynx and the palate is created.[8] Figure 33.10 illustrates the widening of the nasopharynx after the midline palatoplasty. The lateral dimension of the palate is usually increased to approximately 4 cm.

TBRF is adjunctively performed in all patients by administering 3000 joules (rapid lesion technique by Gyrus™, Gyrus ENT, Memphis, TN), which are distributed to ten points along the midline of the tongue behind the circumvallated papillae. This initial treatment is followed by monthly sessions, as needed. The addition of TBRF has been shown to provide significantly better subjective and objective improvement in stage II and III patients undergoing UPPP, when compared to patients that undergo UPPP only.[9]

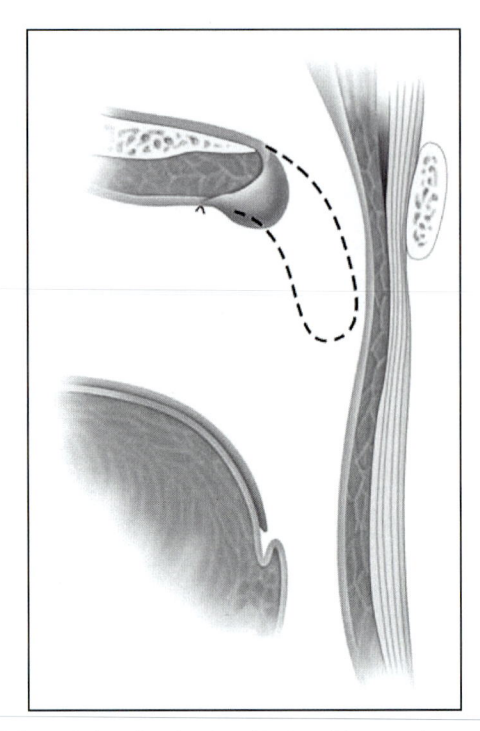

**Fig. 33.10** Lateral view showing the widening of the nasopharynx after ZPP.

**Table 33.1** Comparison of complications between ZPP and classic UPPP, based on a series of 25 matched patients that underwent each procedure

|  | ZPP (n = 25) | UPPP (n = 25) |
|---|---|---|
| Tongue base infection | 1 (4%) | 2 (8%) |
| Bleeding | 0 | 0 |
| Postnasal drip | 3 (12%) | 4 (16%) |
| Dysphagia | 1 (4%) | 11 (44%)* |
| Foreign body sensation | 11 (44%) | 17 (68%) |
| Temporary VPI | 12 (48%) | 7 (28%) |
| Permanent VPI | 0 | 0 |

*$P < 0.001$
Modified from Friedman et al.[3]

## 4 POSTOPERATIVE MANAGEMENT AND COMPLICATIONS

As with any intervention that involves resection of the soft palate, significant morbidity is observed in the first 24 to 72 hours postoperatively in the form of significant pain and dysphagia. The ability of the patient to tolerate at least a liquid diet, oral pain medications, antibiotics and steroids determines the moment when the patient can be safely discharged home. While the discharge could in theory be on the same day of the surgery, most patients will need 1 or 2 days of intravenous fluids and medications before they can start taking an oral diet. Prior to discharge, patients are prescribed acetaminophen with codeine elixir as needed for pain. Pain medication requirements average 6.5 days, and so does the progression from liquid or soft diet to normal diet. Postoperative antibiotics and steroids are also recommended, for a total of 7 days. Additional TBRF sessions may be necessary, depending on the improvement of symptoms of each individual patient.

Complications of the procedure are comparable to classic UPPP (Table 33.1). Bleeding is always a potential complication and the risk is, again, comparable to classic UPPP. Typically, patients can eat a normal diet after 2 weeks. Mild VPI may become manifest when drinking quickly and may persist for up to 3 months. After 3 months, patients have a normal deglutition. Severity of VPI symptoms diminish with time and are expected to progressively resolve. Permanent VPI is a potential complication that must be considered in every patient. Additional morbidity of the procedure is usually related to throat discomfort symptoms, including globus sensation, mild dysphagia, dry throat, and inability to clear the throat. These symptoms are almost universal after any form of uvulopalatopharyngoplasty.

Other complications are related to the adjunctive procedures performed. Tongue base infection is related to TBRF and requires antibiotic treatment. In rare cases, it may lead to tongue base abscess formation, which may require incision and drainage.

## 5 SUCCESS RATE OF THE PROCEDURE

### 5.1 SUBJECTIVE AND OBJECTIVE SYMPTOM ELIMINATION

The subjective success is based on comparative improvement on snoring level, daytime sleepiness and overall well-being. Patients that underwent ZPP were compared to patients who had previously undergone UPPP for the treatment of OSAHS and the results achieved in these parameters were far superior with ZPP, particularly with adjunctive TBRF. Quality of life scores improve significantly more after ZPP than after UPPP.[8]

When focusing on objective success, ZPP shows considerable improvement over UPPP. Objective cure rates for stage II patients treated with ZPP and TBRF are close to 70%, compared to about 30% for classic UPPP with TBRF.

Limitations of this technique include a higher risk of temporary VPI due to a more aggressive modification of the palatal anatomy, even though the resection is limited to the mucosa. While VPI was only temporary, should permanent VPI ensue, this procedure is probably not reversible. There are also no clear anatomic landmarks to assist in describing the size of the flaps and, ultimately, the guidelines outlined in this chapter do not substitute for the surgeon's judgment. The procedure is significantly more difficult technically and takes longer to perform. A learning curve, as with any other procedure, leads to progressively better results.

## 5.2 WHAT TO DO IF THE PROCEDURE FAILS

The treatment, as any other, may fail. Failure can be defined as a persistence of symptoms, which would demand additional treatment. Failure can also occur when symptoms of snoring and daytime sleepiness are eliminated but polysomnography (PSG) scores indicate persistent disease. Typically, patients that fail will show a pattern of elimination of apneas but persistent hypopneas. In spite of an abnormal PSG, however, many patients will have a lower C-reactive protein, indicating a possible reduction of cardiovascular risk[10] (see also Chapter 13: The Impact of Surgical Treatment of OSA on Cardiac Risk Factors). Failure in achieving satisfactory results may in some cases convince the patient to accept CPAP therapy. When CPAP is not accepted by the patient, further evaluation and treatment are essential. The first step should be a thorough investigation in order to identify the site of failure. Sleep endoscopy evaluation may be a valuable test at this point. If the level of obstruction continues to be retropalatal, a transpalatal advancement pharyngoplasty can be considered.[11] If the persistence of obstruction is at the tongue base or hypopharyngeal level, then genioglossus advancement alone or in combination with thyrohyoid suspension could be an option.[12] Bimaxillary advancement should be kept in mind as a second-line procedure if the above interventions fail. This procedure will correct failures at both the retropalatal and retrolingual levels.[13]

## 6 CONCLUSION

No single procedure is effective in treating all OSAHS patients. Treatment should be tailored to the anatomy of each patient. Laterally rerouting the uvula together with the soft palate improves the airway characteristics by enlarging the retropalatal space, which is a distinct advantage over the traditional UPPP. This acquires even more importance when addressing the obstruction at the level of the palate in patients without tonsils.

## REFERENCES

1. Sher AE, Schechtman KB, Piccirillo JF. The efficacy of surgical modifications of the upper airway in adults with obstructive sleep apnea syndrome. Sleep 1996;19:156–77.
2. Fujita S, Conway W, Zorick F, Roth T. Surgical correction of anatomic abnormalities in obstructive sleep apnea syndrome: uvulopalatopharyngoplasty. Otolaryngol Head Neck Surg 1981;89:923–34.
3. Friedman M, Landsberg R, Tanyeri H. Submucosal uvulopalatopharyngoplasty. Op Tech Otolaryngol Head Neck Surg 2000;11:26–9.
4. Fairbanks DN. Operative techniques of uvulopalatopharyngoplasty. Ear Nose Throat J 1999;78:846–50.
5. Senior BA, Rosenthal L, Lumley A, Gerhardstein R, Day R. Efficacy of uvulopalatopharyngoplasty in unselected patients with mild obstructive sleep apnea. Otolarynol Head Neck Surg 2000;123:179–82.
6. Friedman M, Ibrahim H, Joseph N. Staging of obstructive sleep apnea/hypopnea syndrome: a guide to appropriate treatment. Laryngoscope 2004;114:454–9.
7. Friedman M, Ibrahim H, Joseph N. Staging of obstructive sleep apnea/hypopnea syndrome: a guide to appropriate treatment. Laryngoscope 2004;114:454–9.
8. Friedman M, Ibrahim HZ, Vidyasagar R, Pomeranz J. Z-palatoplasty (ZPP): a technique for patients without tonsils. Otolaryngol Head Neck Surg 2004;131:89–100.
9. Friedman M, Ibrahim H, Lee G, Joseph NJ. Combined uvulopalatopharyngoplasty and radiofrequency tongue base reduction for treatment of obstructive sleep apnea/hypopnea syndrome. Otolaryngol Head Neck Surg 2003;129:611–21.
10. Friedman M, Bliznikas D, Vidyasagar R, Woodson BT, Joseph NJ. Reduction of C-reactive protein with surgical treatment of obstructive sleep apnea/hypopnea syndrome. Otolaryngol Head Neck Surg 2006;135:900–5.
11. Woodson BT, Toohill RJ. Transpalatal advancement pharyngoplasty for obstructive sleep apnea. Laryngoscope 1993;103:269–76.
12. Powell NB, Riley RW, Guilleminault C. The hypopharynx: upper airway reconstruction in obstructive sleep apnea syndrome. In: Snoring and Obstructive Sleep Apnea, 2nd edn. Fairbanks DNF, Fujita S, eds. New York: Raven Press; 1994, pp. 193–209.
13. Li KK, Riley RW, Powell NB, Guilleminault C. Maxillomandibular advancement for persistent OSA after phase I surgery in patients without maxillomandibular deficiency. Laryngoscope 2000;110:1684–8.

# SECTION I  PALATAL SURGERY

## CHAPTER 34

# The uvulopalatal flap

*Tod C. Huntley*

## 1 INTRODUCTION

This book includes a number of chapters which describe a variety of palatal surgical procedures for sleep disordered breathing, including traditional uvulopalatopharyngoplasty (UPPP) techniques, Z-palatoplasty (ZPPP), transpalatal advancement pharyngoplasty, laser-assisted uvulopalatoplasty (LAUP), pillar implantation, etc. Most of these procedures can be divided into two mutually exclusive groups based upon several different criteria: by their action on the palate, the setting in which they are performed, and how the surgeon is reimbursed. First, these various procedures usually work by one of two different ways: by either shortening the soft palate or by stiffening it. They also differ in where they are performed: those that are more invasive and which are used for more significant obstructive sleep apnea (OSA) are generally done in the operating room under general anesthesia, and those that are less invasive and which are advocated for less severe forms of sleep disordered breathing (such as primary snoring) are done in the office under local anesthesia. Furthermore, the insurance industry makes a distinction between these two groups of procedures in regards to reimbursement: those done in the OR for OSA are generally reimbursed by insurance, while those done in the office for primary snoring and mild OSA are relegated to self-pay status.

This chapter describes a palatal surgical technique which in many regards bridges these divides, with applicability in both the operating room as an OSA procedure and in the office setting for primary snoring or mild OSA. It is a variation of UPPP which is easily learned, gives reproducible results, and which can be done under local anesthesia in the office in select cases. The procedure can be performed as a limited palatal procedure for snoring or mild OSA, or can be extended to more effectively treat the palate and tonsillar fossas for more significant OSA. In addition, it forms the basis for another effective palatal procedure, the Z-palatoplasty, as described elsewhere in this atlas.

## 2 THE PROCEDURE

The uvulopalatal flap (UPF) procedure involves the shortening of the soft palate by folding the distal soft palate with uvula forward upon itself. The intervening mucosal surfaces of the folded palate are removed, and the palate is sutured in its new position in two layers with interrupted sutures. The resultant palatal shortening creates a surgical result virtually indistinguishable from a traditional UPPP, but with several important potential differences over UPPP and some of the other procedures, as outlined below.

1. The procedure is potentially adjustable or even reversible. If the palatal shortening appears to have been too aggressive, suture placement may be altered and the demucosalized gap can be allowed to heal secondarily. Alternatively, if velopharyngeal insufficiency (VPI) is suspected postoperatively, the sutures may be removed to allow the palate to fall back into its original position to remucosalize. This remucosalization process allows for healing similar to what is seen with a cautery-assisted palatal stiffening operation (CAPSO), and if persistent palatal-associated sleep disordered breathing is identified later, the procedure could be repeated more conservatively.
2. The UPF procedure has the theoretical advantage over traditional UPPP of less scar contracture and nasopharyngeal stenosis, as the suture line lies proximal to the free margin of the soft palate, as diagrammed later in this chapter.
3. The procedure spares the palatal and uvular muscles. Because the uvular muscle is not only preserved, but is repositioned and stabilized more anteriorly, palatal dynamics should not only be maintained but might even improve during sleep. Though unproven, it has been suggested that the contraction of the uvular and distal palatal muscles in their new positions during respiration might assist in maintaining patency of the central retropalatal region during sleep, thus improving airway patency.

4. In select cases, the UPF procedure can be performed in the office setting in one stage under local anesthesia, in a fashion similar to the modified LAUP procedure, pillar implant procedure, etc. Yet the UPF offers several potential advantages over these and other office procedures for sleep disordered breathing. First, it does not require the purchase of a laser, tissue implants, etc, and generally does not even require electrocautery for hemostasis. Secondly, since it is technically a form of UPPP (involving tissue removal, palatal shortening, and suturing), it is more likely to be reimbursable by insurance (with CPT code 42145) in cases that mean criteria for UPPP, even when performed in the office setting, which is not generally the case with LAUP, pillar implantation, etc. at the time of this writing.
5. There is the potential for less pain with the UPF than with other available techniques that involve more extensive tissue destruction or ablation, such as LAUP or UPPP.[1,2]

The UPF procedure was first described by Powell et al.[2] in 1996 as a UPPP variation for the operating room. A similar technique was described in 1993 by Bresalier and Brandes,[3] referred to as the imbrication technique of UPPP in 1999. In 2000, I described the use of this technique in the office under local anesthetic,[4] which was presented in more detail in 2003 by Neruntarat.[5] The procedure can also be expanded under general anesthesia to include greater effects in the laterally, by including concurrent tonsillectomy with tonsillar pillar closure[4,6] or by extending incisions superolaterally from the apices of the tonsillar fossas toward the third molar region;[4] Li et al.[7] call this modification an extended uvulopalatal flap. The principles of the UPF have been further extended by Friedman with the Z-palatoplasty,[8] which is the subject of Chapter 33. The Z-palatoplasty is essentially a UPF procedure in which the uvula and distal soft palate are split in the midline. This creates two flaps which are advanced not only anteriorly but laterally to further augment the retropalatal airway in its lateral dimensions. Because of the versatility of the procedure, therefore, the UPF is a useful tool which should be part of the armamentarium of all surgeons who treat sleep disordered breathing.

## 3 TECHNIQUE

### 3.1 AWAKE, LOCAL ANESTHESIA, OFFICE PROCEDURE

The procedure can be performed with the patient sitting in an examination chair in the upright or recumbent position. Topical local anesthetic is applied to the entire soft palate and uvula, and additional anesthesia to the nasal surface of the palate can be obtained by spraying the nasal cavities with a 1:1 mixture of tetracaine hydrochloride and phenylephrine hydrochloride. After allowing sufficient time for the topical anesthetic to take effect, the surgical site is infiltrated with 2–4 ml of injectable anesthetic with adrenaline. It is important not to distort the tissue or create blebs of submucosal anesthetic by injecting too much solution or by injecting too superficially. In addition to making the patient more comfortable during the procedure, meticulous injection of anesthetic results in enough vasoconstriction that the surgical field is surprisingly bloodless; any oozing can easily be controlled with a battery-operated ophthalmic cautery unit. Electrosurgical cautery should not be necessary except when the procedure is performed under general anesthesia with concurrent tonsillectomy.

The extent of reflection of the uvula and distal palate and the extent of resection of the uvular tip are then determined by grasping the uvula with medium-length forceps and reflecting it cephalad toward the junction of the hard and soft palate while simultaneously examining the retropalatal airway diameter with a number 5 laryngeal mirror. The uvula is retracted sufficiently to create a crease between the intervening mucosal edges. Standard UPPP principles are used to determine the extent of shortening desired. Because the patient is awake and able to phonate, the palatal dimple point is easily identified; VPI is more likely if the palate is shortened much beyond this point. Though varying significantly between patients, the final position of the repositioned uvular tip is generally 5–10 mm from the hard–soft palate junction.

If necessary, relaxing incisions can be made extending cephalad from the apices of the tonsillar fossas. This might be necessary if the palate is very low hanging or is tethered to the lateral pharynx by post-tonsillectomy scarring. Note that these incisions, which can measure 5–10 mm, are made further laterally than are the vertical trenches that are part of the classic LAUP. Additional advancement of the lateral soft palate can be achieved by increasing the amount of mucosal resection at the lateral aspect of the incision. Furthermore, the uvula and distal soft palate can be divided in the midline, as described by Friedman,[8] to create two separate uvulopalatal flaps, which when rotated superolaterally open the oropharyngeal inlet greater in side to side dimensions. Note that though I have done many Z-palatoplasties in the operating room setting, I have done just one in the office setting under local anesthesia.

While still grasping the uvula in its new position, the planned incision is outlined with a marker or with a number 12 blade, as shown in Figure 34.1. This gothic arch-shaped incision generally has its apex within 5–10 mm of the hard–soft palate junction and flares laterally to allow for advancement of the lateral palate. The farther laterally these incisions extend, the greater the elevation of the lateral aspects of the palate. The incision will be carried caudally onto the uvula in a mirror image of the palatal incision. Unless vertical relaxing incisions are necessary, as described previously, it is recommended that the incisions be kept away from the free edge of the palate, to lessen the chance of scar contracture.

SECTION I  PALATAL SURGERY

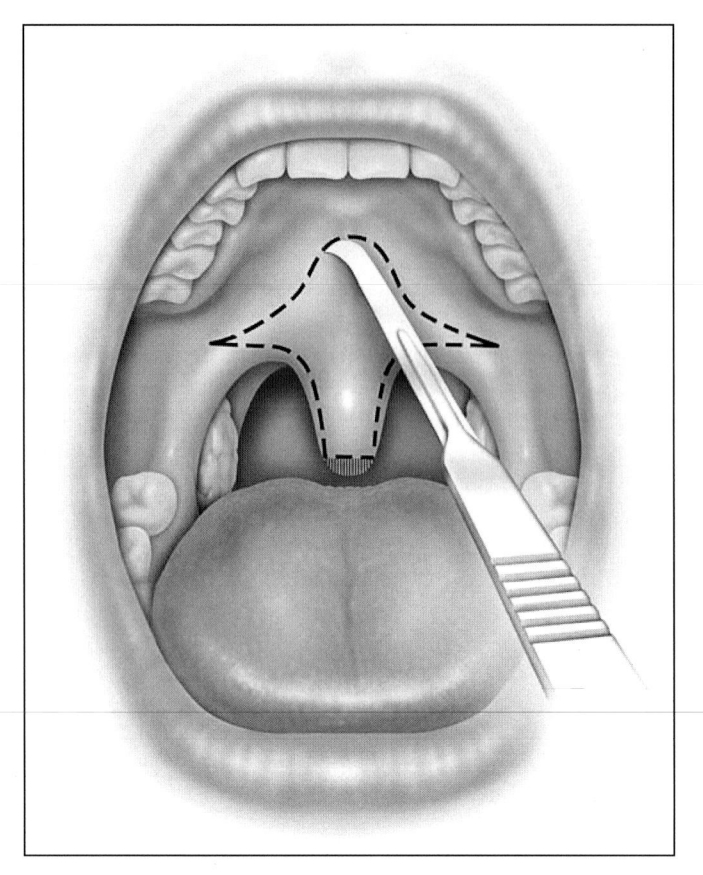

**Fig. 34.1** The surgical site has been outlined and injected with local anesthetic with adrenalin. The dissection is begun with a #12 blade at the apex of the incision. The tip of the uvula is shaded to mark the area to be amputated to aid in closure of the palate.

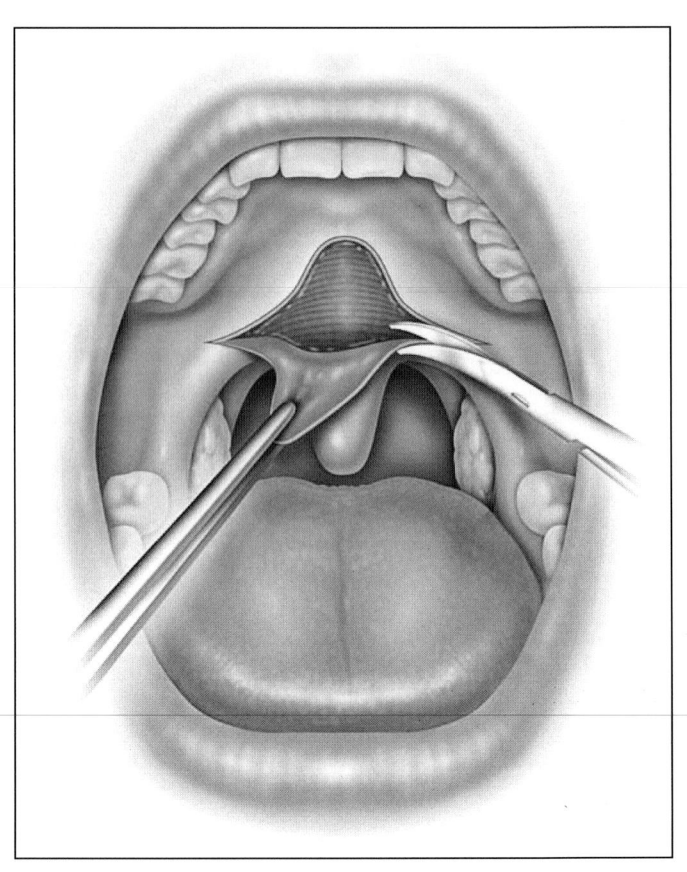

**Fig. 34.2** The mucosa is removed with scissors. Bleeding from the underlying palatal muscle is usually minimal, and can be controlled with a hand-held ophthalmic cautery unit.

The dissection can be performed entirely with a scalpel and with scissors; Metzenbaum or long Iris scissors are adequate. Though the procedure could also be performed acceptably with a needle point cautery unit, the additional expense, tissue destruction, and postoperative pain do not warrant its use, particularly since electrocautery should rarely be necessary for hemostasis if local anesthetic injection and surgical dissection have been meticulous. It is easiest to begin with the scalpel at the apex of the palatal incision and extend inferolaterally on each side. The mucosa within this outlined area is then carefully removed with sharp pointed scissors, as shown in Figure 34.2. As the dissection reaches the tip of the uvula, the tip is usually amputated to reduce the length of tissue brought up to the palate.

The distal soft palate and uvular remnant are then reflected superiorly and sutured in place with 3–0 or 2–0 polyglycolic acid (Vicryl; Ethicon, Somerville, NJ) suture on a tapered (SH) needle. Though these sutures last longer than needed, they can usually be easily removed 2 weeks postoperatively if the patient desires and if healing is sufficient. Note that the sutures could be removed before healing is complete if symptoms of significant VPI (such as voice change or nasal regurgitation) are noted, thus allowing the flap to fall back down inferiorly to either remucosalize or to be repositioned in a less aggressive position.

The initial suture is a mattress suture that first passes through the mucosa and underlying muscle at the apex of the palatal incision and then passes through the tip of the uvular muscle and adjacent mucosa from the nasopharyngeal side of the uvula. This is shown in Figure 34.3. Tension of this mattress suture can be adjusted to allow for proper positioning of the soft palate edge. Additional mucosa on the palate or flap may now be trimmed, if necessary. The closure is then completed in a two layered interrupted surgical technique. It is highly recommended that this closure be done in layers to minimize the chance of postoperative dehiscence.

Note that the advanced uvula and distal palate are a different color than the rest of the palate. This tissue, which originated on the nasopharyngeal surface of the palate, is brighter red than the oral palatal mucosa. This is explained to the patient preoperatively, as is the fact that the folded-over central palate may be somewhat thicker for some time postoperatively. This seems to thin out somewhat postoperatively, and should not require subsequent thinning or revision. Note that patients who have excessively thick and beefy palates may not be optimal candidates for this procedure, however.

CHAPTER 34 · The uvulopalatal flap

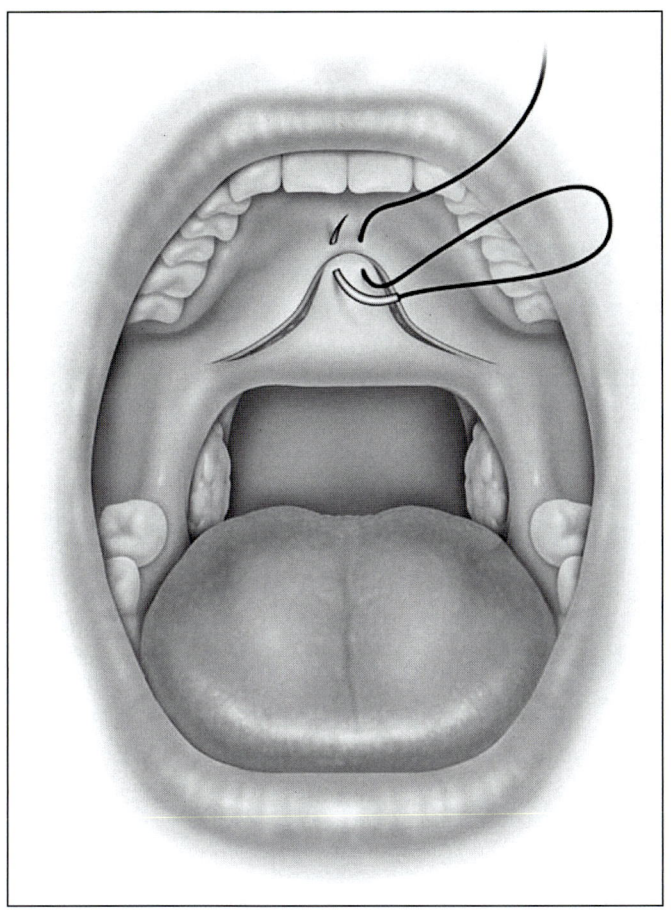

**Fig. 34.3** The uvula and distal soft palate are folded forward and sutured in place. The first suture is a horizontal mattress suture at the apex of the surgical site. The remainder of the closure is accomplished in layers with interrupted sutures.

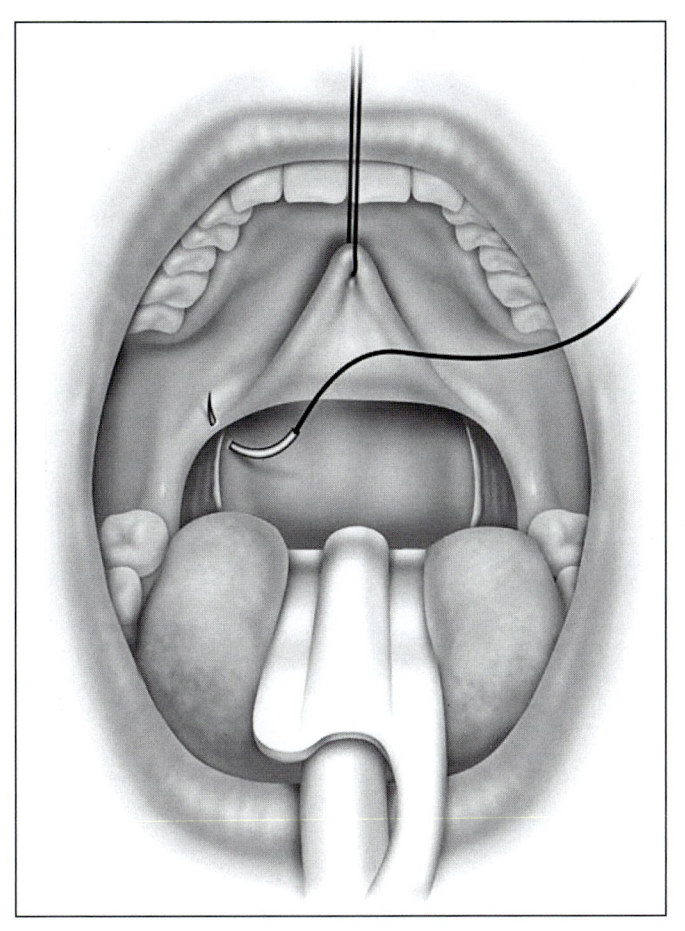

**Fig. 34.4** When performed under general anesthesia, the procedure is performed with a tonsillectomy, as is the case with other variations of UPPP. It is recommended that the tonsillectomy and tonsillar fossa closure be completed before performing the UPF portion of the surgery. The tip of the uvula can be reflected superiorly with a retraction suture to help in surgical planning.

## 3.2 GENERAL ANESTHESIA, WITH CONCURRENT TONSILLECTOMY

The uvulopalatal flap also can be combined with more aggressive pharyngeal mucosal tightening via a tonsillectomy with tonsillar pillar resection, as is generally done with the traditional UPPP. It is performed with the patient in the Rose position with a Crowe–Davis mouth gag and an appropriate sized tongue blade in place.

It is recommended that the tonsillectomy be performed first with care taken to spare as much tonsillar pillar mucosa as possible. Hemostasis is improved by injecting the tonsillar fossas with a total of 5–10 ml of the same local anesthetic with adrenalin as was used to inject the palate previously. This also helps with initial postoperative analgesia. The tonsillar pillar sutures are then placed before the palate is dissected, as illustrated in Figure 34.4. This closure is preferably performed in two layers to obliterate any dead space and to minimize the chance for postoperative dehiscence.

A stay suture held by a hemostat can be placed through the tip of the uvula to retract the distal palate cephalad during the tonsillar fossa closure to help align the tissues properly and aid in correct suture placement. This can also help in determining if relaxing incisions extending cephalad from the apices of the tonsillar fossas are necessary (Fig. 34.5), which would be performed next.

After approximation of the tonsillar pillars, the uvulopalatal flap is made as described before, and is sutured in place in a two-layered interrupted surgical technique. If at this point it is determined that the lateral dimensions of the oropharyngeal inlet at the palatal level should be augmented even more, the distal soft palate and uvula could be split in the midline at this point to convert the procedure to a Z-palatoplasty, as described elsewhere in this text.

## 4 POSTOPERATIVE MANAGEMENT

When performed in the outpatient setting in the office, patients are sent home with prescriptions for an appropriate

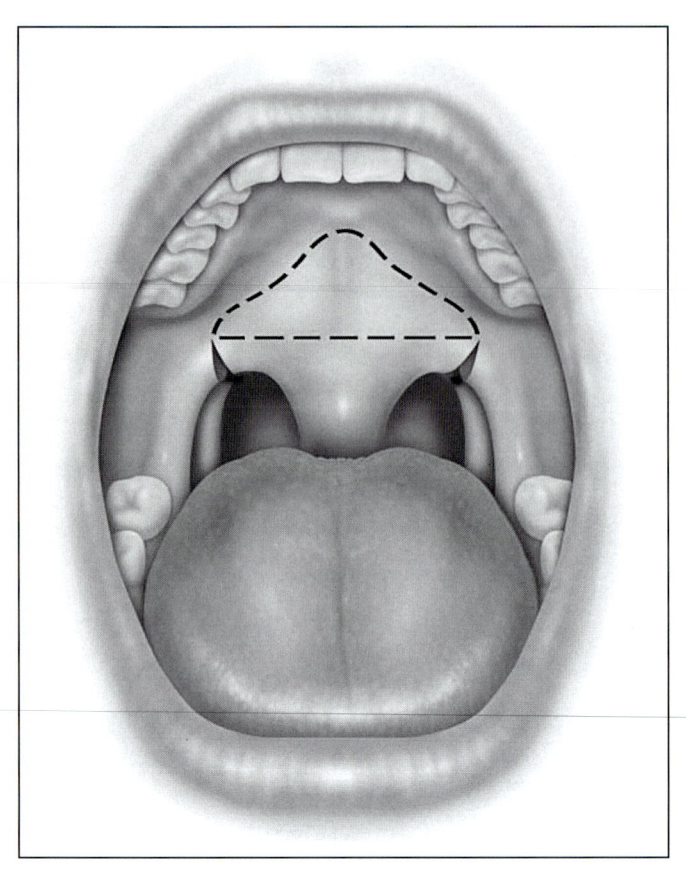

**Fig. 34.5** The UPF procedure can be extended by incising the distal soft palate superolaterally from the apices of the tonsillar fossas to aid in more aggressively shortening the palate.

In addition to wound dehiscence, minor bleeding can be encountered, particularly when combined with a tonsillectomy. Again, if VPI is encountered postoperatively, the suture line may be taken down and the palate may be either re-sutured in a less aggressive position, or may be dealt with again later, once it has remucosalized. On occasion, the bulge of the repositioned uvula may appear prominent enough in the first few weeks that the surgeon is tempted to consider postoperative revision, but this seems to diminish with time. Nevertheless, the use of this technique in a patient with an excessively thick palate or uvula might be inadvisable if the resultant thickness might be considered problematic.

## 6 SUMMARY

The UPF is easy to perform and is a potentially reversible treatment for the palatal obstruction that can accompany snoring with or without OSAS. It may be accomplished at a single session either in the office setting or under general anesthesia in the operating room. It offers several potential advantages over other variations of the UPPP, though some of these perceived advantages require further study for confirmation.

The original procedure as described by Powell et al.[2] has been modified by extending incisions into the lateral distal soft palate[4,7] to allow for augmented flap elevation laterally; when an incision is placed in the midline of the uvula to create two flaps (the Z-palatoplasty) as discussed by Friedman,[8] the lateral dimensions of the oropharyngeal inlet at this level can be augmented even more. This latter modification is thought to provide significant benefit in many cases.

Complications specifically related to the UPF are uncommon. The general surgical complications should be similar to those encountered in traditional UPPP surgery.

antibiotic for several days and a narcotic pain medication. If edema is thought to be problematic, a short course of steroids may be offered. Anxiolytics, sleep aids, or other sedating medications are not recommended in the immediate postoperative period. A regular diet is resumed as soon as the patient is comfortable. Residual sutures may be safely removed after 2 weeks.

When the UPF is performed under general anesthesia in the operating room, either solely or in conjunction with tongue base advancement or resection, nasal surgery, etc., the postoperative management is no different than with the traditional UPPP. If performed as part of the treatment of significant OSAS, postoperative continuous positive airway pressure is recommended until a subsequent polysomnogram shows resolution of the problem.

## 5 COMPLICATIONS

Rare complications can include wound separation, which can be minimized by avoiding chromic sutures that may resorb prematurely and by closing the incisions in two layers. The use of a 2-0 or 3-0 polyglycolic acid suture, as noted before, is recommended.

### REFERENCES

1. Huntley T. Uvulopalatal flap (UPF) vs. LAUP in the treatment of snoring. Presented at the AAO-HNS annual meeting, Washington, DC, 2000 (unpublished data).
2. Powell N, Riley R, Guilleminault C, et al. A reversible uvulopalatal flap for snoring and sleep apnea syndrome. Sleep 1996;19:593–9.
3. Bresalier H, Brandes W. Uvulopalatopharyngoplasty: prevention of complications with the imbrication technique. Ear Nose Throat J 1999;78:920–22.
4. Huntley T. The uvulopalatal flap. Op Tech Otolaryngol Head Neck Surg 2000;11(1):30–35.
5. Neruntarat C. Uvulopalatal flap for snoring on an outpatient basis. Otolaryngol Head Neck Surg 2003;129:353–9.
6. Hormann K, Erhardt T, Hirth K, et al. [Modified uvula flap in therapy of sleep-related breathing disorders]. HNO 2001;49(5):361–66. (article in German).
7. Li H-Y, Li K, Chen N-H, et al. Modified uvulopalatopharyngoplasty: the extended uvulopalatal flap. Am J Otolaryngol 2003;24(5):311–16.

# SECTION I  PALATAL SURGERY

## CHAPTER 35
# Modified uvulopalatopharyngoplasty with uvula preservation

*Han Demin, Ye Jingying and Wang Jun*

## 1 INTRODUCTION

A narrow upper airway is one of the main causes of obstructive sleep apnea/hypopnea syndrome (OSAHS). Uvulopalatopharyngoplasty (UPPP), which ablates both the two tonsils and part of the redundant soft palate to decrease the oropharyngeal obstruction, is still the most widely used surgery. Unfortunately there are about 50% non-responders to UPPP for unselected patients and the classic UPPP has complications such as palatopharyngeal incompetence and palatopharyngeal stenosis. To reduce the UPPP complication rate without compromising the surgical response, the first author designed a new method of UPPP, in which the uvula is preserved, a larger portion of the soft palate is removed, and the basic structure of the oropharyngeal cavity is maintained. This revised UPPP with uvula preservation was first introduced by Han Demin in 2000 and was named Han-UPPP (H-UPPP). H-UPPP is widely used in China and has been proved to be an effective surgical method, causing fewer complications compared with classic UPPP.

## 2 PATIENT SELECTION

### 2.1 INDICATIONS

1. OSAHS patients with the main collapsing sites at the level of oropharynx, which are induced by hypertrophic tonsils, long and enlarged soft palate, and redundant lateral pharyngeal mucosa. For severe OSAHS patients, continuous positive airway pressure (CPAP) should be used in the perioperative period to assure good ventilation.
2. Non-apneic snorers and patients with upper airway resistance syndrome who have oropharyngeal obstruction.

### 2.2 CONTRAINDICATIONS

1. Oropharynx is not the obstruction site.
2. Acute tonsillitis or acute upper airway infections within 2 weeks.
3. Evident risk factors of general anesthesia.
4. Tendency to developing scars.
5. Unstable cardiovascular status or severe cerebrovascular disease.
6. Severe chronic obstructive pulmonary disease.

#### 2.2.1 RELATIVE CONTRAINDICATIONS

1. Severe hypoxemia.
2. Special demands on phonation or speech.
3. Morbid obesity.
4. Older than 65 or younger than 18 years old.

## 3 CLINICAL EVALUATION AND PREOPERATIVE MANAGEMENT

1. An overnight polysomnogram (PSG) should be included to identify the OSAHS patients.
2. Clinical evaluation should include routine vital signs, overall body habitus, facial skeletal pattern and anatomy of the airway. Age, Body Mass Index (BMI), PSG parameters, and anatomy of the pharynx should be documented to help predict responses to the surgery.
3. A detailed upper airway examination should be performed to identify the potential sites of upper airway obstruction. The regions of nose, palate and the tongue base should be highlighted. A computer-assisted fiberoptic pharyngoscopy can be used to evaluate the upper airway characteristics more accurately. Complete occlusion of the upper airway at Mueller's maneuver is a criterion to determine obstruction site. If the obstruction sites are hard to identify by fiberoptic pharyngoscopy

SECTION I PALATAL SURGERY

and radiographic evaluation, an overnight upper airway pressure monitoring and concurrent PSG could be considered to determine the obstruction sites.

4. For severe OSAHS patients (Apnea/Hypopnea Index (AHI) = 40, or the lowest oxygen saturation = 70%), CPAP should be used as early as possible to improve patients' tolerance to anesthesia and surgery. Preoperative CPAP treatment can significantly reduce surgical risks and complications. For those with stubborn hypertension, combined treatment of CPAP and drugs may be effective.

## 4 TECHNIQUES

H-UPPP was carried out under general anesthesia with nasal intubation. The characteristics of H-UPPP are as follows.

- **Anesthesia and tonsillectomy:** Bilateral tonsillectomy is performed first and the redundant bilateral pharyngeal mucosa and submucosal tissue are trimmed or resected to enlarge the oropharyngeal lumen.
- **CO$_2$ laser incision:** Two inverted 'V'-shaped incisions are made on the ventral surface of the soft palate, along both sides of the uvula (see Fig. 35.1).

The upper border of incision and the length of soft palate that should be removed are determined as follows.

1. We found that there are two velum plati spatium along the two sides of palato-uvularis, and the velum plati spatium is between palato-uvularis and the lower margin of both tensor palatini and levator palatini. The spatium is filled with adipose tissue, which is evidently increased in OSAHS patients. The location of velum plati spatium and its adjacent structures is shown in Figures 35.2 and 35.3. On the ventral side of the soft palate, the casting of velum plati spatium borders are about 1–1.5 cm lower than the junction of the hard palate and soft palate, 0.8 cm lateral from the base of uvula.

2. The length of soft palate that should be removed is determined preoperatively according to the anatomy of the patients' pharynx and the severity of sleep apnea (Fig. 35.4). For a moderate sleep apnea patient (AHI 20–40 times/h), the upper border should be as high

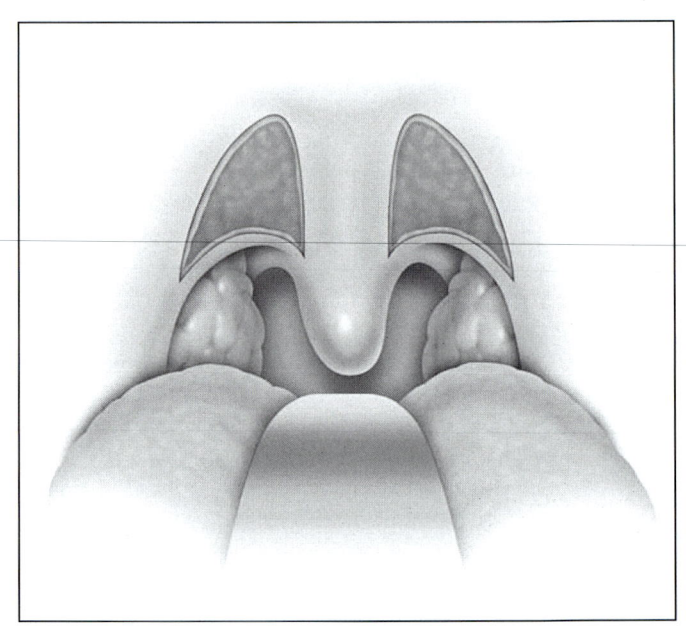

Fig. 35.2 Location of velum plati spatium.

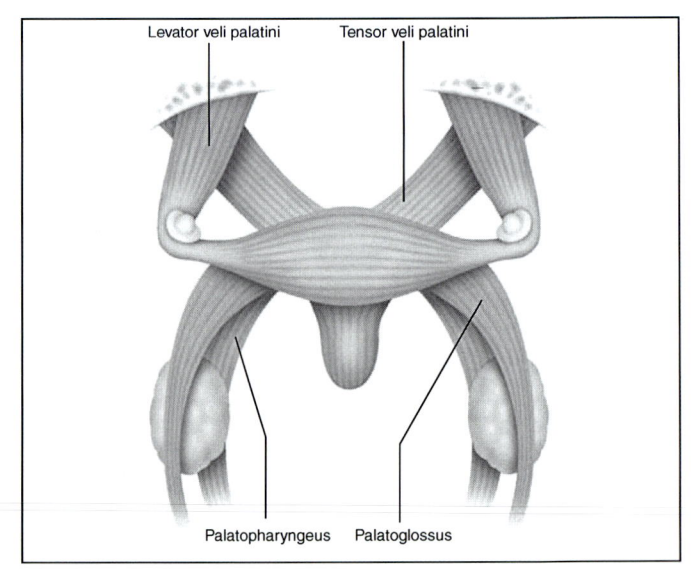

Fig. 35.3 Adjacent structures of velum plati spatium.

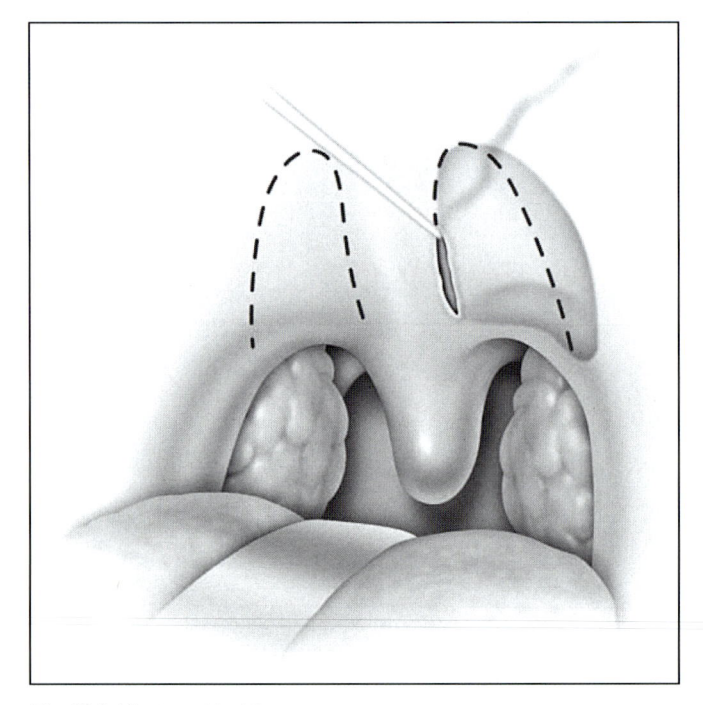

Fig. 35.1 'V'-shaped incisions.

Modified uvulopalatopharyngoplasty with uvula preservation

as the second molar. The incision should be higher in severe patients and lower in mild ones.

3. Once the membrane of the soft palate ventral surface is incised by using the $CO_2$ laser, blunt dissection is used to remove surplus submembranous adipose tissue (Fig. 35.5), i.e. adipose tissue in velum plati spatium. Therefore the tensor palati and palato-uvularis are not damaged.

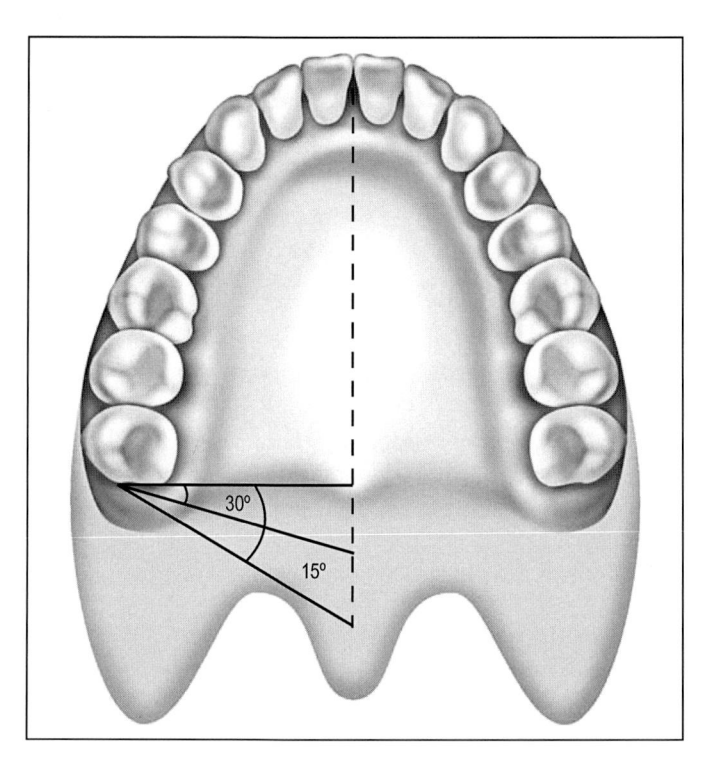

4. The intact margins of the levator palatini and tensor palatini are preserved. The dorsal surface of the soft palate is incised and then trimmed along the uvula bilaterally (Fig. 35.6). The redundant adipose tissue and surplus mucous membrane along the uvularis are removed.

5. The dorsal and ventral margins of the preserved mucosal membrane of the uvula are closed with interrupted sutures, forming a long new uvula. The palatoglossal arch, the soft tissue of the tonsillar fossa and palatopharyngeal arch are also closed with interrupted sutures, so the oropharyngeal cavity is enlarged and the lateral pharyngeal wall is stabilized (Fig. 35.7).

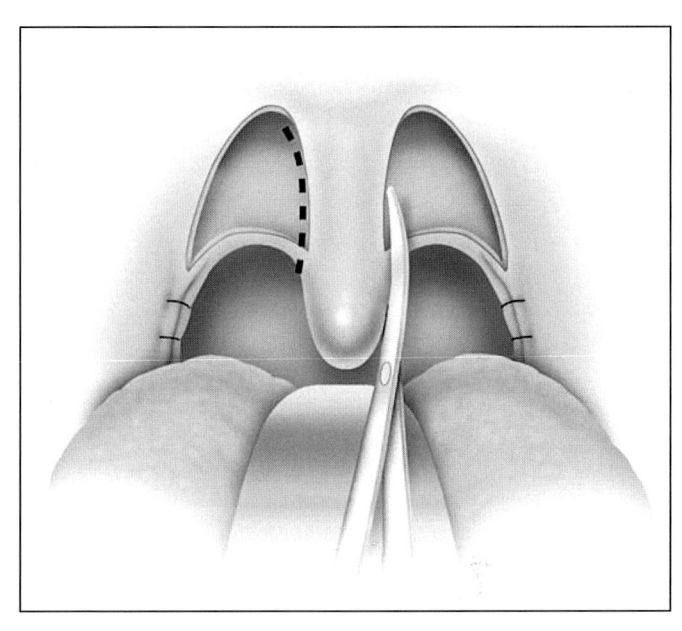

**Fig. 35.4** The upper border of incision in mild, moderate and severe patients.

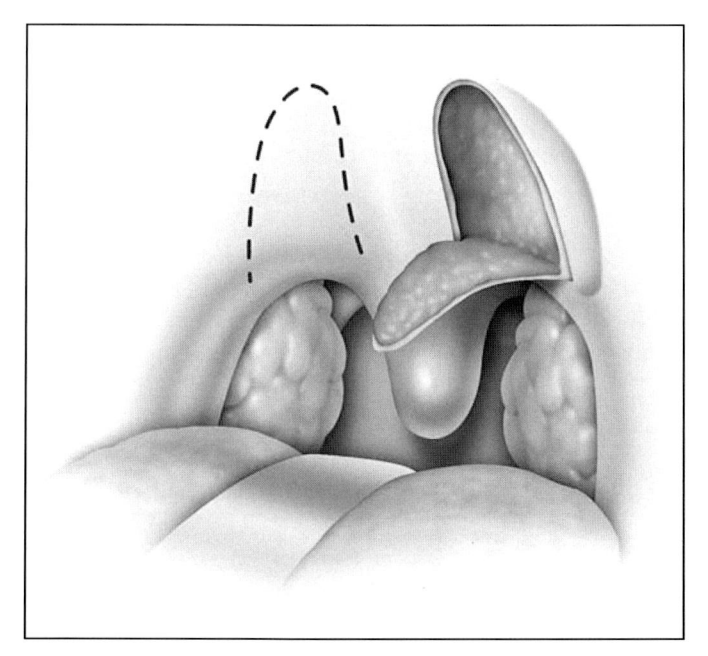

**Fig. 35.5** Removal of surplus submembranous adipose tissue.

**Fig. 35.6** Incision of the dorsal surface of the soft palate.

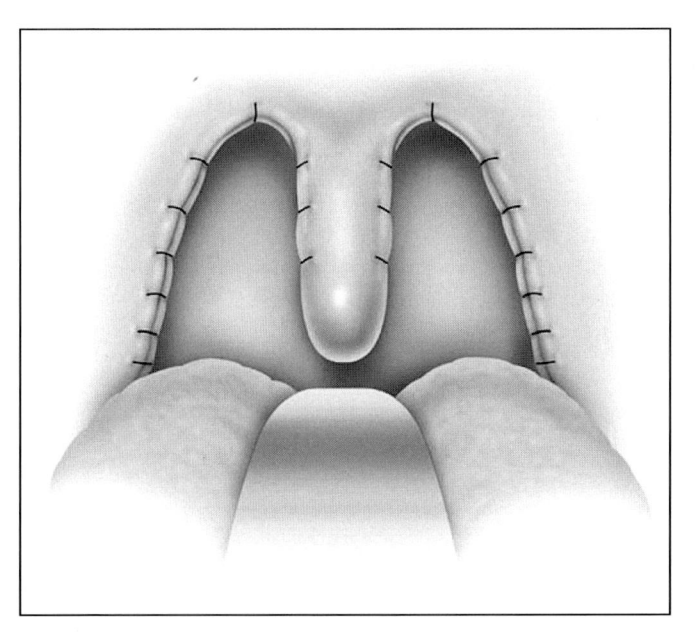

**Fig. 35.7** Oropharyngeal cavity after suture.

# SECTION I: PALATAL SURGERY

## 5 POSTOPERATIVE MANAGEMENT

1. **Medication:** Antibiotics are needed to defend against infection; short-term use of corticosteroids during operation or postoperatively can reduce edema mucosal. Patients who have hypertension should receive antihypertension treatment postoperatively.
2. **Postoperative upper airway obstruction:** Postoperative airway obstruction and asphyxia can be caused by airway edema, bleeding and redundant secretion. The risk of decrease of arterial saturation in oxygen could be enhanced, especially in the first postoperative night. Appropriate monitoring should be employed including vital signs, arterial saturation in oxygen and airway. Secretions should be extracted regularly, and tracheotomy should be performed if needed. Considering their effect of inhibition of ventilatory control, narcotics should be used with caution after general anesthesia for OSAHS patients.
3. **Patients expected to be monitored in the intensive care unit (ICU) postoperatively:**
   - Preoperative lowest oxygen saturation = 70%.
   - AHI = 40 times/h.
   - BMI = 30.1 kg/m$^2$.
   - Tongue base obstruction approved by fiberoptic scope or cephalometry study preoperatively.
   - History of hypertension grade 2 (systolic pressure higher than 150 mm Hg or diastolic pressure higher than 100 mm Hg), angina, or any disorders in hemaglutination.
   - Preoperative electrocardiograph indicated arrhythmia, S-T segment or T wave changes.

   After 24 hours observation in ICU, patients could be transferred to the normal ward if there are no other risk factors. For those who have a severe airway edema or who bleed severely during the operation, the intensive monitoring period should be prolonged.
4. **Postoperative CPAP:** CPAP can improve oxygen saturation, reduce AHI, and reverse sleep debt in OSAHS patients. It also plays a role in expanding the pharynx. If CPAP can be tolerated, CPAP therapy should be started as early as possible and continue for 1–2 months after surgery.
5. **Other measures:** Behavior change has a major role in management and it also affects the long-term surgical outcomes. All obese patients with OSAHS should be counseled about weight loss and cutting down alcohol.

## 6 CLINICAL OUTCOMES AND COMPLICATIONS

### 6.1 THE CONCEPT OF VELUM PLATI SPATIUM

There are two velum plati spatium along the two sides of palato-uvularis, and the velum plati spatium is between palato-uvularis and the lower margin of both tensor palatini and levator palatini. The spatium is filled with adipose tissue, which is evidently increased in OSAHS patients. The clearance of the tissue in velum plati spatium is essential to the improvement of sleep apnea.

### 6.2 THE SIGNIFICANCE OF UVULA PRESERVATION

Fujita first reported the UPPP for treating OSAHS in 1981, and the UPPP has remained the main surgery for OSAHS. Velopharyngeal insufficiency and nasopharyngeal stenosis are two dreaded postoperative complications of UPPP. H-UPPP was designed to allow maintenance of the normal anatomy of the soft palate and the uvula's functions when a larger portion of the soft palate is removed.

The long uvula becomes a 'normal' one through contraction of scar tissue of the soft palate and the bilateral sides of the palato-uvularis and the lower margin of the tensor palatini (Fig. 35.8 A&B). The uvula has important functions like deglutition, respiration, speech and pharyngeal airway dilation. Zakkar found that there is highly concentrated neutral endotryptase in the uvula of normal subjects, but decreased levels in the membrane of the uvula in OSAHS patients, and it is speculated that the uvula is where airflow receptors are distributed. The preservation of the uvula would seem to be very important to maintain the pharyngeal airway muscular tension and normal physiologic functions. To safeguard these important functions, the intact uvularis and its corresponding mucosal membrane (both dorsal and ventral) are preserved. The results show that H-UPPP effectively enlarges the oropharyngeal cavity and avoids some major postoperative complications of classic UPPP.

Velopharyngeal insufficiency can occur if too much tissue is removed. Since the tensor palatini has the function of enlarging the oral cavity, and the levator palatini's function is to pull the soft palate upward and backward, closing the nasopharyngeal cavity during deglutition and phonation, it is important to identify the adipose tissue and muscle, and to keep the levator palatini and the tensor palatini intact. The results of our study show that the uvula's preservation will effectively avoid many significant postoperative complications.

### 6.3 CLINICAL OUTCOMES AND FACTORS INFLUENCING SURGICAL EFFECTIVENESS

It has been reported that successful responders to UPPP amount to 33–77%, but the criteria for patient selection and successful surgical response definitions are not the same between studies. The response rate of H-UPPP

## CHAPTER 35
Modified uvulopalatopharyngoplasty with uvula preservation

degree of the hypertrophic tonsil are relevant to the effectiveness of surgical treatment. Morbid obesity, older age, and tongue base obstruction may play important roles in the failure of H-UPPP. For patients with multilevel obstructive sites, an isolated procedure of H-UPPP may be insufficient. Other surgical techniques should be adopted, such as nasal reconstruction, temperature-controlled radiofrequency tongue base reduction, genioglossus advancement and maxillomandibular advancement.

## FURTHER READING

Demin H, Jingying Y, Jun W, et al. Determining the site of airway obstruction in obstructive sleep apnea with airway pressure measurements during sleep. Laryngoscope 2002;112(11): 2081–85.

Dickson RI, Mintz DR. One-stage laser assisted uvulopalatoplasty. J Otolaryngol 1996;25:155–62.

Esclamado RM, Glenn MG, McCulloch TM, et al. Perioperative complications and risk factors in the surgical treatment of obstructive sleep apnea syndrome. Laryngoscope 1989;99:1125–29.

Fujita S, Convey W, Zorick, F, et al. Surgical correction of anatomic abnormalities in obstructive sleep apnea syndrome: uvulopalatopharyngoplasty. Otolaryngol Head Neck Surg 181:89:923–34.

Han Demin, Ye Jingying, Lin Zhonghui, et al. Revised uvulopalatopharyngoplasty with uvula preservation and its clinical study. J Otorhinolaryngol Relat Spec 2005;67(4):213–19.

Han DM, Ye JY, Li YR, et al. Preoperative overnight airway pressure measurement for predicting the outcome of revised uvulopalatopharyngoplasty. Zhonghua Er Bi Yan Hou Tou Jing Wai Ke Za Zhi 2006;41(10):753–58.

Huang MH, Lee ST, Rajendran K. Structure of the musculus uvulae: functional and surgical implications of an anatomic study. Cleft Palate Craniofac J 1997;34(6):466–74.

Isono S, Remmers JE. Anatomy and physiology of upper airway obstruction. In: Principles and Practice of Sleep Medicine, 3rd edn. Kryger MH, et al., eds. Philadelphia: WB Saunders; 2000, pp. 840–58.

Li YR, Han DM, Ye JY, et al. Sites of obstruction in obstructive sleep apnea patients and their influencing factors: an overnight study. Zhonghua Er Bi Yan Hou Tou Jing Wai Ke Za Zhi 2006;41(6): 437–42.

Loube DI. Uvulopalatopharyngoplasty may compromise nasal CPAP therapy in sleep apnea syndrome. Am J Respir Crit Care Med 1996;154:1759–62.

Meiljetaig H, Mataika S, Haight JS, et al. Subjective and objective assessment of uvulopalatopharyngoplasty for treatment of snoring and sleep apnea. Is J Respir Crit Care Med 1994;150:1286–90.

Mortimore IL, Bradley PA, Murray JAM. Uvulopalatopharyngoplasty may compromise nasal CPAP therapy in sleep apnea syndrome. Is J Respir Crit Care Med 1996;154:1759–62.

Powell N, Riley R, Guilleminault C, Troell R. A reversible uvulopalatal flap for snoring and sleep apnea syndrome. Sleep 1996;19(7): 593–9.

Rennotte MT, Baele P, Aubert G, et al. Nasal continuous positive airway pressure in the perioperative management of patients with obstructive sleep apnea submitted to surgery. Chest 1995;107: 367–74.

Riley RW, Powell NB, Li KK, et al. Surgical therapy for obstructive sleep apnea–hypopnea syndrome. In: Principles and Practice of Sleep Medicine, 3rd edn. Kryger MH, et al., eds. Philadelphia: WB Saunders; 2000, pp. 913–28.

Series F, Cote C, Simoneau JA, Gelinas Y, et al. Physiologic, metabolic, and muscle fiber type characteristics of musculus uvulae in sleep apnea hypopnea syndrome and in snorers. J Clin Invest 1995; 95(1):20–25.

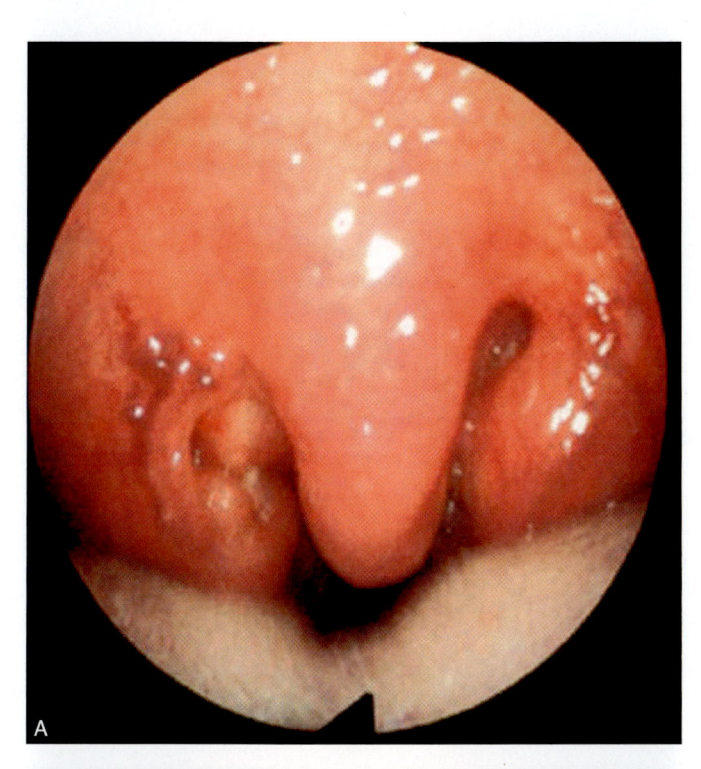

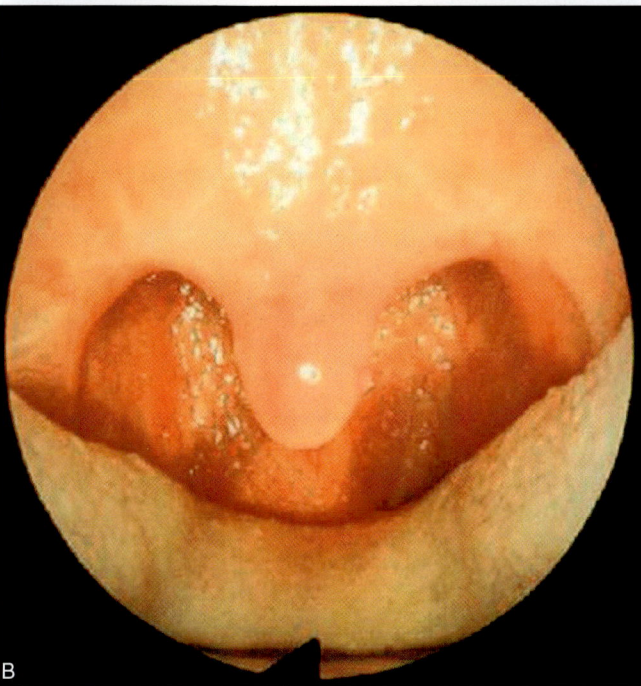

**Fig. 35.8** Comparison of the oropharyngeal cavity before and after H-UPPP. A, Before H-UPPP; B, 3 months after H-UPPP.

was 51.9–69.12%, defined as a >50% reduction of the AHI or AHI < 20/h postoperatively. In patients who have been carefully selected for upper airway reconstruction and whose site of primary obstruction is at the oropharyngeal level, the surgical response rate is 68.57–90%.

Among the non-responders, most are severe OSAHS patients. Some anatomical features of the pharynx such as

Series F, Simoneau JA, St Pierre S. Muscle fiber area distribution of musculus uvulae in obstructive sleep apnea and non-apneic snorers. Int J Obes Relat Metab Disord 2000;24(4):410–15.

Van Duyne J, Coleman JA Jr. Treatment of nasopharyngeal inlet stenosis following uvulopalatopharyngoplasty with the $CO_2$ laser. Laryngoscope 1995;105(9 Pt 1):914–18.

Wang J, Han D, Lin Z, et al. Clinical study of uvulopalatopharyngoplasty treatment for middle degree of obstructive sleep apnea syndromes. Lin Chuang Er Bi Yan Hou Ke Za Zhi 2003;17(2):84–85.

Ye JY, Han DM, Wang J, et al. Computer assisted fiberoptic pharyngoscopy in obstructive sleep apnea syndrome. Chin Arch Otolaryngol Head Neck Surg 2004;11:371–5.

Zakkar M, Sekosan M, Wenig B, et al. Decrease in immunoreactive neutral endopeptidase in uvula epithelium of patients with obstructive sleep apnea. Ann Otol Rhino Laryngol 1997;106:474–77.

# SECTION I PALATAL SURGERY

## CHAPTER 36

# Transpalatal advancement pharyngoplasty

*B. Tucker Woodson*

## 1 INTRODUCTION

The ultimate goal of surgical treatment for obstructive sleep apnea (OSA) is to improve symptoms and eliminate disease morbidity and mortality. This is accomplished by altering airway size, compliance and shape. Successful surgery eliminates collapse, airflow limitation and airway obstruction during sleep. The precise features of successful versus unsuccessful surgery remain poorly understood.

The retropalatal airway segment is a major contributor to airway obstruction in sleep apnea. Although uvulopalatopharyngoplasty (UPPP), as described by Fujita, remains the most common OSA surgery, it suffers from technical failures including inexact patient selection, incorrect and flawed technique, and external factors such as infection. To address palatal failure, a different approach is required.

Transpalatal advancement pharyngoplasty alters the retropalatal airway by advancing the palate forward. Hard palate is excised and a palatal advancement flap is created. It does not require excision of the soft palate. The palate is pulled forward and superior which conceptually is similar to maxillary advancement.

The procedure used alone or in combination with other soft tissue surgeries is indicated for sleep apnea patients having narrowing in the retropalatal airway. It is particularly useful when there is narrowing of the pharyngeal isthmus proximal to the point of palatal excision using traditional UPPP techniques. A transpalatal approach and advancement is also useful for obstructions in the nasopharynx (such as enlarged adenoids) that cannot be accessed through traditional techniques due to the difficult OSA anatomy.

## 2 SURGICAL TECHNIQUE

### 2.1 EVALUATION

Preoperatively, nasopharyngeal endoscopy is currently the primary method of airway evaluation and is performed in both a sitting and supine body position. Features evaluated include size, shape, areas of collapse, and pharyngeal swallow. During endoscopy, close attention is focused on the size and the shape of the proximal pharyngeal isthmus. Narrowing of the airway proximal to this point of estimated excision of traditional UPPP is an indication for primary transpalatal advancement pharyngoplasty. The shape of the pharyngeal isthmus indicates whether narrowing is from anterior–posterior compression (transversely shaped) or from collapse of the lateral walls (sagittally shaped). The locations of the levator muscle and palatopharyngeal sphincter are identified by visualizing the anterior fold of the torus tubarus (torus levatorius) which leads to the position of the levator muscle in the soft palate (Fig. 36.1). A narrow anterior to posterior airway at this level indicates retromaxillary airway narrowing. Such an abnormality cannot be addressed by traditional palatopharyngoplasty without aggressive excision of the levator muscle.

The retropalatal and retromaxillary airway is a fundamental abnormality of adults with sleep apnea. Normal upper airway shape and size must be learned, as well as patterns of stenosis and scarring of the retropalatal segment following palatal or tonsil surgeries. Swallow is also evaluated while performing endoscopy with specific attention to lateral wall motion. Impaired lateral wall motion may increase the risk of swallow dysfunction with any palatal surgery. Patients at high risk of pharyngeal swallowing dysfunction (abnormal endoscopic exam, symptomatic dysphagia, velopharyngeal insufficiency, presbyesophagus, severe reflux and anterior cervical spine surgery) need further swallow evaluation. Fortunately, even in patients who have had prior UPPP, palatal and maxillary advancement are not usually associated with worsening of dysphagia.

Evaluation of the oropalatal airway is also needed. Since the palate relative to the tongue base is pulled forward a small oropalatal airway space may be worsened. This requires additional surgery even if the pharyngeal retroglossal airway space is not severely abnormal. The oropalatal airway is assessed initially with routine oral examination. A modified Malampatti 1 or 2 position indicates excellent oropalatal airway space. Modified Malampatti 3 and 4 have a

# SECTION I
## PALATAL SURGERY

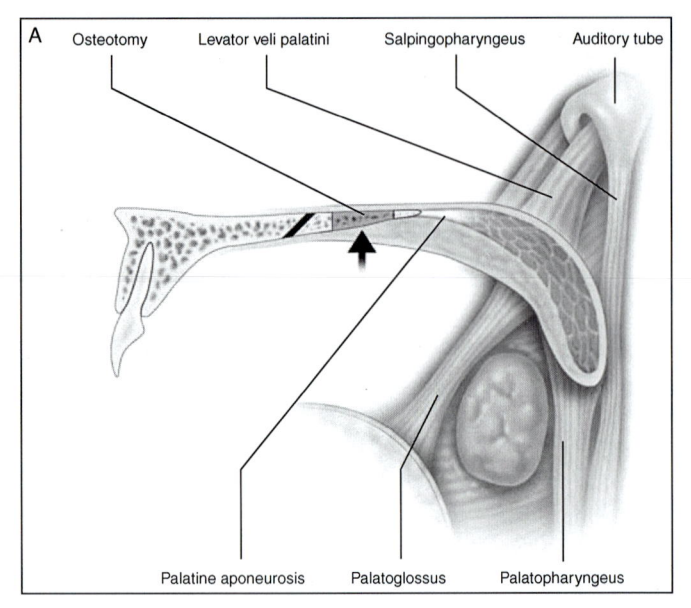

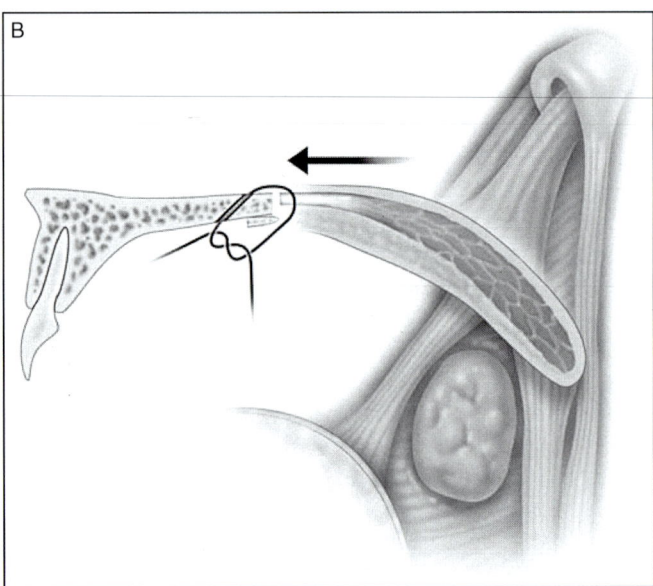

**Fig. 36.1** A, Mid-sagittal depiction of palate anatomy and demonstrating palatal advancement. The location of the palatal aponeurosis close to nasal mucosa is shown. The levator palatine muscle originates at the skull base and passes through the anterior fold of the Eustachian tube (torus levatorius) and into the palate and is a key determinant of palate position relative to the posterior pharyngeal wall. For advancement, drill holes are placed from the oral cavity to the nose anterior to osteotomy. A strong rim of bone supports sutures. The thicker posterior mucosa is shown. The anterior tip of the mucosal incision should be proximal to this and should be placed slightly proximal in the thinner palatal mucosa. B, Mucosa. After osteotomy, sutures are placed through the drill holes and the bone fragment with attached tendon and ligaments is advanced.

compromised oropalatal airway. Those patients with very small oral airways who are primarily mouth breathers need this segment treated prior to palatal surgery.

Contraindications for the procedure include partial or complete cleft palate, swallowing dysfunction with poor lateral wall movement, a large torus palatini (requiring removal prior to advancement), velopharyngeal insufficiency, obligate mouth breathers (may worsen oral breathing), those who have severe gag, or patients unable to accept the recovery from a complication. Maxillary advancement with LeFort osteotomies may in rare circumstances damage the greater palatine vessels and the blood supply to the maxilla. Palatal and tonsil surgery may also impair collateral blood flow to the maxilla and, in the rare event this occurs, increase the risk of avascular necrosis. Those likely to undergo maxillofacial surgery should have this issue discussed. Prior radiation, tissue ablation (sclerotherapy or radiofrequency), and patients with extensive small vessel disease (diabetes, heavy smokers) may increase the risk of wound breakdown. Surgeons should also have adequate resources to address oronasal fistula.

## 2.2 THE PROCEDURE

The procedure may be divided conceptually into steps including: (1) incision; (2) flap elevation; (3) palatal osteotomy; (4) tendinolysis; (5) palate advancement; (6) wound closure; and if needed (7) distal palatopharyngoplasty or tonsillectomy.

The procedure is performed under general anesthesia delivered oro-endotracheally. Patients are placed supine in the Rose position if tonsillectomy is also to be performed, and operative exposure is obtained with a Dingman mouth gag (Pilling Instrument Co., Philadelphia, PA). The Dingman mouth gag facilitates handling of multiple sutures during parts of the procedure, but is not needed for exposure and a normal 'tonsil gag' may also be used. Perioperative antibiotics (cephazolin 1–2g and metronidaizole 500mg) and dexametasone 10mg are administered. For hemostasis, 1% lidocaine with 1:100,000 epinephrine is infiltrated into the exit of the greater palatine foramen, the planned incision sites, the junction of the hard and soft palate, and into the lateral tensor aponeurosis medial to the hamulus. In addition to the injection of the hard and soft palate, nasal mucosa is augmented with oxymetazoline soaked pledgets placed along the floor of the nose which reduce bleeding from the nasal mucosa when placing drill holes and sutures.

### 2.1.1 INCISION, FLAP ELEVATION

See Figure 36.2.

A palatal incision is outlined beginning at the central hard palate posterior to the alveolus. The anterior extent of the flap should extend approximately 5mm anterior to the planned osteotomy. The incision is at the junction of the thinner palatal mucosa and the thicker fibroadipose and muscular layer (Fig. 36.1). The incision goes immediately medial to the greater palatine foramen and is then flared laterally at the junction of the hard and soft palate to

CHAPTER 36 Transpalatal advancement pharyngoplasty

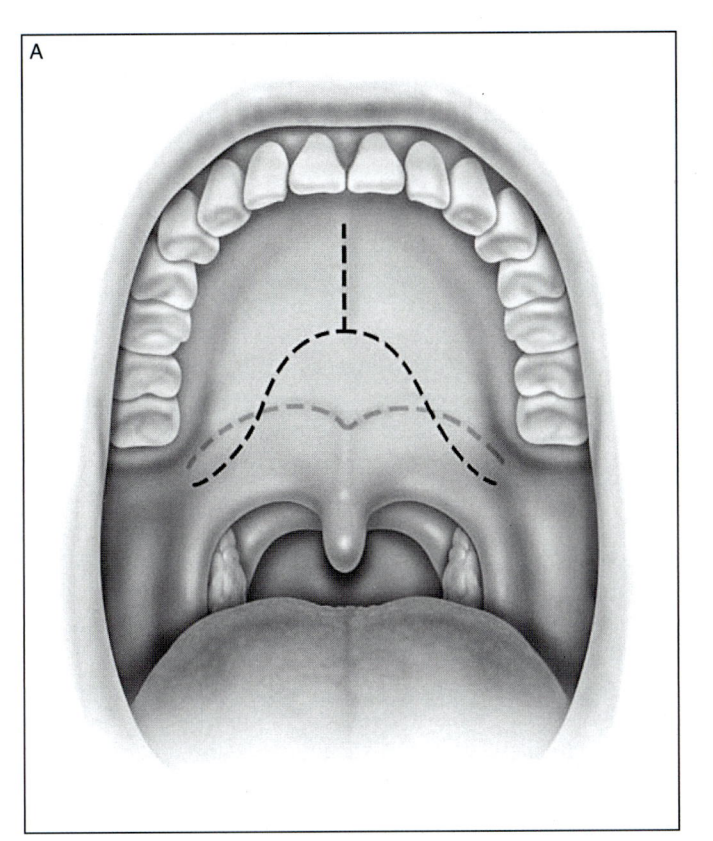

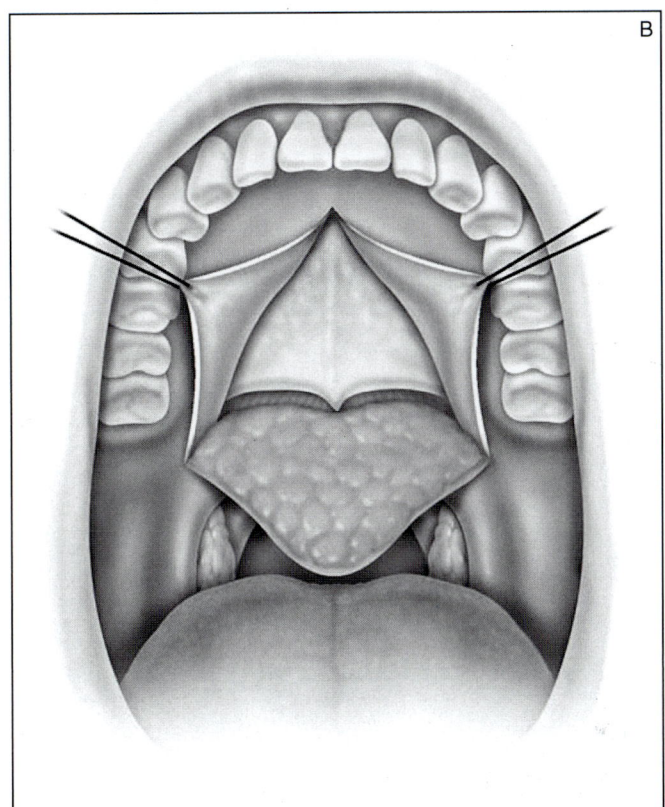

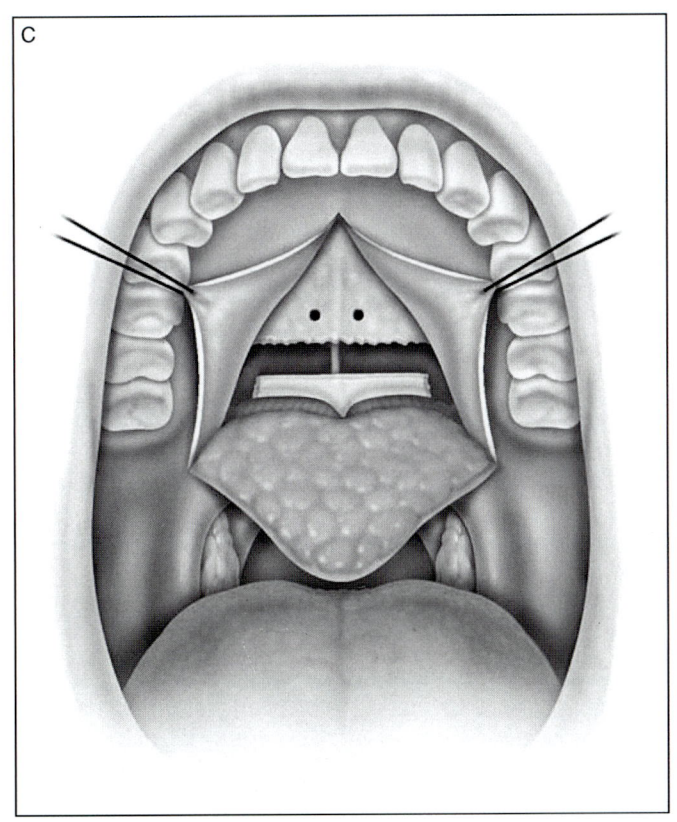

**Fig. 36.2** Diagram of palatal advancement pharyngoplasty. A, Incision placement with the omega shaped incision. Anteriorly, the incision is in thin palate mucosa proximal to anticipated bone removal. The incision is then placed medial to the greater palatine foramen and flares laterally posterior to alveolus towards the hamulus. B, Lateral flaps are elevated. The tip of the midline flap is planned to be 5 mm anterior to bone removal and is elevated just to the junction of the hard and soft palate. Care is taken to not separate the tendon attachments to the hard palate. Posterior elevation is exaggerated in the figure to depict anatomy. C, Sites of osteotomy are shown.

219

extend laterally over the area of the hamulus. This results in a curvilinear 'omega arch' appearance. An additional incision extends vertically up the midline of the hard palate ('T' incision). This allows for laterally based flaps which allow for more lateral and anterior exposure of the hard palate and reduce the need for a longer midline flap which is at risk of tip necrosis.

Lateral flaps are elevated off the bone to expose the proximal hard palate. The midline mucoperiosteal flap is elevated back to the junction of the hard and soft palate. During elevation, the central mucosa is usually thin and care must be taken to avoid tearing it. Laterally and posteriorly, the flap is thicker. Medial and posterior to the greater palatine foramen, the fibroadipose tissue is thicker and it is best bluntly dissected to avoid damage to the greater palatine vessels (a small mastoid curette which has both a curved blunt surface and sharp edge works well). The lesser palatine vessels and nerves may be transected with flap elevation. Bleeding is usually minimal if adequate time for hemostasis has been allotted and postoperatively sensation to the palate returns. Elevation of the flap beyond the border of the soft and hard palate to expose the soft palate is avoided. Care is taken to preserve the tendon and periosteal attachments of the soft palate to the posterior edge of the hard palate. Flap elevation must remain superficial to the tensor aponeurosis.

## 2.1.2 OSTEOTOMY, MOBILIZATION, TENDINOLYSIS, ADVANCEMENT AND CLOSURE

See Figure 36.3.

Two methods have been used to divide the hard and soft palate by separation with an osteotomy. The current method creates a small osteotomized segment that retains the periosteal and ligamentous attachments of the hard and soft palate. This osteotomy take a small additional time to perform but results in a stronger closure. Older methods that simply cut the soft tissue from the bone of the hard palate posterior junction using electrocautery required four to six sutures to close the wound and to advance the palate and were more traumatic to soft tissues. Oronasal fistula rates in the older technique were up to 10% or more. The 'osteotomy method' leaves 1 or 2 mm of bone at the posterior edge with attached periosteal and ligamentous fibers. Closure is stronger with only two sutures.

The hard and soft palates using a distal transverse osteotomy of the posterior hard palate 1–2 mm anterior to the soft palate using a small sagittal saw or drill. Lateral osteotomies are performed far laterally and as close to the alveolus as possible. A dorsal osteotomy with drill or heavy scissors separates the segment from the septum. The lateral and dorsal osteotomies are done with a small rotary burr, small sagittal saw, or heavy scissors. The tensor aponeurosis remains solidly attached to bone.

After the distal osteotomy is performed a posterior 0.5–1.0 cm margin of the hard palate (palatine bone) is removed to provide space to move the soft palate anteriorly.

Bone removal is performed with a rotary drill to remove residual bone and exposes the posterior nasal septum. Mucosa of the floor of the nose is kept intact at this point to allow for easier backwards elevation of the nasal mucosa off the floor of the nose. This elevation allows for the transpalatal sutures to remain submucosal. If not submucosal, there is a small risk of nasal granuloma in the postoperative period. Palatal drill holes are placed at a 45° angle to the palate, extending from the oral surface of the palate into the nasal cavity. A strong segment (3–4 mm) of bone must be left between these drill holes and the excised bony margin. If the procedure is performed with nasotracheal intubation, a small malleable retractor is placed in the floor of the nose for protection and drill holes and use of electrocautery must be done with caution to avoid damage to the tube.

The soft palate must be mobilized, to allow palate advancement. The tensor tendon is incised laterally medial to the insertion on the hamulus. Tendonolysis includes both the tensor tendon and if needed fascial bands of the anterior belly of the levator palatini muscle (Fig. 36.4). Visualizing the nasopharynx is important to identify the lateral nasopharyngeal walls and other landmarks and to avoid inadvertent dissection and trauma into the lateral wall of the nasopharynx. Nasal mucosa is incised (with electrocautery) proximal and lateral to the osteotomy. Fibroadipose tissue is dissected medial to the hamulus to identify the white fibers of the tensor tendon. These are in close proximity to the nasopharyngeal muscosa and tendonolysis is best approached from the dorsal (nasopharyngeal) surface. With sharp or judicious electrocautery dissection, the tensor tendon is identified and cut.

Two sutures (braided) are passed through the drill holes into the nasopharynx and around the osteotomy. Enough soft tissue is grasped with the suture to prevent slippage while tying. Two separate lateral sutures are placed in the tendon and lateral wound. These re-approximate the tensor tendon to the tissues around the hamulus. Identifying and placing sutures in the tendon (aponeurosis) and not just the fibroadipose tissue is critical. Sutures are tied while an assistant pulls the palate forward with a curved blunt instrument.

Excess or redundant tissue of the palate is present after advancement. The posterior flap is thicker than the original hard palate mucosa. Extra mucosa is not trimmed and is preserved for closure. The midline flap may be pulled anteriorly such in a 'V' and 'Y' advancement flap. Since central mucosa is thin and the posterior flap is thick, wide back elevation of the palate mucosa is needed to close the wound. If the midline flap is too thick, a small amount of palatal fibroadipose tissue may be sharply cut to thin the flap. The midline flap is closed with absorbable sutures and this closure especially with an arched hard palate may be technically challenging.

## 2.1.3 DISTAL PALATOPHARYNGOPLASTY

In patients with an anatomically normal palate and uvula, no surgery of the uvula and distal palate is required. In

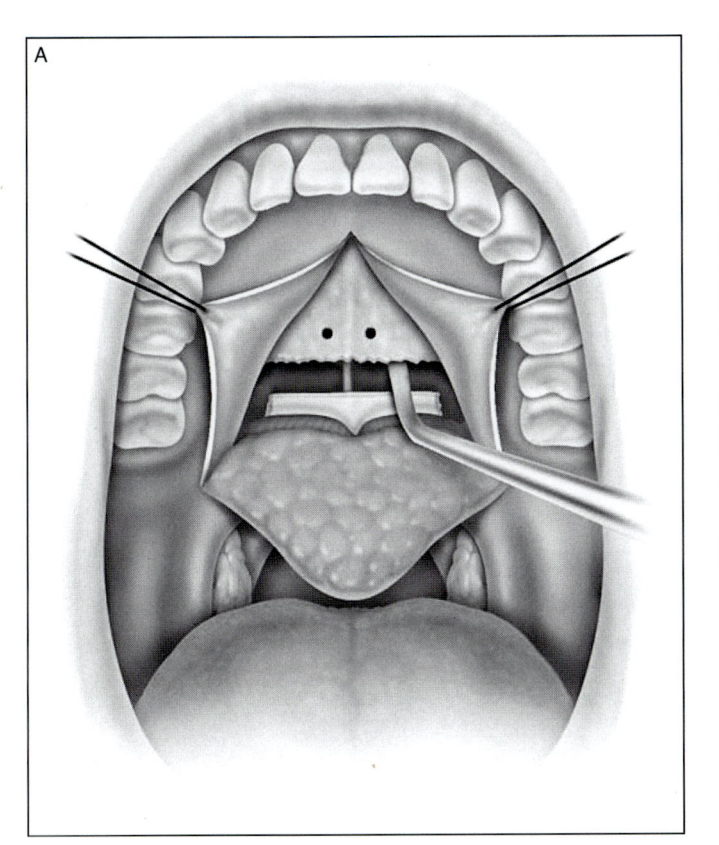

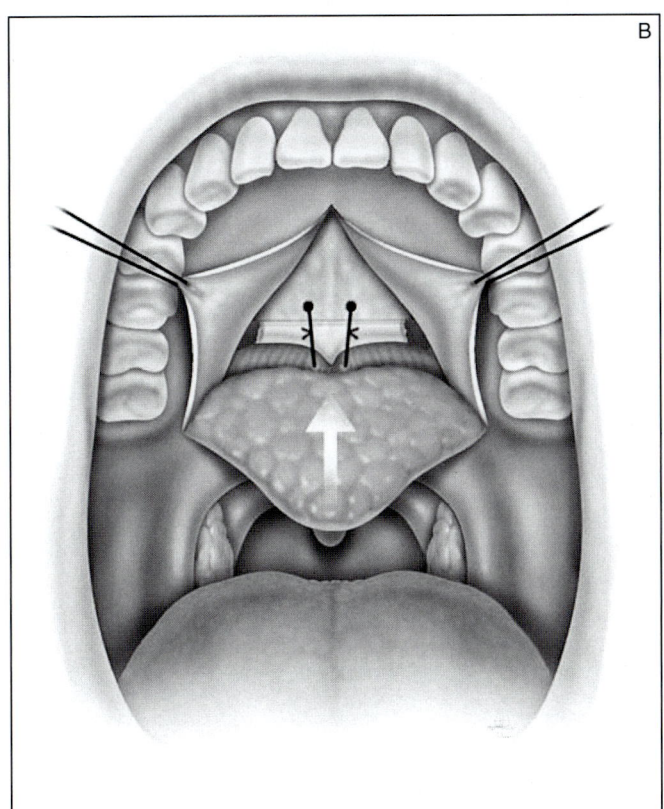

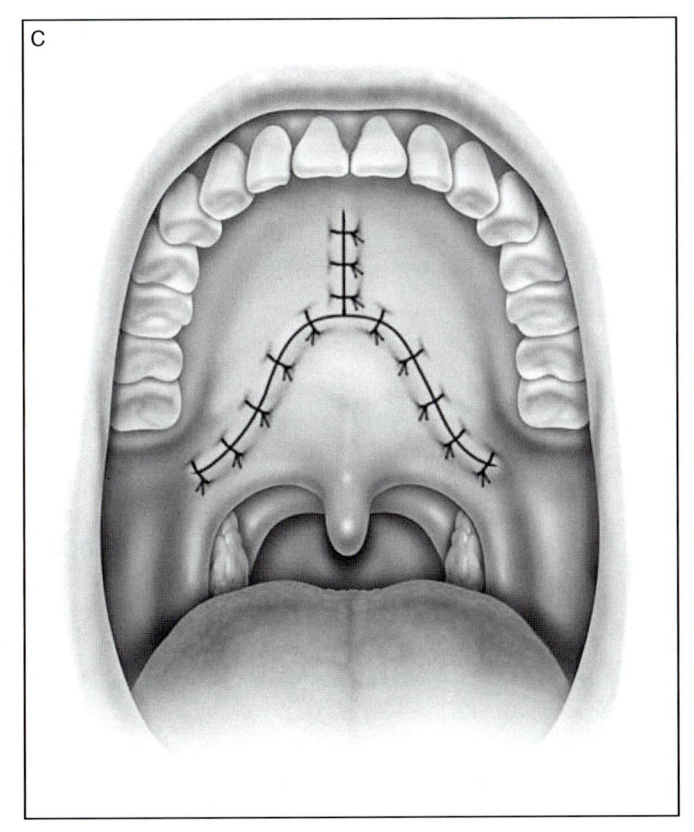

**Fig. 36.3** Diagrammatic procedure of transpalatal advancement pharyngoplasty (continued). A, A posterior osteotomy is performed leaving a 1–2 mm rim of bone. Nasal mucosa is preserved at this point. Proximal drill holes are placed lateral to the septum and medial to the inferior turbinates. The soft and hard palate are separated exposing nasopharynx. The osteotomy is separated from the posterior nasal septum and lateral tendinolysis is performed. B, Sutures are placed through palatal drill holes and around the palatal osteotomy and into the tensor aponeurosis laterally. Posterior traction is used to advance the flap and sutures are tied. C, Mucosa is approximated with multiple interrupted sutures.

# SECTION I  PALATAL SURGERY

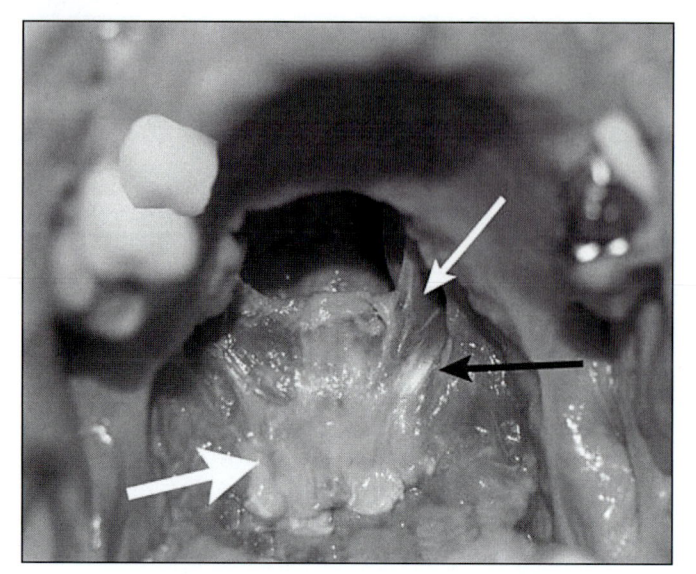

**Fig. 36.4** Anatomical photograph of the tensor tendon. Dissection has incised the hard and soft palate junction and has cut the lateral soft palate attachments. The soft palate has been pulled down (inferiorly) into the oral cavity and nasal and nasopharyngeal mucosa removed. The dorsal nasopharyngeal surface is viewed. Structures include: main belly of levator tensor palatini muscle (small white arrow) emanating from the torus levatorius, anterior belly of the levator muscle (black arrow) with fascial bands inserting on the palatine aponeurosis (large white arrow).

patients with redundant palate, pillar mucosa, uvula, or tonsils, conservative surgery to tighten or remove this tissue may be needed with or without a tonsillectomy. In many patients, palatal advancement is performed after UPPP failure. In these or other cases pharyngeal stenosis may be present and scar release with conservative lateral pharyngoplasty or Z-plasty pharyngoplasty may be needed.

## 3 POSTOPERATIVE CARE AND COMPLICATIONS

A soft diet is begun on the first day. The use of an upper denture is avoided for at least 4 weeks, or until healing is completed. If wound breakdown is noted, an upper palatal splint to cover all or even part of the defect is used. If a splint is used, fistulas close. Attempts at secondary closure without a splint do not succeed. Splints may be easily fashioned (dentist, dental lab, other) and worn with minimal impairment until healing has been achieved. Temporary sutures placed in the office using only local anesthesia may hold for several days and will relieve tension on the wound and speed closure. These can be placed through the transpalatal drill holes and into the soft palate in the office and can be replaced as needed.

Broad-spectrum perioperative antibiotics are used for 3–7 days. Perioperative steroids are given to reduce pain, postoperative nausea, and edema for 1–3 days. To avoid compressions of the palatal flap, dentures are avoided for 4–6 weeks. Due to the change in palatal shape with advancement, dentures likely need to be refit, modified, or replaced. A soft diet for 2 weeks decreases tension with swallow and gag. Close observation for development of oronasal fistula allows for early intervention and use of palatal splint.

Postoperatively, velopharyngeal insufficiency (VPI) has been rare. One case following aggressive UPPP is known to have occurred and was resolved with partial suture release. As with UPPP, transient symptoms of mild nasopharyngeal reflux or dysphagia may occur immediately postoperatively. Changes in pharyngeal volume or shape may alter triggering of swallow or may decrease bolus pressures and contribute to delayed pharyngeal clearance. Palatal flap necrosis and oronasal fistula may occur.

## 4 RESULTS

Early experience observed significant reductions in Apnea/Hypopnea Index (AHI) and Apnea Index (AI). A 67% successful response rate with a Respirators Disturbance Index (RDI) of less than 20 events/hour was observed in patients who only underwent transpalatal advancement.[1–4] RDI in the responder group decreased from 52.8 to 12.3 events/hour. Seven of 11 patients (64%) had RDI reduced to less than 20 events/hour. Increased retropalatal size and decreased compliance have been observed. Photographic evaluation demonstrated increased velopharyngeal anterior posterior dimension and enlargement of the lateral pharyngeal ports.

More recently a controlled study compared a cohort of patients with palatal advancement to a matched historical group of UPPP patients who were all staged as Friedman stage 3. This group would be predicted to have an 8% success rate with UPPP alone. The palatal advancement group demonstrated significant improvement over UPPP. Controlling for Body Mass Index, tongue base surgery, age, and presurgical AHI, the odds ratio of success using palatal advancement over UPPP was 5.77 (95% CI of 1.80–17.98).

Scar tissue formation is less with palatal advancement and acute changes in snoring may also be less than UPPP or laser-assisted palatopharyngoplasty. In many cases, when apnea and airflow limitation are resolved snoring dramatically improves. If snoring persists, this has been successfully treated postoperatively with ancillary snoring procedures such as radiofrequency or implants.

## 5 CONCLUSIONS

Transpalatal advancement pharyngoplasty offers a potential alternative to aggressive UPPP in an attempt to enlarge the upper oropharyngeal airway and improve respiratory function. With this procedure the soft palate is mobilized, not excised, and enlargement occurs with advancement. This advancement affects both the upper and lateral pharyngeal airway. Since palatal advancement alters only a portion of the airway, comprehensive treatment is still required.

## REFERENCES

1. Zohar Y, Finkelstein Y, Strauss M, et al. Surgical treatment of obstructive sleep apnea: comparison of techniques. Arch Otolaryngol Head Neck Surg 1993;119:1023–9.
2. Ryan CF, Love LL. Unpredictable results of laser assisted uvulopalatoplasty in the treatment of obstructive sleep apnoea. Thorax 2000;55:399–404.
3. Blumen MB, Dahan S, Wagner I, et al. Radiofrequency versus LAUP for the treatment of snoring. Otolaryngol Head Neck Surg 2002;126:67–73.
4. Riley RW, Powell NB, Guilleminault C. Obstructive sleep apnea syndrome: a review of 306 consecutively treated surgical patients. Otolaryngol Head Neck Surg 1993;108:117–25.

## FURTHER READING

Aboussouan LS, Bolish JA, Wood BG, et al. Dynamic pharyngoscopy in predicting outcome of uvulopalatopharyngoplasty for moderate and severe obstructive sleep apnea. Chest 1995;107:941–46.
Caballero P, Alvarez-Sala R, Garcia-Rio F. CT in the evaluation of the upper airway in healthy subjects and in patients with obstructive sleep apnea syndrome. Chest 1998;113:111–16.
Friedman M, Ibrahim H, Bass L. Clinical staging for sleep-disordered breathing. Otolaryngol Head Neck Surg 2002;127:13–21.
Fujita S, Conway W, Zorick F, et al. Surgical correction of anatomic abnormalities of obstructive sleep apnea syndrome: uvulopalatopharyngoplasty. Otolaryngol Head Neck Surg 1981;89:923–34.
Ikematsu T. Palatopharyngoplasty and partial uvulectomy method of Ikematsu: a 30 year clinical study of snoring. In: Snoring and Sleep Apnea, 1st edn. Fairbanks DNL, Fujita S, Ikematsu T, Simmons FB, eds. New York: Rivlin Press; 1987, pp. 130–34.
Katsantonis GP, Moss K, Miyazaki S, et al. Determining the site of airway collapse in obstructive sleep apnea with airway pressure monitoring. Laryngoscope 1993;103:1126–31.
Li KK, Troell RJ, Riley RW, Powell NB, Koester U, Guilleminault C. Uvulopalatopharyngoplasty, maxillomandibular advancement, and the velopharynx. Laryngoscope 2001;111:1075–78.
Morrison DL, Launois SH, Isono S, et al. Pharyngeal narrowing and closing pressures in patients with obstructive sleep apnea. Am Rev Respir Dis 1993;148:606–11.
Shepard JW, Thawley SE. Localization of upper airway collapse during sleep in patients with obstructive sleep apnea. Am Rev Respir Dis 1990;141:1350–55.
Sher AE, Schechtman KB, Piccirillo JF. The efficacy of surgical modifications for the upper airway in adults with obstructive sleep apnea syndrome. Sleep 1996;19:156–77.
Skatvedt O. Continuous pressure measurements in the pharynx and esophagus during sleep in patients with obstructive sleep apnea syndrome. Laryngoscope 1992;102:1275–80.
Skatvedt O, Akre H, Godtlibsen OB. Continuous pressure measurements in the evaluation of patients for laser assisted uvulopalatoplasty. Eur Arch Otorhinolaryngol 1996;253:390–94.
Woodson BT. Retropalatal airway characteristics in UPPP compared to transpalatal advancement pharyngoplasty. Laryngoscope 1997;107:735–40.
Woodson BT. Acute effects of palatopharyngoplasty on airway collapsibility. Otolaryngol Head Neck Surg 1999;121:82–86.
Woodson BT, Toohill RJ. Transpalatal advancement pharyngoplasty for obstructive sleep apnea. Laryngoscope 1993;103:269–76.
Woodson BT, Wooten MR. Manometric and endoscopic localization of airway obstruction after uvulopalatopharyngoplasty. Otolaryngol Head Neck Surg 1994;111:38–43.
Woodson BT, Robinson S, Lim HJ. Transpalatal advancement pharyngoplasty outcomes compared to uvulopalatopharyngoplasty. Otolaryngol Head Neck Surg 2005;133:211–17.

SECTION I  PALATAL SURGERY

# CHAPTER 37
# Expansion sphincter pharyngoplasty

*Kenny P. Pang and B. Tucker Woodson*

## 1 INTRODUCTION

Snoring results from the vibration of the soft tissues in the oral cavity – the soft palate, uvula, tonsils, base of tongue, epiglottis and lateral pharyngeal walls. These vibrating soft tissues when subjected to negative pressure within the upper airway may lead to collapse of the upper airway. It is known that when inspiratory transpharyngeal pressure exceeds the pharyngeal dilating muscle action, apneas and hypopneas occur.[1] Collapse of the upper airway is usually multilevel, at the level of the velopharynx, the base of tongue, and the lateral pharyngeal walls. Many patients with obstructive sleep apnea (OSA) have bulky thick lateral pharyngeal walls that vibrate and contribute to the collapse of the upper airway in these patients. The level of collapse is assessed using the Mueller maneuver recorded with fiberoptic flexible nasopharyngoscopy. The Mueller maneuver is usually graded on a five-point scale, 0 to 4.[2] Terris et al. described the Mueller maneuver finding based on three levels: soft palatal collapse, lateral pharyngeal wall collapse and base of tongue collapse.[3] Lateral pharyngeal muscle wall collapse has been demonstrated to be important in the pathogenesis of OSA in imaging studies.[4,5] It is well known that lateral pharyngeal wall collapse plays a significant role in the pathogenesis of OSA. Most authors concur that it is difficult to create, surgically, adequate lateral pharyngeal wall tension to prevent its collapse.

Lateral pharyngoplasty, first described by Cahali,[1] was aimed at addressing lateral pharyngeal wall collapse in patients with OSA. The procedure showed promising results; however, many patients had prolonged dysphagia postoperatively.

The ideal procedure would involve one that is easy to perform, with low morbidity, minimal complications and not requiring any special equipment.

Orticochea[6] first described the construction of a dynamic muscle sphincter, by isolating the palatopharyngeus muscle and transposing it bilaterally, superiorly in the midline, for treatment of velopharyngeal incompetence in patients with cleft palates. Christel et al.[7] modified Orticochea's procedure, by isolating the palatopharyngeus muscle bilaterally, apposing it more superiorly and closing the lateral pharyngeal defects with Z-plasty sutures. Utilizing these procedures, the authors present an innovative technique in creating this tension in the lateral pharyngeal walls, preventing its collapse and reducing the number of apneic episodes. The expansion sphincter pharyngoplasty basically consists of a tonsillectomy, expansion pharyngoplasty, and rotation of the palatopharyngeus muscle, a partial uvulectomy and closure of the anterior and posterior tonsillar pillars.

## 2 PATIENT SELECTION

The authors conducted a prospective randomized clinical trial in 45 adults, age above 18 years old, who have mainly type I Fujita (retropalatal obstruction) and lateral pharyngeal wall collapse. The inclusion criteria included patients with small tonsils (tonsil size 1 and 2), Body Mass Index (BMI) < 30, and Friedman clinical stage II and III who had failed or cannot tolerate nasal continuous positive airway pressure (CPAP) therapy. The clinical examination included height, weight, neck circumference, BMI, and assessment of the nasal cavity, posterior nasal space, oropharyngeal area, soft palatal redundancy, uvula size and thickness, tonsillar size and Friedman tongue position. Flexible nasoendoscopy was performed for all patients, and collapse during a Mueller's maneuver was graded for the soft palate, lateral pharyngeal walls and base of tongue on a five-point scale.[3] These patients were randomized into either the traditional uvulopalatopharyngoplasty (UPPP) procedure or the expansion sphincter pharyngoplasty (ESP). The mean follow-up time was 6.5 months. All patients had a postoperative polysomnogram at 6 months.

## 3 SURGICAL TECHNIQUE

The procedure is done under general anesthesia, with the patient in the supine position. The authors perform the procedure with orotracheal intubation, and a Boyle–Davis mouth gag within the oral cavity keeping the mouth open, and isolating the endotracheal tube forwards. A bilateral tonsillectomy is performed (Fig. 37.1). The palatopharyngeus muscle is identified; its inferior end is transected horizontally (Fig. 37.2). The muscle is isolated and left with its posterior surface partially attached to the posterior horizontal superior pharyngeal constrictor muscles (Fig. 37.3). It is rotated superolaterally with a figure 8 suture, through the muscle bulk itself, with a Vicryl 3/0 round body needle. A superolateral incision is made on the anterior pillar arch bilaterally, identifying the arching fibers of the palatoglossus muscles (Fig. 37.4). The palatopharyngeus muscle is then attached to the arching fibers of the soft palate anteriorly and a partial uvulectomy is then performed (Fig. 37.5). The anterior and posterior tonsillar pillars are then apposed with Vicryl sutures (Fig. 37.6). The same steps are repeated on the opposite side. This new technique of expansion sphincter pharyngoplasty was modified from the Orticochea procedure and lateral pharyngoplasty. The principle of this technique is to isolate the palatopharyngeus muscle (the main part of the lateral pharyngeal wall bulk) and rotate this muscle supero-anterolaterally, in order to create the lateral wall tension and remove the bulk of the lateral pharyngeal walls. The key is to not completely isolate the muscle into a tube and rotate it, but rather to keep part of its fibrous attachment to the superior pharyngeal constrictor muscle, so as to create the necessary

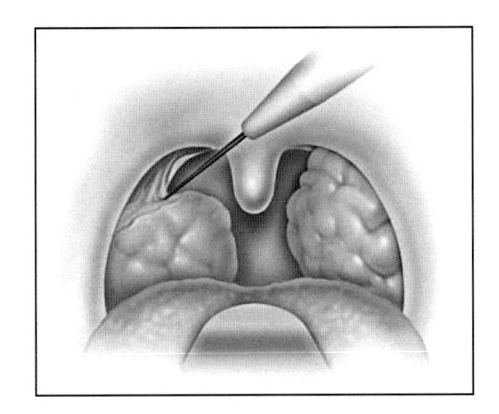

**Fig. 37.1**

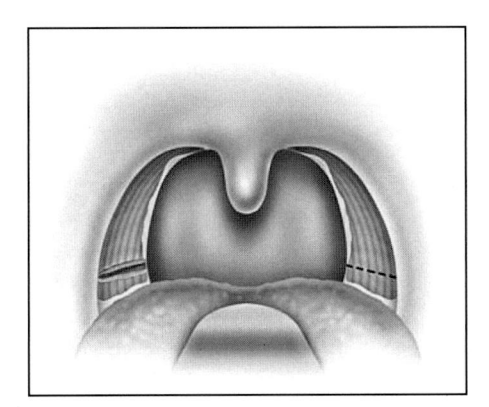

**Fig. 37.2**

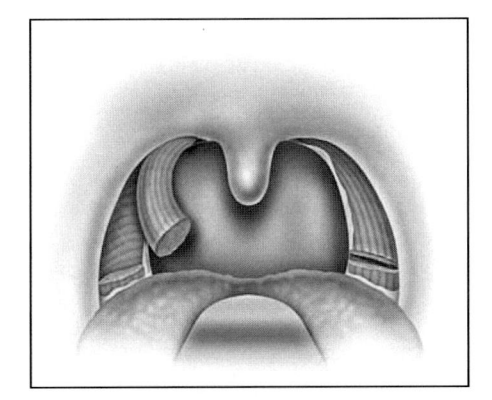

**Fig. 37.3**

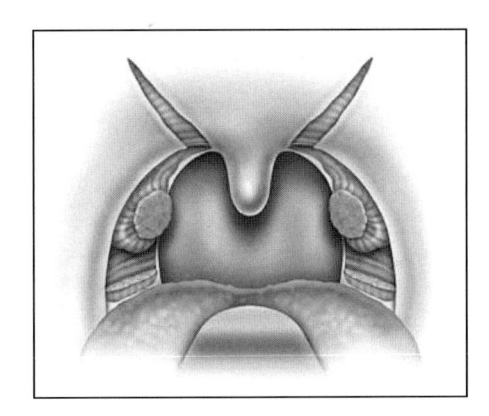

**Fig. 37.4**

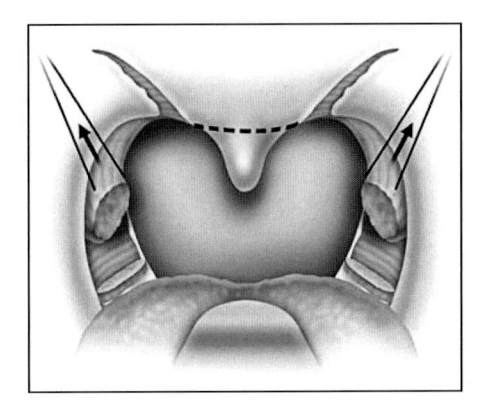

**Fig. 37.5**

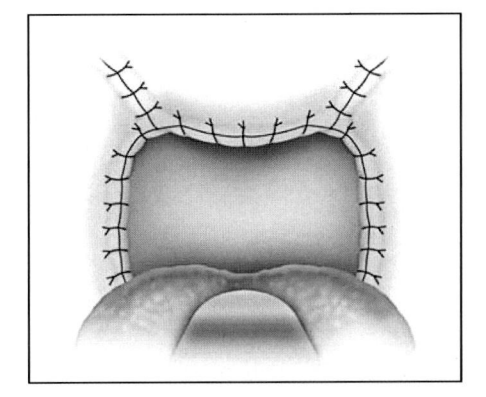

**Fig. 37.6**

tension and pull supero-anterolaterally. A complete or partial uvulectomy is performed together with this procedure.

There are no significant complications; primary or secondary hemorrhages are not increased and are rare; fistulations of the soft palate and oral infections hardly occur.

## 4 POSTOPERATIVE MANAGEMENT AND COMPLICATIONS

All patients were monitored in the postanesthesia care unit for 4 hours before being transferred to the high-dependency ward for overnight monitoring. Monitoring included continuous pulse oximetry, blood pressure and pulse rate. They were given adequate analgesia, in the form of anesthetic gargles (Difflam) and lozenges (Difflam), non-steroidal anti-inflammatory agents (naproxen sodium), and cyclo-oxygenase-2 inhibitors. Most patients were discharged on the first postoperative day. All patients were advised to have adequate oral fluid hydration and a soft blended diet in the first postoperative week. There were no complications from this procedure; there was no primary or secondary hemorrhage; and there were neither fistulae of the soft palate nor any oral infections.

## 5 SUCCESS RATE OF PROCEDURE

There were 45 patients enrolled (22 UPPP, 23 ESP). Forty-one patients were men and four were women. The mean age was 42.1 years (range of 24 to 47 years), the mean BMI was 28.7 (range of 21.7 to 29.8). The mean preoperative Apnea/Hypopnea Index (AHI) for the entire group improved from $42.3 \pm 17.1$ to $19.2 \pm 12.0$ postoperative with a mean follow-up of 6.5 months. The AHI improved from $44.2 \pm 10.2$ to $12.0 \pm 6.6$ ($P < 0.005$) following ESP and from $38.1 \pm 6.46$ to $19.6 \pm 7.9$ in the UPPP group ($P < 0.005$). Mean change was $27.5 \pm 8.4$ in ESP and $18.5 \pm 7.6$ in the UPPP group. Lowest oxygen saturation improved similarly from $78.4 \pm 8.52$ to $85.2 \pm 5.1$ in the ESP group ($P = 0.003$) and from $75.1 \pm 5.9$ to $86.6 \pm 2.2$ in the UPPP group ($P < 0.005$). Selecting an arbitrary threshold of a 50% reduction in AHI and AHI < 20, success was 82.6% in ESP compared to 68.1% in UPPP ($P < 0.05$). Of great interest, when selecting an arbitrary threshold of a 50% reduction in AHI and AHI < 15, the ESP success rate was at 78.2%, compared to that of the UPPP group at only 45.5%. Postoperative endoscopic findings demonstrated significant reduction of lateral pharyngeal wall collapse in the ESP group.

The lateral pharyngoplasty technique, described by Cahali, showed that ten patients with moderate to severe OSA, and who had mainly lateral pharyngeal wall collapse noted on clinical endoscopic examination, had promising results.[1] All ten patients had improvements in their AHI, with a mean of 45.8, reducing to 15.2 ($P = 0.009$) postoperatively, with a mean follow-up of 8 months. There was also improvement in Apnea Index (AI), with a reduction from a mean of 22.4 to 4.8 ($P = 0.005$). There were, however, significant swallowing problems in all ten patients who underwent this procedure. All patients had dysphagia; this ranged from 8 days to 70 days postoperatively (mean 20.4 days). One patient had persistent velopharyngeal insufficiency for up to 6 weeks. Another patient had permanent loss of taste for chocolate for 6 months. Cahali et al.[9] compared lateral pharyngoplasty with the traditional uvulopalatopharyngoplasty in 27 patients with OSA. All 15 patients who underwent lateral pharyngoplasty achieved significant reduction in excessive daytime sleepiness, AHI and AI. There were also improvements in the REM sleep percentage and morning headaches in patients who had lateral pharyngoplasty, compared to those who underwent the traditional uvulopalatopharyngoplasty. They concluded that patients who underwent the lateral pharyngoplasty technique have better clinical and polysomnographic results.

This new technique of expansion sphincter pharyngoplasty may offer benefit over traditional methods of UPPP in a selected group of OSA patients with small tonsils, Friedman Stage II and III and lateral pharyngeal wall collapse noted on endoscopic examination. The procedure has promising results, it is anatomically sound, and has minimal complications.

## REFERENCES

1. Cahali MB. Lateral pharyngoplasty: a new treatment for OSAHS. Laryngoscope 2003;113:1961–68.
2. Borowiecki BD, Sassin JF. Surgical treatment of sleep apnoea. Arch Otolaryngol 1983;109:506–12.
3. Terris DJ, Hanasono MM, Liu YC. Reliability of the Mueller maneuver and its association with sleep-disordered breathing. Laryngoscope 2000;110:1819–23.
4. Remmers JE, De Groot WJ, Sauerland EK, Anch AM. Pathogenesis of upper airway occlusion during sleep. J Appl Physiol 1978;44:931–8.
5. Schwab RJ, Gefter WB, Hoffman EA, et al. Dynamic upper airway imaging during awake respiration in normal subjects and patients with sleep disordered breathing. Am Rev Respir Dis 1993;148:1385–400.
6. Orticochea M. Construction of a dynamic muscle sphincter in cleft palates. Plast Reconstr Surg 1968;41:323–27.
7. Christel SR, Georges B, Christel D, Jacques L, Bernard R, Patrick L, Jean-Louis P. Sphincter pharyngoplasty as a treatment of velopharyngeal incompetence in young people. Chest 2004;125:864–71.
8. Schwab RJ, Gupta KB, Gefter WB, et al. Upper airway and soft tissue anatomy in normal subjects and patients with sleep disordered breathing: significance of the lateral pharyngeal walls. Am J Respir Crit Care Med 1995;152:1673–89.
9. Cahali MB, Formigoni GG, Gebrim EM, Miziara ID. Lateral pharyngoplasty versus uvulopalatopharyngoplasty: a clinical, polysomnographic and computed tomography measurement comparison. Sleep 2004;27(5):844–6.

SECTION I   PALATAL SURGERY

CHAPTER 38

# Lateral pharyngoplasty

*Michel Burihan Cahali*

## 1 INTRODUCTION

We call lateral pharyngoplasty (LP) the surgical splint of the lateral pharyngeal walls, achieved by turning the superior pharyngeal constrictor muscles (SPC) into dilating flaps. The lateral pharyngeal muscular walls are thickened and exceedingly collapsible during respiration in patients with obstructive sleep apnea/hypopnea syndrome, causing narrowing of the pharynx. The SPC muscles envelop all the collapsible segment of the pharynx and form the outer pharyngeal muscular layer.

## 2 PATIENT SELECTION

Currently, we are using the LP procedure to treat patients with increased upper airway resistance during sleep, either socially unacceptable simple snorers, or patients with obstructive sleep apnea/hypopnea syndrome who failed to tolerate or refused non-surgical therapy. The severity of the disease does not influence the selection.

Good candidates for the procedure are those who have a clearly defined, bulky posterior tonsillar pillar (palatopharyngeus muscle) with a soft palate that does not touch the posterior pharyngeal wall while the subject is sitting and awake. In addition, modified Malampatti type 1 or 2, large tonsils and easily visible vocal folds when the tip of a fiberoptic endoscope is positioned in the nasopharynx represent favorable anatomic conditions for this approach. The longer the distance between the soft palate and the tongue, the easier the surgical approach to the SPC muscles.

So far, morbid obesity and gross maxillary or mandible deformities are exclusionary criteria for the procedure. Patients with a Body Mass Index between 35 and 40 kg/m$^2$ should have favorable anatomic conditions present to be considered for the procedure.

We have only carried out LP in individuals over 18 years of age. We speculate that this procedure might be suitable for adolescents presenting an adult pattern of upper airway resistance during sleep.

## 3 SURGICAL TECHNIQUE

The procedure is performed with the patient under general anesthesia, using a mouth gag with a long tongue blade to give adequate exposure (Fig. 38.1). We use 4.0 Vicryl for all sutures. LP is performed as a stand-alone treatment for snoring and sleep apnea. When the patient needs nasal surgery to improve nasal breathing, this can be done in combination with LP. Fourteen per cent of our cases were treated with both LP and nasal surgery together.

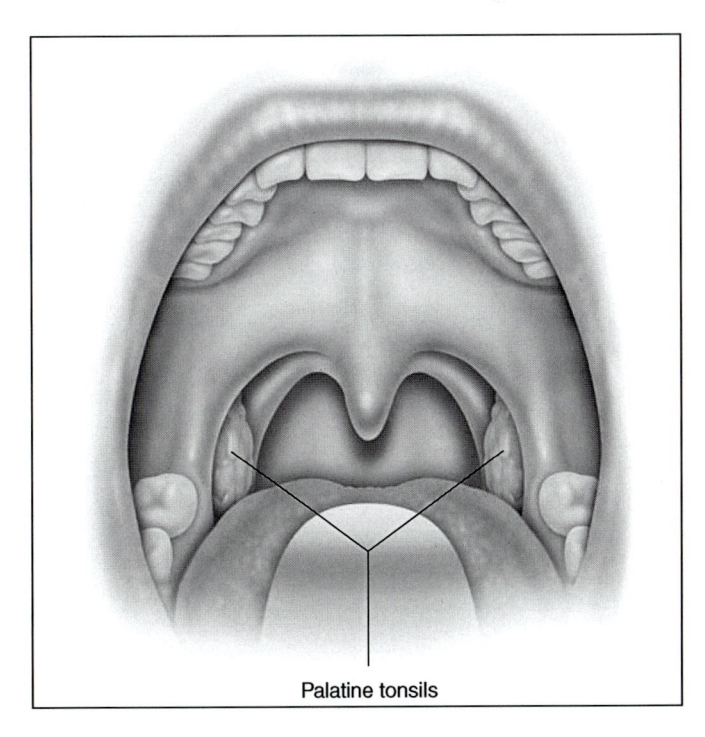

**Fig. 38.1** Initial exposure.

# SECTION I PALATAL SURGERY

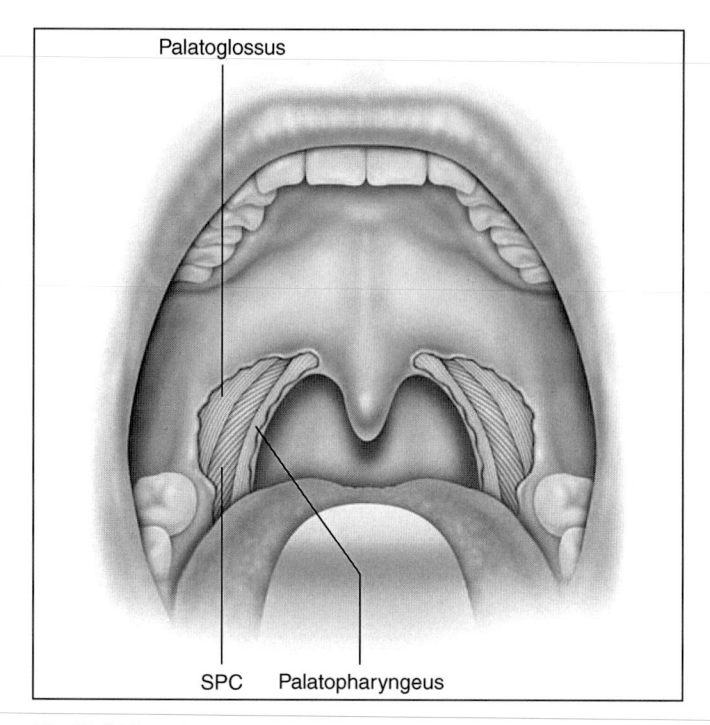

**Fig. 38.2** View after bilateral tonsillectomy, showing palatoglossus muscle, superior pharyngeal constrictor (SPC) muscle and palatopharyngeus muscle.

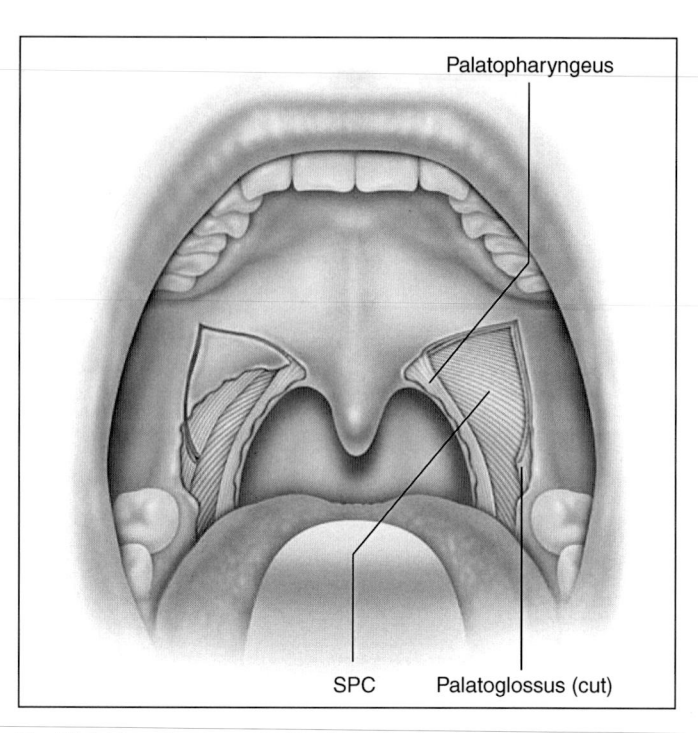

**Fig. 38.4** View after removal of the incised soft palate and palatoglossus muscle, showing SPC muscle, palatopharyngeus muscle, and the remnants of the palatoglossus muscle.

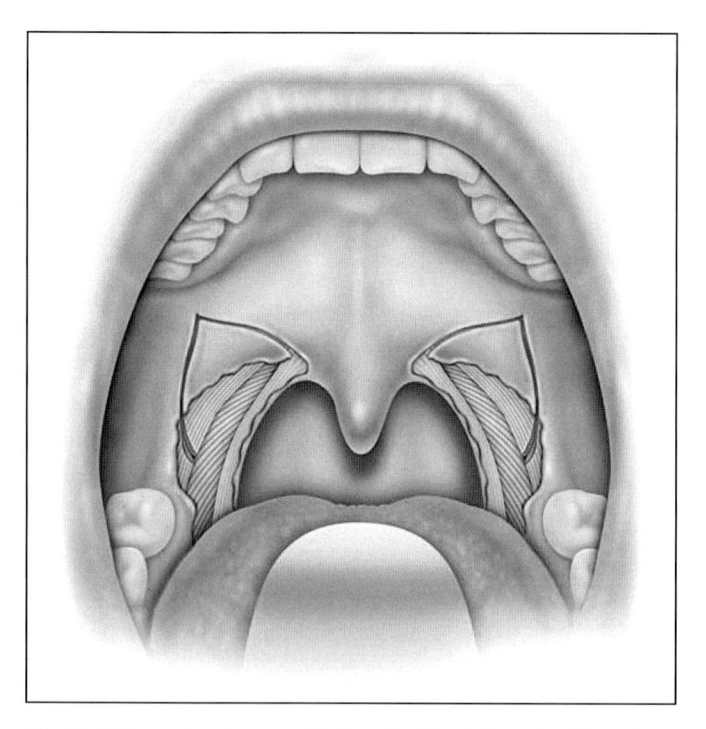

**Fig. 38.3** Bilateral upside down 'V-shape' incision in the soft palate and palatoglossus muscle.

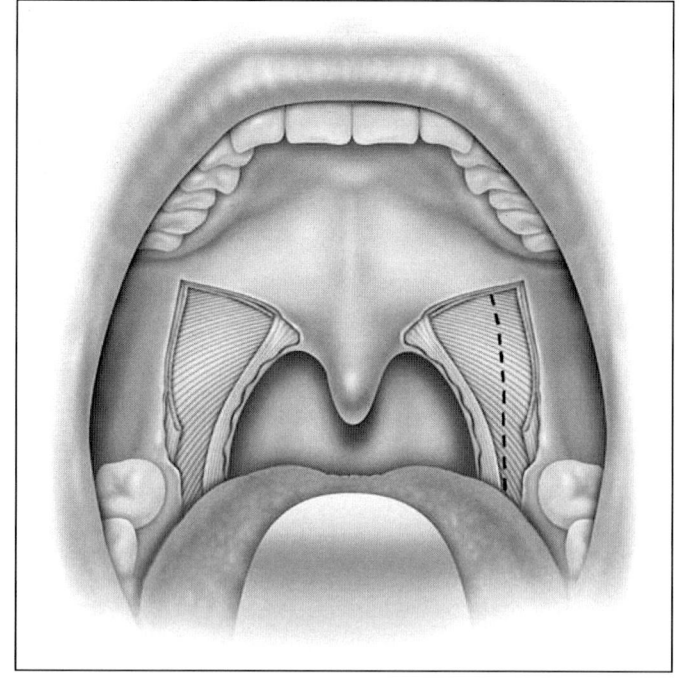

**Fig. 38.5** Wide exposure of both SPC muscles. Area of the left SPC muscle to be elevated and cut (dashed line, see text).

LP starts with a bilateral tonsillectomy (Fig. 38.2). If that has already been done, we undermine and remove the tonsillar fossa lining until we can identify the palatoglossus and palatopharyngeus muscles. Next, with an upside down 'V-shape' incision (Fig. 38.3), we remove a triangle of mucosa and muscle (palatoglossus) from the lateral oral free margin of the soft palate and anterior pillar. That provides a wide exposure of the SPC muscle, including its pterygopharyngeal (partially), buccopharyngeal and mylopharyngeal parts (Figs 38.4 and 38.5). The height

CHAPTER
Lateral pharyngoplasty  **38**

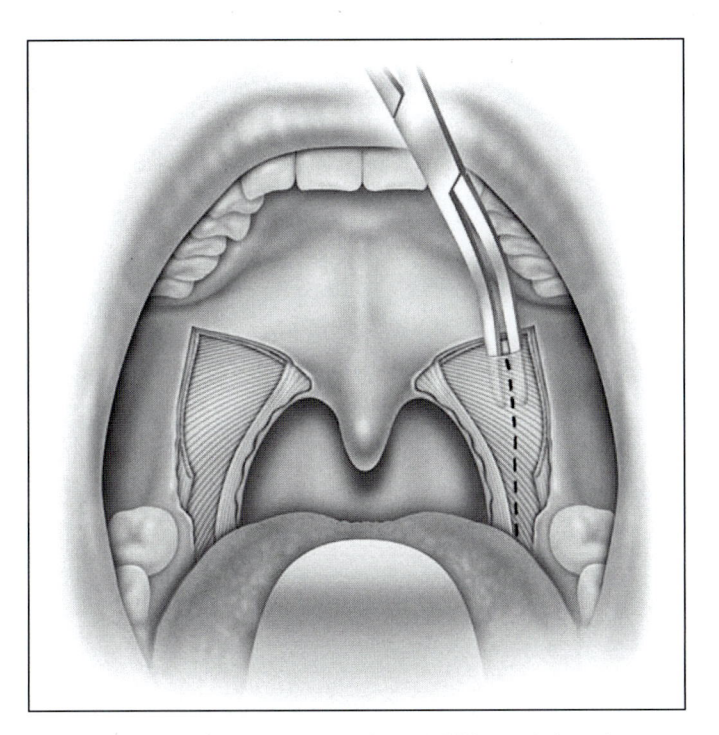

**Fig. 38.6** Undermining and elevation of the left SPC muscle from the peripharyngeal space, preserving the buccopharyngeal fascia.

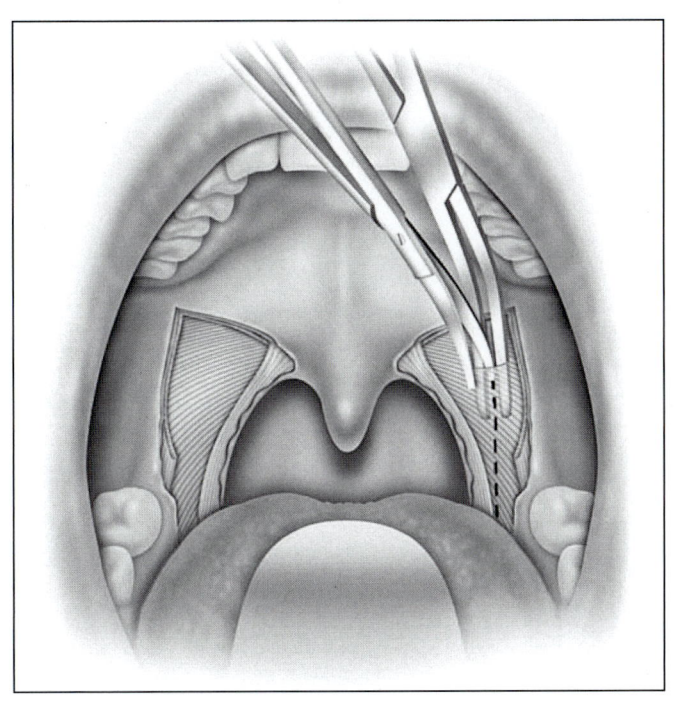

**Fig. 38.7** Section of the left SPC muscle.

of this incision corresponds to that reached by the lateral superior traction (see Fig. 38.10) of the upper part of the palatopharyngeus muscle, which will be used to close this wound.

Once fully exposed, we undermine and elevate the SPC muscle from the peripharyngeal space (Fig. 38.6), starting from its most cranial visible part, and separate it from its fascia (buccopharyngeal fascia). It is very important to preserve this fascia, avoiding injury to cranial nerves IX and X and to other pharyngeal muscles, which could delay swallowing recovery. The SPC muscle is elevated from the pharyngeal wall in its posterior but not lateral aspect, near the palatopharyngeus muscle, since this region has fewer blood vessels, and once you reach the right plane of dissection there, the muscle can be easily detached from its fascia. Usually, the vertical fibers of the palatopharyngeus muscle have to be pulled medially at the start of the dissection, to expose better the horizontal fibers of the SPC. Once detached, we cauterize the SPC with a bipolar and section its fibers in a cranial to caudal direction (Fig. 38.7). We keep this dissection near the palatopharyngeus, using this muscle as a guide to avoid injuring vessels and nerves at the lateropharyngeal space. This dissection extends as far as the caudal end of the SPC muscle (glossopharyngeal part, where it originates from the side of the tongue). To accomplish this, we have to create a submucosal tunnel inferiorly to the tonsillar fossa to preserve and separate the mucosa from the SPC muscle that is being sectioned. This usually extends from 1 to 1.6 cm beyond the tonsillar fossa, depending on the anatomy, and relates to the retroglossal area.

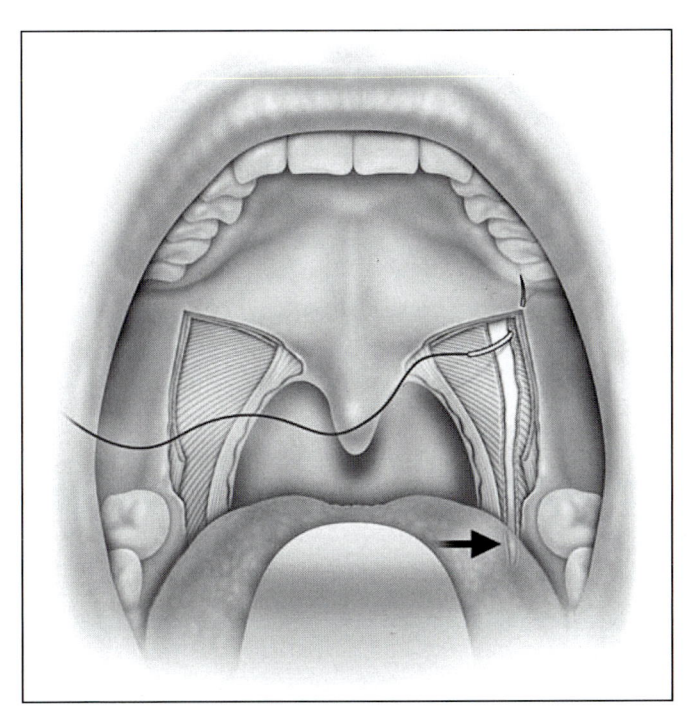

**Fig. 38.8** Suture of the lateral flap of the SPC muscle to the same-side palatoglossus muscle. The arrow indicates the extension of the SPC dissection as far as its glossopharyngeal part.

When the section of the SPC is complete, we get two muscle flaps: one medially based flap that is not manipulated any further, and one laterally based flap that is sutured anteriorly to the same-side palatoglossus muscle with four or five separate stitches (Fig. 38.8). The glossopharyngeal part of the SPC does not need to be sutured. At the end of this suturing line, the peripharyngeal space is

229

SECTION I PALATAL SURGERY

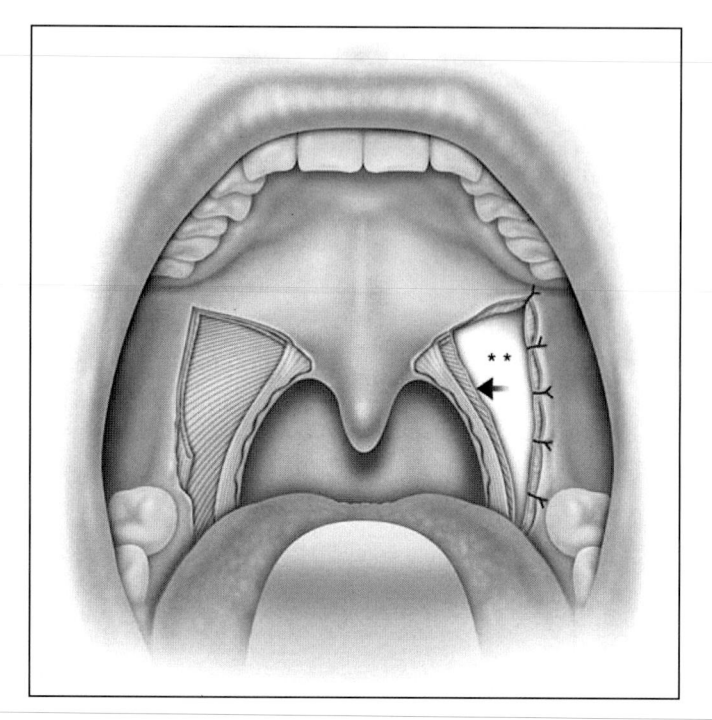

**Fig. 38.9** Aspect after completion of the suture of the SPC muscle to the palatoglossus muscle. The arrow indicates the medial flap of the SPC muscle, which retracts. ** Peripharyngeal space (buccopharyngeal fascia) widely exposed.

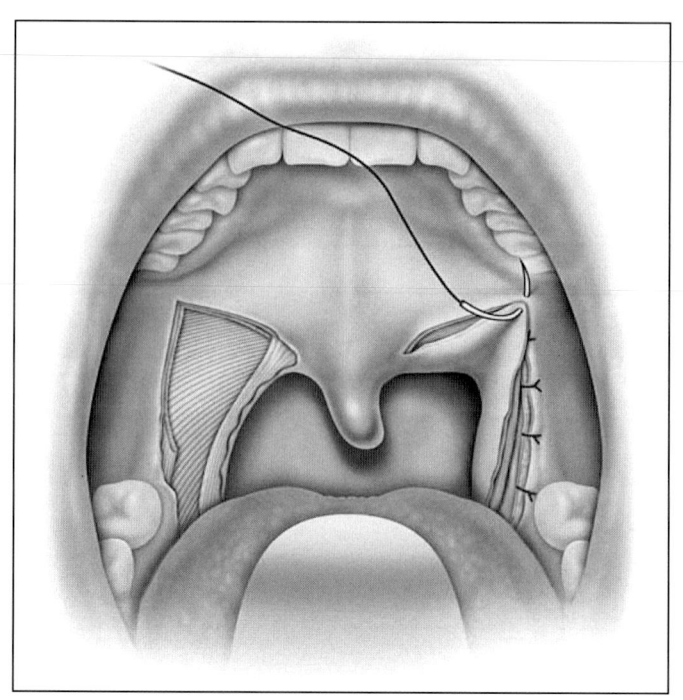

**Fig. 38.11** Closure of the surgical wound with separate stitches.

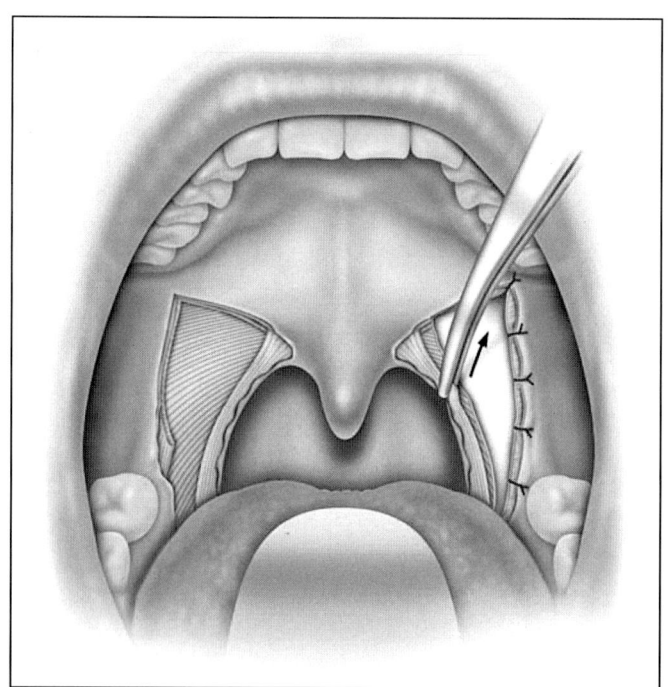

**Fig. 38.10** Grabbing of the palatopharyngeus muscle, leaving the medial flap of the SPC muscle. The arrow indicates the direction of the pull.

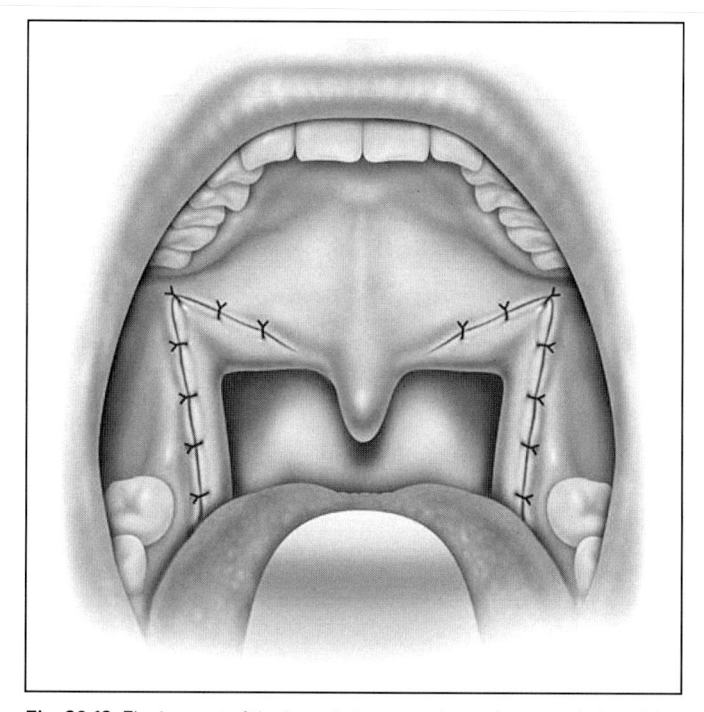

**Fig. 38.12** Final aspect of the lateral pharyngoplasty after completion of the procedure at the opposite side.

widely exposed and the lateral wall is splinted along all of the collapsible pharynx (Fig. 38.9). This surgical wound is then closed by pulling and suturing the palatopharyngeus to the remnants of the palatoglossus muscle (Figs. 38.10 and 38.11). The medial flap of the SPC is not included in this pull. Every step is then repeated on the opposite side (Fig. 38.12). At the end, due to the bilateral pull of the palatopharyngeus muscles, the uvula stays in the midline and sometimes it bends upwards, returning to normal within hours or days.

## 4 POSTOPERATIVE MANAGEMENT AND COMPLICATIONS

Extubation is delayed until the patients are wide awake with good muscle tone. The patients stay monitored in the recovery room for 1–2 hours before going to the ward, with the head of the bed elevated (usually 60°). When respiratory discomfort occurs, it is usually noted immediately after extubation. We have not observed this with this technique, but it did happen in some cases in which we used a Z-plasty instead of our current method of pulling the palatopharyngeus muscles in the lateral port areas. Also, we noted that the use of atropine at the end of the surgery produced a comfortable recovery, with reduced salivation.

The hospital stay usually lasts 1 or 2 days and discharge criteria include pain control and adequate oral intake of fluids. We use antibiotic coverage for 7 days (amoxicillin or azithromycin) and steroids (hydrocortisone, 200 mg intravenously every 8 hours during hospitalization. Additionally, we use painkillers (dypiron, 500 mg orally every 6 hours and, if needed, tramadol hydrochloride, 75 mg orally every 8 hours) and topical anesthetics (benzocaine 0.4%, four sprays in the throat up to four times daily), usually for 10 days after the procedures. The patients also receive gastric acid anti-secretory agents (pantoprazole or esomeprazole, 40 mg orally daily for 1–2 months).

Wound dehiscence typically occurs in the region of the caudal stitch of the tonsillar fossa some days after the surgery, requiring no attention. There is actually a dead space in the pharyngeal wall after LP, which is already drained to the airway lumen and heals during the first week. Postoperative pain is usually moderate and if abnormal, excessive pain arises, it should be treated with removal of the stitches in the area that hurts. Mild velopharyngeal insufficiency is common after LP, reducing gradually and usually disappearing after 2–4 weeks. Swallowing difficulties usually last 2–3 weeks and, after that, the patients are usually able to eat any kind of food with the eventual aid of liquids. Normal swallowing sensation usually takes 2 months to be restored. The majority of patients return to work 10–12 days after the procedure.

## 5 SUCCESS RATE OF PROCEDURE AND WHAT TO DO IF THE PROCEDURE FAILS

So far, we have operated on 69 cases with the concept of lateral pharyngoplasty (66 with sleep apnea and three primary snorers). The success rate of the procedure as it is presented here ('extended LP') is still under investigation. In our initial 30 cases, we did a limited turn of the SPC muscle, only at the tonsillar fossa and retroglossal area, leaving the retropalatal area to be treated with a palatopharyngeal Z-plasty, without pulling the palatopharyngeus muscle laterally, and also adding a partial uvulectomy (which we have abandoned now). We felt that the failures in that initial series were due to persistence of constrictor forces at the retropalatal area. Overall, the Apnea/Hypopnea Index (AHI) decreased from 41.6 to 13.1 ($P < 0.001$) in these 30 cases, with a follow-up polysomnogram done 6–12 months postoperatively. Considering a reduction in the AHI of at least 50% with a final AHI of less than 15, the success rate in that series was 68.4% for Friedman stage 2 patients (moderately favorable anatomy) and 45.5% for Friedman stage 3 cases (unfavorable anatomy).

Treatment options for failures include oral appliances for mild disease and CPAP or bimaxillary advancement for moderate and severe cases.

## ACKNOWLEDGMENTS

I wish to thank Mr J. Falcetti from Arte e Comunicação Médica for the illustrations.

## FURTHER READING

Cahali MB. Lateral pharyngoplasty: a new treatment for obstructive sleep apnea hypopnea syndrome. Laryngoscope 2003;113: 1961–8.

Cahali MB, Formigoni GGS, Gebrim EMMS, Miziara ID. Lateral pharyngoplasty versus uvulopalatopharyngoplasty: a clinical, polysomnographic and computed tomography measurement comparison. Sleep 2004;27(5):942–50.

Friedman M, Tanyeri H, La Rosa M, et al. Clinical predictors of obstructive sleep apnea. Laryngoscope 1999;109:1901–7.

Friedman M, Ibrahim H, Bass L. Clinical staging for sleep-disordered breathing. Otolaryngol Head Neck Surg 2002; 127:13–21.

Isono S, Remmers JE, Tanaka A, et al. Static properties of the passive pharynx in sleep apnea. Sleep 1996;19(Suppl):S175–7.

Li KK, Guilleminault C, Riley RW, Powell NB. Obstructive sleep apnea and maxillomandibular advancement: an assessment of airway changes using radiographic and nasopharyngoscopic examinations. J Oral Maxillofac Surg 2002;60:526–30.

Morrison DL, Launois SH, Isono S, et al. Pharyngeal narrowing and closing pressures in patients with obstructive sleep apnea. Am Rev Respir Dis 1993;148:606–11.

Schellenberg JB, Maislin G, Schwab RJ. Physical findings and the risk for obstructive sleep apnea: the importance of oropharyngeal structures. Am J Respir Crit Care Med 2000;162:740–48.

Schwab RJ, Gefter WB, Hoffman EA, et al. Dynamic upper airway imaging during awake respiration in normal subjects and patients with sleep disordered breathing. Am Rev Respir Dis 1993;148: 1385–400.

Schwab RJ, Gupta KB, Gefter WB, et al. Upper airway and soft tissue anatomy in normal subjects and patients with sleep-disordered breathing: significance of the lateral pharyngeal walls. Am J Respir Crit Care Med 1995;152:1673–89.

Schwab RJ, Pack AI, Gupta KB, et al. Upper airway and soft tissue structural changes induced by CPAP in normal subjects. Am J Respir Crit Care Med 1996;154:1106–16.

Winter WC, Gampper T, Gay SB, Suratt PM. Lateral pharyngeal fat pad pressure during breathing. Sleep 1996;19(Suppl):S178–9.

Woodson BT, Wooten MR. Manometric and endoscopic localization of airway obstruction after uvulopalatopharyngoplasty. Otolaryngol Head Neck Surg 1994;111:38–43.

SECTION J — MINIMALLY INVASIVE HYPOPHARYNGEAL PROCEDURES

# CHAPTER 39
# Fundamentals of minimally invasive radiofrequency applications in ear, nose and throat medicine

*Kai Desinger*

Ear, nose and throat (ENT) medicine currently has several different systems at its disposal for minimally invasive treatments which apply high frequency electric current to achieve a therapeutic effect. This chapter is intended to provide a survey of the technical fundamentals and tissue effects of such systems.

With the purpose of deepening the understanding of the use of high-frequency current for medical applications, an overview of the basics of high-frequency surgery is included in the second section.

## 1 SYSTEM OVERVIEW

The therapy systems currently available on the market are distinguished in terms of their types of application, their therapy effects and the technology of the equipment used.

### 1.1 TYPE OF APPLICATION

Four types of application of high-frequency energy can be distinguished:
- Submucous coagulation.
- Superficial vaporization.
- Submucous vaporization.
- Electrotomy (electroexcision).

#### 1.1.1 SUBMUCOUS COAGULATION

In the process of submucous coagulation, needle-shaped electrodes puncture the surface of the organ and are subsequently positioned inside the organ (Fig. 39.1). When energy is applied, thermally induced coagulation builds up around the electrode, usually of ellipsoid shape, depending on the construction of the electrode. If positioning and energy dose are correct, the organ's surface is conserved and the application is almost entirely free of pain. The body's own decomposition and discharge of the necrotic tissue leads to a reduction in volume in the region treated.

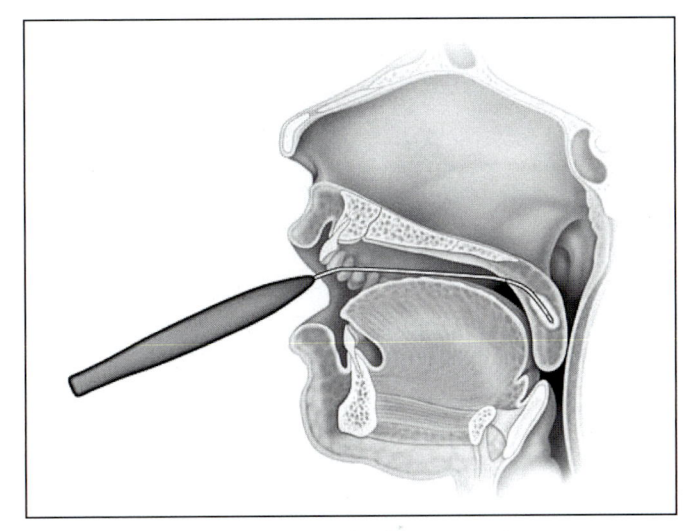

**Fig. 39.1** Submucous coagulation, soft palate.

#### 1.1.2 SUPERFICIAL VAPORIZATION

The reduction in size of an organ, e.g. a tonsil, may also be accomplished by means of direct tissue ablation via vaporization (tissue vaporization) on the surface (Fig. 39.2).

#### 1.1.3 SUBMUCOUS VAPORIZATION

In the process of submucous vaporization, so-called 'channeling', channels are bored in the affected organ. For this purpose, a special bipolar electrode is necessary, at the tip of which a plasma ignition process takes place. When the tip comes into contact with tissue, the latter vaporizes immediately. A channel is generated by pushing the electrode forward in the tissue. More details on so-called plasma applications are to be found in Section 2.4.3.

#### 1.1.4 ELECTROTOMY

Electrotomy is also related to superficial vaporization methods. Contrary to plane vaporization at the surface, however, cuts are generated using fine needle-shaped electrodes with the objective of separating tissue (Fig. 39.3).

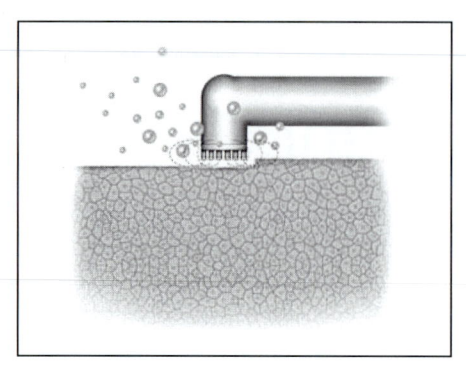

# SECTION J — MINIMALLY INVASIVE HYPOPHARYNGEAL PROCEDURES

**Fig. 39.2** Superficial vaporization.

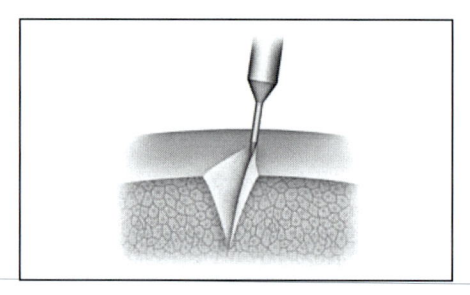

**Fig. 39.3** Electrotomy: tissue separation with high-frequency current.

## 1.2 THERAPY EFFECT

Various different therapy effects are derived from the four types of application mentioned above: the delayed reduction in volume caused by the body's own discharge of thermo-necrotic tissue, the stiffening and tightening of a region of tissue by scar formation as well as the removal of layers of tissue by superficial vaporization and the resection of parts of organs (e.g. uvula or tonsils) using electrotomy.

### 1.2.1 VOLUME SHRINKAGE BY THE BODY'S OWN DISCHARGE OF COAGULATION NECROSIS/TISSUE STABILIZATION BY SCAR FORMATION AFTER COAGULATION NECROSIS

Submucous coagulation shows two time-delayed effects: volume shrinkage caused by the body's own discharge of the coagulated tissue as well as stabilization of a region of tissue by the scarring process.

Following thermo-coagulation several phases take effect in the volume of tissue involved.

- Tissue coagulation becomes apparent immediately after its production by a lighter color resulting from the induced protein denaturation.
- After one day, a clearly defined lesion is evident, bordered by a hyperemic edge surrounding the destroyed tissue.
- About 10 days after treatment, the lesion is surrounded with connective tissue.
- After approximately 3 weeks, the dead muscle tissue has been replaced completely by connective tissue (collagen deposits). The scarring process is complete; the region of tissue involved has decreased in size and hardened.

### 1.2.2 TISSUE ABLATION BY MEANS OF VAPORIZATION

Superficial ablation of tissue at the surface is used, for example, in tonsillotomy – the partial resection of hyperplastic tonsils. In this case, the tissue is removed by vaporization in layers using a special arrangement of electrodes.

### 1.2.3 TISSUE RESECTION BY MEANS OF ELECTROTOMY

In the process of electrotomy, a high current density is generated at the point where the tissue is touched by means of electrodes of small surface area in the form of needles or slings. The tissue is heated to well above 100°C in a very short period of time, leading to vaporization of the cell fluid and bursting of the cells concerned. If the electrode is moved through the tissue a cut is the result. Depending on the cutting power and speed of the cut, a more or less deep coagulation seam is produced at the edges of the cut, with the result that bleeding is reduced or can be avoided.

## 1.3 EQUIPMENT TECHNOLOGY

Radiofrequency systems can be fundamentally divided into monopolar and bipolar systems with regard to the equipment or applicator technology used. Further subdivision relates to the possibilities of therapy monitoring and power regulation.

### 1.3.1 MONOPOLAR AND BIPOLAR APPLICATION TECHNOLOGY

**Monopolar technology**
Monopolar technology, where one of the two electrodes required to close the circuit is connected to the patient as a large-surface return path, is most commonly used in radiofrequency surgical applications to date. The actual working or active electrode is in the shape of a small-surface surgical instrument, e.g. in the form of a needle, a lancet or a ball. It is from the latter electrode that the radiofrequency alternating current from the generator is conducted into the patient, producing the desired surgical effect as a result of high current density at the point where the tissue is touched. The radiofrequency current disperses rapidly in the tissue and flows with lower current density through the body of the patient to the neutral electrode, whence it flows back to the generator (Fig. 39.4).

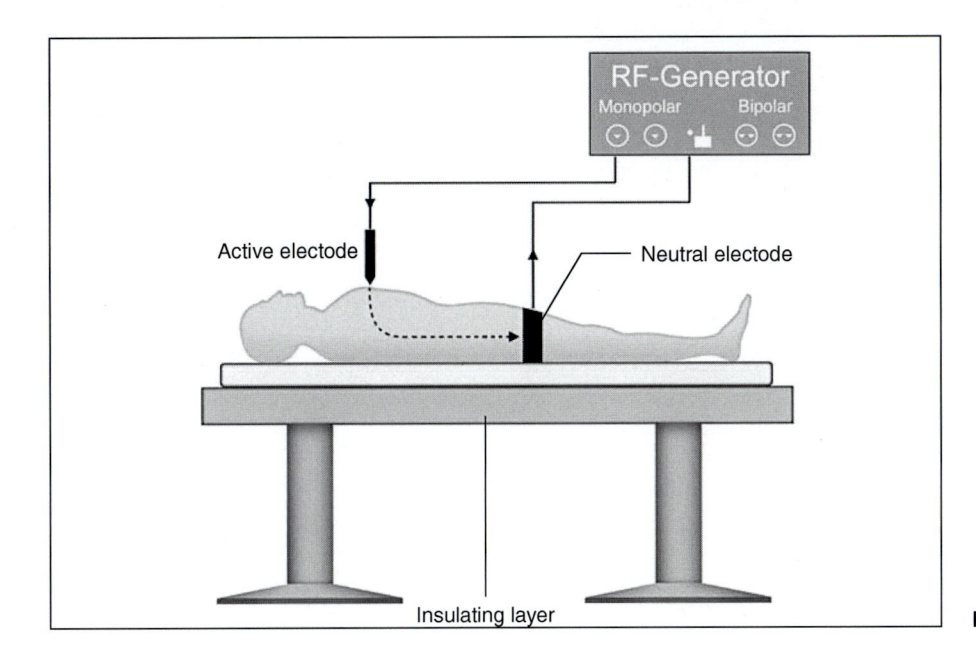

**Fig. 39.4** Monopolar application technology.

A considerable number of complications may arise from the use of radiofrequency surgery, which are excluded when bipolar technology is applied.[1]

*Problem: neutral electrode*
Attachment of a neutral electrode to the patient is necessary when monopolar technology is used. In this context, attention must be paid to the certainty of low contact resistance. The current density has to be evenly distributed over the entire surface of the neutral electrode. Perspiration, hairs or fatty substances between skin and the electrode surface may mean the current is unable to utilize the entire transfer surface, leading to current densities which are too high in certain places and which may in turn lead to burns.[2]

*Problem: current flow through the body between active and neutral electrode*
Thermal tissue damage may occur in parts of the body between the active and neutral electrodes where the cross-section available for current flow is small and electrical resistance high.[2] The current flow is particularly problematic in the region of head and neck: the greater part of the volume concerned here consists of bone as well as air-filled nasal and oral cavities or paranasal sinuses. In certain places only the thin mucous membrane layer remains as conducting residual cross-section.

The application of monopolar high-frequency technology for patients with cardiac pacemakers or catheters may only be carried out in exceptional cases. The specialist literature contains different documented opinions and research results on the interaction between radiofrequency current and pacemakers.[3]

**Bipolar technology**
Although bipolar technology has been known for some considerable time,[4] it was only in the mid-1980s that renewed efforts were made to press ahead and further develop bipolar radiofrequency technology for reasons of safety, both for coagulation and cutting purposes.

Bipolar application technology (Fig 39.5) is characterized in that both electrodes, integrated in an application handset, are brought as close together as possible. The current only passes immediately between the two electrodes, meaning that secondary thermal damage to the patient, both internal and external, caused by leakage currents or marked changes in impedance (cross-sections with a high percentage of bone or fat and poorly conducting residual cross-sections) can be avoided. Since the attachment of a neutral electrode is not required in bipolar radiofrequency surgery, and the current flow is restricted to the point of surgical intervention, the risks involved in monopolar technology as described above can principally be avoided (Fig. 39.6).

## 1.3.2 PROCESS MONITORING AND POWER REGULATION

Superficial coagulation, e.g. using bipolar forceps to stop bleeding, can be directly monitored by the eye of the attending physician. Where submucous coagulation is concerned, however, the physician no longer has this possibility since no visual contact exists with the coagulation taking place underneath the tissue surface. In such a case, technical monitoring of therapy relevant parameters via the power unit is all the more important.

The size of a submucous coagulation (Fig. 39.7) depends on numerous parameters. Worth mentioning in this case are

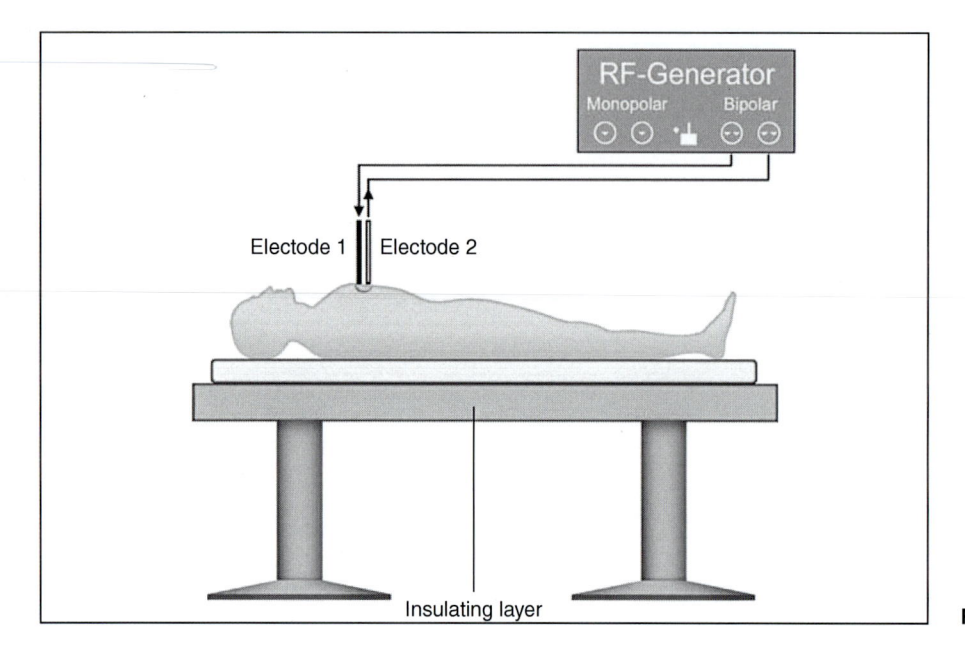

| SECTION J | MINIMALLY INVASIVE HYPOPHARYNGEAL PROCEDURES |

**Fig. 39.5** Bipolar application technology.

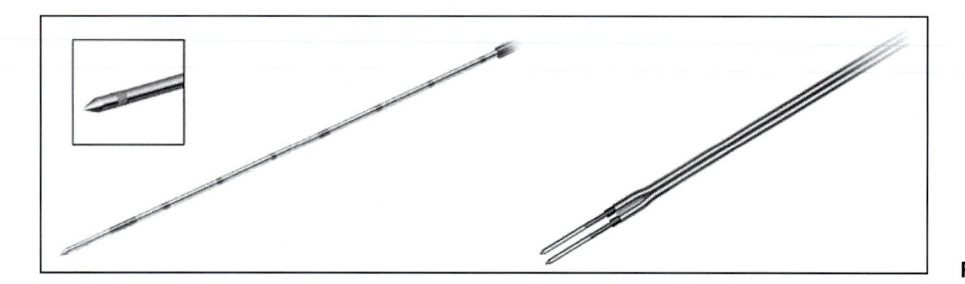

**Fig. 39.6** Bipolar electrodes.

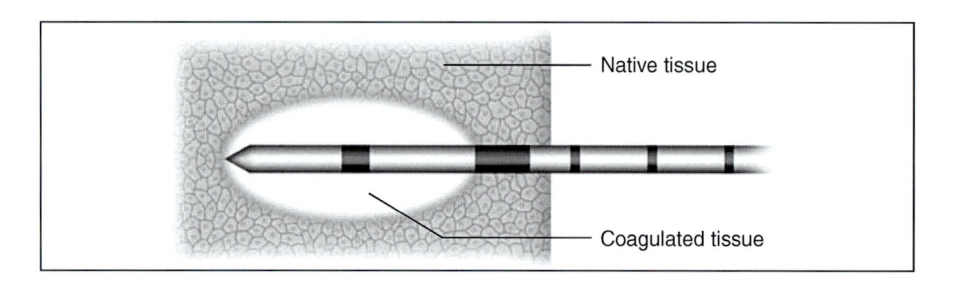

**Fig. 39.7** Ellipsoid submucous coagulation of a bipolar electrode (Celon AG).

the electrode geometry, the power and the application time. Tissue resistance, tissue temperature or the energy input provide information on the tissue changes achieved.

### Tissue resistance measurement
Tissue change can be determined by measurement of the electrical resistance of the tissue (impedance). Protein denaturing during the coagulation process results in destruction of the cell membranes, which in turn induces an improvement of the electrical conductivity. The tissue drying out process on reaching the boiling point, on the other hand, reduces the electrical conductivity of the tissue. These processes make it possible to monitor the coagulation process from start to finish. Tissue resistance provides direct information on the tissue change itself, in contrast to the temperature or energy input, physical parameters which induce the said tissue change.

### Temperature measurement
Tissue destruction is dependent on the tissue temperature and the time the tissue was exposed to this temperature (dose). Measurement of the tissue temperature permits an indirect assessment of the tissue destruction for this reason.

### Determination of energy input
A correlation exists between energy input and coagulation volume in the process of submucous tissue coagulation. If a certain quantity of electrical energy is introduced into the

tissue under treatment, using a particular electrode geometry, a reproducible coagulation volume is the result. This only applies, however, as long as the marginal conditions of the coagulation process do not change. A change in the electrode position (distance from tissue surface or from larger vessels), in the temperature of the tissue or in the blood perfusion rate has the result that a different coagulation volume is produced from a certain quantity of energy.

### Measurement of the application time

If no possibility exists in a radiofrequency therapy system for the measurement of parameters accompanying the coagulation process, such as tissue impedance, temperature or energy input, makeshift help may be provided by estimation of the expected size of coagulation using time measurement. For this purpose, reference is made to experimentally determined data. A power level is selected and the spread of coagulation determined after certain time intervals for certain types of tissue. Where clinical applications are concerned, it is assumed that a particular combination of power and application time will always achieve the same effect in the tissue. Changes in the position of the electrodes affecting the coagulation result, tissue temperature, blood perfusion rate and changes in performance associated with tissue impedance cannot be taken into account with this procedure.

### Power regulation

An optimal coagulation result can be achieved where radiofrequency power is adapted to the current condition of the tissue during the coagulation process. This way, overdosing or even carbonization can be avoided since a power input best suited to the desired result of the treatment is supplied as a function of each moment in time.

## 1.4 THERAPY SYSTEMS CURRENTLY ON THE MARKET

### 1.4.1 CELON AG MEDICAL INSTRUMENTS

*Application:* submucous coagulation and electrotomy.

*Technology:* bipolar.

*Power control therapy monitoring:* impedance-dependent power regulation, automatic end of therapy on reaching target impedance, acoustic control of treatment status.

*Other features:* axial 'in-line' – electrode arrangement for submucous coagulation.

### 1.4.2 GYRUS ENT (SOMNUS)

*Application:* submucous coagulation.

*Technology:* monopolar.

*Power control therapy monitoring:* temperature-dependent power regulation, end of therapy on reaching targeted energy, optical control of temperature and energy input.

### 1.4.3 COBLATOR (ARTHROCARE)

*Application:* submucous vaporization ('channeling')/coagulation and superficial vaporization.

*Technology:* bipolar.

*Power control therapy monitoring:* not present (manual time measurement).

*Other features:* procedures based on so-called plasma technology (sparking at the tip of the applicator caused by very high voltages).

### 1.4.4 DIVERSE RADIOFREQUENCY SURGICAL EQUIPMENT

*Application:* coagulation and cutting (excision).

*Technology:* monopolar, bipolar.

*Power control therapy monitoring:* not present (mainly manual time measurement).

*Other features:* conventional radiofrequency surgical equipment. Different working frequencies through to 4 MHz; direct contact between neutral electrode and tissue is unnecessary at this high frequency. The high-frequency current is also able to flow over so-called capacitive stretches, e.g. thin layers of air or clothing.

## 2 BASICS OF RADIOFREQUENCY SURGERY

Reidenbach has defined radiofrequency surgery as follows[5]: 'radiofrequency surgery is understood as the application of radiofrequency energy for the purpose of changing or destroying tissue cells and of cutting through or removing tissue in combination with mechanical operation techniques'.

### 2.1 HISTORICAL RETROSPECTIVE

The history of the development of radiofrequency surgery goes back as far as Hippocrates, a Greek physician of antiquity, who used a red-hot iron, the so-called 'ferrum candens', to arrest the flow of blood (hemostasis) during amputations around 400 BC.

In the middle of the 19th century, the so-called 'Paquelin burner' was developed as a thermocauter (instrument for thermocautery) and the so-called 'galvanic cauter' as an electrocauter. The first of these consisted of a metal pin heated to over 1000°C by a fuel/air mixture and used for the destruction of tumorous tissue. The electrocauter, on the other hand, made it possible to separate or slough off biological tissue by means of a knife or platinum sling raised to red heat by direct current. Prior to the introduction of high-frequency technology at the beginning of the 20th century, such 'cauterization' was the method usually applied in the field of surgery.

# SECTION J — MINIMALLY INVASIVE HYPOPHARYNGEAL PROCEDURES

In 1891, the French physicist d'Arsonval reported on thermal effects induced in biological tissue by using alternating current at frequencies above 250 kHz without stimulation of muscles or nerves (so-called 'Faradic effect').[6] At the beginning of the 20th century needle electrodes which were inserted into the tissue (so-called 'electro-desiccation') were used by Clark for the first time. Between 1907 and 1910 'coagulation' was developed as a method for tissue destruction, particularly against cancer, by Doyen, Czerny and Nagelschmidt.[4,7–9] In 1929, radiofrequency technology found its way into brain surgery with the development of suitable tube generators by Gulke and Heymann.[10] At this time, a physicist, Bovie, and a surgeon, Cushing, were mainly responsible for the development of one of the first radiofrequency generators for the cutting and coagulation of tissue.[11,12]

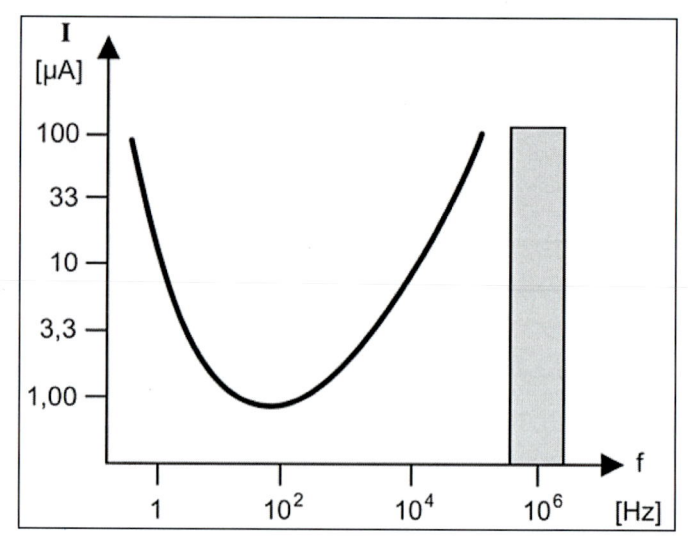

**Fig. 39.8** Stimulating current curve.

## 2.2 PHYSICAL AND TECHNICAL BASICS

Biological tissue comprises a system of different electrolytes, represented as different salt solutions in intracellular and extracellular space. These ions are responsible for electron transport and so for transcellular current flow in tissue. The cell membranes separate the electrolytes from each other, leading to their inhomogeneous distribution in the tissue. As a result of these dissociated salt solutions, depending on their individual concentrations, biological tissue becomes more or less electrically conductive. Where current flows through living biological tissue, three fundamental effects can be described: the Faradic effect, the electrolytic effect and the thermal effect.

### 2.2.1 FARADIC EFFECT

The Faradic effect is apparent using alternating currents of lower and middle frequency between 10 Hz and 10 kHz, which induce motor stimulation of muscle and nerve cells. Figure 39.8 shows the stimulation threshold curve where current is plotted against frequency. It can be seen that the threshold current possesses a minimum between 50 and 100 Hz, meaning that very low currents are enough to cause serious damage to humans within the range of the usual power frequencies. At 50 Hz even small currents may cause ventricular fibrillation.

Nernst[13] has defined the 'physiological stimulation' of alternating currents as a function of the electric current $I$ and the frequency $f$ with the equation:

$$\text{Phys. stim.} = \frac{I}{\sqrt{f}}$$

The Faradic stimulation effect increases with increasing current at constant frequency. If the current is constant and the frequency increases (from approximately 100 Hz onwards), the stimulation effect diminishes. The cellular ionic concentration gradient is reduced since ever smaller amounts of electricity can be transported within the individual half-waves of the alternating current. For frequencies in the range $f > 200...300$ kHz, freedom from stimulation is assumed according to studies carried out by Gildemeister.[14] If high-frequency alternating currents in the range between 300 kHz $< f <$ 2 MHz are used, the Faradic stimulation effect can be eliminated in the widest sense, even at higher currents. At frequencies of >2 MHz, uncontrolled 'vagabond activity' has to be reckoned with as a result of capacitive leakage currents, even over widely insulated stretches and beyond. The arising cable and radiation problems come into the foreground and should be avoided for safety reasons.

### 2.2.2 ELECTROLYTIC EFFECT

The electrolytic effect occurs mainly when direct current and low-frequency alternating currents are used. In such cases, intracellular as well as transcellular ionic migration occurs, with movement towards both electrodes, depending on the ionic charge. Cell membranes possess different permeability towards different electrolytes, with the effect that concentration tailbacks accumulate in these zones. Congestion of this nature destroys isotonia among the cells on the one hand and may lead to serious cell and tissue damage, such as tissue burns, on the other (Fig. 39.9).

Ionic migration of this kind diminishes with increasing frequency on account of the ever-diminishing time between two successive current alternations until ultimately no reactive concentration changes take place which could cause a motor stimulation effect. For this reason polarization no longer occurs and stimulation effects disappear.

### 2.2.3 THERMAL EFFECT

Radiofrequency surgery uses the thermal effect based on Joule's law. Joule's law states that the overall electrical output

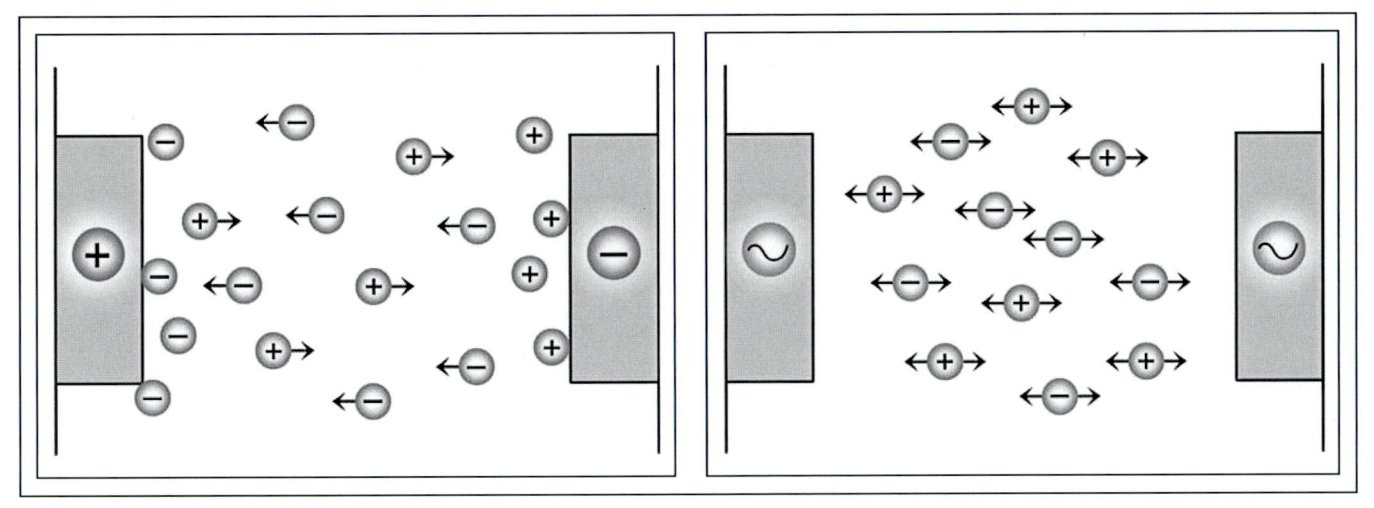

**Fig. 39.9** Cellular ionic migration using direct current (left) and high-frequency alternating current (right).

power $P$ is released in the form of heat when an electric current $I$ flows through an electrical resistance $R$. The relationship between power, resistance and current is as follows:

$$P = R \times I^2 \quad (1)$$

If a current $I$ flows through a resistance $R$ for a time interval $\Delta t$, the amount of heat $\Delta Q$ arises, where:

$$\Delta Q = R \times I^2 \times \Delta t \quad (2)$$

The quotient of current $I$ and surface $A$ is designated as electric current density $J$, where:

$$J = I/A \quad (3)$$

The smaller the cross-sectional area $A$, the larger is the current density. This means that for the same current $I$ a higher current density $J$ is generated by a small electrode than by an electrode with a large surface area.

The electrical resistance $R$ of a cylinder-shaped tissue element as shown in Figure 39.10 can be calculated from the specific resistance $\rho$, the surface area $A$ through which the current passes and the cylinder length $L$, where:

$$R = \rho \times L/A \quad (4)$$

By setting equations (4) and (3) into equation (2) and taking into account that the cylindrical volume is given by $V = A \times L$, the heat generated per volume and time unit can be calculated from $\Delta Q/(V \times \Delta t)$. This tissue heating is directly proportional to the product of the specific resistance $\rho$ and the square of the electric current density $J$.

$$\Delta Q/(V \times \Delta t) = \rho \times J^2 \quad (5)$$

(heating $\sim \rho \times J^2$)

In other words, if current flows into the biological tissue from an active electrode with a small cross-section the current density immediately in front of the electrode is large. In accordance with Joule's law a large heat quantity is created here.

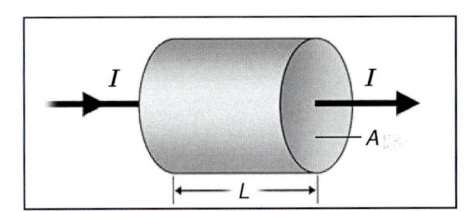

**Fig. 39.10** Cylinder-shaped tissue model with resistance $R$.

Equation (5) also shows that the heating is larger, the larger the specific resistance $\rho$ of the conductor through which the current passes. In other words, if an electric current flows from a metal electrode into biological tissue, the heating takes place almost exclusively in the tissue itself since the specific resistance of the metal is many times smaller than that of the tissue.

## 2.3 TISSUE EFFECTS IN RADIOFREQUENCY CURRENT APPLICATIONS

No cell damage arises from heating the tissue to about 40°C. Further heat input and increasing temperature lead to reversible tissue damage, depending on the duration of exposure. Temperatures above 49°C lead to irreversible cell damage as a result of protein denaturation. This thermal destruction process is markedly dependent on time. The actual coagulation effect starts at a temperature between 60°C and 70°C. Macroscopically viewed, coagulation is accompanied by a white/yellow discoloration and shrinkage of the affected tissue matrix (Fig. 39.11).

If the temperature is raised to 100°C in a short period of time, the vaporization process is accelerated. The internal cell pressure increases to such an extent that the cell bursts, with subsequent tissue dissipation (Fig. 39.12).

# SECTION J — MINIMALLY INVASIVE HYPOPHARYNGEAL PROCEDURES

At temperatures around 200°C, carbonization of the tissue takes place (Fig. 39.13). The carbonized layer has the effect of a thermal insulation shield, leading to a reduction of convective thermal conductivity after coagulation at too high a power level, and to inadequate hemostasis as a consequence. The wound healing process is considerably delayed in the carbonized tissue. At this location a 'foreign body reaction' occurs. The mutagenic effect of carbonized tissue is also a subject of discussion.

## 2.4 TYPES OF RADIOFREQUENCY CURRENT APPLICATION

The types of application of radiofrequency surgery are radiofrequency excision or electrotomy and radiofrequency or electrocoagulation. The methods of radiofrequency fulguration such as the stripping of tissue by a shower of sparks, as well as radiofrequency desiccation using fine needle electrodes, are not discussed here on account of their relatively low usage. So-called 'plasma' surgery is considered in more detail at the end of this chapter since this concept is encountered more frequently at present.

### 2.4.1 ELECTROTOMY

In electrotomy (Fig. 39.14), the cutting of tissue, a high current density is generated by means of small-surface electrodes at the point of transfer to the tissue. The electric power required for this purpose must be sufficient to heat the tissue above 100°C in the shortest time. As a result of this rapid heating or vaporization of the cell fluid, cell rupture, the actual cutting effect, occurs. In the above process, the electric power introduced generates a coagulation seam of greater or lesser depth at the cutting edges, which in turn seals smaller vessels and leads to a reduction of bleeding as a result.

As a result of the almost explosive nature of cell fluid vaporization immediately after starting the flow of current, an electrically insulating steam cushion is created which effectively lifts the cutting electrode away from the tissue. At sufficiently high generator voltage, this steam layer is penetrated by an electric arc. The arc concentrates the total

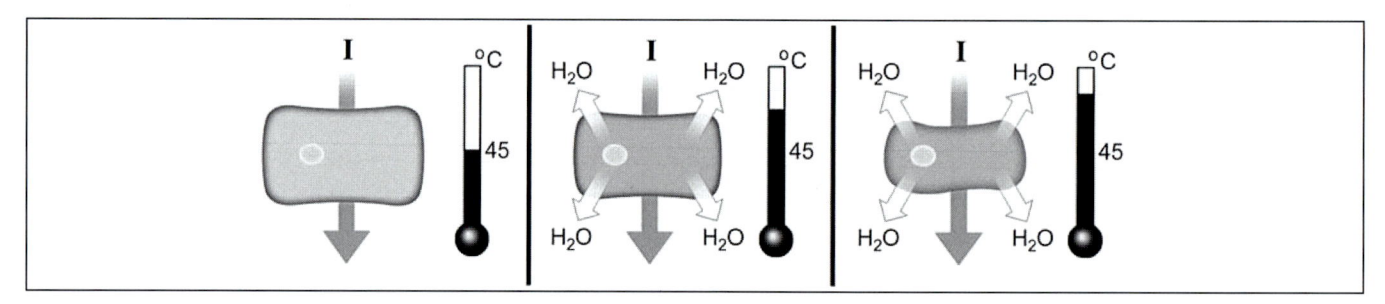

**Fig. 39.11** Influence of slow heating on biological tissue.

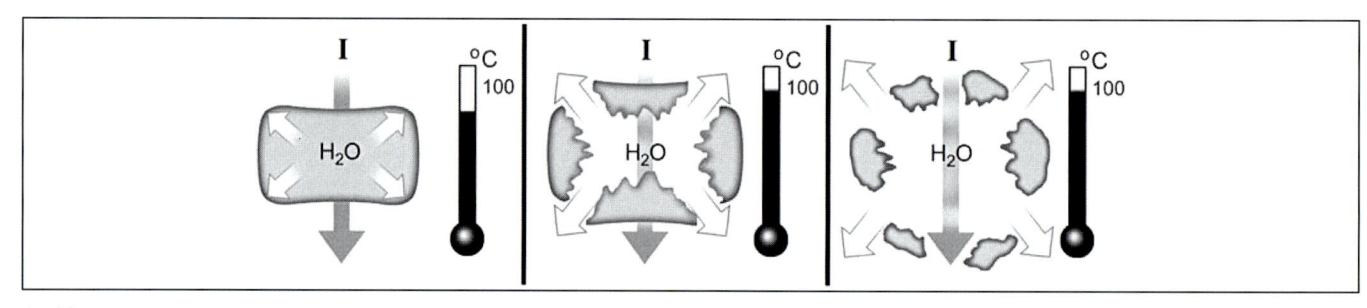

**Fig. 39.12** Cell bursting on rapid heating.

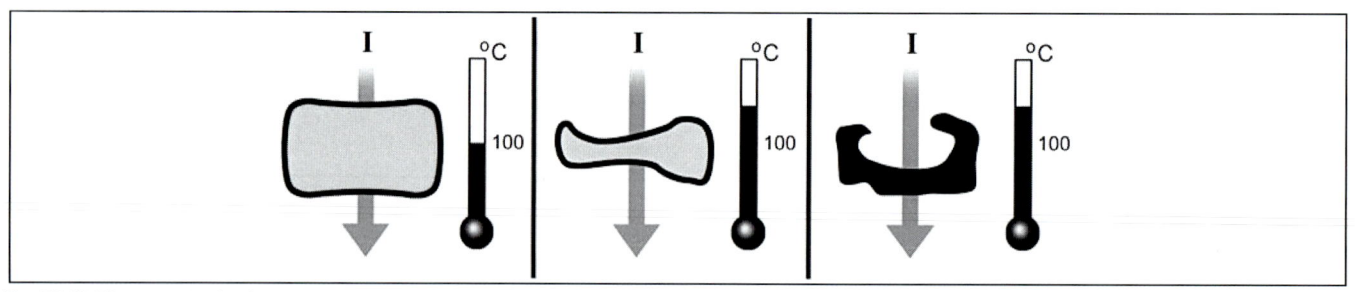

**Fig. 39.13** Tissue carbonization.

electrical energy on a point in such a way that the tissue in the vicinity of the arc's impact point either vaporizes or burns. In this process, more steam is created at the said location with the result that the insulating layer becomes much thicker here and the distance between electrode and tissue correspondingly larger. The result of this is that another point on the electrode reaches higher field strength and the spark flashover now takes place at another location. Over the entire length of the contact zone, tiny arcs are set off wherever the distance between electrode and tissue is momentarily least. In this way, the overall effective tissue contact surface is scanned by flashovers during the cutting process. Such flashovers occur predominantly in the cutting direction, making tissue excision possible as a result of the circumstances described above.

## 2.4.2 COAGULATION

In the process of electrocoagulation large-surface (several mm$^2$) electrodes of cylindrical or conical shape are used as a rule (Fig. 39.15). The contact surfaces between electrode and tissue are larger and the high-frequency voltage smaller than those used in electrotomy, with the result that lower current densities are involved. It is a matter of good sense that the current densities worked with are such that the tissue is gradually heated above the coagulation temperature (approximately 60°C) and do not lead to vaporization (>100°C). The objective of coagulation is hemostasis by the closure of vessels, superficial coagulation or in-depth coagulation, by means of which the large-volume destruction of benign or malignant tumor tissue is usually carried out.

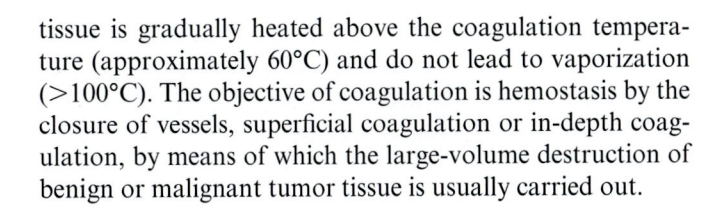

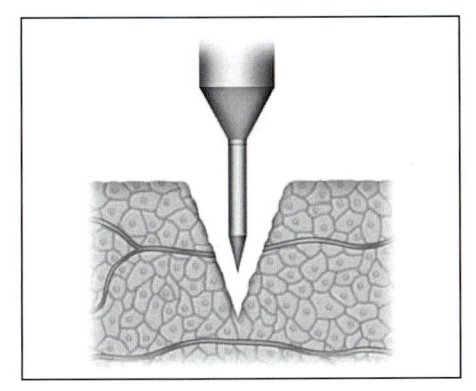

## 2.4.3 'PLASMA' SURGERY

Plasma is understood as a partially or fully ionized gas wherein the electrons and ions present are separated from each other. This means that plasmas are electrically conductive.

If the expression 'plasma' is referred to in radiofrequency surgery, this concerns a gas discharge in the form of a spark discharge. Electrons are torn from their atomic union and accelerated by the high electric field strength prevailing at the electrode. Collision with further atoms generates further electrons. This process, similar to that of an avalanche, creates a spatially restricted discharge channel, generally referred to as a spark or lightning.

Superficial plasma vaporization as well as so-called 'plasma channeling' is comparable to the spark erosion used in metal processing. Ignition to form a visible spark can occur in two ways.

### 1 The electrode is located in the air and approaches the tissue

A high voltage exists between electrode and tissue after activation of the high-frequency generator. When electrode and tissue are brought closer together, the electric field strength increases as a result of their shorter distance apart until it has reached a value leading to a spark discharge. Temperatures of over 1000°C prevail in the sparks, which in turn leads to immediate vaporization of the tissue at the impact point of the spark.

### 2 The electrode is located inside the tissue or is surrounded by a conductive fluid

With this arrangement, a gas discharge may occur if a radiofrequency generator with sufficient power is available and

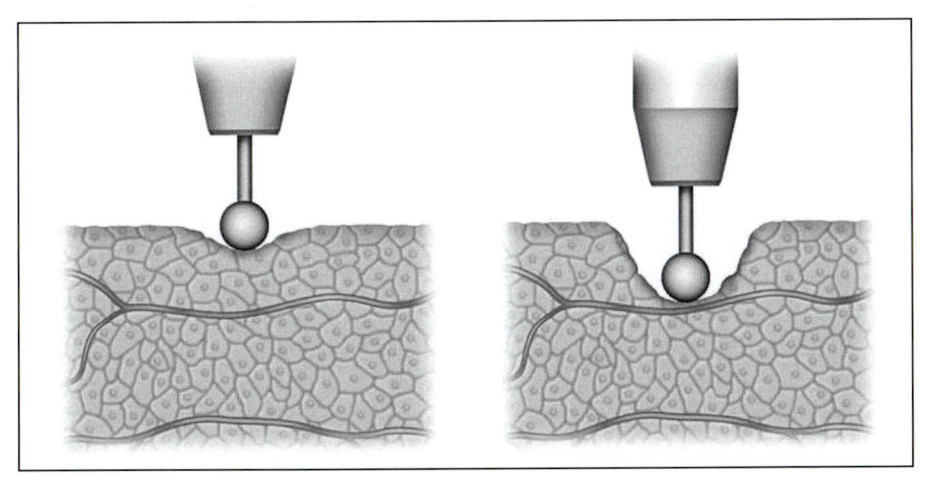

**Fig. 39.14** Principle of electrotomy.

**Fig. 39.15** Coagulation using spherical electrode.

impedances are low. The conductive fluid has to be heated in the shortest time by high currents to such an extent that it vaporizes. In this dehydrated zone at sufficiently high field strength a gas discharge occurs as described in the previous section. Once the spark has been ignited, tissue may be effectively vaporized as a result of the very high temperatures at its impact point. The electric current can continue to flow in order to maintain the spark as a result of the electrical conductivity of the plasma. The spark is only extinguished again if the generator is deactivated or too large a distance arises between electrode and tissue.

Plasma surgery may also be viewed as a special modification of electrotomy. The physical basics and the necessary generator technology are the same. Only the electrode geometry and arrangement in those systems referred to as plasma surgery are different from that of conventional electrotomy electrodes.

## REFERENCES

Mueller W. The advantage of laparoscopic assisted bipolar high-frequency surgery. Endosc Surg Allied Technol 1993; 1:91–6.

Reienbach HD. Fundamentals of bipolar high-frequency surgery. Endosc Surg Allied Technol 1993;1:85–90.

Jung W, Neubrand M, Lüderitz B. Einsatz von Hochfrequenzstorm in der Endoskopie bei Patienten mit Herzschrittmachern. Endopraxis 1995;2:22–5.

Doyen E. Bipolaire Voltaisation. Münch Med Wochenschr 1908;48:2516.

Reidenbach HD. Hochfrequenz und Lasertechnik in der Medizin. Berlin: Springer-Verlag; 1983.

d'Arsonval A. Action physiologique des courants alternatifs. C R Soc Biol 1891;43:283–6.

Doyen E. Traitment local des cancers accessibles par l'action de la chaleur au-dessus de 55°C. Rev Thér Méd Chir 1910;77:551–77.

Czerny V. Über Operationen mit dem Lichtbogen und Diathermie. Dtsch Med Wochenschr 1910;35(11):489–93.

Nagelschmidt F. Über Hochfrequenzströme. Fulguration und Transhermie. Z Phys Diat Ther 1909;3.

Heymann E. Chirurgische Eingriffe mit Hochfrequenzströmen. Med Klin 1930;15:539–45.

Bovie WT. New electro-surgical unit with preliminary note on new surgical current generator. Surg Gynecol Obstet 1928;47:751–84.

Cushing H. Electrosurgery as an aid to the removal of intracranial tumors. Surg Gynecol Obstet 1928;47:751–84.

Nernst W. Zur Theorie des elektrischen Reizes. Pflügers Archiv 1908;122:275–315.

Gildemeister M. Über die im tierische Körper bei elektrischer Durchströmung entstandenen Gegenkräfte. Pflügers Archiv 1912;149:389–400.

SECTION J   MINIMALLY INVASIVE HYPOPHARYNGEAL PROCEDURES

# CHAPTER 40
# Radiofrequency tongue base reduction in sleep-disordered breathing

*Robert J. Troell*

## 1 INTRODUCTION

### 1.1 PREOPERATIVE EVALUATION

Sleep-disordered breathing is caused by collapse or obstruction of the upper airway during sleep. This obstruction may occur at any site along the upper airway passages to include the nasal cavity, oropharynx, hypopharynx and larynx. Once the presence of sleep-disordered breathing is documented by a nocturnal polysomnogram and the patient is intolerant of medical therapy, the presurgical evaluation preceeds. The preoperative evaluation includes a comprehensive head and neck physical examination, fiberoptic nasopharyngoscopy and an optional lateral cephalometric radiograph to determine the site or sites of upper airway obstruction. Other diagnostic avenues, such as sleep endoscopy, may also be performed by the surgeon in directing surgical therapy in a site-specific approach. If the base of tongue is determined to be a causative factor in the upper airway collapse, then adding radiofrequency tongue base reduction to the therapeutic regime is contemplated. Numerous surgical procedures have been developed to address each of the sites of obstruction and have offered the surgeon an armamentarium of options, each with its own set of advantages, disadvantages and success rates.

### 1.2 TECHNIQUE BACKGROUND

Radiofrequency tissue volumetric reduction (RF) was developed to reduce the size of upper airway tissues (nasal turbinate, soft palate and tongue base) as an outpatient, minimally invasive procedure using local anesthesia causing minimal discomfort with a low complication rate. The technique works by using radiofrequency at 460 KHz, by a high-frequency alternating current flow into the tissue creating ionic agitation, resulting in protein coagulation and tissue necrosis. This is followed by chronic inflammation, and fibrosis and tissue volume reduction from scar contracture. The scar contracture causes a decrease in the volume of the tongue, enlarges the diameter of the posterior airway space, and thus, should decrease the amount of upper airway obstruction. The physics behind this technique using the medical RF device (Gyrus ENT LLC, Memphis, TN) enables optimal energy delivery to generate larger yet more consistent lesion volumes. The submucosal lesions created using temperature control features in the probe prevent superficial mucosal injury by controlling the temperature at the mucosa to <40°C.

## 2 PATIENT SELECTION

Patients diagnosed with obstructive sleep apnea in whom the preoperative evaluation confirms or suggests tongue base collapse as the cause of the hypopharyngeal obstruction are candidates for RF. Patients need to be in stable medical condition, understand that the procedure may be a multiple stage process, and appreciate the potential complications. Patients with preoperative complaints of dysphagia or dysarthria should undergo a modified barium swallow and/or a speech therapy evaluation prior to considering these therapeutic options, so as not to exacerbate these complaints post treatment. Those patients with underlying diabetes mellitus should be counseled regarding the increased risk of tongue abscess formation.

Two treatment approaches exist: (1) performing RF alone; (2) performing RF with other base of tongue procedures, such as genioglossus advancement, hyoid suspension or repose procedure.

## 3 OUTLINE OF PROCEDURE: TONGUE BASE RADIOFREQUENCY

The technique can be performed as an outpatient or as an inpatient. Depending on the severity of the patient's

# SECTION J
## MINIMALLY INVASIVE HYPOPHARYNGEAL PROCEDURES

sleep-disordered breathing, post-treatment airway monitoring and/or protection with nasal continuous positive airway pressure (CPAP) or a tracheotomy may be considered.

First, the oral cavity is prepped by the patient gargling with approximately 30 ml of 0.12% oral chlorhexidine (Peridex). Oral or parenteral cephalexin is administered prior to placing the electrode. If under local anesthesia, the tongue may be sprayed with 20% benzocaine as a topical anesthetic. In addition, a local anesthetic as a gel (2% lidocaine) may be placed on a sterile cotton tipped applicator at the tongue injection sites. A 25-gauge needle injects 5.0 ml of local anesthesia such as 0.25% bupivacaine (Marcaine) with 1:200,000 epinephrine into each site. A different sterile needle is used at each site of injection. Lingual nerve blocks may be used, but are not necessary. The author does not inject saline into the treatment area. There is an increased risk of infection with each additional injection at the lesion site by bringing potential superficial tongue debris and bacteria into the area to be ablated.

Currently, a dual 22-gauge RF needle electrode with a 10 mm active length and a 10 mm protective sheath in a custom-fabricated device allows placement of the electrode under the superficial tongue musculature in the area selected for treatment. Potential sites of treatment include the midline and paramedian dorsal base of tongue areas and the anterior ventral tongue areas (Figs 40.1 and 40.2). Treatment sites should be spaced a minimum of 1.5 cm apart if a single needle probe is used or at least 2.5 cm using the dual needle probe device (Fig. 40.3). Continual pressure on the electrode and visualization that the insulation sheath is not retracting out of the tongue tissue reduce the risk of superficial tissue injury. Using the most current Gyrus radio

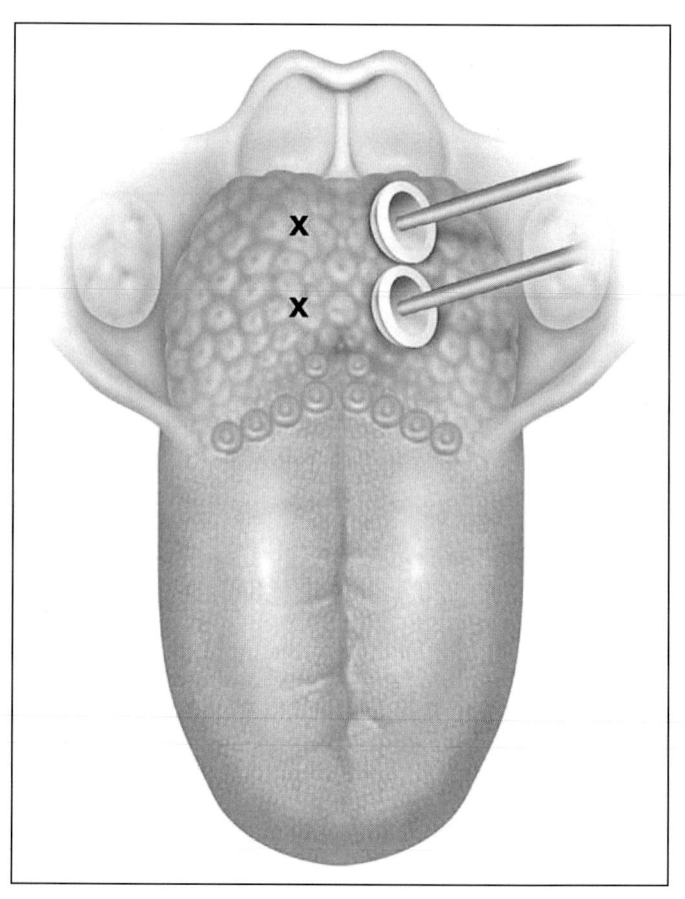

**Fig. 40.2** Tongue dorsum view. Note the position of the probe is at the midline or paramedian position of the dorsal tongue. The probe can be placed at the base of tongue, middle tongue area or ventral surface of the tongue to achieve tongue reduction.

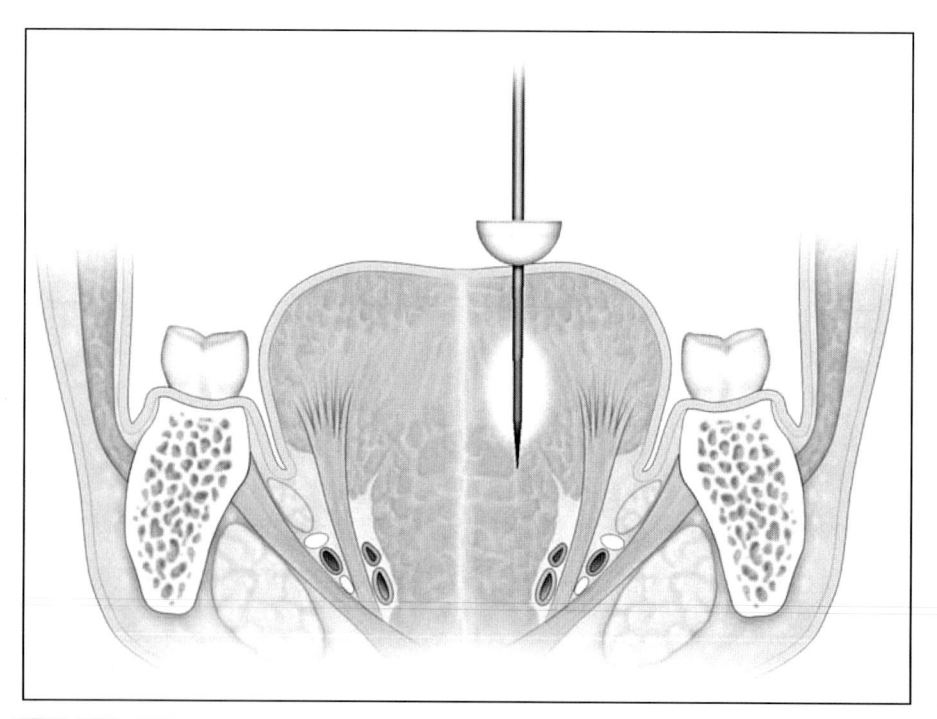

**Fig. 40.1** Tongue cross-sectional view. Note that the probe should be seated firmly against the dorsal tongue tissue to prevent withdrawal of the probe and injury to the superficial tissue. Also, the hypoglossal neurovascular bundle is located approximately 2.0–2.5 cm deep from the dorsum and should be safe from injury if the probe is placed no more lateral than the paramedian position.

# Radiofrequency tongue base reduction in sleep-disordered breathing
## CHAPTER 40

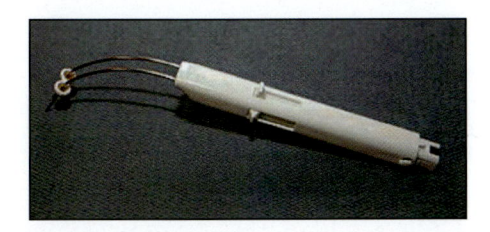

**Fig. 40.3** Tongue radiofrequency handpiece – double or dual probe. Each probe has a 1 cm distal active tip and a 1 cm proximal insulated component.

**Table 40.1** Technical factors to decrease the risk of infection

1. Give prophylactic oral antibiotics.
2. Recommend 0.12% oral chlorhexidine (Peridex) gargle prior to treatment.
3. Use sterile technique.
4. Use a new sterile needle for each local anesthetic injection site.
5. Avoid corticosteroids.
6. Ensure the electrode is seated into the tongue to prevent a superficial ulceration.
7. Do not deliver more than 600 J of rapid energy per treatment site with the dual probe.
8. Consider other treatment alternatives in diabetic mellitus patients.

frequency generator machines and a dual probe at 85°C, 600 joules (J) of rapid energy radiofrequency is delivered to two base of tongue sites with a total of 1200 J delivered. Treatment sessions may be repeated every 4–6 weeks.

Internal Gyrus research comparing the lesions created by the previous generator equipment and the new generators revealed comparable lesion sizes with 1500 J delivered at the two single probe sites from the previous machine compared to 600 J delivered using the dual probe with the new generator. If tongue base RF is being performed simultaneously with other base of tongue procedures, such as the genioglossus advancement, the surgeon must understand that additional tongue swelling will occur. Appropriate airway monitoring and airway protection should be considered perioperatively.

## 4 POSTOPERATIVE MANAGEMENT AND COMPLICATIONS

Patients undergoing the procedure under local anesthesia, who have a prominent gag reflex, may benefit from a 10–20 mg oral dose of oral diazepam. Corticosteroids may be used postoperatively, but the author does not use them, because of the concern of tongue abscess formation. If postoperative swelling and airway compromise are a concern, the surgeon can consider using nasal CPAP or auto-titrating positive airway pressure devices and/or monitoring the patient as an inpatient with pulse oximetry or intensive care monitoring. Ice by mouth is recommended for the first 2 days to decrease tongue edema. Pain as a result of this technique is usually mild with a 2–3 day duration treated with acetaminophen, non-steroidal anti-inflammatory medications or low-dose opioid narcotic analgesics.

The main potential postoperative complications are superficial tongue ulceration, tongue abscess formation, upper airway obstruction from immediate post-treatment swelling or hypoglossal nerve injury. This later complication can result in temporary or permanent dysphagia and dysarthria.

To diminish the risk of infection in patients undergoing tongue base radiofrequency, a number of precautions and directions can be followed (Table 40.1). The incidence of tongue abscess formation in nearly every study ranges from 0 to 1.5%. Following the recommendations in Table 40.1 may limit the incidence of tongue superficial ulcerations and infection.

To avoid hypoglossal nerve injury, it is best to limit the ablation sites to no more than 2 cm lateral to midline. The neurovascular bundle is approximately 2–3 cm from the surface epithelium and approximately 2–3 cm lateral from midline in a normal sized tongue (Figs 40.1 and 40.2).

Tongue discomfort, odynophagia and dysphagia may occur for 3–5 post treatment. To lower the incidence of significant post treatment discomfort one should follow these recommendation: (1) limit the rapid energy delivery per each dual probe to 600 J; (2) limit the treatment to two dual probe sites per treatment session; (3) use crushed ice by mouth as much as possible for the first 24–48 hours; and (4) follow the treatment techniques to limit the risk of infection.

## 5 TONGUE BASE RADIOFREQUENCY RESULTS

In the first published study evaluating RF for sleep-disordered breathing, a porcine study[1] evaluated the relationship of lesion size to total RF energy delivery and subsequent tissue volume reduction. The study showed that tongue musculature volume could be safely reduced using RF energy in a precise and controlled manner with minimal risk of mucosal injury or infection. As the total energy delivered increased from 500 to 2400 J the lesion cross-sectional area increased from 0.7 cm$^2$ to 1.4 cm$^2$. After 3 weeks of scar formation and subsequent contraction the overall tissue volume reduced by 26.3%.

The first human tongue pilot study[2] investigated the feasibility, safety, and possible efficacy in the treatment of sleep-disordered breathing. Eighteen patients were enrolled in the study. These patients were incompletely treated with upper airway reconstruction procedures, all of which underwent at least an uvulopalatopharyngoplasty. The mean preoperative Apnea/Hypopnea Index (AHI) of 39.6 improved to a mean of 17.8 (55%) post treatment; the mean Apnea Index (AI) of 22.1 improved to a mean of 4.1 (80%); and the mean preoperative SAO$_2$ nadir of 81.9% improved to 88.3% (12%) post treatment. The mean energy delivery per treatment session was 1543 J for a mean total energy delivery of 8490 J. Magnetic resonance imaging revealed a tongue volume reduction of 17% with an improvement of the posterior airway space by 15%. Speech and swallowing evaluated by VAS scores were unchanged. The only complication was one tongue abscess in 181 treatment sessions, which resolved after incision and drainage.

A long-term follow-up study[3] on the patients in the initial human study revealed 16 patients completed the follow-up at a mean of 28 months after the initial treatment. Sleep studies were performed using a new nasal cannula by Sleep Solutions (Redwood City, CA), which can quantitate airflow. This technology is thought to be more accurate in identifying hypopneas. The follow-up data revealed that the AI remained the same at 5.4, but the overall AHI relapsed to 28.7. The $SAO_2$ nadir relapsed to 85.8%. There were no changes in the quality of life scale (SF36), Epworth Sleepiness Scale, speech or swallowing VAS scores. The conclusion of the authors was that the success of tongue base RF may reduce with time with the primary relapse in the AHI. The limitation of the study was the use of different monitoring devices to document hypopneas.

A prospective, non-randomized study[4] evaluated 10 patients who underwent uvulopalatopharyngoplasty (UPPP), nasal surgery and tongue base RF as an inpatient. Two additional RF sessions were performed postoperatively in an outpatient setting. Nine of the ten patients received a cumulative dose of approximately 12,000 J. Five of these patients were successfully treated, defined as an AHI <20 with at least a 50% reduction in AHI. The mean preoperative AHI of 29.5 ± 14.8 improved to a mean AHI 18.8 ± 14.6 and the mean AI of 8.7 ± 6.4 improved to a mean AI of 3.7 ± 4.9.

Another study[5] compared the results of treatment with UPPP alone compared to tongue RF along with UPPP showing that the combined approach significantly improved the success rate in patients with level II and III sites of upper airway obstruction. The success rate increased in level II patients by 17.2% (37.9% vs. 55.1%) and in level III patients by 24.9% (8.1% vs. 33.0%) with the addition of tongue base RF to the UPPP procedure.

A multi-institutional study[6] evaluated 73 patients with underlying obstructive sleep apnea; 56 (76.7%) of these patients completed tongue base RF and follow-up polysomnography. Sixty-five (92.9%) had prior pharyngeal surgery. A mean of 5.4 ± 1.8 treatment sessions were performed with a mean of 3.1 ± 0.9 lesions per treatment session and an overall energy delivery of 13,394 ± 5459 J. The mean AHI of 40.5 ± 21.5 decreased to a mean of 32.8 ± 22.6 post treatment. The authors concluded that RF diminishes the severity of obstructive sleep apnea with subjective outcomes comparable to nasal CPAP.

In an investigation to utilize higher energy levels, 20 patients under local anesthesia were treated with two treatment sessions delivering 2800 J per session (700 J to each of four tongue base sites) for a total of 5600 J.[7] The results revealed a reduction of the mean AHI of 27.7 to 22.6 and showed a 45% success rate, defined as an AHI less than 20 with at least a 50% improvement. A subsequent study by the same authors using 2800 J per treatment session and a mean number of 3.4 treatment sessions revealed a mean reduction of the AHI from 32.1 to 24.9 and a 33% success rate.[8]

Steward[9] evaluated 22 patients who underwent both palatal and tongue RF treatments (mean 4.8 tongue and 1.8 palate sessions) and revealed statistical improvement in daytime sleepiness, and a significant improvement in the AHI from 31.0 to 18.7. The surgical success was 59% defined as an AHI less than 20 with at least a 50% improvement. There were no significant postoperative complications.

Twenty-six patients with mild to moderate sleep apnea were randomized to RF therapy for three tongue treatments and then two additional tongue and palate treatments.[10] The initial three tongue treatments significantly improved the quality of life and the additional two tongue and palate RF treatments further significantly improved the quality of life as determined by the Functional Outcomes of Sleep Questionnaire (FOSQ), daytime sleepiness and reaction times.

A study evaluating the efficacy of ventral tongue probe placement combined with dorsal RF delivery in 20 patients revealed no significant complications and a mean AHI decreased from 35.1 ± 18.1 to 15.1 ± 17.4.[11] The authors noted the limitations of the study with lack of a control group, small sample size and short-term follow-up, but had significant results of the combined treatment of the ventral and dorsal surfaces of the tongue.

A randomized trial compared tongue and palatal RF and nasal CPAP to sham-placebo. Both nasal CPAP and multi-level RF revealed improvement in quality of life parameters as compared to placebo and there were no differences between the RF and nasal CPAP groups.[12]

Tongue base radiofrequency has been shown to improve the amount of obstructions in patients with sleep-disordered breathing. The technique can be performed as an outpatient or inpatient, under local or general anesthesia with minimal risks of complications and minimal quality of life changes. Tongue radiofrequency volumetric tissue reduction yields improvement in the AHI of obstructive sleep apnea patients in all studies to date and is usually a low-risk procedure; however, following the preceding recommendations will aid in minimizing possible complications.[13] If there is persistent obstructive sleep apnea confirmed by a postoperative sleep study, other stand-alone surgical procedures or in combination with tongue RF may be considered.

## REFERENCES

1. Powell NB, Riley RW, Troell RJ, et al. Radiofrequency volumetric reduction of the tongue: a porcine pilot study for the treatment of obstructive sleep apnea syndrome. Chest 1997;111:1348–55.

2. Powell NB, Riley RW, Guilleminault C. Radiofrequency tongue base reduction in sleep-disordered breathing: a pilot study. Otolaryngol Head Neck Surg 1999;120:656–64.
3. Li KK, Powell NB, Riley RW, et al. Temperature-controlled radiofrequency tongue base reduction for sleep-disordered breathing: long-term outcomes. Otolaryngol Head Neck Surg 2002;127(3):230–34.
4. Nelson LM. Combined temperature-controlled radiofrequency tongue reduction and UPPP in apnea surgery. ENT J 2001;80(9):640–44.
5. Friedman M. Combined UPPP and radiofrequency tongue base reduction for treatment of OSAHS. Otolaryngol Head Neck Surg 2003;129(6):611–21.
6. Woodson BT, Nelson L, Mickelson S, et al. A multi-institutional study of radiofrequency volumetric tissue reduction for OSAS. Otolaryngol Head Neck Surg 2001;125(4):303–11.
7. Stuck BA, Maurer JT, Horman. Tongue base reduction with radiofrequency tissue ablation: preliminary results after two treatment sessions. Sleep Breath 2000;4(4):155–62.
8. Stuck BA, Maurer JT, Verse T, et al. Tongue base reduction with temperature-controlled radiofrequency volumetric tissue reduction for treatment of obstructive sleep apnea syndrome. Acta Otolaryngol 2002;122:531–6.
9. Steward DL. Effectiveness of multilevel (tongue and palate) radiofrequency tissue ablation for patients with obstructive sleep apnea syndrome. Laryngoscope 2004;114:2073–84.
10. Steward DL, Weaver EM, Woodson BT. A comparison of radiofrequency treatment schemes for obstructive sleep apnea syndrome. Otolaryngol Head Neck Surg 2004;130(5):579–85.
11. Riley RW, Powell NB, Li KK, et al. An adjuvant method of radiofrequency volumetric tissue reduction of the tongue for OSAS. Otolaryngol Head Neck Surg 2003;129(1):37–42.
12. Woodson BT, Steward DL, Weaver EM, et al. A randomized trial of temperature-controlled radiofrequency, continuous positive airway pressure, and placebo for obstructive sleep apnea syndrome. Otolaryngol Head Neck Surg 2003;128(6):848–61.
13. Pazos G, Mair EA. Complications of radiofrequency ablation in the treatment of sleep-disordered breathing. Otolaryngol Head Neck Surg 2001;125(5):462–67.

SECTION J — MINIMALLY INVASIVE HYPOPHARYNGEAL PROCEDURES

# CHAPTER 41
# Minimally invasive submucosal glossectomy

*Sam Robinson*

## 1 INTRODUCTION

The major contributing factors to retrolingual collapse in sleep apnea are macroglossia, hypotonia, retrognathia and lingual tonsillar hyperplasia. Any or all of these may contribute to varying degrees in any given individual. All current low morbidity options have limitations in treating the macroglossia component. The ideal procedure for macroglossia would be low morbidity, allow large tissue volume reduction, have low risk of alteration in tongue function and be single stage. Submucosal glossectomy techniques aim to fulfill these criteria, with preservation of mucosa causing minor pain postoperatively. Although the external submucosal glossectomy with hyoid advancement technique discussed in Chapter 47 meets these criteria, disruption of floor of mouth musculature with open dissection (which then must be repaired) is potentially a disadvantage, and is avoidable with minimally invasive techniques.

Critical to safe dissection with limited access is the ability to safely identify vital structures in the tongue. The use of real-time ultrasound to locate the neurovascular bundles (lingual artery and hypoglossal nerve) and guide submucosal dissection was first reported by myself and co-workers in 2003, via a percutaneous approach.[1] A bipolar plasma wand ('coblation') is used to hemostatically dissect tissue at low temperatures. More recently, several variations of this technique have been used via an intraoral approach, also using coblation and ultrasound guidance. The techniques to be discussed are:

1. percutaneous submucosal glossectomy under general anesthesia (S. Robinson).
2. intraoral submucosal minimally invasive lingual excision ('SMILE') using submucosal endoscopic guided dissection under general anesthesia (E. Mair).
3. intraoral submucosal midline glossectomy under local anesthesia (or 'local glossectomy') (B.T. Woodson).
4. intraoral submucosal lingualplasty under general anesthesia (S. Robinson).

## 2 PATIENT SELECTION

The indication for minimally invasive submucosal glossectomy is macroglossia, and the discussion of patient selection for the external approach (see Chapter 47) applies equally to minimally invasive approaches.

## 3 OUTLINE OF PROCEDURES

### 3.1 PERCUTANEOUS APPROACH

Following induction of general anesthesia, the airway is secured with nasotracheal intubation. Dexametasone and broad-spectrum antibiotic are administered intravenously. Two milliliters of 1% lignocaine + 1:100,000 adrenaline are infiltrated in the midline at a level just above the hyoid. An aseptic technique is used with a suprahyoid stab incision, and the surgeon's dominant hand remains sterile. A bipolar radiofrequency probe is passed into the neck in the midline, while the surgeon's non-dominant hand palpates the tongue base mucosa intraorally (Fig. 41.1). A mouthguard on the upper teeth protects the surgeon's knuckles. The probe can be easily felt through the tongue mucosa to determine depth of dissection. Initially a Reflex 55™ wand was used, which was replaced by a Spinevac™ wand. Currently an Evac T&A™ wand is preferred (ENTec division of ArthroCare Corp, Austin, TX, USA). Real-time ultrasound is used throughout the procedure with a Philips (ATL) HDI 5000 SonoCT system and L 12-5 broadband linear array transducer in a sterile cover (Philips Medical Systems, DA Best, The Netherlands), scanning from the neck. A dedicated sonographer is used to simultaneously identify the radiofrequency probe and lingual neurovascular bundles (hypogossal nerve and lingual artery) in the tongue, allowing a minimum of 5 mm clearance between the tip of the probe and the bundles at all times. Progressive

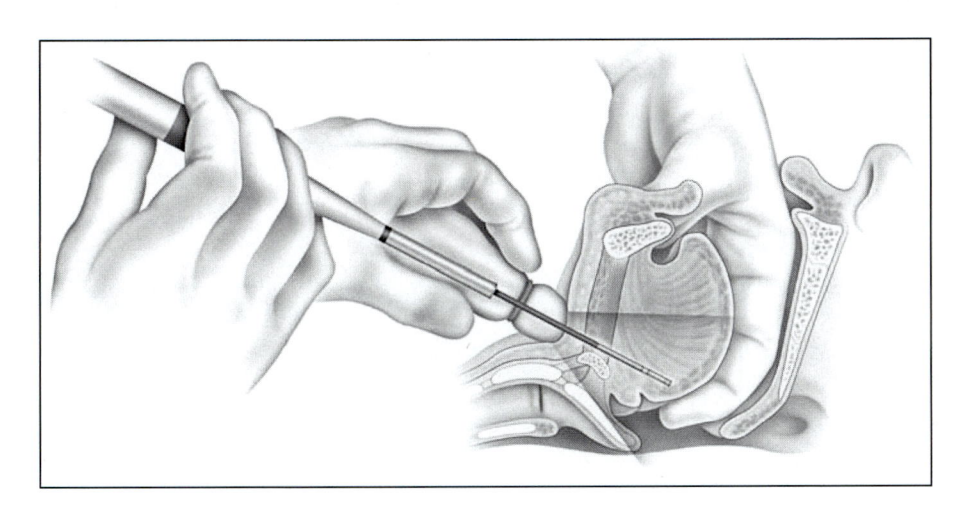

Fig. 41.1 Percutaneous submucosal glossectomy.

hemostatic submucosal resection of the tongue base musculature proceeds from 1–2 cm above valleculae to foramen cecum (or just anterior to foramen cecum) on power setting seven (for T&A wand), with the depth of treatment gauged by continuous intraoral palpation through intact tongue mucosa and ultrasound guidance. The midline is initially treated, with dissection then carried laterally, to a limited degree, between mucosa and neurovascular bundles.

If intraoperative bleeding occurs, initial management is by ultrasound-guided aspiration of blood and bimanual pressure. In more than 30 of these procedures, I have been able to obtain hemostasis with this method; however, if bleeding were to persist, injection of Floseal® (Baxter International Inc., Deerfield, IL, USA) into the cavity, as suggested by Maturo and Mair,[2] or open exploration of the cavity for hemostasis from the neck or dorsal tongue would have been required.

Extramucosal suturing is performed utilizing an Endostitch™ 10 mm disposable suturing device and 0 polysorb suture (Autosuture, Connecticut, USA) inserted after tract dilation, and a glove change prior to tying the knots. This is thought to obtain a more favorable contour of the dorsal tongue mucosa with a central concavity to maximize airway expansion. The incision is initially left open to drain the cavity, and is then closed with a Steristrip the next day.

Several limitations of this operation make it difficult to perform, and I now prefer alternative variations of submucosal tongue reduction.

- Ultrasound guidance from the neck is more difficult than using a transducer on the dorsal tongue and requires a skilled sonographer to maintain orientation of the coblation probe in relation to the neurovascular bundle.
- Hemostasis is reliant on the hemostatic effects of the coblation probe and residual bleeding vessels must be managed by bimanual pressure rather than targeted coagulation, as bleeding sites cannot be visualized.
- Access to dissect between the neurovascular bundle and mucosa into the lateral thirds of the tongue is limited from the percutaneous midline approach with a straight coblation probe. Bending the coblation probe does not solve this issue, as this makes ultrasound localization of the tip extremely difficult.
- The extramucosal stitches are difficult to securely purchase on the undersurface of mucosa by feel, and their reliability in maintaining a 'V'-shaped dorsum is uncertain.

My current preference is for the submucosal lingualplasty approach for tongue reduction (see below).

## 3.2 INTRAORAL SUBMUCOSAL ENDOSCOPIC ASSISTED APPROACH ('SMILE')

This variation has been described by Maturo and Mair and named the 'SMILE' procedure. The small case series reported were all pediatric patients; however, the technique is equally applicable to adults.

After nasotracheal intubation and general anesthesia, the oral cavity is gently brushed with 0.12% chlorhexidine and a 2-0 silk retraction suture is placed through the anterior midline tongue tip. Intravenous steroid and broad-spectrum antibiotic are given in appropriate pediatric doses. An ultrasound with a 'hockey stick' probe in a sterile cover then delineates the course of the lingual arteries, which is marked in pen on the dorsal tongue mucosa bilaterally (Figs 41.2 and 41.3). A 1 cm midline incision is made approximately 2 cm from the tongue tip in pediatric cases, which approximates the junction of anterior and middle thirds of the tongue (anteroposteriorly), and blunt dissection is used to open the incision. An Evac T&A Plasma Wand attached to the Coblator II Surgery System (ArthroCare Corporation, Austin, TX, USA) with coblator ablation at a setting of 9 is then inserted into the

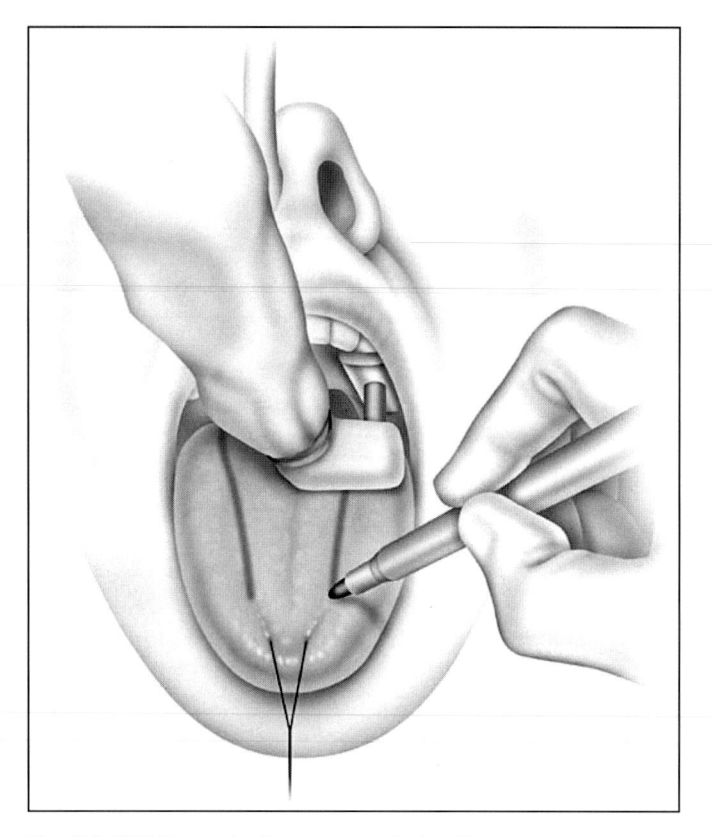

# SECTION J  MINIMALLY INVASIVE HYPOPHARYNGEAL PROCEDURES

**Fig. 41.2** SMILE: mapping the neurovascular bundles.

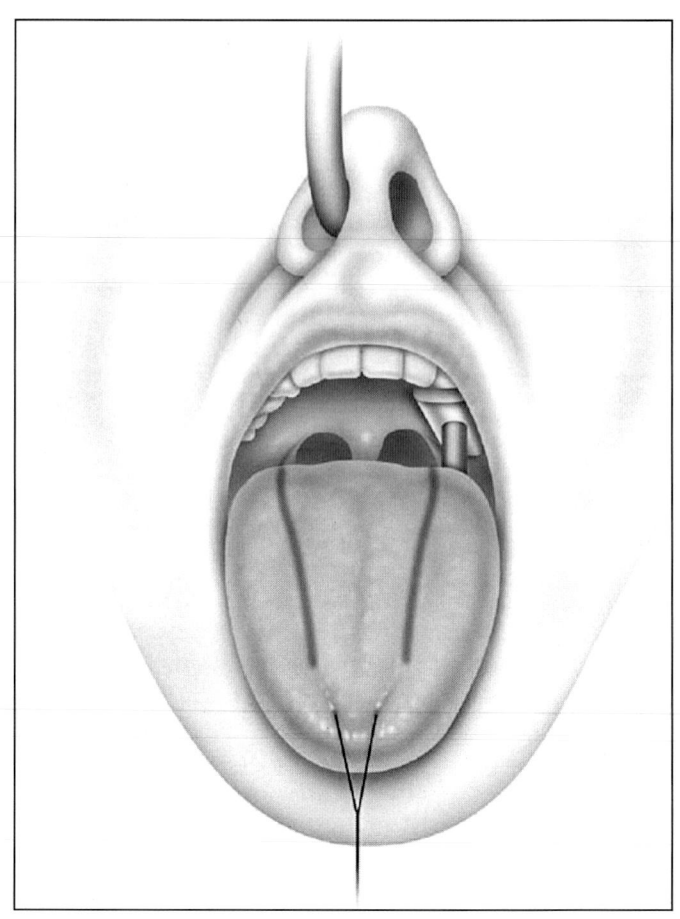

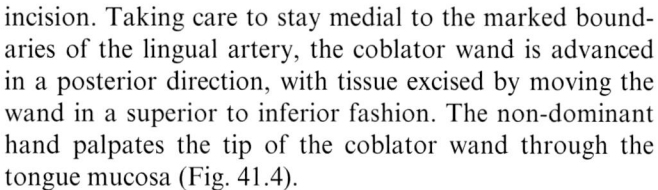

**Fig. 41.3** SMILE: neurovascular bundles marked.

incision. Taking care to stay medial to the marked boundaries of the lingual artery, the coblator wand is advanced in a posterior direction, with tissue excised by moving the wand in a superior to inferior fashion. The non-dominant hand palpates the tip of the coblator wand through the tongue mucosa (Fig. 41.4).

Progress is monitored by intermittently removing the wand and inserting a 0° irrigating endoscope (Clear ESS, SLT, Montgomeryville, PA, USA) into the created cavity. A pressure bag on the saline irrigation of the Clear ESS aids vigorous irrigation of the cavity and therefore identification of bleeding vessels in a clear field. Alternatively, the incision may be extended to allow simultaneous endoscopy and dissection (Fig. 41.5). This facilitates removal of residual strands of undissected muscle, and coagulation of any residual bleeding vessels with the coagulation mode of the wand under endoscopic visualization. I find a second 1 cm midline stab incision, 1 cm further posterior, more convenient for nasendoscope insertion than enlarging the coblator probe incision. This separates the entry points of the nasendoscope and the coblator probe into the tongue, which avoids the instruments crossing, thus avoiding restriction of their movement during dissection.

The light from the nasendoscope in the saline-filled cavity transilluminates the cavity and aids the surgeon in

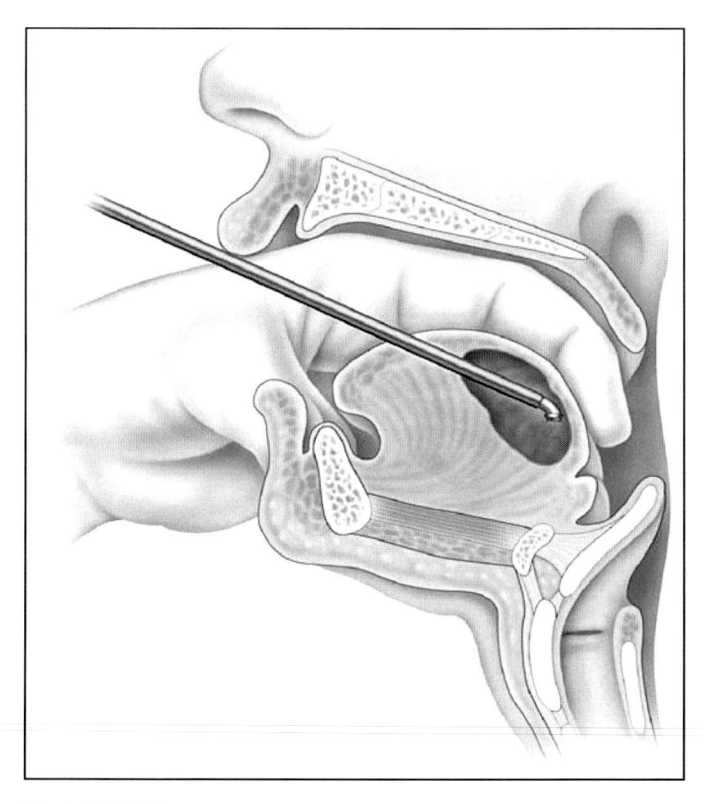

**Fig. 41.4** SMILE: dissection submucosally.

Minimally invasive submucosal glossectomy  CHAPTER 41

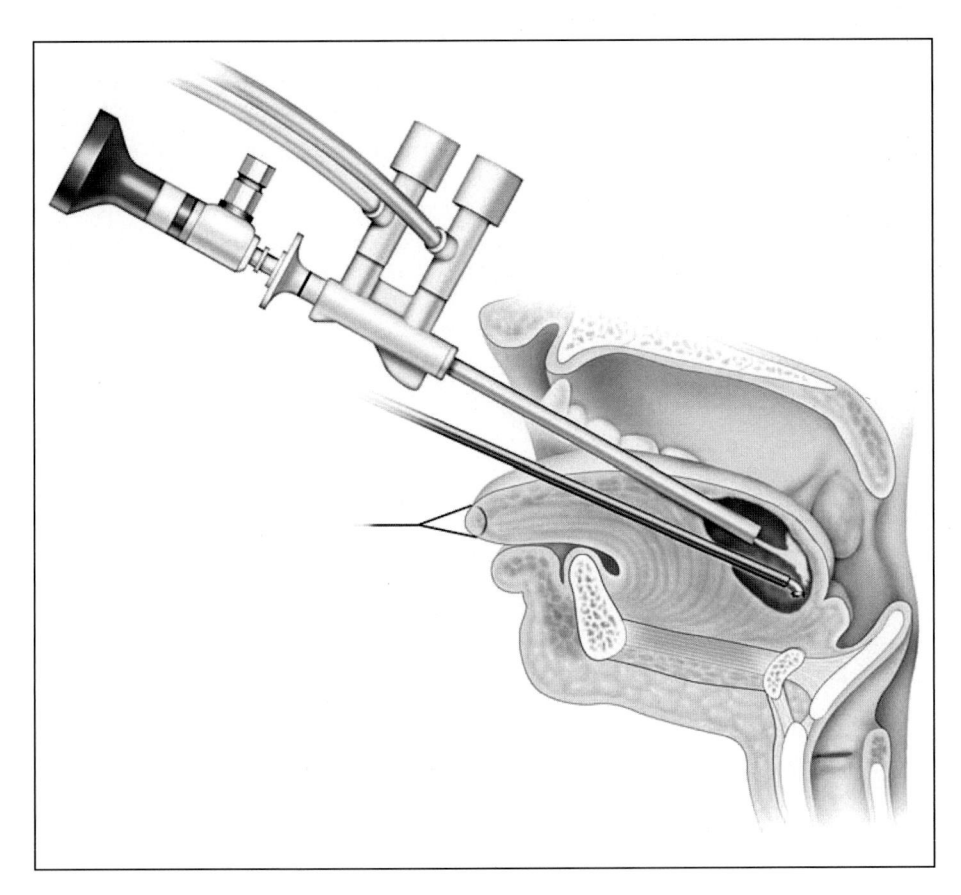

**Fig. 41.5** SMILE: dissection with endoscopic guidance.

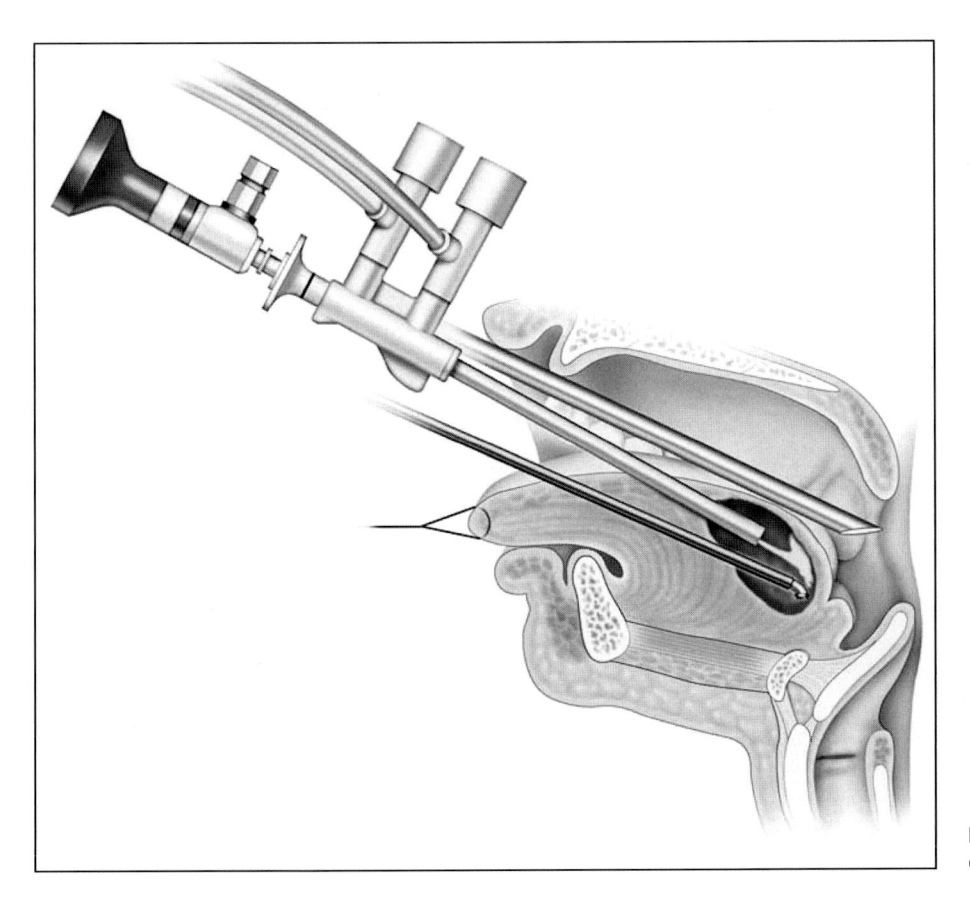

**Fig. 41.6** SMILE: checking posteroinferior limit of cavity with 70° endoscope.

251

determining the posterior limit of dissection relative to surface markings, which should be roughly no lower than opposite the tip of the epiglottis. This posteroinferior extent of dissection can be determined by palpation, or visualized by a second 30° or 70° nasendoscope, placed between soft palate and dorsal tongue mucosa to view the epiglottis (Fig. 41.6). The anterior tongue incision is left open to allow passive drainage of any tissue fluid or blood.

## 3.3 SUBMUCOSAL MIDLINE GLOSSECTOMY

B. Tucker Woodson has developed a submucosal midline glossectomy technique under local anesthesia, which is described in more detail in the following chapter. In brief, the patient is seated in the operating theater and voluntarily protrudes their tongue. The initial steps of the procedure are as for the SMILE procedure, with IV antibiotics and steroids, and marking the location of the neurovascular bundles on the dorsal tongue mucosa with an ultrasound machine and 'hockey stick' hand piece using color Doppler mode, covered in a sterile cover (see Figs 41.2 and 41.3).

Local anesthesia and adrenaline infiltration are performed to obtain an anesthetized and vasoconstricted field medial to the marked neurovascular bundles. Any weakness of tongue protrusion warns of infiltrating too close to the neurovascular bundle, and dissection in that area should be avoided. A 5 cm midline incision between the anterior and posterior extent of the middle third of the tongue with a Bovie enables direct open access to the tongue musculature (Fig. 41.7). This can be extended into the posterior third of tongue if required.

The wound edges are retracted by an assistant with stay sutures, and a submucosal midline glossectomy is performed using an Evac T&A Plasma Wand attached to the Coblator II Surgery System, with coblator ablation at a setting of between 7 and 9 (Fig. 41.8). The lateral limits of dissection are around 5 mm medial to the marked location of the lingual artery. Any vessels not sealed with the ablation mode during dissection are sealed with the coag mode under direct vision. A 30° or 70° nasendoscope held between the palate and the tongue dorsum aids dissection posteriorly, and is viewed on a monitor via a camera attachment. The anterior tongue incision is partly closed with absorbable sutures, but posteriorly part of the wound is left open to allow drainage of any tissue fluid or blood.

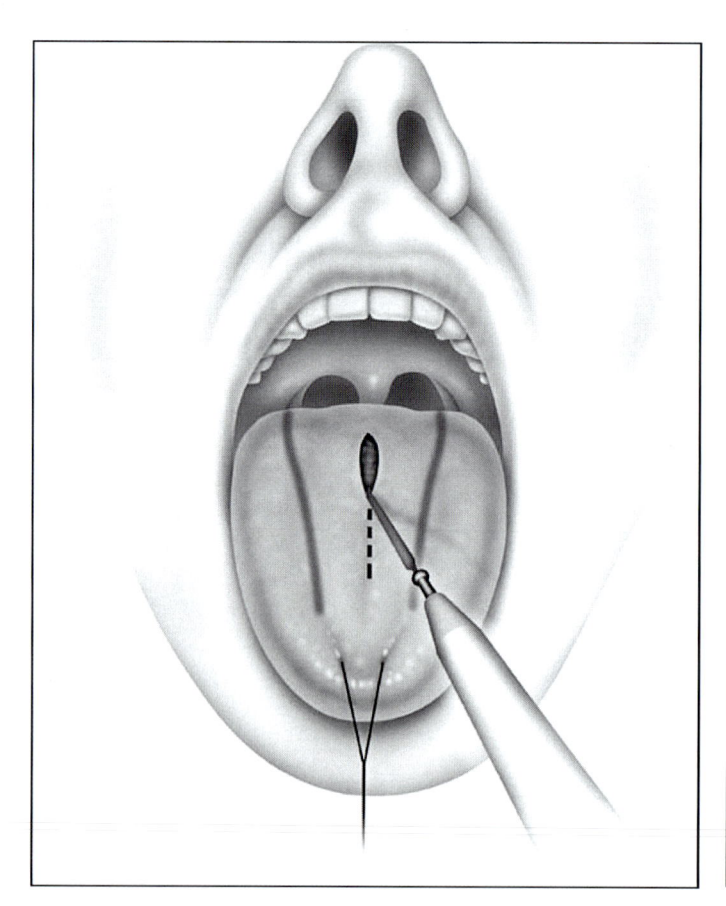

**Fig. 41.7** Submucosal midline glossectomy: incision.

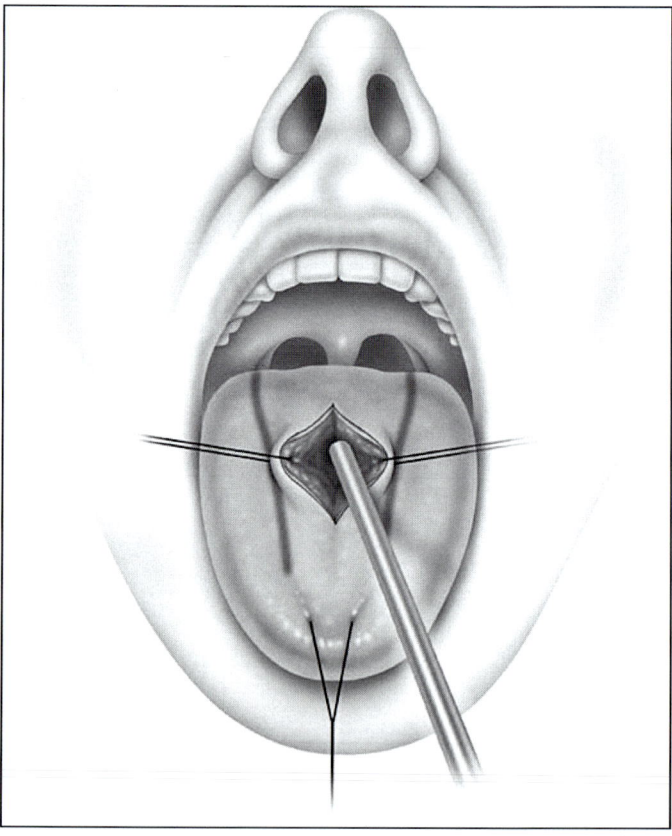

**Fig. 41.8** Submucosal midline glossectomy: dissection.

# CHAPTER 41 — Minimally invasive submucosal glossectomy

## 4 SUBMUCOSAL LINGUALPLASTY

I have extended these above concepts from submucosal midline glossectomy between the neurovascular bundles, to a submucosal lingualplasty which also accesses the lateral thirds of the tongue. The submucosal lingualplasty procedure is performed under general anesthesia. The initial steps involve a midline incision on the dorsal tongue mucosa, from the junction of the anterior and middle thirds of the tongue to 1–2 cm anterior to the circumvallate papillae (see Fig. 41.7). The wound edges are retracted by stay sutures and the mucosa is undermined to expose the underlying tongue musculature (Figs 41.8 and 41.9). The tongue muscles are then split in the midline down to a depth where transverse muscles meet genioglossus. Intraoperative ultrasound is used via the dorsum of the tongue to expose a plane just superficial to the lingual artery with a large hemostat (Fig. 41.10). A 'hockey stick' probe for scanning the dorsum of the tongue as suggested by Mair and Woodson can be used, but access is limited to the anterior half of the tongue, as the probe cannot be moved past the teeth to contact the posterior half of the dorsal tongue. To address this issue, I use a portable ultrasound machine (Portable Logiqbook XP, GE Medical Systems, Milwaukee, WI, USA) with a T-shaped probe (T739-RS intraoperative probe), which can be slid along the tongue mucosa from anteriorly back to the valleculae, to trace the entire course of the lingual artery within the tongue.

Once the plane superficial to the neurovascular bundle is identified with the hemostat, the midline cavity is connected to it by dividing the muscle between the cavity and hemostat, cutting onto the hemostat with a Bovie. A gently curved malleable retractor is inserted into the plane and is pushed posteriorly. This malleable retractor tends to slide in the plane just superficial to the neurovascular bundle via blunt dissection when gentle pressure is applied postero-inferiorly (Fig. 41.11). The ultrasound can then be used again via the dorsal tongue mucosa to ensure the malleable retractor is just superficial to all major vessels (particularly the main lingual artery with accompanying hypoglossal nerve), scanning in a sagittal plane parallel to the midline. The vascular structures can be visualized, and then shielded from the ultrasound if the retractor is moved from a medial to lateral position in the plane superficial to the bundles while scanning in a parasagittal plane. This confirms that excision of tongue musculature superficial to the retractor is safe.

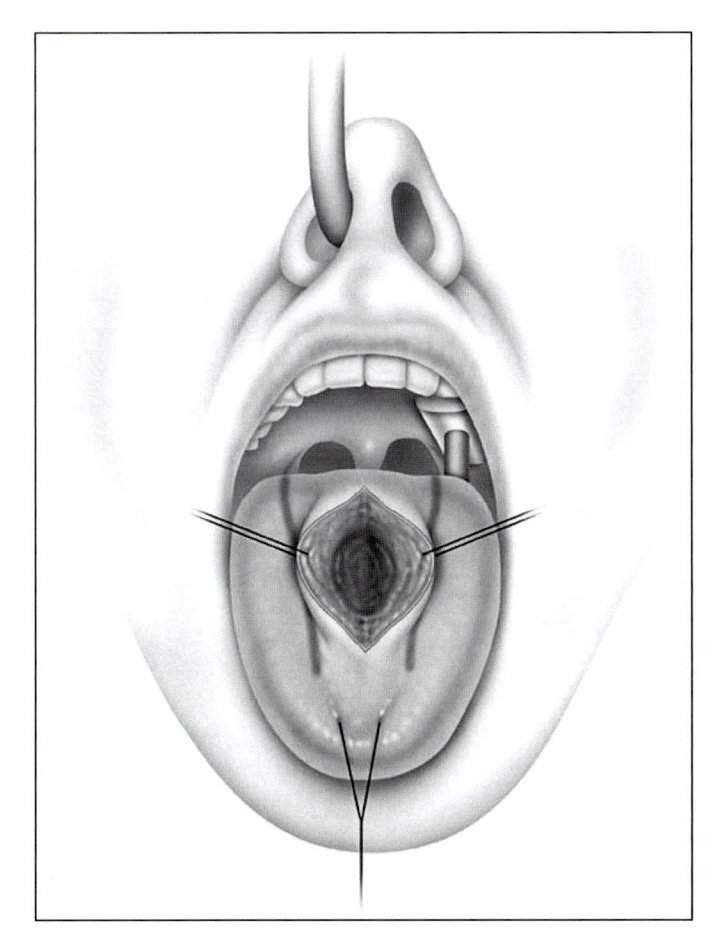

**Fig. 41.9** Submucosal lingualplasty: ultrasound-guided blunt dissection superficial to neurovascular bundles.

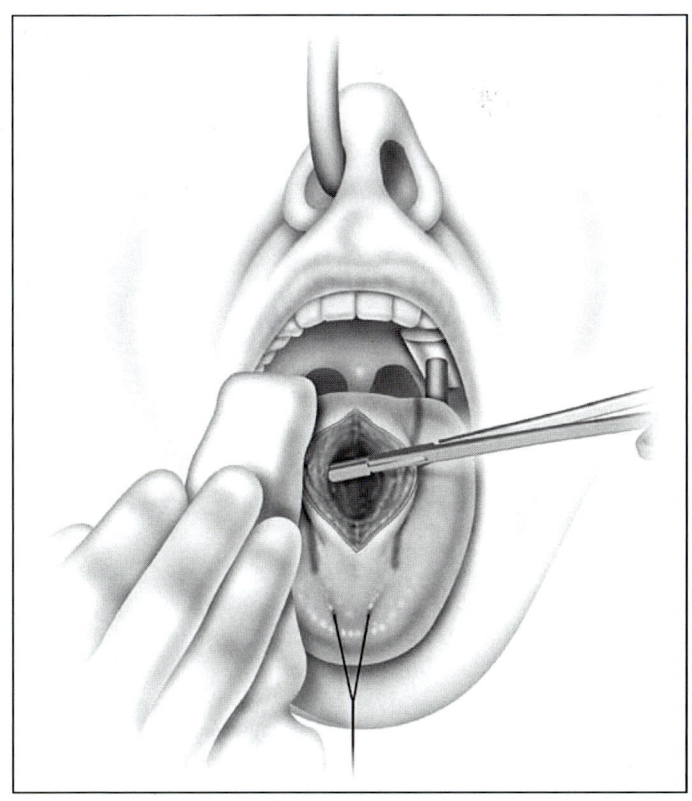

**Fig. 41.10** Submucosal lingualplasty: posterior extension of plane superficial to neurovascular bundles with malleable retractors.

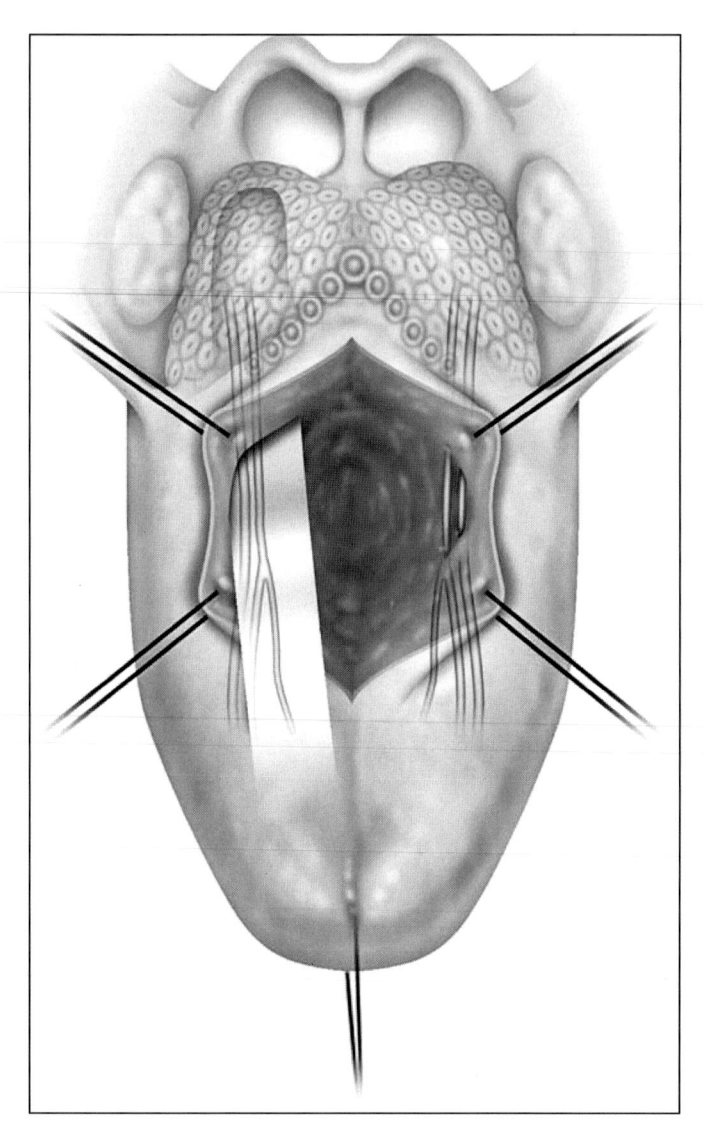

# SECTION J — MINIMALLY INVASIVE HYPOPHARYNGEAL PROCEDURES

**Fig. 41.11** Submucosal lingualplasty: submucosal excision of muscle superficial to malleable retractors.

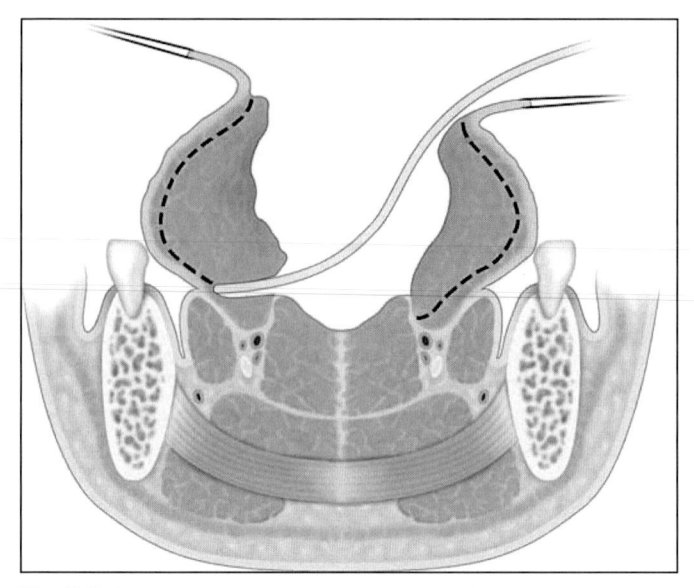

**Fig. 41.12** Submucosal lingualplasty: coronal view of muscle excision.

The dissection is performed with an Evac T&A Plasma Wand setting 7–9 with copious irrigation of saline by using a pressure bag over the irrigation bag. Alternatively an Argon beam coagulator (Conmed ABC system 7500, Conmed Corporation, USA) with a 5 cm tungsten ExplorAr® needle point argon plasma cutting electrode (Surgical Technology Pty Ltd, Carlton Nth, Victoria, Australia) coag setting 50 and gas flow 6 l/min offers even faster dissection with excellent hemostasis, as long as constant traction is maintained on the dissected tissues. Submucosal dissection extends from the midline, to superficial and lateral to the neurovascular bundles in the middle and posterior thirds of the tongue (anteroposteriorly) (Fig. 41.12). Posteriorly medially between the neurovascular bundles and hyoglossus muscles, a further cuff of posterior genioglossus is excised. The posteroinferior limit of dissection is opposite the tip of the epiglottis, and this can usually be judged by palpation. If palpation of the epiglottic tip is difficult, a 70° nasendoscope can be placed between the soft palate and dorsal tongue to determine the inferior limit of dissection.

The tongue musculature superficial and lateral to the neurovascular bundles is more vascular compared to the medial tongue between the bundles, and although dissection in this lateral area with the submucosal lingualplasty allows more aggressive tongue removal, the risk of hematoma and edema is also increased. For this reason, at the completion of dissection, hemostasis is obtained at a mean arterial pressure of 110 mm Hg and using the Valsalva maneuver (as with the external submucosal glossectomy technique). In the posterior tongue, arterial branches 1–2 mm in diameter may be found which are characteristically tortuous, and are situated between the lingual arteries, or branch from the dorsal surface of lingual artery. It is *critically important to ligate any small arterial branches* (I use ligaclips), rather than cauterize these vessels, to avoid serious delayed bleeding on days 3–4 postoperatively.

I have found that, unlike for the submucosal midline glossectomy or SMILE technique, passive intraoral drainage is unreliable after submucosal lingualplasty and results in an unacceptably high rate of postoperative tongue swelling. Therefore a soft 10-gauge suction drain (e.g. Jackson–Pratt drain) is used in preference to relying on passive intraoral drainage. Passive external drainage with a Penrose drain is satisfactory, but results in more tongue swelling than suction drainage. First the trocar is cut off the drain (as the trocar is not curved enough to insert the drain directly through the mouth and out the neck). After vasoconstrictor infiltration, a suprahyoid midline skin crease stab incision admits a large, slightly curved clamp inserted from the neck (e.g. Howard–Kelly clamp). This is

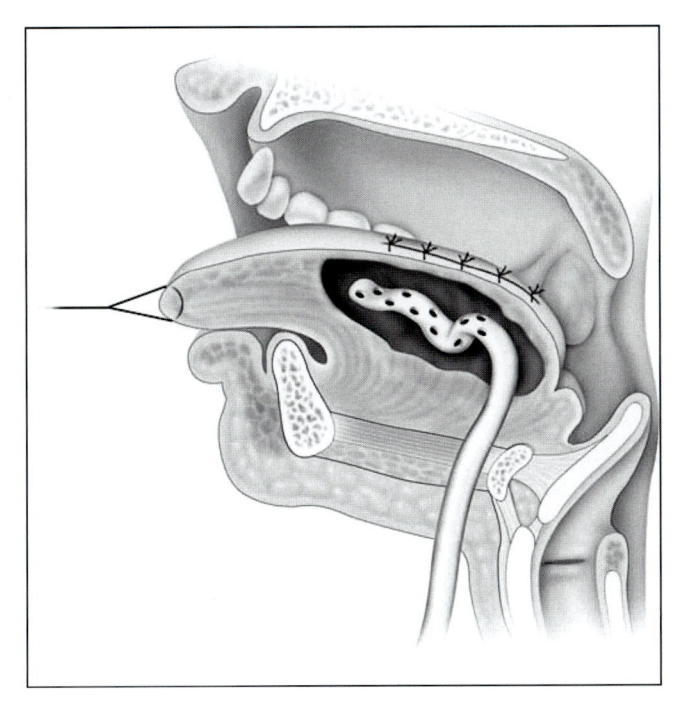

**Fig. 41.13** Submucosal lingualplasty: completed additional posterior cuff genioglossus excision, drain insertion and mucosal closure.

pushed bluntly through the floor of mouth musculature in the midline to enter the cavitated tongue, which allows the drain to be pulled through from the mouth to exit in the neck (Fig. 41.13).

As a large volume of muscle is typically resected (around 20–25 ml), redundant dorsal mucosa is excised conservatively to allow tension-free closure. The posterior mucosal flap is sutured to the remnant genioglossus muscle with a buried 1 Vicryl stitch to decrease dead space. The intraoral incision is closed with interrupted heavy absorbable sutures (e.g. 1 Vicryl) submucosal (with the knots buried beneath mucosa), and a superficial mucosal closure with many interrupted 1 silk stitches to be airtight (which are removed 2 weeks postoperatively in the clinic). The drain can usually be removed on the morning after surgery. If more than 30 ml drains in 24 hours, it may be advisable to leave the drain another day. Due to the large shearing forces in this region, all dorsal tongue mucosal wounds have the potential to break down, thus increasing pain. Work is ongoing to define the ideal closure method.

## 5 POSTOPERATIVE MANAGEMENT

The discussion of postoperative management for the external approach applies equally to minimally invasive approaches (see Chapter 47). Airway protection, blood pressure control and analgesia without respiratory depression are critical.

## 6 COMPLICATIONS

Surgeons restricting dissection to medial of the neurovascular bundles (E. Mair and B.T. Woodson) have not stressed the need to control hypertension; however, early in my experience with the percutaneous approach, I experienced a case of rapid tongue swelling within the hour after surgery when hypertension was uncontrolled.[1] This precipitated an airway emergency necessitating cricothyroidotomy under local anesthesia. Therefore, I feel that maintaining the mean arterial pressure below 100 mm Hg with routine arterial line monitoring adds a margin of safety, and advise this in every case of submucosal glossectomy, regardless of the extent of dissection. I have seen a recent severe tongue hematoma in a patient with a previously undiagnosed bleeding disorder. This was recognized with excessive bleeding intraoperatively and postoperatively from the operative field, and from IV cannula and arterial line sites. Clotting factors and platelet transfusions were required to stop the generalized oozing and ever-increasing tongue size. The patient was not extubated at the end of surgery due to concerns over tongue size, and an evacuation of hematoma and tracheotomy were performed on the third postoperative day. The tongue returned to normal size and function over 10 days, allowing decannulation. As a large raw surface is created in the tongue, it is critical to ensure aspirin is held for 2 weeks prior and NSAID drugs are held for several days prior to surgery, and that a history of previous bleeding or a familial tendency towards bleeding is carefully sought.

As mentioned previously, the posterior third of the tongue contains small-caliber arterial branches. Although these are controllable at the time of initial surgery with diathermy, I have seen two cases of serious delayed bleeding, one at day 3, and one at day 4 postoperatively. Tongue swelling and bleeding into the airway were precipitate and life-threatening, requiring operative intervention within 2 hours. The airway of one patient was secured with awake fiberoptic intubation, as in the operating theater there was tamponade of the bleeding inside the tongue (although slowly increasing tongue size) allowing adequate visualization. The other patient required emergency tracheotomy under local anesthesia to secure the airway, as active bleeding would have made fiberoptic visualization impossible. Once the tongue was explored and the arterial bleeding vessel ligated with clot evacuation, the tongue wounds were resutured and healed uneventfully with minimal pain. It is theorized that one of these arterial branches may also have caused the one case of pre-epiglottic space/tongue base hematoma in the external submucosal glossectomy series reported in Chapter 47. No more bleeding of this nature has occurred since carefully searching for arterial branches during dissection (aided by loupe magnification) and using ligaclip hemostasis. This highlights the need for the surgeon to be always mindful of the potential serious complications which may occur with tongue reduction surgery, and therefore only surgeons comfortable in dealing with airway emergencies should attempt this kind of surgery. My current postoperative protocol keeps the patient nasotracheally intubated on ICU for 2 hours postoperatively to observe for swelling, and then in or near the hospital for the first 5 days following surgery in case of delayed bleeding. The risk of delayed bleeding is now thought to be very low with the use of ligaclips; however, the seriousness of this potential complication warrants caution.

The initial selection of a percutaneous approach for the minimally invasive technique was based on theoretical concerns of infection risk from intraoral contamination of the cavitated tongue 'sump' with an intraoral approach. Early clinical experience to date, however, suggests the infection rate for an intraoral approach is relatively low, although this has not been accurately quantified as yet. In the event infection occurs, this discharges through the intraoral incision and is managed with oral antibiotics as an outpatient.

In contrast to glossectomy techniques involving open mucosal defects, the pain after submucosal glossectomy techniques is minor, and usually controllable with paracetamol only from the first postoperative day. Dehiscence of the wound is sometimes seen in submucosal lingualplasty and local anesthetic midline glossectomy, and this will increase pain significantly, although will usually heal by secondary intention without the need for wound resuturing. This is not such an issue with the small wound of the 'SMILE' operation.

Tongue function is minimally affected by all the procedures described in this chapter, at least subjectively. Speech, swallowing and taste all appear to be unaffected after the first few weeks; however, the risk of damage to the hypoglossal nerve exists and needs to be borne in mind throughout the dissection. All these approaches have been performed on relatively few numbers of patients with no long-term follow-up or objective swallowing measurements as yet, so the apparent lack of impact on tongue function needs to be interpreted with caution. Obviously, excessive excision of tongue musculature would be expected to cause impaired function, but this has not been observed to date with excision limited to the areas described above.

Early in the percutaneous approach series, a temporary tongue weakness was seen when a Reflex 55 wand passed inadvertently within approximately 3 mm of the neurovascular bundle. This resolved spontaneously over months. The long return electrode of the Reflex 55 wand design, coupled with the percutaneous approach, predisposed to this complication when attempting to access tongue tissue lateral to the neurovascular bundle. The Spinevac, or more recently the Evac T&A wands have not caused any more cases of hypoglossal nerve weakness. Intraoral scanning makes orientation of the tip of the coblator probe easier, particularly with the T-shaped GE probe described, and the intraoral approach for dissection makes nerve injury very unlikely with careful technique. However, caution must be used at all times when dissecting near the neurovascular bundles, particularly by surgeons with limited experience in this type of surgery, to avoid the possibility of permanent tongue paralysis.

## 7 OUTCOMES

The initial percutaneous technique yielded a 40% response overall in the first 15 consecutive patients. This was higher when combined with additional phase 1 procedures (80%), and lower when combined with uvulopalatopharyngoplasty (UPPP) alone (20%).[1] Limitations of this small series are two different types of probe being used, and suboptimal volume reduction in many of these cases early in my experience.

In the SMILE procedure, three of the four reported cases had sleep apnea and all these three were pediatric cases associated with syndromal macroglossia (Down's or Beckwith–Wiedemann syndrome). One young child was tracheotomy dependent, and following the procedure could be decannulated without symptoms of sleep apnea. The two older children had their preoperative Respiratory Disturbance Index (RDI) reduced from 10 to less than 1, with marked improvement in symptoms of sleep-disordered breathing. It appears that children with syndromal macroglossia tend to have displacement of their neurovascular bundles laterally, leaving a large area of potentially resectable tongue medial to the bundles. Adults with macroglossia, however, often have a midline furrow, with the major extent of the tongue bulk situated superficial and lateral to the neurovascular bundles. This tongue base shape requires a technique to safely access the lateral tongue to allow adequate volume reduction (e.g. submucosal lingualplasty).

Interpreting the success rate of a single surgical intervention in a disease with multiple causes of airway collapse is difficult. The best results for tongue reduction surgery can be expected when macroglossia is the major or only cause of retrolingual obstruction (with little contribution from hypotonia, lingual tonsillar hyperplasia or retrognathia), retropalatal obstruction is absent or adequately treated, and technically adequate volume reduction is achieved by the surgery. This is well illustrated by the small but highly successful SMILE series. Data for the intraoral submucosal midline glossectomy under local anesthesia and submucosal lingualplasty under general anesthesia are not yet available. However, these are likely to be similar to other glossectomy results of 40% for midline glossectomy alone,[3] and 70–80% response rates if lateral tongue is also resected.[4–6] They are also likely to be influenced by both patient selection and degree of tongue reduction achieved.

## 8 SALVAGE OPTIONS

Failures may be at the palatal level, and success rates of airway reconstruction have been demonstrated to be improved by palatal advancement, or ZPP, rather than UPPP in patients with small or absent tonsils, when controlled for tongue base surgery.[7,8] Lingual tonsillar hyperplasia large enough to obscure the root of epiglottis as viewed on supine nasendoscopy mid-respiration is seen in around a third of adult surgical sleep apnea patients (S. Robinson, unreported data, 2006), and is recommended to be removed if of a significant size.[9] Patients with gross retrognathia (SNB < 75°) are better suited to mandibular advancement rather than tongue reduction techniques, as the airway crowding seen in these cases is due to a relative, rather than absolute macroglossia, and the amount of tongue volume which can safely be resected within the anatomical constraints of the neurovascular bundles is limited. Occasionally patients are seen with co-existing gross retrognathia and true macroglossia who will have severe sleep apnea, and may well require both tongue reduction and maxillomandibular advancement (as staged procedures) to gain adequate control of their disease.

Inadequate volume reduction may be seen, in which case revision submucosal glossectomy is required. Ongoing retrolingual hypotonia during sleep, particularly in the supine position, is not well treated by glossectomy techniques, as was demonstrated in the external submucosal glossectomy series (see Chapter 47). My current protocol for this situation is a second stage geniotubercle advancement; however, (mortised) high sliding genioplasty or a tongue base suture technique (e.g. Repose system) are reasonable alternatives. I do not currently combine submucosal glossectomy procedures with geniotubercle advancement concurrently for fear of the acute edema and impact on tongue function immediately after surgery. This policy will be reviewed after more experience, as it is felt that many patients would have an optimal result from both a volume reduction and tensioning procedure.

Failure due to a posteriorly tilted epiglottis which prolapses into the supraglottis during sleep is uncommon if the palate and tongue are stable during sleep. In my opinion, this situation would be most suitably treated by a hyoid suspension to mandible with fascia lata (see Chapter 47). Although hyothyroidopexy would also seem a reasonable alternative, the anterior vector required to verticalize the epiglottis appears unlikely to be sustained in the longer term due to remodeling of the underlying superior thyroid cartilage, which I have noted on all of my patients (six of six) having reversal or revision of hyothyroidopexy. I prefer to avoid partial epiglottectomy for fear of aspiration, and have found endoscopic glossoepiglottopexy unreliable.

As an alternative to further surgery, a mandibular advancement splint could be reconsidered in cases of both residual bulk and/or hypotonicity. Maxillomandibular advancement is a powerful salvage option, but is considered as a last resort in the skeletally normal patient as it is usually rejected by the patient.

## 9 CONCLUSIONS

Minimally invasive submucosal glossectomy strategies offer the potential for aggressive reduction of macroglossia with little pain and minimal risk to tongue function. Careful perioperative care is crucial in avoiding serious complications. The role of the minimally invasive intraoral submucosal versus the open external submucosal approach needs to be defined, but it seems likely that mucosal sparing techniques will replace traditional mucosal sacrificing options for glossectomy whether an external or intraoral approach is chosen. As most adult sleep apnea patients appear to have some degree of macroglossia and hypotonia contributing to their retrolingual obstruction during sleep, parameters need to be sought to predict which patients would do best with bulk reduction strategies versus tongue tensioning strategies, and which patients will require both. Work is ongoing in this area.

## REFERENCES

1. Robinson S, Lewis R, Norton A, et al. Ultrasound-guided radiofrequency submucosal tongue-base excision for sleep apnoea: a preliminary report. Clin Otolaryngol 2003;28:341–45.
2. Maturo SC, Mair EA. Submucosal minimally invasive lingual excision (SMILE): an effective, novel surgery for pediatric tongue base reduction. Ann Oto Rhino Laryngol 2006;115(8):624–30.
3. Fujita S, Woodson BT, Clark J, Wittig R. Laser midline glossectomy as a treatment for obstructive sleep apnea. Laryngoscope 1991;101:805–9.
4. Robinson, S. External submucosal glossectomy (Chapter 47 in this book).
5. Woodson BT, Fujita S. Clinical experience with lingualplasty as part of the treatment of severe obstructive sleep apnea. Otolaryngol Head Neck Surg 1992;107(1):40–48.
6. Chabolle F, Wagner I, Blumen M, et al. Tongue base reduction with hyoepiglottoplasty: a treatment for severe obstructive sleep apnea. Laryngoscope 1999;109:1273–80.
7. Woodson BT, Robinson S, Lim HJ. Transpalatal advancement pharyngoplasty outcomes compared with uvulopalatopharyngoplasty. Otolaryngol Head Neck Surg 2005;133:211–17.
8. Friedman M, Ibrahim HZ, Vidasagar R, et al. Z-palatoplasty (ZPP): a technique for patients without tonsils. Otolaryngol Head Neck Surg 2004;131(1):89–100.
9. Robinson S, Ettema SL, Brusky L, Woodson BT. Lingual tonsillectomy using bipolar radiofrequency plasma excision. Otolaryngol Head Neck Surg 2006;134(2):328–30.

# SECTION J — MINIMALLY INVASIVE HYPOPHARYNGEAL PROCEDURES

## CHAPTER 42

# A minimally invasive technique for tongue base stabilization

*B. Tucker Woodson*

## 1 INTRODUCTION

Obstructive sleep apnea syndrome (OSAS) results from a complex scenario initiated with airway collapse and obstruction, loss of compensatory wake and sleep reflexes, increased ventilatory effort, arousal, hypoventilation, and asphyxia during sleep. In adults, a structurally small upper airway may be a primary contributing factor. Enlarging this airway may prevent the cascade into sleep apnea and snoring.

The etiology of the small upper airway in adults may include an abnormal craniofacial structure, excessive soft tissue for the available space, and obesity. These abnormalities are not isolated to the upper pharynx and involve multiple upper airway segments. It has long been speculated that failure to treat these other areas of obstruction and collapse has been a cause of failure of isolated treatment with palatal surgery such as uvulopalatopharyngoplasty (UPPP). Hypopharyngeal levels of obstruction may include the structures of the tongue base, lateral hypopharynygeal walls, lingual tonsils and supraglottis. To treat these areas multiple procedures have been described. Each has varying levels of potential effectiveness and risks of morbidity. For surgeons the dilemma has been to adequately treat these observed sites of obstruction with the least morbidity.

Appropriate surgical treatment options require an understanding of the underlying airway abnormality. The pharyngeal wall is the posterior tongue. Its position stabilizes the hypopharynx, the lateral pharyngeal walls, and even the epipharynx. The tongue which in most mammals is an oral structure, in humans is unique and is also a pharyngeal structure. The human pharynx is potentially collapsible and is unique in requiring these muscles to maintain patency during sleep. The genioglossus and other tongue musculature do not just sustain speech and swallowing, but are ventilatory muscles supporting the airway during sleep.

Increasing stability of the tongue and lower pharynx may stabilize the airway during sleep and may effectively treat sleep-disordered breathing. Surgical procedures stiffen the airway, change shape, or increase volume of the airway. Procedures directed at the anterior wall of the pharynx include posterior glossectomy and advancement and suspension procedures. Skeletal osteotomies of the mandible may increase volume of the airway by advancing tissue or may stiffen by traction, muscle tension and stiffening. Glossectomy or tissue volume reduction procedures decrease tongue volume and proportionally increase airway size.

Most of these procedures are not widely applied. The absolute effect of any single procedure is variable. This combined with the perceived or actual morbidity discourages use to a relatively small population. The goal of surgery of the lower pharynx is to improve effectiveness, better define the surgical population, and decrease surgical morbidity. The procedure of tongue base suspension is an option to treat lower pharyngeal obstruction and reduce morbidity compared to alternative procedures.

## 2 RATIONALE

Airway collapse during sleep is both dynamic and passive. Dynamic collapse occurs during inspiration. Passive collapse occurs during expiration. Both are the result of a combination of applied forces that collapse and dilate the airway. In a structurally small airway during sleep, when dilating forces that stabilize the airway are greater than the collapsing forces, the airway is obstructed.

Obstruction during sleep is the result of a complex cascade. During inspiration, upper (pharynx) and lower (chest wall and diaphragm) airway muscles are activated. The lower airway muscles create a negative intraluminal force balanced by upper airway muscles that stiffen and dilate the airway. Increases in negative airway pressure or loss of muscle dilation will obstruct the airway. In sleep-disordered breathing both occur. Increased upper airway resistance leads to more negative intraluminal pressure and activation of upper airway dilator muscles is delayed

CHAPTER
Minimally invasive technique for tongue base stabilization  **42**

is an intraluminal dilating force. This is accomplished by passing a submucosal suture into the posterior midline tongue. The suture prevents passive collapse while not interfering with anterior and superior tongue movements which are involved with swallowing and speech. Placement is directed towards the level of the foramen cecum (Fig. 42.1).

## 3 TONGUE SUTURE SUSPENSION TECHNIQUE

### 3.1 STEP ONE (BONE ANCHOR)

The procedure is performed under general or local anesthesia. Local anesthesia requires an external approach. Technically, the procedure may be combined with other pharyngeal procedures. Due to tethering and edema of the tongue, this procedure may augment the pain and dysphagia of other procedures. Benefits of combined procedures must be balanced with risks of increased perioperative morbidity and increased side effects. Using the procedure as an isolated intervention is recommended until clinical experience is adequate. Since a foreign body is placed, preoperative broad-spectrum antibiotics to cover and intraoral closed wound are given Decadron 10 mg reduces tongue pain and swelling and postoperative nausea. Intubation may be oral or nasal depending on the surgeon's experience and preference. With oral intubation, care must be taken to protect the endotracheal tube from damage or displacement. The oral cavity is prepped with antibacterial solutions such as chlorhexidine oral solution. Exposure is facilitated by using a shoulder roll. Local anesthesia is infused into the anterior midline floor of mouth anterior to Wharton's ducts.

When performing the intraoral approach, an intraoral incision is made posterior to the salivary papillae (Fig. 42.2). The incision should be generous. An excessively long linear incision is easily closed with excellent healing. An incision too small for the device may result in mucosal tearing that may damage the papillae and create an intraoral scar. If an external incision is used an incision is made 1 cm posterior to the gnathion in a convenient skin crease or shadow.

### 3.2 STEP TWO

The suture is anchored to the bone. Two methods may be used. One method is an intraoral approach using the Repose (Influ-ENT Ltd, Concord, NH) bone screw anchoring device. Alternatively the suture may be anchored externally using the Repose device or other methods to anchor the suture to the inferior mandible. The Repose

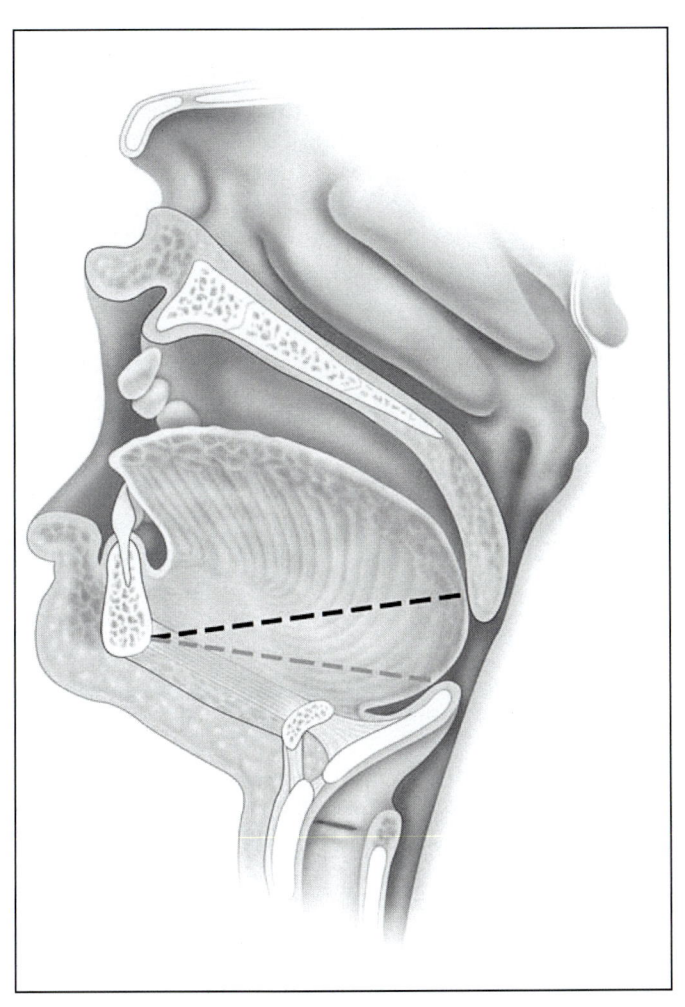

**Fig. 42.1** The angle of insertion of the tongue suspension suture is depicted (solid dotted line). This is directed towards the foramen cecum at the base of tongue. Placement too inferiorly may result in increased pain and paradoxical posterior rotation of the more superior tongue.

or decreased. During expiration, positive pressure forces dilate the airway, and upper airway muscle tone is reduced. If the balance is unfavorable and the effects of tissue mass are not compensated, collapse and obstruction occur.

The tipping point for apnea is poorly understood, but is likely initiated by passive expiratory collapse. It is this collapse that triggers the dynamic events during inspiration. Without passive airway collapse, the cascade of progressive inspiratory flow limitation, increased negative luminal pressure and increased upper airway resistance may be aborted. If adequate airway size is maintained during expiration, inspiratory obstruction is prevented.

Since during expiration the largest decreases in airway size occur in the hypopharynx, treatment of this segment may be critical for most if not all individuals with sleep-disordered breathing. The tongue suspension procedure was conceived as a means of providing an extraluminal dilating force to the lower pharyngeal airway in contrast to nasal Continuous Positive Airway Pressure (CPAP) which

259

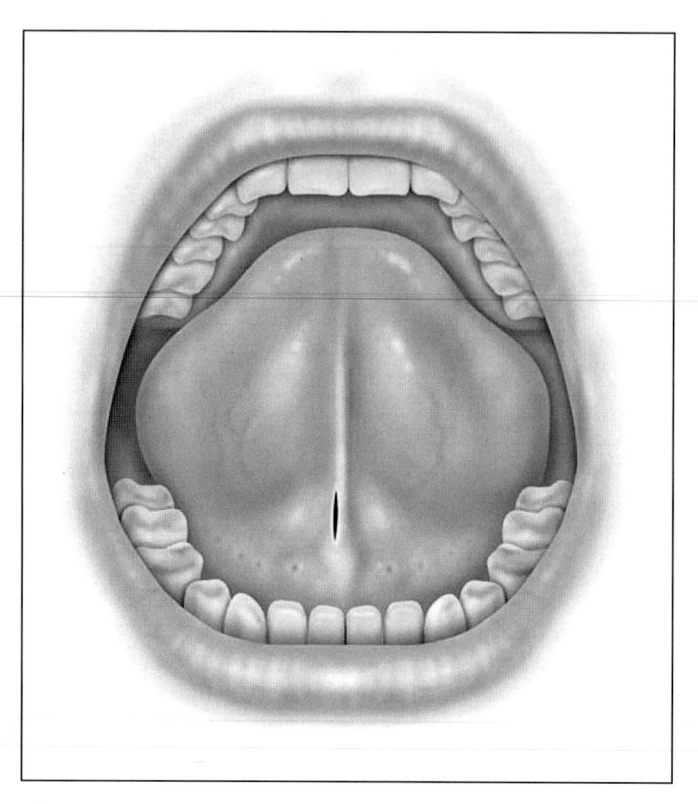

# SECTION J  MINIMALLY INVASIVE HYPOPHARYNGEAL PROCEDURES

**Fig. 42.2** Placement of intraoral incision is shown. The midline incision should be generous in length to avoid trauma and possible tearing of mucosa. Alternatively, an extraoral approach may be performed (not shown).

bone screw system consists of the U-shaped bone screw inserter that is used to place the bone screw onto the lingual surface of the mandible through an incision in the floor of mouth. It also includes the self-tapping titanium screw which is attached to two 1-0 Prolene sutures (Ethicon Endo-Surgery, Inc., Cincinnati, OH) at its base. Lastly, a suture passer is included to pass the suture through the tongue base.

A tunnel is created by dissecting between the genioglossus muscle bellies in the midline with a curved or right angle mixture hemostat. Intraorally, dissection is posterior and deep to Wharton's ducts and is carried palpably to bone. Soft tissue may be gently scraped from the bone at this juncture. If using the Repose device intraorally, placement of the bone screw inserter into the mouth may be difficult in an OSA patient. The back blunt end of the distal device may first be placed into the mouth. The bone-anchoring screw may then be placed into the intraoral incision and then through the midline tunnel down to bone. Care must be taken to place the bone screw below the tooth roots. Using force and orienting the screw perpendicular to the mandibular cortex, the driver is placed against the mandible and inserted with the battery-operated inserter (Fig. 42.3). Alternatively, a Prolene suture may be directly anchored by drilling two parallel holes in the inferior mandible. The end (s) of the suture may then be looped through this attachment.

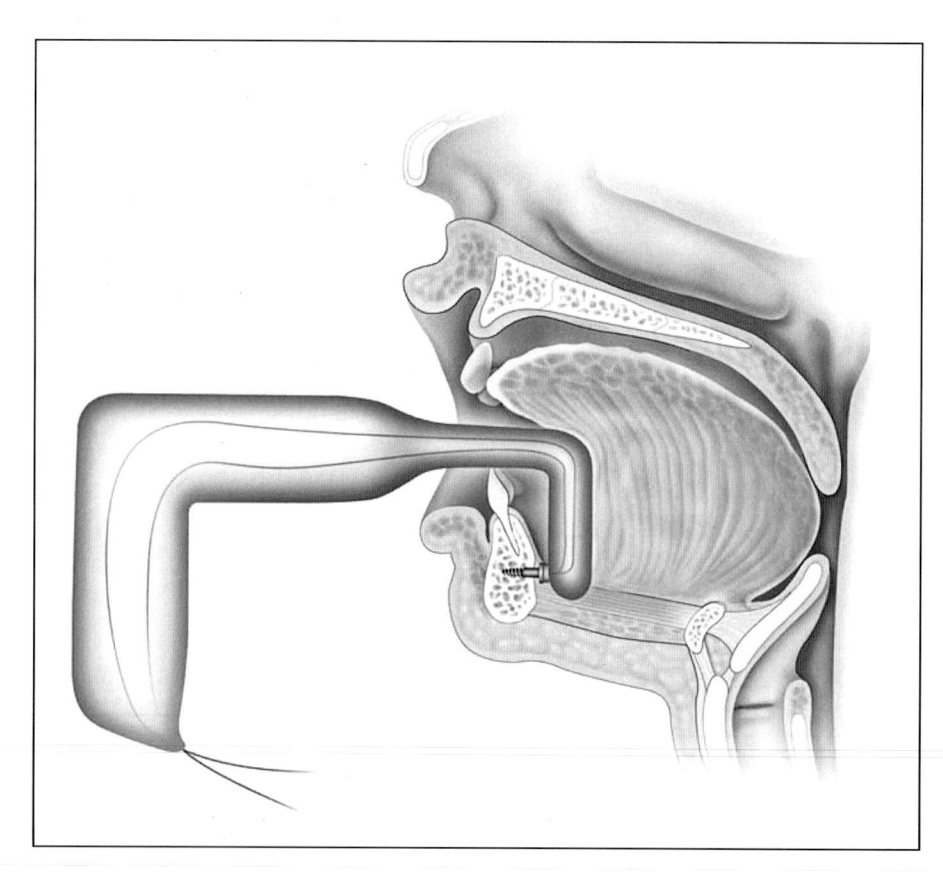

**Fig. 42.3** Repose anchoring on the mandible is depicted. Care must be taken to stay below the level of the incisor teeth. Screw insertion must be perpendicular to the cortical bone to engage bone.

## 3.3 STEP THREE

The suture that is attached to the mandible is then advanced to the tongue base about 1–1.5 cm lateral to the midline with an awl or a suture passer (Fig. 42.4). An empty suture loop is passed in a similar manner on the opposite side of the tongue taking care to avoid the neurovascular bundle that lies laterally. The suture attached to the screw is then threaded onto an empty Mayo needle, inserted into its own exit site on the tongue base and passed submucosally to the exit site of the second suture so that it is threaded into the loop of the second suture (Fig. 42.5). The second suture (the empty suture loop) is then pulled back to the anterior attachment. The Prolene suture attached to the mandible now is in a triangular configuration (Fig. 42.6). The suture is tied to itself and the knot is buried (Fig. 42.7). It is important that the tension on this suture be enough to feel a dimple on the posterior tongue base, but not so great as to cause strangulation. The correct angulation is undetermined and whether effectiveness is altered based on an intraoral or external approach is not known.

## 4 PATIENT SELECTION

Selection of the best candidates for this technique is based on anecdotal reports, clinical experience, and a few surgical case

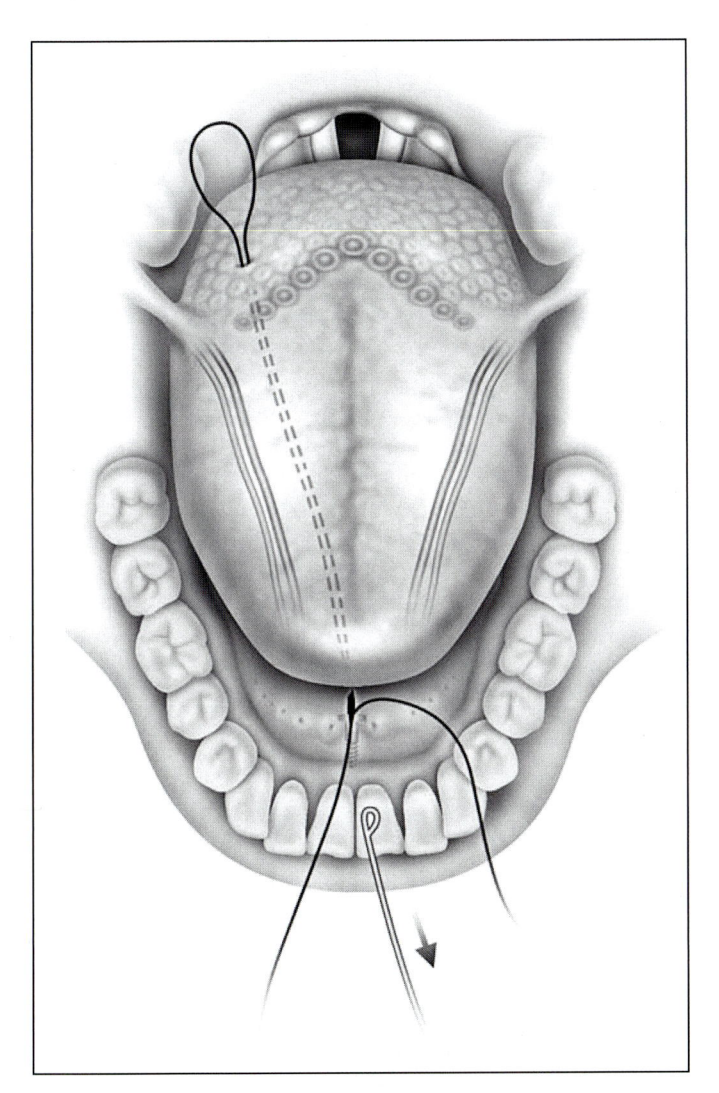

**Fig. 42.4** Direction of the suture loop placement is depicted as view from above to an axial section of the tongue. Passing the suture loop on the patient's right side is favorable for the right-handed surgeon to make passing the suspension suture across the tongue base easier in step 5. The internal anatomy of the tongue neurovascular pedicle is shown in shadowed grey. The first segment of the lingual artery and hypoglossal nerve run obliquely in the neck. The second segment courses more medially and vertically in the tongue and the third segment runs anteriorly. By keeping the sutures in the midline until well posterior, the neurovascular pedicle is avoided. The depth of passage should be superiorly towards the foramen cecum and not inferiorly into the valleculae.

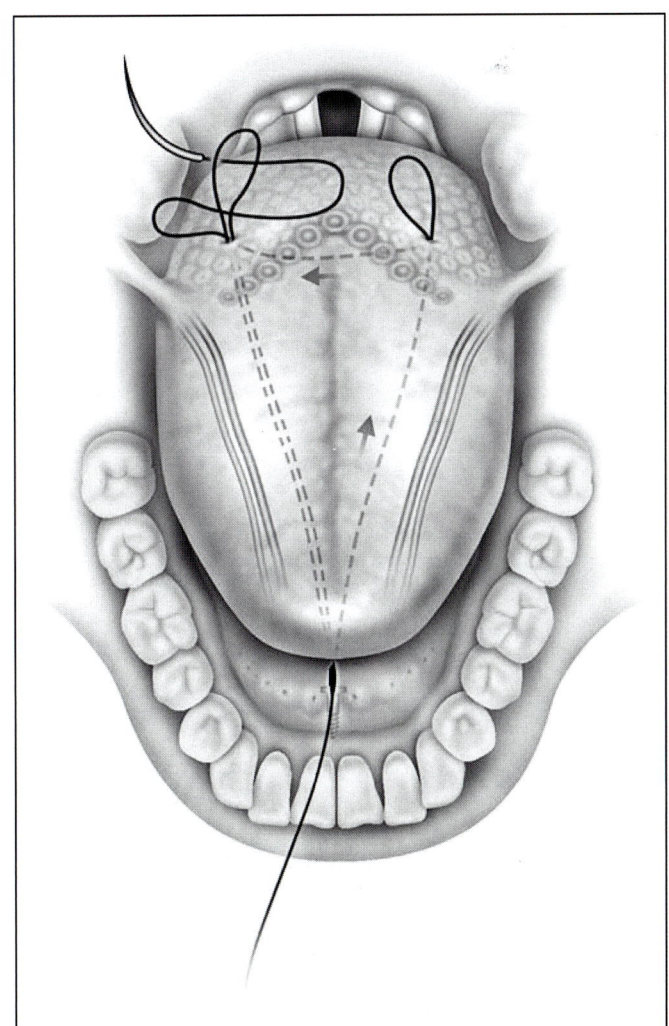

**Fig. 42.5** Placement of suspension suture on left side of patient's tongue. This is then passed to right suture loop by a submucosal suture pass.

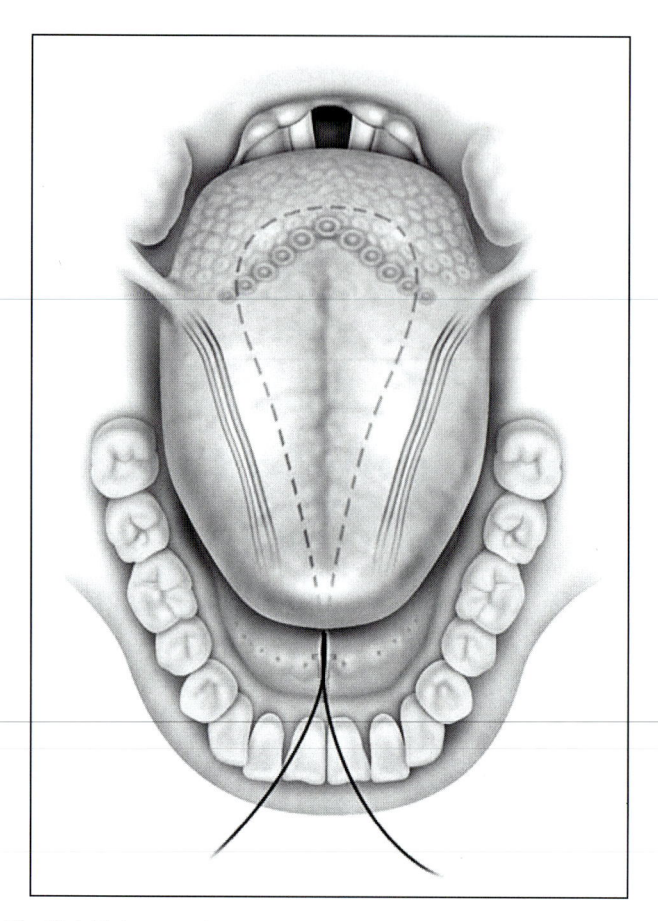

**Fig. 42.6** Right suture loop pulls the suspension suture to complete the suture loop.

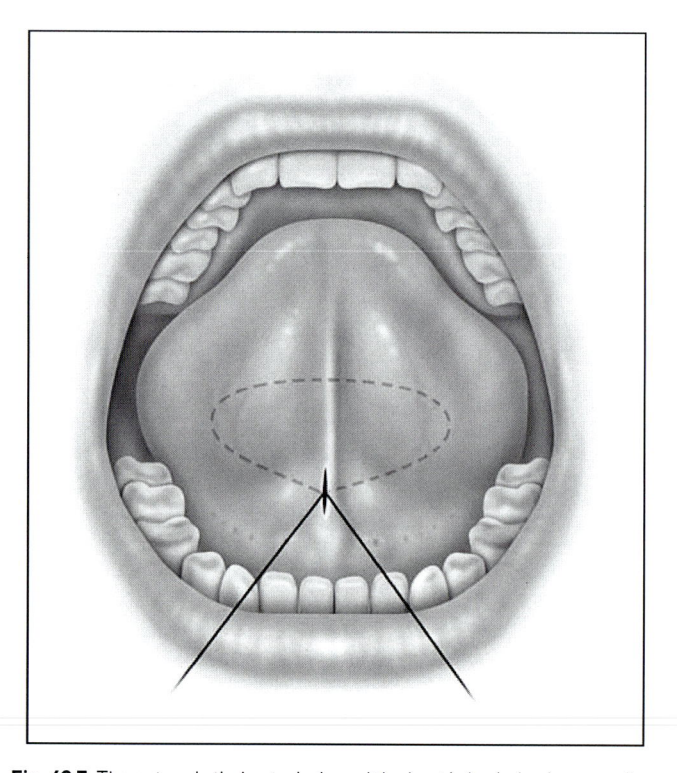

**Fig. 42.7** The suture is tied anteriorly and the knot is buried submucosally.

series. Contraindications to this procedure include poor general medical health or primary upper airway obstruction in the retropalatal region. In addition, relative contraindications include macroglossia, abnormal mandible bone, poor oral hygiene, and severe periodontal disease, history of radiation or history of root canal procedures in the mandibular midline incisors. Since this procedure conceptually does not actively advance tissues, patients with severe obstruction due to excessive tissue volume of the tongue or lateral walls will probably not respond. Patients who have personally responded the best were those without significant macroglossia or lateral wall collapse, and whose posterior airspace dramatically decreased in size going from the sitting to supine position (observed endoscopically).

## 5 DISCUSSION

Tongue suspension has been performed using various techniques. Suture suspension using the proprietary Repose™ device was introduced by DeRowe. The procedure's concept is that the tongue suspension suture decreases compliance of the tongue. Airway space is not increased but posterior displacement is decreased during sleep. This stitch does not clinically alter normal tongue movement although limited anterior movement (such as with licking an ice cream cone) can be decreased. Complication rates of 15–20% have been reported and include edema, hematoma and infection. The suture is removable and reversible.

Published studies of tongue suspension to treat sleep apnea are primarily non-randomized, uncontrolled case series with short-duration follow-up. Most combine UPPP as part of the treatment. Extrapolating results is difficult (Table 42.1). In general, snoring and sleep-related outcomes improve. Snoring may still be bothersome. Postoperative morbidity includes moderate to severe pain, difficulty with speech, swallowing and drooling and transient VPI. Duration has been reported from 7 to 28 days. No long-term speech or swallowing problems were reported in the initial studies.

Complications include delayed floor of mouth sialadenitis, dehydration, delayed gastrointestinal bleeding, floor of mouth hematoma, and prolonged pain/infection leading to removal or loosening of the suture. Other complications include damage to the neurovascular bundle (lingual artery and hypoglossal nerve), osteomyelitis and damage to dental structures. To reduce the risk of these problems, perioperative antibiotics and steroids are recommended. A meticulous technique should be used to ensure that the neurovascular bundle and Wharton's ducts are avoided and the suture buried.

## Table 42.1 Results of studies of tongue suspension to treat sleep apnea

| Reference | DeRowe (2000) | Terris (2002) | Kuhnel (2005) |
|---|---|---|---|
| Level (design) | 4 (cohort) | 4 (cohort) | 4 (cohort) |
| Sample size[†] | 16 | 19 | 28 |
| Procedures | 14 UPPP TS | 16 patients UPPP TS | 28 UPPP TS |
| Follow-up | 3 months | 6 months | 1 year |
| Inclusion criteria | All OSA with multilevel obstruction, Fujita 2, failed CPAP. | AHI > 15 (OSA), moderate and severe OSA, Fujita II, failed CPAP. | Failed CPAP, multilevel obstruction, Fujita 2. |
| Exclusion criteria | Fujita 1 | AHI < 15, BMI > 34 | BMI > 40, age > 70 years |
| Results | AHI improved. ESS improved. Success rate of about 51.4% noted in the TS treated patients. | AHI decreased in OSA, $P < 0.01$. ESS improved, $P < 0.005$. AHI dropped by 51.7%, AI dropped by 81.4%, success rate 67%. | Posterior airway space widened by 2 mm in 60% on patients. 67% Epworth 19 to 9, 55% improved AHI. |
| Morbidity/complications | Pain, limited tongue protrusion, mouth floor cyst. | Transient VPI, limited tongue movement. | Not reported. |
| **Reference** | **Thomas (2003)** | **Woodson (2001)** | **Vincente (2006)** |
| Level (design) | 1 (randomized controlled trial) | 4 (cohort) | 4 (case series) |
| Sample size[†] | 16 | 28 | 55 |
| Procedures | 17 9 TS, 8 TA | TS alone | 55 UPPP TS |
| Follow-up | 6 months | 2 months | 3 years |
| Inclusion criteria | Moderate and severe OSA, multilevel obstruction, Fujita 2, failed CPAP. | AHI < 15 (snorers); AHI > 15 (OSA). | AHI > 30, severe OSA, failed CPAP, multilevel obstruction, Fujita 2. |
| Exclusion criteria | Fujita 1, mild OSA. | AHI > 60, LSAT < 80%, BMI > 34. | BMI > 40, age > 70 years. |
| Results | TS slight advantage over TA. Success rate of about 60% noted in the TS group, slight advantage over the TA group. | AHI decreased in OSA, $P < 0.009$, multi-institutional 7 sites, effect size for total FOSQ 0.74–0.79, ESS 1.23–1.00. | 21 patients also had septoplasty, 78% success rate at 3 years (AHI 50% reduction and <15). Epworth 12.2 to 8.2. Improved $P < 0.02$. |
| Morbidity/complications | Pain, limited tongue protrusion. | 15% (4 with sialadenitis, 1 dehydration, 1 GI bleed). | Not reported. |

[†]Sample size: numbers shown for those not lost to follow-up and those (initially recruited). AHI, apnea/hypopnea index; CPAP, continuous positive airway pressure; ESS, Epwarth Sleepiness Scale; FOSQ, functional outcomes of sleep; LSAT, lowest oxygen saturation; NS, not significant; OSA, obstructive sleep apnea; TA, tongue advancement; TS, tongue suspension; UPPP, uvulopalatopharyngoplasty; VPI, velopharyngeal insufficiency.

## 6 ADVANTAGES AND DISADVANTAGES

The procedure's advantages include that it is a lesser procedure than traditional osteotomies with potentially fewer complications. It is relatively non-invasive and does not require extended general anesthesia time. Placement of the suture above the level of the hyoid allows the tongue to move normally as the patient swallows. It is potentially reversible and does not prohibit later tongue base procedures.

The disadvantages include minimal long-term follow-up data, questions of durability and migration over time of the suture, and the technique's learning curve with respect to the tension required on the fixed suture. Lastly, since Prolene sutures are not radio-opaque, it is not possible to follow the suture over time except by monitoring changes in the patient's clinical status.

Much needs to be learned about the effect and mechanism of the procedure. A better understanding will allow a far more rational selection of patients, an understanding of possible relapse, and the development of improved technology and techniques. Possible modifications could include a radio-opaque suture which would aid in long-term monitoring, adjustability and easier placement, and allow for evaluation of the durability and possible migration of the suture itself. It would provide suture elasticity to act more dynamically rather than as a static sling, and be a less costly and invasive means of placement.

## REFERENCES

1. DeRowe A, Gunther E, Fibbi A, et al. Tongue-base suspension with a soft tissue-to-bone anchor for obstructive sleep apnea: preliminary clinical results of a new minimally invasive technique. Otolaryngol Head Neck Surg 2000;122:100–3.
2. Woodson BT, DeRowe A, Hawke M, et al. Pharyngeal suspension suture with Repose bone screw for obstructive sleep apnea. Otolaryngol Head Neck Surg 2000;122:395–401.

3. Woodson BT. A tongue suspension suture for obstructive sleep apnea and snorers. Otolaryngol Head Neck Surg 2001;124:297–303.
4. Terris DJ, Kunda LD, Gonella MC. Minimally invasive tongue base surgery for obstructive sleep apnea. J Laryngol Otol 2002;116(9):716–21.
5. Miller FR, Watson D, Malis D. Role of the tongue base suspension suture with The Repose System bone screw in the multilevel surgical management of obstructive sleep apnea. Otolaryngol Head Neck Surg 2004;126(4):392–8.
6. Thomas AJ, Chavoya M, Terris DJ. Preliminary finding from a prospective, randomized trial of two tongue-base surgeries for sleep-disordered breathing, Otolaryngol Head Neck Surg 2003;129(5):539–46.
7. Kuhnel TS, Schurr C, Wagner B, et al. Morphological changes of the posterior airway space after tongue base suspension. Laryngoscope 2005;115(3):475–80.
8. Omur M, Ozturan D, Elez F, Unver C, Derman S. Tongue base suspension combined with UPPP in severe OSA patients. Otol Head Neck Surg 2005;133:218–23.
9. Vicente E, Marin JM, Carrizzo S, Naya MJ. Tongue-base suspension in conjunction with uvulopalatopharyngoplasty for treatment of severe obstructive sleep apnea: long-term follow-up results. Laryngoscope 2006;116(7):L1223–7.

SECTION J  MINIMALLY INVASIVE HYPOPHARYNGEAL PROCEDURES

# CHAPTER 43
# Endoscopic coblation lingual tonsillectomy

*Peter G. Michaelson and Eric A. Mair*

## 1 INTRODUCTION

For the clinician and surgeon treating patients with obstructed sleep apnea and related maladies, the retrolingual airway is of much importance. This area, often difficult to examine and identify as an area of concern, has recently been the site of much academic and surgical attention. For with its difficult location comes increased complexity in surgical cure, plagued with both intraoperative and postoperative challenges. Although the palatal–pharyngeal area is often the site of primary obstruction in patients with sleep apnea, there are often areas of secondary blockage, and the tongue base may be an area of interest with the added concern of hypertrophic lingual tonsils.

## 2 PATIENT SELECTION

Obstruction may not be the only presenting sign of hypertrophic lingual tonsils. Symptoms may be classified into two main categories, resulting from problems with either inflammation and infection or hypertrophy and hyperplasia. Inflammation may present with dysphagia and odynophagia with complaints originating at the tongue base or suprahyoid region. These symptoms may occasionally result in lingual tonsillar abscess and recurrent epiglottitis.[1–3] Hypertrophic or hyperplastic tonsils may plague the patient with dysphagia and globus. These patients may have increased symptoms in the supine position, with those afflicted with obstructive sleep apnea having a worsening obstructive process in the deeper stages of sleep. Interestingly, lingual tonsil enlargement is a relatively common finding in children with persistent obstructive sleep apnea following adenotonsillectomy,[4] further intensifying the finding of compensatory lingual tonsil hypertrophy after such a procedure.

The differentiation of lingual tonsil and tongue base pathology is often difficult. Furthermore, the very definition of lingual tonsil hypertrophy has not been standardized. However, if the lingual tonsils are greater than '10 mm in diameter and abutting both the posterior border of the tongue and the posterior pharyngeal wall,' they may be considered clearly enlarged, due to a known relationship to patients with obstructive sleep apnea.[5] Determination between lingual tonsil hypertrophy and an enlarged tongue base is critical, for these two entities often require different therapies with both needing attention. Careful history taking and physical examination when combined with ancillary studies may help the surgeon successfully treat the patient with retrolingual pathology.

There are multiple descriptions of how to surgically address the lingual tonsils, including scalpel, electrocautery, snares, laser and removal with the suction debrider.[6–8] However, these procedures are often fraught with difficult exposure, painstaking dissection, poor visualization, difficult hemostasis, excessive postoperative pain and possible airway edema. A recent report from Robinson et al. describes the novel technique of utilizing bipolar radiofrequency plasma excision, or the coblator, for direct visual removal of the lingual tonsil pad using suspension laryngoscopy and an operating microscope.[9] Advantages of this technique include improved exposure, visualization and hemostasis with decreased postoperative edema and pain when compared to previously described techniques. However, after multiple cases, we find the suspension laryngoscopy and the use of the operating microscope to be burdensome and unnecessary. Of note, the laryngoscope is bulky, distorts the lingual anatomy and requires intraoperative adjustment and re-suspension. Also, even bivalved laryngoscopes may restrict full surgical access to the lateral portion of the tonsil, and may increase the risk of laryngoscope associated complications, including injury to the patient's dentition, temporary dysgeusia and altered tongue mobility. Adding to the difficulty, use of the microscope is tedious and it only works in the straightforward position. Here, we offer our experience with endoscopic coblation lingual tonsillectomy. Being otolaryngologists, already comfortable with the increased visualization and applications offered from our endoscopes, why not apply these superior optics to surgery in a difficult spot?

Lingual tonsillectomy may be indicated for those patients with complaints of hypertrophy or repeated infection. Concerning history, as previously discussed, may alert the clinician to the lingual tonsil as a source of concern. These patients may be pediatric or adult, and our surgical approach applies to both patient types.

Due to the difficulty in examining the retrolingual airway by the front-line primary care health provider, it is critical that the otolaryngologist be familiar with the different tools of preoperative assessment. Examination with laryngeal mirror and flexible endoscopy is critical, for these are the best methods of visualization. Finger palpation is also standard, for tongue base concerns may occasionally stem from foreign bodies or tumor. Visualization is also important in the clinical differentiation of lingual tonsil and tongue base musculature hypertrophy. Since these entities are treated differently, incorrect identification of the area of concern may lead to decreased treatment success. Enlarged lingual tonsils may appear with multiple enlarged follicles, soft to the touch and occasionally filling the vallecula to the point of glottis concealment from a posterior pushed epiglottis. One must characterize the space between the lingual tonsils posterior extent to the posterior oral and hypopharyngeal wall. The Mueller maneuver may add additional clues to the responsible levels of obstruction.[10] Lateral neck radiographs may offer information on tongue position and relative size of the lingual tonsils;[11] however, when in question, we find magnetic resonance imaging (MRI) with gadolinium enhancement to be crucial in imaging the tongue base. This modality, which characteristically enhances the lingual tonsils from tongue base musculature, helps to determine the nature of retrolingual obstruction, be it lingual tonsil hypertrophy or tongue base enlargement, while appropriately exposing other possibilities, such as tumor.[12] If lingual tonsil hypertrophy is suspected, and there are no clinical contraindications, a short burst of oral steroids with re-examination in one week is another way to determine culpability of the lingual tonsil; if the retrolingual airspace widens, the lingual tonsils are likely the perpetrator. If there is no difference, suspect the tongue base. This method may provide a quicker and less expensive clinical method than MRI; however, the chosen modality is ultimately up to the clinician.

In addition, great care must be given to addressing the non-surgical treatments of lingual tonsil hypertrophy which is often due to allergies, sinusitis and gastroesophageal reflux, of which hypertrophy may be a presenting sign with the latter.[5] Often, after appropriate medicinal treatment, such as with an empiric trial of proton pump inhibitors and/or topical nasal steroids, clinical improvement over 4–6 weeks may eradicate the need for surgery. Finally, polysomnogram is the gold standard exam for evaluating concerns of sleep disorder breathing. Extra caution must be given to patients with suspected neuromuscular abnormalities; hypotonia and related disorders (such as cerebral palsy and Down's syndrome) may suffer from obstructive as well as central apnea.

## 3 OUTLINE OF PROCEDURE

Our method of lingual tonsillectomy synergies the technique recently described by Robinson[9] (see Chapter 41) with the otolaryngologist's utilizing endoscopic-assisted surgery. If dealing with obstructive retrolingual anatomy, standard anesthesia precautions are employed. Perioperative antibiotics and steroids are given. After placing the patient in proper Rose position, nasotracheal intubation is employed, and after proper position, a retraction 2.0 silk suture is placed in the anterior tongue. Multiple stitches may ultimately be necessary for improved retraction and visualization; these may even be placed later during the procedure. A standard rubber bite block keeps the mouth open and one or two rubber oronasal catheters may be placed to retract the soft palate if needed. A standard 70° sinus endoscope is placed periorally to directly view the lingual tonsil. The malleable Evac 70 tonsil and adenoid coblation wand is gently bent. The lingual tonsils are ablated under endoscopic guidance (setting 9 on ablate; Arthrocare Corp, ENTec Division, Sunnyvale, CA). The endoscope alone provides an excellent panoramic view of the lingual tonsil with virtually any patient body type. The procedure is dynamic; small changes in amount and direction of tongue retraction change the view and tension of the lingual tonsil and aid in a complete excision. The tonsil is ablated until the tongue musculature is encountered, and care is taken to avoid coblation of the epiglottis or other supraglottic structures. The addition of the endoscopic view enables intraoperative photos and video to be taken, as well as allowing others in the operating room the opportunity to observe the procedure. The ability of the anesthetist to see the resection adds extra benefits. Visualization of the airway often reveals a larger, improved airway at the conclusion of the case and may add confidence to involved providers if extubation is decided upon at the conclusion of the case.

## 4 POSTOPERATIVE MANAGEMENT AND COMPLICATIONS

We routinely extubate at the completion of the tonsillectomy, though this decision must be determined by the surgeon based on the individual characteristics of the patient, the observational hospital setting as well as one's own preference. This decision may also change if other procedures are performed such as tongue base reduction or palatal procedures. Patients are observed for at least 24 hours postoperative in an intensive care setting, being given postoperative antibiotics and steroids. Close follow-up, as well as continued allergy and gastroesophageal reflux medicines, may be continued, as patients are symptomatically followed. If a complete excision is performed, regrowth is unlikely. Success depends on completeness of excision as well as the lingual tonsil's role in preoperative symptoms such as globus or obstruction.

## REFERENCES

1. Elia JC. Lingual tonsillitis. Ann NY Acad Sci 1959;82:52–6.
2. Newman RK, Johnson JT. Abscess of the lingual tonsil. Arch Otolaryngol Head Neck Surg 1979;105:277–8.
3. Lewis M, McClay JE, Schochet P. Lingual tonsillectomy for refractory paroxysmal cough. Int J Pediatr Otorhinolaryngol 2000;53:63–6.
4. Fricke BL, Donnelly LF, Shott SR, et al. Comparison of lingual tonsil size as depicted on MR imaging between children with obstructive sleep apnea despite previous tonsillectomy and adenoidectomy and normal controls. Pediatr Radiol 2006;36(6):518–23.
5. Carr MM, Nagy ML, Pizzuto MP, et al. Correlation of findings at direct laryngoscopy and bronchoscopy with gastroesophageal reflux disease in children: a prospective study. Arch Otolaryngol Head Neck Surg 2001;127(4):369–74.
6. Yonekura A, Kawakatsu K, Suszuki K, et al. Laser midline glossectomy and lingual tonsillectomy as treatments for sleep apnea syndrome. Acta Otolaryngol Suppl 2003;550:56–8.
7. Wouters B, van Overbeek JJ, Buiter CT, et al. Laser surgery in lingual tonsil hyperplasia. Clin Otolaryngol Allied Sci 1989;14:291–6.
8. Conache ID, Meikle D, O'Brien C. Tracheostomy. lingual tonsillectomy and sleep-related breathing disorders, Br J Anaesth 2002;88:724–6.
9. Robinson S, Ettema SL, Brusky L, et al. Lingual tonsillectomy using bipolar radiofrequency plasma excision. Otolaryngol Head Neck Surg 2006;134(2):328–30.
10. Faber CE, Grymer L. Available techniques for objective assessment of upper airway narrowing in snoring and sleep apnea. Sleep Breath 2003;7(2):77–86.
11. Bower CM. Lingual tonsillectomy. Operative Tech Oto 2005;16:238–41.
12. Shott SR, Donnelly LF. Cine magnetic resonance imaging: evaluation of persistent airway obstruction after tonsil and adenotonsillectomy in children with Down syndrome. Laryngoscope 2004;114:1724–9.

# SECTION K — MULTILEVEL PHARYNGEAL SURGERY

## CHAPTER 44

# Multilevel pharyngeal surgery for obstructive sleep apnea

*Kenny P. Pang and David J. Terris*

## 1 INTRODUCTION

Obstructive sleep apnea (OSA) is the commonest sleep disorder. It is characterized by repetitive apneas and hypopneas during sleep. These events are due to partial or complete collapse of the upper airway, resulting in decreased oxygenation and sympathetic overdrive. Frequent arousals occur, causing sleep fragmentation leading to excessive daytime sleepiness, morning headaches, poor concentration, memory loss, frustration, depression and even marital discord. The mechanism of upper airway collapse in OSA is usually multifactorial. Many authors concur that most patients with moderate and severe OSA are very likely to have multilevel obstruction involving the level of the palate and base of tongue. Endoscopic examination with Mueller's maneuver can grade airway collapse at three levels, namely the velopharynx, lateral pharyngeal wall and the base of tongue.[1] There are surgical procedures that can address the various levels of collapse in these patients. Recently, lateral pharyngeal wall collapse has also been dealt with by creating tension in the lateral walls by lateral pharyngoplasty[2] or expansion sphincter pharyngoplasty.[3] Palatal collapse can be treated by traditional uvulopalatopharyngoplasty, Z-plasty or transpalatal advancement; tongue base can be reduced by a glossectomy or a suspension sling suture.

The site of obstruction is unimportant when the modality of therapy is a tracheostomy or nasal continuous positive airway pressure, which indiscriminately overcomes all collapsible airway segments, much like a 'pneumatic splint'. When upper airway surgery is contemplated, it is critical to tailor the approach according to the site of obstruction noted preoperatively on Mueller's maneuver. The type of surgery employed would depend on the type of palatal and tongue base collapse.

Although a staged approach to the upper airway reconstruction is acceptable, and even endorsed by the American Sleep Disorders Association,[4] when the likelihood of multilevel obstruction is high, the chances of surgical success may be nearly doubled by addressing multiple anatomic sites at a single surgical sitting,[5,6] thereby avoiding additional general anesthetic. The initial staged approach was described by Fujita, when he introduced uvulopalatopharyngoplasty for OSA[7]; he recognized that the upper airway may collapse at multiple levels. Hence, he described the laser midline glossectomy for patients who failed UPPP and who were diagnosed to have retrolingual obstruction.[8] It was Riley et al.[6] who first advocated simultaneous multilevel pharyngeal surgery for patients with multilevel obstruction noted clinically on Mueller's maneuver. They showed promising success with minimal complications. Many authors have reported minimal complications with one-stage multilevel pharyngeal surgery for patients with OSA.[9–11]

## 2 PATIENT SELECTION

The key to surgical success is patient selection. Patients with OSA must be treated in a holistic manner, as many of these patients are overweight or obese, and have associated co-morbidities like hypertension, ischemic heart disease or cerebrovascular disease. The overweight patient should be put on a strict weight loss and dietary regime, while being on nasal continuous positive airway pressure, until ideal body weight is attained. Bariatric surgery should also be considered part of the surgical armamentarium in the management of these obese patients. Nasal continuous positive airway pressure (CPAP) has always taken the lead in the treatment of OSA. It is undoubted that nasal CPAP is effective in most OSA patients, if used properly. However, it is also universally known that patient compliance is a major problem in the use of nasal CPAP.

Surgical techniques for the treatment of OSA have long been criticized and frowned upon, especially uvulopalatopharyngoplasty (UPPP). Uvulopalatopharyngoplasty remains the most common surgical procedure performed for sleep disordered breathing (SDB). Traditionally, UPPP was used mainly for patients with collapse/obstruction of the soft palate during Mueller's maneuver (MM). Mueller's maneuver was first described by Borowiecki and Sassin for the preoperative assessment of OSA.[12] According to Fujita's three types of collapse of the upper airway during sleep,[13] Mueller's maneuver was able to identify Fujita type I (soft palatal) collapse, and hence, isolate patients suitable for UPPP. This, unfortunately, was not always the case, as there are multiple factors involved in the dynamics of OSA, and many patients have multilevel obstructions. Due to the varied clinical indications for this procedure, many authors have found unfavorable postoperative results. Sher et al. reviewed a meta-analysis of reported UPPP procedures and found an overall success rate of only 40%.[14] In an attempt to improve surgical success rates, Friedman et al. devised a clinical staging system for SDB in order to better select patients for the UPPP.[15] They described three stages based on Friedman tongue position, tonsil size and BMI.

- Stage I: Friedman tongue position 1 and 2. Tonsil size 3 and 4. BMI < 40.
- Stage II: Friedman tongue position 1, 2, 3 and 4. Tonsil size 1, 2, 3 and 4. BMI < 40.
- Stage III: Friedman tongue position 3 and 4. Tonsil size 1 and 2. BMI (any).

Friedman reported an overall success rate of 80.6% for stage I, 37.9% for stage II and 8.1% for stage III. It is well accepted that patients with Friedman tongue position 3 and 4 are indicative of a large tongue, suggesting that if surgery is contemplated, some form of tongue base surgery would be appropriate as well. Most authors concur that patients who are noted to have multilevel collapse with Mueller's maneuver on endoscopy (of both the palate and tongue base) should have both levels addressed at the same surgical sitting. Friedman et al. showed that selected patients with stage II and stage III disease treated with UPPP and tongue base reduction using a radiofrequency technique (TBRF) had remarkably improved results.[16] Follow-up at 6 months showed successful treatment of patients with stage II disease with success rate improving from 37.9% to 74.0%, and stage III disease improving from 8.1% to 43.3%.[16]

Severity of OSA has also been noted to correlate with clinical examination, namely Mueller's maneuver.[17] It was demonstrated in 102 patients that OSA severity strongly correlated with Mallampati grade ($r = 0.389$, $P < 0.0001$), Friedman clinical staging ($r = 0.331$, $P = 0.0007$) and Mueller's grades of collapsibility, at all three levels. Of significance, only 6.9% of patients with mild OSA had a >50% collapse of the base of tongue region, as compared to 65.9% of patients with severe OSA.[17] This illustrates that patients with severe OSA are 10 times more likely to have tongue base collapse than patients with mild OSA. Hence, patients with severe OSA and with tongue base collapse noted on Mueller's maneuver, falling into Friedman stage II or III, should have multilevel surgery in order to achieve the best possible results. In the uncommon event that a single, severely obstructed site in the upper airway is identified, a staged approach may be considered even if the OSA is severe.

Nasal surgery is offered when the patient has significant nasal obstruction that has failed medical therapy (topical nasal steroids), especially when the patient would want correction of the nasal obstruction independent of its effect on their sleep. However, it is reported that nasal surgery alone has only a 15.8% success rate as a treatment of OSA.[18] The debate would be the safety of multilevel surgery, addressing all three levels: the nose, palate and tongue base at the same surgical sitting. Most authors concur that there is no evidence of increased complication rate or morbidity with these procedures performed together.[11,19–21]

## 3 OUTLINE OF PROCEDURES

### 3.1 HYOID MYOTOMY (SUSPENSION)

Riley et al.[22] first reported a skeletal approach to hypopharyngeal obstruction by using an adaptation of the laryngeal suspension procedure originally developed to minimize aspiration in patients who had had a supraglottic laryngectomy. In their original description, the infrahyoid musculature was removed from the hyoid bone, which was then suspended from the anterior mandibular arch using fascia lata. The technique was later simplified[23] by approximating the hyoid bone antero-inferiorly to the thyroid cartilage (Figs 44.1 to 44.5). Essentially, the hyoid is released from its inferior attachments and advanced anteriorly and inferiorly over the thyroid cartilage. This applies tension to the hyoepiglottic ligament, enlarging the hypopharynx (see figures).

### 3.1.1 TECHNICAL HIGHLIGHTS

- The hyoid bone is exposed as in a thyroglossal cyst excision (Sistrunk procedure).
- The infrahyoid musculature is released from the body of the hyoid (Figs 44.1 and 44.2).
- The strap muscles are divided in the midline, and the thyroid cartilage exposed.
- Four non-absorbable #1-0 Ethibond (Johnson and Johnson) sutures are placed around the hyoid, through the thyroid cartilage to advance the hyoid bone (Fig. 44.3)
- Passive drainage (Penrose soft drain), and closure in layers.

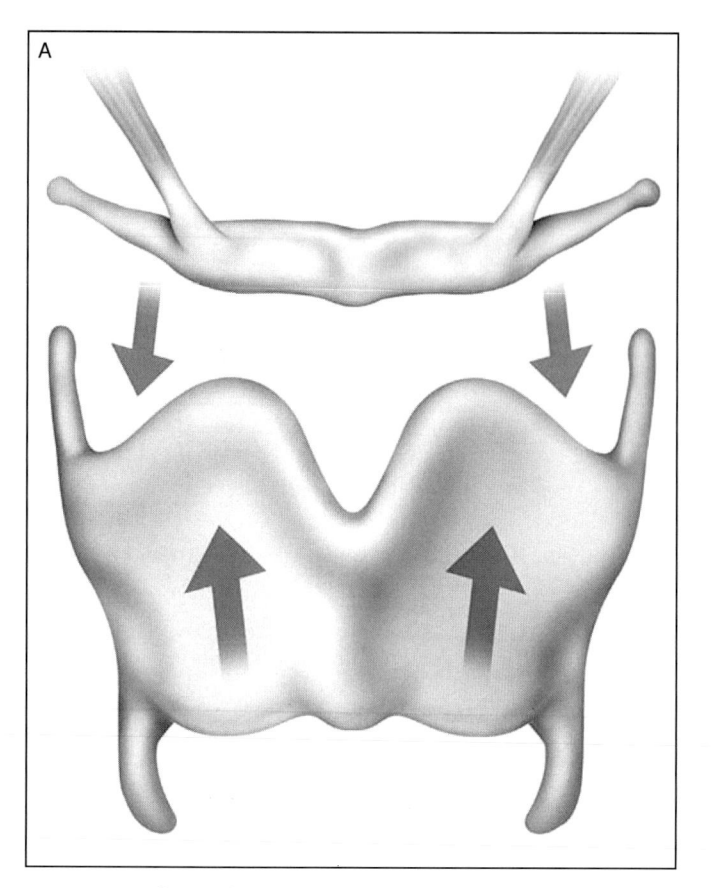

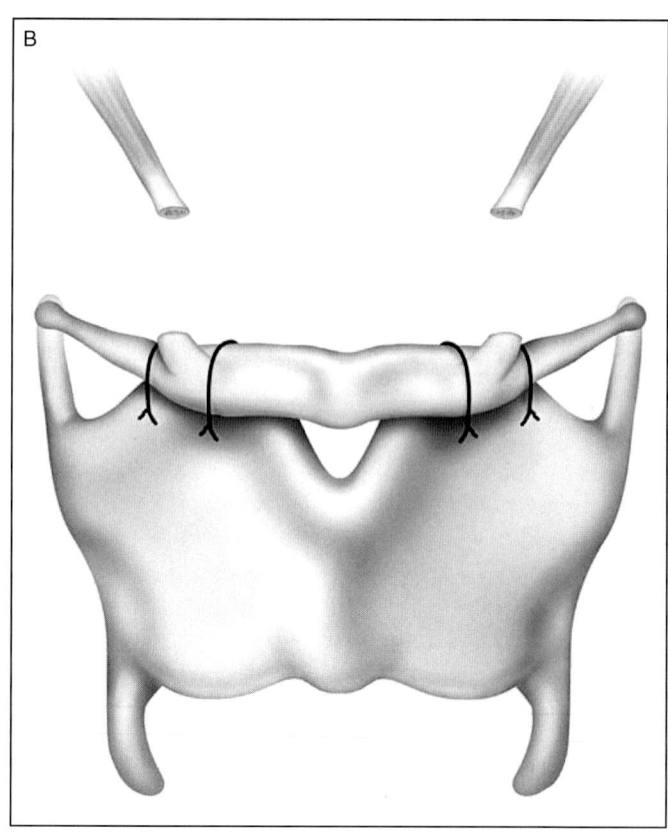

# SECTION K
## MULTILEVEL PHARYNGEAL SURGERY

**Fig. 44.1** A&B, (Hyoid 2). Horizontal skin crease incision made over the hyoid bone.

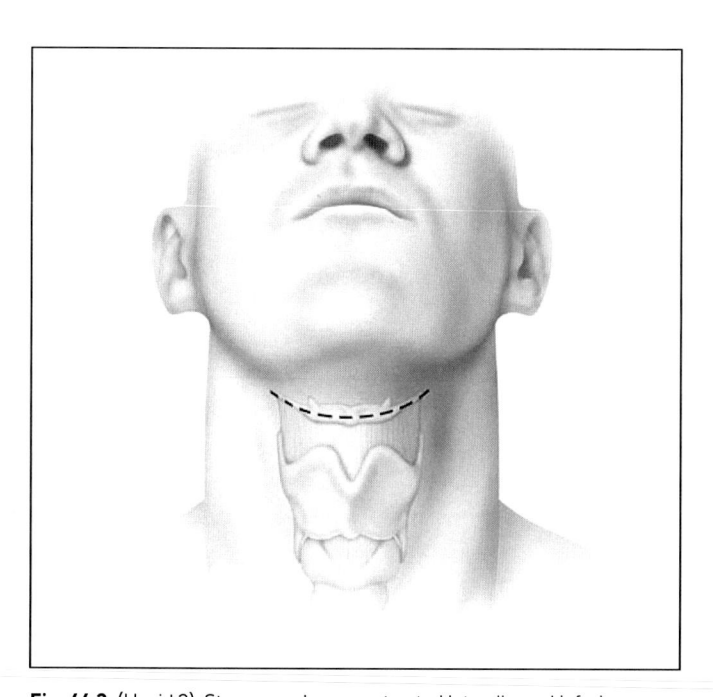

**Fig. 44.2** (Hyoid 3). Strap muscles are retracted laterally, and inferior attachments of the hyoid bone released.

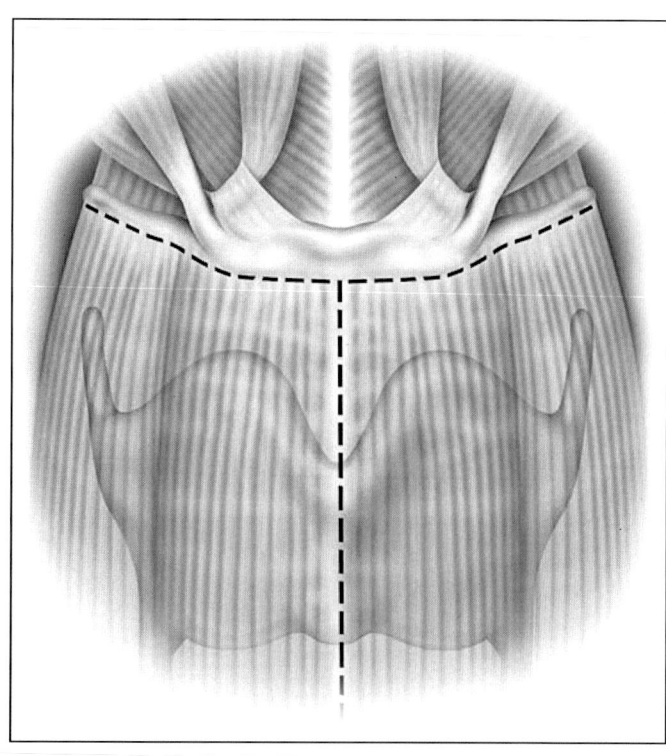

**Fig. 44.3** (Hyoid 1 A). The hyoid bone is approximated down to the thyroid cartilage.

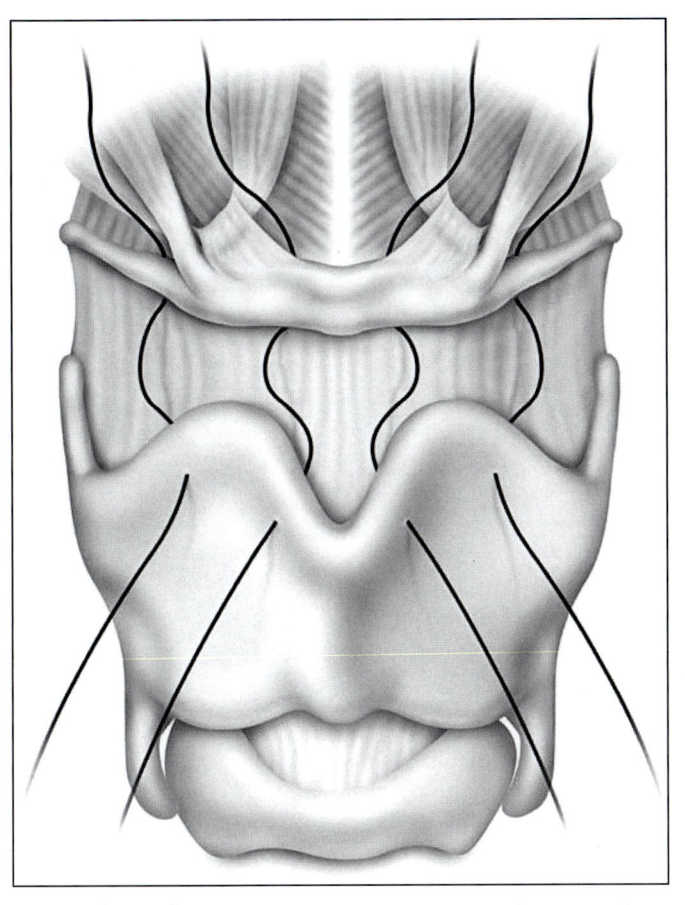

CHAPTER 44 — Multilevel pharyngeal surgery for OSA

**Fig. 44.4** (Hyoid 4). Four non-absorbable sutures are used to appose the hyoid bone down to the thyroid cartilage.

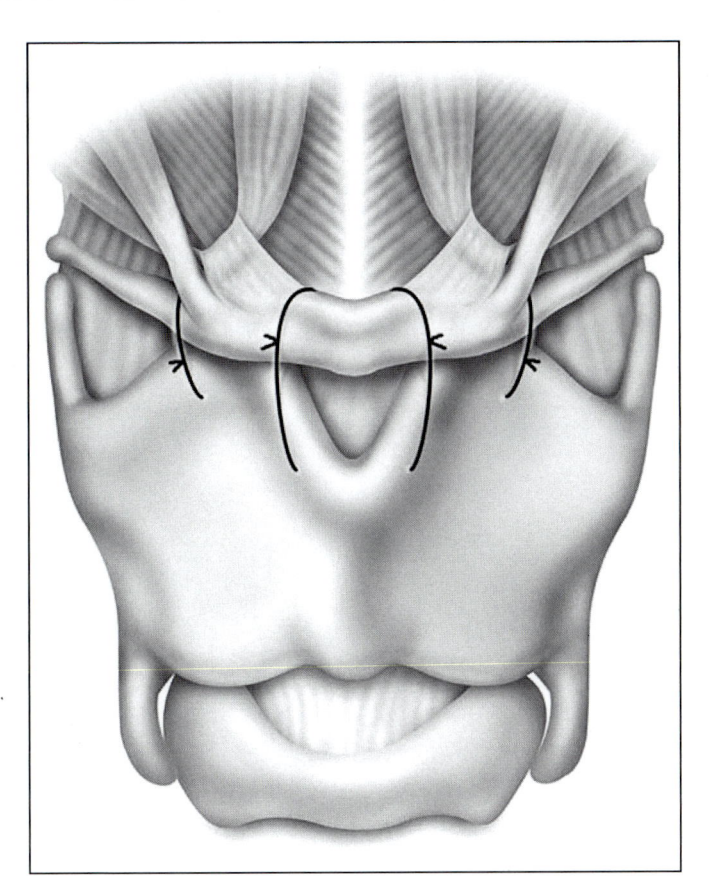

**Fig. 44.5** (Hyoid 5). The thyrohyoid apposition in place.

## 3.2 MANDIBULAR OSTEOTOMY WITH TONGUE ADVANCEMENT

A limited rectangular mandibular osteotomy has replaced the originally described sliding inferior sagittal osteotomy[22] as the preferred approach to advancing the genioglossus muscle anteriorly, thereby enlarging the retrolingual space. Powell et al.[24] first described this technique that made the surgery safer and more practical for the general otolaryngologist to perform. This procedure can be done in combination with the hyoid myotomy.

### 3.2.1 TECHNICAL HIGHLIGHTS

- A gingivolabial sulcus incision favoring the lip side to minimize the risk of dehiscence (Fig. 44.6).
- Exposure of the entire height of the mandible, with measurements made to center the osteotomies over the genial tubercle.

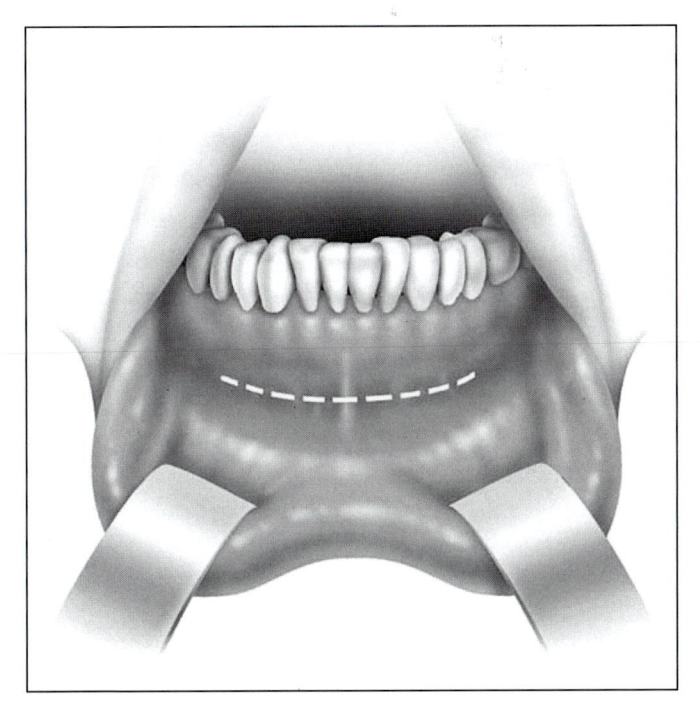

**Fig. 44.6** (GGA 1). Inferior gingivolabial incision made for exposure of the anterior table of the mandible.

# SECTION K — MULTILEVEL PHARYNGEAL SURGERY

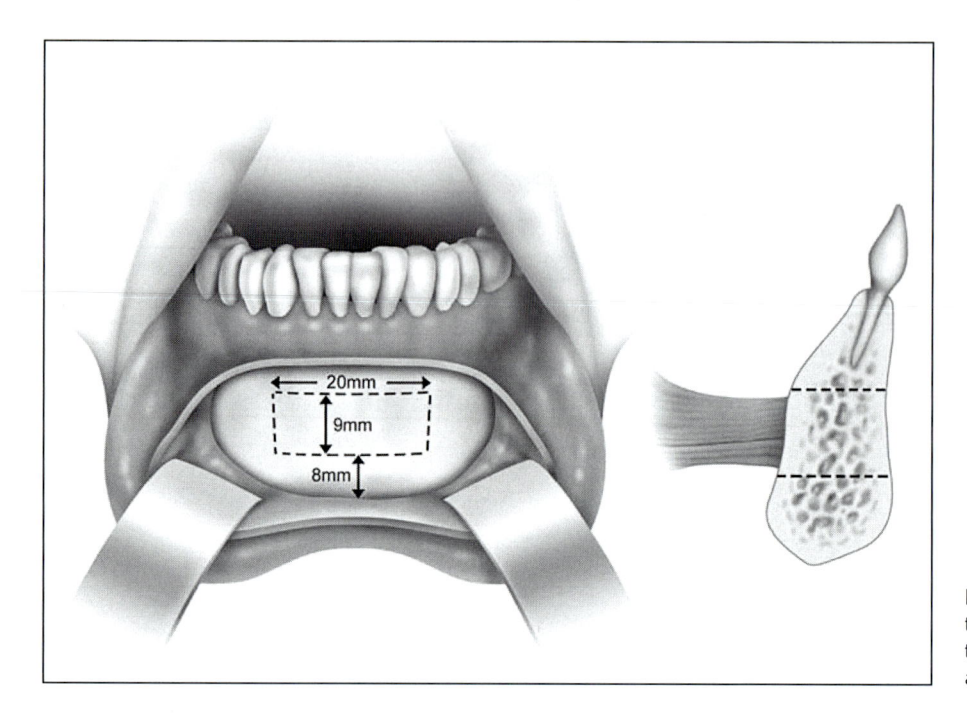

**Fig. 44.7** (GGA 2). Rectangular window made through-and-through on the mandible, ensuring the mandibular menti, genioglossus muscle attachment is included.

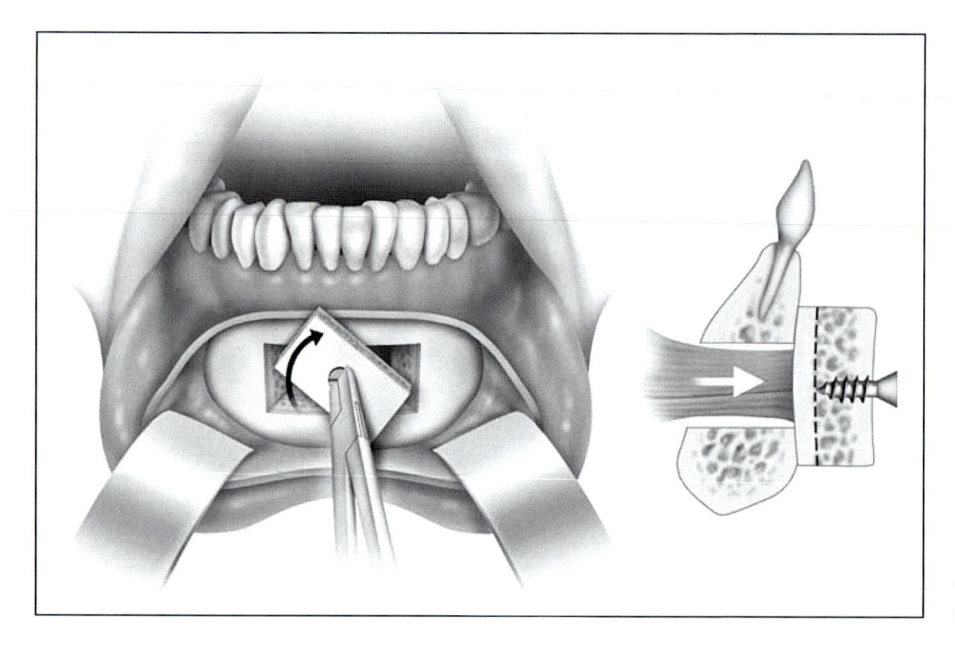

**Fig. 44.8** (GGA 3). Rectangular window is pulled anteriorly and twisted 90° in order to secure it.

- Osteotomies made through the inner and outer cortex of the mandible using 2-hole saw, with particular attention to the corners (Fig. 44.7).
- Advancement of the fragment with a clamp to advance the window anteriorly (Fig. 44.8).
- Rotation of the advanced window fragment.
- Removal of the outer table of the mandible and the marrow space.
- Securing of the fragment to the lower edge of the mandible with a screw (Figs 44.9 and 44.10).

## 3.3 TONGUE SUSPENSION

The principle is based on passing a non-absorbable Prolene suture through the tongue in an inverted triangle, with the apex at the inner table of the mandible, and the base of the triangle at the base of tongue region. The suture acts as a sling or hammock that creates a dimple at the base of tongue and prevents the tongue from falling posteriorly. The dimple in the base of tongue acts to allow a passage

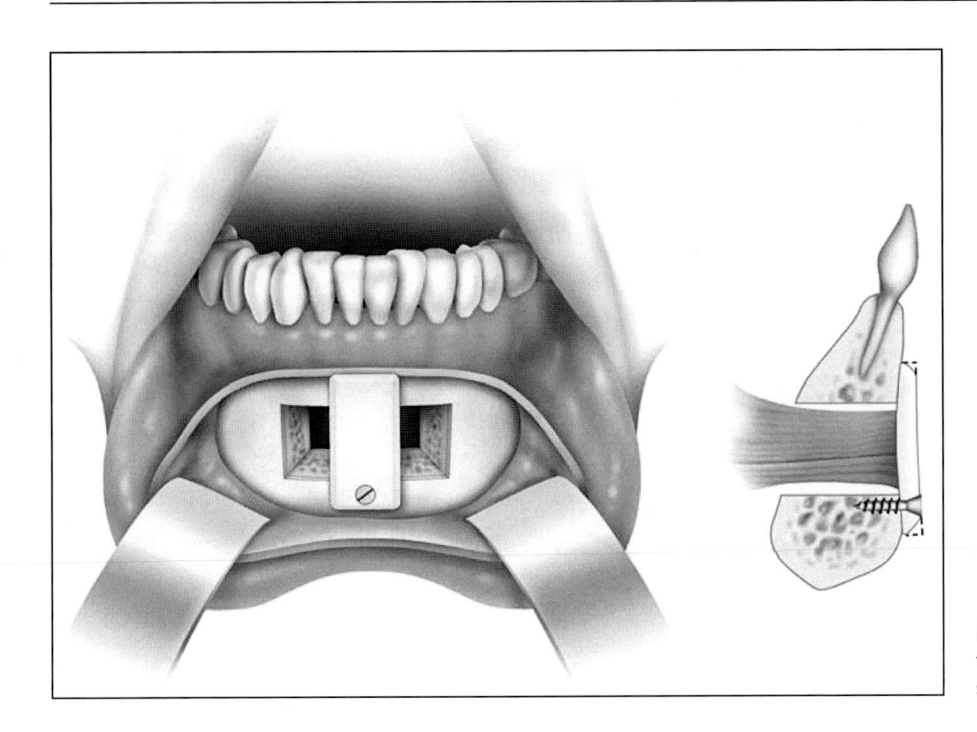

CHAPTER 44
Multilevel pharyngeal surgery for OSA

**Fig. 44.9** (GGA 4). Rectangular window anterior table is removed and the rectangular bone is secured with a screw.

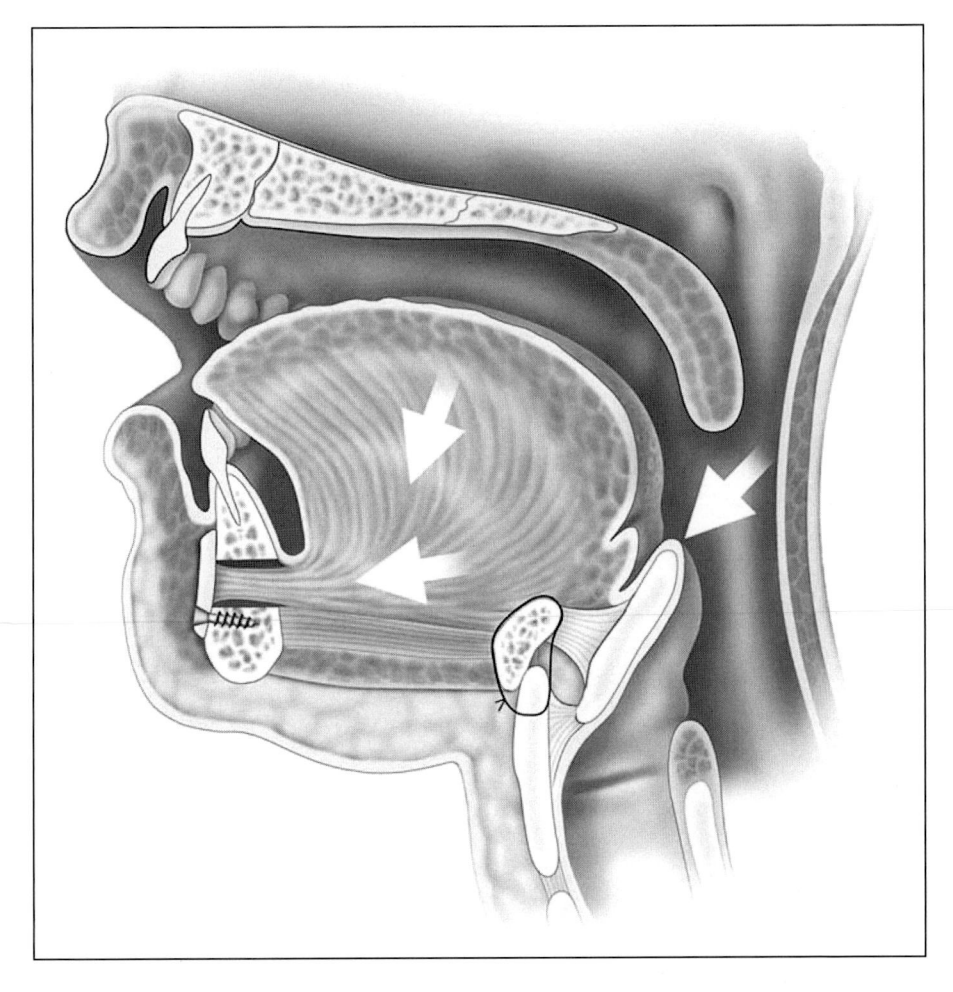

**Fig. 44.10** (GGA 5). Net effect of the hyoid suspension and genioglossus advancement procedure. The retrolingual space is increased.

273

# SECTION K — MULTILEVEL PHARYNGEAL SURGERY

of air through, thus keeping the airway patent. This procedure is usually done in combination with a palate procedure and/or the hyoid myotomy.

- An incision is made on the floor of the mouth, at the frenulum of the tongue, above the two Wharton's ducts.

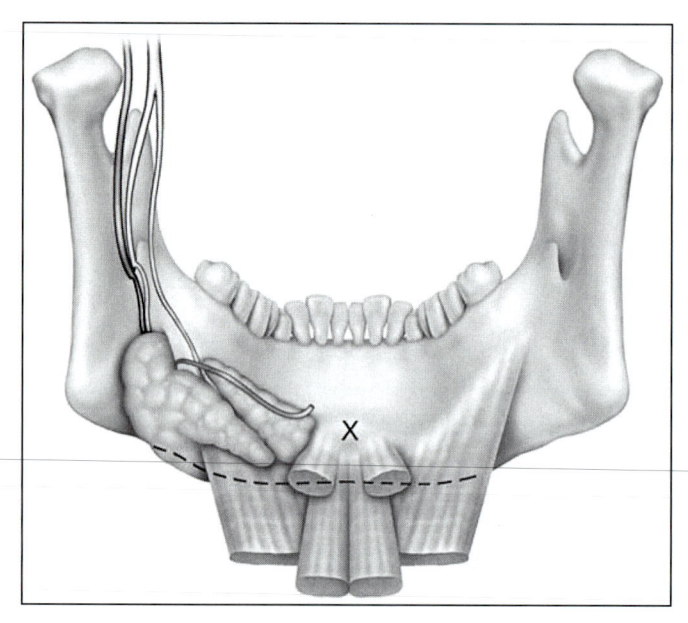

**Fig. 44.11** (Repose 1). Inner view of the mandible, showing ideal position of screw placement (marked X) for the Repose screw.

- With an artery forceps, a plane is created to the inner table of the mandible.
- The periosteum is raised from the inner table of the periosteum.
- The right-angled drill is introduced and activated to secure the screw into the inner table of the mandible (Figs 44.11 and 44.12).
- A suture loop is passed to the patient's right side to the base of the tongue from the frenulum incision (Fig. 44.13).
- The same is done with one end of the Prolene suture attached to the screw, to the left base of tongue (Fig. 44.14).
- A free large curve needle is used to pass the Prolene suture from one side of the tongue base at the exit point of the Prolene suture to the exit point of the suture loop (Fig. 44.15).
- The Prolene suture is then passed through the suture loop and pulled to the front.
- The Prolene suture is secured and tightened, while feeling the dimple in the base of tongue region (Figs 44.16 to 44.18).
- The incision in the frenulum is then closed with Vicryl 4/0 suture.

## 4 POSTOPERATIVE MANAGEMENT AND COMPLICATIONS

Intraoperative intravenous dexametasone is administered to all patients undergoing the tongue base procedure.

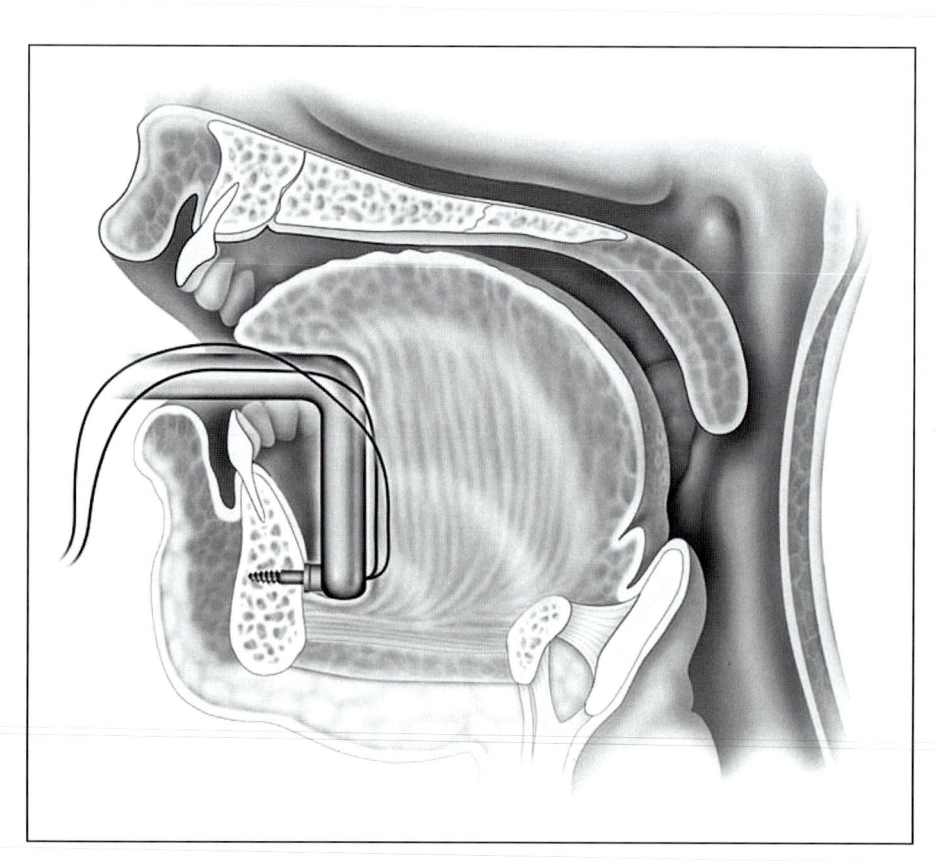

**Fig. 44.12** (Repose 2). Backward drilling device introducing the screw into the inner table of the mandible.

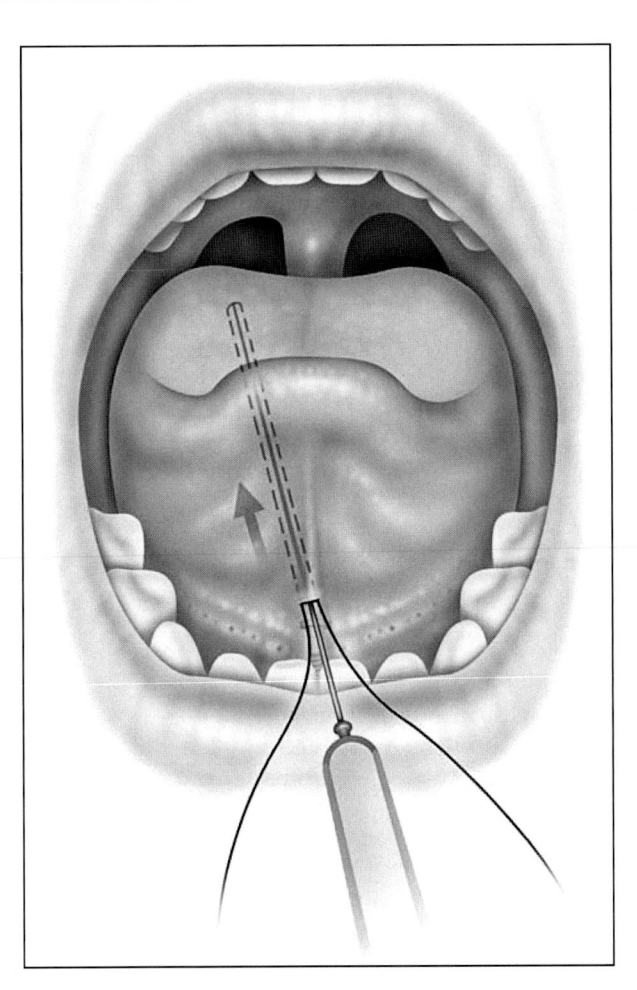

CHAPTER 44 — Multilevel pharyngeal surgery for OSA

**Fig. 44.13** (Repose 3). Suture passer used to pass the suture loop from the floor of the mouth to the base of tongue region at the circumvallate papillae.

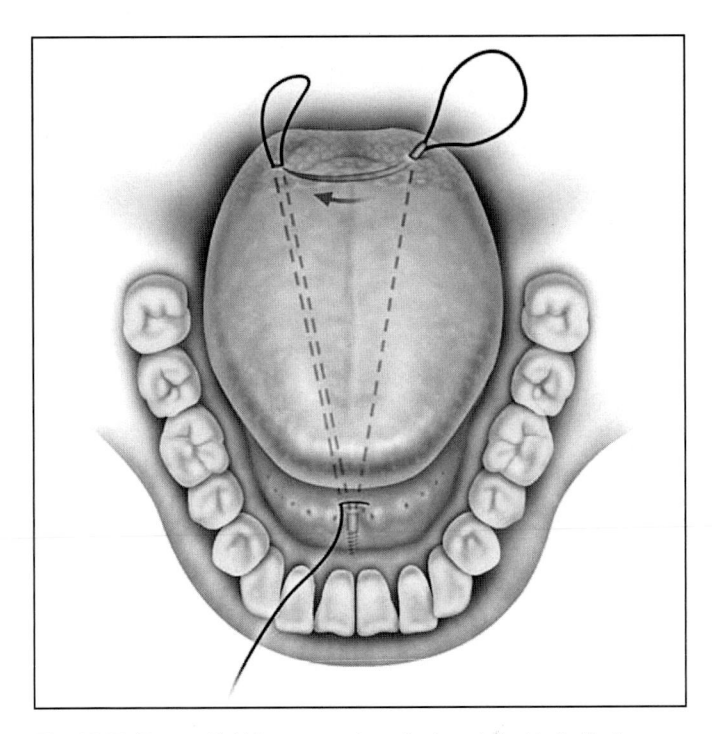

**Fig. 44.15** (Repose 5). Using a curved needle threaded with the Prolene suture, it is passed submucosally from the suture exit hole to the suture loop exit hole and placed through the loop.

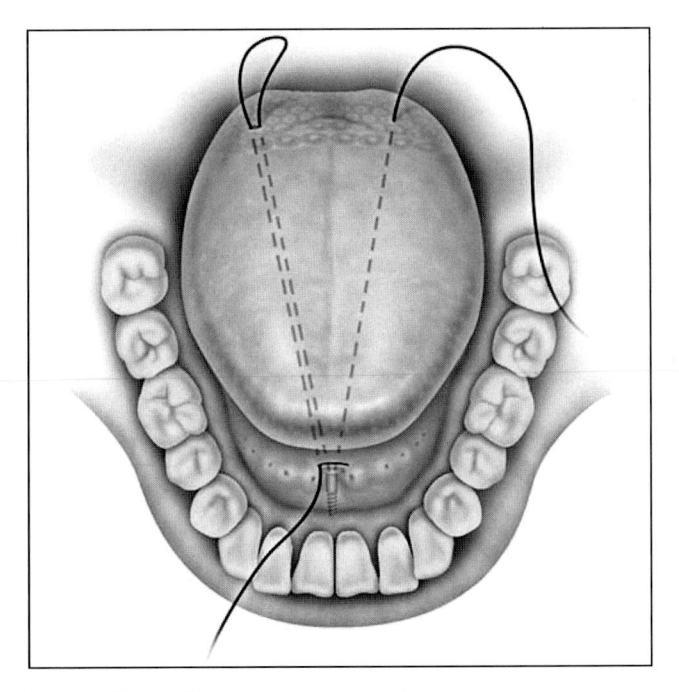

**Fig. 44.14** (Repose 4). Prolene suture passed through the tongue on the opposite side.

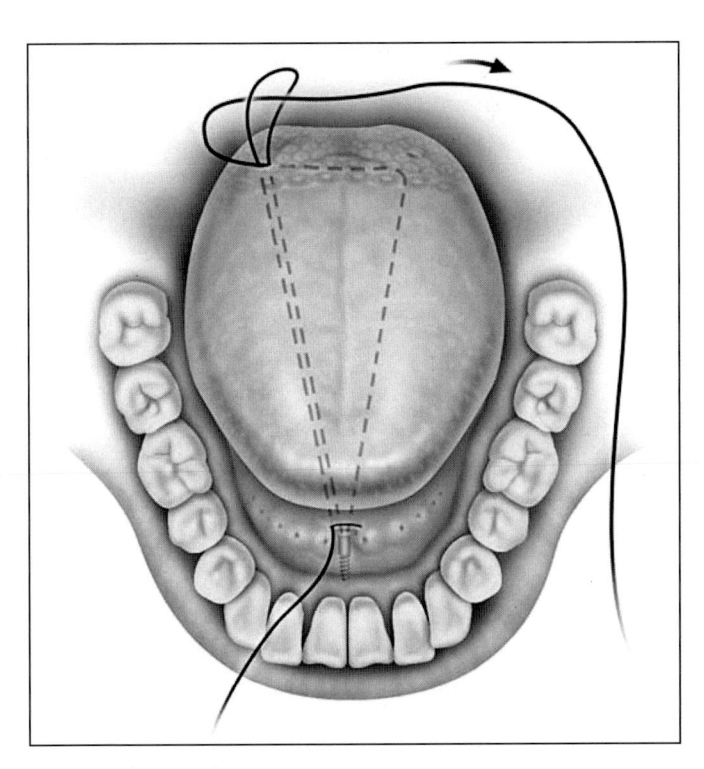

**Fig. 44.16** (Repose 6). The suture loop is then pulled through the tongue dragging the Prolene suture with it to the floor of the mouth.

275

# SECTION K — MULTILEVEL PHARYNGEAL SURGERY

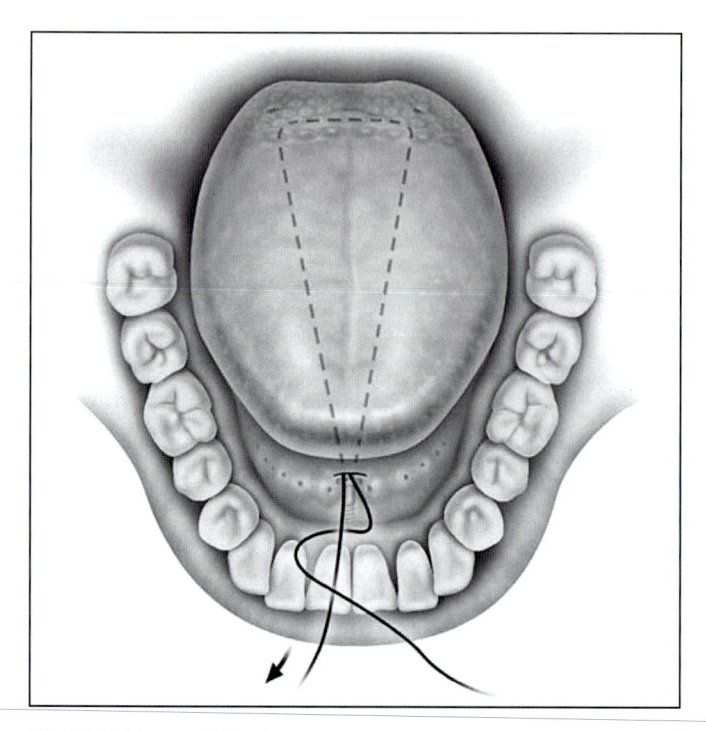

**Fig. 44.17** (Repose 7). The Prolene suture is tied and the knot buried. Tension should be adequate to create a dimple.

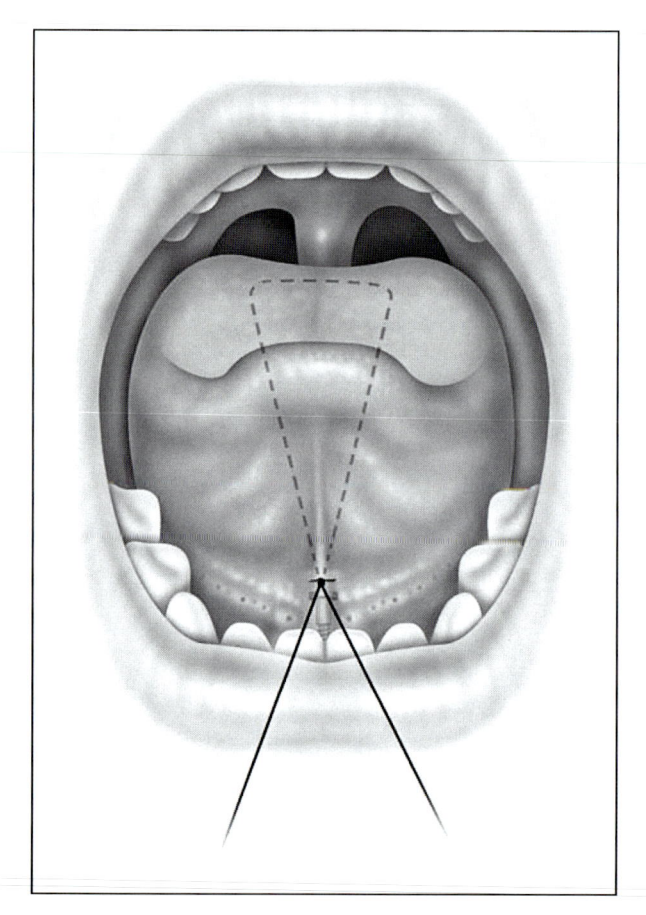

**Fig. 44.18** (Repose 9). Final result of the tongue Repose suture showing the suture holding the tongue base forwards and preventing collapse posteriorly.

Perioperative use of nasal CPAP is strongly encouraged. Patients who undergo multilevel surgery for OSA are monitored in the high-dependency unit overnight. All patients should be monitored closely in the postanesthesia care unit (PACU) for at least 4 hours postoperatively. Many authors believe that the postoperative complications are low, but if they were to occur, they would occur within the first 3 hours.[5,9,10]

Complications of these tongue procedures inadvertently include edema of the tongue, floor of the mouth and palate. A nasal airway is frequently used to stent the upper airway for the first day postoperatively. Trauma to the Wharton's ducts may occur in the tongue suspension procedure. It has also been documented that discoloration of the lower incisors occurs in the genioglossus advancement procedure if the teeth roots are involved.

## 5 SUCCESS RATES OF THE PROCEDURES

As most patients with OSA have multilevel obstruction, most of these tongue procedures are done in combination with a palate procedure. Success rates vary from one study to another; most authors define success as a reduction of Apnea/Hypopnea Index (AHI) by 50% of the preoperative value and below 20.

### 5.1 GENIOGLOSSUS ADVANCEMENT AND HYOID MYOTOMY

These two procedures are frequently done together and hence, most data are of these two procedures combined. Riley et al.[25] were first to report a 60% success rate in 133 patients who underwent the combined UPPP, genioglossus advancement and hyoid myotomy procedure. Riley et al.[26] validated the hyoid procedure as a single operation in 15 patients who had failed UPPP, and found a success rate of 75%. Since the mid-1990s, many authors have reported a success rate of 60–70% for the multilevel procedures with UPPP, genioglossus advancement and hyoid myotomy procedure.[25,27–29] Hormann et al.[30] showed that there was significant increase in the retrolingual space after the hyoid suspension procedure. Neruntarat demonstrated an impressive 78% success rate for combined UPPP and hyoid suspension technique.[31] He also showed a 70% success rate for combined UPPP, genioglossus advancement and hyoid suspension.[32] Hormann et al.[33] in 2004 revealed a 78.8% response rate (defined as a reduction of preoperative AHI by at least >20%) and 57.6% success rate (defined as a 50% reduction of preoperative AHI and <15) in 66 patients who underwent UPPP, hyoid suspension and some other form of tongue base procedure. A small prospective trial showed that genioglossus advancement and the tongue suspension method were useful in patients with severe OSA, with tongue suspension having a slight advantage.[34] Verse et al.[35] also had a 69.6% response rate in 46 patients who underwent the hyoid myotomy procedure. Baisch et al.[36] in 2006 revealed an overall success rate (defined as a 50% reduction of preoperative AHI and <15) of 59.7% in 83 patients who underwent UPPP and the hyoid suspension procedure.

## 5.2 TONGUE SUSPENSION

The tongue suspension suture was first introduced in the late 1990s; the procedure showed promising results and improvements in both subjective and objective outcomes.[37] Subsequent reports also revealed fair improvements in objective polysomnography results.[38] Thomas et al.[34] demonstrated that the success rate of the tongue suspension device was near 60%, and tongue suspension had a slight advantage over the genioglossus advancement procedure. Kuhnel et al.[39] showed in 28 patients that while tongue suspension had benefits in both subjective and objective results, there were no obvious cephalometric changes noted postoperatively. Omur et al.[40] had an impressive 81.8% success rate in 22 patients with severe OSA who had undergone a combined UPPP and tongue suspension procedure. Long-term follow-up at 3 years also showed impressive outcomes of a success rate of 78% in 55 patients with severe OSA.[41]

## 6 CONCLUSION

Moderate to severe OSA usually involves multiple levels of obstruction in the collapsible upper airway. Multilevel pharyngeal surgery, therefore, is usually required to surgically overcome the several sites of obstruction. Modifications of the skeletal technique have made the procedures safe and effective. Many research papers are reporting long-term and promising results for the surgical correction of the upper airway.

## REFERENCES

1. Terris DJ, Hanasono MM, Liu YC. Reliability of the Muller maneuver and its association with SDB. Laryngoscope 2000;110:1819–23.
2. Cahali MB. Lateral pharyngoplasty: a new treatment for OSAHS. Laryngoscope 2003;113:1961–68.
3. Pang KP, Woodson BT. Expansion sphincter pharyngoplasty: a new technique for the treatment of obstructive sleep apnea. Otolaryngol Head Neck Surg 2007;137:110–4.
4. Standards of Practice Committee of the American Sleep Disorders Association. Practice parameters for the treatment of obstructive sleep apnea in adults: the efficacy of surgical modifications of the upper airway. Sleep 1996,19,152–5.
5. Utley DS, Shin EJ, Clerk AA, et al. A cost-effective and rational surgical approach to patients with snoring, upper airway resistance syndrome or obstructive sleep apnea. Laryngoscope 1997;107:726–34.
6. Riley RW, Powell NB, Guilleminault C. Obstructive sleep apnea syndrome: a review of 306 consecutively treated surgical patients. Otolaryngol Head Neck Surg 1993;108(2):117–25.
7. Fujita S, Conway W, Zorick F, et al. Surgical correction of anatomic abnormalities in OSAS: uvulopalatopharyngoplasty. Otolaryngol Head Neck Surg 1993;108:117–25.
8. Fujita S, Woodson BT, Clark JT, et al. Laser midline glossectomy as a treatment of OSA. Laryngoscope 1991;101:805–59.
9. Pang KP. Identifying patients who need close monitoring during and after upper airway surgery for obstructive sleep apnoea. J Laryngol Otol 2006;120:655–60.
10. Terris DJ, Fincher EF, Hansonon MM, Fee WE Jr, Adachi K. Conservation of resources: indications for intensive care monitoring after upper airway surgery on patients with obstructive sleep apnea. Laryngoscope 1998;108(6):784–8.
11. Pang KP. One-stage nasal and multilevel pharyngeal surgery for obstructive sleep apnoea: safety and efficacy. J Laryngol Otol 2005;119(4):272–6.
12. Borowiecki BD, Sassin JF. Surgical treatment of sleep apnoea. Arch Otolaryngol 1983;109:506–12.
13. Fujita S. Surgical treatment of OSA: UPPP and lingualplasty (laser midline glossectomy). In: Obstructive Sleep Apnea Syndrome: Clinical Research and Treatment. Guilleminault C, Partinen M, eds. New York: Raven Press; 1990, pp. 129–51.
14. Sher AE, Schechtman KB, Piccirillo JF. The efficacy of surgical modifications of the upper airway in adults with OSAS. Sleep 1996;19:156–77.
15. Friedman M, Ibrahim H, Bass L. Clinical staging for sleep-disordered breathing. Otolaryngol Head Neck Surgery 2002;127:13–21.
16. Friedman M, Ibrahim H, Joseph NJ. Staging of obstructive sleep apnea/hypopnea syndrome: a guide to appropriate treatment. Laryngoscope 2004;114(3):454–9.
17. Pang KP, Terris DJ, Podolsky R. Severity of OSA: correlation with clinical examination and patient perception. Otolaryngol Head Neck Surg 2006;135:555–60.
18. Verse T, Joachim TM, Pirsig W. Effect of nasal surgery on sleep related breathing disorders. Laryngoscope 2002;112:64–8.
19. Busaba NY. Same-staged nasal and palatopharyngeal surgery for OSA: is it safe? Otolaryngol Head Neck Surg 2002;126:399–403.
20. Rubin AHE, Eliaschar I, Joachim Z, et al. Effects of nasal surgery and tonsillectomy on sleep apnoca. Bull Eur Physiopathol Respir 1983;19:612–15.
21. Dayal VS, Phillipson EA. Nasal surgery in the management of OSA. Ann Otol Laryngol 1985;94:550–54.
22. Riley RW, Powell NB, Guilleminault C. Inferior sagittal osteotomy of the mandible with hyoid myotomy suspension: a new procedure for OSA. Otolaryngol Head Neck Surg 1986;94:589–93.
23. Riley RW, Powell NB, Guilleminault C. OSA and the hyoid: a revised surgical procedure. Otolaryngol Head Neck Surg 1994;111:717–21.
24. Powell NB, Riley RW, Guilleminault C. The hypopharynx: upper airway reconstruction in OSAS. In: Snoring and Obstructive Sleep Apnea, 2nd edn. Fairbanks DNF, Fujita S, eds. New York: Raven Press; 1994, pp. 193–209.
25. Riley RW, Powell NB, Guilleminault C. Obstructive sleep apnoea syndrome: a review of 306 consecutively treated surgical patients. Otolaryngol Head Neck Surg 1993;108(2):117–25.
26. Riley RW, Powell NB, Guilleminault C. Obstructive sleep apnea and the hyoid: a revised surgical procedure. Otolaryngol Head Neck Surg 1994;111(6):717–21.
27. Hendler BH, Costello BJ, Silverstein K, Yen D, Goldberg A. A protocol for uvulopalatopharyngoplasty, mortised genioplasty, and maxillomandibular advancement in patients with obstructive sleep apnea: an analysis of 40 cases. J Oral Maxillofac Surg 2001;59(8):892–7.
28. Silverstein K, Costello BJ, Giannakpoulos H, Hendler B. Genioglossus muscle attachments: an anatomic analysis and the implications for genioglossus advancement. Oral Surg Oral Med Oral Pathol Oral Radiol Endod 2000;90(6):686–8.
29. Vilaseca I, Morello A, Montserrat JM, Santamaria J, Iranzo A. Usefulness of uvulopalatopharyngoplasty with genioglossus and

29. hyoid advancement in the treatment of obstructive sleep apnea. Arch Otolaryngol Head Neck Surg 2002;128(4):435–40.
30. Hormann K, Hirth K, Erhardt T, Maurer JT, Verse T. Modified hyoid suspension for therapy of sleep related breathing disorders. operative technique and complications. Laryngorhinootologie 2001;80(9):517–21.
31. Neruntarat C. Hyoid myotomy with suspension under local anesthesia for obstructive sleep apnea syndrome. Eur Arch Otorhinolaryngol 2003;260(5):286–90.
32. Neruntarat C. Genioglossus advancement and hyoid myotomy under local anesthesia. Otolaryngol Head Neck Surg 2003;129(1):85–91.
33. Hormann K, Maurer JT, Baisch A. [Snoring/sleep apnea – surgically curable]. HNO 2004;52(9):807–13.
34. Thomas AJ, Chavoya M, Terris DJ. Preliminary findings from a prospective, randomized trial of two tongue-base surgeries for sleep-disordered breathing. Otolaryngol Head Neck Surg 2003;129(5):539–46.
35. Verse T, Baisch A, Hormann K. [Multilevel surgery for obstructive sleep apnea. Preliminary objective results]. Laryngorhinootologie 2004;83(8):516–22.
36. Baisch A, Maurer JT, Hormann K. The effect of hyoid suspension in a multilevel surgery concept for obstructive sleep apnea. Otolaryngol Head Neck Surg 2006;134(5):856–61.
37. Woodson BT, Derowe A, Hawke M, et al. Pharyngeal suspension suture with repose bone screw for obstructive sleep apnea. Otolaryngol Head Neck Surg 2000;122(3):395–401.
38. Woodson BT. A tongue suspension suture for obstructive sleep apnea and snorers. Otolaryngol Head Neck Surg 2001;124(3):297–303.
39. Kuhnel TS, Schurr C, Wagner B, Geisler P. Morphological changes of the posterior airway space after tongue base suspension. Laryngoscope 2005;115(3):475–80.
40. Omur M, Ozturan D, Elez F, Unver C, Derman S. Tongue base suspension combined with UPPP in severe OSA patients. Otolaryngol Head Neck Surg 2005;133(2):218–23.
41. Vicente E, Marin JM, Carrizo S, Naya MJ. Tongue-base suspension in conjunction with uvulopalatopharyngoplasty for treatment of severe obstructive sleep apnea: long-term follow-up results. Laryngoscope 2006;116(7):1223–27.

# SECTION K — MULTILEVEL PHARYNGEAL SURGERY

## CHAPTER 45

# Open tongue base resection for OSA

*Tod C. Huntley*

## 1 INTRODUCTION

Surgical treatment of sleep disordered breathing can be difficult for both the patient and the surgeon. The most common surgical treatment for the disorder, uvulopalatopharyngoplasty, is effective as a stand-alone procedure less than half the time,[1] and though the tongue base is recognized as a significant contributing factor in many if not most cases of, Obstructive Sleep Apnea (OSA) it is not often treated sufficiently, for two main reasons: first, most surgeons are not trained to treat this area; second, the results of many of the available procedures for tongue base obstruction are often unpredictable.

It could be argued that if the perfect tongue base operation existed, it would be widely adopted by surgeons. Yet the difficulty in treating the tongue base is exemplified by the multiplicity of available procedures – including genioglossus advancement, hyoid advancement, tongue base suspension, radiofrequency treatment, transoral midline glossectomy, submucosal coblation-assisted tongue base resection, and maxillofacial surgical techniques.

Case reports of tongue base surgery for obstructive sleep apnea date back to the 1980s,[2,3] but it was Fujita[4] in 1991 who is credited with the first significant work in this arena. He resected the midline of the tongue base transorally with a laser, as discussed elsewhere in this atlas; other variations on this type of procedure have since been published.[5–8]

However, these transoral procedures have some inherent drawbacks. Chief among them is the lack of visualization of the neurovascular supply to the tongue. Injury to the hypoglossal nerve and/or the lingual vessels can have devastating consequences regarding articulation, swallowing and quality of life. Because of the location of the hypoglossal–lingual neurovascular bundle, these blind transoral resections are limited to the midline third of the tongue, and do not address the lateral tongue base. An open approach through the neck, however, could include direct visualization of these important structures, thereby allowing for resection of the target tissue while preserving the neurovascular supply to the tongue.

This was the rationale that led Chabolle to develop a novel technique for the treatment of sleep apnea-related tongue base obstruction. First published in the English literature in 1999,[9] his tongue base resection with hyoepiglottoplasty (TBRHE) employs an open suprahyoid dissection of the tongue base through the midline of the neck with identification of the hypoglossal/lingual neurovascular bundle, coupled with a full thickness resection of $24 + 6\,g$ of tongue base extending as far laterally as the palatoglossal folds. This wide excision is afforded by the dissection and lateral retraction of the hypoglossal nerve and lingual vessels, with resection of the tongue base tissue deep to and lateral to them. The procedure concludes with hyoid advancement to the lower border of the mandible and shortening of the suprahyoid musculature. Because of the aggressive nature of the procedure, TBRHE also includes a temporary tracheotomy. The procedure can be combined with UPPP for one-stage OSA treatment, which was reiterated by Sorrenti et al.[10] in a 2006 article documenting additional experience with this procedure.

This chapter describes the surgical steps involved in this procedure in more detail than previously reported. Chapter 41 by Robinson in this atlas details a variation of this procedure that includes a less aggressive resection of the tongue base in an extramucosal plane with avoidance of tracheotomy, in the hope that this is accompanied by faster recovery and less morbidity.

## 2 ANATOMY

Because this surgery in essence is a transcervical suprahyoid dissection of the tongue base, it is important to review some salient points of the region's anatomy, particularly as it relates to the neurovascular structures. The first muscles encountered through the incision are the fan-shaped mylohyoid muscles separated by a relatively avascular midline raphe. The digastric muscles are located more laterally in the surgical field, just superficial to the mylohyoids.

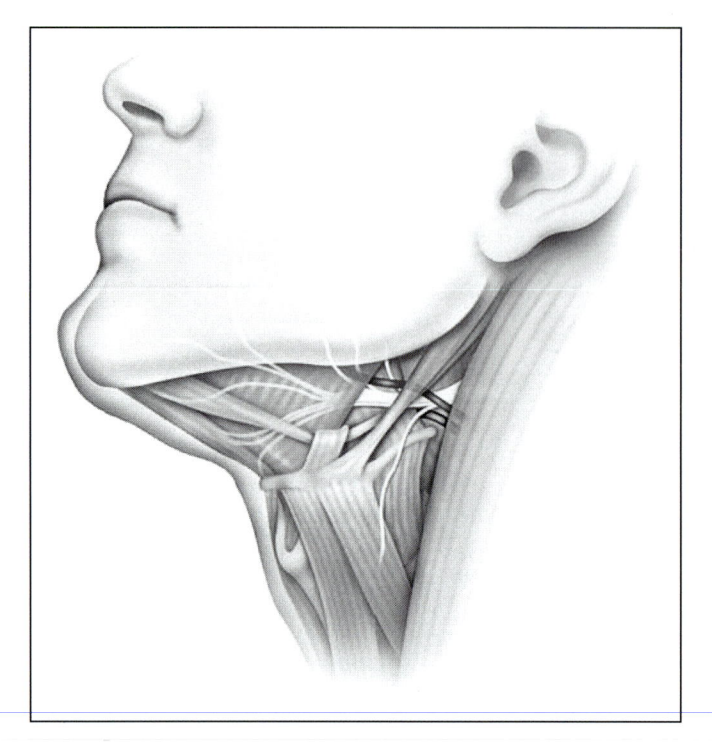

**Fig. 45.1** This illustration shows the relevant anatomy of the region, including the relationships of the suprahyoid muscles and the neurovascular supply to the tongue. Note that the hypoglossal nerve and the lingual vein course superficial to the hyoglossus muscle and the lingual artery runs deep to this muscle on its way to the tongue base.

At the lateral aspects of the mylohyoids are the hyoglossus muscles, arising from the greater horn of the hyoid. These fibers run at a roughly 60° angle to the fibers of the mylohyoid. The importance of the hyoglossus muscles is their relationship to the tongue's neurovascular supply. As shown in Figure 45.1, the hypoglossal nerves and the lingual veins course superficial to the hyoglossus muscles. They are readily seen after releasing the mylohyoid and geniohyoid muscles from the hyoid bone during the surgery. The lingual artery courses deep to the hyoglossus muscle and emerges along its anterior border to parallel the hypoglossal nerve and lingual vein on each side as they enter the tongue base. Also noteworthy is the fact that the hypoglossal nerve is not just a solitary cable that passes over the hyoglossus on its course to the tongue base; it instead gives off a number of small fibers to the portion of the tongue base that is to be resected, which must be divided during the procedure.

## 3 PRESURGICAL EVALUATION

All TBRHE patients should undergo the usual preoperative work-up, as discussed in more detail elsewhere in this atlas. In addition to a polysomnographic evaluation and a complete upper airway/head and neck physical examination, all patients should undergo flexible fiberoptic laryngopharyngoscopy and should have craniofacial skeletal abnormalities ruled out by lateral cephalometric radiography. Those who are skeletally deficient per published cephalometric norms, generally defined as a sella-nasion-subspinale (SNA) angle measuring less than 79° and/or a sella-nasion-supramentale (SNB) angle less than 77°, should probably be considered for a maxillofacial surgical protocol instead.

In addition to these usual cephalometric parameters, Chabolle[9] has published other radiographic criteria that he uses to define abnormalities of tongue size and hyoid position, or the 'hyolingual complex'. This includes measurement of tongue surface area via a T1-weighted mid-sagittal MRI; hyolingual complex abnormalities documented on this MRI include total lingual surface area greater than 28 cm$^2$ and submandibular lingual surface area greater than 4 cm$^2$. The other criterion used by Chabolle is a cephalometric measurement of a quadrilateral space defined as follows: posteriorly by the posterior pharyngeal wall, inferiorly by a perpendicular line extending from the posterior pharyngeal wall to the most anterosuperior point of the hyoid body (H point), anteriorly by a line between H and the posterior nasal spine (PNS), and superiorly by an extension of the line joining the anterior nasal spine to PNS, starting from PNS to the posterior pharyngeal wall. Chabolle contends that a value of more than 25 cm$^2$ within this quadrilateral oropharyngeal space is consistent with hyolingual complex abnormalities.

Sorrenti does not rely on Chabolle's MRI and cephalometric measurements to define the hyolingual complex abnormalities for his cases. He instead relies on the more typically described cephalometric parameters of SNA, SNB, mandibular plane to hyoid distance (with a value of >25 cm considered abnormal) and posterior airway space (<11 mm abnormal).

## 4 RESULTS

Only two published papers were available by the time of this writing for review. The first of these, by Chabolle,[9] details results on 10 patients treated from 1994 through 1997. All underwent full thickness TBRHE with a mean resected lingual volume of 24 + 6 cm$^2$, as measured by the displacement method. All patients underwent concurrent tracheotomy, with decannulation after a mean of 7 + 2.5 days. Eight of the patients underwent concurrent primary or revision UPPP and three had concurrent septoplasty and turbinectomy. Overall surgical success, as defined by the usual criteria of postoperative Apnea/Hypopnea Index (AHI) <20 and reduction in the preoperative AHI by 50% or more, was 80%. The mean AHI improved from 70 to 27. Other indices, including subjective snoring and daytime somnolence, likewise improved in all but one patient. Lateral cephalometry showed elevation of the hyoid by a mean distance of 11.5 + 7 mm (2–26 mm), and this hyoid position remained stable at 3 months despite removal of the hyoid suspension sutures in three patients up to 3 months postoperatively. Oral feeding began at 15 + 4.5

days, and patients remained hospitalized for 19.5 + 4 days. No clinical abnormalities with lingual mobility, speech, or swallowing were encountered, and there was no postoperative bleeding. There were five neck abscesses in the first six cases, and these were felt to be related to the use of nonabsorbable rather than absorbable sutures for the hyoid suspension in those patients.

Sorrenti[10] has published data on 10 additional patients treated from 2001 to 2005. All of these patients underwent concurrent UPPP and TBRHE with concurrent tracheotomy, with decannulation after a mean of 7 + 3 days. The volume of resected tissue was not reported. Success, again defined by the usual Polysomnography (PSG) criteria, was 100%. The mean AHI decreased from 54.7 + 11.5 to 9.4 + 5.4 and the mean low saturation improved from 77% + 6.2 to 90.7 + 3. The hyoid position improved by a mean of 12.1 cm, as measured by the cephalometric change in the mandibular plane to hyoid distance, which improved from 30.4 + 4.1 cm preoperatively to 18.3 + 2.4 cm afterwards. The mean hospital stay was 16 + 2 days and oral feeding began at 13 + 2 days. There were no infections or postoperative bleeds. Barium swallow examinations were done 6–19 months postoperatively, with abnormal results noted in three patients, including premature spillage over the tongue base, vallecular pooling, and incomplete epiglottic excursion, but there was no penetration or aspiration. All patients resumed a normal diet and the patients' families reported no subjective changes in speech quality.

My data[11] are likewise encouraging. At the time of writing, this includes 26 patients treated from 2000 through 2006. Of these, 14 were treated with TBRHE alone for isolated tongue base obstruction (13 had undergone apparently successful UPPP and one had a normal palate on exam); seven patients with both palatal and tongue base obstruction underwent concurrent TBRHE with UPPP. All of these 22 full thickness TBRHE cases included concurrent tracheotomy. An additional five patients have undergone extramucosal tongue base resections without tracheotomy.

Of the 14 patients with presumably normal or successfully treated palates who underwent TBRHE with tracheotomy alone, a mean volume of 26 g (23–30) was resected. Decannulation occurred at a mean of 5 + 3 days; oral feeding commenced at 6 + 5 days; and the mean hospital stay was 8 + 3 days. Success by the usual PSG criteria was 79% (11 of 14), and an additional 14% (two patients) met one of the parameters but not both (one with an AHI drop from 38 to 21.2, the other with AHI improvement from 56 to 27). Complications included persistent but self-limited drainage from the incisions in 10 patients (lasting from 14 to 52 days); extruded hyoepiglottoplasty sutures in two (presenting to 4 years postoperatively); and subjective dysphagia in three (though no patients had aspiration or penetration on modified barium swallows postoperatively). None had objective speech changes as determined by a postoperative speech pathology evaluation, though two reported subjective minor changes.

Of the additional seven of my patients who underwent concurrent UPPP, TBRHE and tracheotomy, success was achieved in six (86%). The mean resected lingual volume in this cohort was 28 g (range 25–33), and all of the patients but one were decannulated within 10 days. Oral feeding commenced within 10 days for all but one (3 weeks), and the mean hospital stay was 9 + 2 days. Complications included one pharyngocutaneous fistula, which closed without treatment within 2 weeks, two patients with persistent drainage to 3 weeks despite no fistula radiographically, and one patient whose hyoepiglottoplasty sutures later extruded. Persistent mild dysphagia for up to 3 months was noted in four patients.

Since mid-2006 I have performed five extramucosal tongue base resections, but these patients have not been followed long enough at the time of writing for discussion of results. Four were done without tracheotomies, and the fifth patient underwent the procedure to allow for decannulation of a pre-existing tracheotomy. None of the other four patients experienced problems related to the lack of concurrent tracheotomy. The mean resected lingual volume (23.3 + 1.7 g) was less with this extramucosal resection than that which was excised in the patients who underwent full thickness TBRHE.

## 6 PROCEDURE

The procedure is performed under general anesthesia without neuromuscular paralysis, so that hypoglossal nerve function can be monitored during the case. In addition to visually inspecting the nerve, I now use a nerve integrity monitoring system (NIM-Response system, Medtronic Xomed, Jacksonville, FLA), with an active electrode placed transorally into the musculature on each side of the tongue. This system should alert the surgeon to subclinical hypoglossal nerve stimulation with an alarm.

The neck and chin are prepped and draped in a sterile fashion. If a tracheotomy is planned, as recommended by Chabolle and by Sorrenti, it is done at this point. This is advisable because of the risk of airway compromise from bleeding, pharyngocutaneous fistula, edema, etc. with full thickness TBRHE; if an extramucosal resection is planned, however, a tracheotomy can be done at the surgeon's discretion, and is not thought to be needed routinely.

A transverse neck incision measuring approximately 5–6 cm is made approximately 1 cm above the hyoid in the midline neck, preferably in a natural skin crease, as shown in Figure 45.2. This incision should be placed high enough so that the lower midline border of the mandible can be reached without difficulty. Skin and subcutaneous tissue can be retracted with handheld retractors or with elasticized fishhooks fastened to the drapes, but my choice is the self-retaining Lone Star retractor system (Lone Star Medical Products, Inc., Stafford, TX). Skin and subcutaneous flaps are developed in a plane just superficial to the mylohyoid muscles, and are elevated to the hyoid inferiorly,

# SECTION K  MULTILEVEL PHARYNGEAL SURGERY

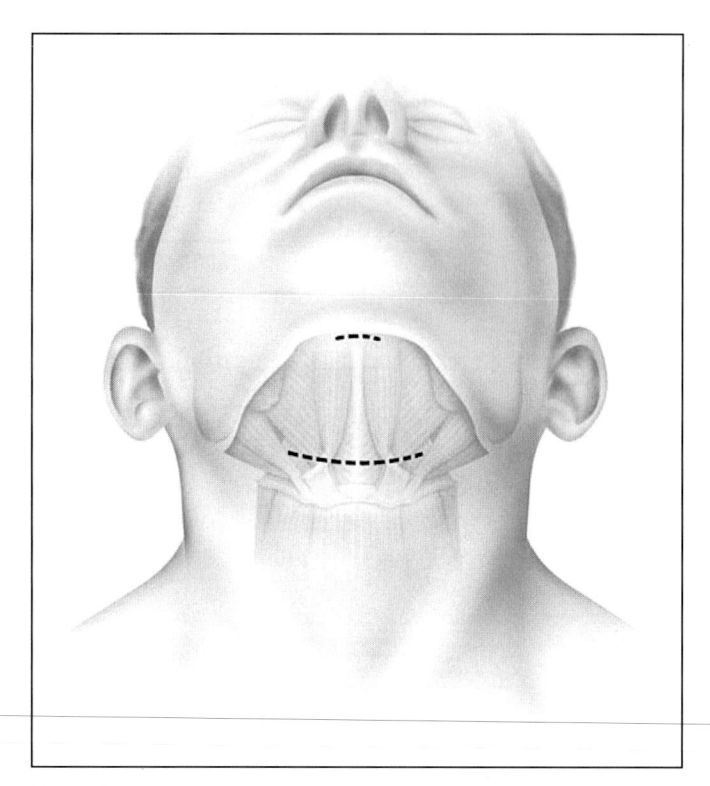

**Fig. 45.2** The patient is prepped and draped for surgery. The transverse suprahyoid incision is placed in a skin crease and measures approximately 5 cm. The optional smaller submental incision is made only if necessary to provide exposure for placement of the drill holes in the lower border of the mandible for the hyoid advancement.

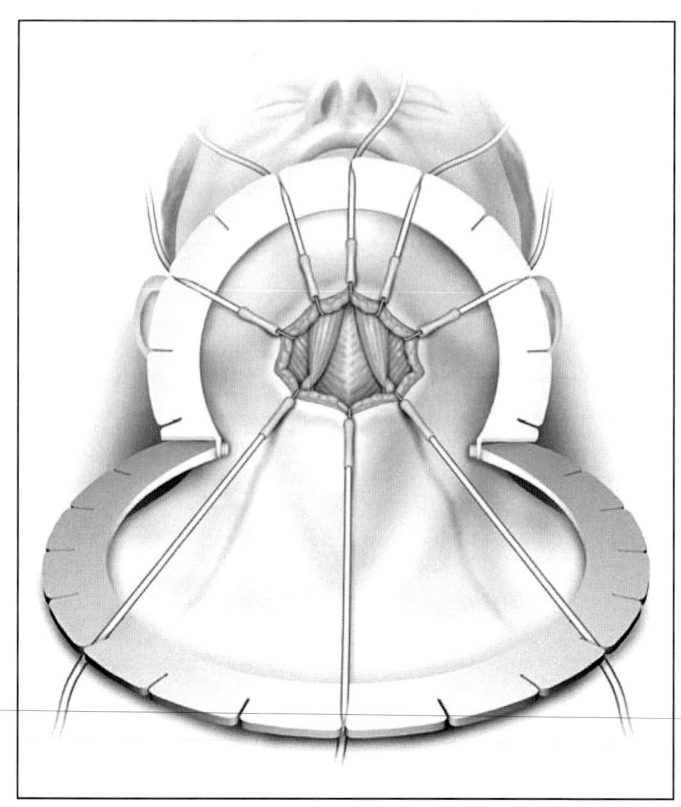

**Fig. 45.3** The skin flaps have been elevated and are secured to the Lone Star retractor. The underlying digastric and mylohyoid muscles are now visible.

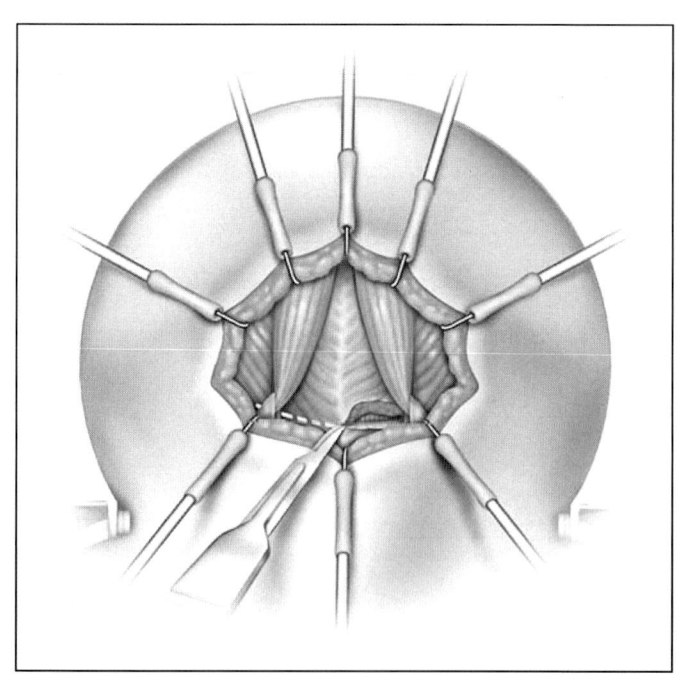

**Fig. 45.4** The mylohyoid myotomy is performed, and the underlying geniohyoid muscle is exposed. The mylohyoid will be retracted cephalad once it is elevated.

to the lower border of the mandible superiorly, and to the medial borders of the submandibular glands laterally. The anterior bellies of the digastric muscles and the underlying flat, triangular bellies of the paired mylohyoid muscles should now be easily visible, as shown in Figure 45.3.

Dissection then continues with a stepwise release of the suprahyoid muscles in order, starting with the digastrics and proceeding through the mylohyoids, geniohyoids and the hyoglossus muscles. These muscles are sectioned approximately 1 cm from their insertions in the hyoid bone, so that a sufficient cuff of muscles is left on the hyoid to allow for layered muscle closure at the conclusion of the case. If a self-retaining retractor such as the Lone Star is used, its hooks can be repositioned to retract these muscles superiorly.

These initial myotomies begin with a release of the digastric tendons from the hyoid bone to allow them to be retracted superolaterally. The underlying mylohyoid fibers run inferomedially from the mandible in a 'hands in pants' configuration and join at a roughly 60° angle at the midline raphe. The mylohyoids are now incised (Fig. 45.4), leaving the midline raphe intact, and are retracted cephalad to expose the underlying geniohyoid muscles.

The geniohyoids are two narrow paired bundles which originate at the posterior mentum and insert on the anterior surface of the lesser cornu of the hyoid. At the lateral aspects of these vertically oriented bundles, the anterior borders of the fan-shaped hyoglossus muscles are seen. The geniohyoid muscles lie medial to and slightly superficial to the hyoglossus muscles, and are carefully incised approximately 1 cm above their insertions on the hyoid bone (Fig. 45.5),

# Open tongue base resection for OSA

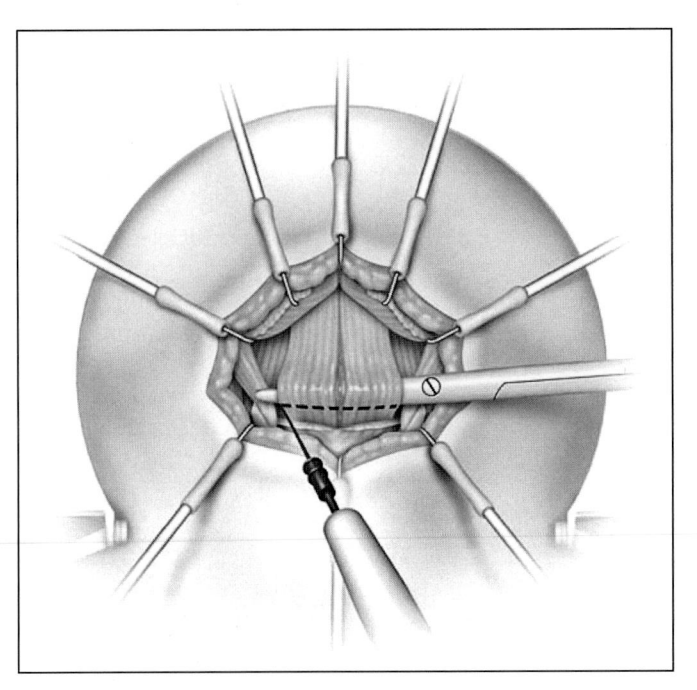

**Fig. 45.5** The geniohyoid muscle is incised approximately 1 cm above its insertion at the hyoid. The mylohyoid and digastric muscles are retracted cephalad in this diagram.

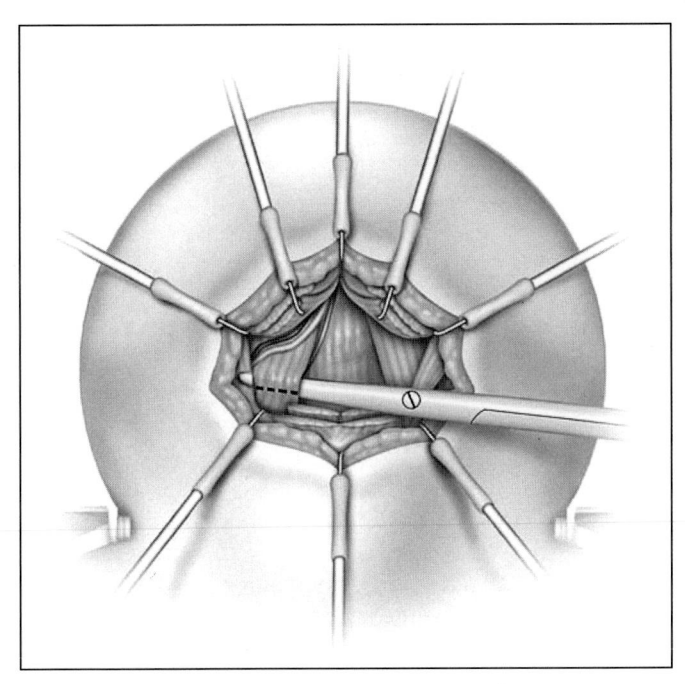

**Fig. 45.6** The hyoglossus myotomy is performed. This is done meticulously to avoid damage to the hypoglossal nerve and lingual vein, which run superficial to the muscle, and the lingual artery, which courses immediately underneath the muscle. It is safest to cut this muscle inferior to the course of the lingual artery.

and are reflected superiorly. This muscle division is done meticulously, as the hypoglossal nerves and lingual veins run superficial to the hyoglossus muscles and may immediately underlie the lateral aspects of the genioglossus muscles at this level, approximately 1 cm cephalad to the hyoid.[12]

Once the geniohyoids are reflected superiorly, the underlying genioglossus muscle is visible. As the genioglossus muscle fibers run in the same direction as the geniohyoid fibers, the differentiation of these muscles can be difficult at times, but there is usually a pretty well-defined plane between these two muscle layers. The paired hyoglossus muscles overlie the lateral aspects of the genioglossus, with the hypoglossal nerve and the lingual vein passing superficially and the lingual artery coursing underneath. If the lingual arteries are not easily identified at this point, they can be located where they emerge at the anterior aspect of the hyoglossus with aid of a Doppler probe. The hyoglossus muscles are then carefully incised with fine scissors, as shown in Figure 45.6, and are retracted superiorly. The lingual vessels and hypoglossal nerves, which now run together to the tongue base, are then gently retracted superolaterally with elastic vessel loops, held with the Lone Star retractor. It is possible to induce hypoglossal neuropraxia if the nerves are too aggressively retracted at this stage. This retraction of the neurovascular bundles, illustrated in Figure 45.7, allows for adequate resection of the underlying tongue base, not just in the midline, but also as far laterally as possible. It is this ability to directly visualize and resect the lateral aspects of the tongue base outside the neurovascular bundles that might give this open procedure

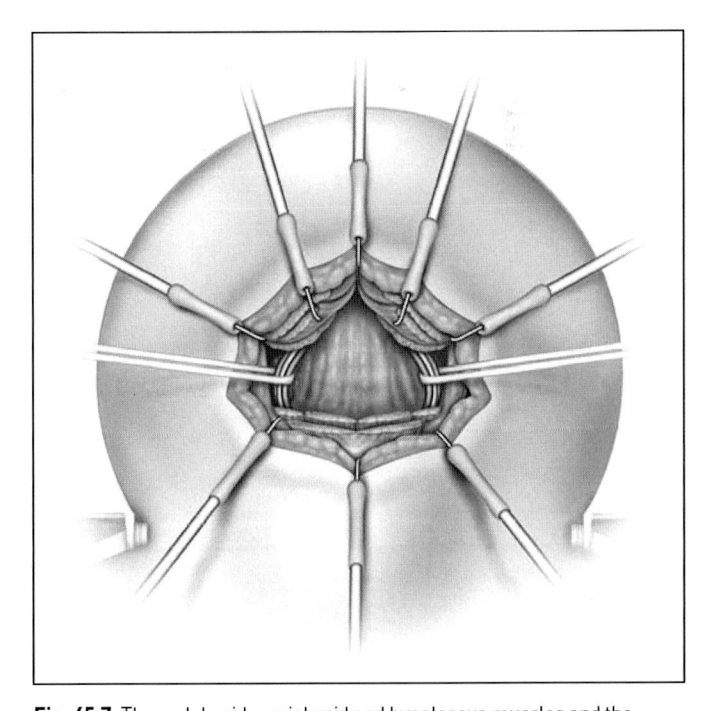

**Fig. 45.7** The mylohyoid, geniohyoid and hyoglossus muscles and the lingual–hypoglossal neurovascular bundles have been retracted, and the underlying genioglossus muscle is now ready for resection. This resection can include either the full thickness of the tongue base as advocated by Chabolle, or just the muscle, sparing the mucosa, as described in Chapter ••. Regardless of which variation is chosen, the approach to this point is the same.

283

a theoretical advantage over other procedures such as the coblation-assisted extramucosal glossectomy. At this stage, the branch(es) of the hypoglossal nerve innervating the portion of the tongue base to be resected are divided, leaving the main trunk unmolested.

Once the suprahyoid muscles have been sectioned and retracted, and once the vessels and nerves have been retracted, exposure is complete and the tongue base resection can begin. At this point, the surgeon has the choice as to whether the resection is to be done in the full thickness fashion described originally by Chabolle, as shown in Figure 45.8, or in an extramucosal fashion, as advocated by Robinson, as outlined in Chapter 41. To this point, however, the approach for both procedures is identical.

If the full thickness resection is chosen, the pharynx is entered from this suprahyoid approach approximately 1 cm cephalad to the hyoid at the same level as the mylohyoid, hyoglossus and geniohyoid myotomies. This suprahyoid pharyngotomy is extended from side to side to the lateral aspects of the tongue base, with dissection deep to the reflected nerve and vessels. The cut tongue base cephalad to this incision is grasped with Allis or Lahey tenaculums, and is reflected through the pharyngotomy to allow for direct visualization of the tissue to be resected. This exposure allows for a wedge-shaped resection of 20–30 g of tongue base.[10] The resection can extend as far laterally as the palatoglossal folds, and as cephalad as the circumvallate papillae; the amount of tissue resected tends to increase as experience with this procedure is gained. The hypoglossal–lingual neurovascular bundles are kept under direct visualization throughout this resection, as the dissection proceeds deep to and lateral to the vessels and nerves. As the cut edge of the tongue base is retracted with Allis or Lahey tenaculums, the vertical cuts through the lateral tongue base are made with heavy Mayo scissors. These vertical cuts can extend as far cephalad as the circumvallate papillae, which are visualized from below. The apices of these cuts are then connected with a horizontal incision at or just inferior to the circumvallate papilla level, made either with scissors, an electrocautery unit, or a #10 blade. The resultant resected tissue – lingual musculature and mucosa – is weighed, with an average resected volume of 20–30 g. It is admittedly difficult – if not impossible – with any technique of lingual resection to know precisely how much tissue should be resected, however.

The defect thus created is impressive looking, and may appear too significant to close, but an accompanying aggressive advancement of the hyoid of up to 2 cm or more toward the lower border of the mandible brings the cut lingual edges close enough together so that closure can be accomplished safely. This hyoepiglottoplasty advances the lower aspect of the resection (including the vallecular mucosa, hyoid, and epiglottis) both superiorly and anteriorly toward the cut margin of the tongue.

The hyoid is anchored with heavy sutures to the lower border of the mandible. Chabolle advocates the use of five 1–0 absorbable sutures (such as Vicryl), around the hyoid and through the base of the epiglottis, anchored through via drill holes in the lower border of the mandible. The placement of the sutures through the base of the epiglottis as they are passed around the hyoid results in a more vertical orientation of the epiglottis postoperatively, and if the epiglottis is excessively long or floppy, one could even resect part of it at this stage, though I have not felt it necessary to do so in my series.

Note that the exposure of the lower border of the mandible for placement of the drill holes and suspension sutures can be difficult through the neck incision, particularly if the incision is placed close to the hyoid. In such cases, a separate small submental incision can be helpful. Alternatively, the Repose® system (InfluENT Medical, Concord, NH) can be used to place several bone anchors with attached sutures to the mandible through the pre-existing neck incision. The Repose® drill and screw system allows for quick anchoring of the sutures to the lower border of the mandible without the need for direct visualization of the mandible, and the use of three doubled-over Repose® sutures knotted on themselves should provide similar

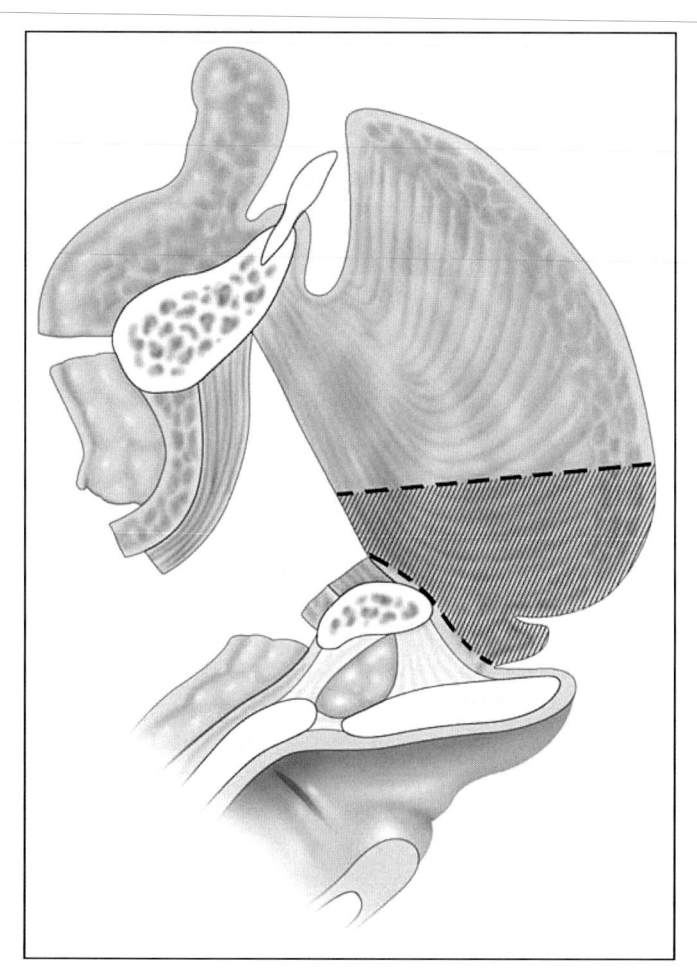

**Fig. 45.8** A full thickness resection of the tongue base is illustrated. The suprahyoid pharyngotomy has been performed, and the cut edge of the tongue base has been grasped and has been retracted cephalad. The more cephalad tongue base is prolapsing into the wound, and can be easily inspected and resected. Note the epiglottis in the inferior aspect of field.

retentive strength compared to the five single thickness sutures placed through drill holes advocated by Chabolle. The Repose® system does add cost to the procedure, but the time saved and the reduced dissection are considered advantageous. Regardless of which technique or suture material is used, the hyoid should be held in its new position with an Allis clamp, a shown in Figure 45.9, while the sutures are tied. Suture placement is demonstrated in Figure 45.10.

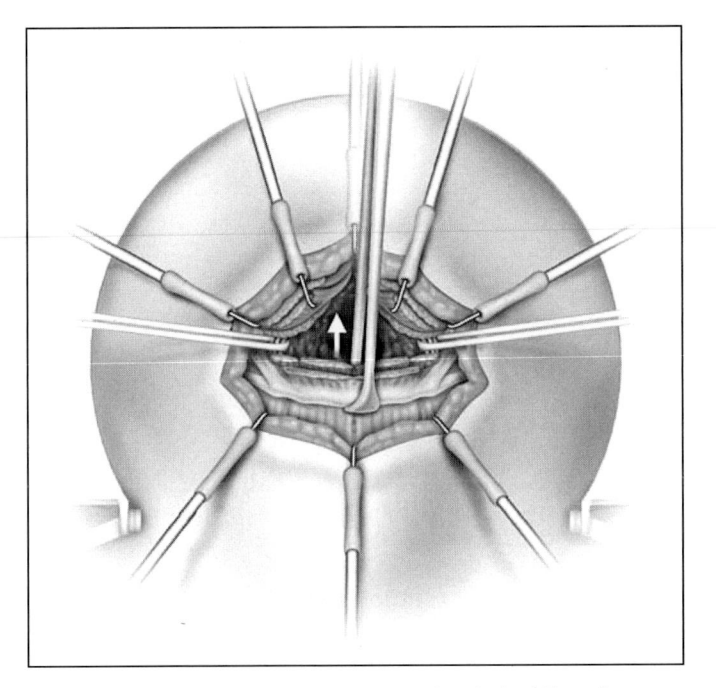

**Fig. 45.9** After completion of the lingual resection, the hyoid bone is grasped with a tenaculum and is retracted superiorly. It will later be anchored to the lower border of the mandible with sutures.

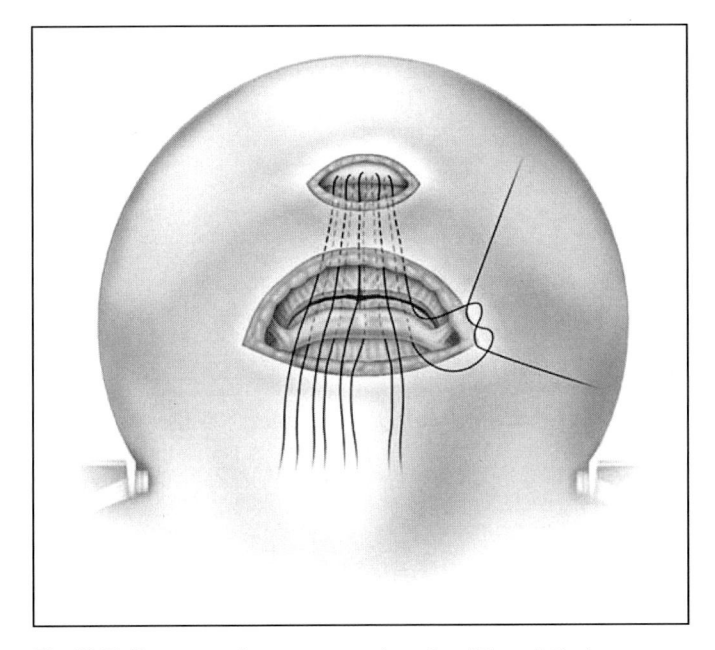

**Fig. 45.10** The suspension sutures are then placed through the lower border of the mandible superiorly and through the base of the epiglottis and around the body of the hyoid inferiorly.

It is also worth noting that the Repose® system utilizes a non-absorbable suture, and runs contrary to Chabolle's contention that the use of non-absorbable sutures increases the risk of infection compared to the use of absorbable sutures. This is based on his feeling that the permanent sutures provide a greater opportunity for colonization of the wound with oropharyngeal flora, based on the five wound infections in his first seven cases in which non-absorbable sutures were used, versus no infections in the next three cases when absorbable sutures were used. Two of Chabolle's abscesses were in the early postoperative period, and the other three were reported as occurring both early and late, though the precise timing of the late abscesses was not discussed. Based on these data, Sorrenti used absorbable sutures only, and experienced no infections. Neither author felt that the use of absorbable sutures resulted in hyoid positional relapse over the long term. I have not found an increased infection risk with non-absorbable sutures, however, having seen wound drainage without pharyngocutaneous fistula in approximately half of my full thickness TBRHE cases, no matter which suture is used.

Once the tongue base has been resected and the hyoepiglottic complex has been suspended to the mandible, the tongue wound is closed. Note that it may not be possible to close the tongue surface mucosa primarily without pulling the tongue posteriorly and tilting the tip posterosuperiorly toward the hard palate, which could adversely affect articulation and the oral phase of swallowing. As long as there is a good layered muscle closure in these cases, however, the mucosal defect appears to heal secondarily without incident and looks normal weeks later when viewed with a fiberoptic endoscope. The hyoepiglottoplasty produces redundancy of the lingual and suprahyoid muscles, and the mylohyoid and geniohyoid muscles can be trimmed to allow for a layered closure free of tension and tissue redundancy. This suprahyoid muscle shortening might help in keeping the hyoid in its new position over the long term, even after resorption or extrusion of any of the sutures used in the hyoid advancement. Note that the hyoid suspension sutures can make for more difficult placement of these underlying muscular sutures, so it can be helpful to trim the mylohyoid and geniohyoid muscles and place the muscular sutures without tying them before knotting the hyoid suspension sutures, as shown in Figure 45.11. Once the hyoepiglottoplasty suspension sutures are tied, the muscular closure sutures can then be knotted.

After closure of the tongue base muscles, a suction drain is placed through a separate stab wound to evacuate the neck wound, and the skin wound is then closed in layers.

As noted previously, a modification of this procedure involves a submucosal resection of the genioglossus muscle without extending the cuts through the full thickness of the tongue. This is outlined in more detail in Chapter 41. There are advantages and disadvantages of each approach, and further study will be necessary before one might be considered superior. However, some general observations

# SECTION K — MULTILEVEL PHARYNGEAL SURGERY

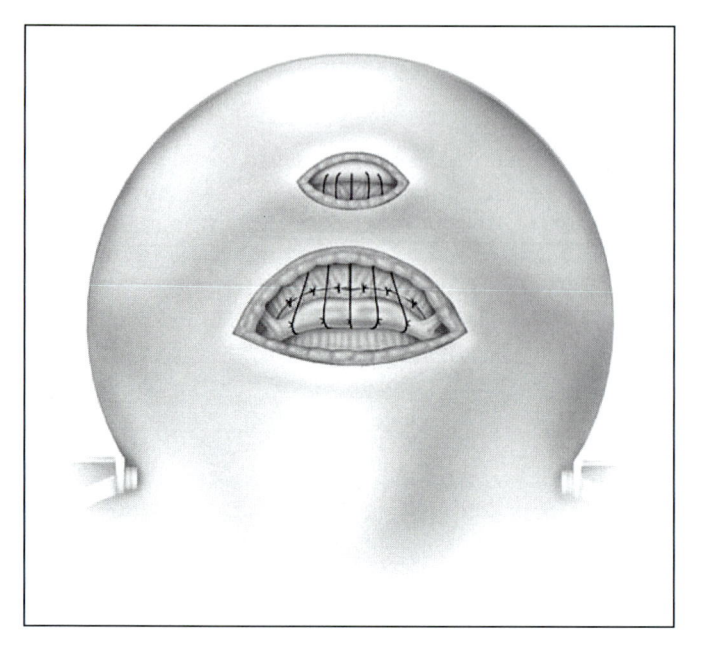

**Fig. 45.11** The redundant portions of the suprahyoid muscles are trimmed and reapproximated. These layered sutures are placed through the muscles but are not tied at this point. They are instead knotted after the hyoid suspension sutures have been secured. For illustrative purposes, the hyoid suspension sutures are not shown in this drawing.

can be made. The advantage of the full thickness resection is improved visibility. Because the tongue's dorsal surface does not lie horizontally when viewed in the coronal or sagittal planes, but instead curves from side to side and from top to bottom, the depth of resection varies from one part of the tongue to another. For this reason, it is more difficult to know the depth of dissection at any given location unless the dorsal surface is seen directly as a reference. As a result of this improved direct visualization, it is certainly possible that a more aggressive resection is possible via the Chabolle approach, but whether this results in a more effective procedure is at this point conjectural. In addition, it is possible to inadvertently enter the pharynx without recognizing it when attempting an extramucosal resection, and if not noted, pharyngocutaneous fistula could result. Yet the risk of wound infection and abscess formation should ultimately be less with the extramucosal modification of this procedure, because of less oropharyngeal bacteria contamination. As previously noted, the Chabolle full thickness resection includes a tracheotomy, which is advisable, given the aggressive nature of the procedure, possibility of bleeding into the airway from the cut edges of the tongue, etc. However, it appears acceptable to perform the extramucosal modification of this procedure without a concurrent tracheotomy, as advocated by Robinson and based on the relatively few of these procedures that I have done at the time of writing.

In summary, open full thickness TBRHE is a viable procedure, and the limited experience reported thus far suggests that it can effectively treat patients with significant abnormalities of the hyolingual complex who are not skeletally deficient. It can be safely combined with palatal surgery for single stage treatment of severe OSA. Yet it is an aggressive operation, utilizing surgical techniques more often seen in head and neck cancer treatment than in the pantheon of sleep surgery. The procedure includes a temporary tracheotomy, with a hospital stay of more than a week. Potential early complications include infection, dysphagia and articulation problems, though long-term complications have not been reported. Further study is certainly warranted to compare this procedure against less invasive alternatives, such as the various methods of tongue base suspension, the extramucosal variation of this open approach, and closed submucosal coblation-assisted tongue base resection techniques.

## REFERENCES

1. Sher AE, Schechtman KB, Piccirillo JF. The efficacy of surgical modifications of the upper airway in adults with obstructive sleep apnea syndrome. Sleep 1996;19(2):156–77.
2. Afzelius LE, Elmqvist D, Laurin S, Risberg AM, Aberg M. Sleep apnea syndrome caused by acromegaly and the treatment with a reduction plasty of tongue. ORL J Otorhinolaryngol Relat Spec 1982;44:142–5.
3. Djupesland G, Lyberg T, Krogstad O. Cephalometric analysis and surgical treatment of patients with obstructive sleep apnea syndrome. Acta Otolaryngol 1987;103:551–7.
4. Fujita S, Woodson BT, Clark JL, Wittig R. Laser midline glossectomy as a treatment for obstructive sleep apnea. Laryngoscope 1991;101:805–9.
5. Woodson BT, Fujita S. Clinical experience with linguoplasty as part of the treatment of severe obstructive sleep apnea. Otolaryngol Head Neck Surg 1992;107:40–48.
6. Faye-Lund H, Djupesland G, Lyberg T. Glossopexia: evaluation of a new surgical method for treating obstructive sleep apnea syndrome. Acta Otolaryngol Suppl 1992;492:46–9.
7. Mickelson SA, Rosenthal L. Midline glossectomy and epiglottidectomy for obstructive sleep apnea. Laryngoscope 1997;107:614–19.
8. Li HY, Wang PC, Hsu CY, et al. Same stage palatopharyngeal and hypopharyngeal surgery for severe obstructive sleep apnea. Acta Otolaryngol 2004;124:820–26.
9. Chabolle F, Wagner I, Blumen M, et al. Tongue base reduction with hyoepiglottoplasty: a treatment for severe obstructive sleep apnea. Laryngoscope 1999;109(8):1273–80.
10. Sorrenti G, Piccin O, Mondini S, et al. One-phase management of severe obstructive sleep apnea: tongue base reduction with hyoepiglottoplasty plus uvulopalatopharyngoplasty. Otolaryngol Head Neck Surg 2006;126:906–10.
11. Huntley T. Unpublished data, submitted for publication.
12. Lauretano AM, Li KK, Caradonna DS, et al. Anatomic location of the tongue base neurovascular bundle. Laryngoscope 1997;107(8):1057–59.

# SECTION K — MULTILEVEL PHARYNGEAL SURGERY

## CHAPTER 46

# Midline laser glossectomy with linguoplasty: treatment of obstructive sleep apnea

*Hsueh-Yu Li*

## 1 INTRODUCTION

Obstructive sleep apnea (OSA) is a disorder characterized by repeated collapse of the pharyngeal airway during sleep.[1] In adult OSA patients the site of obstruction is roughly evenly split between the palatal level and the hypopharyngeal level.[2] Therefore, simultaneous oropharyngeal and hypopharyngeal surgery was conducted to treat multilevel obstruction in adult OSA patients. Uvulopalatopharyngoplasty (UPPP) is the most commonly utilized surgical modality for treating OSA with palatopharyngeal obstruction. Glossectomy has been used to reduce the volume of the tongue base, with resultant increase of the hypopharyngeal airway. Because of the lateral location of important neurovascular bundles in the tongue base, glossectomy is sometimes performed at the midline position to prevent major morbidity.[3] The literature described two different surgical approaches.[4,5] The transcollar technique to date has been less popular because it involves an open surgery with neck wound. Traditional transoral procedures are performed using $CO_2$ laser.[6] However, the inconvenience of using a large $CO_2$ laser handpiece in a narrow oral cavity and the poor capability of hemostasis have limited the clinical application of this procedure.[7] This chapter describes the outcomes of performing UPPP plus midline laser glossectomy (MLG) in severe OSA patients, with a specially designed handpiece comprising Nd:Yag laser fiber and suction tube being used to facilitate midline glossectomy.

## 2 PATIENT SELECTION

Indications for MLG were determined via anatomical structure (Friedman staging),[8] but this study only enrolled patients with Friedman stage III or IV. Disease severity is not the main concern of this study. However, to date the procedures of MLG have been reserved for patients with severe OSA who cannot be adequately treated with continuous positive airway pressure (CPAP) therapy, owing to invasiveness and potential morbidities such as bleeding, airway compromise, dysphagia and taste disturbance.

No rigid contraindications to MLG exist. However, patients with certain conditions (namely, morbid obesity, poor cardiovascular or pulmonary function) are empirically considered to be poor respondents or high risk for surgical treatment for OSA, so glossectomies have not been performed on such patients.

## 3 SURGICAL PROCEDURE

MLG was regularly performed in combination with UPPP for simultaneously enlarging the oropharyngeal and hypopharyngeal airway. MLG was implemented immediately following UPPP. An endotracheal tube was moved from the middle (UPPP position) to the right side and was re-fixed to the right mouth angle. None of the study cohort required tracheostomy. Nd:Yag laser was delivered via laser fiber which was fixed to a metallic suction tube with tape to create a novel excision-suctioned handpiece (Fig. 46.1). Moreover, Nd:Yag laser (Contact Laser™, Surgical Laser Technologies, Montgomeryville, PA, USA) (Fig. 46.2) was set in a continuous mode with a power of 10 watts. The tongue was pulled out as far as possible using MacGill forceps to expose its base (Fig. 46.3). A tongue blade was

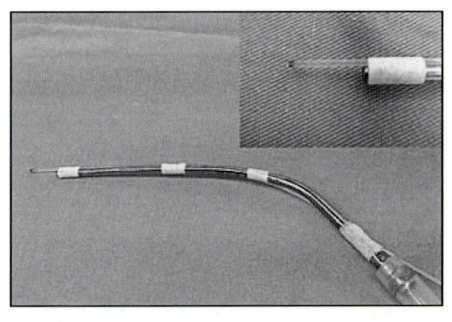

**Fig. 46.1** Nd:Yag laser was delivered via laser fiber which is fixed to a metallic suction tube using tape to establish a novel excision-suctioned handpiece.

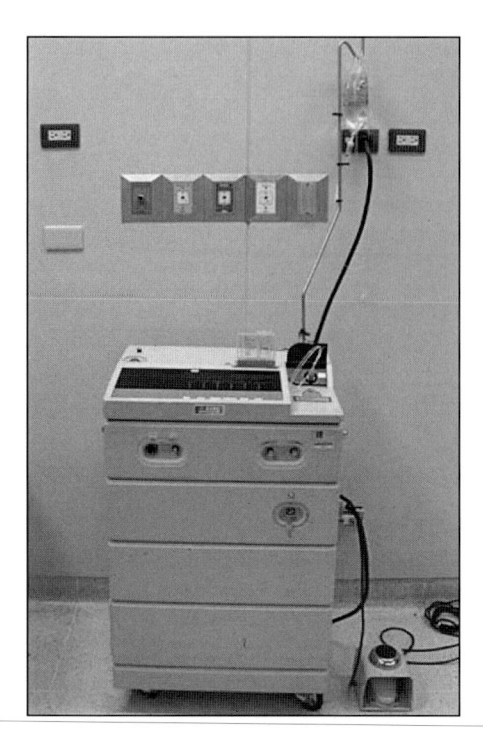

# SECTION K MULTILEVEL PHARYNGEAL SURGERY

**Fig. 46.2** Nd:Yag laser (Contact Laser™, Surgical Laser Technologies, Montgomeryville, PA, USA) was set to a continuous mode at a power of 10 watts.

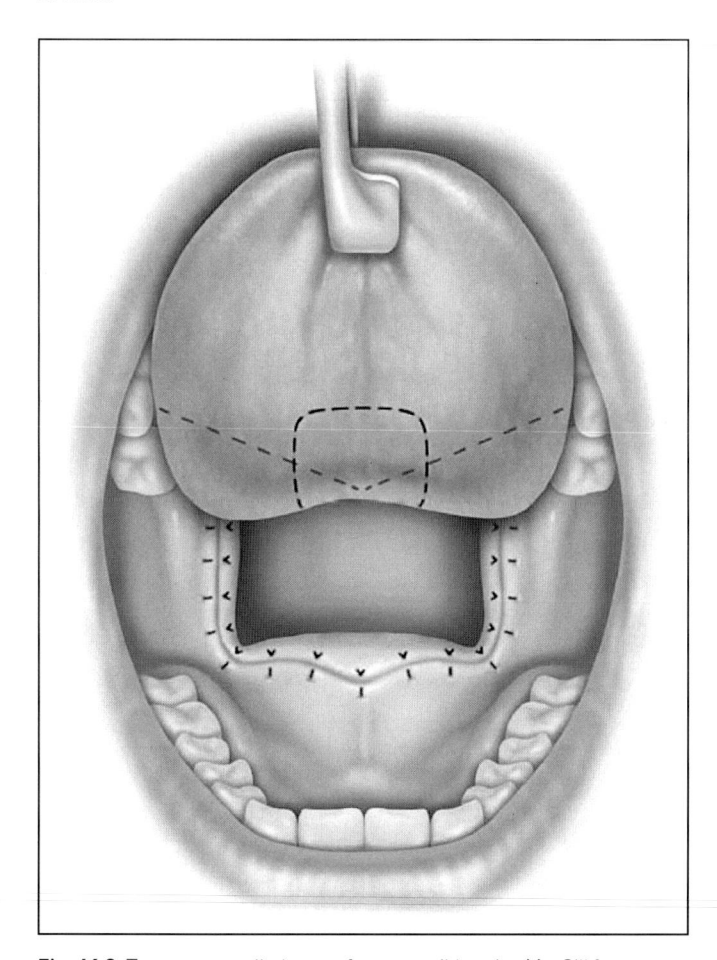

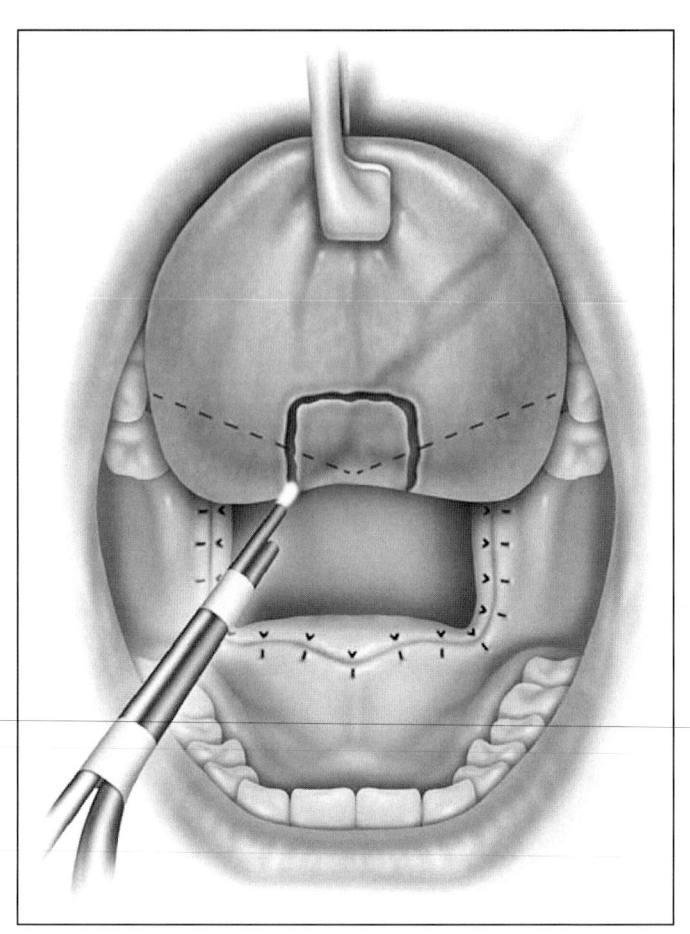

**Fig. 46.4** A rectangular midline section line of the dorsum of the tongue was marked, approximately 1 cm anterior to the papilla and extending posterior into the vallecula.

**Fig. 46.3** Tongue was pulled out as far as possible using MacGill forceps to expose the base of the tongue.

not used to facilitate prolapsing of the tongue base into the surgical field owing to previous experience showing that the tongue base wound made via this technique was always anterior to the position required. A rectangular midline section line of the dorsum of the tongue was marked, roughly 1 cm anterior to the papilla and extending posterior into the vallecula (Fig. 46.4). Laser cutting of the tongue base began from the left side of the tongue, ran across the dorsum of the tongue, and turned to the right side of tongue. After creating the excision border, teeth forceps were used to grip the dissected tissue to facilitate excision (Fig. 46.5). Bleeding from the lateral border of the wound was not unusual and was stopped by electrocautery. A rectangular wound in the tongue base (2 cm in width, 2–2.5 cm in length and approximately 1–1.5 cm in depth) was created after tissue removal (Fig. 46.6). Additional lingual tonsils were not removed since our previous investigation revealed that hypertrophic lingual tonsil, despite having an obscure laryngeal structure, did not contribute significantly to adult OSA.[7] The laser char in the tongue base wound was carefully cleaned using a cotton soaked with $H_2O_2$. Finally, the wound was approximated in the tongue base using 2–0 Dexon via mattress suture (2–3 stitches) (Figs 46.7 and

CHAPTER 46

*Midline laser glossectomy with linguoplasty*

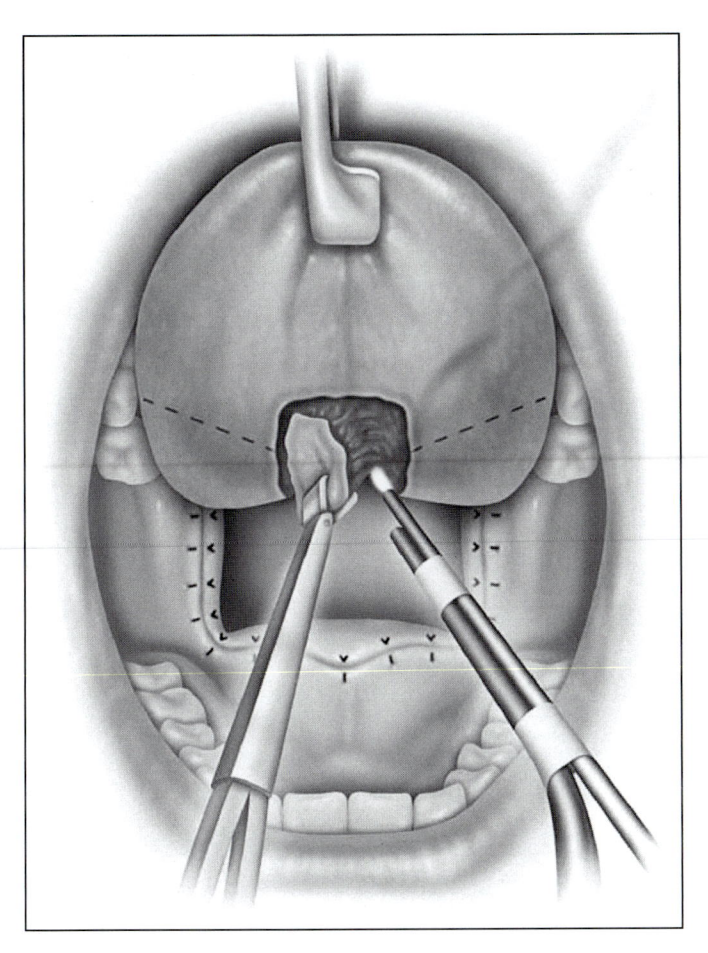

**Fig. 46.5** After creating the excision border, teeth forceps were used to grip the dissected tissue to facilitate excision.

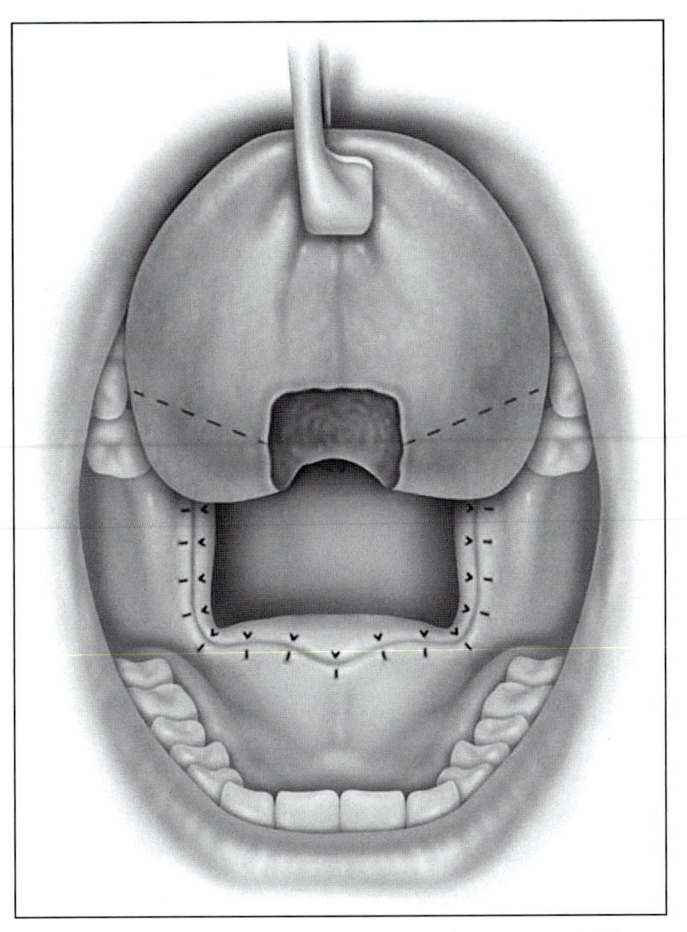

**Fig. 46.6** A rectangular wound in the tongue base (2 cm in width, 2–2.5 cm in length and approximately 1–1.5 cm in depth) was created following tissue removal.

46.8). This study demonstrates a case showing the area of the tongue base resected before and after MLG (Figs 46.9 and 46.10).

The technique of UPPP used in our hospital has been modified and contains the following key steps: bilateral tonsillectomy, removal of supratonsillar adipose tissue, box-shape incision of soft palate, dissection and stripping of submucosal adipose tissue, developing uvulopalatal flap, imbricating and suturing the flap to soft palate, closure of tonsillar fossa and maximized lateralization of posterior pillar. The detailed procedures have been published elsewhere.[9]

## 4 POSTOPERATIVE MANAGEMENT

For each patient, intravenous dexametasone (10 mg) was administered immediately before the completion of surgery to reduce postoperative airway edema. Ice was applied to the upper neck for one day following surgery. Elevation of the bed head by 45° was proposed to reduce postoperative swelling. Prophylactic systemic antibiotic (ampicillin 500 mg) was administered postoperatively at 6-hour intervals for 3 days. A humid oxygen mask was used to reduce throat discomfort during sleep. Patients received intravenous ketorolac (30 mg) every 6 hours during the daytime and an additional 30 mg of ketorolac dissolved in 500 ml of normal saline as a drip after midnight to minimize disturbance of sleep from pain during hospitalization. It was recommended to patients that they begin a liquid diet 6 hours following surgery, and then advance to solids as they were able to tolerate. The standard hospitalization period for patients receiving UPPP plus MLG was 4 days. No patient was retained in an intensive care unit for observation.

## 5 COMPLICATIONS

No intraoperative complications occurred. All patients were extubated after regaining full consciousness in the operating theater. No patients required reintubation or tracheostomy to secure their airway during the perioperative period.

289

# SECTION K — MULTILEVEL PHARYNGEAL SURGERY

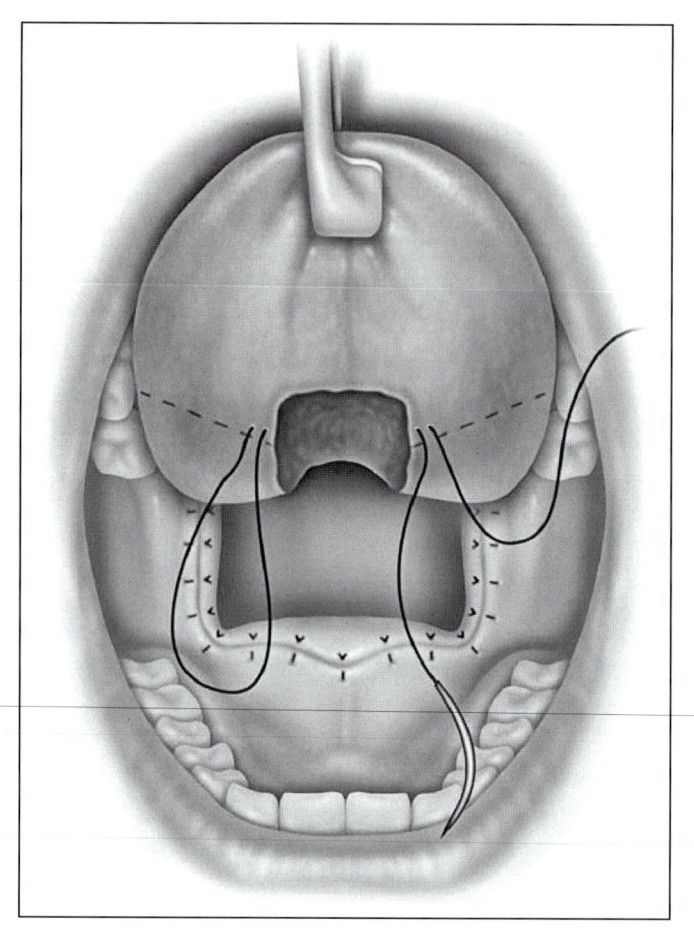

**Fig. 46.7** The wound in the tongue base was approximated using 2-0 Dexon.

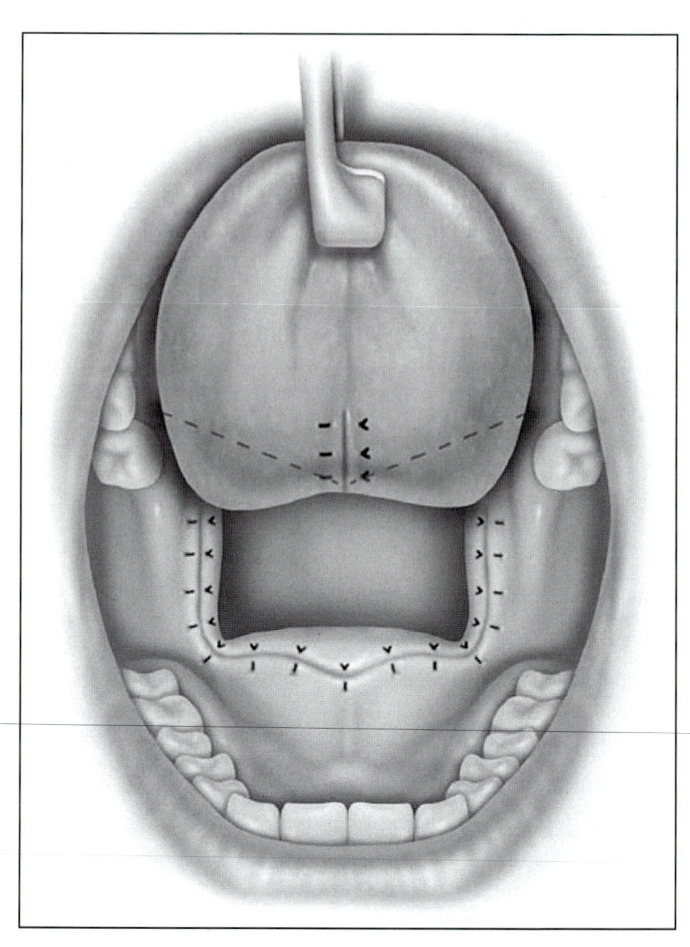

**Fig. 46.8** The closure was completed with mattress sutures (2–3 stitches).

One patient developed postoperative bleeding on the seventh day postoperatively. The bleeding was self-limited following ice packing over submental area without using electrocautery in the operation theater. Sixty-four percent (14/22) of patients classified their postoperative pain as 'mild' during hospitalization. However, one patient reported taste disturbance 3 months following surgery, and recovered his taste function 9 months postoperatively.[10] Additionally, two patients experienced intense hiccups following surgery, which resolved after 2 days. No other permanent complications have yet been observed in this work.

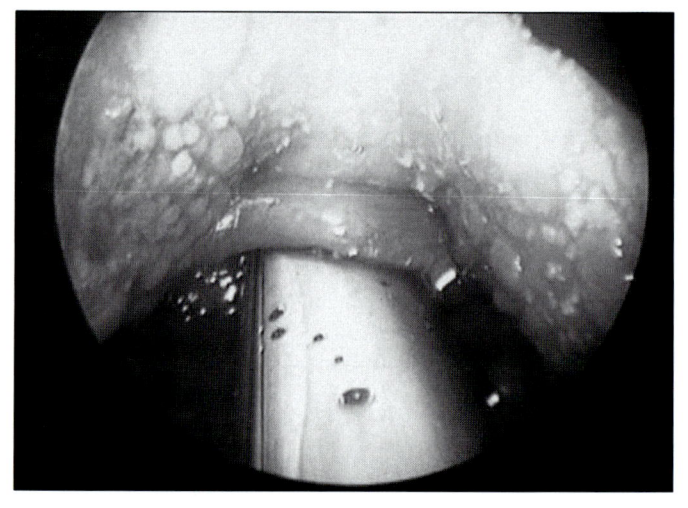

**Fig. 46.9** The tongue base before surgery.

## 6 RESULTS AND SUCCESS RATE

Surgical success was defined as a 50% reduction of the preoperative AHI and a postoperative AHI of <20/h. Preliminary results demonstrated a success rate of 63.6% (14/22). Furthermore, the mean Apnea/Hypopnea Index (AHI) decreased from $62.5 \pm 17.8$/h to $27.0 \pm 21.5$/h ($P < 0.001$, paired $t$-test) and the minimal oxygen saturation increa-sed from $74.5 \pm 11.8\%$ to $84.6 \pm 8.6\%$ ($P < 0.001$, paired $t$-test).

# CHAPTER 46
Midline laser glossectomy with linguoplasty

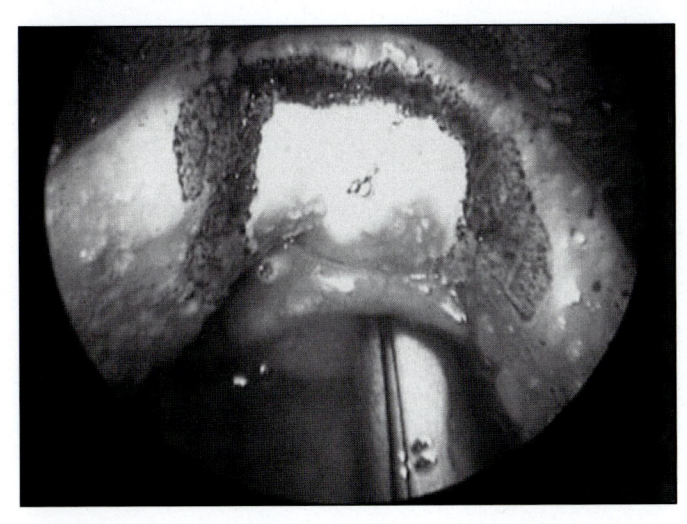

**Fig. 46.10** The tongue base was resected following midline laser glossectomy.

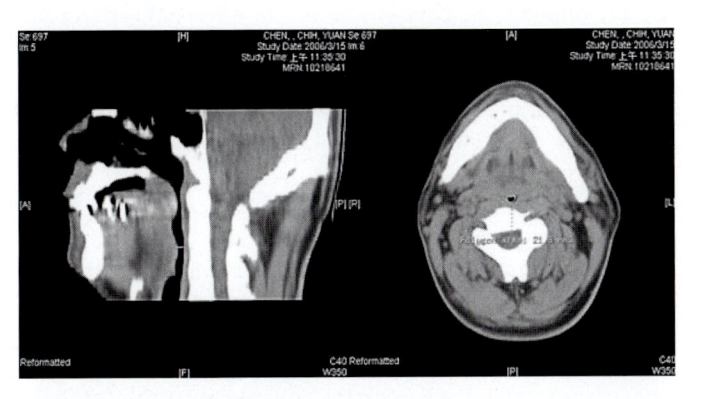

**Fig. 46.11** Three-dimensional computed tomography reveals narrowing of the retroglossal space (21.9 mm$^2$).

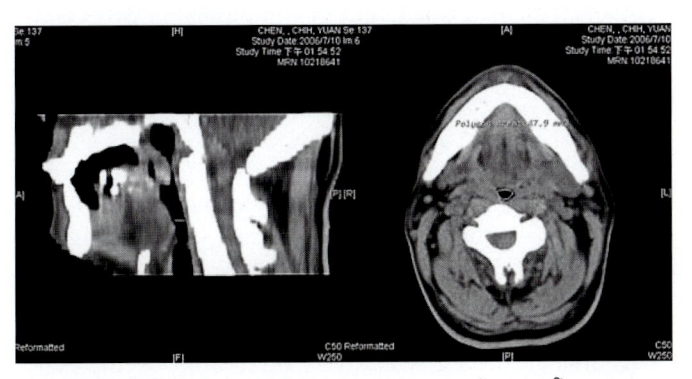

**Fig. 46.12** Significant widening of retroglossal space (47.9 mm$^2$) occurred 6 months following midline laser glossectomy.

Three-dimensional computed tomography in one of the cases presented here showed a significant widening of the hypopharyngeal space from 21.9 to 47.9 mm$^2$ (Figs 46.11 and 46.12). Detailed image techniques were published elsewhere.[11]

## 6.1 FURTHER TREATMENT OF THE FAILED CASE

Oral appliances were recommended to patients with persistent high AHI and excessive daytime sleepiness.

## REFERENCES

1. Douglas NJ, Polo O. Pathogenesis of obstructive sleep apnoea/hypopnea syndrome. Lancet 1994;344:653–55.
2. Woodson BT, Fujita S. Clinical experience with lingualplasty as part of the treatment of severe obstructive sleep apnea. Otolaryngol Head Neck Surg 1992;107:40–8.
3. Lauretano AM, Li KK, Caradonna DS, Khosta RK, Fried MP. Anatomic location of the tongue base neurovascular bundle. Laryngoscope 1997;107:1057–9.
4. Fujita S. Surgical treatment of obstructive sleep apnea: UPPP and lingualplasty (laser midline glossectomy). In: Obstructive Sleep Apnea Syndrome: Clinical Research and Treatment. Guilleminault C, Partinen M, eds. New York: Raven Press; 1990, pp. 129–51.
5. Chabolle F, Wagner I, Blumen M, Sequert C, Fleury B, de Dieuleveult T. Tongue base reduction with epiglottoplasty: a treatment for severe obstructive sleep apnea. Laryngoscope 1999;109:1273–80.
6. Fujita S, Woodson BT, Clark JL, Wittig R. Laser midline glossectomy as a treatment for obstructive sleep apnea. Laryngoscope 1991;101:805–9.
7. Li HY, Wang PC, Hsu CY, Chen NH, Lee LA, Fang TJ. Same-stage palatopharyngeal and hypopharyngeal surgery for severe obstructive sleep apnea. Acta Otolaryngol 2004;124:820–26.
8. Friedman M, Ibrahim H, Bass L. Clinical staging for sleep-disordered breathing. Otolaryngol Head Neck Surg 2002;127:13–21.
9. Li HY, Li KK, Chen NH, Wang PC. Modified uvulopalatopharyngoplasty: the extended uvulopalatal flap. Am J Otolaryngol 2003;24:311–6.
10. Li HY, Lee LA, Wang PC, et al. Taste disturbance after uvulopalatopharyngoplasty for obstructive sleep apnea. Otolaryngol Head Neck Surg 2006;134:985–90.
11. Li HY, Chen NH, Wang CR, Shu YH, Wang PC. Use of 3-dimensional computed tomography scan to evaluate upper airway patency for patients undergoing sleep-disordered breathing surgery. Otolaryngol Head Neck Surg 2003;129:336–42.

# SECTION K — MULTILEVEL PHARYNGEAL SURGERY

## CHAPTER 47

# External submucosal glossectomy

*Sam Robinson*

## 1 INTRODUCTION

The major contributing factors to retrolingual collapse in sleep apnea are macroglossia, hypotonia, retrognathia and lingual tonsillar hyperplasia. Any or all of these may contribute to varying degrees in any given individual. All current low morbidity options have limitations in treating the macroglossia component. The ideal procedure for macroglossia would be low morbidity, allow large tissue volume reduction, have low risk of alteration in tongue function and be single stage. Submucosal glossectomy techniques aim to fulfill these criteria, with preservation of mucosa causing minor pain postoperatively.

## 2 PATIENT SELECTION

Patients with macroglossia are candidates for submucosal glossectomy techniques (with appropriate palatal surgery for any co-existing retropalatal collapse). The larger the tongue, the more tissue is potentially resectable in the medial tongue between the neurovascular bundles, with or without extension of excision to the lateral tongue superficial to the neurovascular bundles and deep to mucosa. The converse is true: if the tongue is not enlarged, little excess muscle tissue will be able to be safely removed within the anatomical constraints of the neurovascular bundles, with only a small improvement in retrolingual airspace. Acromegaly may cause macroglossia, therefore patients with normal or near normal body weight and a large tongue should be screened with a growth hormone assay, particularly if they have coarse facial features. Patients with a Body Mass Index (BMI) >40 are more appropriately treated with bariatric surgery rather than airway reconstructive surgery, although morbidly obese patients may be offered airway reconstructive surgery if bariatric surgery fails or is refused.

Clinical indicators of macroglossia are most commonly used, but are subjective. Flexible nasendoscopic observation (supine, standardized for phase of respiration) is commonly used to examine the retrolingual airway.[1] Variation in muscle tone changes airway size during quiet breathing. If the retrolingual airspace is reduced in mid-respiration (and particularly if reduced on end inspiration when muscle tone is greatest), and there is no co-existing retrognathia (defined as sella-nasion-supramentale (SNB) <76° on cephalostat) or lingual tonsillar hyperplasia, it can be assumed that macroglossia exists.

Tongue size, as visualized orally, has been shown (when considered with tonsillar size) to predict uvulopalatopharyngoplasty outcomes.[2] Friedman tongue positions 3 and 4 are potential candidates for submucosal glossectomy techniques. Untreated tongue bulk of the middle third of the tongue (measured antero-posteriorly) may precipitate or exacerbate retropalatal collapse by prolapse onto the oral side of the palate during sleep, which is not readily perceived by nasendoscopic examination (awake or sedated). In addition, a bulky dorsal tongue will reduce the oropalatal airway, which may be symptomatic, particularly if palatal surgery has advanced the free edge of the soft palate anteriorly to treat retropalatal obstruction (with or without scarring of the free palatal edge). Symptoms of a reduced oropalatal airway typically include globus pharyngeus (which can be localized to the free edge of soft palate on examination), reduced exercise tolerance (less oral airway), and sometimes frequent gagging. These symptoms can be expected to resolve with adequate separation of the tongue dorsum and the free edge of soft palate as a result of successful tongue reduction surgery.

Radiological parameters offer more objective measures of tongue size. Chabolle et al. have published anatomical data (in French) from a midsagittal MRI, demonstrating a lingual area of $25.8 \pm 4.6$ cm$^2$ in sleep apneic patients, compared to $20.2 \pm 3.2$ cm$^2$ in normal patients ($P < 0.001$).[3] I use a midsagittal reconstruction from a spiral multislice CT scan to define the same area and thus quantify tongue size. Chabolle suggested tongue reduction surgery if the lingual area was greater than 26 cm,[2,3] which was later revised to >28 cm$^2$ in relation to open tongue base reduction with hyoepiglottoplasty.[4] I consider submucosal glossectomy techniques in patients with a lingual area greater than 26 cm$^2$, but the ideal parameters to define which patients with retrolingual collapse need bulk reduction, which need tensioning of the tongue and which need both strategies are, at present, unknown.

## 3 OUTLINE OF PROCEDURE

The external submucosal glossectomy procedure follows Chabolle's principles,[4] but mucosal preservation significantly reduces pain, delay of oral intake and hospital stay. Hyoid advancement toward the mandible with mylohyoid shortening is incorporated, but epiglottic suture verticalization is omitted, as adequate verticalization is planned to be achieved from hyoepiglottic ligament pull alone.

General anesthesia is induced, and the airway secured with nasotracheal intubation. An arterial line is routinely used to measure intraoperative and postoperative blood pressure. Broad-spectrum antibiotics and 8 mg dexamethasone are administered IV. The neck is extended with a rolled sheet beneath the shoulders. Skin crease incisions over the hyoid and in the submental crease are marked (Fig. 47.1). The incisions are injected with 1% lidocaine + 1:100,000 adrenaline, with a 10-minute delay for vasoconstriction to take effect, during which time routine preparation of a sterile field is performed. The incision over the hyoid is extended from the medial edge of one sternomastoid muscle to the other, and a subplatysmal plane is developed to expose the suprahyoid and strap muscles (Fig. 47.2).

Bovie dissection onto the hyoid bone is performed, with a small pocket created above and below the hyoid in the midline so the bone can be gently grasped with an Allis clamp. Leaving a cuff of a few millimeters of muscle on the superior surface of the hyoid, an incision is made transversely from the midline to the level of the lesser cornu. Intermittent gentle anterior traction on the hyoid helps to define the stylohyoid muscle inserting into lesser cornu, which should not be cut.

The cut edge of mylohyoid is shortened by 8–10 mm and retracted anteriorly. The anterior belly of digastric and stylohyoid are retracted laterally with Lagenbeck retractors (Fig. 47.3). This exposes the key anatomical landmark to the dissection, which is the hyoglossus muscle. The surgeon will see first the rounded anterolateral edge of hyoglossus, as the muscle is approached obliquely from the anterior direction. Running *superficial* to hyoglossus is the hypoglossal nerve, with accompanying lingual vein. These structures are gently mobilized with a curved clamp (e.g. a Gemini), and a colored loop of vascular tape is placed around the nerve and vein together, and clipped. Any bleeding is controlled with careful bipolar diathermy. Magnification of the operative field with loupes is helpful, but is not essential.

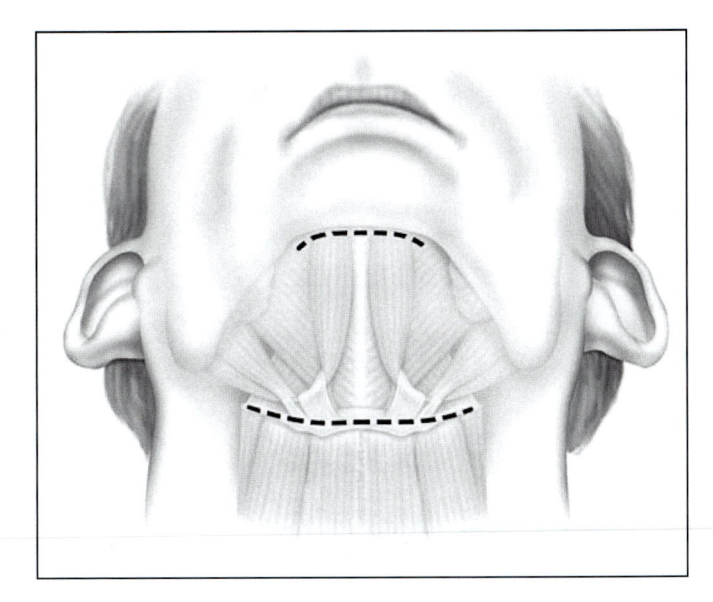

**Fig. 47.1** Skin incisions marked.

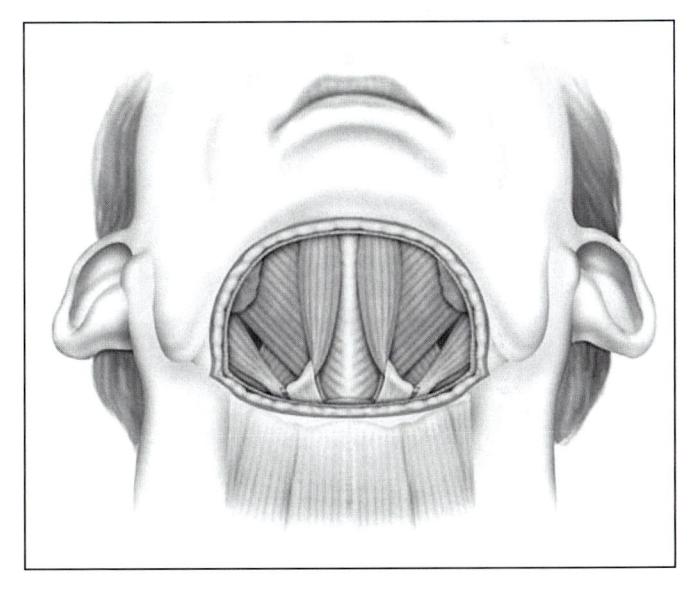

**Fig. 47.2** Subplatysmal flap elevation.

Lagenbeck retractors are now used to retract the hyoglossus laterally, and geniohyoid medially to expose the lingual artery lying *deep* to hyoglossus (Fig. 47.4). If difficulty is encountered in finding the artery, digital palpation in this area for pulsations can be helpful, as can use of a Doppler or ultrasound machine. Another loop of vascular tape is placed around the artery.

With the neurovascular structures identified and gently retracted laterally, geniohyoid, genioglossus and intrinsic tongue muscles are sectioned until the undersurface of tongue mucosa is reached, beveling approximately 30° superior to the axial plane from hyoid, to avoid dissection of

# SECTION K — MULTILEVEL PHARYNGEAL SURGERY

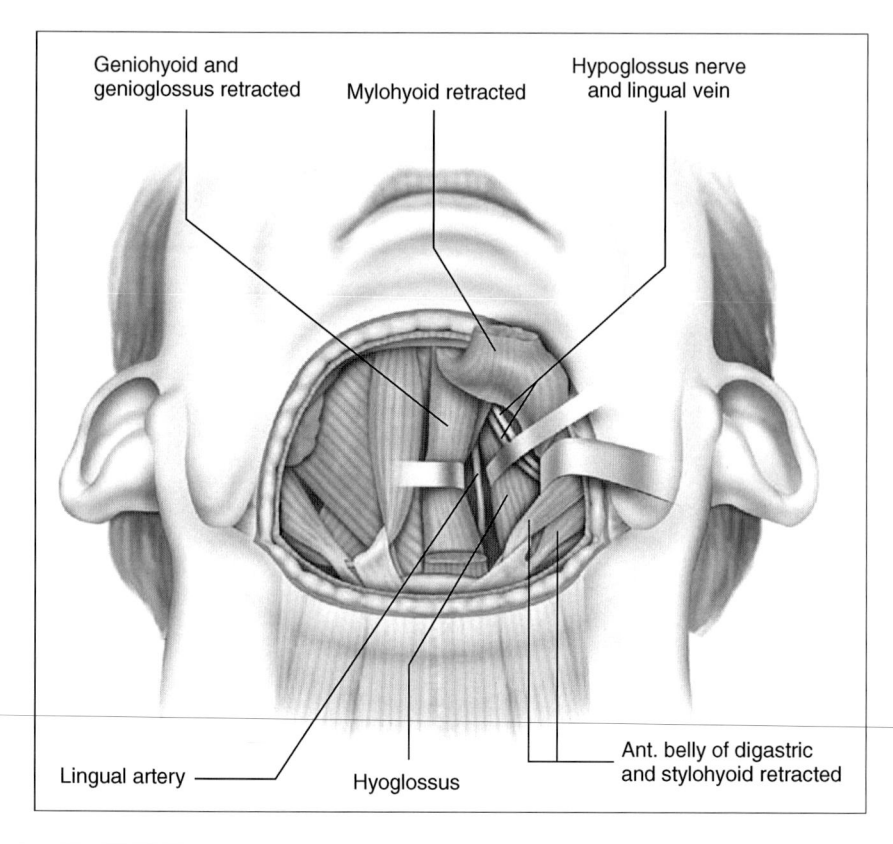

**Fig. 47.3** Exposure of hyoglossus muscle, with hypoglossal nerve/lingual vein.

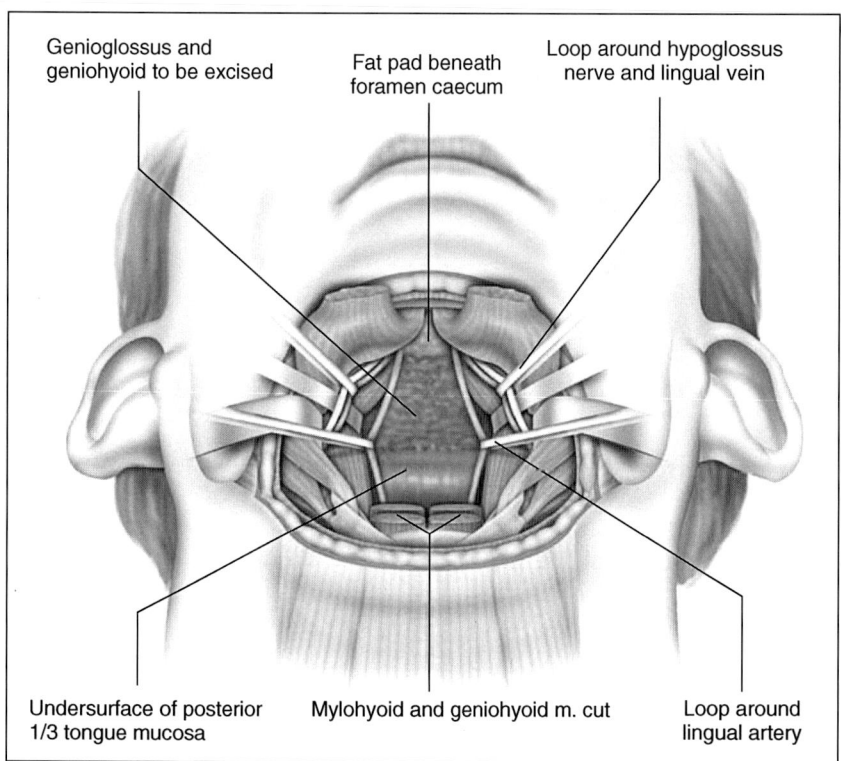

**Fig. 47.4** Lateral retraction of neurovascular bundles and submucosal excision of posterior third of tongue musculature.

the pre-epiglottic space and hyoepiglottic ligament (Figs 47.4 and 47.5). The extent of dissection is tailored to the patient's anatomy, but at a minimum includes muscle between the neurovascular bundles from above hyoid to the level of foramen cecum superiorly. The foramen cecum is identified by palpation from the undersurface of mucosa and a 'sentinel' fat pad beneath it. Lateral extension of the dissection between the neurovascular bundles and mucosa

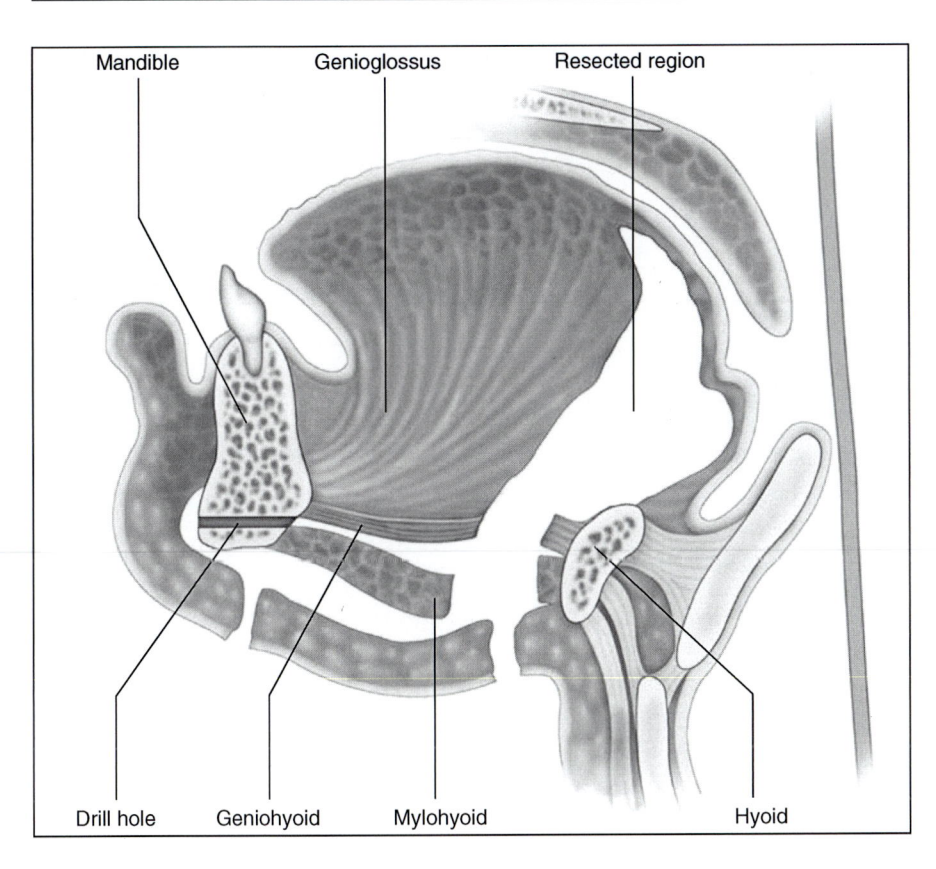

**Fig. 47.5** Submental incision performed to place inferior mandibular drill hole; sagittal view of completed dissection.

is frequently desirable, particularly in patients with a bulky lateral tongue base. Extension of the dissection anterior to the foramen cecum is also frequently desirable (into the middle third of the tongue antero-posteriorly), which is the area of bulk assessed by oral examination (Friedman tongue size).[2] Enough genioglossus must be left anteriorly for normal tongue function, which is most easily decided by palpation, and is roughly defined by a coronal plane through the foramen cecum. A surgeon starting this technique should err on the side of caution, and it is usual for the extent of muscle excision to increase with increased experience. Therefore, if viewed in a sagittal plane, the cavity dissected is submucosal and crescenteric (Fig. 47.5).

A second 3 cm incision is performed in the submental skin crease with a knife, and Bovie dissection continues onto the inferior border of mandible. Periosteal elevation for 1 cm on the anterior and posterior surface of mandible is performed, and a drill hole is made through the inferior mandible with a 2 mm K wire driver, or a fissure burr. A subplatysmal tunnel is fashioned to connect the two operative sites.

Hemostasis with the mean arterial blood pressure at 120 mm Hg, and a Valsalva maneuver with hand ventilation are advised at this point while wide access to the muscle bed is available. Small arterial branches should be ligated rather than diathermied (see below). Cavity closure of the undersurface of mucosa to remnant tongue muscle is performed with 4 × 2-0 Vicryl. Two 0 Vicryl sutures are looped around the hyoid, passed through the subplatysmal tunnel while grasped in a clamp, passed backward through the mandibular drill hole, and returned through the subplatysmal tunnel to be clipped and cut. The cut edges of mylohyoid are stitched with 4 × 2-0 Vicryl (all clipped and cut). A 15-gauge suction drain is placed between mucosa and genioglossus remnant, but should also be placed so that some holes drain the subcutaneous space superficial to mylohyoid. This is removed the morning after surgery (unless there is ongoing drainage). The heavy 0 Vicryl sutures are tied to suspend the hyoid from mandible anteriorly, then the 2-0 Vicryl is tied to close mylohyoid (Fig. 47.6). 3-0 Vicryl is used to platysma and staples to skin.

In contrast to Chabolle's experience when all muscle and mucosa of the posterior third of the tongue was also excised,[4] the anteriorly advanced hyoid position was not maintained over time with absorbable sutures in this operation. In view of this, a variation with suspension of the hyoid from mandible with two fascia lata strips, secured to the inferior mandible with a four-hole miniplate, is suggested (Fig. 47.7). The ability of fascia lata to resist stretching when used for this purpose has not yet been demonstrated conclusively, but in a large series of hyoid suspension with fascia lata to mandible done at Stanford University in the 1980s and early 1990s,[5] the hyoid position anecdotally appeared stable in most cases over years

SECTION K — MULTILEVEL PHARYNGEAL SURGERY

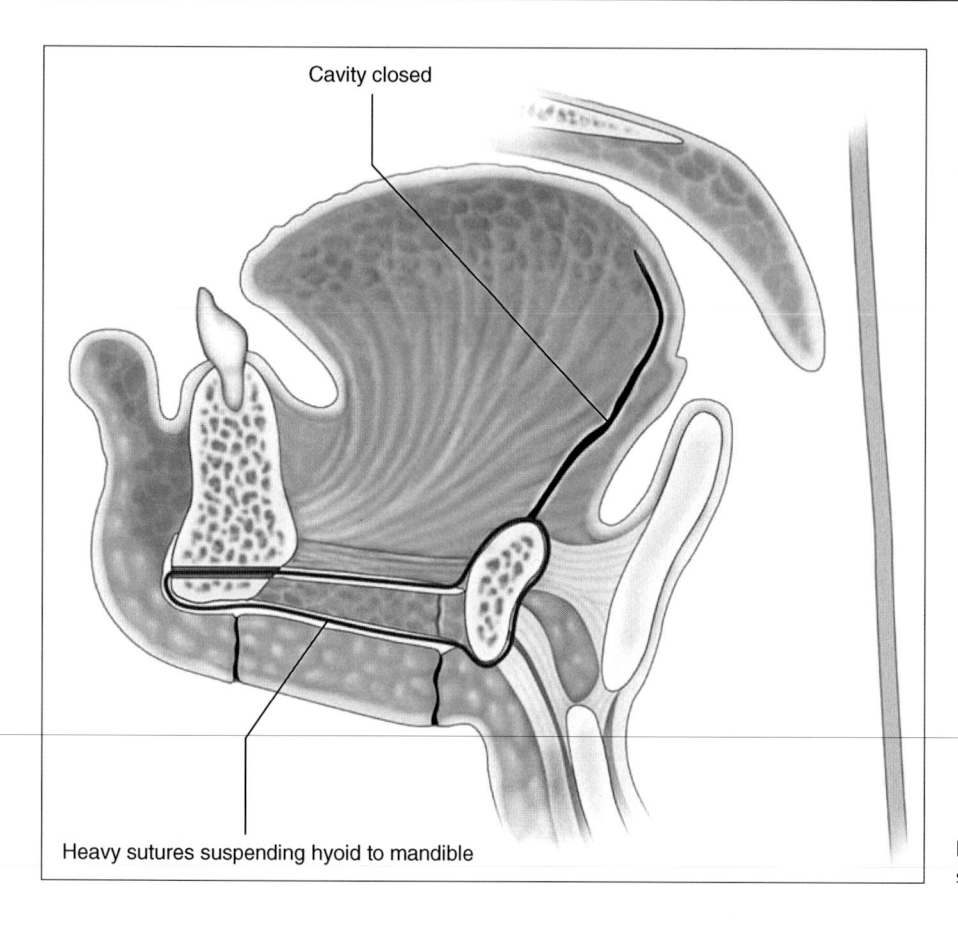

Cavity closed

Heavy sutures suspending hyoid to mandible

**Fig. 47.6** Closure and hyoid suspension with sutures (drain not shown).

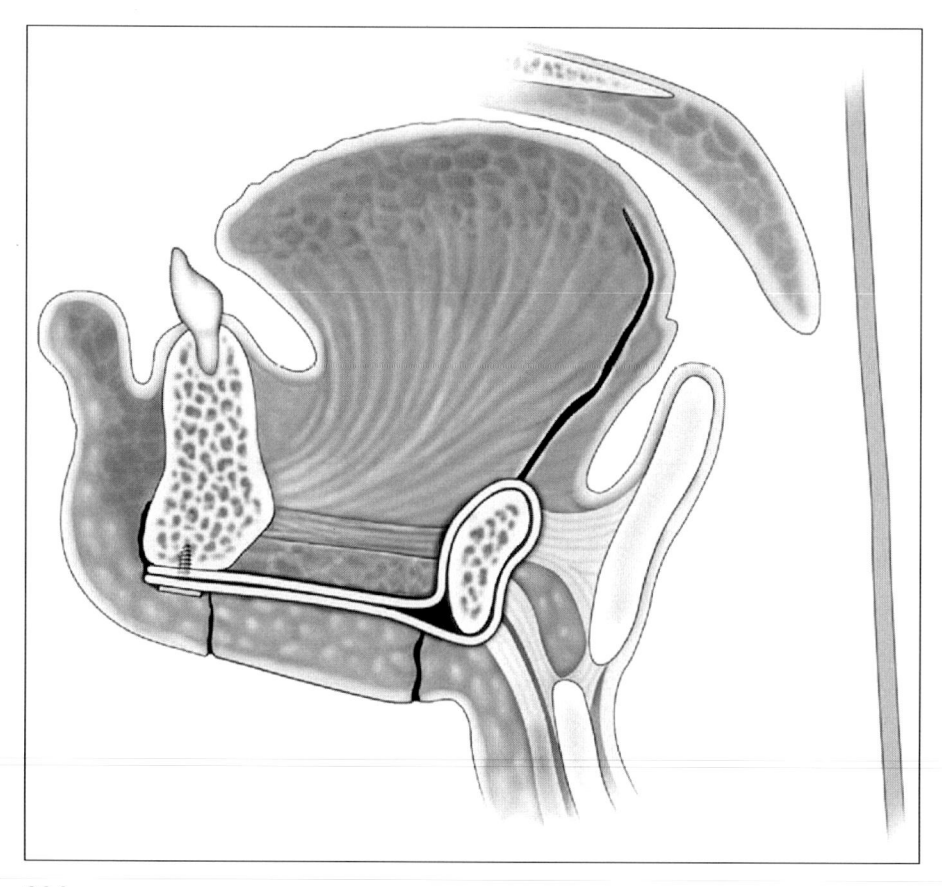

**Fig. 47.7** Alternative (and currently recommended) suspension of hyoid to mandible with fascia lata (drain not shown).

CHAPTER 47 External submucosal glossectomy

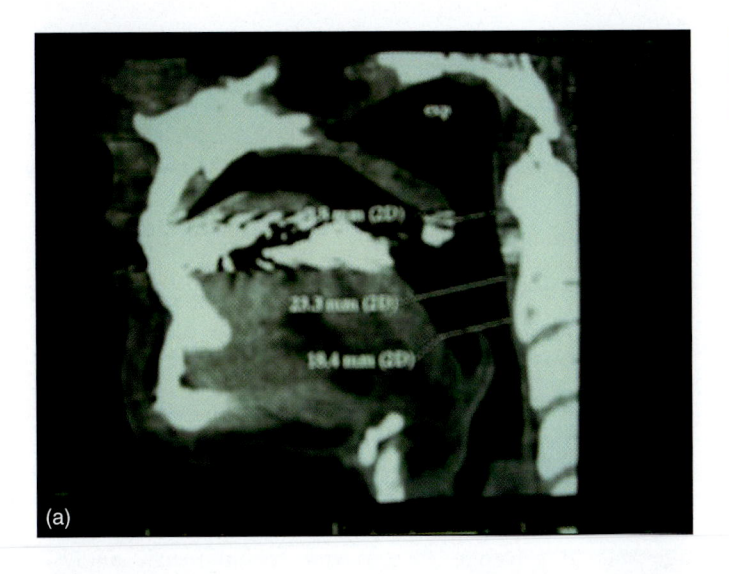

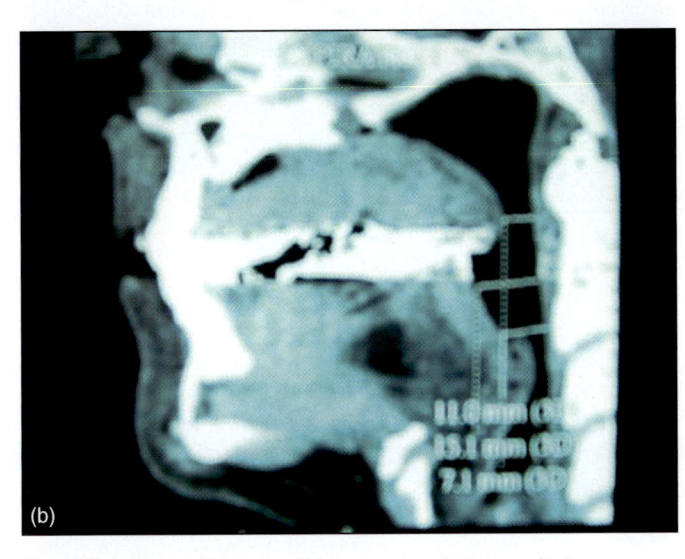

**Fig. 47.8** A, Pre- and B, postop CT scan, end expiration, sagittal reconstruction showing increased retrolingual airway. Note also increased retropalatal airspace now tongue mucosa no longer contacting the soft palate (no palatal surgery performed between the two scans).

(N. Powell, personal communication, 2006). Some authorities have found autologous gracilis tendon or cadaveric semitendinosis tendon more reliable than fascia lata for hyomandibular suspension (K. Moore, personal communication, 2006). An example of changes in airway size is demonstrated by pre- and postoperative spiral CT scan sagittal reconstructions (Fig. 47.8).

## 4 POSTOPERATIVE MANAGEMENT

Tongue base surgery for sleep apnea has three major considerations for postoperative care, which have been previously well described by Riley et al.[6]

### 4.1 RESPIRATORY COMPROMISE FROM THE EFFECTS OF ANESTHETIC OR ANALGESICS

Intubation and extubation are performed with the surgeon present. The preoperative assessment of airway anatomy should be discussed with the anesthetist to allow anticipation of any intubation difficulties, and a tracheotomy tray is always available in case of airway emergency. The patient is nursed in a monitored setting for the first postoperative night to allow narcotic analgesia, if required, with continuous oximetry monitoring to detect any respiratory depression.

### 4.2 HYPERTENSION WITH HEMATOMA

In the large series of upper airway surgeries reported from Stanford, around 40% of patients had baseline hypertension, but 70% needed postoperative antihypertensives.[6] *It is essential to keep the mean arterial pressure < 100 mm Hg postoperatively* (after securing hemostasis during surgery at a MAP of 110–120 mm Hg with Valsalva). Our initial experience was with beta-blocker and clonidine intraoperatively, and postoperative hydralazine boluses, as required. Although many strategies for blood pressure control exist, our current preference is for a dexmeditomidene infusion intraoperatively, which is continued postoperatively, with dose titration to control blood pressure. The characteristics of antihypertension, analgesia and sedation without respiratory depression make this an ideal drug for use in any tongue base surgery for sleep apnea. The danger time for postoperative surges in blood pressure is in the first 6 hours postoperatively which, if not avoided, may result in sudden tongue base hematoma and rapid airway obstruction requiring emergency reintubation or cricothyrotomy/tracheotomy.

### 4.3 POSTOPERATIVE EDEMA

Dexametasone (8 mg), with broad-spectrum antibiotics, is administered on induction of anesthesia, and both are continued for 24–48 hours. Any concurrent palatal surgery is advised to be performed first, with re-scrub and re-preparation of a sterile field prior to commencing the external submucosal glossectomy procedure, as prolonged pressure from the tongue blade of a mouth gag on a dissected tongue will increase the risk of edema. Due to the risk of tongue edema with glossectomy techniques, it is advisable to observe the patient while still nasotracheally intubated on ICU for the first 2 hours postoperatively, then extubate the patient if there is no significant tongue swelling. If there is any doubt regarding tongue size, it is preferable to leave the patient intubated overnight while steroids diminish edema. If the patient is able to use nasal continuous positive airway pressure (CPAP) (but wishes to discontinue in the longer term), CPAP should be worn whenever asleep for at least 2 weeks postoperatively (and preferably until just before the postoperative sleep study at 3–6 months) to minimize edema.

## 5 COMPLICATIONS

The morbidity of the procedure in terms of pain and return to oral intake was markedly lower than mucosal sacrificing glossectomy techniques.[4,7] Analgesia was achieved with regular paracetamol (from the day of surgery) and ibuprofen (commencing on the first postoperative day). Oxycodone 5–10 mg 4-hourly as required was given as a breakthrough pain control medication, and was often needed very little, or not at all (average number of 5 mg tablets used was six, range 0–20). The length of stay was 1–2 days (except one patient with a complication who stayed 6 days). No infections or subjective significant alteration to swallowing, speech or taste were noted at 3 months.

Two significant complications occurred. One patient developed a feeling of a lump in his throat and onset of stridor 30 hours after surgery, progressing over 30 minutes. A tracheotomy under local anesthesia was performed, followed by endoscopy under general anesthesia, which revealed a large hematoma of the inferior tongue base/pre-epiglottic space. He was treated with steroids and was decannulated 4 days later, with discharge the following day. In retrospect, this may have been avoided by not dissecting adjacent to the pre-epiglottic space. Since beveling the dissection 30° superior from the axial plane above hyoid bone, we have not encountered any more patients with this complication. This delayed bleed may have been caused by a small arterial branch; these are more prevalent in the tongue close to the hyoid bone (see Chapter 41 on Minimally invasive glossectomy). If encountered, *small arterial branches must be ligated* (with ligaclips) rather than diathermied to minimize the risk of delayed bleeding in the 5 days following surgery.

The second type of complication occurred in three patients in whom the hyoid suspension to mandible step was omitted. They were thought not to require shortening of their mandibular plane to hyoid distance (two had had previous hyothyroidopexy, and one had a normal MP-H distance); therefore after submucosal partial glossectomy, the mylohyoid was simply closed. All developed significant swallowing problems, manifesting during the first postoperative week, and not responding to conservative management over months. On re-exploration of the neck, dehiscence of mylohyoid to hyoid was seen in all cases, and a suspension of the hyoid to mandible was performed (with reapproximation of the ends of mylohyoid). The swallowing difficulties resolved immediately. This is avoidable if one always resuspends hyoid from mandible, even if mylohyoid is not shortened.

## 6 OUTCOMES

An audit was conducted of 13 consecutive (male) adult OSA patients from private practice having external submucosal partial glossectomy with hyoid advancement. The mean age was 51.7 (range 33–63), and cephalometric analysis showed normal jaw projection with sella-nasion-subspinale (SNA) measurement of 83.4° + 2.6 and SNB 80.8° + 1.7. All patients were assessed as Friedman stage III on physical examination. The operation was performed as a primary procedure with concurrent palatal advancement + uvulopalatopharyngoplasty (UPPP) in 5/13 (= 38%), and as a second stage procedure (previous UPPP/palatal advancement/geniotubercle advancement/+ hyothyroidopexy) in 8/13 (62%). Postoperative in lab sleep studies were performed in all patients at 3 months.

Snoring resolved in all patients. The Epworth Sleepiness Scale fell (non-significantly) from a mean of 8.5 to 6.2 ($P = 0.3$) (Table 47.1). The Apnea Index (AI) fell from $27.3 \pm 19.2$ to $9.2 \pm 15.2$ ($P = 0.08$). 'Clinical success' by AI criteria of AI < 10 and fall > 50% was 10/13 = 77%.

The total Respiratory Disturbance Index (RDI) fell from 54 + 16.8 to $28.7 \pm 22.9$ ($P = 0.004$) (Table 47.2). A total of 69% of patients achieved RDI < 30 measuring hypopneas with pressure transducers, which corresponds to the same target of RDI < 20 when hypopneas are measured with thermistors.[8] This corresponds to mild disease, and is slightly less, but in a similar range to the outcomes of around 80% success with mucosal sacrificing glossectomy techniques, by either endoscopic[7] or external[4] approaches.

The lateral RDI fell from $40.6 \pm 28.2$ to $18.5 \pm 24.1$ ($P = 0.014$) (Table 47.3). A total of 82% of patients achieved a lateral RDI < 30. The results for supine sleep were far inferior, with supine RDI falling from $75.3 \pm 29.5$ to $57.9 \pm 29.4$ ($P = 0.2$) (Table 47.4). Only 33% of patients achieved a supine RDI < 30. The fact that most patients achieved a satisfactory RDI overall is due to the majority of sleep time being in the lateral position (which was similar pre- and postoperatively). The lowest oxygen saturation rose from $80\% \pm 8.6$ to $84.7 \pm 6.5$ ($P = 0.16$). The Body Mass Index (BMI) fell slightly from $30.9 \pm 3.7$ to $29.6 \pm 2.9$ ($P < 0.001$).

Anatomically, the posterior airspace (supine, end expiration) increased from $6.7 mm \pm 3.7$ to $10.8 \pm 4.3$ ($P = 0.008$). The mandibular plane to hyoid distance (MP-H) increased

**Table 47.1** External submucosal glossectomy

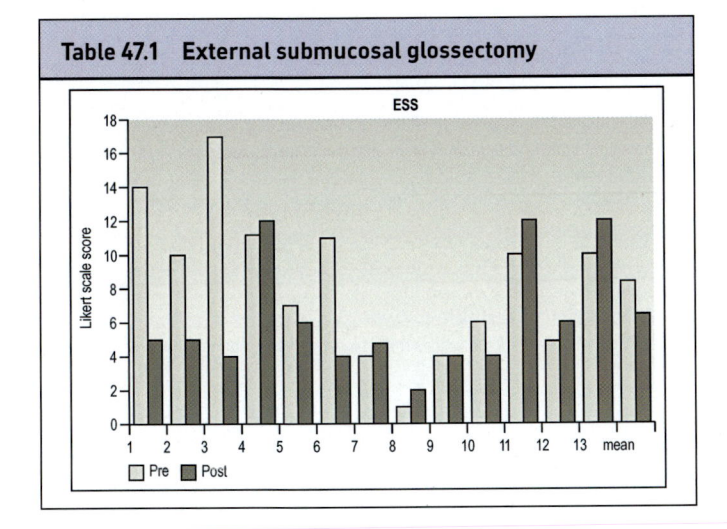

*(Bar chart: ESS, Likert scale score, Pre vs Post, patients 1–13 and mean)*

**Table 47.2** Total Respiratory Disturbance Index

*(Bar chart: Total RDI, Pre vs Post, patients 1–13 and mean)*

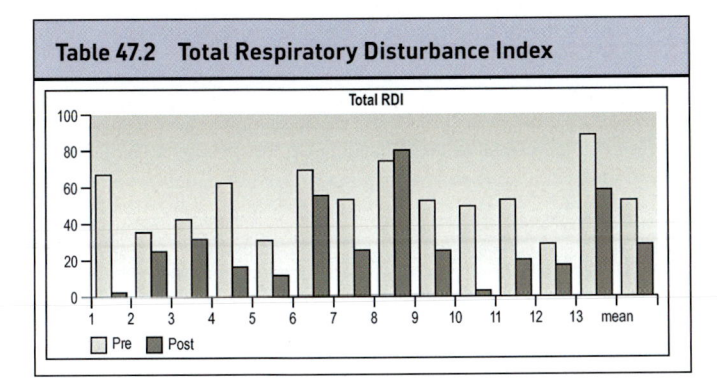

**Table 47.3** Lateral Respiratory Disturbance Index

*(Bar chart: Lateral RDI, Pre vs Post, patients 1–13 and mean)*

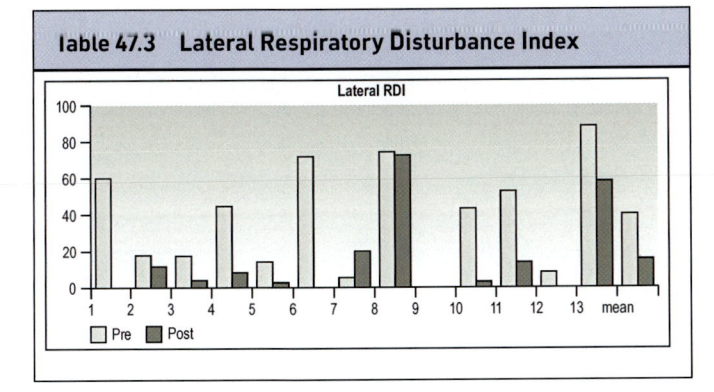

**Table 47.4** Supine Respiratory Disturbance Index

*(Bar chart: Supine RDI, Pre vs Post, patients 1–13 and mean)*

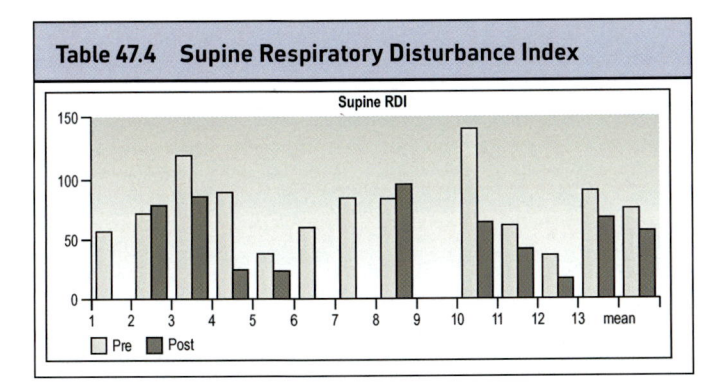

slightly from 22.1 mm ± 7.4 to 22.8 mm ± 7.2 ($P < 0.001$), which is an adverse anatomical change. The hyoid advancement towards mandible component of the surgery aimed to shorten this distance, thus shortening the airway length, advancing the lower tongue base forwards and verticalizing the epiglottis via tension on the hyoepiglottic ligament. Although the hyoid was repositioned anterosuperiorly during the operation, it was concluded that the 0 Vicryl hyomandibular suspension sutures with mylohyoid shortening were not adequate to maintain this new position over time. As noted in the operative description section, instead of the 0 Vicryl sutures, it is now recommended to use fascia lata to resuspend the hyoid to mandible (Fig. 47.7).

## 7 SALVAGE OPTIONS

No patients failed at the palate with a combination of palatal advancement and conservative UPPP. Palatal advancement +/− UPPP has been shown to be 5.8 times more powerful than UPPP alone when controlled for severity of sleep apnea, age, BMI and tongue base pathology,[9] and is therefore my standard palate intervention in patients with absent, 1+ or 2+ sized tonsils. The failures were analyzed, and most were thought to be due to insufficient tongue bulk reduction, particularly early in the series when minimal lateral extension beyond the neurovascular bundles and minimal anterior extension beyond the foramen cecum were performed. Increasing experience allowed more aggressive tongue reduction. Another cause of failure was hypotonicity, particularly in the supine position when the tongue tends to retrodisplace under the influence of gravity. It is postulated that a more durable hyoid advancement with fascia lata may improve this factor, and an additional fascia lata strip anchored from the mandible to submucosally loop around the genioglossus remnant at the level of foramen cecum (as a sling to counter hypotonicity during sleep) may also be helpful, but is yet to be evaluated.

If failure is seen due to inadequate tongue reduction, further bulk reduction may be undertaken. If postural sleep apnea is the cause due to genioglossus hypotonia during sleep (diagnosed with the awake hypotonic method and/or sedation nasendoscopy) despite a widely patent retrolingual airspace in mid respiration, tongue tensioning strategies should be employed. Options would include geniotubercle advancement or (mortised) high sliding genioplasty, a tongue base suture technique (e.g. Repose system), or the proposed experimental fascia lata sling technique discussed above. As an alternative to further surgery, a mandibular advancement splint could be reconsidered in cases of residual bulk and/or hypotonicity. Maxillomandibular advancement is a powerful option, but is considered as a last resort.

If posterior epiglottic tilt position precipitates supraglottic obstruction during sleep, despite a stable and normal size tongue base, further hyoid advancement towards mandible could be considered. Although hyothyroidopexy[10] would also seem a reasonable alternative, the anterior vector required to verticalize the epiglottis appears unlikely to be sustained in the longer term due to remodeling of the underlying superior thyroid cartilage, which I have noted on all patients (6 of 6) having reversal or revision of hyothroidopexy (unreported data). I prefer to avoid partial epiglottectomy for fear of aspiration, and have found endoscopic glossoepiglottopexy unreliable.

## 8 CONCLUSIONS

Open submucosal partial glossectomy achieves significant tongue reduction with minimal pain and minimal impact on tongue function. Control of apneic events is excellent, but hypopneas are far more easily controlled in the lateral position than supine. This may be addressed with future refinements in technique. The degree of macroglossia at which bulk reduction techniques are more appropriate than tongue tensioning techniques is yet to be clearly defined, and many patients may need both strategies to yield optimal results.

More aggressive bulk reduction and therefore better results are likely to be achieved with increased experience. Perioperative attention to analgesia, airway edema and blood pressure control in a monitored setting are mandatory. Standard surgical equipment and dissection skills are required for the procedure, making it straightforward to learn.

## REFERENCES

1. Woodson BT, Naganuma H. Comparison of methods of airway evaluation in obstructive sleep apnea syndrome. Otolaryngol Head Neck Surg 1999;120(4):460–63.
2. Friedman M, Ibrahim H, Bass L. Clinical staging for sleep-disordered breathing. Otolaryngol Head Neck Surg 2002;127:13–21.
3. Chabolle F, Lachiver X, Fleury B, et al. Intérêt physio-pathologique d'une etude céphalométrique par téléradiographis et IRM dans le syndrome d'apnée du sommeil; déductions thérapeutiques. Ann Oto Laryng (Paris) 1990;107:159–66.
4. Chabolle F, Wagner I, Blumen, et al. Tongue base reduction with hyoepiglottoplasty: a treatment for severe obstructive sleep apnea. Laryngoscope 1999;109:1273–80.
5. Riley RW, Powell NB, Guilleminault C. Obstructive sleep apnea syndrome: a review of 306 consecutively treated surgical patients. Otolaryngol Head Neck Surg 1993;108(2):117–25.
6. Riley R, Powell N, Guilleminault C, et al. Obstructive sleep apnea surgery: risk management and complications. Otolaryngol Head Neck Surg 1997;117(6):648–52.
7. Woodson BT, Fujita S. Clinical experience with lingualplasty as part of the treatment of severe obstructive sleep apnea. Otolaryngol Head Neck Surg 1992;107(1):40–48.
8. Aguirregomoscorta JI, Altube L, Menendez I, et al. Comparacion entre las normativas de la SEPAR de 1993 y 2002 en la lectura de los eventos respiratorios de las mismas polisomnografias (Comparison between the 1993 and 2002 Guidelines of the Spanish Society of Pulmonology and Thoracic Surgery (SEPAR) for identifying respiratory events in polysomnography tests). Arch Bronconeumol (Spain) 2005;41(12):649–53.
9. Woodson BT, Robinson S, Lim HJ. Transpalatal advancement pharyngoplasty outcomes compared with uvulopalatopharyngoplasty. Otolaryngol Head Neck Surg 2005;133:211–17.
10. Riley RW, Powell N, Guilleminault C. Obstructive sleep apnea and the hyoid: a revised surgical procedure. Otolaryngol Head Neck Surg 1994;111:717–21.

SECTION K — MULTILEVEL PHARYNGEAL SURGERY

# CHAPTER 48

# Genioglossus advancement in sleep apnea surgery

*Kasey K. Li*

Obstructive sleep apnea syndrome is associated with airway obstruction due to a decrease in upper airway muscle tone during sleep. Because the genioglossus muscle is a major pharyngeal dilator, it has long been suggested to play a major role in nocturnal airway obstruction. Genioglossus advancement is a surgical procedure which places the genioglossus muscle under tension, thus restricting the collapse of the tongue into the airway during sleep-induced hypotonia. This chapter describes my technique.

## 1 INTRODUCTION

Hypopharyngeal obstruction is a major contributing factor in obstructive sleep apnea (OSA). Hypopharyngeal obstruction stems from the prominence or relaxation of the base of the tongue, lateral pharyngeal wall collapse, and occasionally involves the aryepiglottic folds or epiglottis.[1–3] Because the genioglossus muscle is a major pharyngeal dilator, it has long been suggested to play a major role in nocturnal airway obstruction.[4,5] Genioglossus advancement is a surgical procedure designed to place the genioglossus muscle under tension, thus restricting the collapse of the tongue into the airway during sleep-induced hypotonia. Multiple studies have demonstrated that genioglossus advancement combined with uvulopalatopharyngoplasty achieves improvement of OSA.[6–8] Several designs of the osteotomy during genioglossus advancement have been described, with each one aimed at minimizing the surgical morbidity while improving the incorporation and the advancement of the genioglossus muscle.[6,9–11]

## 2 PRESURGICAL EVALUATION

The presence of hypopharyngeal obstruction is confirmed by physical examination as well as utilizing fiberoptic evaluation and lateral cephalometric radiograph. The operation is designed to reposition the genial tubercle forward, thus improving the tension of the tongue musculature and limiting its posterior displacement during sleep. Preoperative radiograph such as a panoramic dental x-ray is also necessary to assist the surgeon in the evaluation of the genial tubercle position and tooth root position. The panoramic radiograph will demonstrate the course of the inferior alveolar nerve canal, the mental foramen, the position of the mandibular tooth roots, as well as the detection of potential pathologic processes of the mandible.

## 3 SURGICAL TECHNIQUE

The procedure is performed under general anesthesia with oroendotracheal intubation. Local anesthetic injection (10 milliliters of 2% lidocaine with epinephrine) is administered at the anterior mandibular vestibule. The procedure begins with a mucosal incision approximately 10 mm below the mucogingival junction (Fig. 48.1). A subperiosteal dissection is performed to expose the mandibular symphysis. Exposure and identification of the mental nerves are unnecessary as the mental foramen is lateral to the surgical site. The genial tubercle and genioglossus muscle can be estimated by finger palpation in the floor of the mouth and with the aid of the lateral cephalometric and panoramic radiographs. A rectangular osteotomy encompassing the estimated location of the genial tubercle is performed under copious irrigation (Fig. 48.2). It is recommended that the superior horizontal bone cut be at least 5 mm below the mandibular root apices to decrease the likelihood of tooth paresthesia. The inferior horizontal bone cut should be designed to preserve approximately 10 mm of the inferior border of the mandible to reduce the risk of a pathologic mandibular fracture. If there is insufficient mandibular symphyseal height, this procedure should not be performed as the risk of pathologic mandibular fracture or tooth root injury is increased. Due to the elongated canine tooth roots that are often present, the vertical bone cuts are made just medial to the canine tooth to avoid root injury. It is crucial

## SECTION K — MULTILEVEL PHARYNGEAL SURGERY

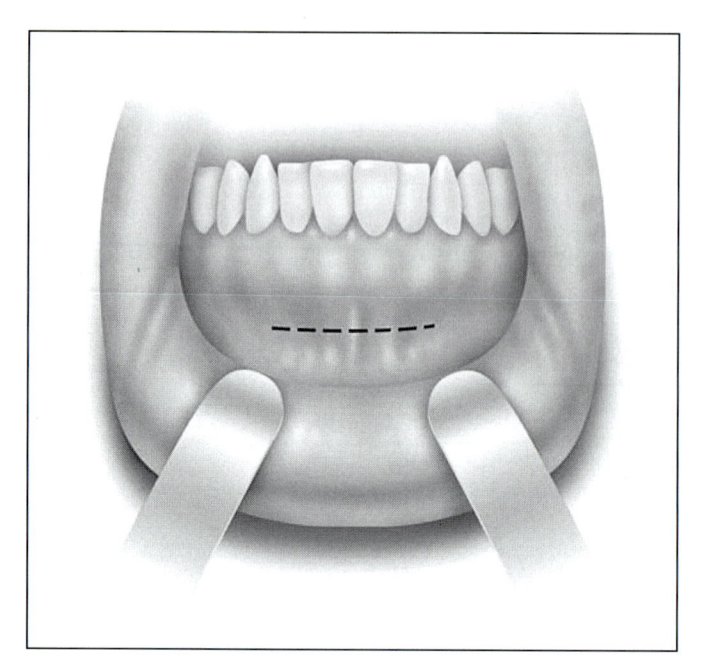

**Fig. 48.1** Mucosal incision made approximately 10mm below the mucogingival junction.

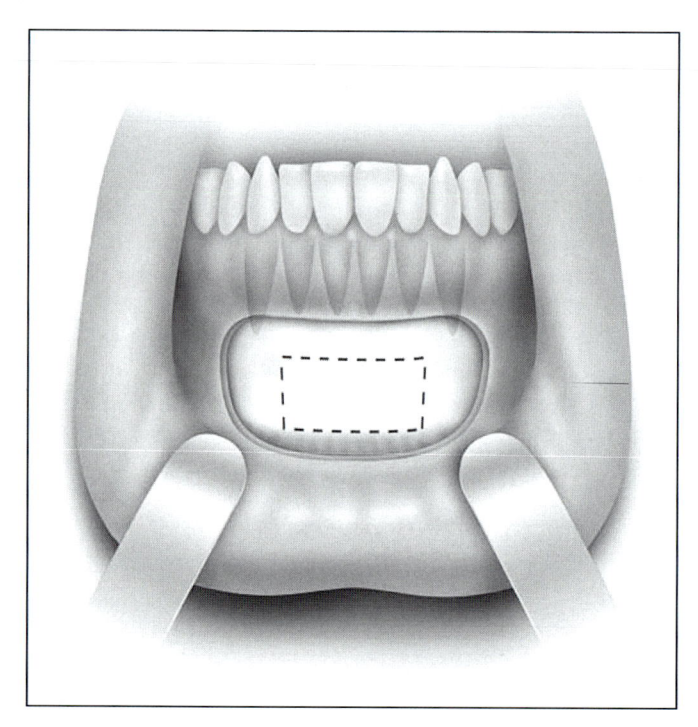

**Fig. 48.2** A rectangular osteotomy encompassing the estimated location of the genial tubercle is performed.

to follow parallelism of the osteotomies to facilitate the ease of releasing the rectangular bone flap. Prior to completing the osteotomy, a titanium screw is placed in the outer cortex to control and manipulate the bone flap. At the completion of the osteotomy, the bone flap is released from the surrounding bone and is advanced and rotated 60° to prevent retraction back into the floor of the mouth. The outer cortex and marrow are removed and the inner cortex is rigidly fixed with a lag screw (Fig. 48.3).

Bleeding is controlled with electrocautery and a hemostatic agent such as Gelfoam® (Pharmacia and Upjohn Company, Kalamazoo, Michigan 49001). Bone wax is not recommended for control of bleeding due to extrusion problems. It is important to irrigate the wound with copious irrigation to eliminate bone dusts. The procedure is completed with layer closure of the wound with re-establishment of the mentalis muscle and mucosa layers. This layered closure is crucial to minimize wound dehiscence.

### 3 PERIOPERATIVE MANAGEMENT

Patients with OSA have an increased risk for postoperative airway compromise. All patients should be extubated awake in the operating room immediately following surgery. ICU monitoring should be considered in patients undergoing multiple procedures (uvulopalatopharyngoplasty combining with genioglossus advancement and/or hyoid myotomy and suspension), or in patients with significant co-existing medical problems such as hypertension and coronary artery disease. Nasal CPAP or humidified oxygen via face tent should be considered in all patients, and oximetry monitoring is performed throughout the hospitalization. Blood pressure should be monitored closely and hypertension treated aggressively with intravenous antihypertensive medications to minimize postoperative bleeding and edema.

### 4 DISCUSSION

It is well recognized that the hypopharyngeal airway often needs to be addressed in order to maximize the surgical response in sleep apnea treatment. Genioglossus advancement has been utilized in the management of hypopharyngeal obstruction since the 1980s.[12] Regardless of the osteotomy design, the principle of the procedure is the same, i.e. advancing of the genioglossus muscle and limiting the tongue base collapse. It should be pointed out that there are advantages and disadvantages with different designs. The rectangular osteotomy described in this article is less invasive when compared to the mortise osteotomy which includes the lower border. It also minimizes the risk of mandibular fracture since the lower border of the mandible is preserved. The genioglossus muscle is routinely captured in the advancement. However, the rectangular design is more technically challenging. Although the mortise design captures more muscle in the advancement, the advancement is usually less. Regardless of the osteotomy design, potential

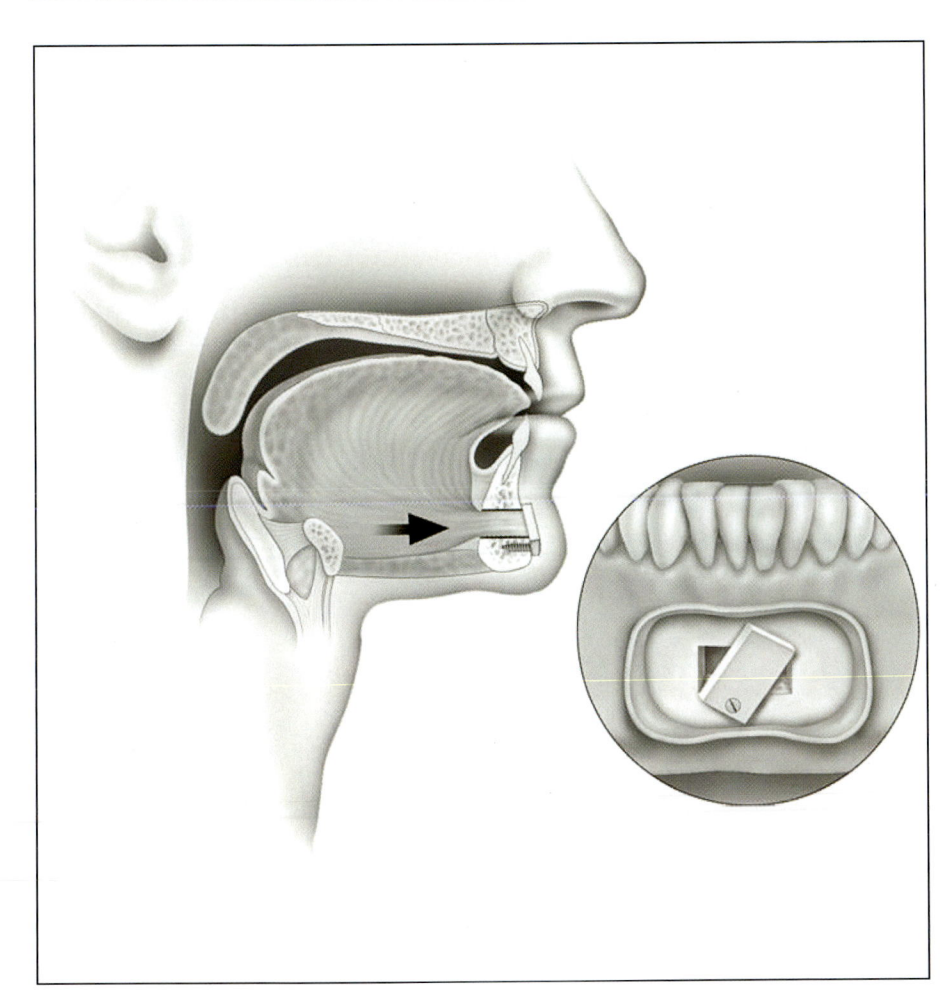

**Fig. 48.3** The bone flap is advanced and rotated 60° to prevent retraction back into the floor of the mouth. The outer cortex and marrow are removed and the inner cortex is rigidly fixed with a lag screw.

complications of genioglossus advancement include bleeding, infection, paresthesia, anesthesia or dysthesia of the chin and teeth as well as mandibular fracture.

Although most studies have shown that combining uvulopalatopharyngoplasty and genioglossus advancement achieves improvement of OSA, the success rate can be quite variable, ranging from 22% to 67%.[6–13] This is likely due to the complexity associated with the etiology of OSA, patient selection and surgical execution.

## REFERENCES

1. Rojewski TE, Schuller DE, Clark RW, et al. Videoendoscopic determination of the mechanism of obstruction in obstructive sleep apnea. Otolaryngol Head Neck Surg 1984;92:127–31.
2. Kletzker GR, Bastian RW. Acquired airway obstruction from histologically normal abnormally mobile supraglottic soft tissues. Laryngoscope 1990;100:375–9.
3. Schwab RJ, Gefter WB, Hoffman EA. Dynamic upper airway imaging during awake respiration in normal subjects and patients with sleep disordered breathing. Am Rev Respir Dis 1993;148:1385–400.
4. Remmers JE, Degroot WJ, Sauerland EK, Anch AM. Pathogenesis of upper airway occlusion during sleep. J Appl Physiol 1978;44:931–8.
5. Mezzanotte WS, Tangel DJ, White DP. Waking genioglossal electromyogram in sleep apnea patients versus normal controls (a neuromuscular compensatory mechanism). J Clin Invest 1992;89:1571–9.
6. Miller FR, Watson D, Boseley M. The role of the genial bone advancement trephine system in conjunction with uvulopalatopharyngoplasty in the multilevel management of obstructive sleep apnea. Otolaryngol Head Neck Surg 2004;130:73–9.
7. Lee NR, Givens CD Jr, Wilson J, Robins RB. Staged surgical treatment of obstructive sleep apnea syndrome: a review of 35 patients. J Oral Maxillofac Surg 1999;57:382–85.
8. Kezirian EJ, Goldberg AN. Hypopharyngeal surgery in obstructive sleep apnea: an evidence-based medicine review. Arch Otolaryngol Head Neck Surg 2006;132:206–13.
9. Li KK, Riley RW, Powell NB, Troell RJ. Obstructive sleep apnea surgery: genioglossus advancement revisited. J Oral Maxillofac Surg 2001;59:1181–4.
10. Li KK. Discussion on 'A protocol for UPPP, mortised genioplasty, and maxillomandibular advancement in patients with obstructive sleep apnea: an analysis of 40 cases'. J Oral Maxillofac Surg 2001;59:898–9.

11. Hendler B, Silverstein K, Giannakopoulos H, Costello BJ. Mortised genioplasty in the treatment of obstructive sleep apnea: an historical perspective and modifications of design. Sleep Breath 2001;5:173–80.
12. Riley R, Guilleminault C, Powell N, Derman S. Mandibular osteotomy and hyoid bone advancement for obstructive sleep apnea: a case report. Sleep 1984;7:79–82.
13. Bettega G, Pepin JL, Veale D, Deschaux C, Raphael B, Levy P. Obstructive sleep apnea syndrome. Fifty-one consecutive patients treated by maxillofacial surgery. Am J Respir Crit Care Med 2000;162:641–9.

SECTION K  MULTILEVEL PHARYNGEAL SURGERY

CHAPTER 49

# Hyoid suspension as the only procedure

*Nico de Vries and Cindy den Herder*

## 1 INTRODUCTION

Obstruction of the airway at the retropalatinal and retropharyngeal airway is the key factor in the pathophysiology of obstructive sleep apnea syndrome (OSAS). Patient selection is crucial in successful surgery of the upper airway in OSAS. In addition to polysomnography, topical diagnostic work-up is of paramount importance in this regard. We routinely perform polysomnography first, and after that in cases of an Apnea/Hypopnea Index (AHI) below 30, schedule patients for sedated endoscopy ('sleep endoscopy') with midazolam (without an anesthetist present), in those patients in whom surgery is considered. In patients with an AHI > 30, who refuse NCPAP treatment upfront, or in patients who cannot accept NCPAP for whatever reason, sedated endoscopy is performed as well, but by an anesthetist, with propofol. In the study period (March 2000 to June 2004), in the case of mainly or only retrolingual obstruction, as assessed by sleep endoscopy and a low AHI (arbitrarily <15–20, snoring up to mild sleep apnea) we usually started with radiofrequent ablation of the tongue base. In this situation, in the case of mild or moderate OSAS, oral devices were offered as an alternative. In cases of a relatively higher AHI (moderate to severe OSAS), the effect of MRA treatment is less efficacious. In the case of an index of 15–30, and mainly retrolingual obstruction, we performed hyoid suspension (a.k.a. hyoidthyroidpexia) as the only procedure. In higher AHI patients we perform multilevel surgery (hyoid suspension, radiofrequency ablation of the tongue base, uvulopalatopharyngoplasty (UPPP), with/or without genioglossal advancement (see Chapter 17, Multilevel surgery). These patients usually have more severe and multilevel obstruction, which explains the higher AHI.

Hyoid suspension involves stabilization of the hyoid bone inferiorly by attachment to the superior border of the thyroid cartilage. The underlying principle for altering the hyoid is that anatomically, the hyoid complex is an integral part of the hypopharynx. Anterior movement of the hyoid complex increases the posterior airway space and neutralizes obstruction at the tongue base. This concept has been supported by several reports. In the United States, hyoid suspension is often performed in combination with genioglossus advancement (GA) and followed by maxillomandibular osteotomy (MMO) as phased surgery in case of failure. The rationale for using hyoid suspension only in our series was to avoid more radical and more extensive unnecessary surgery in well-selected patients. In this chapter we report our experiences with this procedure.

## 2 PATIENTS AND METHODS

Surgery was offered to symptomatic patients with moderate to severe OSAS for whom UPPP was unsuccessful or who rejected or could not accept CPAP and preferred surgical therapy.

All patients had full polysomnography and underwent upper airway examination using physical examination and sleep endoscopy under midazolam or propofol.

### 2.1 POLYSOMNOGRAPHY

For sleep registration, patients stayed one night in the hospital. A CNS-Sleep I/T-8 recorder was used. This records sleep architecture (derived from an electroencephalogram, electro-oculogram and submental electromyogram); respiration (thoracic and abdominal measurement); airflow (mouth and nose thermistors); oxygen saturation (finger probe); movements of limbs; and the intensity of snoring.

### 2.2 UPPER AIRWAY ASSESSMENT

Hyoid suspension was performed in the case of obstruction at the base of tongue (Fig. 49.1), assessed by physical examination and flexible sleep endoscopy. A high suspicion

# SECTION K: MULTILEVEL PHARYNGEAL SURGERY

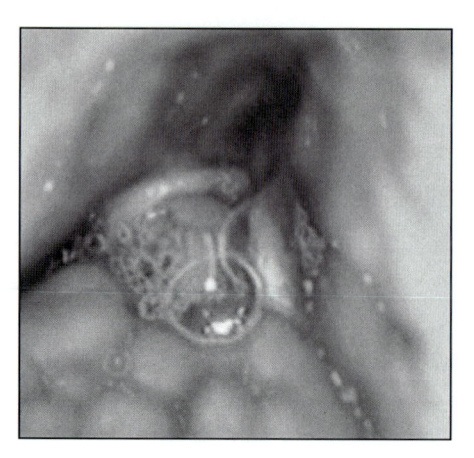

**Fig. 49.1** Obstruction at tongue base level during sleep endoscopy with midazolam.

of mainly retropalatal obstruction (large tonsils and long uvula) excluded patients for hyoid suspension. Candidates for surgery were categorized into two groups: those who did not have prior surgery at oro- or hypopharyngeal level (primary hyoid suspension); and those for whom UPPP was inadequate or detrimental (secondary hyoid suspension). In the latter group hyoid suspension was offered as salvage treatment. Multilevel obstruction (Fujita II) occurred in 20 patients; slight obstruction at retropalatal level in nine patients (primary hyoid suspension, $n = 14$) and residual retropalatal obstruction after UPPP in 12 patients (secondary hyoid suspension, $n = 17$). Only four patients who underwent primary hyoid suspension showed simple tongue base obstruction (Fujita III). Prior to UPPP, 15 patients showed

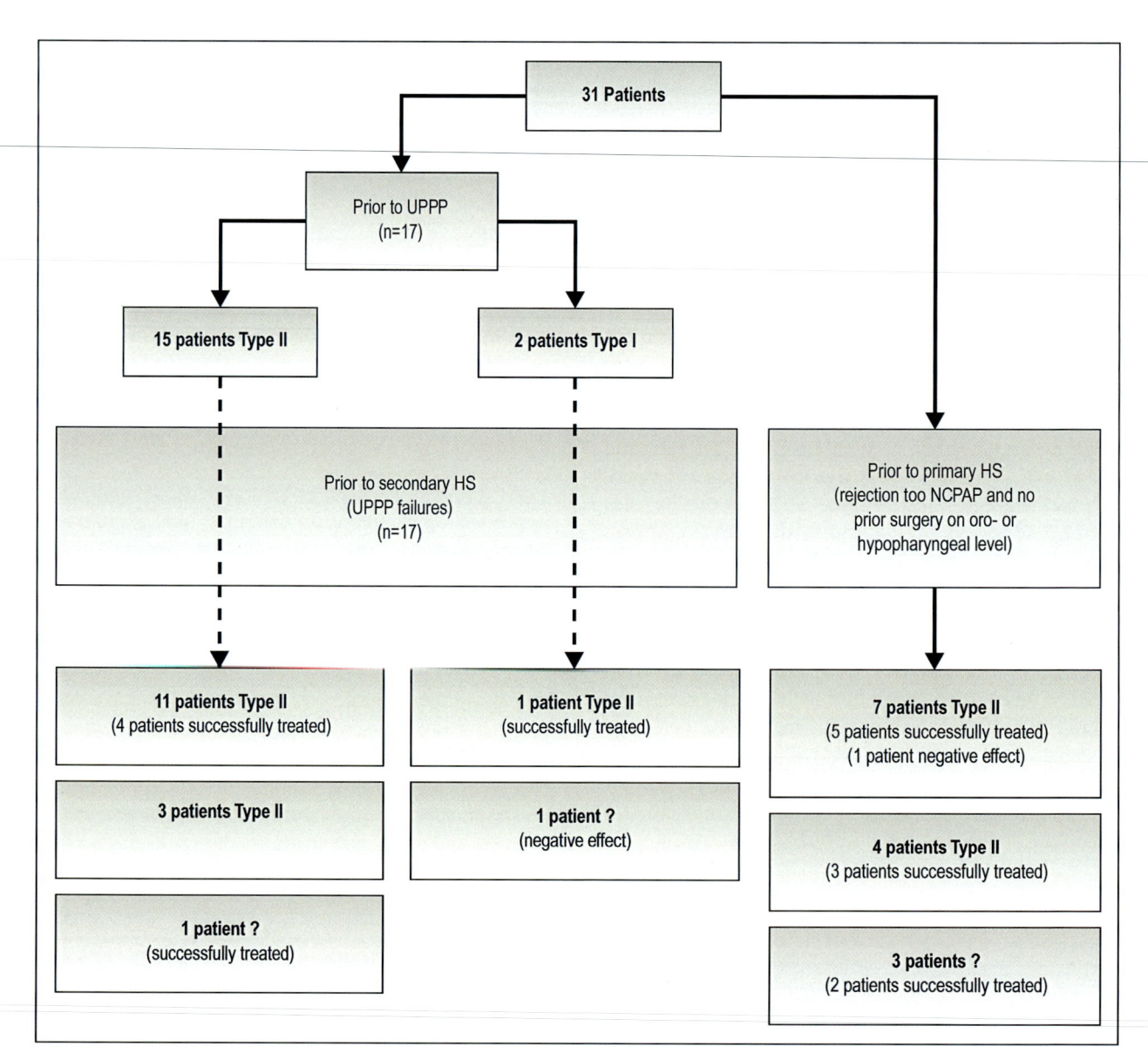

**Fig. 49.2** Endoscopic work-up using Fujita's classification and detailed synopsis of surgical success. Type I: Palate obstruction (normal base of tongue), Type II: Palate and base of tongue obstruction. Type III: Base of tongue obstruction with normal palate. HS, hyoid suspension.

multilevel obstruction (Fujita II), with emphasis on the palatal level; two patients showed retropalatal obstruction only (Fujita I). Sleep endoscopy work-up according to the Fujita classification is shown in Figure 49.2.

## 3 SURGICAL TECHNIQUE

### 3.1 HYOIDTHYROIDPEXIA AND POSTOPERATIVE MANAGEMENT

Under general anesthesia, with the head in a slightly extended position, a horizontal incision of approximately 5 cm is made in a relaxed skin tension line at the level between hyoid and thyroid cartilage (Fig. 49.3). Excessive fat tissue is excised, if helpful for better visualization. In the case of a further posterior positioned hyoid, removal of fat is recommended also, since otherwise the anterior placement of the hyoid will result in a somewhat turkey-like neck contour.

Second, the strap muscles are severed just below the attachment to the hyoid. Partial removal of the severed strap muscles at the level between hyoid and thyroid cartilage is sometimes also considered for the same cosmetic reasons, while there is no point in leaving the non-functional cut strap muscles in situ.

The tendon of the stylohyoid muscle is cut only if after release of the strap muscles insufficient mobilization is gained. Otherwise the stylohyoid tendon is preserved. By mobilizing the hyoid bone in an anterocaudal direction and fixing it to the thyroid with two permanent sutures per side through the thyroid cartilage and around the hyoid bone, more space is created retrolingually. Although with increasing age ossification of the thyroid will take place, in more than 80 cases we have never needed to make drill holes. A sharp cutting needle has so far always been sufficient to pierce the thyroid cartilage.

Antibiotics are not routinely applied. A surgical drain is placed and usually removed after 24–72 hours postoperatively if drainage was less than 10 ml per 24 hours. Nocturnal oximetry is monitored throughout the first postoperative night in the intensive care unit and non-opioid analgesics are used for pain relief, if necessary.

## 4 POSTOPERATIVE EVALUATION

All patients had a second polysomnography 3 months after surgery. The AHI, Epworth Sleepiness Scale (ESS), desaturation index and visual analogue scores (VAS) for hypersomnolence and snoring and pain sensation were compared pre- and postoperatively, per patient and between the two groups. Success was defined as when AHI indexes decreased at least 50% or dropped below the threshold of 20, or AI indexes decreased below 10 and responders as when AHI has decreased.

### 4.1 STATISTICAL ANALYSIS

Tests between groups on continuous variables were performed with a Wilcoxon rank sum test. Categorical variables were tested with a Fisher's exact test. All results are shown as mean ± SD. Significance was accepted for $P < 0.05$.

## 5 RESULTS

Between March 2000 and June 2004, 31 patients: (29 males and two females) underwent hyoid suspension. Secondary hyoid suspension was performed in 17 patients. Fourteen patients underwent primary hyoid suspension: 12 had difficulties using NCPAP, two refused NCPAP. Patient baseline characteristics are shown in Table 49.1. No differences were found preoperatively for AHI, Body Mass Index (BMI), age, ESS, desaturation indexes and VAS scores. The BMI did not change significantly postoperatively and all polysomnographies were considered valid.

Changes in AHI score are shown in Table 49.2. Twenty-five of the 31 (81%, 95% confidence interval 63–93%) patients showed a decrease in AHI; after secondary hyoid suspension, the mean AHI decreased from 31.5 to 26.2 ($P = 0.059$) (Fig. 49.4) and after primary hyoid suspension the AHI decreased from 32.9 to 17.5 ($P = 0.0067$). The decrease was significantly greater in the primary hyoid suspension group compared to the secondary hyoid suspension group ($P = 0.037$) (Fig. 49.5). In terms of success, 16 of the 31 (52%, 95% confidence interval 33–70%) patients showed a reduction of the AHI of more than 50%, or a post-AHI value below 20 and post-AI below 10. Although almost twice as many patients showed success in the primary hyoid suspension group (35% versus 71%), the difference was not significant ($P = 0.073$).

In contrast to the primary hyoid suspension group, the desaturation index in the secondary hyoid suspension group decreased significantly from 23.6 to 17.5 ($P = 0.017$).

Reduction of snoring in the primary hyoid suspension group (VAS: 8.5 to 5.6, $P = 0.009$) and secondary hyoid suspension group (VAS: 8.8 to 5.6, $P = 0.002$) was significant. No difference in snoring reduction was observed between both groups ($P = 0.80$). VAS scores for hypersomnolence showed a significant decrease from 6.6 to 4.3 ($P = 0.027$) and 5.8 to 3.4 ($P = 0.002$) after primary and secondary hyoid suspension respectively; again, no difference was found between the groups ($P = 0.88$). All patients

*Body Mass Index (BMI)

# SECTION K
## MULTILEVEL PHARYNGEAL SURGERY

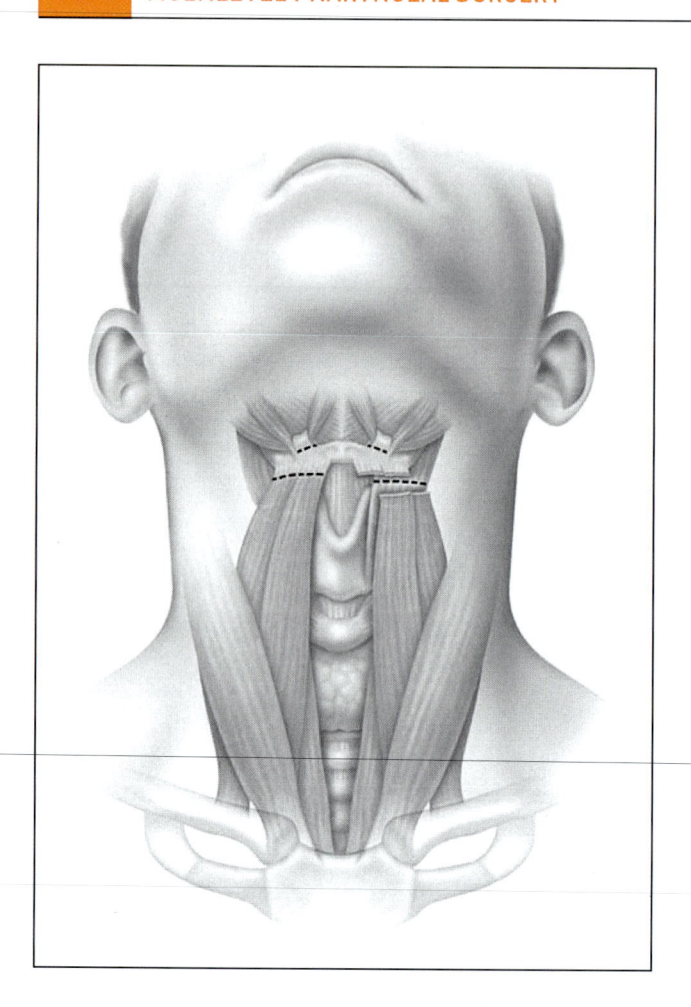

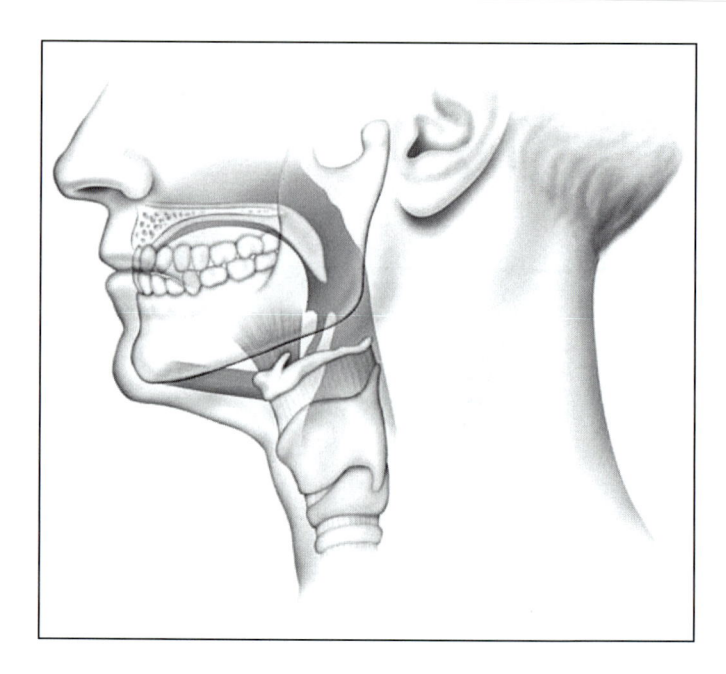

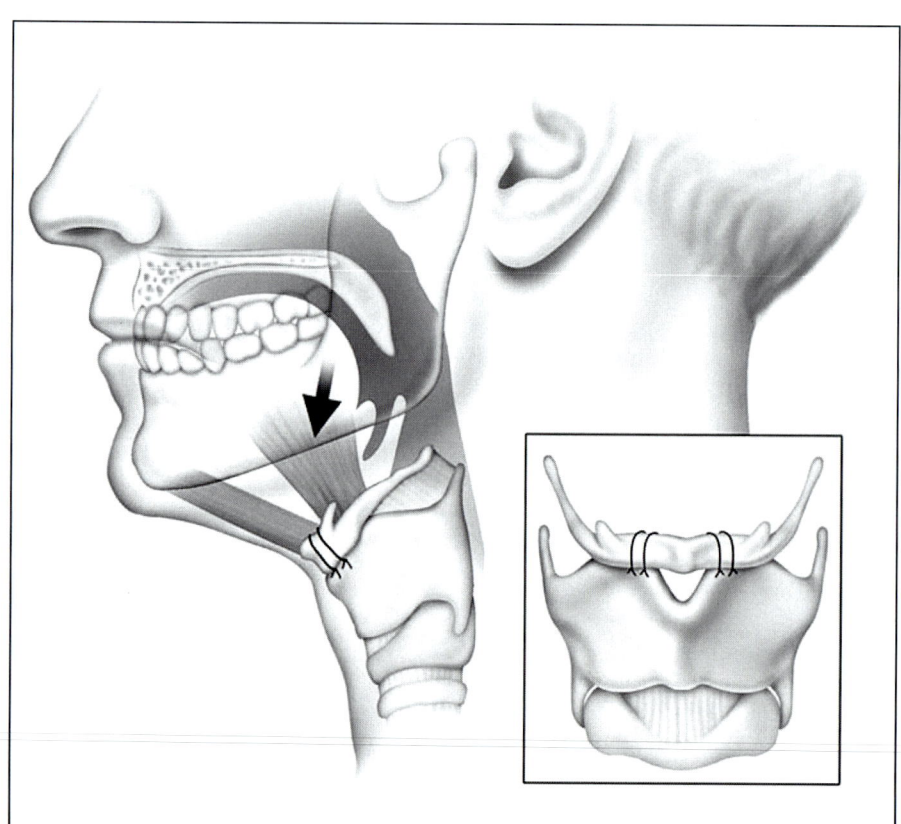

**Fig. 49.3** A, Anterior view. After exposure via a horizontal incision at the level of the thyroid membrane, the strap muscles (sternohyoid, omohyoid and thyrohyoid) are divided just below the hyoid and the tendons of the stylohyoid are divided from the hyoid bone, superior to the hyoid. B, Before hyoid suspension. C, After hyoid suspension. Permanent sutures are inserted through the thyroid cartilage and around the hyoid bone with subsequent antero-caudal mobilization and permanent fixation of the hyoid to the thyroid.

### Table 49.1 Baseline characteristics

| Measurement | Subjects HTP after previous UPPP (n = 17) | Subjects primary HTP (n = 14) | P value |
|---|---|---|---|
| BMI (kg/m$^2$) | 27.7 ± 4.3 | 26.3 ± 2.0 | 0.370 |
| AHI pre-HTP, events per hour | 31.5 ± 8.9 | 32.9 ± 11.9 | 0.717 |
| Desaturation index, events per hour | 23.62 ± 18.0 | 14.55 ± 8.3 | 0.294 |
| ESS pre-HTP | 6.7 ± 5.6 | 8.6 ± 7.0 | 0.537 |
| Age, year | 46.3 ± 8.3 | 47 ± 9.0 | 0.659 |
| Ratio male : female | 16 : 1 | 13 : 1 | 1.000 |

AHI, Apnea/Hypopnea Index; BMI, Body Mass Index; ESS, Epworth Sleepiness Scale.

### Table 49.2 Apnea/Hypopnea Index

| | Pre-AHI | Post-AHI | Impr. AHI | P* (WR) | P* (FE) | Responders | P (FE) |
|---|---|---|---|---|---|---|---|
| Primary HTP (n = 14) | 32.9 ± 11.9 | 17.5 ± 17.1 | 15.4 ± 16.6 | 0.006* | 0.037* | 71% (10/14) [95% C.I. 35–87%] | 0.073 |
| Secondary HTP (n = 17) | 31.5 ± 8.9 | 26.2 ± 12.8 | 5.3 ± 10.9 | 0.059 | | 35 % (6/17) [95% C.I. 14–62%] | |
| Total HTP (n = 31) | 32.1 ± 10.2 | 22.2 ± 15.2 | 9.9 ± 14.5 | 0.0005* | | 52% (16/31) [95% C.I. 33–70%] | |

Mean and deviation, Wilcoxon signed rank (WR) and Fisher exact test (FE) are recorded for the difference in response between both groups. AHI: Apnea/Hypopnea Index; C.I., confidence interval; Corr, correlation; Impr, improvement.

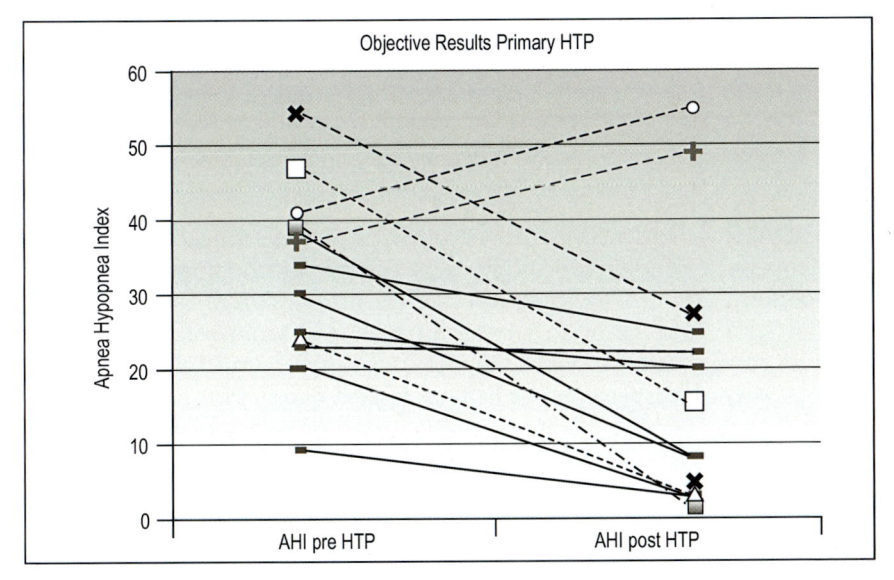

Fig. 49.4 AHI post-UPPP and post-HTP.

experienced less morbidity after hyoid suspension than after UPPP. The VAS pain score after UPPP (with paracetamol 1000 mg four times daily) was 7.0; after hyoid suspension patients' marked (without painkiller) 2.2. ESS scores significantly dropped for both primary and secondary hyoid suspension ($P = 0.001$ and $P = 0.031$ respectively). No difference was found between the two groups ($P = 0.13$). Statistical details are shown in Table 49.3.

No significant correlations between ESS scores and AHI indexes pre- and postoperatively, ESS scores and

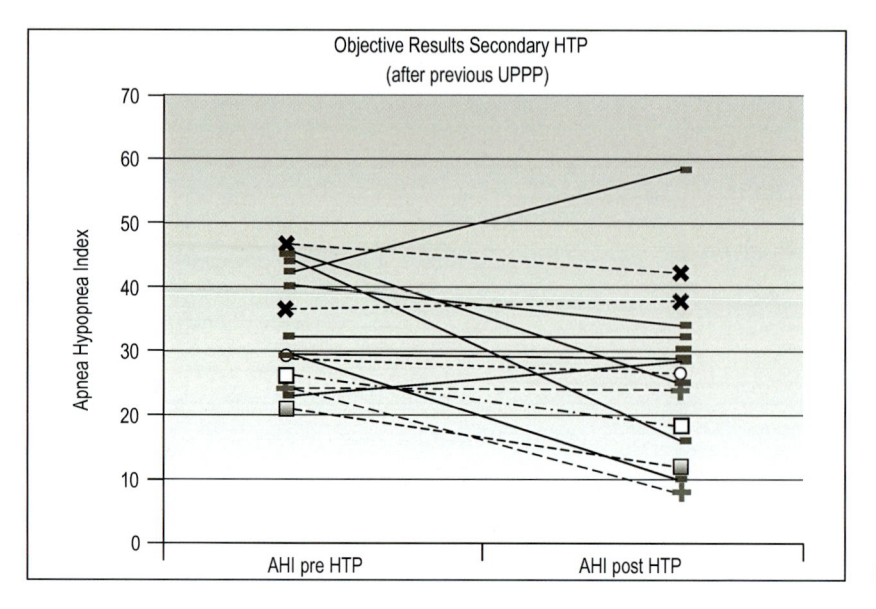

**Fig. 49.5** AHI pre- and post-primary HTP.

**Table 49.3  Secondary indices for improvement**

|  | Subjects HTP after previous UPPP | N | P* (WR) | Subjects primary HTP | N | P* (WR) | P (FE) | Total HTP | N | P* (WR) |
|---|---|---|---|---|---|---|---|---|---|---|
| ESS impr. | 2.4 ± 3.5 | 15 | 0.031* | 4.4 ± 5.2 | 14 | 0.001* | 0.131 | 3.3 ± 4.5 | 19 | <0.0001* |
| Desaturation index impr. | 6.2 ± 10.8 | 17 | 0.017* | −1.1 ± 16.3 | 8 | 0.757 | 0.256 | 3.8 ± 12.9 | 25 | 0.129 |
| VAS snoring impr. | 3.2 ± 3.2 | 14 | 0.002* | 2.9 ± 3.2 | 13 | 0.009* | 0.801 | 3.0 ± 3.1 | 27 | <0.0001* |
| VAS hypersomn. impr. | 2.4 ± 3.2 | 16 | 0.002* | 2.3 ± 3.6 | 14 | 0.027* | 0.876 | 2.4 ± 3.3 | 30 | <0.0001* |
| Follow-up, days | 98 ± 54.0 | 17 |  | 105 ± 50.0 | 14 |  |  |  |  |  |

Mean and deviation, Wilcoxon signed rank (WR) and Fisher exact test (FE) are recorded for the difference in response between both groups.
ESS, Epworth Sleepiness Scale; Impr, improvement; Hypersomn, hypersomnolence during the day; VAS, visual analogue scale.

VAS scores for hypersomnolence preoperatively and AHI indexes and VAS scores for hypersomnolence preoperatively were seen. However, a positive correlation between postoperative VAS scores for hypersomnolence and AHI indexes as well as ESS scores postoperatively (Pearson correlation coefficient 0.48, $P = 0.006$ and 0.52, $P = 0.004$) was detected.

## 6 COMPLICATIONS

Up to July 2006, >80 patients underwent hyoid suspension, alone or in combination with other procedures. Tracheotomy (in the third patient) was performed once because of a compromised airway due to postoperative bleeding. There is a definite learning curve here. A few patients had swallowing problems for a few days; re-intervention for post-operative bleeding was necessary in two patients; fistulas occurred in three patients. In these cases one or two stitches were removed with good result, and in one case (multilevel treatment) a lesion of the hypoglossal nerve occurred (see Chapter 17, Multilevel surgery). No other serious complications were observed. Overall, hyoid suspension was better tolerated than UPPP.

## 7 DISCUSSION

Short-term experiences with hyoid suspension only, especially as primary treatment, in this small series of patients with retrolingual obstruction as assessed by sedated endoscopy, with moderate to severe OSAS, are favourable. Our results show that hyoid suspension only can be efficacious: 71% of the patients did not need further treatment. Only four patients were not successfully treated. Alternative treatment was offered to hyoid suspension failures, including a new attempt with NCPAP treatment or oral device and revision surgery of relative palatal stenosis after UPPP. A floppy epiglottis caused airway obstruction at hypopharyngeal level in two other cases; these patients were considered non-responders. One patient underwent partial epiglottectomy. Clinical improvement in those patients, in terms of reduced snoring and improvement in general well-being, was such that further therapy was not regarded as necessary by both patient and physician.

Secondary hyoid suspension showed a reduction in AHI, but was occasionally unsatisfactory and definitely inferior to primary hyoid suspension, although the improvement of desaturation index was significant. Relative stenosis at soft palate level after UPPP, objectified after sleep endoscopy, might explain the lack of improvement of OSAS. Improvement of the airway at the base of tongue level by secondary hyoid suspension is less effective or sometimes ineffective. It goes without saying that this group is complex and might not at all be comparable to patients undergoing primary hyoid suspension. Twelve patients with UPPP failure ($n = 17$) had multilevel obstruction, with emphasis at the base of the tongue, in addition to the preoperatively assessed obstruction at palatal level with sleep endoscopy prior to UPPP. In the primary hyoid suspension group, nine of the 14 patients also had a slight obstruction at palatal level. The latter patients clearly responded better in terms of a stronger decline in AHI. A strong reduction in the amount of soft palate tissue (UPPP) might cause the tongue to drop back more easily, especially in cases of multilevel obstruction, because of lack of support by the soft palate. These patients might be better candidates for more invasive and aggressive treatments; in the case of a very high AHI, MMO should be considered. The overall success rate was 52%; overall the AHI significantly decreased ($P = 0.0005$). Some patients with UPPP failure were cured by hyoid suspension, but it remains hard to predict which patients will do well in the future.

Comparison with other series is difficult, because in almost all other series hyoid suspension was combined with other procedures, with the exception of a series from Stuck et al. from Mannheim, Germany, who found an AHI reduction of 35 to 27 in a group of 14 patients. Treatment outcome of surgery is further negatively affected by an increasing BMI. Patients with BMI > 25 are considered overweight, in the case of BMI > 30, obese. Bowden et al. in a paper with a somewhat misleading title ('Outcomes of hyoid suspension for the treatment of obstructive sleep apnea') in fact included UPPP in most patients. Their results were very disappointing, probably due to the very high BMI (34) in their series. It is our belief that performing sedated endoscopy would probably have prevented surgery in these patients, because in the case of a very high AHI usually a circumferential collapse (anterior–posterior as well as lateral wall collapse) is seen, making such patients unsuitable for hyoid suspension.

Although our experiences are encouraging, we have changed our policy after the reported series. Since it has been shown that radiofrequency of the tongue base as the only procedure has a moderate effect, and since we have found that radiofrequency of the tongue base is almost without adverse events and side effects (applying antibiotics, but no steroids) we now more or less routinely ('why not' intervention) combine it with hyoid suspension. Results will be reported elsewhere.

We conclude that hyoid suspension, in particular as primary treatment in cases of obstruction at tongue base level, is a valuable addition to the therapeutic armamentarium of moderate to severe OSAS. It is clear that experience with more patients is needed, while long-term results are lacking. In patients with UPPP failure or patients who refuse, or have difficulties using NCPAP, hyoid suspension should be considered. Selection criteria are: moderate to severe OSAS with preferably a BMI < 28, major obstruction at the base of the tongue, small tonsils and normal uvula, without a floppy epiglottis or a palatal stenosis after UPPP.

## FURTHER READING

Bowden MT, Kezirian EJ, Utley D, Goode RL. Outcomes of hyoid suspension for the treatment of obstructive sleep apnea. Arch Otolaryngol Head Neck Surg 2005;131:440–45.

Den Herder C, Schmeck J, Appelboom DJ, de Vries N. Risks of general anaesthesia in people with obstructive sleep apnoea. BMJ 2004;329:955–9.

Den Herder C, van Tinteren H, de Vries N. Hyoidthyroidpexia: a surgical treatment for sleep apnea syndrome. Laryngoscope 2005;115(4):740–45.

Den Herder C, van Tinteren H, de Vries N. Sleep endoscopy versus modified Mallampati score in sleep apnea and snoring. Laryngoscope 2005;115(4):735–9.

Den Herder C, van Tinteren H, Kox D, de Vries N. Bipolar radiofrequency induced thermotherapy of the tongue base: its complications, acceptance and effectiveness under local anesthesia. Eur Arch Otolaryngol 2006;263:1031–40.

Fujita S, Conway W, Zorick F, Roth T. Surgical correction of anatomic abnormalities in obstructive sleep apnea syndrome: uvulopalatopharyngoplasty. Otolaryngol Head Neck Surg 1981;89:923–34.

Hessel NS, de Vries N. Diagnostic work-up of socially unacceptable snoring II Sleep endoscopy. Eur Arch Otorhinolaryngol 2002;259:158–61.

Hessel NS, Laman M, van Ammers VCPJ, de Vries N. Diagnostic work-up of socially unacceptable snoring. I History or sleep registration. Eur Arch Otorhinolaryngol 2002;259:154–7.

Kezirian E, Goldberg AN. Hypopharyngeal surgery in obstructive sleep apnea. Arch Otolaryngol Head Neck Surg 2006;132:206–13.

Schmidt-Nowara W, Lowe A, Wiegand L, Cartwright R, Perez-Guerra F, Menn S. Oral appliances for the treatment of snoring and obstructive sleep apnea: a review. Sleep 1995;18:501–10.

Sher AE, Schechtman KB, Piccirillo JF. The efficacy of surgical modifications of the upper airway in adults with obstructive sleep apnea syndrome. Sleep 1996;19:156–77.

Stuck B, Neff W, Hörmann K, et al. Anatomic changes after hyoid suspension for obstructive sleep apnea: a MRI study. Otolaryngol Head Neck Surg 2005;133:397–402.

# SECTION K — MULTILEVEL PHARYNGEAL SURGERY

## CHAPTER 50

# Multilevel surgery (hyoid suspension, radiofrequent ablation of the tongue base, uvulopalatopharyngoplasty) with/without genioglossal advancement

*Nico de Vries, Wietske Richard, Dennis Kox and Cindy den Herder*

## 1 INTRODUCTION

Severe obstructive sleep apnea syndrome (OSAS) is preferably treated by nasal continuous positive airway pressure (NCPAP). Unfortunately, 30–50% of patients refuse or cannot accept NCPAP for a variety of reasons. Approximately 25% of patients refuse upfront or cannot pass the test period, others cannot accept or refuse it in the long run, or use it for only a few hours per night and/or less than 5 nights per week. It is our experience that increasingly many – especially young – patients refuse NCPAP therapy upfront and ask how realistic surgical alternatives are. Whatever the reason for not using NCPAP, treatment remains indicated in patients with severe OSAS and NCPAP refusal/failure. Many invasive alternatives are being explored. Various surgical interventions are available, such as uvulopalatopharyngoplasty (UPPP), Z-PP, uvula flap and other variations, in case of palatal obstruction, and hyoid suspension (HS) and genioglossal advancement (GA), in retrolingual obstruction. Maxillomandibular advancement (MMA) and tracheostomy are usually very effective, but the morbidity of these two modalities limits their application in the first line of surgery. In addition to surgical modalities, minimally invasive interventions exist, such as radiofrequent thermotherapy of palate and/or tongue base (RFTB). Surgery can be divided into unilevel (at palatinal or tongue base level only) and multilevel (surgery at both these levels), and can be performed either staged, or in one surgical event. Nose and nasopharynx in this regard are less important, in that where no nasal blockage is present, it has been shown that there is little use in increasing nasal airflow.

## 2 PATIENT SELECTION

In severe OSAS, the likelihood that obstruction is present on both a palatinal as well as a retrolingual level is high; in fact, obstruction at both levels is usually responsible for the high Apnea/Hypopnea Index (AHI). This is confirmed by sleep endoscopy of large series of patients with OSAS, who showed retropalatinal and retrolingual obstruction in a large percentage of cases. For this reason, the effect of unilevel surgery is often disappointing in severe OSAS. A therapeutic dilemma is whether these patients should undergo intervention (and what form of surgery), at both levels staged (and in which sequence) or simultaneously. Performing multilevel surgery in a staged sequence will in the case of multilevel obstruction often lead to a prolonged path to success. Eliminating obstruction at one level while leaving the other obstruction untreated is useless. In this paper we present our experience of one tempo multilevel surgery (hyoid suspension, radiofrequent ablation of the tongue base, UPPP, with/without genioglossal advancement) in severe OSAS and NCPAP failure or refusal, and compare it with the literature. We focus in this chapter on literature concerning UPPP and hyoid suspension with/without radiofrequency of the tongue base; experiences with UPPP and genioglossal advancement without hyoid suspension are covered elsewhere in this book (see Chapter ••)

## 3 PATIENTS AND METHODS

All patients who visited our department from July 2003 to June 2005 because of habitual snoring and/or suspicion of sleep apnea syndrome were evaluated by history, physical examination, full overnight polysomnography and either by midazolam or propofol-induced sedated endoscopy. Patients with moderate to severe OSAS, both retrolingual and retropalatinal narrowing or collapse at sedated endoscopy, and refusal or non-acceptance of NCPAP treatment were offered a multilevel surgical approach. Full night sleep registration was performed preoperatively and 3 months postoperatively (see Chapter 49: Hyoid suspension as only procedure).

Surgical success was defined as AHI < 20 and >50% reduction in AHI and response rate as reduction of AHI between 20 and 50%. The overall response rate was defined as more than 20% reduction in AHI.

## 3.1 TREATING OBSTRUCTION AT PALATINAL LEVEL

Uvulopalatopharyngoplasty was performed according to Fujita's technique; the anterior and posterior tonsillar pillars were trimmed and reoriented, and the uvula was excised to create more retropalatinal space (Fig. 50.1). Tonsillectomy was performed if it had not been done previously (in 15 of 22 [68%] patients). In patients who had had tonsillectomy previously, with a short anterior posterior diameter at retropalatinal level, Z-PP according to Friedman was performed (see Chapter 33).

## 3.2 TREATING OBSTRUCTION AT TONGUE BASE LEVEL

### 3.2.1 RADIOFREQUENT ABLATION OF THE TONGUE BASE (BIPOLAR, CELON®)

This was used for stiffening of the base of tongue. Energy was delivered with an exclusive needle device through the dorsal surface of the tongue. Evidence-based criteria for technical adjustment and optimal energy dosage according to relevant increase in lesion size were used. After the initial surgical procedure, on indication a second and sometimes third additional RFTB was performed (Fig. 50.2).

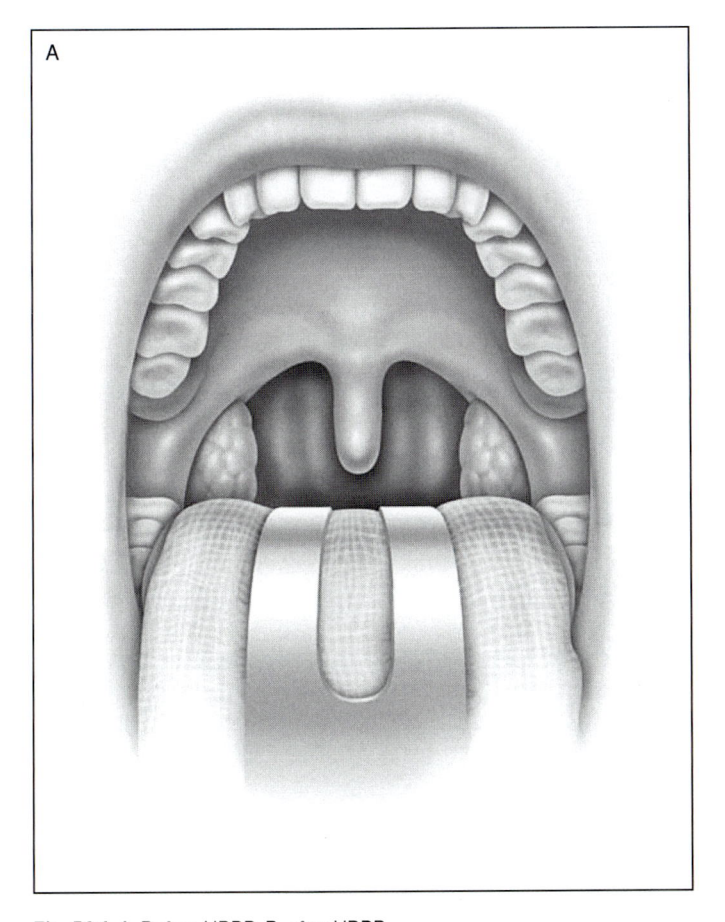

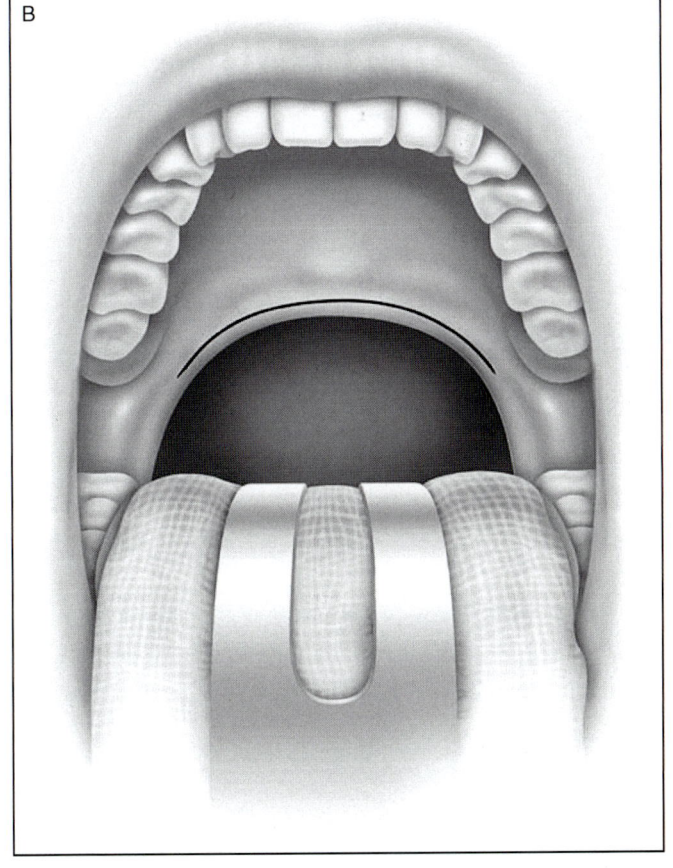

**Fig. 50.1** A, Before UPPP; B, after UPPP.

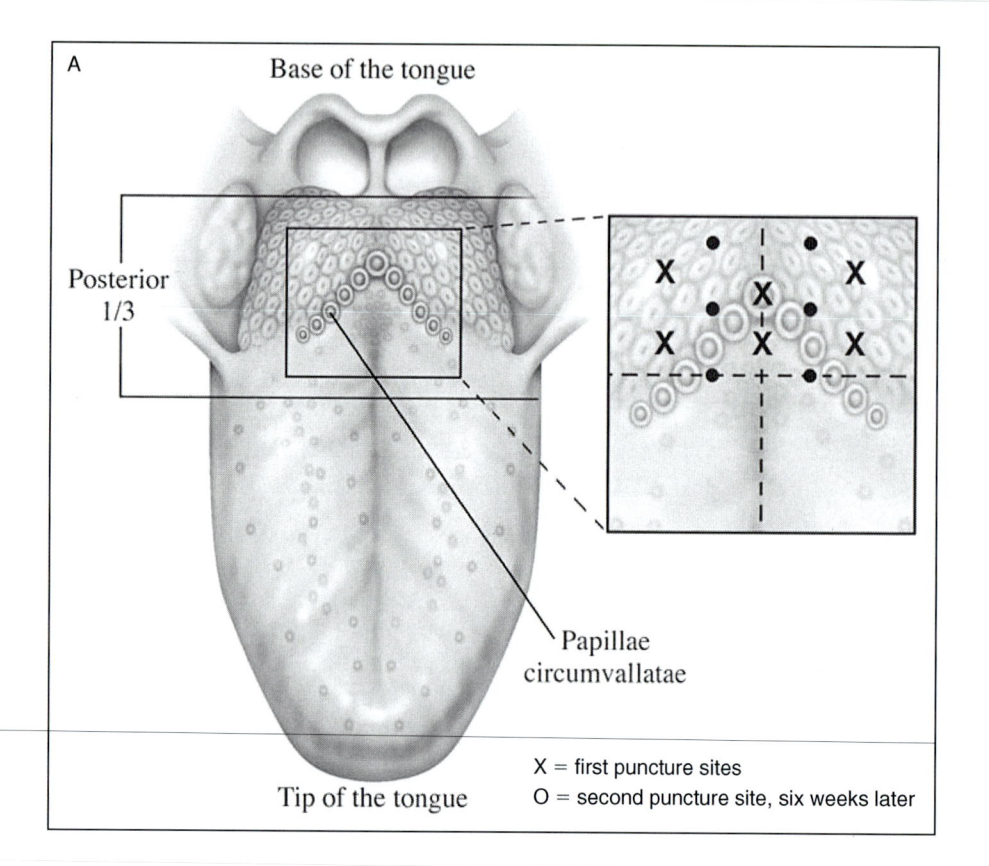

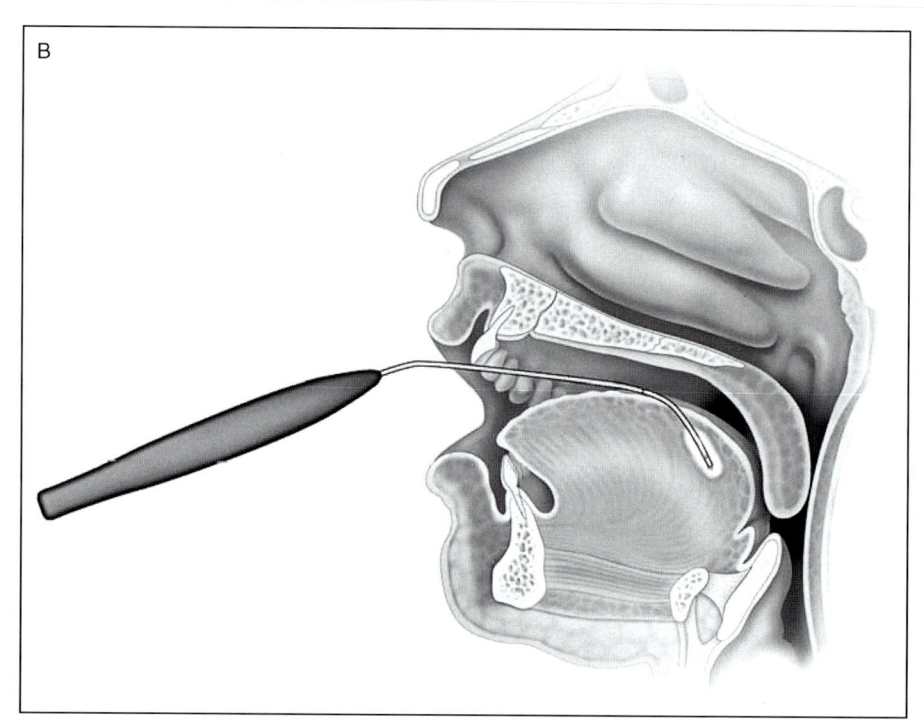

**Fig. 50.2** Radiofrequency ablation puncture sites.

### 3.2.2 HYOID SUSPENSION

After exposure via an external horizontal incision at the level of the membrana thyrohyoidea, the strap muscles (M. sternohyoideus, M. omohyoideus and M. thyrohyoideus) were divided just below the hyoid and superior to the hyoid the tendon of the stylohyoideus was divided from the hyoid bone (Fig. 50.3) (for details see Chapter 49: Hyoid suspension as only procedure).

Multilevel surgery with/without genioglossal advancement  CHAPTER 50

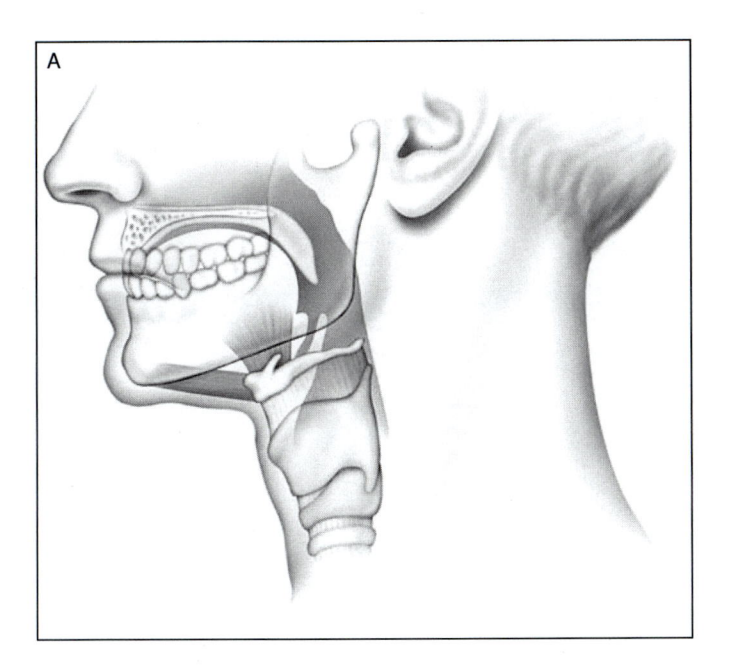

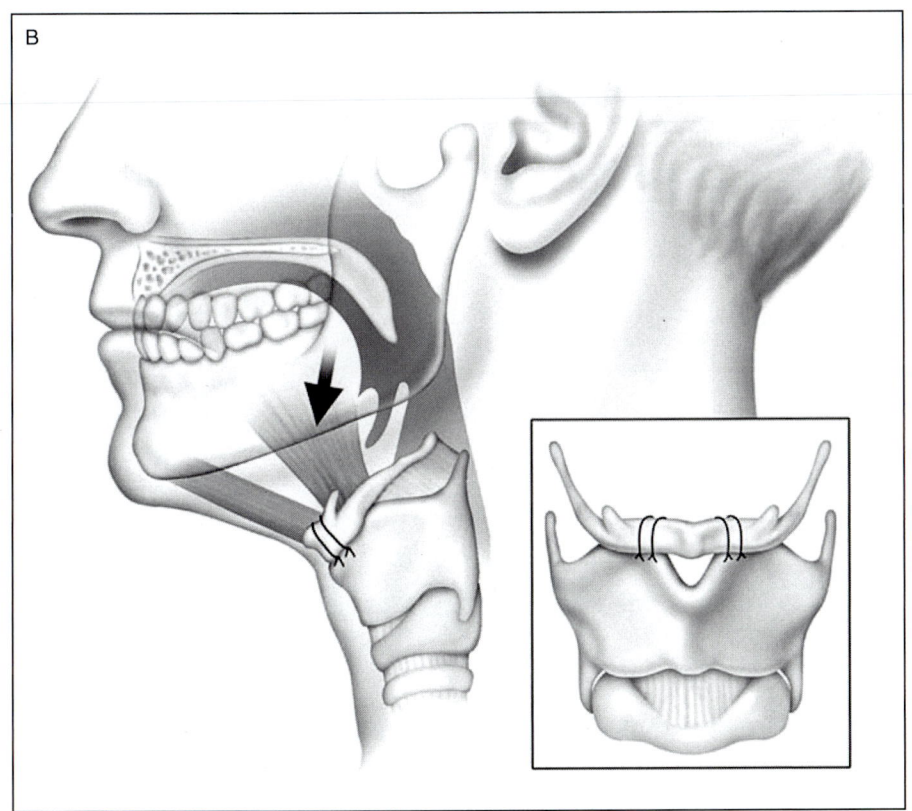

**Fig. 50.3** A, Before hyoid suspension; B, after hyoid suspension.

### 3.2.3 GENIOGLOSSUS ADVANCEMENT

A standard anterior mandibular osteotomy, limited to advancement of a rectangular window of the mandible including the genial tubercle and genioglossus musculature, but without rotation of the segment, was performed. The outer cortex and medulla were removed, the lingual cortical plate advanced and fixed with bone screws (Fig. 50.4).

## 4 PRE- AND POSTOPERATIVE CARE

Conscientious monitoring of oxygen saturations in an intensive care unit for one night after surgery is mandatory because of the risk of a compromised airway due to postoperative bleeding or edema. All patients received 2 grams of amoxicillin IV during surgery, and 625 mg three times a day

315

SECTION K  MULTILEVEL PHARYNGEAL SURGERY

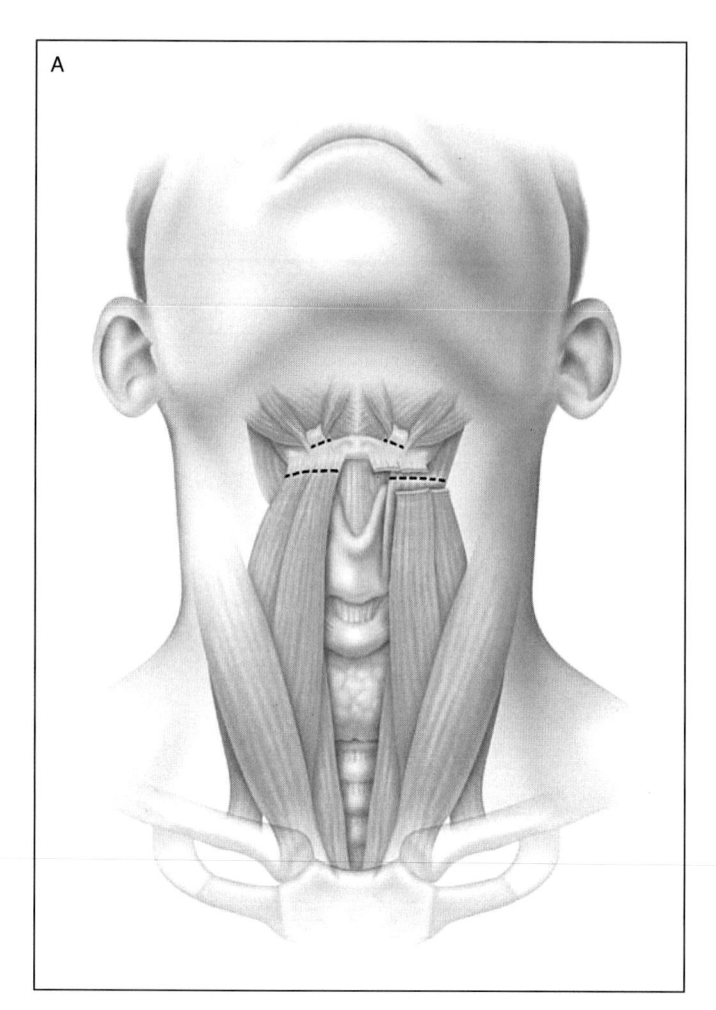

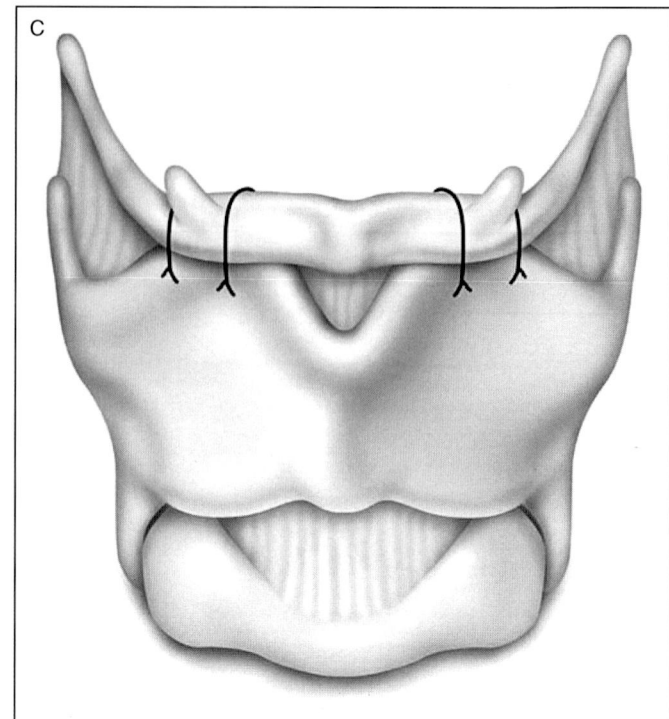

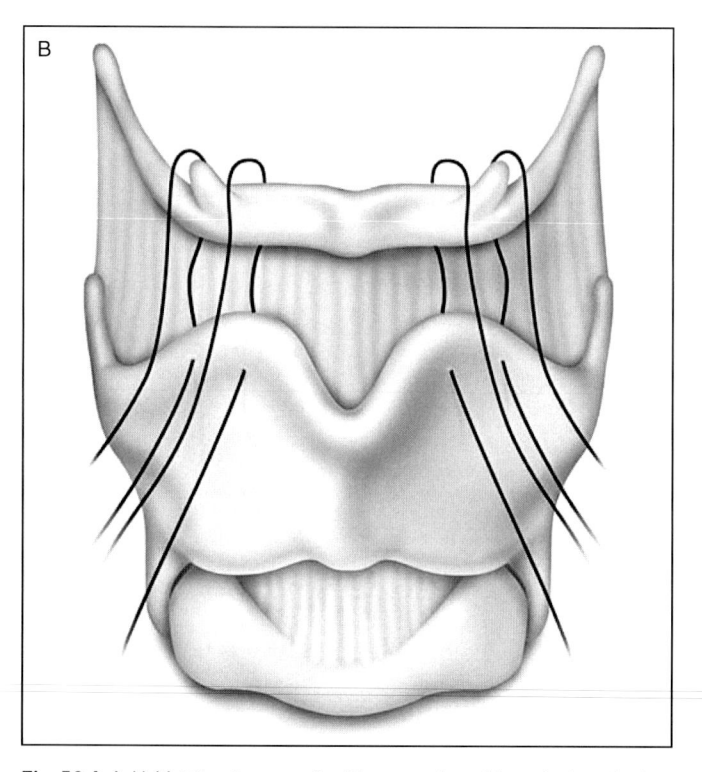

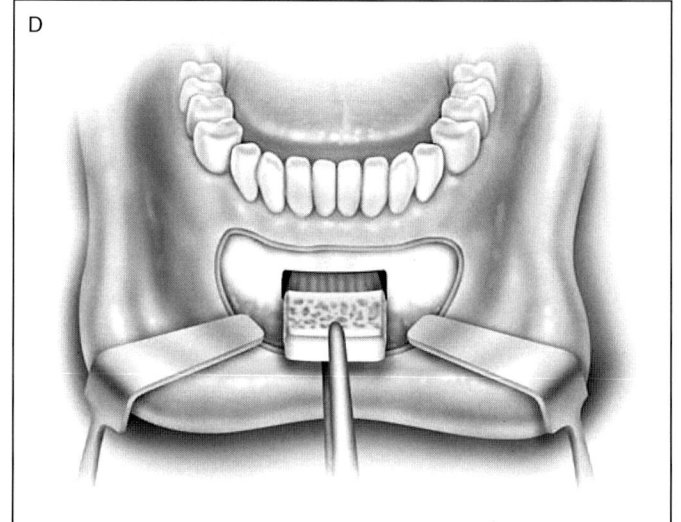

**Fig. 50.4** A–H, Multilevel surgery hyoid suspension with genioglossal advancement.

## Chapter 50 — Multilevel surgery with/without genioglossal advancement

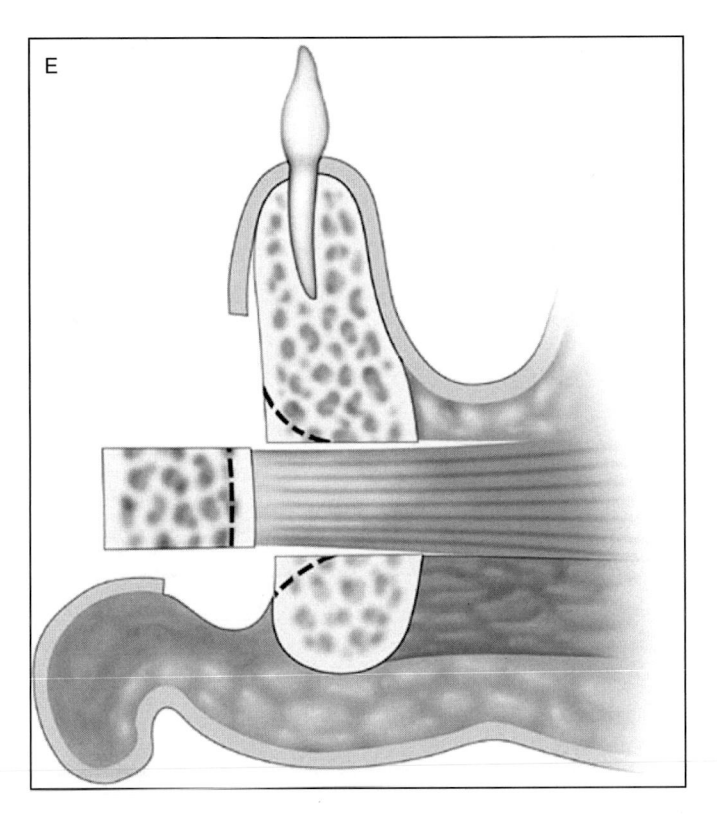

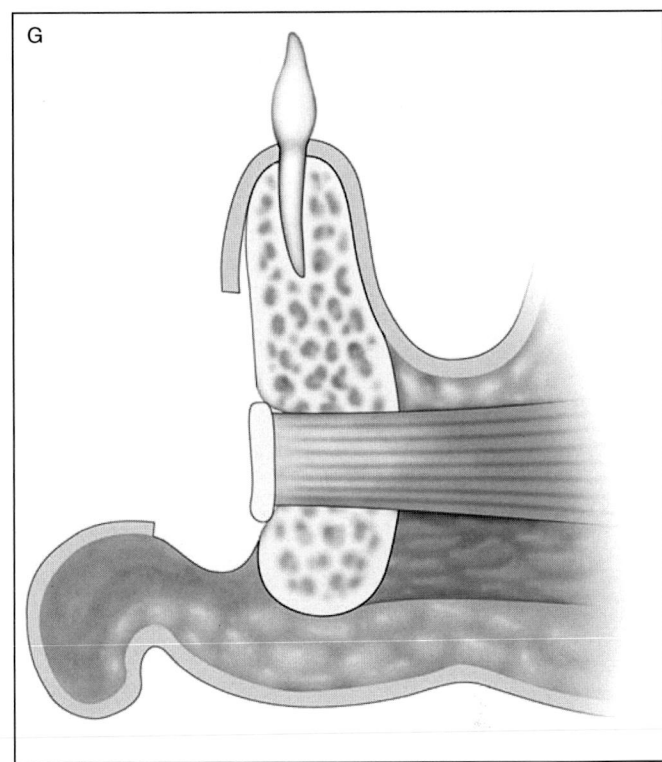

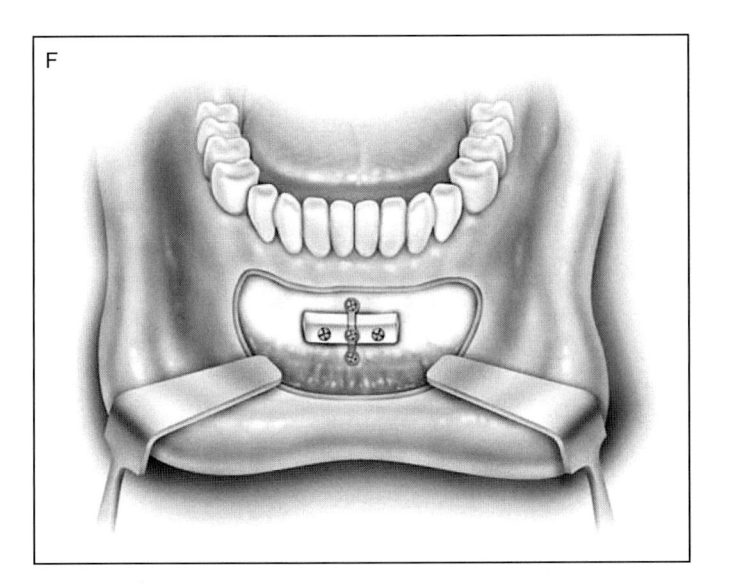

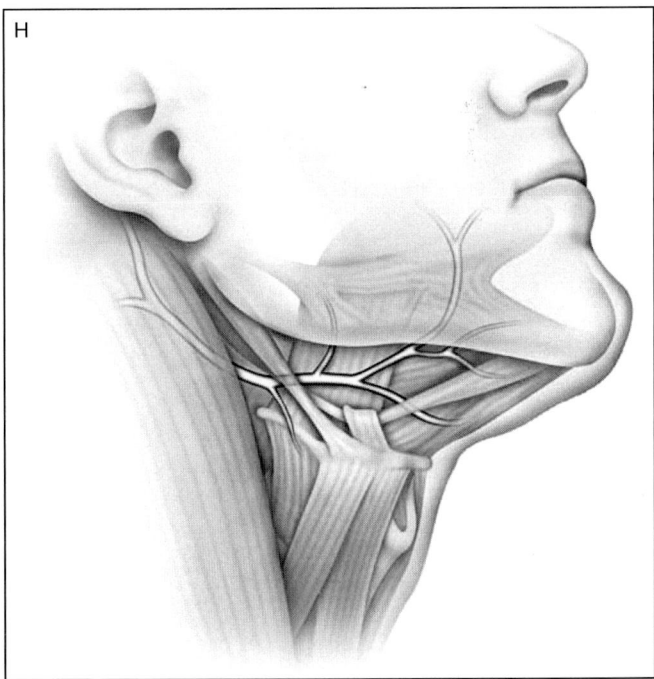

**Fig. 50.4** (Continued)

orally for one week postoperatively. Oral painkillers were administered. Steroids were not used routinely. Patients were usually discharged 48–72 hours postoperatively.

## 4.1 STATISTICS

Changes in parameters before and after intervention were compared by means of a Wilcoxon signed rank test (paired analyses). Differences in parameters between interventions (with or without genioglossal advancement) were tested with a Wilcoxon rank sum test. For the binomial proportions (responses) exact 95% confidence intervals were calculated.

## 5 RESULTS

Twenty-two patients underwent multilevel surgery, 14 with genioglossal advancement and eight without. Patient characteristics are shown in Table 50.1. Between the groups with and without genioglossal advancement, there were no significant preoperative differences in AHI, AHI supine, Desaturation Index (DI), Body Mass Index (BMI), total sleeping time (TST), Epworth Sleepiness Scale (ESS) and Visual analogue score (VAS) scores. Also in treatment outcome there were no significant differences.

The mean AHI for the total group decreased significantly from 48.7 (range 17.4–100.9) to 28.8 (diff 19.9, SD 18.5, $P < 0.0001$). Surgical success, defined as AHI < 20 and >50% reduction in AHI, was seen in 45% (95% CI 24–68%) of patients. Reduction of AHI between 20% and 50%, response rate, was seen in 16 patients (27%). The overall response rate was 72% (95% CI 49–89).

Dividing patients into three groups on the basis of the AHI, the success rates decreased with increasing AHI (Table 50.2). The success rates of patients with an AHI < 55 and >55 were 56% and 0% respectively. Overall, four patients increased in AHI after surgery. The AHI in supine position decreased significantly from 63.3 to 35.6 ($P = 0.0055$). The DI decreased from 31.9 to 17.6 ($P < 0.0001$). In 83.3% of the patients without surgical success the DI did increase. In Figures 50.5 and 50.6 the relative differences in AHI and DI pre- and post-surgery for each patient are shown respectively.

We did not see differences in preoperative BMI (range 23.8–39) between the successful group and the non-successful group. BMI and TST did not change substantially before and after surgery (respectively $P = 0.2292$ and $P = 0.3855$).

Hypersomnolence during daytime and snoring complaints pre- and postoperatively decreased from 8.6 to 3.6 ($P < 0.0001$) and 8.6 to 3.8 ($P < 0.0001$) respectively. The Epworth Sleepiness Scale improved significantly from 7.4 to 3.9 ($P < 0.0001$).

Table 50.1  Baseline characteristics

| Measurement | Total subjects ($n = 22$) |
|---|---|
| Age (years) | 50.3 ± 7.7 |
| BMI (kg/m$^2$) | 27.7 ± 3.4 |
| AHI | 48.7 ± 19.7 |
| Ratio male : female | 20 : 2 |

BMI: Body Mass Index; AHI: Apnea/Hypopnea Index.

Table 50.2  Success rates on basis of preoperative AHI

| AHI | |
|---|---|
| <40 | 60 |
| 40–55 | 53.8 |
| >55 | 0 |

## 6 COMPLICATIONS

We did not encounter infection, postoperative hemorrhage, tongue base abscess, compromised airway, or velopharyngeal insufficiency postoperatively. Only one serious complication was seen: a long-lasting hypoglossal nerve paresis. It is unclear whether this was caused by the sutures around the hyoid used for hyoid suspension or by one of the lesions of the radiofrequency in the tongue.

## 7 DISCUSSION

A variety of interventions, both minimally invasive (RF of palate and tongue base) and surgical (UPPP, Z-PP, uvula-flap, laser glossectomy, hyoid suspension (HS), geniogossal advancement (GA)) have been reported as part of multi-level treatment in severe OSAS and NCPAP failure or non-acceptance, both staged and in one session. We decided to perform multilevel surgery (UPPP, RFTB, HS with/without GA) in one procedure. In a staged surgical procedure, patients are more prone to become discouraged in completing the advised treatment and will be treated only partly.

The application of this surgical approach has resulted in a success rate of 45% and overall response rate of 72%. In eight of the 22 patients we added GA to the UPPP, HS and RFTB. This was not designed as a randomized trial; GA simply became available to us. There were no differences between the groups with and without GA for AHI or BMI. Intriguingly, we found no difference in effect for

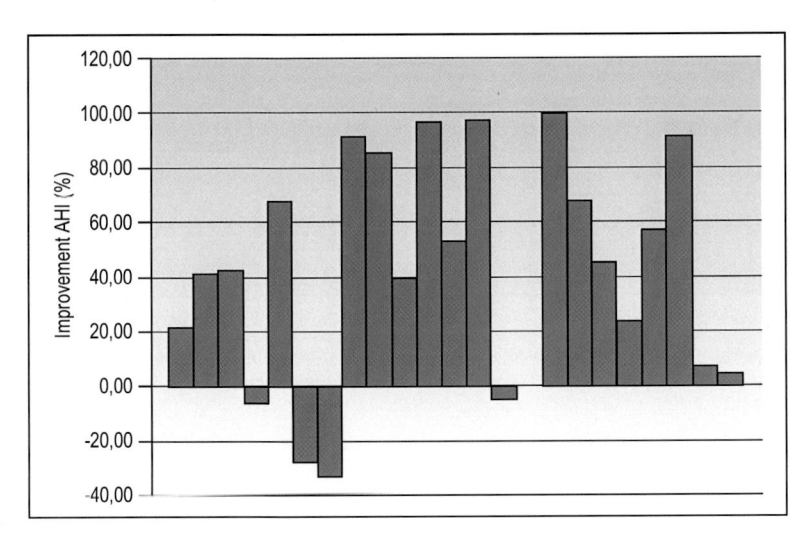

**Fig. 50.5** Relative difference in AHI pre- and post-surgery.

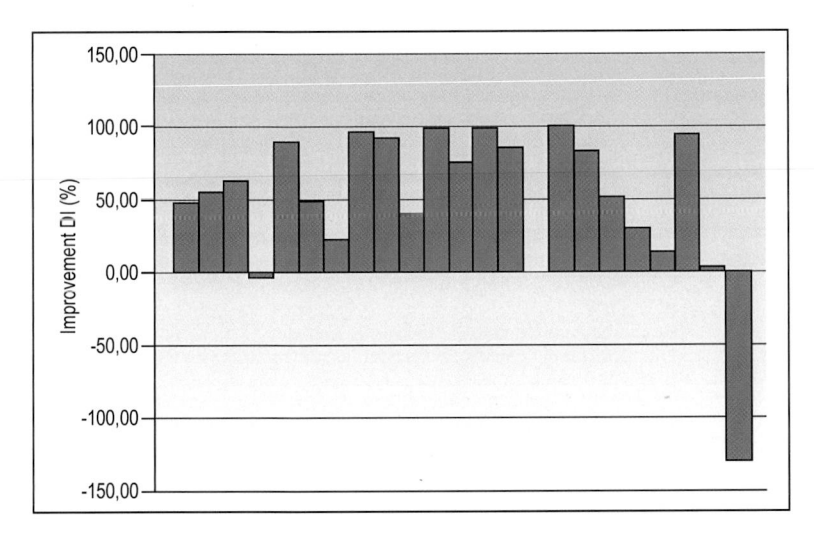

**Fig. 50.6** Relative difference in DI pre- and post-surgery.

the groups with and without GA. Since GA can have several complications such as mandible fracture and necrosis, hematomas and infection of the floor of mouth and injury of tooth roots, we presently tend to limit multilevel surgery to UPPP, HS and RFTB, although we are aware that positive results of GA have been reported in the literature (and are discussed elsewhere in this book).

Table 50.3 shows data of reported similar one-stage multilevel surgical interventions (at least UPPP and HS, but not UPPP and GA without HS), with success rates of 42–78% and overall response rates to approximately 73%. Differences in success rates are probably due to variations in study design and patient selection. The severity of OSAS preoperatively differs between the studies. The chance of surgical success is inversely related to the AHI: the higher the AHI preoperatively, the lower the success rate (Table 50.2). Also the definition of success is different between the studies.

For those patients for whom NCPAP therapy is no longer an option an alternative treatment is indicated and even when success (AHI reduction > 50%, below 20) is not reached, response (AHI reduction of 20–50%) can still be of significant value in terms of both increased quality of life and reduction in risk of morbidity and mortality. The sometimes significant discrepancy between subjective impressive improvement and subjective moderate improvement (reduction in AHI) in some patients remains fascinating.

In our series, the AHI of four patients increased after intervention. It is known that 56% of patients with sleep apnea syndrome are position dependent. Two of these four patients were positional and slept more in a supine position postoperatively. One patient had a subtotal nasal septal perforation – too large to attempt to close it – with decreased nasal passage. It is tempting to speculate that this might have played a role in the failure. Another patient had a significant weight gain of almost 10%, which may explain the postoperative higher AHI. Peppard et al. showed that a 10% weight gain predicts an approximate 32% increase in AHI.

## SECTION K — MULTILEVEL PHARYNGEAL SURGERY

**Table 50.3** Reported series on one-stage multilevel surgery, including at least HS and UPPP

| Authors | Procedure | N | AHI pre | AHI post | Success rate (%) | Response rate (%) | BMI |
| --- | --- | --- | --- | --- | --- | --- | --- |
| Riley et al. | UPPP, HS, GA | 223 | 48.3 | 9.5 | 60 | ? | 29.2 |
| Hsu and Brett | UPPP, HS, GA | 13 | 52.8 | 15.6 | 76.9 | ? | 31 |
| Datillo and Drooger | UPPP, HS, GA | 42 | 36.5 | 14.5 | 78 | ? | ? |
| Neruntarat | UPPP, HS, GA | 46 | 47.9 | 18.6 | 65.2 | ? | 27.1 |
| Verse et al. | UPPP, HS | 31 | 38.9 | 20.7 | 51 | 26 | 28 |
| Bowden et al. | HS, UPPP | 29 | | | 17 | | 34 |
| Present series | UPPP, HS, RFTB ± GA | 22 | 48.7 | 28.8 | 45 | 72 | 27.7 |

UPPP: uvulopalatopharyngoplasty; HS: hyoid suspension; GA: genioglossal advancement; RFTB: radiofrequent ablation tongue base; MMA: maxillomandibular advancement. Success rate was defined as AHI < 50% and AHI < 20 or equal with CPAP in Riley et al. and Hsu and Brett; in Neruntarat et al. as AHI < 50%; and AHI < 15 in Verse et al. and Datillo and Drooger.

When the success rate was elevated according to the severity based on preoperative AHI, there was a clear trend. No patients with an AHI > 55 met the criteria for success. Based on these experiences we have abandoned multilevel surgery (and thus the phased Stanford protocol) in patients with an AHI > 55–60. In these patients MMA is offered upfront, with tracheotomy in reserve as last refuge. The invasiveness of these modalities with significant morbidity indicates that these procedures should be kept for patients with an AHI above 55 as primary surgical treatment, and for non-responders to multilevel surgery with an AHI < 55.

We conclude that one-stage multilevel surgery, in which genioglossal advancement in our hands is not of additional value, can be a valuable addition to the therapeutic armamentarium and can be considered a viable alternative, objective as well as subjective, to NCPAP or as primary treatment in well-selected patients with severe OSAS with an AHI < 55.

## FURTHER READING

Bettega G, Pepin JL, Veale D, et al. Obstructive sleep apnea syndrome. Fifty-one consecutive patients treated by maxillofacial surgery. Am J Respir Crit Care Med 2000;162:641–9.

Bowden MT, Kezirian EJ, Utley D, Goode RL. Outcomes of hyoid suspension for the treatment of obstructive sleep apnea. Arch Otolaryngol Head Neck Surg 2005;131(5):440–45.

Datillo DJ, Drooger SA. Outcome assessment of patients undergoing maxillofacial procedures for the treatment of sleep apnea: comparison of subjective and objective results. J Oral Maxillofac Surg 2004;62:164–8.

Den Herder C, Kox D, van Tinteren H, de Vries N. Bipolar radiofrequency induced thermotherapy of the tongue base: its complications, acceptance and effectiveness under local anesthesia. Eur Arch Otorhinolaryngol 2006;263:1031–40.

Hsu PP, Brett RH. Multiple level pharyngeal surgery for obstructive sleep apnoea. Singapore Med J 2001;42(4):160–64.

Li KK, Powell NB, Riley RW, Troell R, Guilleminault C. Overview of phase I surgery for obstructive sleep apnea syndrome. Ear Nose Throat J 1999;78(11):836–7, 841–5.

Neruntarat C. Genioglossus advancement and hyoid myotomy: short-term and long-term results. J Laryngol Otol 2003;117(6):482–6.

Oksenberg A, Silverberg DS, Arons E, Radwan H. Positional vs. nonpositional obstructive sleep apnea patients. Chest 1997;112:629–39.

Peppard PE, Young T, Palta M, et al. Longitudinal study of moderate weight change and sleep-disordered breathing. JAMA 2000;284:3015–21.

Richard W, Kox D, den Herder C, et al. The role of sleep position in obstructive sleep apnea syndrome. Eur Arch Otolaryngol 2006;263:946–50.

Riley RW, Powell NB, Guilleminault C. Obstructive sleep apnea and the hyoid: a revised surgical procedure. Otolaryngol Head Neck Surg 1994;111(6):717–21.

Riley RW, Powell NB, Guilleminault C. Obstructive sleep apnea syndrome: a review of 306 consecutively treated surgical patients. Otolaryngol Head Neck Surg 1993;108(2):117–25.

Stuck BA, Köpke J, Maurer JT, et al. Lesion formation in radiofrequency surgery of the tongue base. Laryngoscope 2003;113:1572–6.

Verse T, Baisch A, Maurer JT, Stuck BA, Hörmann K. Multi-level surgery for obstructive sleep apnea. Short-term results. Otolaryngol Head Neck Surg 2006;134:571–7.

Vilaseca I, Morillo A, Monserrat JM, et al. Usefulness of uvulopalatopharyngoplasty with genioglossus and hyoid advancement in the treatment of obstructive sleep apnea. Arch Otolaryngol Head Neck Surg 2002;128:435–40.

SECTION K   MULTILEVEL PHARYNGEAL SURGERY

# CHAPTER 51

# Hyo-mandibular suspension and hyoid expansion for obstructive sleep apnea

*Yosef P. Krespi*

## 1 INTRODUCTION

Upper airway obstruction results from excess and/or collapse of soft tissue in the soft palate, tonsillar pillars, tongue, tongue base, and hypopharyngeal walls. Specific anatomic risk factors predisposing to obstructive sleep apnea/hypopnea syndrome (OSAHS) include long soft palate, shallow palatal arches, large tongue base, narrow mandibular arches, and mandibular hypoplasia.[1] Other general anatomic factors often associated with OSAHS include obesity, large Body Mass Index (BMI), shortened thick neck, anterior larynx location, enlarged tonsils and/or adenoids, lingual tonsils, thickened pharyngeal walls, elongated uvula, redundant soft palate, large tongue volume, deviated nasal septum, turbinate hypertrophy, and redundant or folded epiglottis.[2] Cephalometric studies employing computed tomography (CT) have correlated increased OSAHS severity with increased BMI, larger tongue and soft palate volumes, and decreased airway space.[3] Diagnostically, Fujita employed endoscopy with the Mueller maneuver (reverse Valsalva) to identify sites of obstruction in the nasopharynx, oropharynx and hypopharynx.[4] Three general profile types were identified based on the predominant areas of obstruction: Type I – retropalatal/velopharyngeal; Type II – retropalatal/velopharyngeal and hypopharyngeal; and Type III – hypopharyngeal. Catheter pressure transducers employed in OSA sleep studies have shown that upper airway collapse occurred at the velopharyngeal/retropalatal level and the hypopharyngeal/postlingual level in comparable frequencies.[5]

The grading system most commonly used to identify retrolingual obstruction is the Friedman tongue position (FTP) (see Chapter 16). Patients with FTP III and IV have a likelihood of retrolingual obstruction contributing to OSAHS.

## 2 OPERATIVE PROCEDURES

### 2.1 HYO-MANDIBULAR SUSPENSION

In the event of severe OSAHS, a hyoid expansion and hyo-mandibular suspension procedure is performed. These surgical methods enhance the anterior superior repositioning of the tongue base, enlarge the pharyngeal airway in a lateral dimension and partially separate the tongue base from the lower airway by an infrahyoid myotomy. Hyoid expansion and hyo-mandibular suspension/myotomy may be performed in conjunction with or following transoral or transcervical tongue suspension.

The anterior neck is prepped and draped. The anterior mandible, hyoid and the thyroid cartilages are then outlined with a skin marker with the neck slightly extended. Lidocaine with epinephrine 1:100,000 is injected into the planned incision sites. Two 0.5 cm incisions are made under the chin off the midline and using blunt dissection, the soft tissues overlying the mandible are cleaned. After insertion of the first screw using the Repose device (Influent, Concord, NH), the screw inserter is loaded with a new spare screw and the inserter is positioned perpendicular to the mandible, firm pressure applied and the screw is inserted into the inferior edge of the mandible. A loop of #1 polypropylene suture is already preloaded to the screw by the manufacturer (Fig. 51.1).

A second horizontal incision is made over the body of the hyoid measuring 5–6 cm. Subcutaneous fatty adipose tissue can be dissected and removed. Electrocautery is used to separate the infrahyoid muscles from the body of the hyoid bone. A single bone hook is placed to retract and stabilize the hyoid during the dissection. The sternohyoid and thyrohyoid muscles are detached from the body of the hyoid between the lesser cornuae (Fig. 51.2). Careful

# SECTION K: MULTILEVEL PHARYNGEAL SURGERY

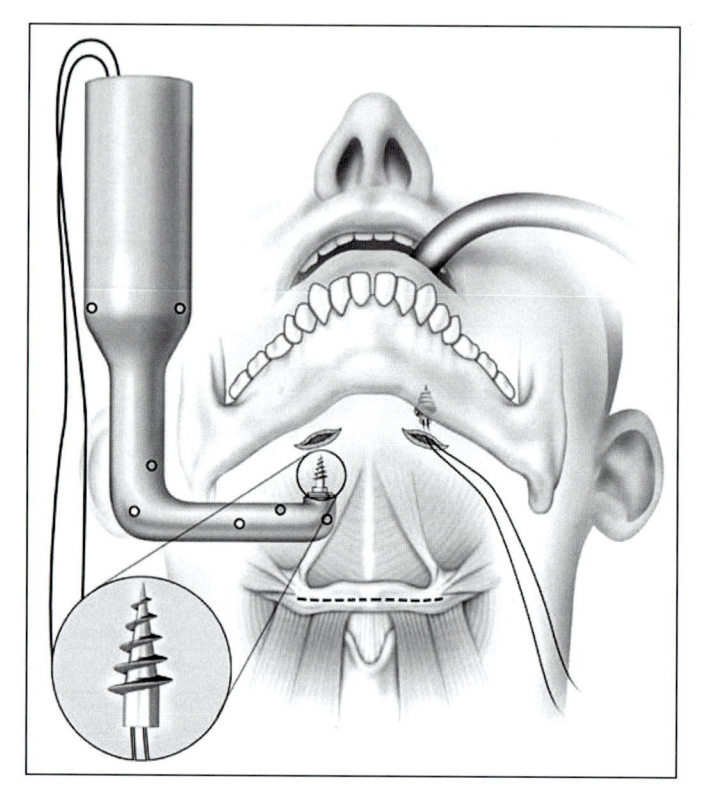

**Fig. 51.1** Insertion of two Repose screws to the mental area of the mandible via stab incision. Insert shows details of the screw with preloaded suture.

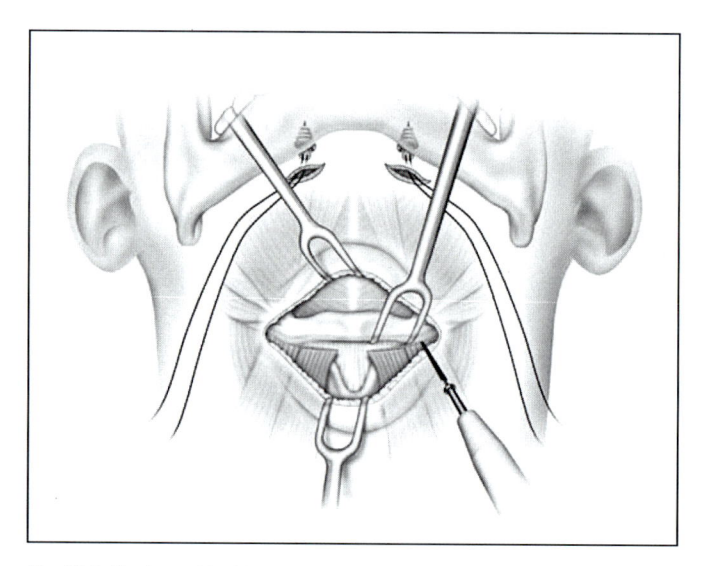

**Fig. 51.2** Horizontal incision exposing the body of the hyoid, separation of infrahyoid muscle with electrocautery.

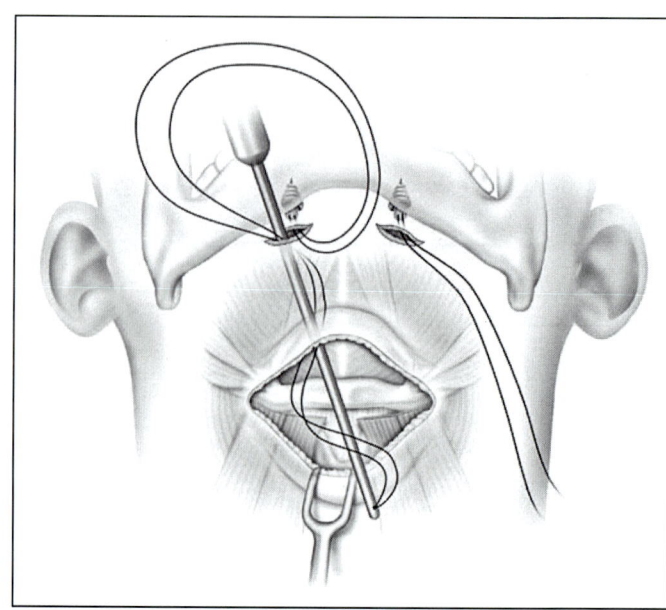

**Fig. 51.3** Delivery of sutures to the lower incision with a suture passer.

dissection around the body of the hyoid eliminates risk of injury to the neurovascular structures. Careful dissection and good hemostasis are mandatory to avoid injury to the pre-epiglottic fat pad. The suture passer is then loaded with the polypropylene suture and tunneled at the subplatysma layer from the mandibular incisions into the lower (hyoid) incision (Fig. 51.3). The suture passer is then removed. One free end of the polypropylene suture is then loaded into a Mayo needle and is passed through the suprahyoid muscles, catching a full thickness bite of the tissue.

## 2.2 HYOID DISTRACTION AND EXPANSION

When the hypopharyngeal airway needs to be enlarged in a lateral direction, as determined by preoperative fiberoptic endoscopy, the hyoid bone is then divided in the midline (hyoid distraction) (Fig. 51.4). Following the division of the hyoid bone the polypropylene suture is passed around both sides of the divided edges in a figure of eight configuration (Fig. 51.5). The distracted hyoid segments are then prepared for suspension toward the mandible. In order to maintain stability of the two hyoid segments an absorbable or non-absorbable rigid or semirigid implant can be placed to keep the two ends of the divided hyoid in expansion (hyoid expansion) (Fig. 51.6).

The two ends of the polypropylene suture are then tied together to achieve a superior anterior pull of the hyoid and tongue base. The inferior wound is drained and both wounds are closed in layers.

All patients were admitted for close observation overnight. Perioperative and postoperative care includes steroids, intravenous antibiotics, anti-reflux medications, humidified oxygen, intravenous fluids, nasal trumpet, and pulse oximetry monitoring.

# Hyo-mandibular suspension and hyoid expansion for OSA

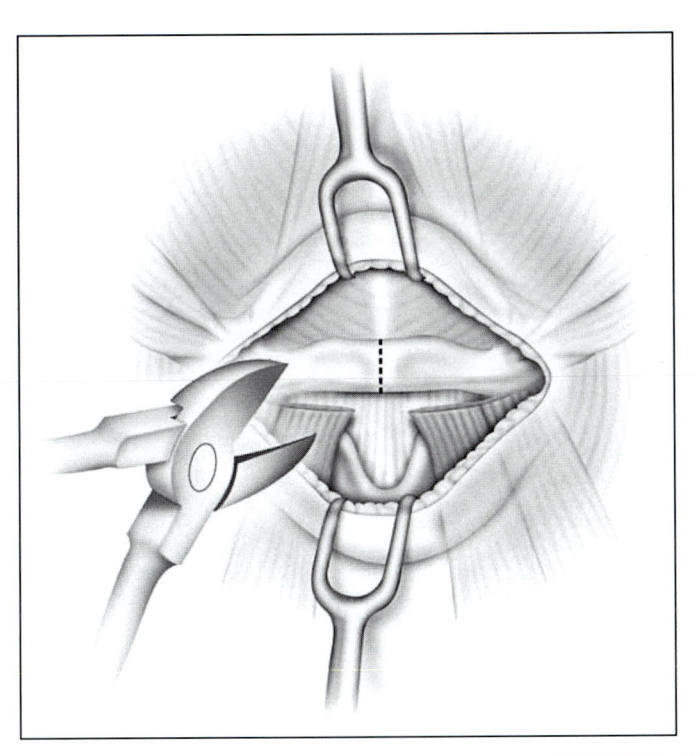

**CHAPTER 51**

**Fig. 51.4** Hyoid distraction, division of the hyoid body in the midline after myotomy using a bone cutter or chisel.

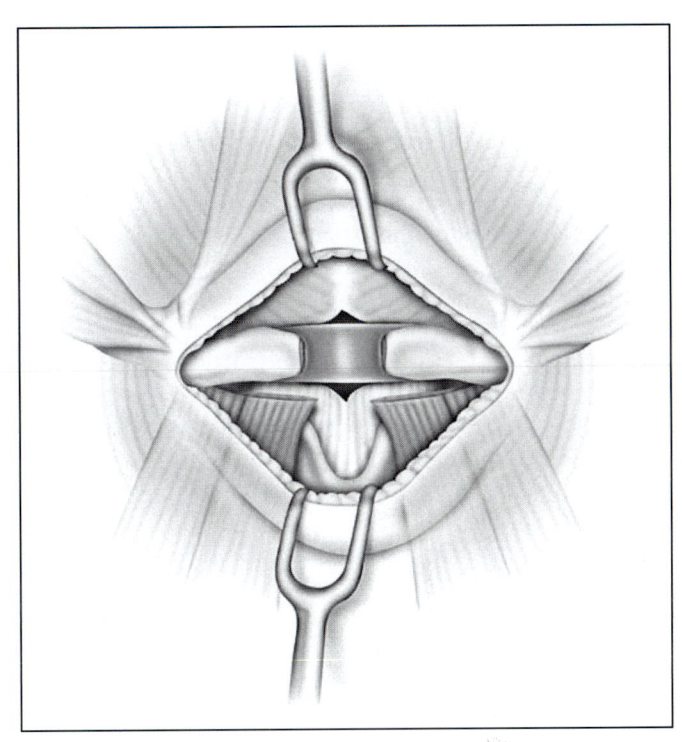

**Fig. 51.6** Hyoid spacer between the two cut ends of the bone, using non-absorbable graft. Hyoid expansion.

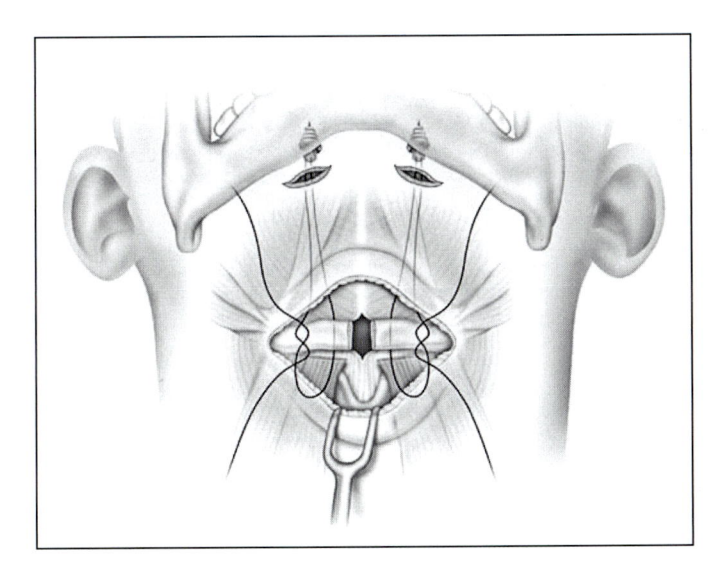

**Fig. 51.5** Division of the hyoid bone in the midline and suspension of the hyoid segments toward the mandible by figure of eight sutures.

## 3 RESULTS

The most common postoperative patient complaints included dysphagia, odynophagia and surgical wound pain. All patients were able to tolerate liquids and a soft diet at the time of discharge. No patients requested or required removal of the suspension sutures.

After 3–12 months of follow-up postoperatively, over 90% of the patients were subjectively improved by patient and/or spouse history. Symptomatic improvement included decrease in snoring, improved quality of sleep, and decreased daytime somnolence. Follow-up polysomnographic studies were performed 3 months to 1 year postoperatively in 52 patients. The patients that underwent hyo-mandibular suspension with or without hyoid expansion showed significant improvement in the mean Respiratory Disturbance Index (RDI) from 71.2 (+/−18.0) preoperatively to 28.4 (+/−16.8) postoperatively.

## 4 DISCUSSION

The most important part of surgical treatment of OSAHS is making a correct diagnosis of the site(s) of obstruction. The difficulty with OSAHS and tongue base obstruction has been the poor ability to grade severity and predict surgical success.

The advantages of the hyoid expansion and suspension are multi-fold. The splitting of the hyoid allows for potential lateral widening of the hypopharyngeal airway. Division of the infrahyoid musculature allows partial separation of the larynx from the hyoid and tongue base. This incomplete laryngeal drop can keep the inferior pulling force of intrathoracic structures from the hypopharyngeal structures separate. The negative pressures that occur

323

during the inspiration phase of respiration in an OSA patient can significantly contribute to further collapsing the flaccid structures of the upper airway.

Potential complications of hyoid suspension and expansion include airway obstruction, prolonged odynophagia, speech problems, neck hematoma, wound infection and intense cervical pain. Our experience, however, has shown very few problems. Pain and dysphagia/odynophagia are the most common complaints, but have all resolved in reasonable time. Patients with prolonged dysphagia/odynophagia may benefit from instructions on a modified supraglottic swallow (tongue push and elevation with throat clearing) as mentioned by Woodson and Fujita.[6,7] It is important to note that there were no airway or bleeding problems in the perioperative period. There were no suture or equipment problems either.

We have found that hyo-mandibular suspension and hyoid distraction–expansion procedures for tongue base obstruction have an important place in the surgical correction of tongue base and hypopharyngeal collapse in patients with severe OSA. We prefer this relatively minor external procedure over multiple stage transoral thermal ablation of the tongue base. Hyoid expansion with interposition of a semirigid spacer implant is the only surgical method that potentially enlarges the pharyngeal airspace in a lateral direction.

## REFERENCES

1. Rojewski TE, Schuller DE, Clarke RW, et al. Video-endoscopic determination of the mechanisms of obstruction in obstructive sleep apnea. Otolaryngol Head Neck Surg 1984;92:127–31.
2. Chervin RD, Guilleminault C. Obstructive sleep apnea and related disorders. Neurol Clin 1996;14(3):583–609.
3. Lowe AA, Fleetham JA, Adachi S, et al. Cephalometric and computed tomographic predictors of obstructive sleep apnea severity. Am J Orthod Dentofac Orthop 1995;107:589–95.
4. Fujita S. Pharyngeal surgery for obstructive sleep apnea and snoring. In: Snoring and Obstructive Sleep Apnea. Fairbanks DNF, et al, eds. Raven Press, New York; 1987, pp. 101–28.
5. Chaban R, Cole P, Hoffstein V. Site of upper airway obstruction in patients with idiopathic obstructive sleep apnea. Laryngoscope 1988;98:641–47.
6. Fujita S, Woodson BT, Clark J, et al. Laser midline glossectomy as a treatment for obstructive sleep apnea. Laryngoscope 1991;101:805–9.
7. Woodson BT, Fujita S. Clinical experiences with lingualplasty as part of the treatment of severe obstructive sleep apnea. Otolaryngol Head Neck Surg 1992;107:40–48.

## FURTHER READING

Aboussouan LS, Golish JA, Dinner DS, et al. Limitations and promise in the diagnosis and treatment of obstructive sleep apnoea. Respir Med 1997;91:181–91.

Chaban R, Cole P, Hoffstein V. Site of upper airway obstruction in patients with idiopathic obstructive sleep apnea. Laryngoscope 1988;98:641–47.

Chervin RD, Guilleminault C. Obstructive sleep apnea and related disorders. Neurol Clin 1996;14(3):583–609.

Crumley RL, Stein M, Gamsu G, et al. Determination of obstructive site in obstructive sleep apnea. Laryngoscope 1987;97:301–8.

DeRowe, A, Gunther, E, Fibbi, A, et al. Tongue-base suspension with a soft tissue-to-bone anchor for obstructive sleep apnea: preliminary clinical results of a new minimally invasive technique. Otolaryngol Head Neck Surg 2000;122:100–3.

Fujita S. Pharyngeal surgery for obstructive sleep apnea and snoring. In: Snoring and Obstructive Sleep Apnea. Fairbanks DNF, et al., eds. Raven Press, New York; 1987, pp. 101–28.

Fujita S, Conway W, Zorick F, et al. Surgical correction of anatomic abnormalities in obstructive sleep apnea syndrome: uvulopalatopharyngoplasty. Otolaryngol Head Neck Surg 1981;89:923–34.

Haraldsson P, Carenfelt C, Lysdahl M, et al. Long-term effect of uvulopalatopharyngoplasty on driving performance. Arch Otolaryngol Head Neck Surg 1995;121:90–94.

Kimmelam CP, Levine SB, Shore ET, et al. Uvulopalatopharyngoplasty: a comparison of two techniques. Laryngoscope 1985;95:1488–90.

Lowe AA, Gionhaku N, Takeuchi K, et al. Three-dimensional CT reconstructions of tongue and airway in adult subjects with obstructive sleep apnea. Am J Orthod Dentofac Orthop 1986;90:364–74.

Lowe AA, Fleetham JA, Adachi S, et al. Cephalometric and computed tomographic predictors of obstructive sleep apnea severity. Am J Orthod Dentofac Orthop 1995;107:589–95.

National Commission on Sleep Disorders Research. A report of the National Commission on Sleep Disorders Research. Wake up America: A National Sleep Alert, vol 2. Washington, DC: US Government Printing Office 1995; p. 10.

Partinen M, Jamieson A, Guilleminault C. Long-term outcome for obstructive sleep apnea syndrome patients: mortality. Chest 1988;94:1200–1204.

Piccirillo JF, Gates GA, White DL, et al. Obstructive sleep apnea treatment outcomes pilot study. Otolaryngol Head Neck Surg 1998;118(6):833–44.

Pollack CP, Chervin RD, Weitzman ED. Symptomatic improvement in 34 of 40 cases of severe hypersomnia–sleep apnea syndrome treated by tracheoplasty. Sleep Res 1982;11:163–66.

Rapoport DM, Garay SM, Goldring RM. Nasal CPAP in obstructive sleep apnea: mechanisms of action. Bull Eur Physiopath Resp 1983;19:616–20.

Riley R, Guilleminault C, Powell N, et al. Palatopharyngoplasty failure cephalometric roentgenograms and obstructive sleep apnea. Otolaryngol Head Neck Surg 1985;93:240–50.

Riley RW, Powell NB, Guilleminault C, et al. Maxillary mandibular and hyoid advancement: an alternative to tracheostomy in obstructive sleep apnea syndrome. Otolaryngol Head Neck Surg 1986;94:584–88.

Riley RW, Powell NB, Guilleminault C. Inferior sagittal osteotomy of the mandible with hyoid myotomy–suspension: a new procedure for obstructive sleep apnea. Otolaryngol Head Neck Surg 1986;94:589–93.

Riley RW, Powell NB, Guilleminault C. Maxillofacial surgery and obstructive sleep apnea: a review of 80 patients. Otolaryngol Head Neck Surg 1989;101:353–61.

Riley RW, Powell NB, Guilleminault C. Maxillary mandibular and hyoid advancement for treatment of obstructive sleep apnea syndrome: a review of 40 patients. J Oral Maxillofac Surg 1990;48:20–26.

Riley RW, Powell NB, Guilleminault C. Obstructive sleep apnea syndrome: a review of 306 consecutively treated surgical patients. Otolaryngol Head Neck Surg 1993;108:117–25.

Riley RW, Powell NB, Guilleminault C. Obstructive sleep apnea syndrome: a surgical protocol for dynamic upper airway reconstruction. J Oral Maxillofac Surg 1993;51:742–47.

Riley RW, Powell NB, Guilleminault C. Obstructive sleep apnea and the hyoid: a revised surgical procedure. Otolaryngol Head Neck Surg 1994;111:717–21.

Rojewski TE, Schuller DE, Clarke RW, et al. Video-endoscopic determination of the mechanisms of obstruction in obstructive sleep apnea. Otolaryngol Head Neck Surg 1984;92:127–31.

Rubin A-HE, Eliaschar I, Joachim Z, et al. Effects of nasal surgery and tonsillectomy on sleep apnea. Bull Eur Physiopath Resp 1983;19:612–15.

Shepard JW, Thawley SE. Localization of upper airway collapse during sleep in patients with obstructive sleep apnea. Am Rev Respir Dis 1990;141:1350–55.

Sher AE, Thorpy AJ, Shprintzen RJ, et al. Predictive value of Mueller maneuver in selection of patients for uvulopalatopharyngoplasty. Laryngoscope 1985;95:1483–87.

Sher AE, Schechtman KB, Piccirillo JF. The efficacy of surgical modifications of the upper airway in adults with obstructive sleep apnea syndrome. Sleep 1996;19:(2):156–77.

Terris DJ, Wang MZ. Laser-assisted uvulopalatoplasty in mild obstructive sleep apnea. Arch Otolaryngol Head Neck Surg 1998;124:718–20.

Waite WP, Wooten V, Lachner J, et al. Maxillomandibular advancement surgery in 23 patients with obstructive sleep apnea syndrome. J Oral Maxillofac Surg 1989;47:1256–61.

Woodson BT, Wooten MR. Comparison of upper-airway evaluations during wakefulness and sleep. Laryngoscope 1994;104:821–28.

Young T, Palta M, Dempsey J, et al. The occurrence of sleep-disordered breathing among middle-aged adults. N Engl J Med 1993;328:1230–5.

Zorick F, Roehrs T, Conway W, et al. Effects of uvulopalatopharyngoplasty on the daytime sleepiness associated with sleep apnea syndrome. Bull Eur Physiopath Resp 1983;19:600–3.

# SECTION L  MAXILLOFACIAL SURGICAL TECHNIQUES

## CHAPTER 52

# Maxillofacial surgical techniques for hypopharyngeal obstruction in obstructive sleep apnea

*Donald M. Sesso, Robert W. Riley and Nelson B. Powell*

## 1 INTRODUCTION

Due to poor patient acceptance of tracheostomy and incomplete treatment of obstructive sleep apnea syndrome (OSA) with palatal surgery, we have explored the use of maxillofacial surgical techniques to alleviate hypopharyngeal obstruction.[1,2] The aim of surgical treatment is to alleviate upper airway obstruction and its associated neurobehavioral symptoms and morbidities.[3,4] No longer is a 50% reduction in the Apnea/Hypopnea Index (AHI) deemed acceptable. Rather, the objective is to treat to cure (normalization of respiratory events and elimination of hypoxemia) and achieve outcomes that are equivalent to those of continuous positive airway pressure (CPAP).[5]

Selecting the appropriate surgery for a patient can be challenging. However, we have created a two-phase surgical protocol (Powell–Riley protocol) as a logically directed plan to treat the specific areas of upper airway obstruction.[6,7] It is imperative that a polysomnogram (PSG) be obtained after any surgery to determine efficacy. Genioglossus advancement and hyoid suspension are considered part of phase I surgery. These are conservative maxillofacial techniques which are often combined with nasal and palatal surgery, should multilevel obstruction exist. Phase II surgery refers to maxillomandibular advancement (MMO). This surgery is usually reserved for those patients who have been incompletely treated with phase I surgery and have documented hypopharyngeal obstruction. MMO is the only surgery which physically creates more room for the tongue by advancing both the mandible and maxilla.

## 2 PATIENT SELECTION

Proper selection of patients is paramount to achieve successful outcomes and to minimize postoperative complications. The presurgical evaluation requires a comprehensive medical history, head and neck examination, fiberoptic nasopharyngolaryngoscopy, radiographic cephalometric analysis and polysomnography (PSG). This systematic approach will aid in determining the severity of OSA and identifying probable anatomic sites of obstruction. Armed with this information, the surgeon can proceed with a site-specific surgical protocol.[8]

Since CPAP is considered the primary treatment of OSA, all patients should be offered this therapy prior to surgical intervention. While the efficacy of CPAP has been clearly documented, a subset of patients struggle to comply with CPAP therapy.[9] In fact, Kribbs et al. reported that only 6% of patients who receive CPAP therapy are able to tolerate the device for at least 7 hours per night on 70% of days.[10]

Typically, surgery is offered to patients with an AHI > 20. However, those patients whose AHI is less than 20 may still be candidates for surgery. Surgery is appropriate if these patients have associated excessive daytime sleepiness which alters daytime performance or comorbidities as recognized by the Center for Medicare and Medicaid Services (including ischemic heart disease and stroke). Certain factors exist which could portend a poor outcome and are considered relative contraindications to surgery. These factors include psychiatric instability, unrealistic expectations of outcome and unstable cardiovascular or pulmonary disease.

As with any surgery, ensuring that a patient is medically stable for the operative procedure is vital. This evaluation includes the appropriate cardiopulmonary, laboratory and radiographic testing. We recommend a comprehensive metabolic panel, complete blood count, thyroid stimulating hormone, electrocardiogram and chest x-ray. In patients with existing comorbid medical problems, consultation with the appropriate medical specialist should be sought.

Our protocol encourages all patients to use their CPAP for 2 weeks prior to surgery, particularly those patients with severe OSA (AHI > 40). Preoperative CPAP can alleviate the risks associated with sleep deprivation and postobstructive pulmonary edema. Furthermore, we recommend the insertion of a temporary tracheostomy in patients with an AHI > 60 and/or a SaO$_2$ < 70% who are intolerant of CPAP.[11]

Despite a thorough preoperative selection process, it is difficult to accurately predict outcomes for an individual patient. While MMO has documented success rates >90%, our studies have demonstrated that a substantial number of patients may not need such extensive surgery.[12–14] In fact, approximately 70% of our patients have obviated the need for MMO by undergoing phase I surgery.[12] Thus, we employ conservative maxillofacial surgical techniques (genioglossus advancement or hyoid suspension) to treat hypopharyngeal obstruction, before proceeding to MMO. There are cases in which MMO may be the initial surgery, as in non-obese patients with marked mandibular deficiency and a normal palate.

## 3 MANDIBULAR OSTEOTOMY WITH GENIOGLOSSUS ADVANCEMENT

When the preoperative evaluation implicates the base of tongue (Fujita Type II–III) as the source of airway obstruction, the genioglossus advancement (GA) procedure is indicated. This procedure is a conservative maxillofacial technique since the osteotomy is created without altering the dental occlusion. The rationale for the GA procedure is to place the primary protrusion muscle of the tongue, the genioglossus, under direct tension. This tension resists the collapse of the tongue into the airway that can occur with sleep-induced hypotonia.[15] Essentially, the genial tubercle and the attached genioglossus muscle are advanced anteriorly. The degree of advancement depends on the thickness of the anterior mandible and the compliance of the genioglossus muscle. Less muscle compliance will provide a greater degree of tension. Unfortunately, there is no objective preoperative study to determine the compliance of the genioglossus muscle.

Surgery may be performed under general anesthesia or, in appropriate cases, with the patient under intravenous sedation. An intraoral incision is made in the gingivolabial sulcus, taking care to preserve a cuff of mucosa to facilitate closure and prevent wound dehiscence. The incision extends between the canine dentition. Dissection is performed submucoperiosteally to expose the inferior border of the mandible. The floor of the mouth is palpated to identify the location of the genial tubercle. A rectangular osteotomy is then outlined along the outer cortex of the mandible with a 2-hole sagittal saw blade. The osteotomy is typically 9 mm × 20 mm in order to capture the genial tubercle. It is recommended that the superior osteotomy be placed at least 5 mm inferior to the root apices to avoid injury.[16] In addition, the inferior osteotomy should be approximately 8 mm above the inferior border of the mandible to avoid a potential fracture (Fig. 52.1). A titanium screw is inserted in the center of the osteotomy to allow manipulation of

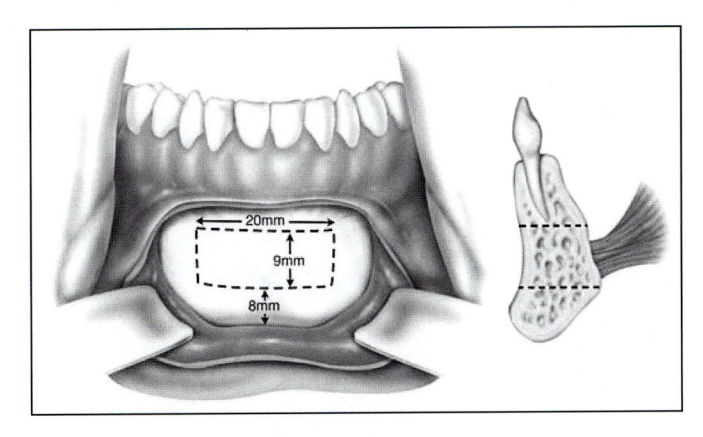

**Fig. 52.1** A 2-hole sagittal saw is used to create the rectangular osteotomy. The osteotomy is typically 9 × 20 mm. Care should be taken to protect the tooth roots. The inferior osteotomy is placed at least 8 mm above the inferior border of the mandible to prevent fracture. (From Terris DJ. Multilevel pharyngeal surgery for obstructive sleep apnea: indications and techniques. Operat Techn Otolaryngol Head Neck Surg 2000;11:12–20.)

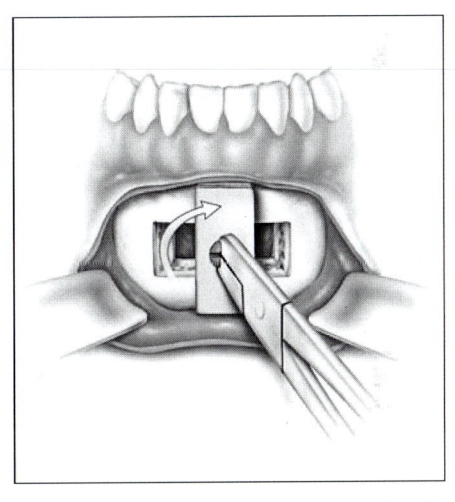

**Fig. 52.2** A, 2 mm screw is inserted in the outer cortex of the fragment. This screw allows manipulation of the fragment. The segment is displaced into the floor of the mouth and hemostasis is achieved. A screw grasping forceps is used to elevate the fragment from the osteotomy site. Steady pressure is applied while advancing the genial tubercle, without avulsing the genioglossus muscle. (From Terris DJ. Multilevel pharyngeal surgery for obstructive sleep apnea: Indications and techniques. Operat Tech Otolaryngol Head Neck Surg 2000;11:12–20.)

the fragment (Fig. 52.2). The cuts are then completed through the inner cortex. It is critical to maintain parallel walls while performing the osteotomies to prevent tapering of the inner cortex. The fragment is displaced into the floor of the mouth and hemostasis is achieved (Fig. 52.3). The titanium screw is then grasped and the bony fragment is gently advanced and rotated 90° in either direction (Fig. 52.4). The outer cortex and marrow are removed with the sagittal saw. A 10 mm × 2.0 mm titanium screw is used to fix the fragment to the mandible inferiorly (see Fig. 52.4).

SECTION L  MAXILLOFACIAL SURGICAL TECHNIQUES

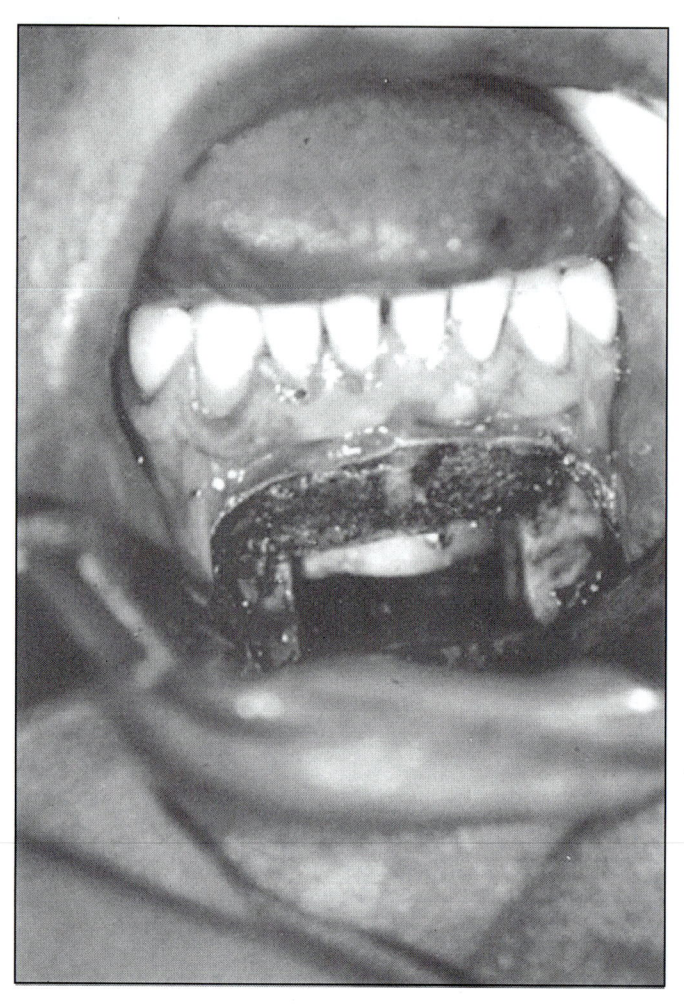

Fig. 52.3 Intraoperative view of the rectangular osteotomy. Note that the fragment has been displaced into the floor of the mouth to achieve hemostasis at the osteotomy site.

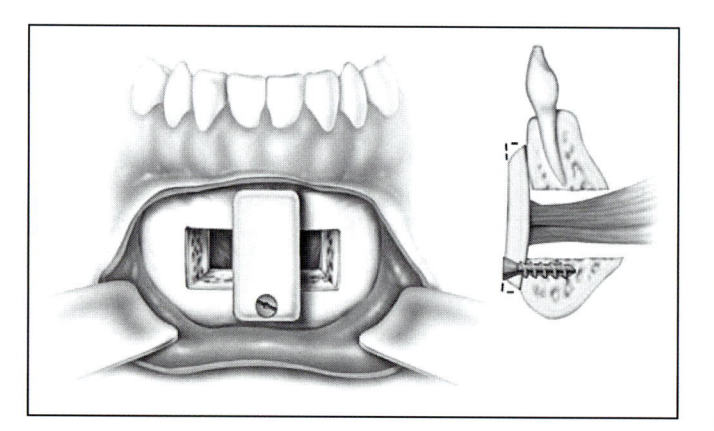

Fig. 52.4 The bone fragment has been rotated 90° to overlap the inferior border of the mandible. The outer cortex and medullary bone have been removed with a sagittal saw. A 10 mm × 2.0 mm titanium screw is used to secure the fragment to the lower border of the mandible. (From Terris DJ. Multilevel pharyngeal surgery for obstructive sleep apnea: indications and techniques. Operat Tech Otolaryngol Head Neck Surg 2000;11:12–20.)

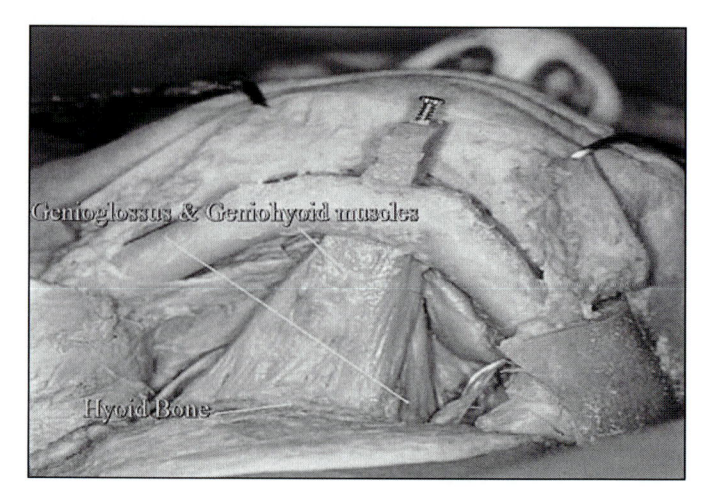

Fig. 52.5 Cadaver dissection demonstrating the tension placed on the genioglossus muscle by advancing the genial tubercle.

A pear-shaped cutting burr may be used to contour the bony fragment. Lastly, the wound is irrigated and closed with interrupted absorbable sutures (Fig. 52.5).

## 4 HYOID MYOTOMY WITH SUSPENSION

The surgical approach for hyoid suspension is similar to thyroglossal duct excision (Sistrunk procedure). Either general or local anesthesia may be utilized. A horizontal incision is placed at the level of the hyoid bone along a natural skin crease. Dissection is continued to expose the body of the hyoid. The infrahyoid musculature is detached. The stylohyoid ligament may need to be sectioned from the lesser cornu to allow adequate mobility, but the suprahyoid musculature remains intact. The strap muscles are divided in the midline to expose the thyroid cartilage (Fig. 52.6). An Allis clamp is placed on the body of the hyoid and the hyoid complex is advanced anteriorly. Constant traction is maintained on the hyoid bone. Three or four #1-0 permanent sutures are passed around the hyoid and through the superior aspect of the thyroid cartilage to advance and stabilize the hyoid bone (Fig. 52.7). Meticulous hemostasis is achieved. A drain is placed and the wound is closed in layers. Placement of a pressure dressing for 24 hours reduces the incidence of hematoma or seroma formation.

## 5 MAXILLOMANDIBULAR ADVANCEMENT OSTEOTOMY (MMO)

Diligent planning in the preoperative period is critical to achieve successful outcomes. Consequently, we fashion a methylmethacrylate splint several weeks prior to surgery

## Hypopharyngeal obstruction in obstructive sleep apnea  CHAPTER 52

and surgeon can expedite this process. 1% Lidocaine with 1:100,000 epinephrine is used to inject the maxillary vestibule and the gingivolabial sulcus overlying both the maxillary and mandibular arches. Vasoconstriction of the nasal mucosa is achieved by placing cottonoids soaked with 4% cocaine hydrochloride along the floor of the nose. The table is rotated 180° away from the anesthesiologist and the patient is sterilely prepped and draped.

Surgery begins with the application of arch bars to the maxillary and mandibular arches. The arch bars are secured to the dentition with 24-gauge wires. Rarely do we maintain patients in intermaxillary fixation (IMF) following surgery. Rather, IMF is utilized intraoperatively to ensure proper occlusion during rigid fixation of the advanced bone segments. In certain instances, a patient may have orthodontic brackets placed prior to surgery, thus precluding the need to place arch bars.

An incision is placed in the gingivolabial sulcus of the maxilla between the second molars. The periosteum is elevated with a periosteal elevator to visualize the root of the zygoma laterally. Care is taken to preserve the infraorbital nerve. A Freer elevator is used to elevate the periosteum of the piriform aperture and floor of the nose. Bleeding commonly occurs while elevating the soft tissue of the piriform aperture and nasal floor. Hemostasis is achieved by placing cottonoids in this dissection plane. The Le Fort I osteotomy is then performed. A reciprocating saw is inserted at the level of the piriform aperture and the osteotomy is carried laterally through the zygomatic maxillary crest to the pterygomaxillary suture. The osteotomy must be placed at a vertical height that will avoid the apices of the teeth. A fenestration is created in the anterior maxillary sinus wall with a pear-shaped cutting burr. This is performed at the level of the osteotomy. A thin osteotome is placed through this fenestration to cut the posterior and medial walls of the maxillary sinus. The osteotomy is completed by placing a curved osteotome into the pterygomaxillary suture to separate the maxilla from the pterygoid plates (Fig. 52.8). This process is completed on the contralateral aspect of the maxilla. An osteotome is used to separate the nasal septum from the maxillary crest. A 24-gauge wire is passed through the anterior nasal spine to allow manipulation of the maxilla. Using gentle, constant pressure the maxilla is down fractured. The descending palatine arteries are identified and, if possible, preserved. If necessary, the arteries may be ligated using vascular clips. Riley–Powell distraction forceps are utilized to mobilize the maxilla anteriorly. While mobilizing the attachments of the pterygoid plates, be careful not to tear the mucosa. It is critical to completely mobilize these attachments to allow for the 10–12 mm of advancement that is needed. The maxilla is advanced and rigid fixation is accomplished with two 24-gauge wires and two titanium mini plates (2.0 mm plates) on each side of the maxilla.

Attention is then turned to the mandible. Advancement is achieved by a sagittal split osteotomy. An incision is

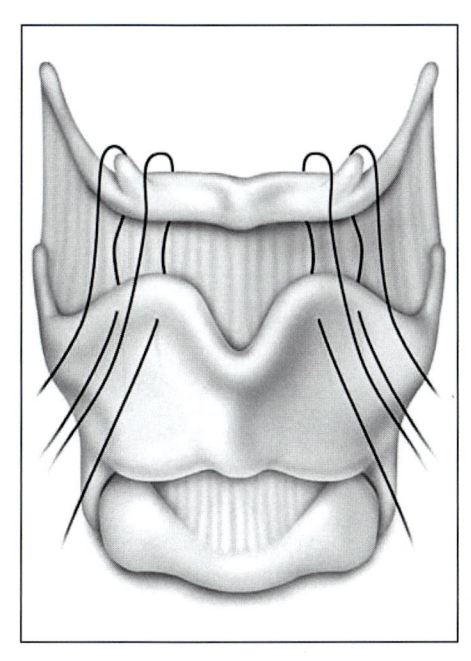

**Fig. 52.6** A horizontal incision is placed over the hyoid bone. The body of the hyoid and the superior border of the thyroid cartilage are skeletonized. The infrahyoid muscles are released.

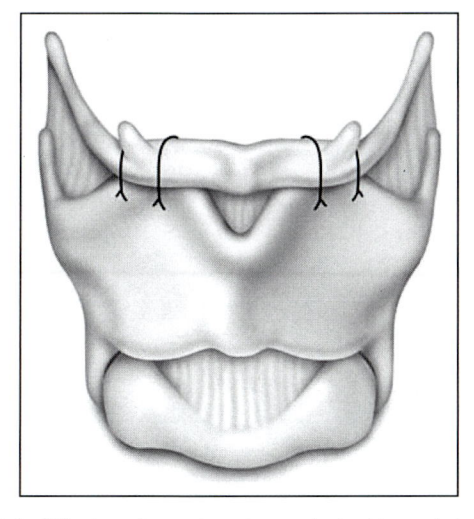

**Fig. 52.7** An Allis clamp is used to advance the hyoid anteriorly. #1.0 Ticron sutures are passed around the body of the hyoid and secured to the superior border of the thyroid cartilage. Usually, four sutures are placed; however, a small thyroid cartilage may only allow placement of three sutures.

to maintain proper dental occlusion postoperatively. Furthermore, we ask all patients to provide one unit of autologous blood in case a transfusion is needed. The surgery is performed under general anesthesia via nasotracheal intubation. It is essential that the surgeon be present during induction of anesthesia in case an airway emergency arises. Frequently, sleep apnea patients can be difficult to intubate, so proper communication between the anesthesiologist

SECTION L  MAXILLOFACIAL SURGICAL TECHNIQUES

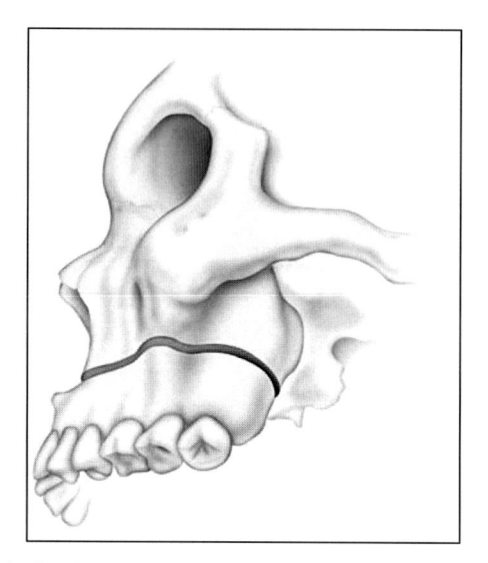

**Fig. 52.8** Le Fort I osteotomy. The osteotomy is placed superior to the apices of the teeth. A curved osteotome is placed into the pterygomaxillary suture to separate the maxilla from the pterygoid plates. The descending palatine arteries are identified and preserved.

made in the mucosa along the external oblique ridge. The incision extends from the third molar to the first molar. Dissection is carried down to the periosteum. The periosteum is reflected to expose the medial and lateral aspects of the mandibular ramus. A V-shaped retractor is used to reflect the periosteum and the muscular attachments of the mandible superiorly to the level of the coronoid process. Subperiosteal dissection continues along the medial border of the ramus in order to identify the lingula. A nerve hook can be used to palpate for the lingula, if it cannot be easily visualized. Identification of the lingula allows one to protect the inferior alveolar neurovascular bundle. A pear-shaped cutting burr is used to create a trough just above and lateral to the lingula (Fig. 52.9). This permits the insertion of a reciprocating saw which carries the sagittal osteotomy to the level of the first molar. Care is taken to stay 5 mm lateral to the molar teeth to prevent injury to the roots. Only the outer cortex is cut with the reciprocating saw. The vertical osteotomy is performed along the inferior border of the mandible at the mesial surface of the first molar with a fissure burr. A channel retractor is very effective in retracting and protecting the soft tissue along the inferior border of the mandible. It is recommended that both the inner and outer cortices of the mandible are cut at the inferior border. Both cortices are cut for approximately 5 mm, at which point the cut only includes the outer cortex as the vertical osteotomy meets the sagittal component (Fig. 52.10). The osteotomy is then completed using osteotomes to gently separate the medial and lateral segments. Once again, the inferior alveolar nerve must be identified and preserved. If necessary, the nerve may need to be dissected from its canal to allow advancement of the distal segment. After a sagittal split osteotomy is performed on

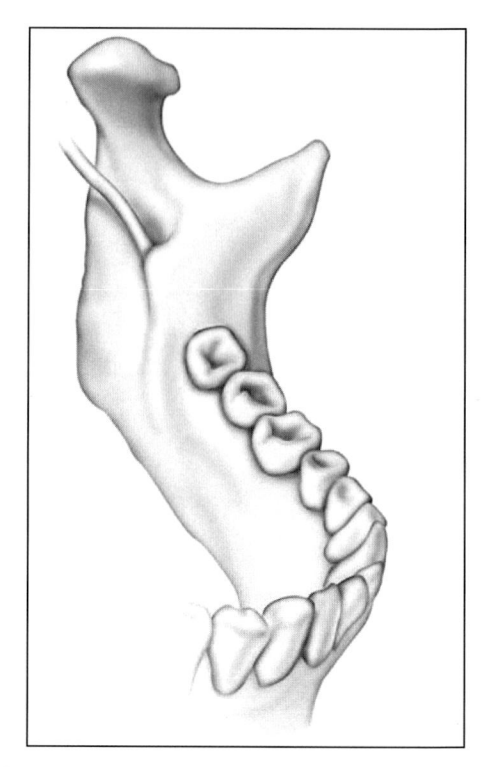

**Fig. 52.9** View of the lingula of the mandible and the inferior alveolar neurovascular bundle. A pear-shaped cutting burr creates a trough above and lateral to the lingula. This permits insertion of the reciprocating saw to begin the sagittal split osteotomy.

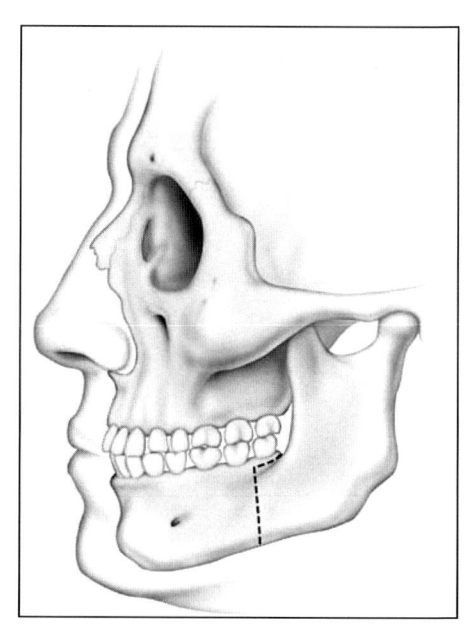

**Fig. 52.10** Outline of sagittal split osteotomy. It is essential to ensure that both the inner and outer cortices of the inferior border of the mandible are cut prior to completing the split.

the contralateral aspect of the mandible, the distal segments can be advanced. The dental splint, which was fashioned preoperatively, is inserted to ensure proper occlusion. IMF is accomplished with 24-gauge stainless steel wires.

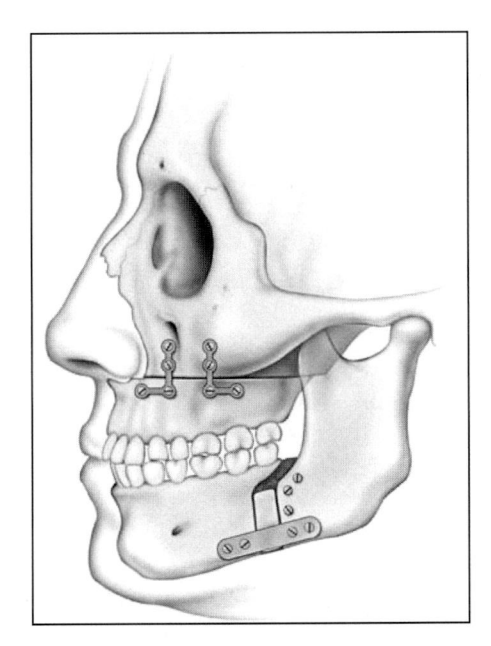

## CHAPTER 52
### Hypopharyngeal obstruction in obstructive sleep apnea

**Fig. 52.11** Maxillomandibular advancement osteotomy with rigid fixation. 2.0 mm titanium plates are used to fix the maxilla. Fixation of the mandible is achieved with bicortical screws and 2.3 mm plates inserted along the inferior border of the mandible.

Rigid fixation is achieved with percutaneous bicortical titanium screws placed in the proximal segments. Additionally, 2.3 mm titanium plates are used to rigidly fix the advanced distal segments of the mandible (Figs 52.11 and 52.12). The IMF wires are released and the patient's occlusion is evaluated. If the occlusion is not correct, the fixation hardware will need to be readjusted to correct this problem. Previously harvested bone grafts may be placed in the osteotomy sites, if the surgeon deems this necessary. Cranial bone grafts may be used; however, more recently, we have been using bone grafts obtained from the maxilla. This reduces the operative time and potential morbidity associated with harvesting cranial bone grafts.[17] All intraoral incisions are closed with interrupted 4-0 Vicryl. The percutaneous incisions are closed with interrupted 5-0 chromic. Rubber bands may be placed on the arch bars to limit jaw opening in the early postoperative period. The upper aerodigestive tract is suctioned. A head wrap is placed for 24 hours to prevent hematoma formation. Finally, the anesthesia is reversed but the patient is not extubated until it is clear that they have the ability to maintain their airway.

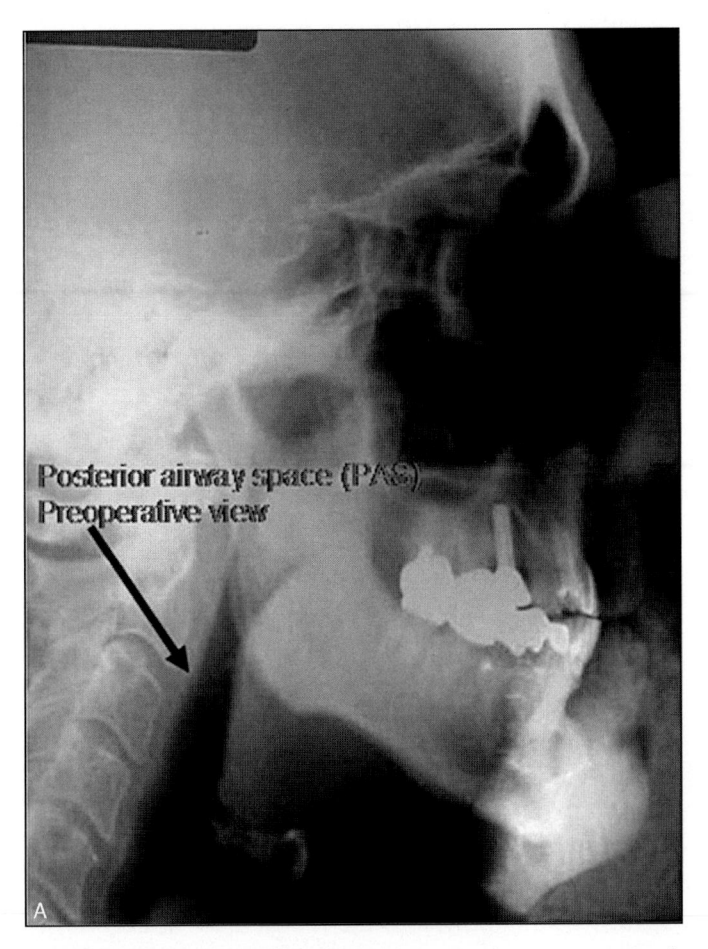

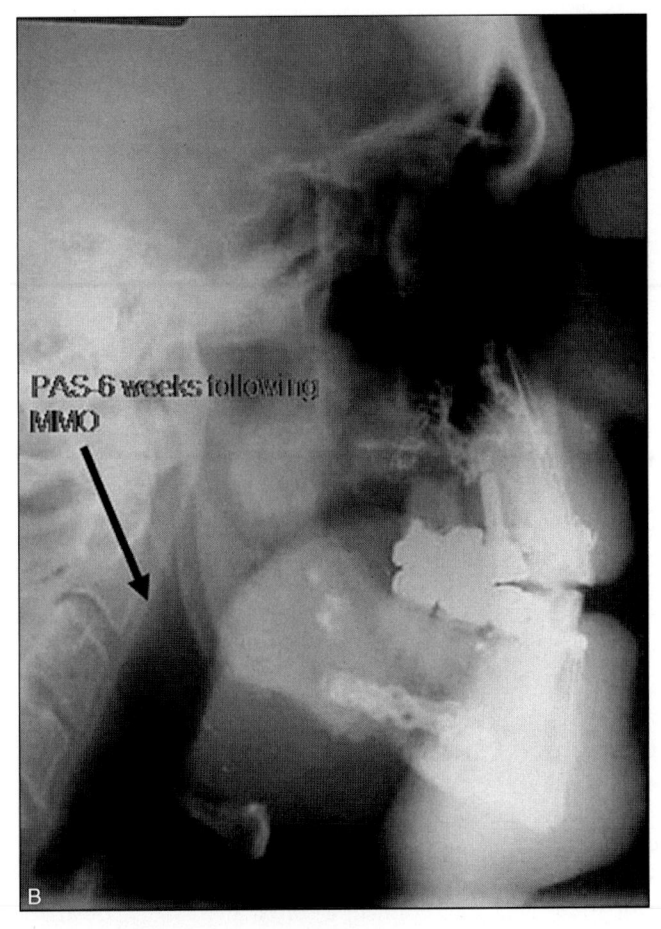

**Fig. 52.12** Lateral cephalograms. Note the narrow posterior airway space (PAS) on this preoperative film (A). Markedly widened PAS following maxillomandibular advancement (B).

331

## 6 POSTOPERATIVE MANAGEMENT AND COMPLICATIONS

Many factors can complicate the postoperative management of OSA patients. Commonly, patients have a medical condition (hypertension, arrhythmias) which increases the risk of surgery. However, preventing airway obstruction remains the priority. Sleep apnea patients already have a compromised airway. The added surgical edema, muscle atonia and respiratory depression from general anesthesia and narcotics further jeopardize the airway. Thus, we have implemented a risk management protocol to ensure patient safety.[18,19]

Admission to the ICU overnight is indicated for patients with comorbid medical conditions, moderate to severe OSA, multilevel surgery and MMO. Continuous pulse oximetry and hemodynamic monitoring are mandatory. Furthermore, we use CPAP immediately after surgery to reduce edema and prevent REM rebound sleep.[19]

Postoperative airway edema is unavoidable; however, every attempt must be made to minimize swelling. This can be accomplished by limiting intravenous fluids administered intraoperatively. Also, meticulous hemostasis during surgery will reduce the chance of hematoma formation. Unless medically contraindicated, all patients receive 24 hours of intravenous corticosteroids. Additionally, hypertension is aggressively treated with intravenous antihypertensive medications to prevent bleeding and edema. Our goal is to maintain the mean arterial pressure (MAP) between 80 and 100. Often, this necessitates placement of an arterial line.

While providing adequate analgesia is important, the medical staff must be educated to avoid excessive sedation of the OSA patient. Intravenous analgesics, such as morphine sulfate, should only be given in the ICU. Small doses are administered and the nursing staff monitors the patient for sedation prior to giving any more medications. Patient-controlled analgesia (PCA) is not recommended because of the risk of over-sedation. Intramuscular meperidene HCl and oral oxycodone elixir may be used on the ward. The patient is discharged with hydrocodone and acetaminophen elixir. Any other medications which can potentially sedate a patient (e.g. benzodiazepines) are contraindicated.

A single dose of antibiotics is administered prior to incision and they are continued for a total of 7 days to prevent infection. The patient is followed closely in the convalescence period to monitor for wound infection. Infection is treated aggressively with debridement, irrigation and culture-directed antibiotics. The hardware rarely needs to be removed if the infection is identified and treated early.

The requirements for discharge from the hospital include reasonable pain control, adequate oral intake and a patent airway. We perform fiberoptic laryngoscopy on all patients prior to discharge to confirm a stable airway.[20] If obstruction is noted, the patient is observed in the hospital until this resolves.

The arch bars are removed 6 weeks following surgery for those patients who undergo MMO. If minor occlusal abnormalities exist, they can be equilibrated at the same time as arch bar removal. All patients are obligated to obtain a PSG 3 months postoperatively to assess their response to surgery.

Obstruction of the airway is the most feared complication following surgery. Hopefully, the prevention strategies previously mentioned will reduce this complication. Each of the maxillofacial procedures has its own risks. Patients must be counseled about these potential complications prior to undergoing surgery.

Mandible fractures can occur as a result of genioglossus advancement surgery. Any technique which violates the inferior border of the mandible increases the risk of fracture. While the rectangular osteotomy technique significantly reduces this risk, a fracture can occur if the osteotomy is poorly designed.[21] Avulsion of the genioglossus muscle is perhaps the most worrisome complication and may not be correctable. Minor complications, such as wound infection, anesthesia of the teeth or lower lip and root injury requiring endodontic therapy, have incidences rates of 2%, 6% and 1% respectively, at our center.

Hyoid suspension is rarely associated with major complications. While injury to the superior laryngeal or hypoglossal nerve is possible, we have not encountered this problem. Seroma formation can occur; however, the placement of surgical drains and pressure dressings has markedly reduced this complication. Transient dysphagia or aspiration can be observed but it usually resolves within 10 days. If these symptoms persist, removal of the suspension sutures should alleviate this problem.[22]

Injury to the descending palatine arteries can occur during the Le Fort I osteotomy. Although rare, avascular necrosis of the palate can occur. If there is any indication that the blood supply to the maxilla is inadequate, the surgeon should place the maxilla in its preoperative position. Injury to the inferior alveolar nerve can cause permanent anesthesia of the dentition and perioral region following sagittal split osteotomy. Typically, the anesthesia is transient and self-limited as a result of edema of the neurovascular bundle. Dental malocclusion may occur despite the use of a dental splint. Usually this can be managed with occlusal equilibration. More complicated problems may warrant orthodontic treatment or surgical correction.[22]

## 7 SUCCESS RATE

As noted previously, genioglossus advancement and hyoid suspension are considered part of phase I surgery. Furthermore, a majority of our patients have multilevel pharyngeal obstruction, which necessitates treating the palate synchronously with the tongue base. Rarely do we perform hyoid suspension or genioglossus advancement as isolated procedures. Exceptions would include those patients who do not have palatal obstruction or those who have previously undergone palatal surgery. Our published data have shown that approximately 70% of patients are cured with phase I surgery.[12]

Incomplete treatment with phase I surgery is related to persistent hypopharyngeal obstruction. Those patients who have been incompletely treated would then be considered for phase II surgery (MMO). Maxillomandibular advancement osteotomy has documented success rates >90%.[12–14] Temperature-controlled radiofrequency of the tongue base or tracheostomy are the only other surgical modalities available if a patient should be incompletely treated with MMO.

## REFERENCES

1. Sher AE, Schechtman KB, Piccirillo JF. The efficacy of surgical modifications of the upper airway in adults with obstructive sleep apnea syndrome. Sleep 1996;19:156–77.
2. Riley RW, Powell NB. Maxillofacial surgery and obstructive sleep apnea syndrome. Otolaryngol Clin North Am 1990;23:809–26.
3. Dincer HE, O'Neill W. Deleterious effects of sleep-disordered breathing on the heart and vascular system. Respiration 2006;73:124–30.
4. Yaggi HK, Concato J, Kernan WN, et al. Obstructive sleep apnea as a risk factor for stroke and death. N Engl J Med 2005;353:2034–41.
5. Riley RW, Powell NB, Guilleminault C. Maxillofacial surgery and nasal CPAP: a comparison of treatment for obstructive sleep apnea syndrome. Chest 1990;98:1421–5.
6. Riley R, Powell N, Guilleminault C, et al. Obstructive sleep apnea syndrome: a surgical protocol for dynamic upper airway reconstruction. J Oral Maxillofac Surg 1993;51:742–7.
7. Powell NB, Riley RW. A surgical protocol for sleep disordered breathing. Oral Maxillofac Surg Clin North Am 1995;7:345–56.
8. Powell NB, Riley RW, Guilleminault C. Surgical management of sleep-disordered breathing. In: Principles and Practices of Sleep Medicine, 4th edn. Kryger MH, Roth T, Dement WC, eds. Philadelphia: Elsevier Saunders; 2005, pp. 1081–97.
9. Sin DD, Mayers I, Man GC, et al. Long-term compliance rates of CPAP in obstructive sleep apnea: a population-based study. Chest 2002;121:430–35.
10. Kribbs NB, Pack AI, Kline LR, et al. Objective measurement of patterns of nasal CPAP use by patients with obstructive sleep apnea. Am Rev Respir Dis 1993;147:887–95.
11. Powell N, Riley R, Guilleminault C, et al. Obstructive sleep apnea, continuous positive airway pressure, and surgery. Otolaryngol Head Neck Surg 1988;99:362–9.
12. Riley R, Powell N, Guilleminault C. Obstructive sleep apnea syndrome: a review of 306 consecutively treated surgical patients. Otolaryngol Head Neck Surg 1993;108:117–25.
13. Waite PD, Wooten V, Lachner J, et al. Maxillomandibular advancement surgery in 23 patients with obstructive sleep apnea syndrome. J Oral Maxillofac Surg 1989;47:1256–61.
14. Hochban W, Brandenburg U, Hermann PJ. Surgical treatment of obstructive sleep apnea by maxillomandibular advancement. Sleep 1994;17:624–9.
15. Troell RJ, Powell NB, Riley RW. Hypopharyngeal airway surgery for obstructive sleep apnea syndrome. Semin Respir Crit Care Med 1998;19:175–83.
16. McBride KL, Bell WH. Chin surgery. In: Surgical Correction of Dentofacial Deformities, 1st edn. Bell WH, Proffit WR, White RP, eds. Philadelphia: WB Saunders; 1980, pp. 1210–81.
17. Powell NB, Riley RW. Facial contouring with outer table calvarial bone. Arch Otolaryngol Head Neck Surg 1989;115:1454–8.
18. Riley RW, Powell NB, Guilleminault C, et al. Obstructive sleep apnea surgery: risk management and complications. Otolaryngol Head Neck Surg 1997;117:648–52.
19. Li KK, Powell N, Riley R. Postoperative management of the obstructive sleep apnea patient. Oral Maxillofac Surg Clin N Am 2002;14:401–404.
20. Li KK, Riley RW, Powell NB, et al. Fiberoptic nasopharyngoscopy for airway monitoring following obstructive sleep apnea surgery. J Oral Maxillofac Surg 2000;58:1342–5.
21. Riley R, Powell N, Guilleminault C. Inferior sagittal osteotomy of the mandible with hyoid myotomy–suspension: a new procedure for obstructive sleep apnea. Otolaryngol Head Neck Surg 1986;94:589–93.
22. Li KK, Riley R, Powell N. Complications of obstructive sleep apnea surgery. Oral Maxillofac Surg Clin N Am 2003;15:297–304.

SECTION L — MAXILLOFACIAL SURGICAL TECHNIQUES

CHAPTER 53

# Modified maxillomandibular advancement technique

*Yau Hong Goh, Winston Tan and Mark Hon Wah Ignatius*

## 1 INTRODUCTION

Orthognathic surgery has been used to treat obstructive sleep apnea (OSA) since the mid-1980s.[1] In the classic phase II surgery for OSA described by Riley and Powell, 10 mm advancement of the maxilla and mandible resulted in an impressive 97% cure rate in patients who had failed phase I surgery and 91% in patients treated solely by phase II surgery.[2] Other studies on bimaxillary advancement techniques have also shown success rates ranging from 75% to 100%, which are superior to other surgical treatments for OSAS.[3-5] Maxillomandibular advancement has now been accepted as an effective modality in the treatment of OSAS.

Many studies that have evaluated the perceived facial changes associated with such advancement surgeries reported favorable perceived aesthetic result from the patients' viewpoint[6-9]; however, all of these studies were done on Caucasian cohorts. There is currently no literature on the aesthetic outcome of maxillomandibular advancement of such a large extent for the treatment of OSA in Asians. The aesthetic outcome after maxillomandibular advancement is different between Caucasians and Far East Asians as there is a greater incidence of bimaxillary protrusion in the Far East Asian face. These and other ethnic differences in the cephalometric parameters between the Far East Asian and the Caucasian have been previously shown.[12,13] Though the soft tissue measurements such as the distance from the mandibular plane to the hyoid bone (MP-H), posterior airway space (PAS), and the distance from the posterior nasal spine to the tip of the soft palate (PNS-P) did not vary significantly, the angle measurement from the sella to nasion to point A, subspinale (SNA), and the angle from sella to nasion to point B, supramentale (SNB), were significantly different between the racial groups.

From a purely aesthetic point of view, profiles that are flat or slightly bimaxillary protrusive are considered more attractive in the Western sense of aesthetics than those which have extreme bimaxillary protrusion.[16] On the contrary, in a comparative study of the perception of Chinese facial profile aesthetics by native Chinese dental professionals, students and lay people, facial profiles that were normal or had bimaxillary retrusion were perceived to be more attractive than profiles that had bimaxillary protrusion, protrusive mandible, retrusive mandible, retrusive maxilla or protrusive maxilla.[17] Therefore considering the relatively greater maxillary and mandibular protrusion in the Asian population and the biased perception by the native Chinese favoring bimaxillary retrusion, the aesthetic effects of increased bimaxillary protrusion after maxillomandibular advancement would be undesirable in the Far East Asian face.

Patients with bimaxillary protrusion may have lip seal problems due to the protrusion as evidenced by upward strain of the mentalis and increased activity of perioral muscles; this may be unfavorably increased after maxillomandibular advancement. The increased tension on advanced maxillary and mandibular segments in a patient with bimaxillary protrusion may also affect the stability of the advancement, which may increase regression and failure rates postop-eratively. The long-term stability of the advanced segments due to decreased tension after an anterior segmental setback was also a factor in the consideration of the development of the modified technique for the Far East Asian face.

## 2 PATIENT SELECTION

Anterior segmental surgeries have been practiced in oral and maxillofacial surgery since the 1960s. It is generally indicated for cases of bimaxillary protrusion. This involves the posterior setback of the anterior maxilla (premaxilla) and the anterior alveolar segment of the mandible, usually after the extraction of a bicuspid from each quadrant of the dental arch. Together with the standard Le Fort I and bilateral sagittal split osteotomies, the surgery, when applied to OSAS patients, achieves the aim of increasing the posterior airway space without significant aesthetic facial alterations.

The indications for modified MMA to treat obstructive sleep apnea are the same as for standard maxillomandibular advancement. The modification is offered in patients with bimaxillary protrusion who do not want their facial profile and appearance altered postoperatively. These patients can be identified on physical examination by the presence of lip closure problems, excessive proclination, wide nasal alar base, excessive show of teeth or gums when smiling and protrusive lips on facial profile examination and cephalometric measurements.

Preoperative model surgery is undertaken to assess suitability. Several dental considerations exist with the maxillary segmental setback surgery. Presurgical orthodontic preparation of the teeth involves arch co-ordination and elimination of dental crowding. When combined with the Le Fort I maxillary advancement procedure, the setback is likely to result in some retroclination of the anterior segment with tipping and reduction of the maxillary to sella–nasion angle. Orthodontic tipping of the canine and premolar teeth away from the osteotomy site will allow for maximum bone removal during surgery and reduce this tendency.

Another dental consideration with the maxillary setback surgery is the superior/upward movement of the upper canine as the segment is moved back. This potentially creates an open bite at the canine/premolar positions and post-surgical orthodontics may be required to track the canine tip down. Care should be taken to reduce this tendency at the planning and surgical phase without compromising the vitality to the canine root tip. Reducing tipping and a conscious attempt to effect a bodily movement of the segment in the posterior direction will allow for maximum corresponding maxillary advancement without compromising facial aesthetics. Occasionally, a careful division of the anterior segment in the midline is useful to help swing the canines into position. It should be stressed that maintenance of the palatal pedicle is paramount, and a careful handling is essential to prevent aseptic necrosis of the small sub-segment.

Smoothing of the arch form at this surgery is also possible, especially if the patient has a pre-existing skeletal/transverse discrepancy. A midline split of the palate is sometimes helpful to co-ordinate the arch to reduce the amount of postoperative orthodontic movement necessary. This, coupled with the division of the anterior segmental component, creates a four-piece Le Fort I osteotomy. We find that transverse expansion beyond 4mm to 5mm is difficult to achieve without risking an oro-nasal perforation and should be avoided in treatment planning. Excessive surgical expansion of the arch usually results in a buccal tipping of the teeth, as opposed to the entire dentoalveolar complex moving laterally. A preformed arch bar should be fabricated, in addition to the occlusal wafer, to control the segments as much as possible. Fixation is otherwise standard with four bone plates for the entire maxilla.

Several considerations exist for the mandibular segmental surgery for the treatment of OSA. The primary concern is that the genial tubercles are attached to the lingual surface of the mandible and the segment should not be too large or gains created by the advancement surgery will be nullified by the anterior segmental setback. In patients who require a concurrent advancement or lengthening genioplasty for facial aesthetics, we find it useful to preserve a bony bridge between the segmental and genioplasty cuts for muscle attachment or plication. Preservation of an intact bony bridge is important (more so in female patients), as this prevents a potential broadening of the mandible with the tendency for opening up of the bone fragments laterally and the creation of a widening of the mandible. This is, however, a welcome side effect, especially in males with an already dolichofacial structure, as it creates a more masculine face form. Advancement genioplasty should be very carefully considered in patients with an already long facial height, as elongation is likely to be magnified with the setback, especially in females where an undesirable 'witch-like' profile may result.

The tooth positions are less critical in the lower segment as the lower teeth are fairly vertical at the canine/premolar position. Again care should be taken with the root positions in the presurgical orthodontic preparation, as this will allow for a maximum set-back of the segment, without jeopardizing tooth vitality. The lower canine root is the longest tooth in that part of the jaw, and care should be taken not to transect the root with the horizontal bone cut.

The lower dental arch form may also be smoothed out with a midline split of the mandible and a reduction in the transverse width of the arch can be carried out to smooth the arch form and eliminate the transverse step created by the extraction of the lower premolar teeth. On occasion, a Lindorf genioplasty may be carried out as it will simultaneously advance the genial tubercles, bringing the tongue forward in the process. The application of bone plates is challenging in situations where many bone fragments are present and a prefabricated arch bar wired to the teeth is imperative in helping to stabilize these segments.

## 3 SURGICAL PROCEDURE

Prior to surgery, a methylmethacrylate occlusal splint and preformed arch bars are fabricated for the alignment of the mobilized dental segments during surgery. The final positions of the dental and bony segments are determined according to model surgeries performed in the laboratory. Intraoperatively, the selected bicuspids are extracted and the segmental (anterior subapical maxillary and mandibular segmental) surgeries are performed (Figs 53.1 and 53.2). The resultant wedges of bone removed from the segmental sites are kept for grafting to the maxillary osteotomy sites during the later part of the surgery. The use of bone from the segmental surgery sites obviates the need for calvarial bone graft harvesting and hence lessens the morbidity

# SECTION L — MAXILLOFACIAL SURGICAL TECHNIQUES

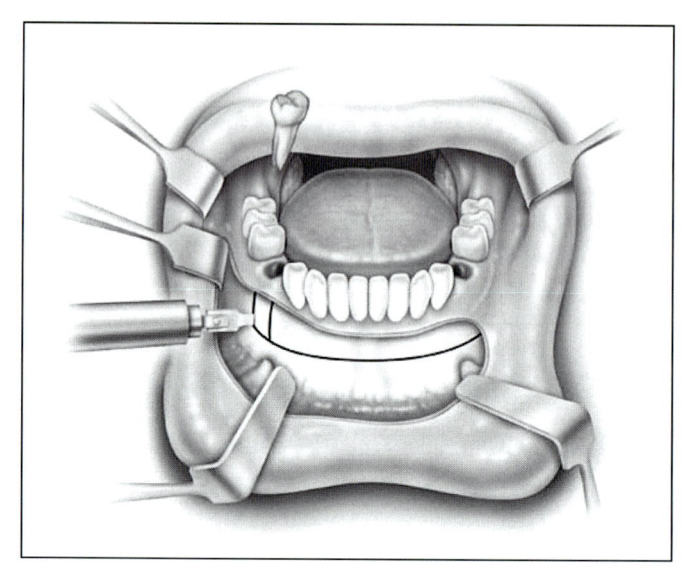

**Fig. 53.1** Following extraction of both bicuspids, a circumvestibular incision is made and the mucosal flap raised to expose the mandible. A horizontal subapical osteotomy is made about 5 mm below the teeth apices and extended bilaterally over the mental foramen. With the use of a cutting burr, interdental osteotomies are made between the bone sockets.

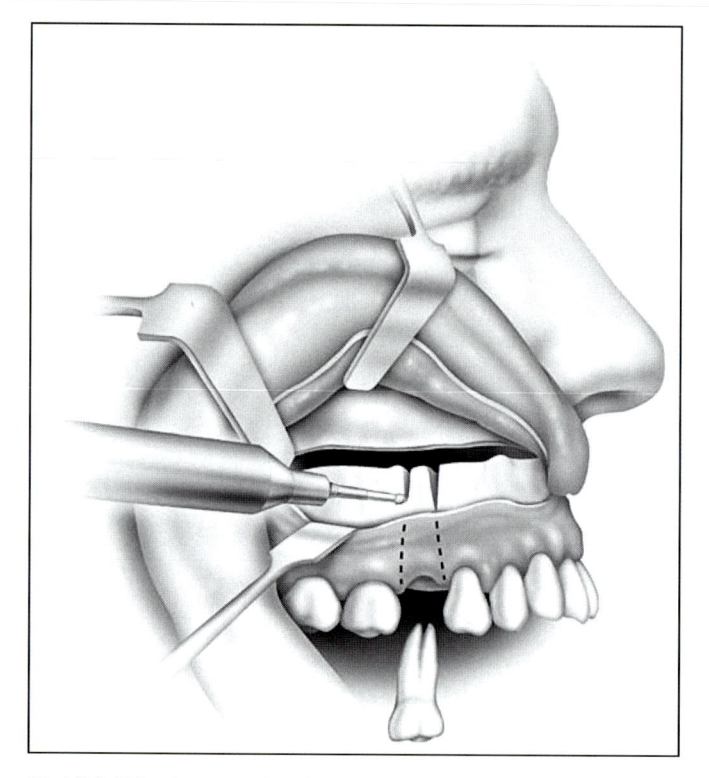

**Fig. 53.2** Following extraction of both bicuspids, a circumvestibular incision is made and the mucosal flap raised to expose the maxilla. After a Le Fort I osteotomy and down-fracturing of the maxilla, a vertical interdental osteotomy is carried out between the sockets. Completion of the transpalatal osteotomies bilaterally will free the premaxilla. Careful burring and reduction of obstructing bony protrusions will facilitate the setting back of the premaxilla segment.

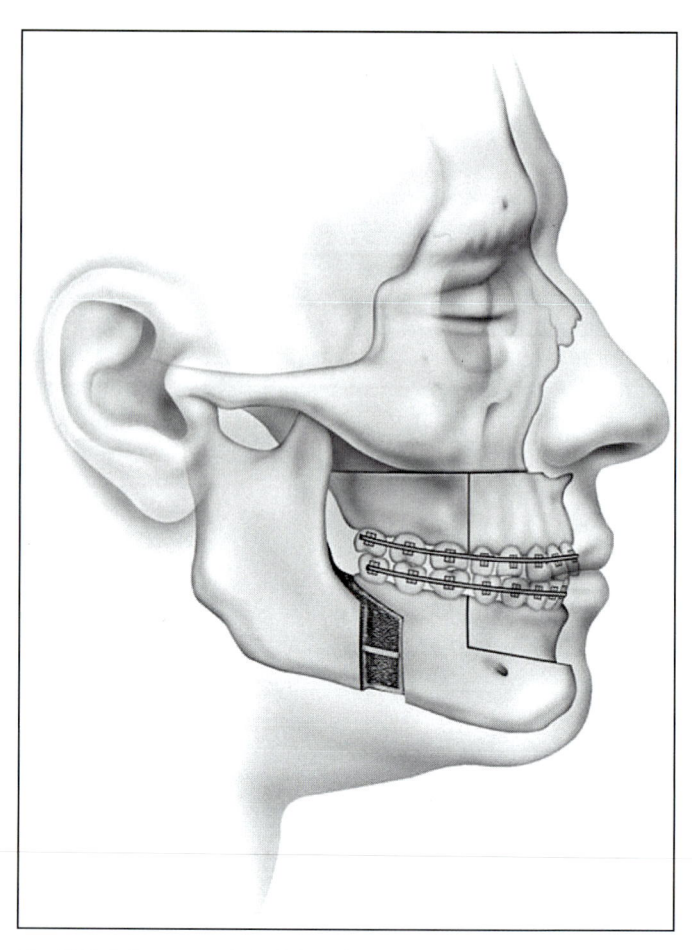

**Fig. 53.3** A diagrammatic depiction of the entire modified maxillomandibular advancement technique: a Le Fort I osteotomy with anterior subapical segmental osteotomy and bilateral sagittal split osteotomies with anterior subapical segmental osteotomy.

of the surgery. After the segments are secured in the final positions with preformed arch bars, the Le Fort I maxillary osteotomy and bilateral sagittal split osteotomies are performed in the standard way (Fig. 53.3). The maxilla and the mandible are advanced 10 mm. Rigid fixation of the maxilla is by way of four bone plates. The free bone grafts are used at this site to promote bony union and also to stabilize the maxilla. The grafts are stabilized with bone screws if necessary. The mandible is positioned by intermaxillary fixation with the preformed interposing occlusal splint and fixed with one bone plate on each side. The occlusal splint is left in situ for stabilization of the occlusion, and intermaxillary fixation is left in place for up to 6 weeks.[12]

## 4 POSTOPERATIVE MANAGEMENT AND COMPLICATIONS

Postoperative management principles include airway control, cardiovascular and hemodynamic stability, prevention of ischemia of segments, prevention of wound infection, maintenance of stability of advanced segments.

The patient should be managed in the intensive care unit overnight inclined head up 30° in bed. A rubber band cutter should be available at the bedside in case the patient develops airway difficulties. The patient is kept on an intravenous drip and fasted overnight. Close monitoring of the blood pressure with an intra-arterial line to keep mean arterial BP within 90–100 mm Hg is essential to prevent ischemia to the mandibular and maxillary segments while reducing hematoma formation. Use of anti-hypertensives and narcotic analgesics must be closely monitored to prevent hypotension and respiratory depression. Anti-emetics are prescribed to treat nausea. The hemoglobin concentration should be normalized if required and the arterial oxygen saturation should be kept normal with the use of supplemental oxygen early postop-eratively. Nasal decongestants used regularly will prevent nasal congestion and improve ventilation. Meticulous oral and nasal toilet will help prevent infections and pulmonary aspiration. Intravenous dexametasone is given for 2 days to reduce edema and intravenous antibiotics are continued for 2 days and then oralized for the next week.

Orthopantomography is undertaken on the first postoperative day to confirm implant placements and segment positions and the patient is allowed to sit up and ambulate. The drains are removed after the first 24 hours and the head bandage after 48 hours. The patient is moved to the general ward on the first postoperative day and discharged on the second to third postoperative day if recovery is uneventful. Outpatient reviews are done weekly and at 3 weeks the heavy rubber bands are changed to lighter ones, depending on the occlusion. The patient is kept on a fluid diet for the next 6 weeks when the preformed arch bars are removed, after which a soft diet is started and progressed up to a normal diet.

Complications unique to the modified maxillomandibular advancement include bleeding, airway difficulties, ischemia and loss of the anterior maxilla and mandibular segments, implant-related problems, paresthesia and settling of segments resulting in malocclusion. Malocclusion has been previously elaborated in the preoperative dental considerations.

Bleeding into the osteotomy sites can track into the airway and potentially cause aspiration or airway obstruction. Bleeding that tracks into the soft tissue around the face will increase facial swelling and may compromise blood supply to the face; this is seen when the skin over the face develops a red and shiny look. Drainage of the hematoma and hemostasis is then required. Ischemia and subsequent necrosis of the osteotomy segments is a catastrophic complication and prevention is better than cure.

Airway difficulties may develop from various causes. Postoperative edema, pooled secretions and blood may accumulate in the airway and cause obstruction. Suctioning of the nose and oral cavity should be done regularly and the nose should be kept patent.

Paresthesia of the upper and lower lips occurs in most patients with sensation recovering between 6 and 12 months. The risk of paresthesia is higher than that from the standard maxillomandibular advancement because of the additional osteotomies and mucosal incisions.

Complications from implants may occur and include pain, sensitivity to pressure or temperature changes and infection. Treatment of these complications may require removal of the implants.

## 5 SUCCESS RATE

Since 2000, a total of 31 modified MMAs have been undertaken in our center. A 4-year review of 11 patients, all men, who underwent surgery was published in 2003.[18] There were five Chinese (45.5%), four Malays (36.3%), one Indian (9.1%) and one Eurasian (9.1%). The mean age was 42.8 years (range: 32–56 years). Two patients underwent previous uvulopalatopharyngoplasty (UPPP), hyoid suspension and genioglossus advancement while another had UPPP alone for the treatment of OSA. All three patients had persistent OSA after the phase I surgery. One patient needed a preoperative tracheostomy (lowest oxygen saturation of 40% with high tracheal intubation risk). The remaining eight patients underwent modified MMA as the primary procedure for the treatment of OSA.

The preoperative polysomnography (PSG) results were as follows: Apnea Index (AI) 55.7 ± 19.8 (SD); Apnea/Hypopnea Index (AHI) 70.7 ± 15.9 (SD); lowest oxygen saturation (LSAT) 58.6 ± 12.3 (SD) %; longest apnea/hypopnea 67.9 ± 23.7 (SD) seconds; arousal index 47.1 ± 18.2 (SD). The mean preoperative Body Mass Index (BMI) was 29.4 ± 4.6 (SD) kg/m$^2$. Four patients had associated hypertension, all of whom were poorly controlled. The mean hospital stay was 4.2 days.

The postoperative PSG results were as follows: AI 3.4 ± 3.4 (SD); AHI 11.4 ± 7.4 (SD); LSAT 83.9 ± 8.8 (SD) %; longest apnea/hypopnea 38.2 ± 24.6 (SD) seconds; arousal index 15.1 ± 7.3 (SD). The mean postoperative BMI was 27.2 ± 3.3 (SD) kg/m$^2$. Of the four patients with hypertension, one was normotensive and without anti-hypertensives 6 months post surgery. The blood pressures of the remaining three patients were better controlled after surgery. The mean BMI change after surgery was 6.5%.

Apart from two patients with minor postoperative wound pain which warranted limited removal of limited titanium screws and plate, there were no significant postoperative complications.

The modified MMA technique for the treatment of OSA is a promising procedure for Asian faces; it is highly effective in treating this challenging nocturnal airway condition without the significant facial profile alteration commonly associated with the classic MMA.

# REFERENCES

1. Riley RW, Powell NB, Guilleminault C, et al. Maxillary–mandibular and hyoid advancement: an alternative to tracheostomy on obstructive sleep apnea. Otolaryngol Head Neck Surg 1986;94:584–8.
2. Li KK, Riley RW, Powell NB, et al. Overview of phase II surgery for obstructive sleep apnea syndrome. Ear Nose Throat J 1999;78:851–7.
3. Hochban W, Conradt R, Brandenburg U, et al. Surgical maxillofacial treatment of obstructive sleep apnea. Plast Reconstr Surg 1997;99:619–26.
4. Bettega G, Pepin JL, Veale D, et al. Obstructive sleep apnea syndrome: fifty-one consecutive patients treated by maxillofacial surgery. Am J Respir Crit Care Med 2000;162:641–9.
5. Prinsell JR. Maxillomandibular advancement surgery in a site-specific treatment approach for obstructive sleep apnea in 50 consecutive patients. Chest 1999;116:1519–29.
6. Li KK, Riley RW, Powell NB, et al. Maxillomandibular advancement for persistent obstructive sleep apnea after phase I surgery in patients without maxillomandibular deficiency. Laryngoscope 2000;110:1684–8.
7. Rosen HM. Maxillary advancement for mandibular prognathism: indication and rational. Plast Reconstr Surg 1991;87:823–32.
8. Rosen HM. Facial skeleton expansion: treatment strategies and rationale. Plast Reconstr Surg 1992;89:798–808.
9. Wolford LM, Chamello PD, Hilliard FW. Occlusal plane alteration in orthognathic surgery. J Oral Maxillofac Surg 1993;51:730–40.
10. Ong KC, Clerk AA. Comparison of the severity of sleep-disordered breathing in Asian and Caucasian patients seen at a sleep disorders center. Respir Med 1998;92:843–8.
11. Li KK, Kushida C, Powell NB, et al. Obstructive sleep apnea syndrome: a comparison between far-East Asian and white men. Laryngoscope 2000;110:1689–93.
12. Lee JJ, Ramirez SG, Will MJ. Gender and racial differences in cephalometric analysis. Otolaryngol Head Neck Surg 1997;117:326–9.
13. Will MJ, Ester MS, Ramirez SG, et al. Comparison of cephalometric analysis with ethnicity in obstructive sleep apnea syndrome. Sleep 1995;18:873–5.
14. Steinberg b, Fraser B. The cranial base in obstructive sleep apnea. J Oral Maxillofac Surg 1995;53:1150–54.
15. Lam B, Ip MSM, Tench E, Ryan CF. Craniofacial profile in Asian and white subjects with obstructive sleep apnoea. Thorax 2005;60:504–510.
16. Wolfe SA, Hu L, Berkowitz S. In search of the harmonious face: Apollo revisited. with an examination of the indications for retrograde maxillary displacement. Plast Reconstr Surg 1997;99:1261–71.
17. Soh J, Chew MT, Wong HB. A comparative assessment of the perception of Chinese facial profile aesthetics. Am J Orthod Dentofacial Orthop 2005;127:692–9.
18. Goh YH, Lim KA. Modified maxillomandibular advancement for the treatment of obstructive sleep apnea: a preliminary report. Laryngoscope 2003;113(9):1577–82.

SECTION L  MAXILLOFACIAL SURGICAL TECHNIQUES

CHAPTER 54

# Distraction osteogenesis and obstructive sleep apnea syndrome

*Kasey K. Li*

Maxillofacial skeletal deficiency in the sagittal and frontal plane has been shown to be a major contributing factor in obstructive sleep apnea syndrome (OSA). Despite the success of conventional surgical procedures in maxillofacial skeletal expansion, increasing interest has been generated in the use of distraction osteogenesis for skeletal expansion for the management of OSA. This chapter will discuss the method as well as relevant results.

## 1 INTRODUCTION

Obstructive sleep apnea syndrome (OSA) results from partial or total obstruction of the upper airway during sleep due to narrowing or total obstruction of the upper airway. The airway narrowing or collapse necessitates the patient to increase his/her negative intrathoracic pressures during sleep which results in sleep fragmentation and excessive daytime somnolence as well as a decrease in life expectancy, increased risk for hypertension, myocardial infarction and cardiac arrhythmia.

Maxillofacial skeletal abnormality is a well-recognized predictor in OSA. Maxillomandibular deficiency results in diminished airway dimension which leads to nocturnal obstruction.[1,2] Currently, the most effective surgical procedure in the management of OSA is the expansion of facial skeleton by advancing the maxilla and mandible, i.e. maxillomandibular advancement (MMA). MMA achieves enlargement of the pharyngeal and hypopharyngeal airway by physically expanding the skeletal framework. In addition, the forward movement of the maxillomandibular complex improves the tension and collapsibility of the suprahyoid and velopharyngeal musculature. Lateral pharyngeal wall collapse, which has been shown to be a major factor in airway obstruction,[3] is also shown to be lessened following MMA.[4] The current MMA technique involves the use of maxillary Le Fort I osteotomy and mandibular sagittal split osteotomy to facilitate the forward movement of the maxillomandibular complex followed by the application of rigid fixation.[5]

Since the early recognition of the role of maxillofacial skeletal deformity in OSA, all of the emphasis of deformity recognition and treatment has been primarily limited to the sagittal plane. The transverse deficiency of the maxilla and/or mandible as a potential contributor and treatment of OSA has received little attention. Recently, the constriction of the maxilla has been suggested as a possible risk factor of OSA. In a comparative study between OSA and control subjects by Seto et al.,[6] OSA subjects were found to have narrower, more tapered and shorter maxillary arches. Kushida et al.[7] found that the intermolar distance of the maxilla is related to the presence of OSA. Cistulli et al.[8] have reported that patients with Marfan's syndrome, in which maxillary constriction is a common finding, have increased incidence of OSA and elevated nasal resistance. The relationship of nasal resistance and maxillary morphology has long been suggested in the orthodontic literature.

Despite the past success in conventional maxillofacial surgery for the treatment of airway obstruction, there is increasing interest in the use of distraction osteogenesis for skeletal expansion in treating OSA due to its feasibility in the pediatric population as well as the less invasive nature of the procedure. This chapter will discuss the method as well as relevant results.

## 2 DISTRACTION OSTEOGENESIS IN THE MAXILLOFACIAL REGION

Skeletal expansion by slow osseous distraction (distraction osteogenesis) is not new and has been previously studied extensively in orthopedic surgery. It has demonstrated acceptable feasibility, efficacy, safety, and reproducibility of its treatment results. In its simplest form, distraction osteogenesis (DO) describes the generation of new bone in the stretched fracture callus. A screw-driven appliance that is firmly attached to the bone fragments slowly pulls apart the cut/or fractured bony edges, and new bone can fill in the stretched callus tissue. DO was first described by

Alessandro Codvilla in 1905, who first published the use of this technique in lengthening the long bone.[9] However, it is Ilizarov who is credited with developing the current methods of DO.[10] DO in the maxillofacial region was first investigated by Snyder et al.[11] in the canine mandible. Karp et al.[12] demonstrated that bone formation during DO in the maxillofacial region is similar to that of long bones, which is predominantly by intramembranous ossification. Surgical lengthening by DO in sagittal plane was first described by McCarthy, who reported on the application of DO of the human mandible in pediatric patients in 1992.[13] The surgical expansion of the maxilla and mandible to increase the width by distraction osteogenesis was reported by Bell and Epker[14] and Guerrero,[15] respectively.

DO is a potentially new approach for the treatment of OSA by slowly expanding the mandible and/or the maxilla in the sagittal or frontal plane, thereby expanding the airway. This technique is less invasive than the traditional technique. It requires less tissue manipulation, less blood loss, and has less skeletal relapse potential.

## 3 BRIEF DESCRIPTION OF MAXILLOMANDIBULAR ADVANCEMENT

See Figure 54.1.

The procedure is performed in the operating room under general anesthesia technique. The maxillary advancement is a Le Fort I osteotomy. The procedure is modified for DO with the placement of bilateral maxillary distraction devices following a limited down-fracturing of the maxilla without extensive mobilization. In the mandible, the procedure consists of performing an osteotomy behind the last molar, followed by application of the intraoral distraction device. Following 5–7 days of latency period, the device will be activated two to four times per day to achieve 1 mm of bone lengthening per day. The total bone lengthening will be determined preoperatively based on the patient's anatomy, dentition, facial appearance and the severity of OSAS. After the completion of distraction (approximately 1–3 weeks), the distraction devices are maintained in place for 2–3 months to allow bone ingrowth and healing. The distraction devices are then removed under either general anesthesia or intravenous sedation technique.

## 4 BRIEF DESCRIPTION OF MAXILLOMANDIBULAR WIDENING

See Figures 54.2 and 54.3.

In the pediatric population, maxillary widening often does not require surgical intervention since the midpalatal suture can be widened and the maxilla is expanded simply with a distractor placed in the palate. However, after the fusion of the midpalatal suture after adolescence, osteotomy is required to facilitate the expansion. The procedure is performed in the operating room under general anesthesia technique. Maxillary widening is achieved by a limited osteotomy in the Le Fort I level without down-fracturing. A limited osteotomy in the midline of the maxilla is also performed. The distraction device is usually placed by the orthodontist before surgery, and it is activated for 0.5 mm at the completion of the operation. In the mandible, a midline osteotomy is made, followed by application of the intraoral distraction device. Following 5–7 days of latency period, the device will be activated two to four times per day to achieve 1 mm of bone lengthening per day. The total widening will be determined preoperatively based on the patient's anatomy, dentition, facial appearance and the severity of OSAS. Typically, a widening of 5–10 mm can be achieved. After the completion of distraction (approximately 1–3 weeks), the distraction device will be maintained for 2–3 months to allow bone ingrowth and healing. The maxillary distraction device is removed by the orthodontist, and the mandibular distraction device is removed under general anesthesia.

## 5 DISCUSSION

DO offers several advantages over the conventional techniques by eliminating the need for bone grafting, and it involves less surgical dissection because bone lengthening is the result of natural bone healing in a gap created by a simple osteotomy. The incremental skeletal movement allows accommodation of the soft tissue, thus enabling large skeletal movement that usually cannot be achieved by conventional techniques. The gradual soft tissue accommodation also improves the stability of the new skeletal position.

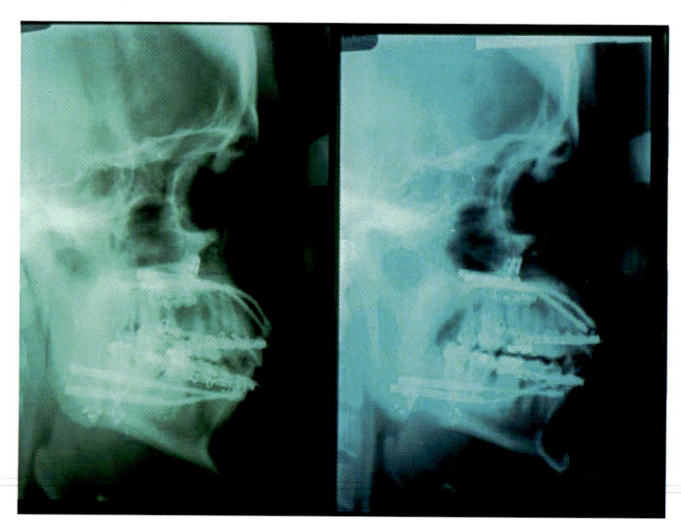

**Fig. 54.1** Pre- and postoperative cephalometric radiographs and panoramic radiographs.

CHAPTER 54
Distraction osteogenesis and obstructive sleep apnea syndrome

mandibular expansion pre

mandibular expansion post

Maxillary expansion pre

Maxillary expansion post

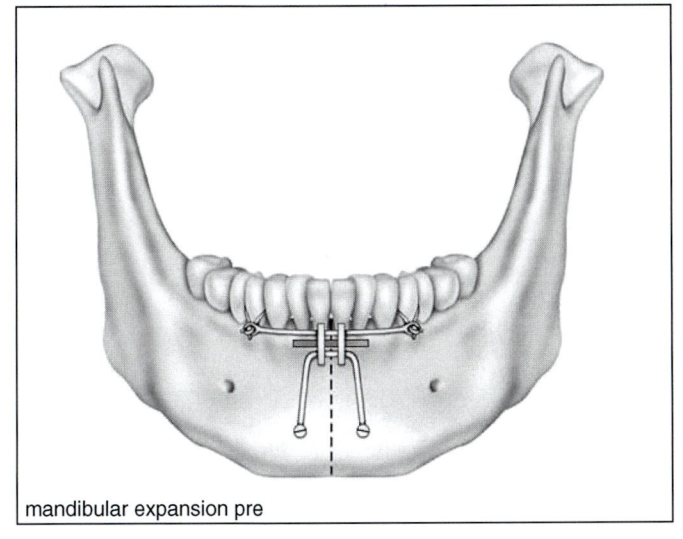

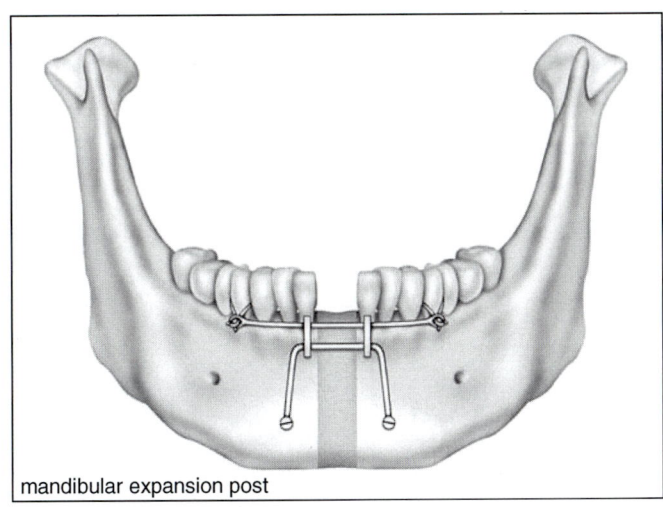

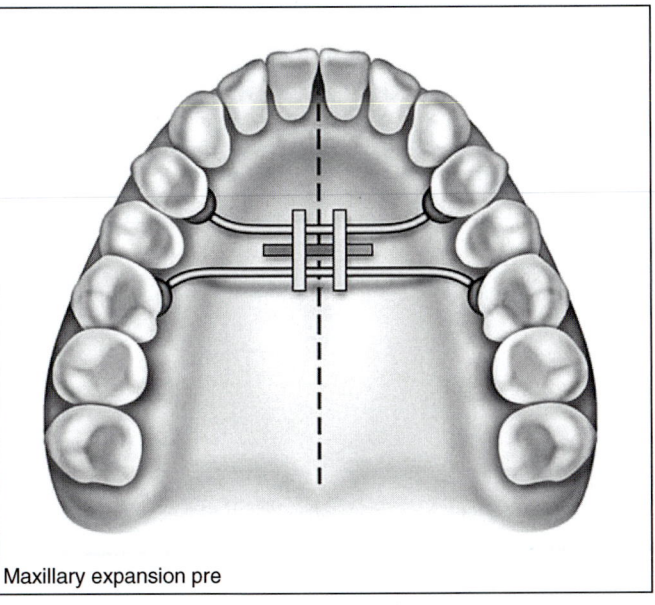

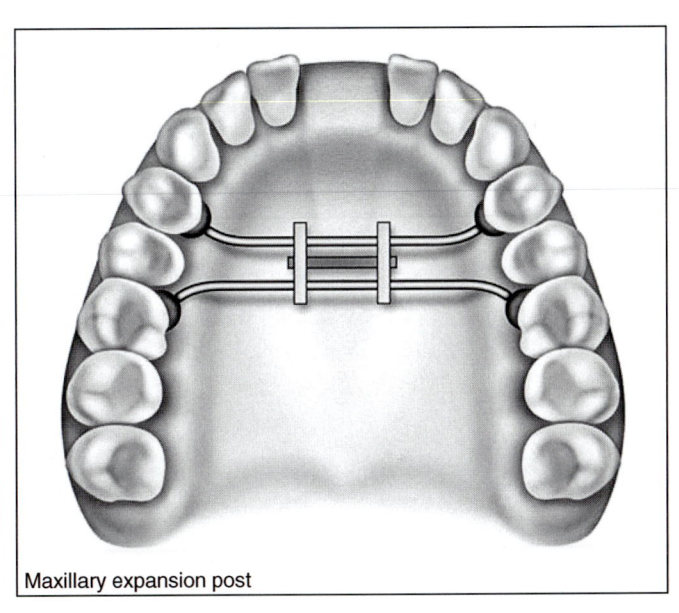

**Fig. 54.2** Progression of maxillomandibular widening.

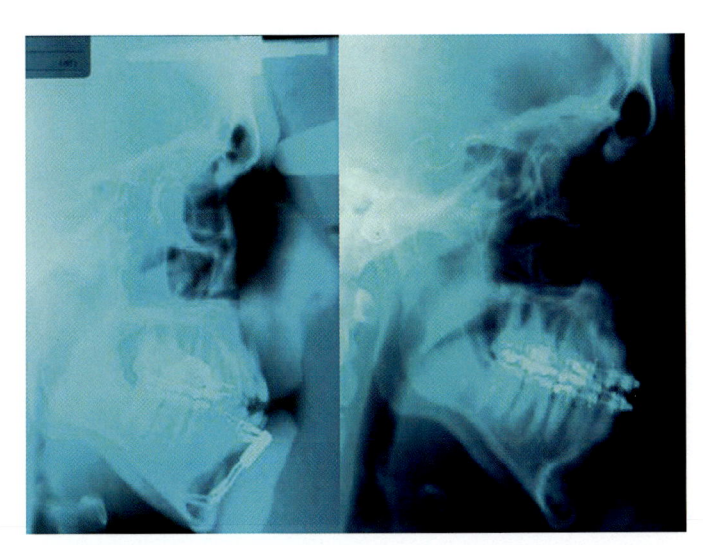

**Fig. 54.3** Pre- and postoperative cephalometric radiograph. Note the increase in airway space behind the tongue base.

The major advantage in the application of DO for maxillofacial skeletal expansion is in the pediatric population where access for the conventional procedure is limited, the volume of bone is insufficient for conventional procedure, there is a need for much greater skeletal expansion than the conventional technique can provide and the potential for surgical scarring by conventional procedure due to the extensiveness of the operation, which can negatively impact future facial growth. Both advancement and widening of the maxilla and mandible have been shown to improve OSA. Maxillary widening improves nasal airway resistance,[16,17] although the beneficial effect of maxillary expansion on nasal resistance may not be uniformly achieved in all patients. It appears that patients with greater degrees of nasal resistance tend to have greater improvement after maxillary expansion.[18,19] Nocturnal enuresis is improved in children.[20,21] Cistulli et al.[22] performed maxillary expansion on 10 OSA patients with maxillary constriction and

341

improvement was achieved in nine of the 10 patients. The mean Apnea/Hypopnea Index (AHI) was reduced from 19 events per hour to seven events per hour, and the mean maxillary expansion achieved was 12.1 mm. It is unknown whether mandibular expansion can be performed with maxillary expansion, and if simultaneous maxillary and mandibular expansion can improve OSA. Pirelli et al.[23] treated 31 children with orthodontic maxillary expansion. Nasal resistance was improved in all patients. The AHI was reduced from 12.2 events per hour to less than one event per hour. The mean expansion was 4.32 mm.

There is extensive literature support for the application of DO to advance the maxilla or the mandible. Since the initial report by McCarthy et al.[13] mandibular advancement by DO in the pediatric population has gained increasing popularity. The majority of the studies have demonstrated impressive success in the management of OSA in pediatric patients with craniofacial syndromes.[24–27] It has become the preferred management in patients who are tracheotomy dependent and the majority of the patients can be decannulated following DO. Contrarily, DO to achieve maxillary or mandibular advancement in the adult population has not gained significant acceptance. Only two centers have reported their experience of DO in the management of adult OSA.[28,29] This is likely due to the increased treatment time required, the presence of distraction devices which significantly affect the patient's mastication, aesthetics and speech. These unfavorable factors have limited the patient's acceptance of DO in the adult population.

## REFERENCES

1. Jamieson A, Guilleminault C, Partinen M, Quera-Salva MA. Obstructive sleep apneic patients have craniomandibular abnormalities. Sleep 1986;9:469–77.
2. DeBerry-Borowiecki B, Kukwa A, Blanks R. Cephalometric analysis for diagnosis and treatment of obstructive sleep apnea. Laryngoscope 1988;98:226–34.
3. Schwab RJ, Gefter WB, Hoffman EA, Gupta KB, Pack AI. Dynamic upper airway imaging during respiration in normal subjects and patients with sleep disordered breathing. Am Rev Respir Dis 1993;148:1385–400.
4. Li KK, Guilleminault C, Riley RW, Powell NB. Obstructive sleep apnea, maxillomandibular advancement and the airway: a radiographic and dynamic fiberoptic examination. J Oral Maxillofac Surg 2002;60:526–30.
5. Li KK. Surgical therapy for adult obstructive sleep apnea. Sleep Med Rev 2005;9:201–9.
6. Seto BH, Gotsopoulos H, Sims MR, Cistulli PA. Maxillary morphology in obstructive sleep apnea syndrome. Eur J Orthod 2001;23:703–14.
7. Kushida C, Efron B, Guilleminault C. A predictive morphometric model for the obstructive sleep apnea syndrome. Ann Int Med 1997;127:581–7.
8. Cistulli PA, Richards GN, Palmisano RG, Unger G, Berthon-Jones M, Sullivan CE. Influence of maxillary constriction on nasal resistance and sleep apnea severity in patients with Marfan's syndrome. Chest 1996;110:1184–8.
9. Codvilla A. On the means of lengthening, in lower limbs, the muscles and tissues which are shortened through deformity. Am J Orthop Surg 1905;2:353–69.
10. Ilizarov GA. The principles of the Ilizarov method. Bull Hosp Joint Dis Orthop Inst 1988;48:1–11.
11. Snyder CC, Levine GA, Swanson HM, Browne EZ. Mandibular lengthening by gradual distraction: preliminary report. Plast Reconstr Surg 1973;51:506–8.
12. Karp NS, McCarthy JG, Schreiber JS, Sissons HA, Thorne CHM. Membranous bone lengthening: a serial histological study. Ann Plast Surg 1992;29:2–7.
13. McCarthy JG, Schreiber J, Karp N, Thorne CHM, Grayson BH. Lengthening the human mandible by gradual distraction. Plast Reconstr Surg 1992;89:1–10.
14. Bell WH, Epker BN. Surgical-orthodontic expansion of the maxilla. Am J Orthod 1976;70:517–28.
15. Guerrero CA, Bell WH, Contasti GI, Rodriguez AM. Mandibular widening by intraoral distraction osteogenesis. Br J Oral Maxillofac Surg 1997;35:383–92.
16. Timms DJ. The effect of rapid maxillary expansion on nasal airway resistance. Br J Orthod 1986;13:221–8.
17. Timms DJ. The reduction of nasal airway resistance by rapid maxillary expansion and its effect on respiratory disease. J Laryngol Otol 1984;98:357–62.
18. White BC, Woodside DG, Cole P. The effect of rapid maxillary expansion on nasal airway resistance. J Otolaryngol 1989;18:137–43.
19. Hartgerink DV, Vig PS, Abbott DW. The effect of rapid maxillary expansion on nasal airway resistance. Am J Orthod Dentofac Orthop 1987;92:381–9.
20. Timms DJ. Rapid maxillary expansion in the treatment of nocturnal enuresis. Angle Orthod 1990;60:229–33.
21. Kurol J, Modin H, Bjerkhoel A. Orthodontic maxillary expansion and its effect on nocturnal enuresis. Angle Orthod 1998;68:225–32.
22. Cistulli PA, Palmisano RG, Poole MD. Treatment of obstructive sleep apnea syndrome by rapid maxillary expansion. Sleep 1998;21:831–5.
23. Pirelli P, Saponara M, Guilleminault C. Rapid maxillary expansion in children with obstructive sleep apnea syndrome. Sleep 2004;15:761–6.
24. Cohen SR, Simms C, Burstein FD. Mandibular distraction osteogenesis in the treatment of upper airway obstruction in children with craniofacial deformities. Plast Reconstr Surg 1998;101:312–18.
25. Monasterio FO, Drucker M, Molina F, Ysunza A. Distraction osteogenesis in Pierre Robin sequence and related respiratory problems in children. J Craniofac Surg 2002;13:79–83.
26. Williams JK, Maull D, Grayson BH, et al. Early decannulation with bilateral mandibular distraction for tracheostomy-dependent patients. Plast Reconstr Surg 1999;103:48–57.
27. Mandell DL, Yellon RF, Bradley JP, et al. Mandibular distraction for micrognathia and severe upper airway obstruction. Arch Otolaryngol Head Neck Surg 2004;130:344–48.
28. Li KK, Powell NB, Riley RW, Guilleminault C. Distraction osteogenesis in adult obstructive sleep apnea surgery: a preliminary report. J Oral Maxillofac Surg 2002;60:6–10.
29. Wang X, Wang XX, Liang C, et al. Distraction osteogenesis in correction of micrognathia accompanying obstructive sleep apnea syndrome. Plast Reconstr Surg 2003;112:1549–57.

# CHAPTER 55

## Tracheostomy for sleep apnea

*Robert H. Maisel*

Tracheostomy historically is the first treatment offered for obstructive sleep apnea. It remains the only surgical option directed at obstructive sleep apnea that uniformly eliminates sleep apnea permanently. Since it was first introduced in 1968[1] and subsequently reported in several large studies,[2,3] newer choices of medical and surgical intervention have reduced the number of people needing a tracheostomy to relieve severe and life-threatening obstructive sleep apnea (OSA).

There remain some patients for whom other treatments have been ineffective, intolerant or refused. Current reports[4,5] have agreed with the long-term success at maintaining an open upper airway by creating a tracheostomy to reduce morbidity and mortality.

Patient selection and counseling are paramount in long-term, uncomplicated success of tracheostomy for OSA. Education of the patient and family, in anticipation of surgery, as well as post-surgical support of the caregivers is needed. The patient and family frequently attend training in stoma and device care. The confidence and the ability to manage a tracheostomy at home achieved by support and good teaching justifies the time and effort of these sessions. The patient must be discharged with a full complement of equipment available, and with the knowledge of how to use this in the home environment. Nurse visits are helpful, but the surgeon and his or her staff are the best source to create a confident patient and family in the management of the tracheostomy. Many patients do very well with infrequent office visits and manage self-care with telephone contact and equipment supplies as the only support needed. We recommend an office visit twice to four times a year in all circumstances once the stoma care is stable.

For the patient with normal body habitus who has failed mechanical devices and stepwise surgery of the palate and tongue, a routine tracheostomy through a horizontal skin incision created midway between the cricoid cartilage and the sternal notch will result in satisfactory stoma maintenance. Blunt and sharp dissection through the platysmal layer is performed and a vertical dissection at the midline of the strap muscles results in an approach to the cricoid with the thyroid gland immediately below. This endocrine gland is divided and ligated to expose the midline of the trachea and a window below the second tracheal ring can be removed as is standard for open tracheostomy. A cuffed double lumen tube (Shiley #8 in males; Shiley #6 in females) is placed through this fenestra and the faceplate is sutured to the skin. Sutures are left in place 3–5 days. Gauze ties of $\frac{1}{4}$ inch (6.35 mm) to secure the tube in place are placed around the neck and secured with one or two fingers laxity between tape and neck skin. Patients with sleep apnea are anticipated to have an active and productive life once sleep apnea has been treated surgically and even with significant co-morbidities, we anticipate an active lifestyle. However, the tracheostomy technique described above does not allow temporary extubation, and under only extraordinary circumstances would allow a tube-free tracheostomy, even for short times during the day or overnight. Therefore, most patients, including many of normal body habitus, who have severe obstructive sleep apnea and have been untreatable with mechanical positive pressure or upper airway surgery are recommended to have a tracheostomy as described below. Most of these patients are severely obese with a Body Mass Index greater than 36 and with sizable adipose tissue between skin and trachea. These people need a more thorough approach to the airway and a better solution to stoma hygiene in what is anticipated as life-long airway and apnea management.

Complications from routine tracheostomies in this population have included granulation, tracheal stenosis, loss of lumen with accidental extubation and low-grade chronic wound infection with pain, malodor, bleeding and a weeping wound.

While tracheostomy for obstructive sleep apnea was reported by Kuhlo in 1968,[1] Fee and Ward[6] described a technique of skin-lined flap tracheostomy to overcome the above complications in the obese patient with obstructive sleep apnea. The goal had been to create a stoma of permanence with a diameter of 8–10 mm.

Their plan was to create a series of vertical and horizontal skin incisions which allow easy access to the fibrofatty

# SECTION M  TRACHEOSTOMY FOR OSAHS

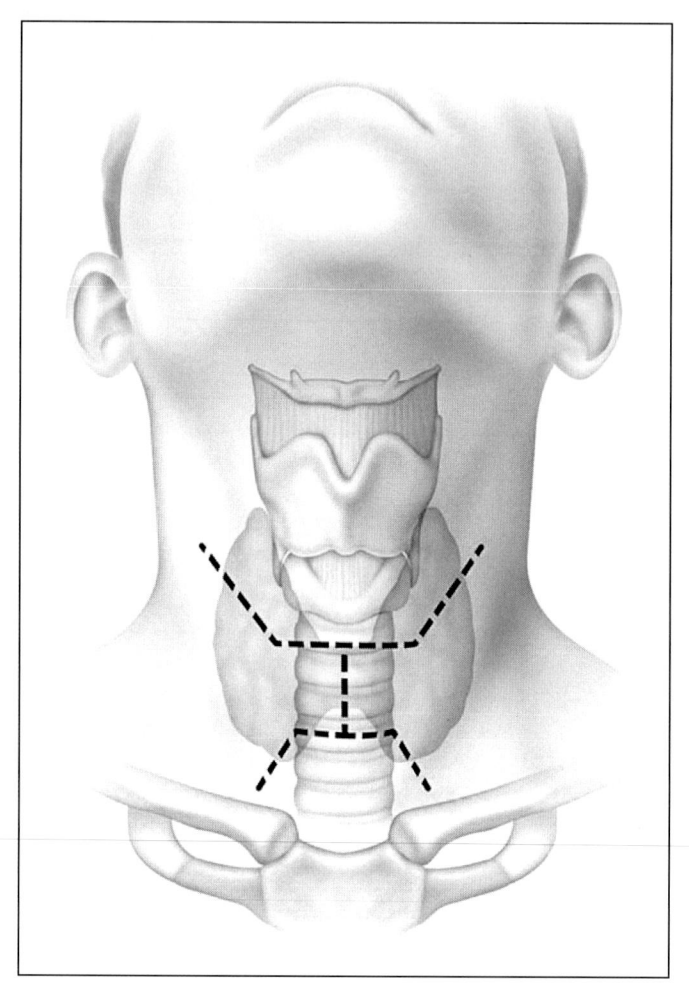

**Fig. 55.1** A horizontally designed 'H' with extension of the flaps superiorly and inferiorly, which allows defatting of the skin flaps and access to the inferior neck from the level of the hyoid bone to the fifth tracheal ring.

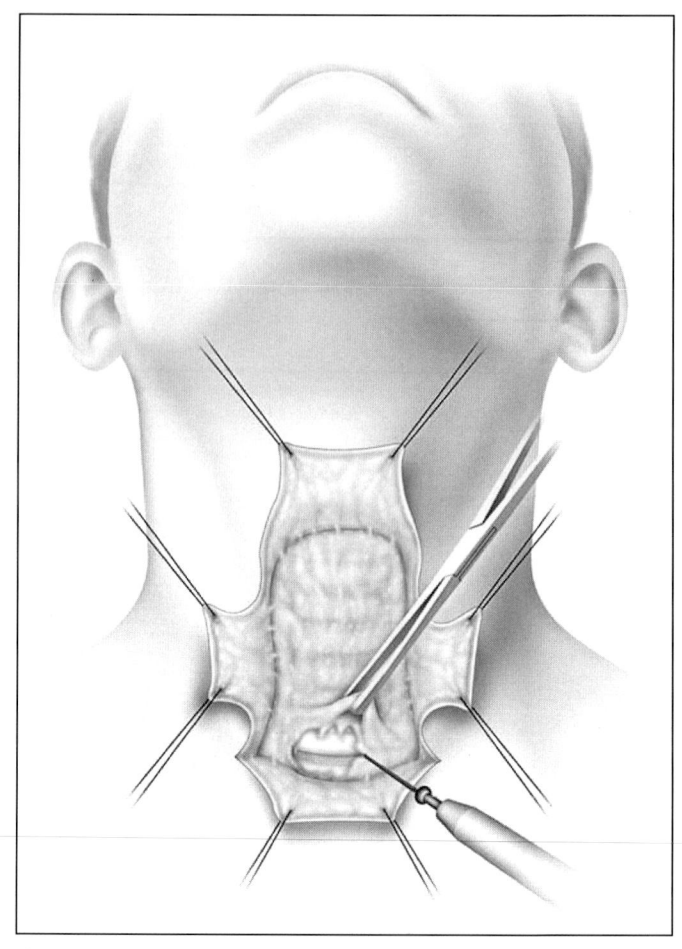

**Fig. 55.2** Lipectomy to remove a panniculus panus in the central compartment of the neck and allowing access to the trachea, as well as permitting the skin flaps to oppose the fascia of the neck with better healing.

pad of tissue overlying the muscles from the level of the hyoid bone above to the sternal notch below (Fig. 55.1). This flap elevation includes defatting the skin flaps safely and creating two vertical and two horizontal skin flaps that will be sutured to the trachea mucosa. Defatting and elevating the skin flaps safely with respect to vitalizing the skin is most important. When elevation is complete, the surgical field is ready for a lipectomy, which is achieved from the level of the hyoid bone often down to the level of the fifth tracheal ring (Fig. 55.2). The skin flap elevation allows access to perform a hyoidopexy to the mandible or thyroid cartilage, if indicated, and allows removal of submental fat which will permit the healed patient to maintain an open tracheal lumen without a submental flap occluding the stoma when the head falls to the chest during sleep.

These skin flaps, two horizontally and two vertically based, must be designed to reach the tracheal mucosa after retracting the strap muscles, which are separated in the midline after lipectomy is complete. The thyroid gland is incised and either cauterized in the midline or ligated with both lobes lateralized off the trachea. Blunt dissection of fascia and retraction of the thyroid permits visualization of the trachea to the level of ring five.

The incision (H-shaped) is made in the trachea with the horizontal limb below ring two (Fig. 55.3). The four skin flaps are then sutured with an inferiorly based flap, which is longer than the superior flap, to allow tension-free opposition of the inferior skin flap with the inferior tracheal flap. The four skin flaps are then sutured with a superior and inferior flap sewn to cartilage that everts into the wound, and the two lateral skin flaps, having been appropriately defatted, are sutured to the lateral tracheal wall.

These operations are performed under general endotracheal anesthesia and co-operation with the anesthesiologist is paramount. Extubation is often unnecessary until the skin flaps are all closed, and suction or Penrose drains placed. It is often necessary for the cuff on the endotracheal

# CHAPTER 55
## Tracheostomy for sleep apnea

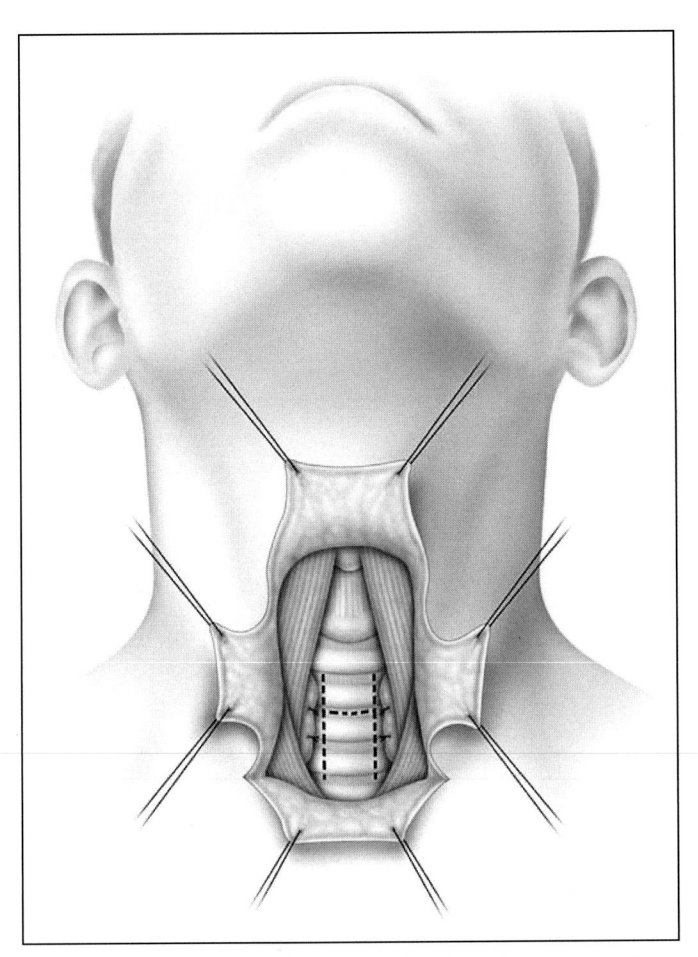

**Fig. 55.3** The vertical 'H' incision used to incise the trachea transversally at tracheal ring three, with an inferior flap slightly longer than the superior to allow tension-free opposition of the epithelial flap. This is designed to be comfortably sutured to the mucosa of the trachea.

tube to be deflated intermittently as sutures are placed in the tracheal lumen. This can avoid puncturing the balloon on the tracheostomy tube which requires replacement of the ventilating tube either through the stoma or by reintubating transorally (Fig. 55.4 A&B).

The stoma, when complete, has a 360° mucocutaneous junction and as this heals without skin necrosis or diastasis, minimizes granulation and maintains a cutaneous tracheal lumen. We always complete the procedure with placement of a cuffed tracheostomy tube. This eases control of secretions from the wound, and ensures adequate mechanical ventilatory support can be rendered in the early postoperative period for these patients. They often have significant cardiopulmonary co-morbidity, which may be exacerbated by converting from transoral respiration to transcervical.[7]

The skin flaps designed as in Figure 55.1 offer viable flaps which reach the trachea with little tension. They allow an open approach to the fibrofatty flap and as described can permit easy access to the level of the mandible and the submental fat pad. However, visible scars are created. These may call unnecessary attention to the neck in these patients, who otherwise look unchanged after complete healing of the incisions and when wearing a high-collar shirt (Fig. 55.4C). Many patients create a necklace that includes a tracheostomy occlusal device of silver or gold, and the patient may be complimented by the casual observer for his attractive jewelry.

For some patients we can create a larger and better vascularized skin flap when designed as depicted in Figure 55.5, with a long collar incision, usually placed at a higher level than a routine thyroidectomy skin incision. The center of the flap near the midline is designed so that a thumbnail sized U-shape elevation of the flap is created that will reach to the tracheal lumen. This flap offers similar exposure to the previously described horizontal H skin incision and usually allows skin flaps to be sutured under minimal tension to the mucosa of the trachea. It enhances the vitality of the inferior skin flap because of its broader base. It is this flap and suture line that are usually at greatest risk of dehiscence and necrosis, creating a granulating wound. When healed, a skin-lined inferior flap allows the tracheostomy to sit on a healed epithelial surface and results in fewer patient complaints of malodorous drainage, bleeding during tracheostomy tube change or cleaning, and minimizes stomal stenosis.[8–10] Another flap, designed by Clayman and Adams, uses superiorly and inferiorly based rectangular flaps united to an inferiorly based U flap of trachea[9] (Fig. 55.4B).

Once complete healing has occurred and the patient is prepared to occlude the tracheostomy tube while active and awake, and to open the lumen only for sleep, we often use an uncuffed plastic (Shiley) or an uncuffed metal (Jackson) tube. We have good success using a Montgomery cannula[11] as a replacement stoma vent after tracheal mucosal healing has occurred and the sutures are absorbed or removed. This cannula (Fig. 55.6A&B) has two flanges which grasp the anterior tracheal wall superiorly and inferiorly, and allow a larger tracheal lumen to permit full activity without dyspnea in these patients. They are often active at work and play, and notice increased air hunger with a plugged standard tracheostomy tube. The tube has been designed at an angle of 27° to fit unobtrusively in the lumen. In general, it extends from the skin more than an uncuffed tracheostomy tube which is built without an Ohio adaptor. Many patients learn to extubate themselves, clean the tracheostomy tube and replace it, plugging it during the day so that they humidify their inspired air transnasally. They can communicate without air escape through the tracheostomy stoma, and lead normal, functional lives. The plug is removed at night or during naps so that no obstructive apnea events will occur.

Custom-molded stoma buttons have been made with co-operation from dental prosthodontists and have been useful to patients with a well-healed stoma. We attempted

## SECTION M TRACHEOSTOMY FOR OSAHS

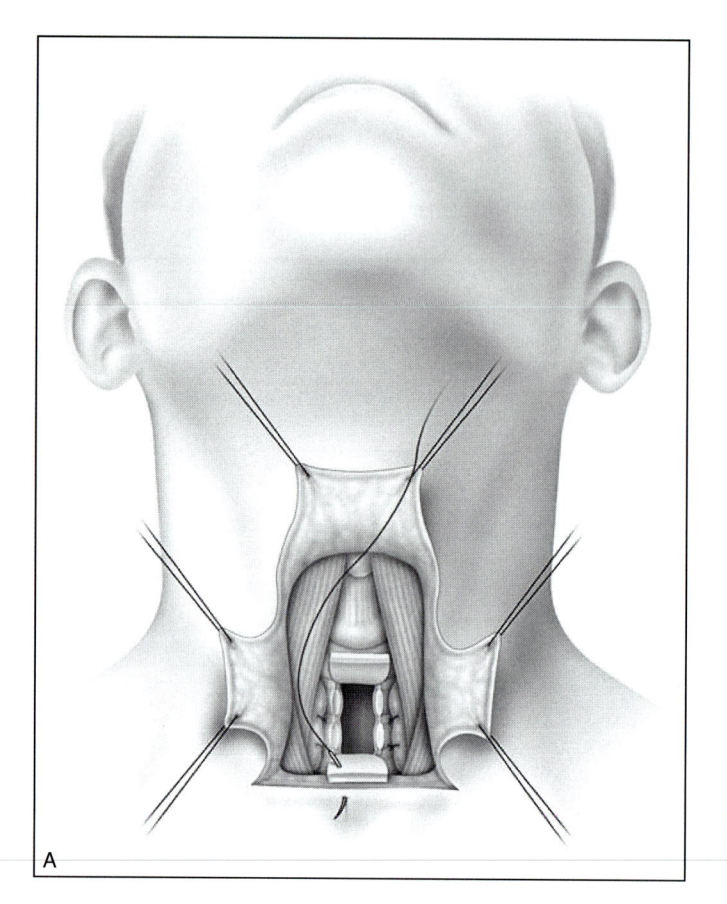

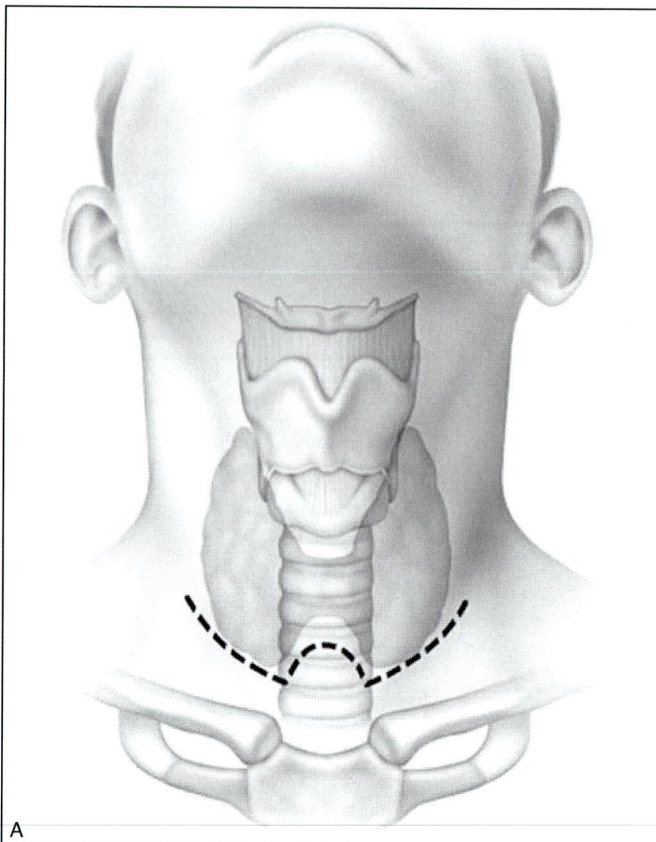

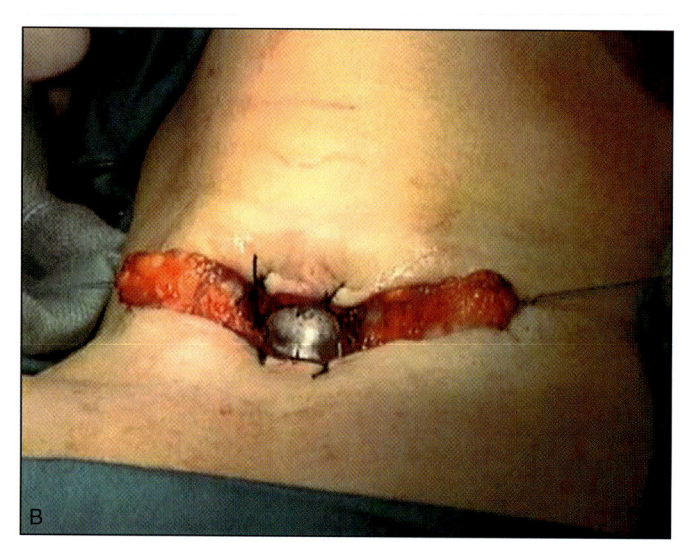

**Fig. 55.4** A&B, Suturing the trachea to the skin flaps creating a healed mucocutaneous junction.

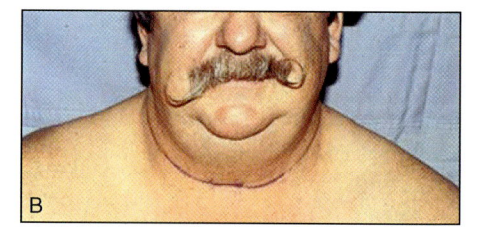

**Fig. 55.5** An alternative skin incision which has been successful in appropriate circumstances.

creating a mold to allow multiple stoma button production. We have found little success at creating a perfect size that fits all patients without an air leak, even as the wound heals and the lumen contracts to fit the button scarred into place.

Therefore, we have not continued to pursue this approach for daytime stoma occlusion in our population of obstructive sleep apnea patients with tracheostomy. Other physicians and their patients continue to work with personalized stoma stents.

Our success with tracheostomy remains excellent, and our complications with this technique, which minimizes granulation and allows the stoma to remain unsupported in many patients overnight, is exemplary. This is in contrast to tracheostomy without skin lining which always requires a stent in place. Our results[4] (Table 55.1) agree with Haapaniemi et al.[12] who noted long-term success and no deaths among seven tracheostomy patients followed for 5 years. Our results also agree with those of

CHAPTER 55
Tracheostomy for sleep apnea

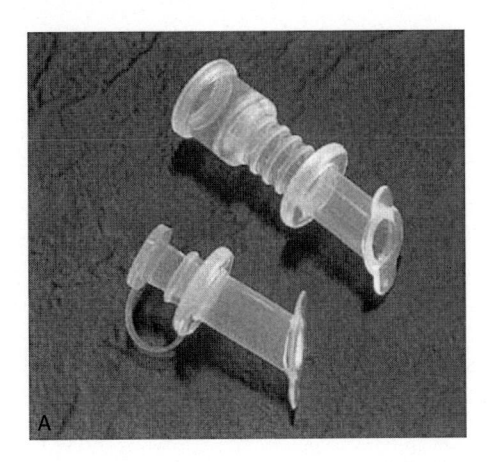

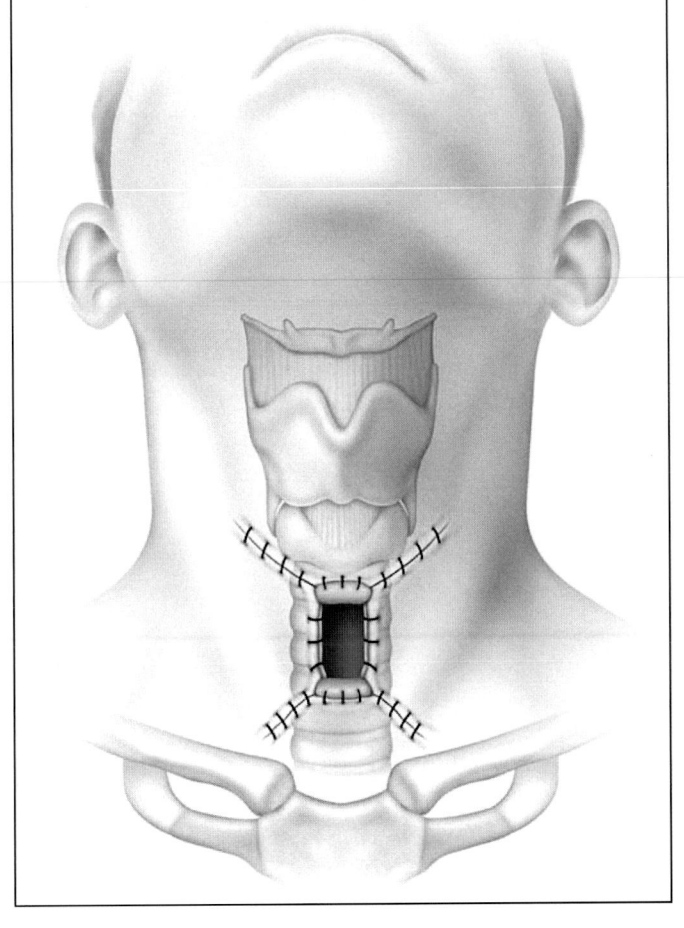

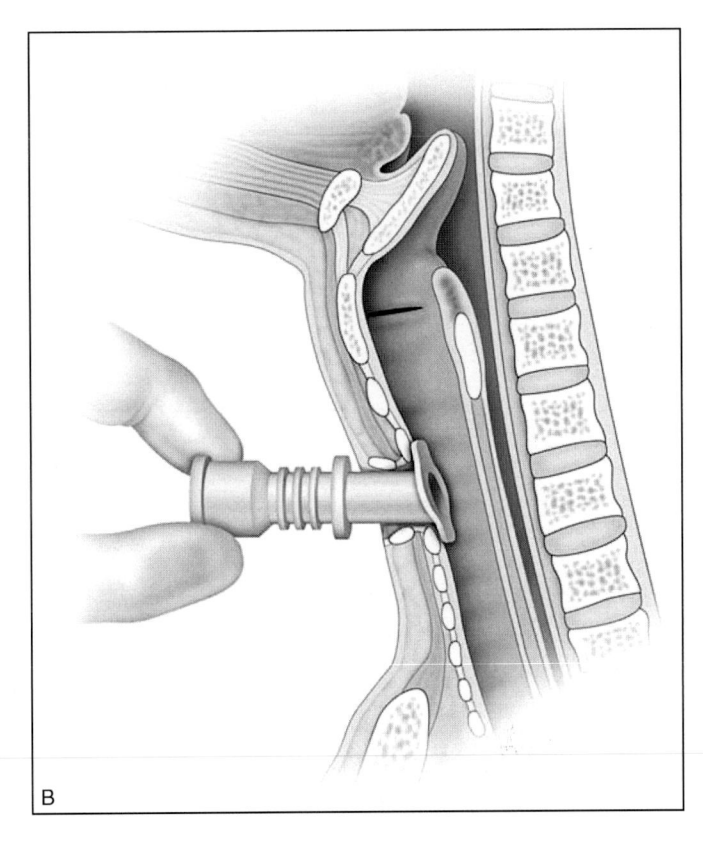

**Fig. 55.6** A, The Montgomery tracheal cannula. B, The tube in place, allowing the entire transverse area of the trachea to provide ventilation during daily activities.

Partinen.[13] He and his co-workers noted no deaths among 33 tracheostomy patients, in contrast to 11 deaths among those who were not treated.[14] The series by Thatcher and Maisel followed obstructive sleep apnea patients long term. This series shows similar encouraging results over a range of up to 20 years for 79 tracheostomy patients.[4]

In conclusion, for patients who are intolerant of mechanical measures or fail upper airway surgery and continue to have severe symptoms or physiologic changes related to obstructive sleep apnea, flap tracheostomy is a reasonable alternative creating a population of alert, awake patients with reduced morbidity and mortality from severe obstructive sleep apnea.

347

# SECTION M: TRACHEOSTOMY FOR OSAHS

| Table 1 | Patient Statistics |
|---|---|
| *No. of patients* | |
| Male | |
| 70 | |
| Female | |
| 9 | |
| *Follow-up* | |
| Mean | |
| 8.3 years | |
| Range | |
| 3 mo–20 y | |
| *Age* | |
| Mean | |
| 47 y | |
| Range 25–70 y | |
| *Body Mass Index* | |
| Mean | |
| 41 | |
| Range | |
| 23–64 | |
| *Respiratory Disturbance Index* | |
| Range 45–146 | |
| Mean 82 | |

## REFERENCES

1. Kuhlo W, Doll E, Frank MC. Successful management of Pickwickian syndrome using long-term tracheotomy. Dtsch Med Wochenschr 1969;13:1286–90.
2. Simmons FB, Guillemainault C, Dement WC, et al. Surgical management of airway obstructions during sleep. Laryngoscope 1976;86:326–38.
3. Weitzman ED, Kahn E, Pollock CP. Quantitative analysis of sleep and sleep apnea before and after tracheostomy in patients with hypersomnia–sleep apnea syndrome. Sleep 1980;3:407–23.
4. Thatcher GW, Maisel RH. The long-term evaluation of tracheostomy in the management of severe obstructive sleep apnea. Laryngoscope 2003;113:201–4.
5. Kim SH, Eisele DW, Smith PL, et al. Evaluation of patients with sleep apnea after tracheotomy. Arch Otolaryngol 1998;124:996–1000.
6. Fee WE, Ward PH. Permanent tracheostomy. Ann Otolaryngol 1977;86:635–8.
7. Sahni R, Blakely B, Maisel RM. 'How I do it' – flap tracheostomy in sleep apnea patients. Laryngoscope 1985;95(2):221–3.
8. Maisel RH, Goding GS. Tracheostomy for obstructive sleep apnea: indications, techniques and selection of tubes. Operat Tech Otolaryngol Head Neck Surg 1991;2:107–11.
9. Clayman GL, Adams GL. Permanent tracheostomy with cervical lipectomy. Laryngoscope 1990;100(4):422–4.
10. Campanini A, De Vito A, Frassineti S, Vicini C. Role of skin-lined tracheotomy in obstructive sleep apnoea syndrome: personal experience. Acta Otorhinolaryngol Ital 2004;24:68–75.
11. Montgomery WW. Silicone tracheal cannula. Ann Otolaryngol 1980;89:521–8.
12. Haapaniemi JJ, Laurikainen EA, Halme P, Antilla J. Long-term results of tracheostomy for severe obstructive sleep apnea syndrome. ORL Relat Spe 2001;63(3):131–6.
13. Partinen N, Jameson A, Guillame C. Long-term outcome for obstructive sleep apnea patients. Chest 1988;94:1200–4.
14. He J, Kryger MH, Zorick FJ, et al. Mortality and apnea index in obstructive sleep apnea. Chest 1988;94:9–14.

SECTION M  TRACHEOSTOMY FOR OSAHS

CHAPTER 56

# Speech-ready, long-term tube-free tracheostomy for obstructive sleep apnea

*Isaac Eliachar, Lee M. Akst and Robert R. Lorenz*

## 1 INTRODUCTION

Obstructive sleep apnea (OSA) is caused by obstacles to the free flow of air through the upper airway from the lips or nasal tip to the larynx and therefore is within the otolaryngologist's sphere of responsibility. Management can involve weight loss, treatment of nasal obstruction, surgery of the pharynx, or the use of various ventilatory assist devices such as continuous positive airway pressure (CPAP). This condition has serious health risks and consequences and should be thoroughly researched and investigated to be treated effectively. Furthermore, it is often multifactorial, requiring a multidisciplinary approach to identify the etiology and optimal treatment for each patient.

Tracheotomy (or tracheostomy) provides the most efficacious bypass of upper airway obstruction and is rightfully considered among the treatments of OSA. Although they can singularly cure OSA, tracheotomy/tracheostomy are regarded as extreme modes of treatment due to associated surgical and postoperative morbidities. In various instances these procedures are reserved for emergencies such as difficult intubation or considered as last resorts in patients with severe, refractory, or life-threatening apnea. Other less frequent indications include morbid obesity, complicated oropharyngeal obstruction with severe hypoxia, failed management attempts, and disabling daytime somnolence.

### 1.1 SEMANTIC CLARIFICATION

In order to understand the role of tracheostomy in the management of obstructive sleep apnea, one must distinguish between *tracheotomy* and *tracheostomy*. These terms are frequently interchanged, mixed or misused. In this chapter, *tracheotomy* refers to an operation in which an opening is made in the trachea for the purposes of short-term cannulation which closes spontaneously when the cannula is removed. On the other hand, *tracheostomy* is derived from the Greek term 'stoma' and is reserved for procedures which are performed with the intent of establishing a patent, long-term or permanent opening between the trachea and the overlying skin.

When this surgically established stoma safely retains its patency, it obviates the dependency on tubes or other devices for support and is designated as a *long-term tube-free tracheostomy*.

With this semantic clarification in mind, one can understand that tracheotomy and tracheostomy have two distinct roles in the management of OSA. For instance, tracheotomy can be performed ad hoc in urgent conditions to *temporarily* secure problematic high-risk airways, making it possible and safe to manage the disease through other techniques. By contrast, tracheostomy may be applied as a primary and definitive treatment of OSA whenever long-term or permanent bypass of the obstructed upper airway is indicated. Once established, tracheostomy is intended to provide safe, complication-free and readily accessible control of the airway during which extended management of a patient's disease with adjunct procedures may be undertaken with minimal risk to the patient's safety. Reversal of both procedures is possible, although with tracheostomy the closure is an operative procedure, while a tracheotomy most often closes spontaneously after cannula removal. This chapter discusses both tracheotomy and tracheostomy, yet the true focus will be upon the use of tracheostomy as a definitive therapy for OSA.

Historically, the documented performance of tracheotomy (semantically misrepresented as tracheostomy) for 'Pickwickian syndrome' was first described in 1969.[1] Since then various modifications of the procedure have evolved into the 'gold standard' for management of OSA because, when successful, it bypasses upper airway obstruction in 100% of the cases in which it is used.[2] Unfortunately, as mentioned above, patients with OSA are often difficult candidates for performance and maintenance of routine tube-dependent tracheotomy; their unfavorable anatomy may be compounded by obesity, diabetes, infection and

# SECTION M: TRACHEOSTOMY FOR OSAHS

cardiopulmonary comorbidity. With each negative experience, lessons were learned that led to modifications of tracheotomy as it related to the treatment of OSA. Through this process, tracheotomy evolved into increasingly refined techniques such as *tube-dependent tracheostomy* and subsequently into the *tube-free tracheostomy* which has been researched, promoted and formulated by the authors. Further classification of these terms is provided below.

## 1.1.1 GLOSSARY

- Short-term procedures:
  Tracheotomy – incisional or percutaneous.
- Long-term procedures:
  Tracheostomy, tube or stent-dependent.
  Tracheostomy, long-term tube-free (LTTFT).
  Speech-ready, LTTFT.

## 2 PATIENT SELECTION

As a treatment option for patients with OSA, tracheotomy/tracheostomy can be performed either as definitive therapy or as a temporary means to control the airway while another upper airway surgery is performed. For instance, the risks of difficult intubation or postoperative airway obstruction due to perioperative edema and hemorrhage may necessitate short-term tracheotomy before, during, or after other surgeries. For most patients, the perioperative risks of such other surgery can be obviated through CPAP or remain low enough that temporary tracheotomy is not necessary. When tracheotomy is performed for this indication, the technique may be in some instances similar to that for any other short-term, tube-dependent procedure. However, as will be further discussed, the degree of obesity and the difficult anatomy that frequently causes OSA may lead to higher rates of intraoperative and/or post-surgical complications that mandate modification of traditional tracheotomy. Furthermore, as patients may fail to lose weight or may not benefit from other surgeries, tracheotomy may not always be as short term as originally planned. For these reasons, traditional tracheotomy has given way to both tube-dependent and tube-free tracheostomy techniques in the management of OSA.

When permanent tracheostomy is considered, it is generally indicated for one of three scenarios. The first scenario is dictated by the patient's abnormal anatomy that cannot be managed under the limitations of traditional tracheotomy, and therefore requires tracheostomy. The second scenario may be encountered in patients with OSA who have failed more conservative medical and/or surgical therapies. As the rest of this book demonstrates, CPAP may not always be applicable, effective, or well-tolerated, and other surgical techniques lack the 100% success rate of bypassing obstruction which is the hallmark of tracheostomy. For patients who fail at weight loss or continue to have medically significant OSA despite conservative medical and/or surgical management, tracheostomy may be considered as the final measure of what is a graduated, step-wise approach to treatment.

In the last scenario, tracheotomy/tracheostomy is performed as the primary procedure for control of severe disease and/or life-threatening cardiopulmonary manifestations of OSA. Polysomnographic indications for tracheo-stomy as a primary treatment modality for OSA include Respiratory Disturbance Index (RDI) $> 50$ and oxygen desaturation to $<60\%$. Additionally, if OSA of any severity causes significant cor pulmonale or cardiac dysrhythmias in association with the apneic episodes, tracheostomy might be warranted as the initial management of choice. For instance, severe bradycardia, asystole, multiple premature ventricular contractions and even runs of ventricular tachycardia in association with apneas may all serve as indications for primary tracheostomy. Lastly, other comorbid states such as impending or recent myocardial infarction, unmanageable hypertension, or diabetes mellitus might serve as indications for immediate and conclusive management through urgent tracheostomy. For example, an epileptic who experiences seizures while apneic or a patient with coronary artery disease who develops nocturnal angina in association with OSA might be promptly and effectively managed with tracheostomy. When indicated, such patients may benefit from the use of modified transtracheal ventilation (e.g. CPAP) at all stages of their treatment (see below).

## 3 TRACHEOTOMY AND TUBE-DEPENDENT TRACHEOSTOMY

'Standard tracheotomy' might be performed in situations in which the duration of cannulation is not expected to exceed several days. These tracheotomies might be performed in OSA if they are used to temporarily secure the airway while other upper airway surgery performed. Even then, the technique may require modifications such as lipectomy or resort to specially designed and constructed tubes in order to be safe and effective. Once postoperative edema is resolved and the risk of perioperative hemorrhage and any other problems have been overcome, the tracheotomy tube may be withdrawn and the tracheotomy site allowed to heal by secondary intent. *If prolonged cannulation is expected, such 'standard tracheotomy' (even when modified) is not the procedure of choice.* Patients with severe obstructive sleep apnea are prone to develop more serious complications as they often have short, thick necks and high incidence of anatomic deformations. Chondritis, granulation tissue, infection, and stenosis make long-term maintenance of a 'temporary standard tracheotomy' undesirable.[2]

Techniques for 'permanent' tracheostomy were developed in order to minimize these complications whenever cannulation is expected to be prolonged.[3] Among the several indications for establishment of a 'permanent' skin-lined tracheostoma are severe laryngeal or laryngotracheal stenosis, bilateral vocal cord fixation (conditions that may cause OSA in and of themselves), neurologic conditions such as myasthenia gravis and amyotrophic lateral sclerosis, and, of course, severe OSA. The first report of permanent tracheostomy for the management of pulmonary disease was by Penta and Mayer[4] in 1960; the technique was subsequently popularized for OSA by Fee and Ward[5] in 1977. These techniques aim to decrease the length of the tracheocutaneous tract and bring the margins of the tracheal fenestration into direct contact and continuity with the cervical skin. Shortening the skin-to-trachea tract limits granulation tissue within the wound bed, promotes primary healing of the mucocutaneous junction, inhibits stomal stenosis, and aims to limit other complications associated with prolonged tracheotomy.

There are several techniques for creating a 'permanent' tracheostoma depending upon the degree of continuity established between the trachea and the cervical skin. One early method for creation of a permanent tracheostomy was the Bjork flap, in which an inferiorly based tracheal flap (generally created from the anterior portion of the second or third tracheal ring) is sutured to the inferior skin margin.[6] Use of this flap relative to standard tracheotomy reduced rates of accidental decannulation and facilitated re-insertion of a displaced tracheotomy tube.[7] Later methods for tracheostomy attempted to further improve the primary attachments between the trachea and the skin. An example is the 'H-flap' technique described by Mickelson.[2] By mobilizing both cervical skin and tracheal flaps, a fully circumferential stoma is created through this technique.

More extensive surgical approaches were researched with the intent to achieve maximal shortening of the tracheocutaneous tract, at the same time producing a tension-free, fully circumferential, permanently patent mucocutaneous junction. These modifications are designed to promote primary healing, ease wound care and facilitate re-cannulation more readily than the Bjork flap or the 'H-flap.' Protracted healing by secondary intent, which is often accompanied by stenosis or scar formation, is thus minimized. In past experiences, even these permanent tracheostomies depended upon prolonged placement of irritating foreign bodies in the form of tracheotomy tubes or designated stoma stents. As will be discussed later, these tube- or stent-dependent tracheostomy techniques, although better tolerated than standard tracheotomy, still develop inevitable tube-related complications which have led to the evolution of the *tube-free* concepts advocated by the authors.

## 4 REVIEW OF THE LITERATURE ON THE EFFICACY OF TRACHEOTOMY AND TRACHEOSTOMY IN OSA

*The reader should be aware that these two terms may be inappropriately interchanged in the following references.*

Once successfully performed, tracheotomy or tracheostomy should provide secure and complete bypass of any ventilatory obstruction proximal to the tracheotomy's point of entry into the trachea. This achievement is unmatched by any other form of therapy for OSA. In one study, for instance, tracheostomy successfully relieved OSA in 24 patients; 22 of these patients had already failed other treatment modalities.[8] Nor does the efficacy of tracheotomy fade with time, provided that local tracheal complications are avoided. A retrospective review of 79 patients with tracheostomies for OSA reveals that, even with a mean follow-up of over 8 years, tracheostomy eliminated the obstructive component in OSA in all cases.[9] Long-term follow-up suggests that tracheostomy improves parameters such as Apnea/Hypopnea Index, snoring, and excessive somnolence with efficacy unmatched by any other therapy.[10]

Another benefit of tracheostomy is the immediacy with which it cures OSA. Obstruction is relieved soon after the tracheostomy is established. Polysomnographic measures of sleep architecture reveal that delta-wave and REM sleep are greatly increased soon after tracheotomy, in a 'rebound' phenomenon in which the body attempts to replenish those stages of deep sleep lost to apneic episodes.[2] Within 1 month following tracheostomy, normal sleep architecture is returned; within weeks after tracheostomy, patients experience resolution of daytime sleepiness and snoring.[11] In association with these improved sleep parameters, Guilleminault et al. also found that tracheotomy resolved the personality changes, erratic behavior, enuresis, morning headache, sleepwalking, and other symptoms related to OSA.[12]

Other studies demonstrate the effectiveness of tracheostomy in reducing the mortality associated with OSA. He et al. found that in patients with apnea indices >20, the 38% 8-year mortality of untreated patients was reduced to 0% in 33 patients with tracheostomy.[13] Partinen et al. report similar findings in their cohort of 198 patients, 71 treated with tracheostomy and 127 treated conservatively with weight loss.[14] All deaths at 5 years were in the weight loss group with a 5-year mortality rate of 11% as compared to 0% for tracheostomy. These differences in mortality are even more remarkable given that the tracheostomy group had, on average, higher apnea and body mass indices than the comparable weight loss group.

One early study on tracheostomy and hemodynamic changes in OSA was published by Motta et al. in 1978.[11] Comparing patients with OSA before and after tracheostomy, these investigators found that during sleep, mean pulmonary and femoral artery pressures were significantly reduced following tracheostomy, while arterial oxygen levels were increased. Although the underlying mechanisms of increased cardiovascular morbidity and mortality are not entirely understood, one postulated etiology is that repeated hypoxic events in OSA initiate oxidative stress, cause endothelial cell dysfunction, and exacerbate atherogenic injury.[15]

Unfortunately, there are some limits to the effectiveness of tracheostomy for treatment of sleep apnea. First, tracheostomy can successfully treat only *obstructive* sleep apnea; central apnea may continue to be a problem for these patients. Indeed, one case report even describes the obstructive apneas corrected by tracheostomy being replaced by central events of similar duration and severity.[16] Second, *tube-dependent tracheostomy* can only provide effective bypass of upper airway obstruction as long as the tube remains patent. In a patient with a large body habitus, excess soft tissue or skin folds over the chest and under the chin may actually obstruct the tube's proximal end. It is for that reason that some authors recommend specially designed tubes in addition to adequate lipectomy in combination with tracheostomy for obese patients.[17] Misalignment between the tube and the trachea may result in impaction of the tube's caudal end against the tracheal wall, causing local ridge formation or stenosis, both of which may be compounded by traumatic suctioning. Unfortunately, patients with OSA compounded by cardiopulmonary decompensation may be more prone to complications including infections and even persistent apnea following tracheostomy (from central events, stenosis or tube obstruction) than patients with 'uncomplicated' OSA.[18]

## 5 COMPLICATIONS OF TUBE-DEPENDENT TECHNIQUES (TRACHEOTOMY OR TUBE-DEPENDENT TRACHEOSTOMY)

The complications of tube-dependent tracheotomy/tracheostomy can generally be divided into short-term and long-term categories. Short-term complications include possible intraoperative consequences such as damage to the great vessels, injury of the tracheo-esophageal party wall, pneumothorax, and pneumomediastinum. Early postoperative consequences of tracheotomy such as tube obstruction, tube displacement, and infection can also be considered short-term complications. Among the long-term complications are such problems as deep tissue infection, granulation tissue and laryngeal and/or tracheal stenosis at the stomal level or at the caudal end of the tube with predisposition to tracheo–innominate artery fistula. In addition to these physical complications, the often persistent morbidity associated with tube-dependent tracheostomy may have emotional consequences (such as depression) as well, for both the patient and the patient's family.[12,19]

Several studies have documented the incidence of short-term complications following tracheotomy/tracheostomy for OSA. Thatcher and Maisel's review of 79 patients counts four instances of peristomal wound infection, four instances of skin flap necrosis, and one fatal episode of cardiac arrest among early complications.[9] Harmon et al. report a 15% incidence of peristomal infection following tracheostomy for OSA,[20] while Guilleminault et al. suggest that the incidence of low-grade infection causing peristomal granulation may be closer to 42%.[12] This same group also reports that a similar percentage (42%) of patients experienced early problems with poorly fitted tracheotomy tubes, such that the tube would become obstructed when the patient's head was flexed, hyperextended or turned to the side.

Postobstructive pulmonary edema has been commonly reported following relief of short-term upper airway obstruction, such as that found with postoperative laryngospasm.[21] However, postobstructive pulmonary edema has also been described as a consequence of OSA, perhaps secondary to effects of OSA on the heart and pulmonary vasculature.[22] Given that tracheostomy for severe OSA provides immediate relief of prolonged upper airway obstruction, it should not be surprising that postobstructive pulmonary edema has been described in this setting as well. Comparing 45 OSA patients to 25 non-OSA patients, Burke et al. found an incidence of pulmonary edema of 67% in the OSA group following tracheotomy as compared to a control group incidence of 20%.[23] While most OSA patients with post-tracheotomy pulmonary edema were graded as 'mild', 8/30 patients with pulmonary edema were graded as 'moderate' or 'severe' and two patients (7% of the overall OSA group) died of complications related to cor pulmonale in the post-tracheotomy period.

Among long-term complications of tracheostomy, tracheo–innominate artery fistula is the most feared. Though rare (only one of 79 patients in Thatcher and Maisel's study[9]), it carries a mortality rate of 73%. One controllable factor which might predispose towards fistula is a 'too low' tracheotomy, and for this reason, tracheotomy is rarely performed beneath the third tracheal ring. Unfortunately, emphysematous, barrel-chested, or overweight OSA patients may have a high innominate artery, mandating modifications in the surgical procedure that may promote additional damage, to the larynx in particular.

A much more common long-term complication of tracheostomy is progressive, tube-related deformation of the trachea itself, including the development of laryngotracheal stenosis. Estimates of long-term tracheal damage following tracheostomy for OSA vary and depend on the surgical technique and endpoint used in each study. For instance, Conway et al.[19] reported on eight patients with standard tracheotomy and found that seven (87.5%) experienced tracheal granuloma or stomal stenosis. Among eight patients (five revision, three primary) with skin-lined permanent tracheostomy, the incidence of tracheal complications decreased to 25%. Thatcher and Maisel do not record the overall

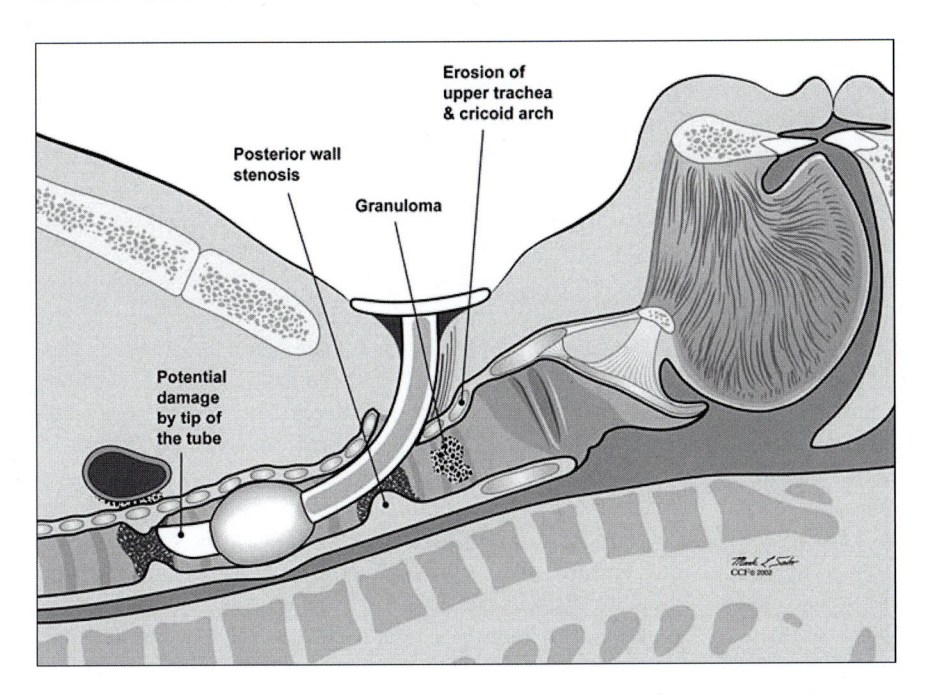

**Fig. 56.1** Prolonged maintenance of a tracheotomy tube causes inevitable tracheal complications, particularly just above the level of the stoma.

proportion of patients who developed granulation tissue, but document that eight of 79 (10%) of their cohort needed to return to the operating room for management of this problem.[9]

Such retrospective studies might underestimate the degree of structural laryngotracheal deformities, infections, chondritis, granulation tissue and stenosis compared to prospective studies. Law et al. review several studies and find that retrospective reviews report obstructive tracheal lesions at rates of 1–11%, while prospective studies find obstructive lesions in 20–64% of patients with long-term tracheostomies.[24] Their own study of 81 patients with long-term tracheotomy (mean duration 4.9 months) utilizing fiberoptic bronchoscopy prior to decannulation discovered obstructive lesions in 54 patients (67%). Of these 54 patients with tracheal obstruction secondary to prolonged tube-dependent tracheotomy, almost half (23 of 54, 43%) had more than one type of obstructing lesion. All of the lesions were located above the level of the stoma, and included 45 obstructing tracheal granulomas (all from the anterior tracheal wall), 19 patients with tracheomalacia, and 10 episodes of tracheal stenosis.

Unfortunately, damage to the trachea and larynx above the level of the stoma is too commonly an unavoidable consequence of prolonged cannulation with a curved tracheotomy tube. The introduction of a mismatched curved foreign body (the routinely used tracheotomy tube) into an otherwise straight airway displaces the suprastomal portion of the anterior tracheal wall inwards (Fig. 56.1). This pathologic buckling of the trachea is an unrelenting dynamic process perpetuated by the movements of the tube relative to the trachea during coughing, breathing, swallowing, and manipulation of the tube for cleaning. In this fashion, progressive deformation of the trachea can erode the anterior superior tracheal wall and lead to suprastomal inflammation,

infection, granulation, perichondritis, chondritis and eventually necrosis, potentially extending to the cricoid arch and conus elasticus. When the tube is withdrawn, various degrees of tracheomalacia and tracheal stenosis may occur. Variations of standard tracheotomy tubes (i.e. tubes that are narrower, smoother, softer, more flexible, shorter, etc.) can help reduce but cannot eliminate the laryngotracheal morbidity associated with prolonged cannulation.[25]

## 6 TUBE-FREE TRACHEOSTOMY

### 6.1 EVOLUTION OF LONG-TERM TUBE-FREE TRACHEOSTOMY

Commitment to minimize the serious consequences of tube-induced damage and its complications prompted extensive research and efforts that brought forward the concept of *long-term tube-free tracheostomy* (LTTFT) as an alternative to tube-dependent tracheostomy.[26] A case report by Eliashar et al. in which an OSA patient with an existing tube-dependent tracheotomy is revised to a LTTFT typifies the efforts to minimize the *tube-induced* complications of long-term tracheotomy and/or tracheostomy.[27] The permanently tube-free patent stoma acquired the descriptive nickname 'third nostril'. LTTFT is currently our recommended procedure of choice for severe and refractory OSA, as well as for other indications which require prolonged tracheostomy.

Just as tube-dependent techniques progressed from standard tracheotomy to the inferiorly based Bjork flap to fully circumferential skin-lined 'permanent tracheostomies', so did long-term tube-free tracheostomy evolve out of previous techniques. The procedure of LTTFT currently practiced by us is not the first tube-free technique to be described. For instance, three of the four patients described by Fee and Ward in 1977 could have been managed without tracheostomy tubes.[5] However, early descriptions of tube-free techniques generally employed plugs, stents or other prostheses to enable speech during daytime even as they maintained a tube-free stoma at night.[28-30] In the staged development leading to the current procedure of LTTFT, the senior author almost routinely applied specially designed Eliachar/Hood stoma stents, often with attached speaking valves, to support the patency of the stoma.[31] This use of a stent, with or without a speaking valve, was practiced in all but seven patients who underwent flap-tracheostomy by the senior author prior to 1992. Of the seven tube-free patients in this group who did not require a stoma stent, five used finger occlusion of their stomata to produce speech and cough. The remaining two patients developed the ability to intentionally constrict the neck muscles around the stoma, temporarily closing it in a voluntary and timely fashion to divert airflow from the stoma through the glottis with ample volume, pressure, and velocity to produce audible voice and almost normal speech. They also succeeded in producing an effective cough which enabled them to clear secretions through the glottis rather than out of the stoma.

These patients had converted a 'third nostril' for respiration into a 'second mouth' which could be alternately opened and closed to redirect the flow of the air and allow for respiration, speech, and cough without any form of prosthesis or finger occlusion.

These two patients with volitional stoma closure formed the impetus for *deliberate* establishment of a truly tube-free speech-ready technique. They clearly enjoyed higher levels of function and comfort than those patients who required use of a stoma stent. The absence of tubes and prostheses in these patients reduced local irritation and improved management of secretions at the same time that it practically eliminated almost all the morbid symptoms and/or complications from tracheostomy. Because of this experience, a prospective study was designed in an effort to intentionally create long-term, tube-free, *speech-ready* tracheostomata in 35 patients from 1992 to 1999.[26] As a consequence of successful outcomes of this study, the updated surgical technique for establishment of speech-ready LTTFT has been routinely employed in over 100 more patients since that time.

## 6.2 TECHNIQUE OF SPEECH-READY, LONG-TERM TUBE-FREE TRACHEOSTOMY

As is the case with most surgical procedures, the technique of speech-ready LTTFT is best performed primarily in patients without previous tracheostomies. A relatively more difficult revision procedure may be applied in patients with pre-existing tube-dependent tracheotomies or tube-dependent tracheostomies. The technique has been described comprehensively in previous articles.[26] Preoperatively the patient's medical condition, prognosis and surgical risks are thoroughly assessed. Flexible bronchoscopy and computed tomography scans with reconstituted sagittal and coronal images contribute to the surgical planning. Additionally, assessing the depth of the trachea relative to the sternal notch with the head both flexed and extended can determine appropriate levels for both intraoperative intubation and the physiologically correct placement of the tracheal fenestration. While this examination may be performed in the office, preoperative endoscopic evaluation in the operating room can be an invaluable tool for satisfactory surgical outcome. The procedure should be thoroughly co-ordinated with the patient's primary managing physicians and the anesthesiologists, covering topics such as the required deep intubation and the need for an extra-long endotracheal tube that will position the cuff deep to the site of the intended fenestra. Plans must be made for possible postoperative consequences such as pulmonary edema and provisions arranged for the immediate availability of specially modified precurved endotracheal tubes needed for safe, atraumatic postoperative management. On the operating table, the patient's neck should not be overextended to ensure physiologic placement of the stoma.

The procedure itself involves a wide horizontal omega-shaped skin incision with the horizontal limbs located approximately a centimeter superior to the clavicles, extending beyond the sternocleidomastoid muscle laterally (Fig. 56.2A). The 'dome' of the omega reaches up to the level of the cricoid arch in the moderately extended neck. This skin incision is carried through the platysma muscle, and subplatysmal flaps are widely undermined in all directions. To achieve full mobilization of the flaps, it is often required to extend the dissection and undermining beyond the margins of the sternocleidomastoid muscles laterally and beneath the sternum caudally.

The dissection continues by separating the strap muscles in the midline (Fig. 56.2B). Similarly, the isthmus of the thyroid gland is divided or excised and the lobes are suture-ligated for hemostasis. The next crucial step is to laterally mobilize and dissect the thyroid lobes off the anterolateral surface of the trachea. By everting the strap muscles and thyroid lobes and then suturing their medial free margins laterally to the sternal tendon of the sternocleidomastoid muscles, a wide trough can be created in the midline so that the skin may be easily mobilized and brought into direct continuity with the tracheal fenestration without any interposing tissue in the way.

A superiorly based flap is created from the anterior tracheal wall, based upon the second and third or third and fourth tracheal rings. This superiorly based tracheal flap complements the design of the inferiorly based skin flap created through use of the omega skin incision. Excess submental fat is trimmed subplatysmally throughout the upper surgical field. The tracheal flap can thus be elevated superiorly in such a fashion as to maintain stomal patency.

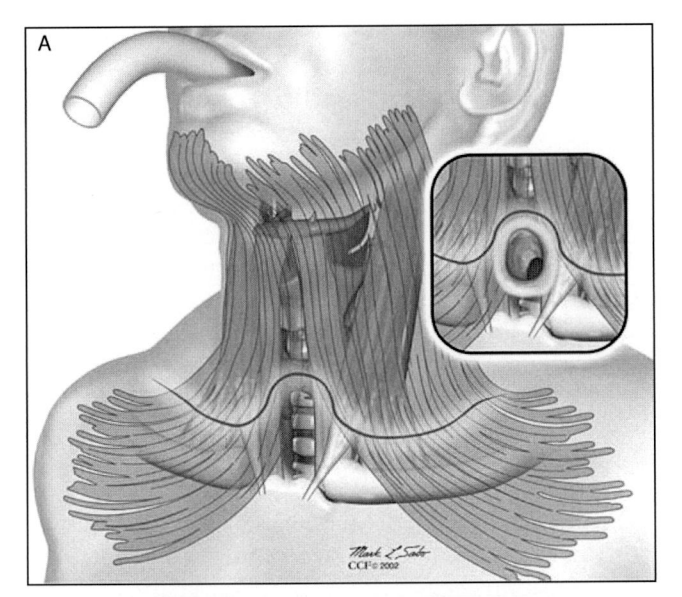

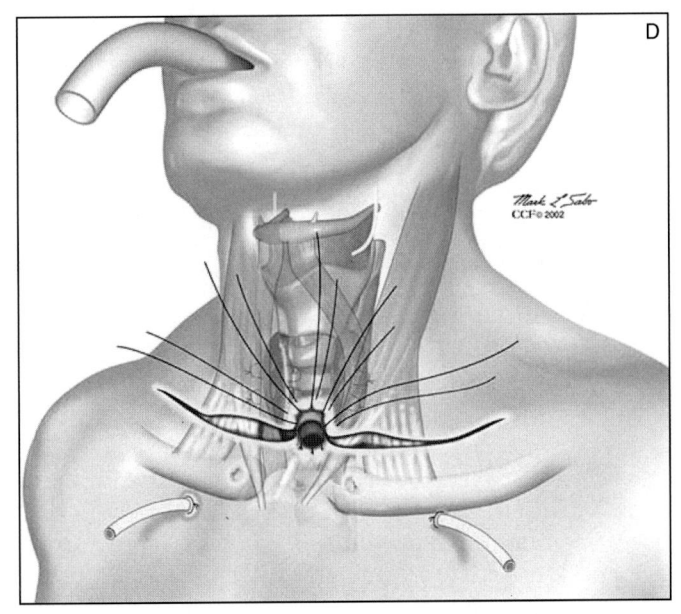

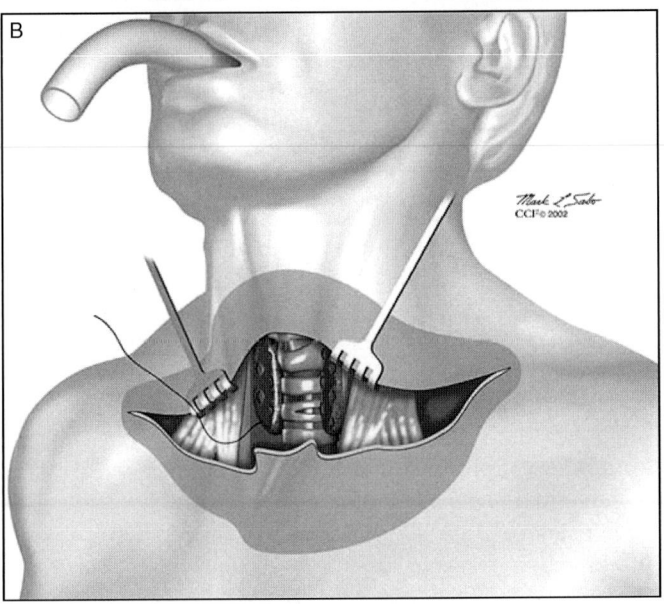

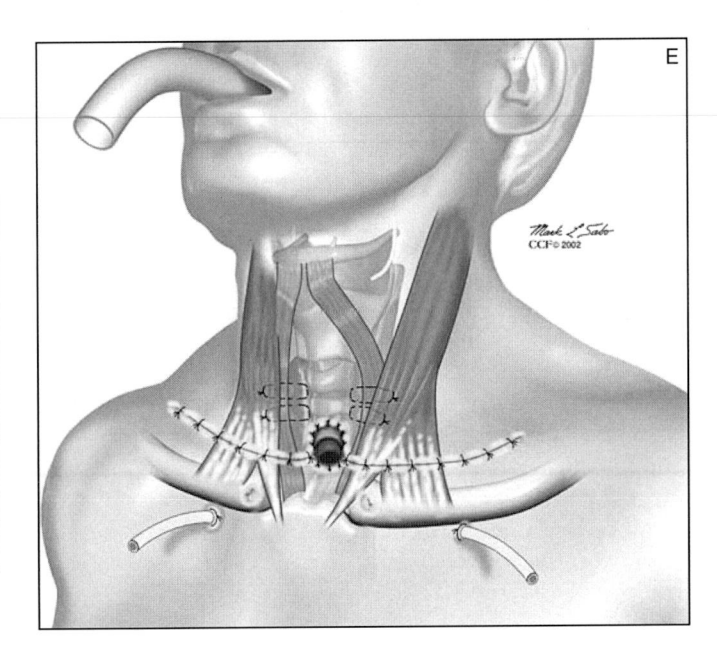

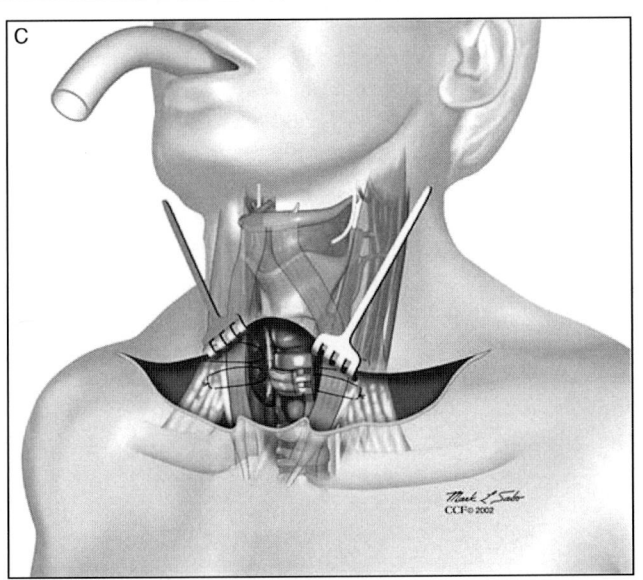

CHAPTER 56
Speech-ready, long-term tube-free tracheostomy for OSA

**Fig. 56.2** A, A curvilinear incision allows for an inferiorly based omega-shaped skin flap. This incision can accommodate pre-existing tracheotomy (inset). B, Midline dissection divides the strap muscles and thyroid lobes in order to expose the trachea. C, Stay sutures lateralize these structures away from a superiorly based tracheal fenestration, so that there is no tissue barrier between the skin flaps and the trachea. D, Drains are placed as the skin flaps are advanced towards the trachea. Suturing of the inferiorly based omega-shaped skin flap to the superiorly based tracheal flap fenestration allows for creation of a circumferentially stable tube-free stoma. E, The end result is a fully circumferential mucocutaneous junction.

355

Meanwhile, excess fat is also trimmed from the undersurface of the inferior peristomal skin flaps so that they can be fully mobilized as well. Care must be taken during the subplatysmal excision of the adipose tissues to avoid compromise of the vascular supply to the skin flaps. Monopolar cautery is used sparingly, as bipolar cautery may reduce collateral tissue damage. Suspension stay sutures placed bilaterally between the inferior skin flap and the tendons surrounding the sternoclavicular joints can help to advance this flap superiorly and facilitate adaptation to the tracheal fenestra for tension-free closure (Fig. 56.2C). Suction drains are placed bilaterally. The tracheal fenestration and margins of the skin flaps are brought together with vertical mattress sutures in order to create a secure skin-tight circumferentially lined stoma (Fig. 56.2D). The superiorly based tracheal flap itself is surrounded by the superior skin flap, while the omega portion of the inferior skin flap is extended tension free to reach the inferolateral aspects of the tracheal fenestration. The overall effect is to create a continuous, airtight, circumferential, tension-free mucocutaneous junction which will mature by primary intent into a secure, patent tube-free stoma with a short tracheocutaneous tract (Fig. 56.2E).

Postoperative care of the suture line and the stoma must be frequent, thorough, careful and routinely performed in order to promote complete healing and aid stoma maturation. Every few hours, trained nurses, employing sterile approach and avoiding the use of tissue irritants such as hydrogen peroxide, remove crusts, gently suction, and apply protective antibiotic ointment to the peristomal suture line. The modified pre-curved, postoperative tube provides secure ventilation during the crucial first postoperative hours. This tube should be removed (unless otherwise indicated) by the end of the first postoperative day, and under no circumstances should a conventional tracheotomy tube be placed through the tracheostoma as it heals. Drains may be removed as necessary. Lateral skin sutures (from the horizontal aspects of the skin incision) can be removed one week postoperatively. Peristomal sutures should be maintained for 10 days or longer, depending upon stoma maturation. After several days in the hospital, the patient and patient's family are trained and encouraged to assume responsibility for stoma care. Home nursing care is provided, and the patient is closely monitored for the first several postoperative weeks as it becomes clear whether the stoma will remain patent or stenose. All efforts are made to maintain the stoma without a tube or stent. It is our experience that once a tube or stent is placed during the healing process, the resulting physical deformation and foreign body-induced inflammatory effects may render its later removal difficult or impossible. In the series of 35 patients with LTTFT published in 2000, all patients were managed in a truly tube-free fashion.[26] At present, we consider use of a stent or tube to be a relatively infrequent and short-lived perioperative setback which is usually encountered predominantly in conversion and in revision cases.

## 6.3 BENEFITS OF LONG-TERM, TUBE-FREE, SPEECH-READY TRACHEOSTOMY

Aside from freedom from the consequential morbidity and tracheal complications described above, there are functional pulmonary benefits to LTTFT. Tracheobronchial mucociliary functions recover postoperatively, and without a tube to disrupt clearance, secretions are transferred naturally up the trachea and through the larynx into the pharynx where they can be cleared by swallowing or coughing with no spewing of the discharge through the stoma. Aspiration is effectively prevented after LTTFT because the normal laryngeal reflexes and cough are not impeded, as they are by tube-dependent techniques. Additionally, airflow from the tube-free stoma circulates both superiorly and inferiorly, and not just inferiorly as it does through a tracheotomy tube. Patients with LTTFT can circulate odorants through the nasopharynx and restore taste and smell. Overall, the tube-free stoma allows for more natural airflow patterns, airway protection, and secretion management than standard tracheotomy.

As patients achieve more control over their stomata, they may also enjoy the benefits of hands-free speech and cough. Although originally conceived as a passive 'third nostril' which maintains patency and provides bypass of upper airway obstruction, *speech-ready* LTTFT has been found to function more as an active 'second mouth' by enabling most patients to voluntarily close their stoma. In this mode, the stoma is opened for ventilation and is closed for speech and cough (Fig. 56.3A&B). Closure of the stoma diverts expiratory airflow through the native larynx and upper airway so that these tasks can be accomplished without the use of prostheses or finger occlusion.

Beyond the benefits of hands-free and prosthesis-free speech and cough, long-term tube-free tracheostomy also offers easier hygiene than tube-dependent tracheotomy/tracheostomy. When nocturnal assisted ventilation is required, patients or family members can easily insert a designated well-tolerated tube through the stoma. Otherwise, there is no need for routine maintenance or care of a tracheotomy tube, suctioning is rarely necessary, and no special nursing care is required. Patients are able to clean their stoma much as they would clean their nostrils and are freed from the responsibility of carrying the burdensome equipment upon which their life might have depended were they maintained with curved tracheotomy tubes. In many ways, switching from a tube-dependent tracheotomy to LTTFT tracheostomy allows patients to regain mobility and freedom along with improved function; together, these changes can improve morale and quality of life. Anecdotally, improved quality of life has certainly been the much appreciated experience of those patients who have been revised from a tube-dependent tracheotomy to a LTTFT. For patients with LTTFT, a turtleneck shirt or a bib worn over the stoma may be the only clue to alert an astute observer to the presence of a successful tube-free stoma.

Speech-ready, long-term tube-free tracheostomy for OSA  CHAPTER 56

## 6.4 THE SUPPLEMENTARY SLING PROCEDURE

In order to divert the flow of air through the larynx rather than the stoma, and thus generate audible hands-free speech and cough, stomal closing pressures must exceed translaryngeal resistance. The ability to volitionally close a stoma sufficiently to direct flow through the larynx and upper airway is a skill that most patients learn innately, though some need encouragement or special exercises. Occasionally, either local muscle weakness or scarring may lead to inadequate voluntary stomal constriction. Also, fixed laryngotracheal stenosis above the stoma, bilateral vocal cord fixation or upper airway obstruction (as found in patients with OSA) may increase upper airway resistance. In these settings where laryngeal resistance exceeds stomal closure, attempts to generate unaided speech encounter a variable degree of air leakage through the intentionally constricted stoma. For these patients, an auxiliary second surgical procedure called the *supplementary sling procedure* may be performed several months after establishment of the tube-free stoma.[32] (The sling procedure should *never* be performed before the tube-free stoma is completely mature.) This procedure repositions neck tendons and muscles in order to help these particular patients to improve stoma closure. The sling procedure has been instrumental in helping to achieve more effective stoma closure with improved voice and tracheal clearance in almost all patients with tube-free stomata who have required this further intervention (Fig. 56.4). Of the 80 LTTFTs performed since 2002, only 22 patients required the sling procedure to gain more effective volitional stomal closure.

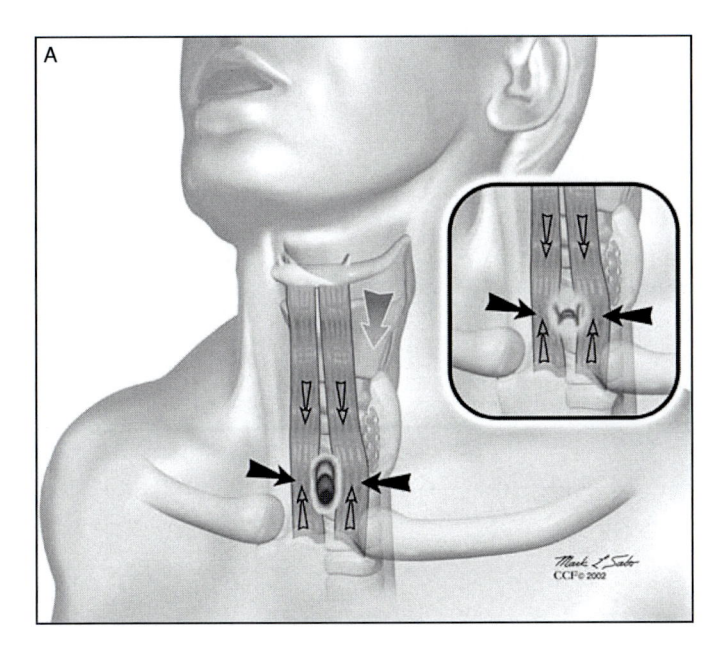

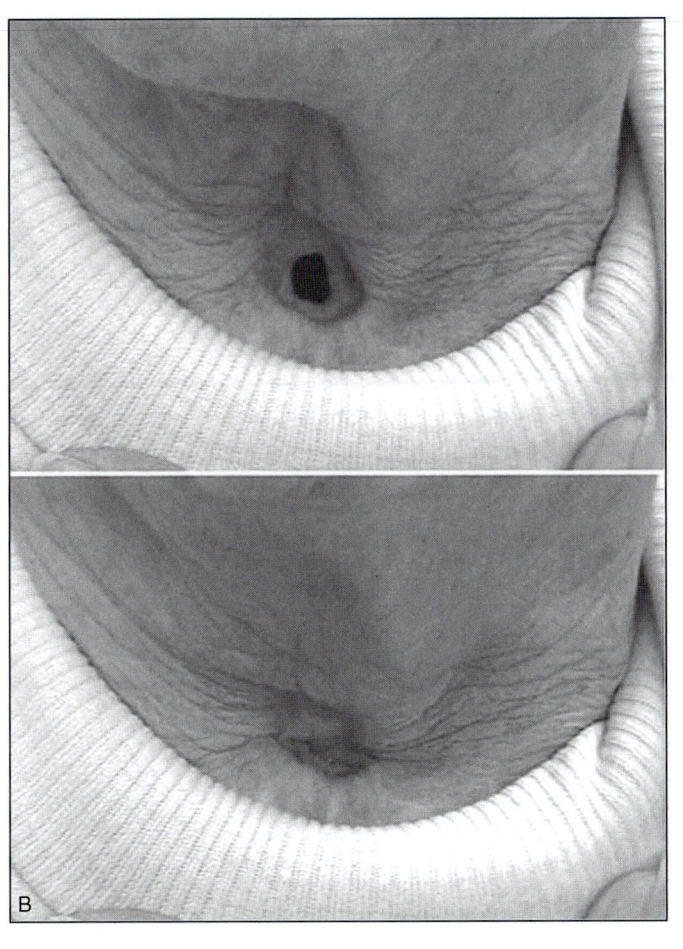

**Fig. 56.3** A, A schematic representation of how a patient can use the neck muscles to voluntarily leave the stoma open for breathing and then close it for effective hands-free speech and cough. B, Actual patient images demonstrate voluntary control of the long-term tube-free tracheostoma.

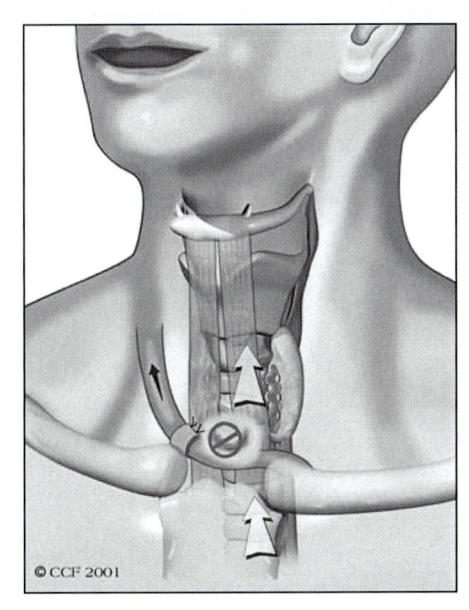

**Fig. 56.4** The sling procedure: a right superiorly based SCM muscle flap is tunneled inferior to the stoma and approximated to the left, inferiorly based SCM muscle. The result is a voluntary closure of the stoma through superior movement of the inferior stomal mucocutaneous margin.

357

# SECTION M  TRACHEOSTOMY FOR OSAHS

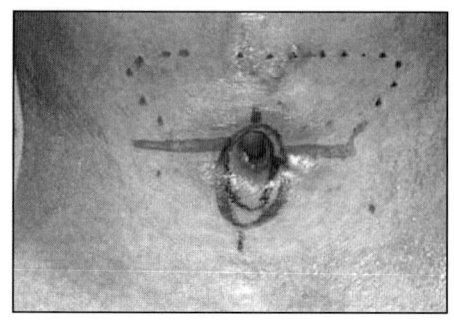

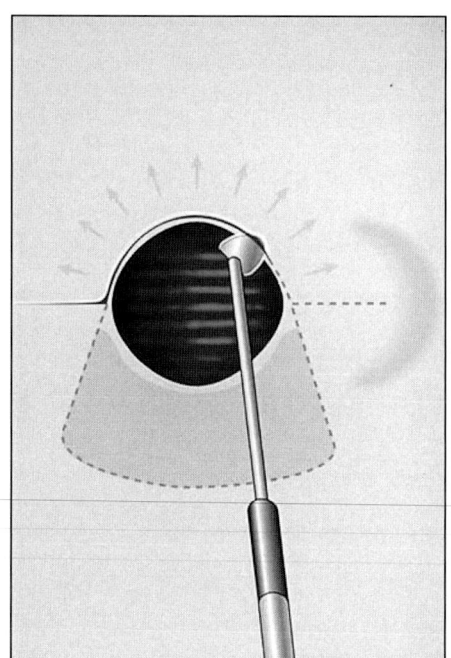

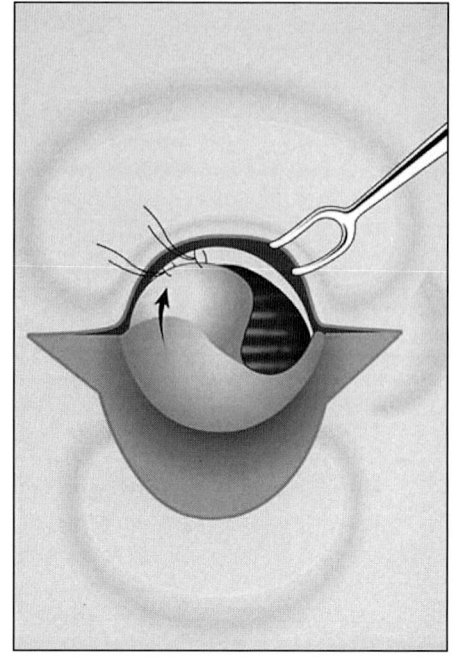

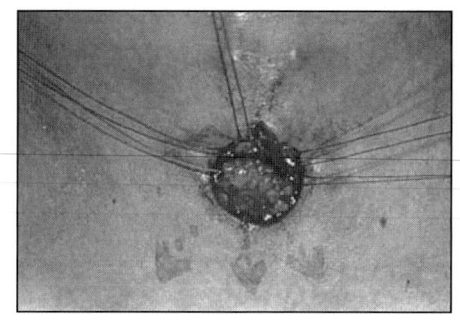

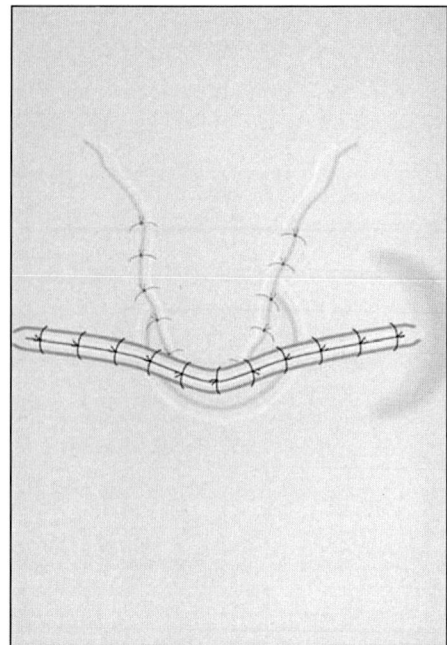

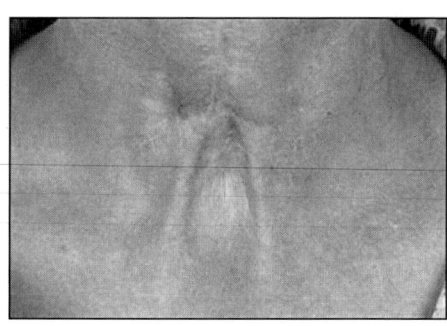

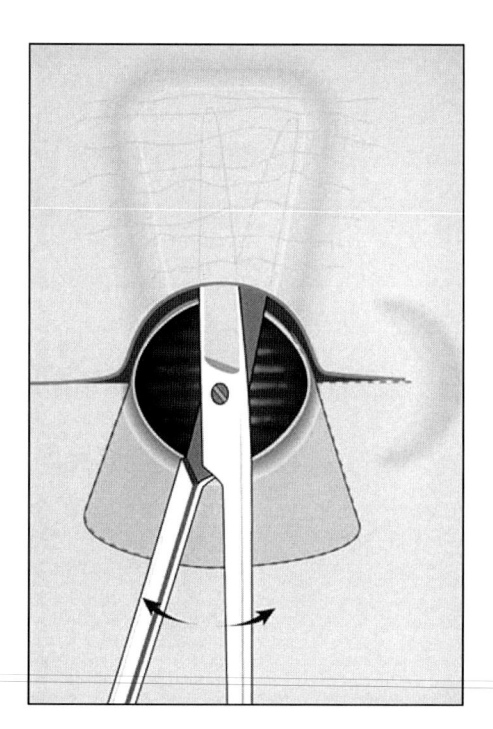

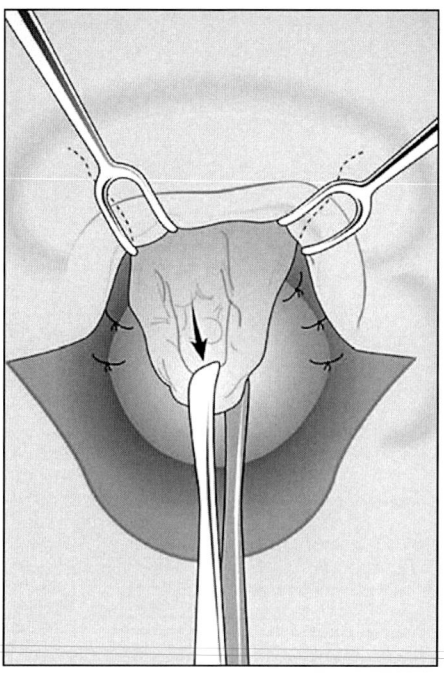

**Fig. 56.5** Tracheostomy closure. A, Planning of incisions (solid lines) and undermining of skin in a horizontal type of stoma closure. B, Superior incision is performed to accept the 'turn-over' flap and create the superiorly based external skin advancement flap. C, Wide superior undermining is a key portion of the procedure to allow the advancement flap. D, The inferiorly based 'turn-over' flap is formed, sized to meet the superior margin of the stoma (overly sized flaps become obstructive in the tracheal lumen). E, Absorbable sutures approximate the turn-over flap to the stomal upper margin. F, Advancement of fibro-fatty tissue creates a soft tissue cushion to the wound, allowing for less dimpling to the postoperative appearance. G, The superiorly based advancement flap is brought down to meet the inferior incision. H, Two-month follow-up result of the horizontally closed stoma.

## 7 TRACHEOSTOMY CLOSURE

The decision to close a tracheostomy must be made very carefully. If a stoma is closed inappropriately, the patient might experience recurrence of OSA. Therefore, closure becomes appropriate only if other surgery, weight loss, or compliance with CPAP can effectively control OSA in lieu of tracheostomy. The degree of OSA which might be present following tracheostomy closure can be assessed by performing polysomnography with the tube plugged or the stoma seal-taped. Thorough endoscopic and, if needed, radiologic examinations must rule out signs of potential laryngotracheal stenosis before closure. Recent studies document the significant effect that gastric bypass may have upon weight loss and subsequent tracheostomy closure in patients with OSA.[33,34] Despite these advances, long-term studies with large numbers of patients demonstrate that relatively few patients with tracheostomy for OSA ever have their stomata closed – 16 of 79 patients for Thatcher and Maisel,[9] and only four of 50 patients for Guilleminault et al.[12]

Mickelson and Rosenthal[35] studied two techniques for closure of skin-lined tracheostomata in 76 patients. Those patients managed with wide undermining and then three-layer closure of the strap muscles and soft tissue overlying the trachea enjoyed good cosmetic results, but 30% of patients experienced complications such as subcutaneous emphysema, stridor, and tracheal granuloma in the immediate post-closure period. An alternative technique, termed 'de-epithelialization', involves decannulation one week prior to planned surgery in order to let the stoma narrow. Epithelium is then excised down to the trachea without undermining, deep tissues are loosely approximated, and no skin sutures are used. This technique is less cosmetically desirable than formal three-layer closure, but complications are reduced.

For LTTFT, there is no tube to begin with, and therefore no possibility that the stoma will narrow down and seal shut after decannulation as described above. Therefore, closure of LTTFT may require a more involved surgical technique. Our technique, which effectively closes LTTFT with minimal complications, combines a turn-over flap, medialization of fibroadipose tissue, and skin closure with an advancement flap.[36] This approach can be performed under either general or local anesthesia, and it balances functional and cosmetic results (Fig. 56.5A–H).

## 8 PEDIATRIC TRACHEOSTOMY AND OSA

Sleep apnea has different presentations and manifestations in children than in adults. For young children, it is less a consequence of elevated Body Mass Index than it is a result of congenital syndromes. For example, craniofacial abnormalities may co-exist with obstructive apnea as a consequence of macroglossia, retrognathia or micrognathia. Also, neurological syndromes may cause abundant central or obstructive apneas. In either case, tracheostomy can be truly life-saving.[37] Given size constraints and the soft flexibility of the skin in the early pediatric age group, tube-free techniques are not recommended in the pre-teen pediatric population. Instead, a preferred pediatric tracheostomy technique is 'starplasty', named for the fashion in which a circumferential tracheocutaneous fistula is created.[38] This fistula is then maintained with a traditional pediatric tracheotomy tube. After age 12, LTTFT may be a viable option.

Unfortunately, long-term pediatric tracheotomy dependence can have severe medical and emotional consequences. In appropriate patients, aggressive surgery (craniofacial skeletal expansion, mandibular distraction, etc.) can help to either avoid tracheostomy altogether or speed decannulation.[39,40] Such surgery may yield improved quality of life relative to tracheostomy in children with OSA.[41]

## 9 CONCLUSION

Long-term tube-free speech-ready tracheostomy, in its present form, has assumed the position of the ultimate 'gold standard' for management of severe chronic upper airway obstructions. Even though the procedure requires extensive surgery and prolonged postoperative care, it is probably the least injurious and the most effective single treatment modality in the management of severe or intractable OSA. The tube-related morbidity inherent to conventional tracheotomy/tracheostomy is avoided, as are most of the complications. Several functional advantages are offered, such as hands-free speech, effective cough, and control of aspiration with improved personal hygiene and comfort. Additionally, it is readily reversible. It provides the benefits of tracheotomy or tube-dependent tracheostomy safely and durably, while avoiding morbidity and promoting better quality of life for patients.

## REFERENCES

1. Kuhlo W, Doll E, Franck MD. Erfolgreiche behandlung eines Pickwick-syndroms durch eine dauertrachealkanule. Dtsch Med Wochenschr 1969;94:1286–90.
2. Mickelson SA. Upper airway bypass surgery for obstructive sleep apnea syndrome. Otol Clin North Am 1998;31:1013–23.
3. Eliachar I, Zohar S, Golz A, et al. Permanent tracheostomy. Head Neck Surg 1984;7:99–103.
4. Penta AO, Mayer E. Permanent tracheostomy in the treatment of pulmonary insufficiency. Ann Otol Rhinol Laryngol 1960;69:1157–69.
5. Fee WE, Ward PH. Permanent tracheostomy: a new surgical technique. Ann Otol Rhinol Laryngol 1977;86:635–8.
6. Bjork VO. Partial resection of the only remaining lung with the aid of respirator treatment. J Thorac Cardiovasc Surg 1960;29:179–88.

7. Weissler MC. Tracheotomy and intubation. In: Head and Neck Surgery–Otolaryngology. Bailey BJ, ed. Philadelphia: Lippincott Williams & Wilkins; 2001, pp. 677–89.
8. Katsantonis GP, Schwitzer PK, Branham GH, et al. Management of obstructive sleep apnea: comparison of various treatment modalities. Laryngoscope 1998;98:304–9.
9. Thatcher GW, Maisel RH. The long-term evaluation of tracheostomy in the management of severe obstructive sleep apnea. Laryngoscope 2003;113:201–4.
10. Ledereich PS, Thorpy MJ, Glovinsky PK, et al. Five-year follow-up of daytime sleepiness and snoring after tracheotomy in patients with obstructive sleep apnea. In: Chronic Rhonchopathy. Chouard CH, ed. Proceedings of the 1st International Congress on Chronic Rhonchopathy. Paris: Libbey Eurotext; 1988, pp. 354–7.
11. Motta J, Guilleminault C, Schroeder JS, et al. Tracheostomy and hemodynamic changes in sleep-induced apnea. Ann Intern Med 1978;89:454–8.
12. Guilleminault C, Simmons FB, Motta J, et al. Obstructive sleep apnea syndrome and tracheostomy. Long-term follow-up experience. Arch Intern Med 1981;141:985–8.
13. He J, Kryger M, Zorick J, et al. Mortality and apnea index in obstructive sleep apnea: experience in 385 male patients. Chest 1988;94:9–14.
14. Partinen M, Jamieson A, Guilleminault C. Long-term outcome for obstructive sleep apnea patients: mortality. Chest 1988;94:1200–4.
15. Lavie L. Obstructive sleep apnoea syndrome – an oxidative stress disorder. Sleep Med Rev 2003;7:35–51.
16. Fletcher EC. Recurrence of sleep apnea syndrome following tracheostomy: a shift from obstructive to central apnea. Chest 1989;96:205–9.
17. Gross ND, Cohen JI, Anderson PE, et al. 'Defatting' tracheotomy in morbidly obese patients. Laryngoscope 2002;112:1940–44.
18. Kim SH, Eisele DW, Smith PL, et al. Evaluation of patients with sleep apnea after tracheotomy. Arch Otolaryngol Head Neck Surg 1998;124:996–1000.
19. Conway WA, Victor LD, Magilligan DJ, et al. Adverse effects of tracheostomy for sleep apnea. JAMA 1981;246:347–50.
20. Harmon JD, Morgan W, Chaudhary B. Sleep apnea: morbidity and mortality of surgical treatment. South Med J 1989;82:161–4.
21. McConkey PP. Postobstructive pulmonary oedema – a case series and review. Anaesth Intensive Care 2000;28:72–6.
22. Chaudhary BA, Nadimi M, Chaudhary TK, et al. Pulmonary edema due to obstructive sleep apnea. South Med J 1984;77:499–501.
23. Burke AJC, Duke SG, Clyne S, et al. Incidence of pulmonary edema after tracheotomy for obstructive sleep apnea. Otolaryngol Head Neck Surg 2001;125:319–23.
24. Law JH, Barnhart K, Rowlett W, et al. Increased frequency of obstructive airway abnormalities with long-term tracheostomy. Chest 1993;104:136–8.
25. Eliachar I, Papay FA. Laryngotracheal devices. In: Complications in Head and Neck Surgery. Krespi J, Ossuf R, eds. Philadelphia: WB Saunders; 1993, pp. 233–56.
26. Eliachar I. Unaided speech in long-term tube-free tracheostomy. Laryngoscope 2000;110:749–60.
27. Eliashar R, Goldfarb A, Gross M, Sichel JY. A permanent tube-free tracheostomy in a morbidly obese patient with severe obstructive sleep apnea syndrome. Isr Med Assoc J 2002;4:1156–7.
28. Weitzman E, Pollak C, Borowiecki B, et al. The hypersomnia–sleep apnea syndrome: site and mechanism of upper airway obstruction. In: Sleep Apnea Syndromes. Guilleminault C, Dement W, eds. New York: Allan R. Liss Corporation; 1978.
29. Olson K, Pearson B. Sleep apnea tracheostomy. Laryngoscope 1984;94:555–6.
30. Sahni R, Blakley B, Maisel R. Flap tracheostomy in sleep apnea patients. Laryngoscope 1985;95:221–3.
31. Miller FR, Eliachar I, Tucker HM. Technique, management, and complications of the long-term flap tracheostomy. Laryngoscope 1995;105:543–7.
32. Eliachar I, Akst LM, Eliashar R. Unaided speech in tube-free tracheostomy: the supplementary sling procedure. Otolaryngol Head Neck Surg 2002;127:213–20.
33. Scheuller M, Weider D. Bariatric surgery for treatment of sleep apnea syndrome in 15 morbidly obese patients: long-term results. Otolaryngol Head Neck Surg 2001;125:299–302.
34. Rasheid S, Banasiak M, Gallagher SF, et al. Gastric bypass is an effective treatment for obstructive sleep apnea in patients with clinically significant obesity. Obes Surg 2003;13:58–61.
35. Mickelson SA, Rosenthal L. Closure of permanent tracheostomy in patients with sleep apnea: a comparison of two techniques. Otolaryngol Head Neck Surg 1997;116:36–40.
36. Eliashar R, Sichel JY, Eliachar I. A new surgical technique for primary closure of long-term tracheostomy. Otolaryngol Head Neck Surg 2005;B2(1):115–18.
37. Cohen SR, Lefaivre JF, Burstein FD, et al. Surgical treatment of obstructive sleep apnea in neurologically compromised patients. Plast Reconst Surg 1997;99:638–46.
38. Koltai PJ. Starplasty. A new technique of pediatric tracheotomy. Arch Otolaryngol Head Neck Surg 1998;124:1105–11.
39. Cohen SR, Simms C, Burstein FD, et al. Alternatives to tracheostomy in infants and children with obstructive sleep apnea. J Ped Surg 1999;34:182–7.
40. Williams JK, Maull D, Graytson BH, et al. Early decannulation with bilateral mandibular distraction for tracheostomy-dependent patients. Plast Reconst Surg 1999;103:48–57.
41. Cohen SR, Suzman K, Simms C, et al. Sleep apnea surgery versus tracheostomy in children: an exploratory study of the comparative effects on quality of life. Plast Reconst Surg 1998;102:1855–64.

## FURTHER READING

Chouard CH, ed. Chronic rhonchopathy. Proceedings of the 1st International Congress on Chronic Rhonchopathy. Paris: Libbey Eurotext; 1988, pp. 354–7.
Conway WA, Victor LD, Magilligan DJ, et al. Adverse effects of tracheostomy for sleep apnea. JAMA 1981;246:347–50.
Eliachar I. Unaided speech in long-term tube-free tracheostomy. Laryngoscope 2000;110:749–60.
Eliachar I, Papay FA. Laryngotracheal devices. In: Complications in Head and Neck Surgery. Krespi J, Ossuf R, eds. Philadelphia: WB Saunders; 1993, pp. 233–56.
Eliachar I, Akst LM, Elaishar R. Unaided speech in tube-free tracheostomy: the supplementary sling procedure. Otolaryngol Head Neck Surg 2002;127:213–20.
Eliachar I, Zohar S, Golz A, et al. Permanent tracheostomy. Head Neck Surg 1984;7:99–103.
Eliachar R, Goldfarb A, Gross M, Sichel JY. A permanent tube-free tracheostomy in a morbidly obese patient with severe obstructive sleep apnea syndrome. Isr Med Assoc J 2002;4:1156–7.
Fee WE, Ward PH. Permanent tracheostomy: a new surgical technique. Ann Otol Rhinol Laryngol 1977;86:635–8.
Gross ND, Cohen JI, Anderson PE, et al. 'Defatting' tracheotomy in morbidly obese patients. Laryngoscope 2002;112:1940–44.
Guilleminault C, Simmons FB, Motta J, et al. Obstructive sleep apnea syndrome and tracheostomy. Long-term follow-up experience. Arch Intern Med 1981;141:985–8.
Katsantonis GP, Schwitzer PK, Branham GH, et al. Management of obstructive sleep apnea: comparison of various treatment modalities. Laryngoscope 1998;98:304–9.
Ledereich PS, Thorpy MJ, Glovinsky PK, et al. Five-year follow-up of daytime sleepiness and snoring after tracheotomy in patients with obstructive sleep apnea. In: Technique, Management, and Complications of the Long-term Flap Tracheostomy. Miller FR, Eliachar I, Tucker HM, eds. Laryngoscope 1995;105:543–7.
Partinen M, Jamieson A, Guilleminault C. Long-term outcome for obstructive sleep apnea patients: mortality. Chest 1988;94:1200–4.
Penta AO, Mayer E. Permanent tracheostomy in the treatment of pulmonary insufficiency. Ann Otol Rhinol Laryngol 1960;69:1157–69.
Sahni R, Blakley B, Maisel R. Flap tracheostomy in sleep apnea patients. Laryngoscope 1985;95:221–3.
Thatcher GW, Maisel RH. The long-term evaluation of tracheostomy in the management of severe obstructive sleep apnea. Laryngoscope 2003;113:201–4.

SECTION N   POSTOPERATIVE MANAGEMENT AND COMPLICATIONS

# CHAPTER 57
# The postoperative management of OSA patients after uvulopalatopharyngoplasty. Inpatient or outpatient?

*Jeffrey H. Spiegel and Yanina Greenstein*

## 1 INTRODUCTION

Obstructive sleep apnea (OSA) is a condition that is estimated to affect up to 4% of the adult population.[1] The OSA syndrome can be defined as the periodic cessation of airflow during sleep. The most common symptoms of this syndrome include loud snoring, daytime sleepiness and cognitive impairment. A variety of surgical procedures, which include tracheotomy, nasal surgery, and uvulopalatopharyngoplasty (UPPP) with or without tonsillectomy, may be performed to alleviate symptoms and improve the patient's quality of life.

Out of the available procedures, UPPP is the most common surgery performed for adult patients with OSA. It was originally introduced by Fujita in 1981.[2] Despite the frequency of this procedure, the appropriate level of postoperative monitoring for complications has become a controversial issue. Initially all UPPP patients were monitored postoperatively in the intensive care unit. It is the opinion of the authors of this chapter that there is no unique danger to uvulopalatopharyngoplasty for obstructive sleep apnea that would require such intensive postoperative observation. Nonetheless, otolaryngology textbooks typically recommend close observation in the recovery area and subsequent transfer to the intensive care unit for the first 24 hours post UPPP.[3] Currently, some surgeons still advocate a 24-hour observation period as a routine part of postoperative management.

On the other hand, others may prefer close monitoring but do not recommend it as a routine practice. Instead they base the need for extended observation on the severity of a patient's OSA, the extent of the operation and the presence of pre-existing medical conditions. In fact, many recent reports have concluded that routine postoperative ICU monitoring is not necessary, stating that intensive care or step-down unit monitoring should not be required for most patients after upper airway surgery for OSA since most complications occur within a few hours of the procedure.[4–6]

While it is clear that a variety of factors may influence a surgeon's decision to prolong postoperative care, studies have shown that most overnight admissions for UPPP are uneventful and in most cases, same-day discharge is advisable.[7] Based on this fact, this chapter seeks to clarify and outline appropriate postoperative management strategies of OSA patients undergoing UPPP.

## 2 POSTOPERATIVE COMPLICATIONS

Inherently, there is no greater risk of postoperative complications with UPPP surgery than with tonsillectomy, which is commonly conducted on an outpatient basis. While complications do occur after UPPP, researchers have shown that they are most common in the immediate, postoperative care period and overnight stay may not be a necessary part of postoperative management of OSA patients undergoing UPPP.[8]

Although the overall incidence of serious postoperative complications after UPPP is low,[9] it is important to review which complications may occur in order to understand how they affect a surgeon's approach to managing patients. In the case of UPPP, complications may be categorized as either early or late events. Early complications can be defined as those that occur either intraoperatively, immediately postoperatively or in the recovery room. Late complications may be observed over the course of the inpatient stay. The most commonly reported early postoperative complications are either respiratory in origin or involve bleeding from the surgical site.[8] Other early complications include arrhythmia, hypertension, pain, dehydration and poor oral intake. All of these possibilities should be addressed before determining the most appropriate postoperative management plan for UPPP patients.

# SECTION N: POSTOPERATIVE MANAGEMENT AND COMPLICATIONS

## 2.1 AIRWAY OBSTRUCTION

The most common serious respiratory complications after UPPP are airway obstruction and oxygen desaturation. Complete and untreated airway obstruction may lead to respiratory arrest, and reintubation or emergency tracheotomy could become necessary and lifesaving.

Although airway obstruction may be considered a common postoperative complication after UPPP, the actual incidence of such an event is quite low. Additionally, there has been a change in the number of serious respiratory complications reported over time, with more recent studies reporting lower rates. For example, in 1989 Esclamado et al.[10] conducted a retrospective chart review of 135 patients surgically treated for OSA and found the incidence of respiratory complications to be 10.3%. Half of these complications were airway obstructions that occurred at extubation, and half were due to failed intubation. It is important in a discussion of postoperative management to note that the onset of all respiratory events occurred in the *early* phase. That is, all respiratory complications occurred during or immediately after intubation. A review in 1994 by Haavisto and Suonpaa[11] of 101 patients undergoing UPPP for OSA showed an incidence of airway complications of 11%. Again all cases occurred in the early phase.

In a 1998 review of 109 patients undergoing UPPP for OSA, Terris et al. reported a 5.5% incidence or early respiratory complications.[6] This rate included one case of airway compromise, and the patient required naloxone, oxygen and suctioning of his airway. This single episode of airway obstruction occurred only 15 minutes after the patient was transferred out of the operating room.

An additional 1998 study by Mickelson and Hakim of 347 patients undergoing UPPP for OSA reported only five patients who had experienced airway-related complications, or 1.4% of all patients.[5] Three of the five suffered shortness of breath either at extubation or immediately after in the recovery room. Two of the five patients experienced complications in the surgical ward. These included one case of pulmonary edema and one case of shortness of breath of unclear origin. No actual cases of airway obstructions were reported.

Spiegel and Raval reviewed 117 patients in 2005 for complications associated with UPPP.[8] Ten patients were discharged the same day as the surgery. The remainder of the patients experienced a 4.3% incidence rate of respiratory complications. While most cases were due to oxygen desaturation, two patients developed airway obstruction from presumed laryngospasm at the time of extubation. Both of these patients developed postobstructive pulmonary edema within minutes of the obstruction.

Overall, the rate of airway obstruction appears to be in the range of 1.4–11%. Most importantly, obstruction events appear to occur immediately after surgery in the early phase of recovery, so it is not likely that an extended period of observation would be a useful way to prevent this type of complication.

## 2.2 OXYGEN DESATURATION

Oxygen desaturation is also often cited as a common complication in OSA patients undergoing UPPP. A value of less than 85–93% is typically considered significant desaturation. In the past, some surgeons have advocated postoperative ICU monitoring for fear of serious desaturation events. However, such monitoring may not be reasonable since most desaturations occur in the early phase of recovery. Additionally, more mild nocturnal desaturations may continue for weeks, since UPPP does not correct OSA immediately.[12]

The fact that most occurrences of desaturations happen relatively early in the recovery process further supports same-day patient discharge for the majority of patients. For example, in a 2006 study by Hathaway and Johnson of 110 patients undergoing UPPP, desaturations in three patients all occurred in the recovery room.[7] In the review by Spiegel and Raval, three desaturations below 90% were reported.[8] The first desaturation occurred in the recovery room, the second on the first postoperative night and the third on the first postoperative day. The third patient likely desaturated on the first postoperative day because he was given narcotic patient-controlled analgesia (morphine) for pain, and narcotic analgesia tends to impede respiratory function.

Advocates of extended postoperative stays after UPPP also claim the need for post-surgical oxygen supplementation on the floor as an important argument for hospitalization. However, there is some evidence that there may not be a direct relationship between oxygen supplementation and lower desaturation rates. For example, Riley et al.[13] found no significant difference in the postoperative low oxyhemoglobin saturation (LSAT) between patients receiving continuous positive airway pressure (CPAP) and the non-CPAP group.

A patient's preoperative Respiratory Distress Index (RDI) may also be a poor predictor of whether or not they may desaturate, as was the case in the review by Hathaway and Johnson.[7] While two of the admitted patients had RDIs over 50 (indicating severe OSA) one patient had an RDI of 22 and still desaturated. Desaturations occurred in the recovery room, and all patients were admitted into the hospital, but none required the ICU. The authors concluded that preoperative polysomnography data such as the RDI may not predict which patients will experience desaturation in the early postoperative period.

Overall, research shows that desaturation, particularly nocturnal desaturation, is a very common complication of UPPP surgery for OSA. In fact, it should be considered more of an expectation than a complication. Giving oxygen postoperatively may or may not make a difference, so admitting all UPPP patients in order to give them oxygen would not be reasonable. Also, preoperative sleep indices may not be an accurate indicator for identifying patients who may desaturate, so it would not be practical to hospitalize all patients due to fear of this complication. The most likely scenario is that if a serious desaturation occurs, it would be in the early phase of recovery, at which point the patient should be admitted to the hospital. Otherwise, minor nocturnal desaturations are to be expected since it may take a few weeks to note improvement in a patient's OSA.

## 2.3 BLEEDING

Bleeding, particularly from the surgical site, is another frequently noted complication of UPPP. The onset of bleeding tends to be biphasic with cases either occurring immediately after surgery or more than 24 hours post operation.[8]

For example, a Haavisto and Suonpaa review of 101 in 1994 had an incidence rate of hemorrhage of 14% or 14 total cases.[11] Out of the 14 cases, nine required surgical management such as electrocautery and ligation while five were managed with conservative treatment or suctioning. All but one of the hemorrhages that required electrocautery occurred within 5 hours of the initial surgery during the early phase of recovery. Three cases occurred much later, at 24 hours or more post procedure. One patient reportedly experienced asystole and died.

In a paper by Esclamado et al., hemorrhage that required return to the OR occurred in 2.2% of patients immediately post operation.[10] Mickelson and Hakim reported a 1.4% incidence of bleeding, or a total of five cases.[6] This included two episodes of epistaxis, one of tracheostomy bleeding, and a third of bleeding from the patient's tonsils. These four cases occurred in the early phase of recovery. However, one patient began to bleed from his tonsillectomy site while out on the surgical ward and required a return to the ICU.

Spiegel's study also illustrated the biphasic nature of bleeding events and reported seven cases of hemorrhage with time of onset ranging between 5 and 14 days postoperatively.[8] No cases of bleeding were reported during the hospital stay.

The biphasic pattern of bleeding after UPPP appears to be a common occurrence and is reported in various studies. Since most complications occur early, and those that do not occur much later than the average period of inpatient monitoring, a short observation period of 2–3 hours should be sufficient for detecting most bleeding events.

## 2.4 CARDIAC COMPLICATIONS

Hypertension, arrhythmia, angina and miscellaneous other cardiac complications are also observed after UPPP, but tend to be relatively rare. Significant hypertension frequently occurs intraoperatively or immediately after surgery. In the Terris et al. study, seven of 125 patients were described as having mild hypertension (systolic pressure greater than 190 mm Hg and diastolic over 100 mm Hg) and did not require intravenous anti-hypertensive drugs or ICU monitoring.[6] Six additional patients experienced severe hypertension and required intravenous treatment, but in all of the cases hypertension manifested in the first 2 postoperative hours.

Hypertension requiring intravenous narcotics was also noted in three cases by Spiegel and Raval.[8] All three cases occurred in the recovery area, and two of the three patients had a medical history of hypertension. Riley et al.[13] reported the highest rate of postoperative hypertension that required intravenous medication at 70.5%. Such elevated rates may be due to the fact that OSA patients tend to experience a higher incidence of postoperative hypertension because they have a greater prevalence of hypertension prior to surgery. Comorbid factors such as elevated Body Mass Index (BMI) and age may account for some of the association, but OSA itself probably presents an independent risk factor as well.[6] Since most cases of postoperative hypertension occur in the early phase of recovery and can be controlled with intravenous narcotics, hypertension alone should not constitute a reason for prolonged inpatient visits of ICU monitoring.

While hypertension is the most common cardiac complication after UPPP, cases of arrhythmia and angina have also been reported. In the review by Riley et al., four out of 182 patients (1.9%) had a postoperative arrhythmia that required treatment despite a negative medical history and work-up.[13] All reported arrhythmias were new-onset atrial fibrillations. One patient had unstable angina.

Terris et al. also noted one arrhythmia, but the patient had a prior history of premature ventricular contractions (PVCs).[6] Haavisto and Suonpaa also reported one case of arrhythmia.[12] A review of 1004 patients by Spiegel and Raval,[8] which included the studies mentioned above, found an average rate of arrhythmia of 0.8%, and 0.2% for angina. Clearly, these complications are very rare and monitoring during the early phase of recovery should be sufficient in detecting the vast majority of such adverse cardiac events.

## 2.5 PULMONARY EDEMA

Postobstructive pulmonary edema (POPE) is a much feared complication for OSA patients undergoing UPPP and is often cited as a justification for admission. One theory is that POPE, also known as negative pressure pulmonary edema, is a non-cardiogenic pathologic process in which the generation of markedly negative intrathoracic pressures that are created by forced inspiration against a closed glottis cause a transudation of fluid into the pulmonary interstitium.[14] Typically, POPE has a benign and rapidly resolving clinical course, assuming it is recognized and treated in a prompt manner.

However, studies reveal that POPE can also result in significant morbidity, with mortality rates ranging from 11% to 40%, so clearly it is of concern to physicians.[14] Why POPE appears in some individuals and not others is unclear. Literature has shown that POPE is usually triggered by laryngospasm during extubation. Again, this serious complication is identified in the immediate postoperative period (early) and a prolonged period of postoperative monitoring would not seem indicated for all patients. In a study by Goldenberg et al.,[14] all six reviewed cases of POPE occurred within 60 minutes after the onset or relief of obstruction.

Also, it is important to note that the incidence of POPE is quite low. In a review of 1004 OSA patients undergoing UPPP, only three cases of POPE were reported.[8] The risk of POPE can be reduced even further by using a bite lock to prevent accidental compression of the endotracheal tube. When POPE does occur, it usually manifests in the immediate part of recovery, typically at the time of extubation, so overnight monitoring would not decrease its incidence. The use of perioperative corticosteroids may help decrease airway edema,[6] but the most important preventive measure possible is immediate recognition and treatment of the problem in the rare circumstances that it does occur.

Laryngospasm as a cause of POPE is not unique to UPPP but can occur with any surgical procedure, though it is more likely in procedures involving blood within or manipulations of the oropharynx. That removing the anatomic site of obstruction causes an immediate and uncompensated pressure change, resulting in fluid shifts, is not logical. If that were the case, certainly individuals with OSA would be at risk of developing POPE every time they wake up and their temporary obstruction is relieved.

## 2.6 PAIN AND DEHYDRATION

Pain, dehydration and poor oral intake may be the most reasonable justification for overnight patient admission, though they hardly warrant observation within an intensive care setting. Physicians familiar with the UPPP procedure undoubtedly are aware of how very uncomfortable patients are postoperatively. We routinely caution patients regarding the significant postoperative pain and review pain management strategies at length during preoperative counseling.

Hathaway and Johnson reported on 90 out of 110 UPPP procedures on an outpatient basis.[7] Of the 20 patients admitted for overnight stay, eight patients were admitted due to limited oral intake and three for nausea. Five patients had a prolonged stay despite having no specific complications. The same was noted by Spiegel and Raval[8] – several patients had a prolonged stay due to inadequate pain control and poor oral intake.

Pain control, poor oral intake and dehydration are important issues to address, though with adequate preoperative preparation and patient selection, outpatient surgery is still recommended for the majority of individuals.

## 3 CONCLUSION

After reviewing the major possible postoperative complications of UPPP, it is safe to conclude that overnight stay is not necessary for most patients. Certainly, routine intensive care monitoring would not seem to be supported by the literature. Serious complications, such as death and the development of POPE, are fortunately extremely rare. When POPE occurs, it tends to occur within the operating room or immediately after; again, prolonged postoperative stay does not appear warranted.

Polysomnogram measurements such as the RDI do not appear to be a valid way to determine who will need to be admitted for overnight stay. Thus, routine admission based on such indices is not recommended. Because multiple surgeries may be associated with a greater number of complications, particularly the combination of nasal surgery and UPPP,[5,7] it is advisable to monitor patients who are undergoing multiple procedures more closely. For example, procedures to reduce the tongue base are particularly worrisome with regard to possible postoperative complications.

A few important general recommendations can be made in terms of postoperative management for all OSA patients after UPPP. First, patients should be monitored immediately after surgery using continuous pulse oximetry and should be provided with supplemental oxygen as needed to prevent desaturation. Second, patients can be encouraged to use humidified CPAP for several days after surgery, particularly if they were on it before surgery, since the improvement in OSA severity after UPPP is not immediate. If they find the CPAP uncomfortable or if the surgeon feels the positive pressure will present the patient with an increased risk of postoperative complication such as hemorrhage, then the patient can simply leave their OSA inadequately treated for a few days. Recall that OSA is harmful to one's health in the long term more than immediately. Additionally, in cases of severe OSA, CPAP should be made available immediately after surgery should the patients require hospitalization. Finally, preoperative counseling should focus on techniques for proper hydration, sufficient oral intake and pain control.

With proper monitoring, a 2–3 hour observation period after UPPP should be sufficient for detecting serious postoperative complications. As reviewed in this chapter, most serious complications, such as airway obstruction, desaturation and POPE, occur immediately after surgery during the early phase of recovery. Other complications, such as bleeding, occur in a biphasic pattern, and take place either early on in, or much later than the typical postoperative monitoring period. With careful monitoring in the early phase of recovery, outpatient surgery for OSA patients undergoing UPPP should become routine.

## REFERENCES

1. Bresnitz EA, Goldberg R, Kosinski RM. Epidemiology of obstructive sleep apnea. Epidemiol Rev 1994;16:210–27.
2. Fujita S, Conway WA, Zorick FJ, et al. Surgical corrections of anatomic abnormalities in obstructive sleep apnea syndrome: uvulopalatopharyngoplasty. Otolaryngol Head Neck Surg 1981;89:923–4.
3. Walker RP. Snoring and obstructive sleep apnea. In: Head and Neck Surgery: Otolaryngology, 3rd edn. Bailey BJ, Calhoun KH, Healy GB, et al, eds. Philadelphia: Lippincott Williams and Wilkins; 2001, p. 539.
4. Gessler EM, Bondy PC. Respiratory complications following tonsillectomy/UPPP: is step-down monitoring necessary? Ear Nose Throat J 2003;82:628–32.
5. Mickelson SA, Hakim I. Is postoperative intensive care monitoring necessary after uvulopalatopharyngoplasty? Otolaryngol Head Neck Surg 1998;119:352–56.
6. Terris DJ, Fincher EF, Hanasono MM, et al. Conservation of resources: indications for intensive care monitoring after upper airway surgery on patients with obstructive sleep apnea. Laryngoscope 1998;108:184–788.
7. Hathaway B, Johnson JT. Safety of uvulopalatopharyngoplasty as outpatient surgery. Otolaryngol Head Neck Surg 2006;134:542–4.
8. Spiegel JH, Raval TH. Overnight stay is not always necessary after uvulopalatopharyngoplasty. Laryngoscope 2005;115:167–71.
9. Kezirian EJ, Weaver EM, Yueh B, et al. Incidence of serious complications after uvulopalatopharyngoplasty. Laryngoscope 2004;114:450–53.
10. Esclamado RM, Glenn MG, McCulloch TM, et al. Perioperative complications and risk factors in the surgical treatment of obstructive sleep apnea syndrome. Laryngoscope 1989;99:1125–9.
11. Haavisto L, Suonpaa J. Complications of uvulopalatopharyngoplasty. Clin Otolaryngol 1994;19:243–7.
12. Burgess LP, Derderian SS, Morin GV, et al. Postoperative risk following uvulopalatopharyngoplasty for obstructive sleep apnea. Otolaryngol Head Neck Surg 1992;106:81–6.
13. Riley RW, Pewell NB, Guilleminault C, et al. Obstructive sleep apnea surgery: risk management and complications. Otolaryngol Head Neck Surg 1997;117:648–52.
14. Goldenberg JD, Portugal LG, Wenig BL, et al. Negative pressure pulmonary edema in the otolaryngology patient. Otolaryngol Head Neck Surg 1997;117:62–66.

# SECTION N — POSTOPERATIVE MANAGEMENT AND COMPLICATIONS

## CHAPTER 58

# Multi-modality management of nasopharyngeal stenosis following uvulopalatopharyngoplasty

*Yosef P. Krespi and Ashutosh Kacker*

## 1 INTRODUCTION

Nasopharyngeal stenosis (NPS) after uvulopalatopharyngoplasty (UPPP) is a serious problem. More palatal procedures are being performed leading to an increased incidence of nasopharyngeal stenosis, but little has been written about this severe complication and its management.

Historically, adult NPS was a consequence of maxillofacial trauma or severe infection such as syphilis. Now NPS is seen as a complication of surgery such as tonsillectomy and adenoidectomy in the pediatric population, and UPPP in the adult population with obstructive sleep apnea. Rhinoscleroma, lupus, diphtheria, tuberculosis, acid burn, scarlet fever and aggressive velopharyngeal repair can also cause nasopharyngeal stenosis.[1,2]

The complication of severe nasopharyngeal stenosis following UPPP is well understood. Most cases are problems of surgical technique. The management of intraoperative or postoperative bleeding with nasopharyngeal packing and electrocautery is an important cause of NPS. Adenoidectomy in conjunction with UPPP carries an increased risk of nasopharyngeal stenosis. Other technical errors include excessive excision and cauterization of the posterior tonsillar pillars or undermining the posterior and lateral pharyngeal walls. Wound dehiscence, infection, necrosis and scarring in keloid-forming patients are some other causes of acquired NPS. Also, the use of KTP (potassium titanyl phosphate) laser to perform adenoidectomy is associated with an extremely high incidence of NPS.[1]

The management of NPS is difficult and reoperation using conventional methods results in only short-term improvement in symptoms with restenosis.

## 2 SURGICAL TECHNIQUE

Nasopharyngeal stenosis is graded as type I (mild) when the lateral aspects of the palate adhere to the posterior pharyngeal wall. Type II (moderate) is the occurrence of circumferential scarring with small central opening of the soft palate. This circumferential opening is between 1 and 2 cm in diameter. Type III (severe) is when the entire palate fuses with the posterior and lateral palatal wall, leaving a residual opening less than 1 cm (Fig. 58.1). Treatment for type I stenosis can be carried out as an outpatient, whereas treatment for type II and III stenosis may require general anesthesia in an inpatient setting. $CO_2$ laser is used in conjunction with a scanning device at 30 watts, with a pharyngeal handpiece in a continuous mode in type I patients. During surgery, two nasopharyngeal tubes (size 6 or 7) are passed and left in place for 3–4 days as temporary stents (Fig. 58.2). A customized nasopharyngeal obturator is used in type II and III patients and inserted after removal of the stents on the third or fourth postoperative day (Figs 58.3 and 58.4). The nasopharyngeal obturator consists of an upper dental appliance with a customized nasopharyngeal extension as an obturator to stent open the nasopharynx. The patients use the stent during the day and remove it at night. The stent is left in place for 3–6 months (Fig. 58.5).

For patients with severe stenosis (type II or III), we have also used a topical 6–8 minute application of 0.04% mitomycin-C to the raw surface area of the nasopharynx.

## 3 DISCUSSION WITH RESULTS AND ALTERNATIVE TREATMENT OPTIONS

UPPP remains the most commonly performed surgical treatment for obstructive sleep apnea/hypopnea syndrome. NPS is a severe complication of UPPP, though its incidence is not known. The incidence of severe type II and type III is estimated to be under 1%. Factors that increase the incidence of NPS include postoperative bleeding, infection, overheated tissues by the use of KTP laser, over-resection or excessive undermining of lateral pillars and combination of adenoidectomy with UPP. No uniform risk factors or surgical errors have been identified in our study.

# Nasopharyngeal stenosis following uvulopalatopharyngoplasty

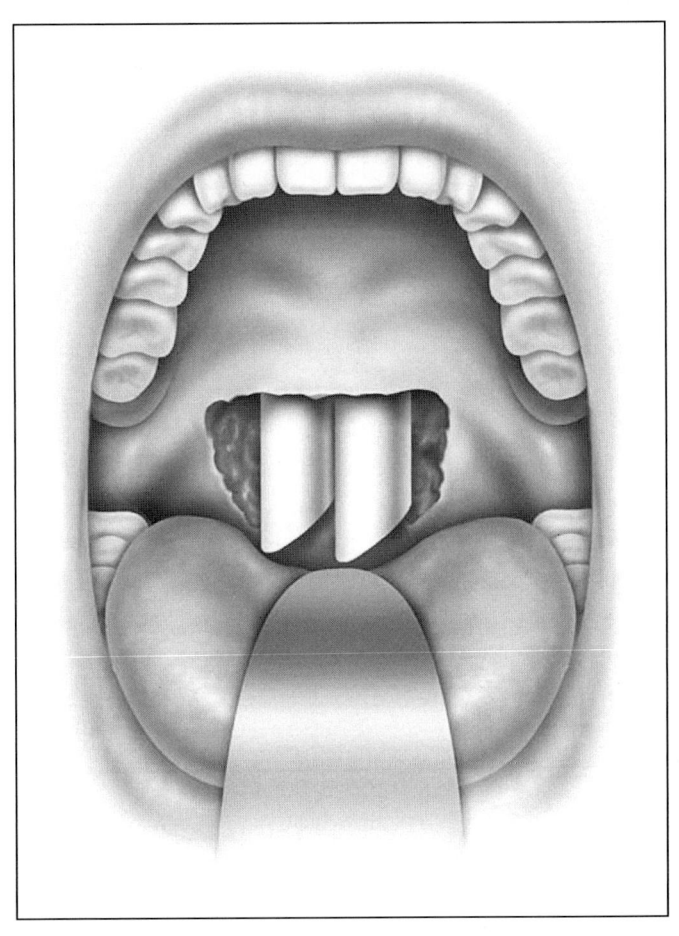

## CHAPTER 58

**Fig. 58.2** Intraoperative view after the release of stenosis with temporary stents in place.

Many methods of repair of NPS have been reported in the literature with variable results. These methods include passage of a heavy silk suture through the stenotic lumen, cervical pedicled skin flap, local rotation and advancement flaps, Z-plasty, intralesional steroid injection, free flaps and $CO_2$ laser.

The type I stenosis is treated under local anesthesia in an office setting using $CO_2$ laser without the use of a nasopharyngeal obturator. Moderate and severe cases of NPS are treated in the operating room under general anesthesia. Most of these patients require prolonged use of the nasopharyngeal obturator. The obturator used has been custom designed by the senior author to treat severe cases of nasopharyngeal stenosis. The nasopharyngeal obturator consists of a standard dental obturator, which is constructed after a dental impression has been taken, and a nasopharyngeal extension with an airway to fill the neo-nasopharynx. This nasopharyngeal extension is contoured to the shape of the neo-nasopharynx using a drill after surgery to tightly fit the neo-nasopharynx after temporary stents have been removed. Use of the nasopharyngeal obturator in conjunction with $CO_2$ laser led to a patent nasopharynx (defined for the purpose of this study

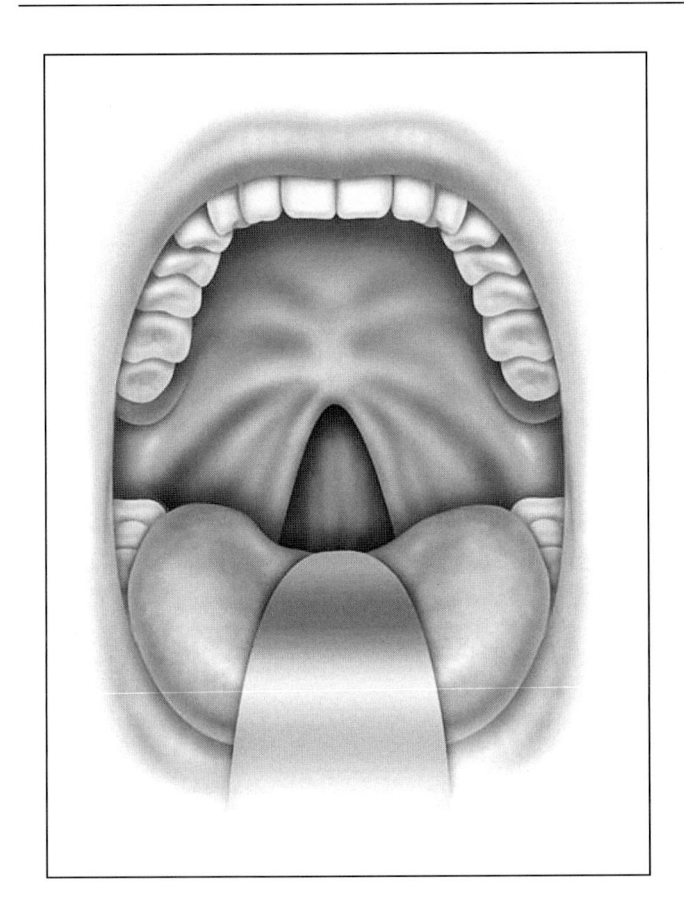

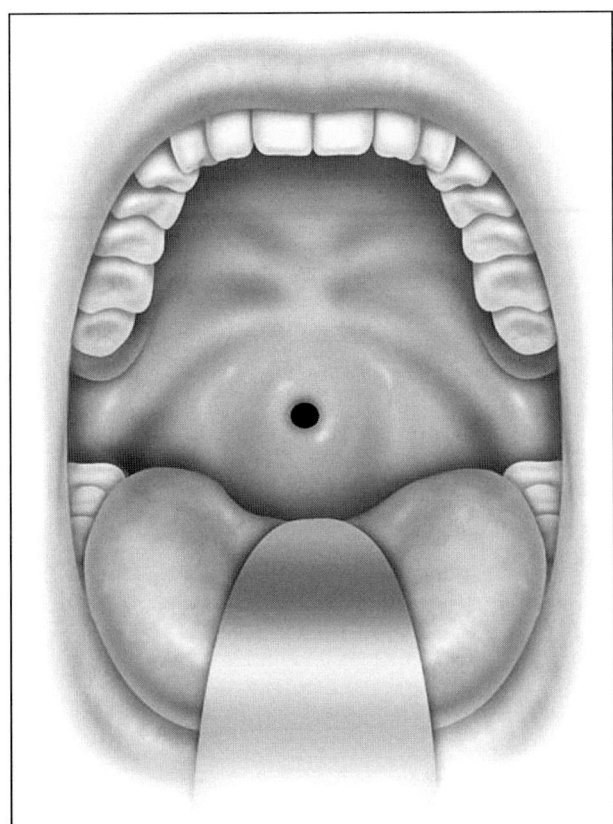

**Fig. 58.1** A, Mild nasopharyngeal stenosis. B, Severe nasopharyngeal stenosis.

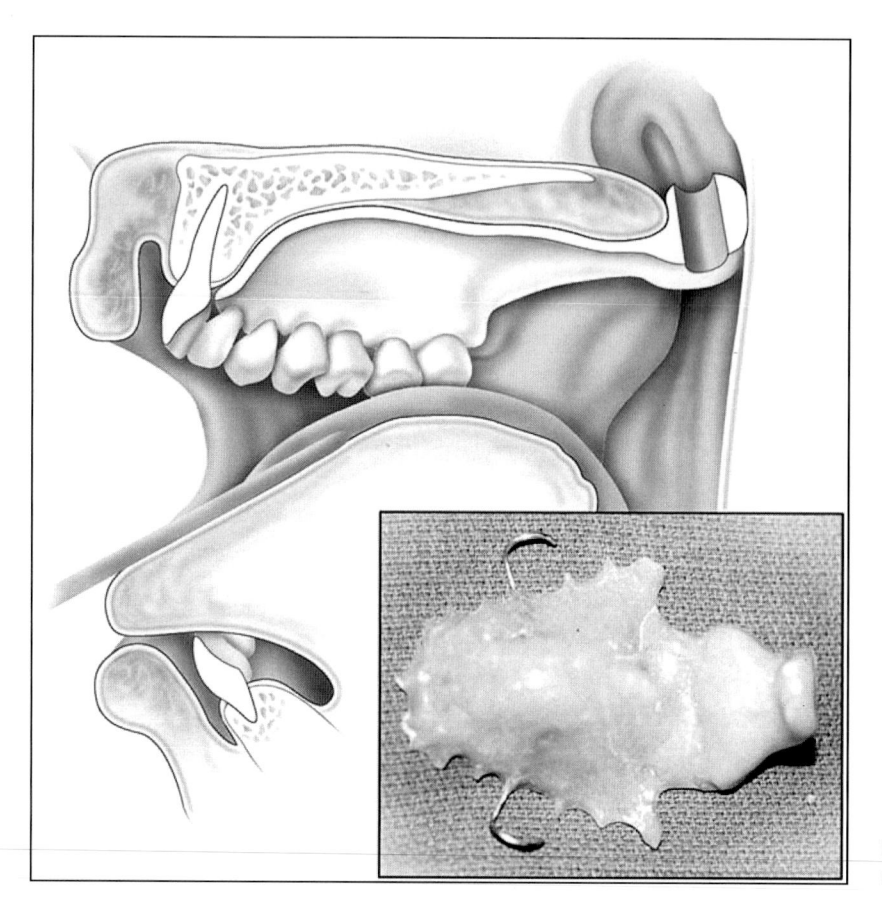

SECTION N  POSTOPERATIVE MANAGEMENT AND COMPLICATIONS

**Fig. 58.3** Customized palate obturator with nasopharyngeal extension.

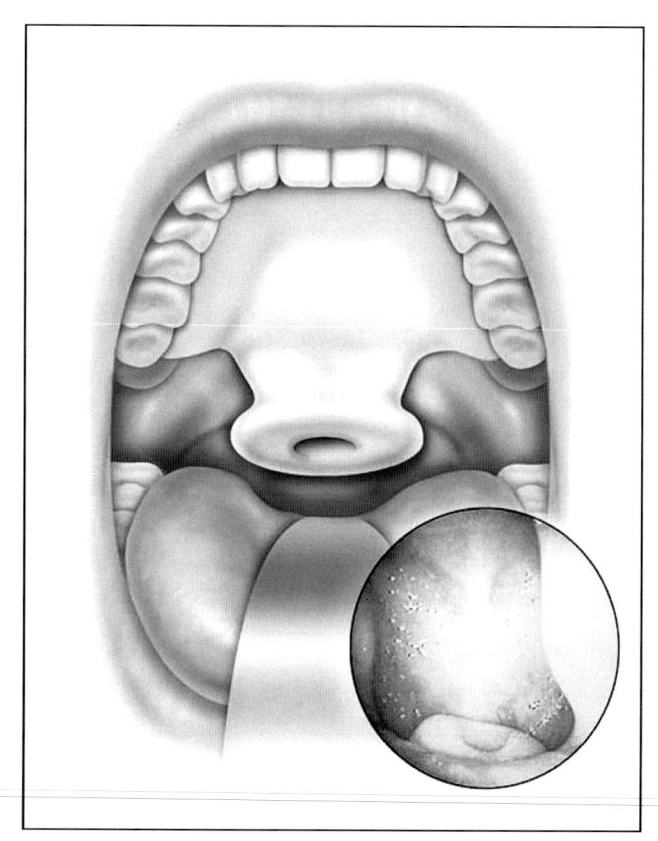

**Fig. 58.4** Palate obturator with nasopharyngeal extension (oral and nasopharyngeal views).

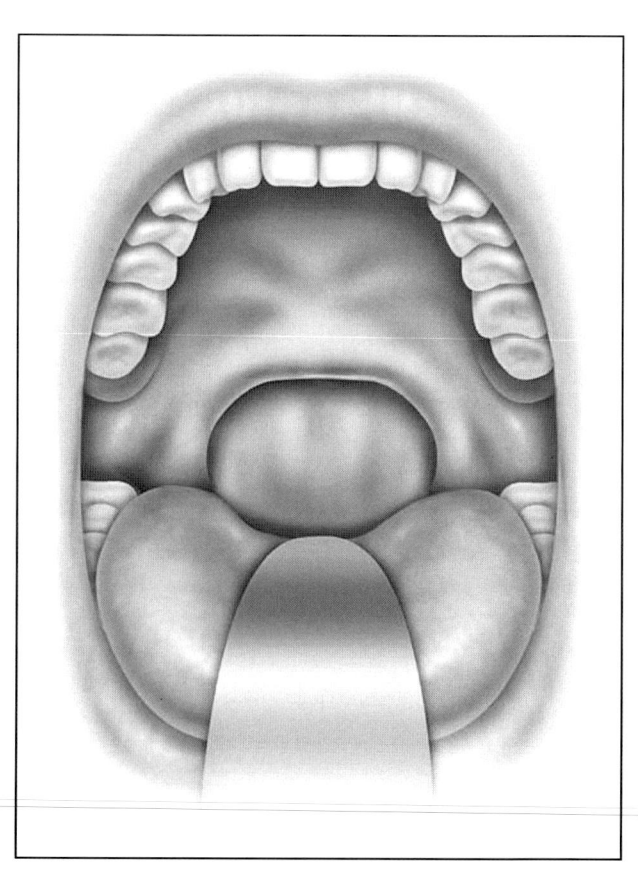

**Fig. 58.5** Postoperative photo showing a widely patent nasopharynx.

as a nasopharyngeal opening of greater than 3 cm with no bands between the lateral pharyngeal wall and the palate in all patients.

In most cases NPS occurred 4–5 weeks postoperatively. The timing of repair is important and repair is usually performed 6–8 months after the primary surgery to allow for the maturation of nasopharyngeal scar tissue and complete re-epithelialization of nasopharyngeal mucosa. Early intervention can lead to restenosis and failure of this procedure, as scar bands continue to contract and reshape the nasopharynx.

The advantages of using the $CO_2$ laser scanning device with high energy density when compared to Nd-Yag laser, KTP laser, electrocautery or radiofrequency ablation devices for repair of NPS include reduced thermal damage to nasopharyngeal tissue and minimal de-epithelialization of nasopharyngeal mucosa. The advantage of the $CO_2$ laser scanner over a surgical knife is improved hemostasis and reduced lateral scanner zone damage with limited tissue slough.

Disadvantages of using the $CO_2$ laser include the increased cost, and expertise needed in using the special handpiece with the surgical scanner.

The success rate of the techniques described in the literature is not known, due to the small number of patients in the various series.

Mitomycin-C (MMC) is an anti-neoplastic agent, which causes inhibition of DNA and protein synthesis. Data are available on the topical application of mitomycin-C (0.4 mg/ml applied for 8–10 minutes) in laryngotracheal reconstruction patients where reduced granulation formation has been reported. The use of MMC to prevent postoperative scarring has been the focus of several recent studies. A natural antibiotic derived from *Streptomyces caespitosus*, MMC has been demonstrated to have both anti-neoplastic and anti-proliferative properties. The former is attributed to its ability to cross-link DNA and inhibit DNA, RNA and protein synthesis while the latter is a result of its suppression of fibroblast activity. Within ophthalmology, MMC has been used with success in glaucoma filtration and strabismus surgery, optic nerve decompression, pterygium excision and dacryocystorhinostomy. Use of MMC in our series has led to less scar formation and reduced the length of time an obturator needs to be worn. This is due to the inhibition of fibroblasts and similar effects have been seen in the nose (choanal atresia repair) and the airway.

## REFERENCES AND FURTHER READING

1. Giannoni C, Sulek M, Friedman EM, et al. Acquired nasopharyngeal stenosis – a warning and a review. Arch Otolaryngol Head Neck Surg 1998;124:163–7.
2. McLaughlin KE, Jacobs IN, Todd NW, et al. Management of nasopharyngeal stenosis in children. Laryngoscope 1997;107:1322–31.
3. Krespi YP. Laser assisted uvulopalatoplasty – result and complications in 1000 patients. In: Office-Based Surgery of the Head and Neck. Krespi YP, ed. Philadelphia: Lippincott-Raven; 1998, pp. 147–53.
4. Coleman JA, Van Duyne J. Treatment of nasopharyngeal inlet stenosis following uvulopalatoplasty with the $CO_2$ laser. Laryngoscope 1995;105:914–18.
5. Randall DA, Hoffer ME. Complications of tonsillectomy and adenoidectomy. Otolaryngol Head Neck Surg 1998;118:61–8.
6. Fairbanks DNF. Uvulopalatopharyngoplasty complications and avoidance strategies. Otolaryngol Head Neck Surg 1990;102:239–45.
7. Katsantonis GP, Friedman WH, Krebs FJ, et al. Nasopharyngeal complications following uvulopalatopharyngoplasty. Laryngoscope 1987;97:309–14.
8. Croft CB, Golding-Wood DG. Uses and complications of uvulopalatopharyngoplasty. J Laryngol Otol 1990;104:871–5.
9. Ingrams DR, Spraggs PD, Pringle MB, et al. $CO_2$ laser palatoplasty: early results. J Laryngol Otol 1996;110:754–6.
10. Stepnick DW. Management of total nasopharyngeal stenosis following UPPP. Ear Nose Throat J 1993;72:86–90.
11. Kazanjian VH, Holmes EM. Stenosis of the nasopharynx and its correction. Arch Otolaryngol 1946;44:376–86.
12. Cotton RT. Nasopharyngeal stenosis. Arch Otolaryngol 1985;111:146–8.
13. Correa AJ, Reinisch L, Sanders DL, Huang S, Deriso W, Duncavage JA, Garrett CG. Inhibition of subglottic stenosis with mitomycin-C in the canine model. Ann Otol Rhinol Laryngol 1999;108(11 Pt 1):1053–60.
14. Holland BW, McGuirt WF Jr. Surgical management of choanal atresia: improved outcome using mitomycin. Arch Otolaryngol Head Neck Surg 2001;127(11):1375–80.

SECTION N — POSTOPERATIVE MANAGEMENT AND COMPLICATIONS

# CHAPTER 59

# Current techniques for the treatment of velopharyngeal insufficiency

*Harlan R. Muntz*

## 1 INTRODUCTION

Velopharyngeal insufficiency (VPI) is a significant speech disorder. This is usually identified and addressed in childhood, but may be seen as a consequence of central nervous system disease or injury, peripheral nerve injury or palate resection with cancer ablation in the adult. VPI can be a result of inappropriate articulation and hence, in these cases, remediable by aggressive speech therapy. All too often the treatment will need to be surgical. In this chapter, the surgical treatment will be addressed. Prosthetic management can be quite useful as well and will be addressed in the patient selection section, but will not be fully described here.

## 2 PATIENT SELECTION

Most children with VPI can be successfully treated by speech therapy. It is therefore imperative that the surgeon work closely with the speech pathologist in reduction of hypernasality, with appropriate phoneme production. In the case of VPI following CNS injury, the speech pathologist may be needed to address both swallowing as well as speech. Because recovery of function may take months, surgical intervention in these cases should proceed only after there seems to be a cessation of improvement in function.

The trained ear may hear the hypernasality, nasal emission and nasal turbulence in structured samples or spontaneous speech. The use of a non-heated mirror beneath the nose may give a reasonable assessment of the leakage of air through the nose during speech tasks. As /m,n,ng/ are normally nasalized sounds, the speech sample should focus on the other consonant non-nasal phonemes including /p,b,t,d,s,sh,z/. If the phoneme is not appropriately articulated it may be hypernasal. If possible the sample should obtain isolated phonemes, single words, phrases, sentences and spontaneous speech. Focus should be on the phonemes that are accurately articulated. The assessment of appropriate articulation is best done by the speech pathologist. This emphasizes the need for team care of the person with VPI. Surgical intervention should not be the order when speech therapy alone could suffice.

Another objective measure of hypernasality is nasometry, also called nasalence testing. The procedure compares the energy coming from the nose versus the mouth in a structured speech environment. With a sample loaded with non-nasal phonemes, hypernasality will be documented as a higher number and is compared to an established normal. It is rated as the number of standard deviations from the mean. If the sample is well articulated and there is good co-operation, this can be a help in deciding the need for surgical intervention.

Occasionally it is felt that the patient needs aggressive intervention, but is not a surgical candidate. These situations include severe airway obstruction, progressive disease, and prior radiation therapy to the airway or medical problems that would reduce the advisability of surgery. In these cases prosthetic management should be considered. An adequately long palate can be lifted to allow velopharyngeal competence or an obturator placed behind the palate can be used. The obturator is especially useful if there is a soft tissue defect from a cancer ablation or if the palate is congenitally short and the palatal lift cannot allow complete closure.

The appliance is clasped to the teeth and may be used during the day, but is removed for cleaning and sleep. This is of special help for both adults and children with a risk of obstructive sleep apnea. Children with other craniofacial syndromes may be at special risk for airway obstruction and prosthetic management may be a good option for them. Endoscopy can help with the determination of the need for prosthesis, as well as its fitting.

If the decision is made that surgery is necessary, endoscopic evaluation of the velopharynx during speech is needed to decide the type and extent of surgery needed.

Though some use only a single surgical procedure for all, there is wisdom in deciding the surgery based on the shape and the size of the 'gap' that needs obturation. A coronal or circular closure pattern may be more successful with sphincter pharyngoplasty than the sagittal closure pattern, as the area needing obturation may be more lateral. A pharyngeal flap that obturates the central velopharynx may be more helpful in these situations. If there is a small central gap, one should consider an augmentation.

If the levator veli palatini muscles are longitudinal in orientation rather than transverse, consideration must be given to either an intravelar veloplasty or a Furlow double opposing Z-plasty. In both of these operations the levator is reoriented to improve palatal motion, thereby correcting the VPI. The Furlow will be described in detail here.

Regardless of which surgical intervention is chosen, there is a potential effect on the airway. The Furlow lengthens and thickens the palate. All of the others to a greater degree reduce the cross-sectional airway area at the velopharynx. This alteration unfortunately may precipitate immediate post-surgical airway obstruction and OSA or sleep-disordered breathing, also. In general it seems the procedures from least to most obstructive are: Furlow, augmentation, sphincter and pharyngeal flap. Of course, each of the latter three may be altered to some extent to increase or decrease nasopharyngeal obturation and hence airway obstruction. This is based on the degree of motion of the velopharynx during speech. Care must be taken in the decision for surgical intervention to offer informed consent with regard to the airway issues.

As one considers surgery for VPI, it is important to plan the procedure based on the endoscopic findings. As was discussed above, one should consider the Furlow for any submucous cleft palate, as one could hope the reorientation of the levator sling would allow improved closure. If there is substantial lateral wall motion, the pharyngeal flap is ideal as it allows obturation without as much airway risk as a wide flap. Sphincter pharyngoplasty works well for most situations, as most people will have a circular or coronal closure pattern and this obturates the lateral and posterior velopharynx.

The association of 22q11 microdeletions (velocardiofacial syndrome) with especially non-cleft VPI makes it imperative to consider cardiac disease in the population of children with VPI. Careful examination and clearance by pediatrics or cardiology are important. Additionally many children with this syndrome will have medialization of the great vessels. This is often seen endoscopically as a pulsatile area in the hypo- or velopharynx. Though usually one may be able to successfully and safely complete the speech surgery even in this setting, it is critical to know this is present and avoid injury to the vertebral or carotid artery. Not only should this be considered at endoscopy, but as the pharynx is inspected as the mouth gag is placed, one should always re-evaluate for pulsation.

## 3 COMMON CONSIDERATIONS FOR THESE PROCEDURES

The surgery is performed under general anesthesia. Usually the use of an oral RAE tube will allow less interference with the field. The Dingmann mouth gag is usually used. It has the advantage of self-retaining lateral retractors and springs to allow suture retention. Other mouth gags used in tonsil surgery can be employed as well. Craig Senders suggested that releasing the pressure on the tongue during the surgery allowed improved blood flow and likely decreased pain.[1]

Local infiltration of the flap areas is necessary for hemostasis and will decrease local pain to make the anesthesia smoother. Lidocaine with epinephrine is good, but has a relatively shorter duration of pain control.

A throat pack is suggested, especially if the endotracheal tube is non-cuffed. This will hopefully prevent both aspiration of blood around the endotracheal tube and also swallowing of blood that could increase the chance of postoperative nausea.

At the end of surgery, a tongue suture can be placed. This is tied loosely and the tail remains long. It is taped to the side of the mouth. In the event of postoperative airway obstruction, pulling the tongue anteriorly with the suture will improve the airway. This is usually removed the following morning if the airway is secure.

## 4 FURLOW DOUBLE OPPOSING Z-PLASTY

The Furlow double opposing Z-plasty is quickly becoming a standard way of repairing a cleft palate. The advantage is the reorientation of the levator. If the levators are longitudinal one must consider the Furlow, or completely dissecting the levators to perform an intravelar veloplasty. In this chapter the focus will be on the Furlow.

A Z-plasty lengthens a scar. In VPI the problem often includes a short palate. The double Z-plasty lengthens the palate. The initial 'Z' can be made in either direction but the right-handed surgeon seems to do better as pictured (Fig. 59.1A). The posteriorly based flaps are always the myomucosal flaps. The anteriorly based flaps are mucosa only. Kathy Sie suggests rounding the tips of the flaps to improve the vascular supply.[2] The incision is carried through the oral cavity mucosa. As the incision is made in the left hemipalate, care must be taken to maintain a small amount of mucosa behind the posterior edge of the hard palate so that suturing is easier. Careful dissection through the levator and tensor veli palatini tendon brings one to the nasal mucosal layer. The plane is usually well defined. Meticulous blunt and sharp dissection separates the undersurface of the muscle bundle from the nasal mucosa.

# SECTION N: POSTOPERATIVE MANAGEMENT AND COMPLICATIONS

The anteriorly based mucosal flap is raised off the palatal muscles. This mucosa is markedly thicker than the nasal mucosa, but is still prone to injury if the dissection is not careful. The midline incision can be made through the palate at the initial step of the operation, or once both oral flaps are raised (Fig. 59.1B).

Approaching the nasal layer, the posterior left hemipalate incision is made to create the anteriorly based mucosal flap. The right hemipalate incision is made anterior near the hard palate edge to allow the myomucosal flap to be posteriorly based. Again it is important to leave a cuff of muscle and mucosa to facilitate the closure.

The nasal layer is closed by rotation of the left nasal mucosal flap across the midline, suturing it to the area of the right posterior hard palate. The nasal layer myomucosal flap is rotated to the left to be sutured to the defect.

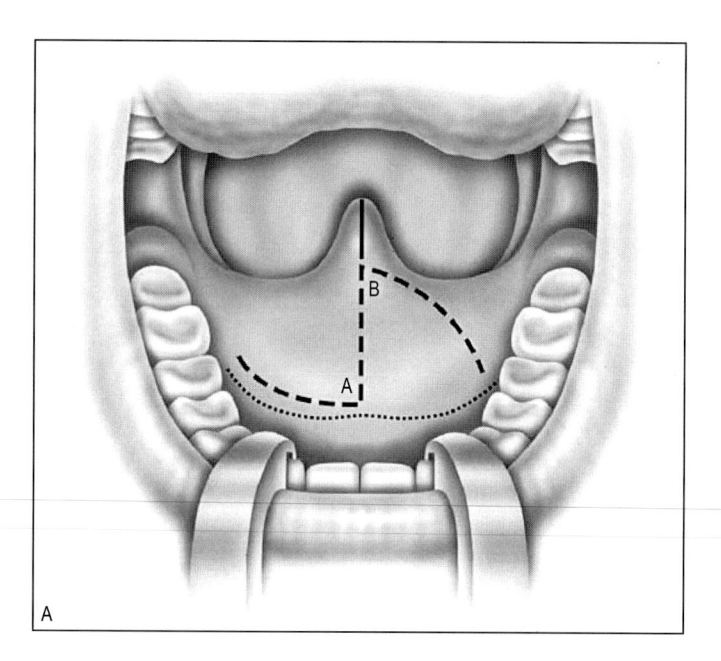

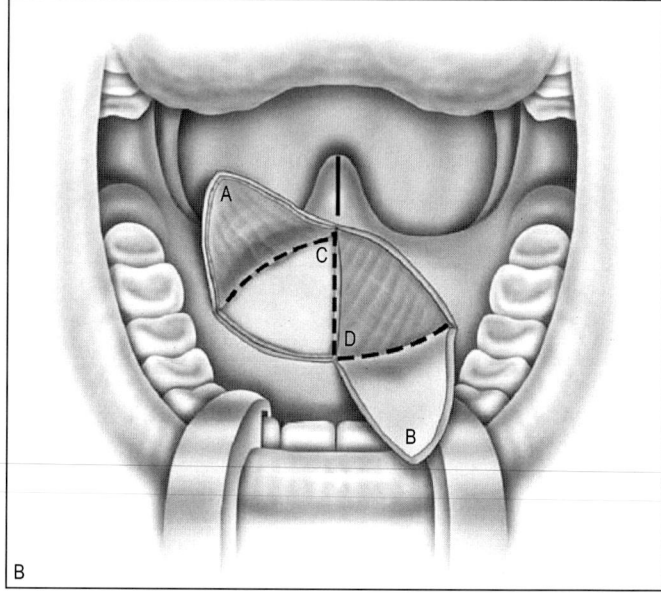

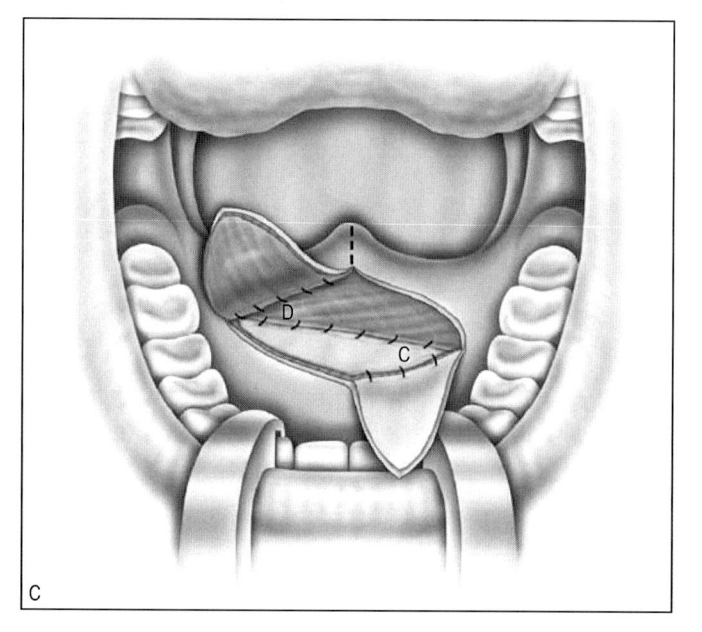

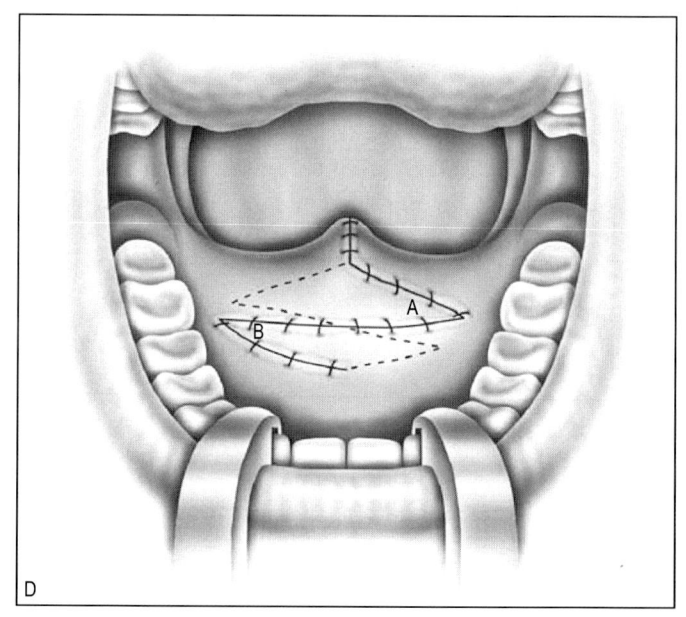

**Fig. 59.1** Furlow. A, The dashed line indicates the location of the incisions for the initial Z-plasty. The dotted line describes the posterior border of the hard palate. Flap (A) is the oral cavity myomucosal flap and flap (B) is the mucosal flap. B, The posteriorly based myomucosal flap (A) has been elevated as has the anteriorly based mucosal flap (B). The dashed lines show the location for the incisions to create the nasal layer myomucosal flap (D) and the nasal mucosal flap (C). C, The flaps (C) and (D) have been rotated and sutured into position. The uvula is often divided at this point to grant more mobility to the flap (D). The flaps (A) and (B) are retracted out of the field to improve the access for suturing the nasal layer. D, The flaps (A) and (B) have been rotated to create the second Z-plasty. They have been sutured into position. The uvula has been closed. The dashed line shows the location of the closure of the nasal Z-plasty.

This places the midline incision at the posterior left hemipalate and the anterior incision along the nasal mucosal flap (Fig. 59.1C).

The oral mucosal flap is now rotated to the left and the myomucosal flap rotated to the right and closed. One can see the muscle bundles are now in a horizontal orientation and posterior in the palate. The mucosal layers are more anterior against the hard palate. The uvula is reapproximated (Fig. 59.1D).

## 5 PHARYNGEAL FLAP

The pharyngeal flap has been the 'workhorse' for years. Though many have abandoned this procedure in favor of sphincter pharyngoplasty, it is still useful and in experienced hands affords excellent results.

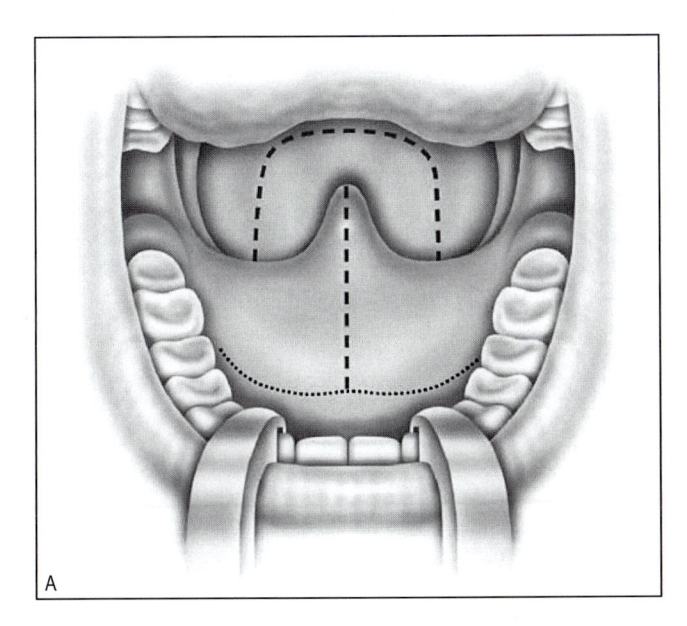

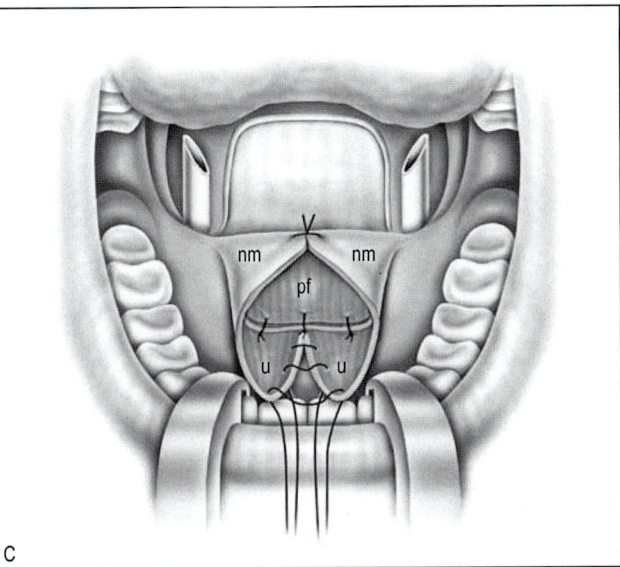

The idea is to bring a superiorly based midline flap from the pharynx and insert this into the palate. The following will describe one approach that allows mucosal covering of the flap to decrease flap contracture.

The surgery is done with a midline split of the soft palate (Fig. 59.2A). The posteriorly based nasal mucosal flap is elevated from the palate with careful blunt and sharp dissection. The nasal mucosa is divided just at the hard–soft palate border. The midline pharyngeal flap is developed from the center of the pharynx. Its width would be determined by the degree of obturation needed, as based on the preoperative endoscopy. This is elevated to the level of the hard palate.

In order to reduce the possibility of lateral port scarring that will increase the risk of postoperative airway obstruction, either an endotracheal tube or other catheter is placed through each nare and brought into the nasopharynx. The catheter size is determined by the desired port size.

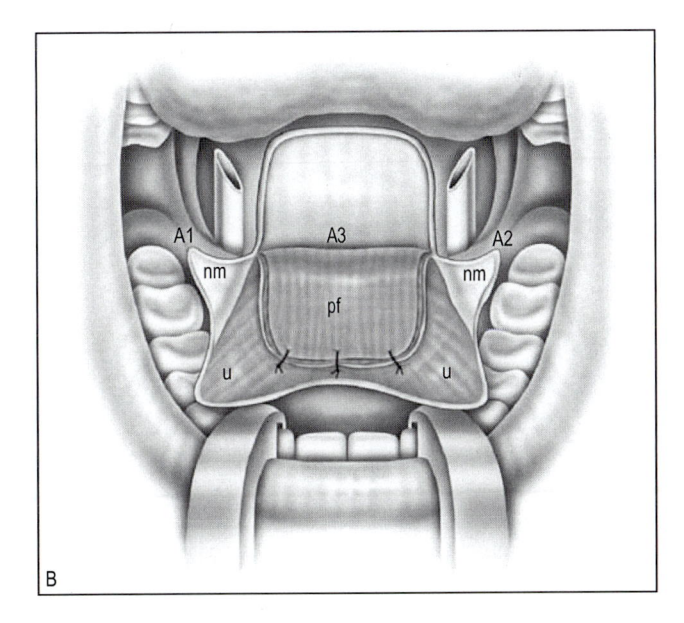

**Fig. 59.2** Pharyngeal flap. A, The incisions for the palatal split and the posterior pharyngeal flap have been outlined with a dashed line. The dotted line defines the posterior border of the hard palate. The initial incision in the palate is carried through the oral cavity and nasal mucosa. The hemipalates can be rotated laterally to improve the exposure to the posterior pharyngeal wall. The incision in the posterior pharyngeal wall is carried to the fascia. Because the flap will retract, it should be made slightly longer than you might expect. This is a myomucosal flap. B, The nasal mucosal layer (nm) has been delicately elevated from the muscle bundle and rotated laterally. The tip on the left is labeled (A¹) and that on the right labeled (A²). The elevated pharyngeal flap (pf) is rotated superiorly and sutured to the posterior aspect of the hard palate. The uvula (u) is, of course, divided. C, The nasal mucosal layer (nm) is sutured over the raw surface of the pharyngeal flap (pf). The remainder of the palate is closed in three layers: oral mucosa and uvula, muscular layer and finally the nasal layer.

# SECTION N: POSTOPERATIVE MANAGEMENT AND COMPLICATIONS

The pharyngeal flap is sutured to the posterior aspect of the hard palate (Fig. 59.2B). The nasal mucosal flaps are then sutured to the pharyngeal flap to cover the raw surface area. The soft palate is then closed in layers, reapproximating the muscle, the oral cavity mucosa and the uvula (Fig. 59.2C).

The defect in the posterior wall may be loosely approximated.

## 6 SPHINCTER PHARYNGOPLASTY

This operation has become a standard surgery for the treatment of VPI. The fundamental design is to create a posterior and lateral ridge. The palate will contact this during speech. Because the coronal and circular closure patterns are the most common, this has been exceptionally useful. Originally the hope was that this would create a functional sphincter because of the myomucosal flaps. This rarely happens.

Superiorly based myomucosal lateral pharyngeal wall flaps are elevated (Fig. 59.3A). The flap can include the posterior tonsillar pillar, or only the lateral pharyngeal wall. If the posterior pillar is used the flap tends to be more obstructive but is very useful in a large gap. The flap design is based on the amount of obturation needed. If little obturation is needed, the flap can be longer and narrower. If the sphincter needs to be tight, the shorter, wider flap creates a much smaller port.

A horizontal incision is made at the point of insertion (Fig. 59.3A). This can be defined by the point of maximal palatal elevation as seen in a lateral x-ray taken during speech, landmarks seen at the time of endoscopy or, as in many cases, placed as high as possible in the nasopharynx. Often this can be problematic if there is adenoid tissue in

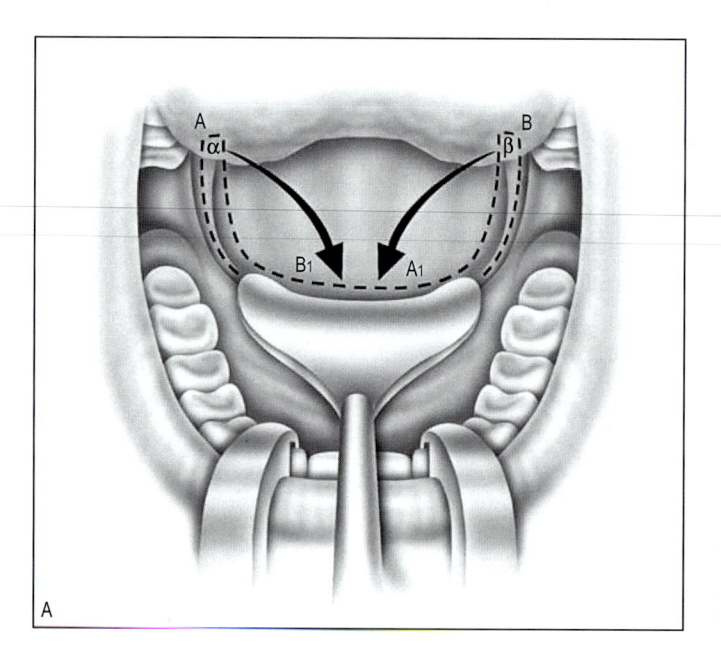

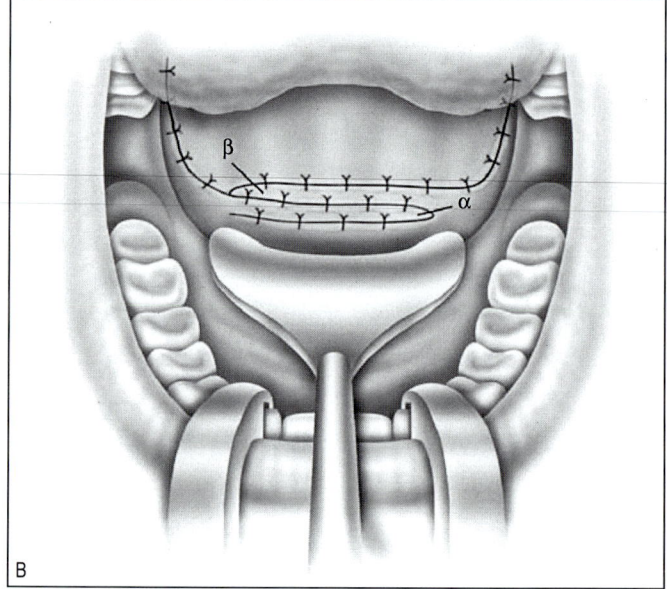

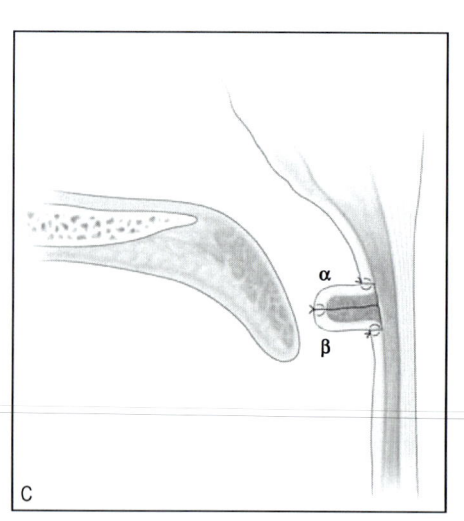

Fig. 59.3 Sphincter pharyngoplasty. A, A uvula retractor is used to retract the palate superiorly. The dashed lines demonstrate the location of the incisions. In this drawing the posterior pillar is included in the flap. The horizontal portion of the incision is made as high in the nasopharynx as possible or at a level determined by the anatomy seen on endoscopy. The left superiorly based myomucosal flap is labeled ($\alpha$) and the right labeled ($\beta$). The distal end of the flap (A) will be rotated to ($A^1$) and (B) will be rotated to ($B^1$). In order to have the raw surfaces juxtaposed the ($\beta$) flap will be rotated on its axis 180° degrees. B, The flaps are sutured into position in the nasopharynx. The lateral wall defects are loosely approximated. C, This sagittal view demonstrates the closure of the ($\alpha$) and ($\beta$) flaps.

the way. Suturing in the adenoids is difficult and increases the risk of bleeding and the flap not holding. De Serres presented a technique to help with this problem.[3] A microdebrider is used to remove the adenoids from the area of the horizontal incision. Hemostasis is assured and the flaps can be sutured into this space.

There are many ways to suture the flaps. The most practical way is to bring the left flap into the nasopharynx, suturing the posterior cut edge to the superior portion of the horizontal incision. The right myomucosal flap must be rotated at its base 180° on axis and then into the nasopharynx so the anterior cut edge is sutured to the inferior aspect of the horizontal incision (Fig. 59.3B). This opposes the raw surfaces (Fig. 59.3C). The degree of overlap and the length and width of the flap determine size of the central port. Exposure of the nasopharynx can be difficult. Retraction of the palate can be done with a uvula retractor as seen in the illustrations or bilateral transnasal red rubber catheters. Adequate visualization for accurate suture placement is a must.

The free edges of the flaps are sutured together (Fig. 59.3C). The defect created as the flaps were raised can be loosely approximated as well.

## 7 POSTERIOR WALL AUGMENTATION

On endoscopy one may see a small gap. If the gap appears to be 7 mm or less one should consider a posterior wall augmentation. This pharyngoplasty will attempt to address just the small area of concern. For decades there have been many augmentation procedures described. A rolled superiorly based pharyngeal flap has achieved some degree of success, but there is concern that scar could reduce the durability. Injections of both man-made and body substances have been tried, but none have had long-term success.

The following is a technique that is easily performed and has been very successful. This technique uses acellular dermis (Alloderm®).

Two vertical incisions are made in the nasopharynx. This area should correspond to the identified area of leak on endoscopy. A pocket is elevated beneath the fascia. A moderate thickness Alloderm sheet is rolled and sutured with absorbable sutures to maintain the shape. One of these sutures is left long, to assist with placement.

A right-angle clamp is placed through the pocket and the long suture is grasped. The Alloderm roll is pulled into the pocket (Fig. 59.4). Firmly holding the graft in position, multiple absorbable sutures are placed through the graft to stabilize it in the nasopharynx during the healing process. The long suture is cut and the vertical incisions closed.

This has less risk of airway obstruction. It can be used to augment a scarred pharyngoplasty. If the augmentation fails it does not preclude the use of any other pharyngoplasty. If the graft becomes exposed it may become infected and need excision. Postoperative antibiotic coverage is a must.

## 8 POSTOPERATIVE MANAGEMENT AND COMPLICATIONS

The use of anti-emetics during and after the operation will hopefully improve the immediate postoperative course.

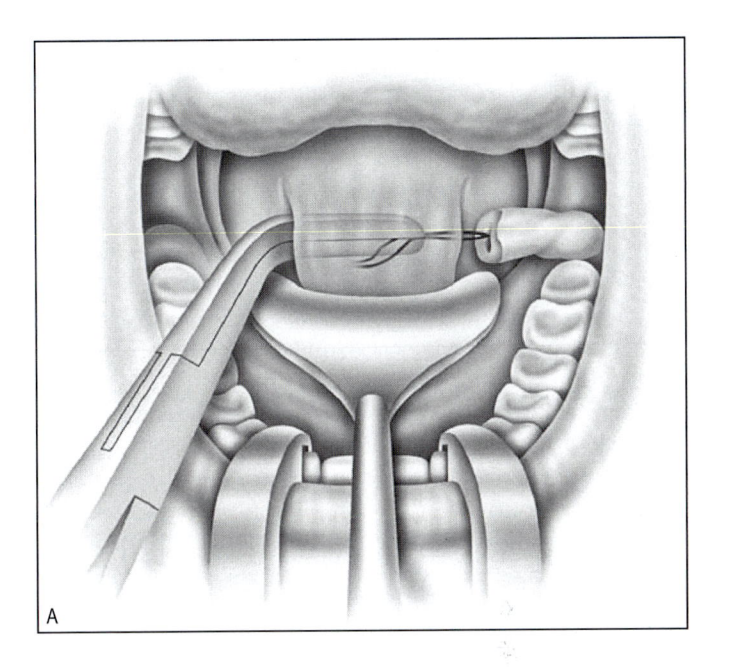

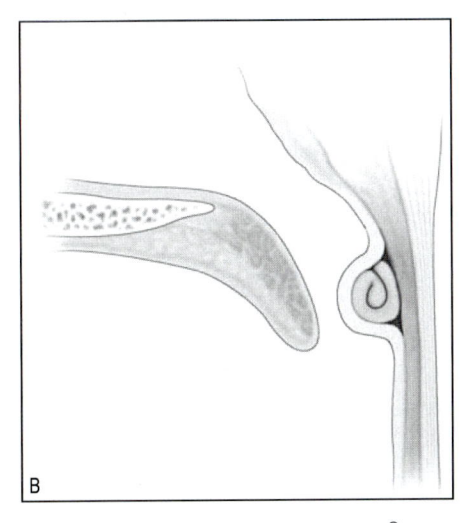

**Fig. 59.4** Posterior wall augmentation. A, The Alloderm® was rolled and sutured to retain its shape. At one end the suture is left long. After the bilateral vertical incisions are made, a tunnel is made beneath the fascia. Inserting a long right-angle clamp, the long suture is grasped and the rolled Alloderm® is pulled into the tunnel. It will be sutured into position and the vertical incisions closed. B, This sagittal view shows the orientation of the rolled Alloderm®.

# SECTION N: POSTOPERATIVE MANAGEMENT AND COMPLICATIONS

Antibiotics during and after the procedure may be helpful in preventing infection and improving healing.

Postoperative pain control is important. IV narcotics should be transitioned to oral as soon as possible. Unfortunately as there is some risk of airway obstruction with these procedures, one must always guard against respiratory depression with narcotics; close monitoring after surgery is important. This is especially important if there is micrognathia. The tongue suture will allow the tongue to be pulled forward to relieve the obstruction. This is important to consider in any child, but especially in those with risk factors for postoperative upper airway obstruction.

Usually hospitalization is necessary after surgery, until the child has adequate oral intake and the airway is assured.

Complications of the surgery include bleeding, airway obstruction, and failure to achieve normal resonance. In general meticulous dissection decreases the risk of bleeding. Intraoperative hemostasis should be achieved with bipolar or low wattage monopolar cautery. This will hopefully decrease unwanted scar formation.

Airway obstruction after these surgeries can be severe or mild. Obstructive sleep apnea is a commonly described complication of pharyngeal flap, but there are reported cases of this as well in sphincter pharyngoplasty. If appropriate, the use of a Furlow or posterior wall augmentation may reduce the risk of postoperative airway obstruction. Even in these cases, there can be obstruction in the child with other risk factors such as micrognathia or other craniofacial anomalies.

Revision of the sphincter and pharyngeal flap is possible to reduce the airway obstruction. This needs to be balanced against the speech concerns, and a repeat endoscopy should be carried out to allow an evaluation of where revision can safely be accomplished without worsening the speech. If there has been significant improvement of speech, continuous positive airway pressure (CPAP) and bi-level positive airway pressure (Bi-PAP) can be considered in the postoperative period. Often over time the need for this pressure-assisted breathing is reduced, whether through the growth of the child or physiologic changes in the velopharynx. There have been multiple reports of taking down a pharyngeal flap without deterioration of speech. This should be considered in the older child.

The endoscopy could also reveal adenoid enlargement or encroachment of the tonsils into the airway. Tonsillectomy should be considered even if the tonsils are small. Adenoidectomy is more difficult, but can be done with a microdebrider through the velopharyngeal port. If the port is too small, a transnasal partial adenoidectomy can be done with a microdebrider. Bearing this in mind, one should consider tonsillectomy and adenoidectomy prior to pharyngoplasty if they are large and endoscopically seem to be a potential for airway obstruction. The speech surgery should be delayed 2–3 months to allow healing of the nasopharynx and oropharynx.

Nasal obstruction can present as mouth breathing, snorting and inability to blow the nose. Occasionally the chief complaint will be hyponasality. Some children and families will be very annoyed with these symptoms. If the endoscopy suggests that a revision would not compromise speech, the flaps can be reduced surgically. Care must be taken to design the surgery based on the endoscopic findings and to make sure mucosal surfaces are closed. Exposed raw surfaces may increase scar formation and make the airway obstruction worse. Often if the obstruction follows a sphincter pharyngoplasty and there is a strong coronal closure pattern, the sphincter can be released laterally. The posterior obturation remains and the airway can often be increased three-fold.

## 9 SUCCESS AND POTENTIAL FAILURE OF THE PROCEDURE

In properly selected patients with good preoperative planning, the improvement in velopharyngeal function should exceed 90%. Syndromic patents will be more difficult to treat, especially those with Nager's and velocardiofacial syndrome. Postoperative evaluation by speech pathology and nasalence testing can be helpful in determining the success of these surgeries.

If the surgery failed to eliminate the hypernasality, one must consider possible reasons. Hypernasality may be related to continued articulation issues. The family needs to know this preoperatively. There is usually a need for ongoing speech therapy to perfect the articulation. This is especially the case in maladaptive or compensatory articulation.

Postoperative endoscopy may show air leakage during appropriately articulated phonemes. If the Furlow has failed, one can use any of the other techniques to eliminate the hypernasal resonance. The use of the posterior wall augmentation does not 'burn bridges' for using either the sphincter or pharyngeal flap. Revision of the sphincter can be more easily undertaken than in the pharyngeal flap. If there is residual VPI, endoscopy will define the area of concern. The resection of a 'V' from the flap followed by a two-layer closure, tightens the port. Raising an additional superiorly based myomucosal flap from the lateral pharyngeal wall and inserting that into the existing sphincter can bulk the area to further obturate the port. After a pharyngeal flap, endoscopy can define which of the ports is the problem and to what extent. The ports can be further obturated with a V–Y advancement flap on the lateral or posterior wall. Additional midline tissue can be added to the lateral aspect of the flap as well.

## 10 CONCLUSION

The treatment of VPI should be based on an understanding of the closure pattern during speech. A major potential risk of the surgery is airway obstruction, often demonstrated as obstructive sleep apnea. Of the procedures discussed, those with the least risk for airway obstruction are the Furlow and posterior wall augmentation. If there is postoperative sleep apnea the pharyngeal flap and sphincter can be revised to open the port and improve breathing, or CPAP or BiPAP can be used.

## REFERENCES

1. Senders CW, Eisele JH. Lingual pressures induced by mouthgags. Int J Pediatr Otorhinolaryngol 1995;33(1):53–60.
2. Sie KC, Gruss JS. Results with Furlow palatoplasty in the management of velopharyngeal insufficiency. Plast Reconstr Surg 2002;109(7):2588–89, author reply p. 2590.
3. de Serres LM, Deleyiannis FW, Eblen LE, et al. Results with sphincter pharyngoplasty and pharyngeal flap. Int J Pediatr Otorhinolaryngol 1999;48(1):17–25.

## FURTHER READING

Antony AK, Sloan GM. Airway obstruction following palatoplasty: analysis of 247 consecutive operations. Cleft Palate Craniofac J 2002;39(2):145–8.

Armour A, Fischback S, Klaiman P, Fisher DM. Does velopharyngeal closure pattern affect the success of pharyngeal flap pharyngoplasty? Plast Reconstr Surg 2005;115(1):45–52.

D'Antonio LL, Eichenberg BJ, Zimmerman GJ, et al. Radiographic and aerodynamic measures of velopharyngeal anatomy and function following Furlow Z-plasty. Plast Reconstr Surg 2000;106(3):539–49, discussion pp. 550–3.

Furlow LT Jr. Cleft palate repair by double opposing Z-plasty. Plast Reconstr Surg 1986;78(6):724–38.

Larossa D, Jackson OH, Kirschner RE, et al. The children's hospital of Philadelphia modification of the Furlow double-opposing Z-palatoplasty: long-term speech and growth results. Clin Plast Surg 2004;31(2):243–9.

Liao YF, Noordhoff MS, Huang CS, et al. Comparison of obstructive sleep apnea syndrome in children with cleft palate following Furlow palatoplasty or pharyngeal flap for velopharyngeal insufficiency. Cleft Palate Craniofac J 2004;41(2):152–6.

Mann EA, Sidman JD. Results of cleft palate repair with the double-reverse Z-plasty performed by residents. Otolaryngol Head Neck Surg 1994;111(1):76–80.

March JL. Management of velopharyngeal dysfunction: differential diagnosis for differential management. J Craniofac Surg 2003;14(5):621–8.

Mehendale FV, Sommerlad BC. Surgical significance of abnormal internal carotid arteries in velocardiofacial syndrome in 43 consecutive Hynes pharyngoplasties. Cleft Palate Craniofac J 2004;41(4):368–74.

Peat BG, Albery EH, Jones K, Pigott RW. Tailoring velopharyngeal surgery: the influence of etiology and type of operation. Plast Reconstr Surg 1994;93(5):948–53.

Perkins JA, Lewis CW, Gruss JS, et al. Furlow palatoplasty for management of velopharyngeal insufficiency: a prospective study of 148 consecutive patients. Plast Reconstr Surg 2005;116(1):72–80, discussion pp. 81–4.

Saint Raymond C, Bettega G, Deschaux C, et al. Sphincter pharyngoplasty as a treatment of velopharyngeal incompetence in young people: a prospective evaluation of effects on sleep structure and sleep respiratory disturbances. Chest 2004;125(3):864–71.

Senders CW, Sykes JM. Modifications of the Furlow palatoplasty (six- and seven-flap palatoplasties). Arch Otolaryngol Head Neck Surg 1995;121(10):1101–4.

Witt PD, Marsh JL, Marty-Grames L, Muntz HR. Revision of the failed sphincter pharyngoplasty: an outcome assessment. Plast Reconstr Surg 1995;96(2):129–38.

Witt PD, Marsh JL, Muntz HR, et al. Acute obstructive sleep apnea as a complication of sphincter pharyngoplasty. Cleft Palate Craniofac J 1996;33(3):183–9.

Witt PD, O'Daniel TG, Marsh JL, et al. Surgical management of velopharyngeal dysfunction: outcome analysis of autogenous posterior pharyngeal wall augmentation. Plast Reconstr Surg 1997;99(5):1287–96.

Ysunza A, Garcia-Velasco M, Garcia-Garcia M, et al. Obstructive sleep apnea secondary to surgery for velopharyngeal insufficiency. Cleft Palate Craniofac J 1993;30(4):387–90.

Ysunza A, Pamplona C, Ramirez E, et al. Velopharyngeal surgery: a prospective randomized study of pharyngeal flaps and sphincter pharyngoplasties. Plast Reconstr Surg 2002;110(6):1401–7.

# SECTION N  POSTOPERATIVE MANAGEMENT AND COMPLICATIONS

## CHAPTER 60
# Uvulopalatopharyngoplasty: analysis of failure

*Nico de Vries and Naomi Ketharanathan*

## 1 INTRODUCTION

Sleep disordered breathing (SDB) encompasses a spectrum of conditions including socially unacceptable snoring (SUS) and obstructive sleep apnea syndrome (OSAS). Where SUS is mostly debilitating in social circumstances, OSAS and its complications pose a major health problem for society.[1] Increased awareness has led to the development of various treatment modalities to combat both these diseases of which uvulopalatopharyngoplasty (UPPP) is without doubt the most widely used surgical intervention.

UPPP was first performed in 1963 by Ikematsu,[2] but modified and formally introduced as a surgical treatment for OSAS in 1981 by Fujita.[3]

Now a quarter century later it is time to do an accounting. Has UPPP lived up to its initial expectations? At this point numerous studies have been performed estimating the outcome of UPPP in both the short and long term. Unfortunately, UPPP as sole (surgical) management is not as uniformly successful as initially hoped for. Growing understanding of the multifactorial and multilevel pathophysiology of OSAS has raised discussions whether the widespread application of UPPP continues to be justifiable, or whether UPPP should be offered only to well-selected patients. This chapter aims to review the current knowledge on factors especially associated with negative UPPP outcome and discuss various ways of selecting patients for UPPP.

## 2 PATIENT SELECTION

The first step in the process of patient selection is diagnosing the severity of the condition. This starts with a thorough history from the patient and possible partner as well as general ENT examination. Body Mass Index (BMI) and neck circumference are noted at this stage too. The severity of disease is important only to determine if the patient is a candidate for surgery or whether the patient should have non-surgical minimally invasive techniques. Severity will not be a guide to determine the type of surgery. The location of the obstruction will determine the correct surgical procedure.

The next step in the work-up of suspected OSAS patients is a *polysomnogram* (PSG). This objective tool allows qualitative and quantitative measurements such as differentiation between SUS and OSAS and evaluation of the degree of disease severity. There are four levels of polysomnographic testing of which level I is the most elaborate, including recordings such as an electroencephalogram, registration of eye movements, submental electromyogram, registration of thoracic and abdominal respiratory movement, limb movements, oxygen saturation and the intensity of snoring all recorded in a clinical setting for the duration of at least 6 hours. The other levels are less extensive and not performed in a clinical setting.[4] Events recorded during PSG and most commonly used to estimate severity and treatment outcome are the Apnea Index (AI), Apnea/Hypopnea Index (AHI), Respiratory Distress Index (RDI), Respiratory Arousal Index (RAI), Respiratory Effort Related Arousals (RERA) and Oxygen Desaturation Index (ODI). Recently the American Academy of Sleep Medicine (AASM) formulated recommendations for clinical and research definitions of PSG studies.[5]

A subjective measuring tool is the *Epworth Sleepiness Scale (ESS)*, a questionnaire regarding hypersomnia. It was originally designed as an easy, non-invasive tool to distinguish SUS from OSAS.[6] Although practical in use, it has been shown to have a low predictive value, and it cannot show the severity of the disease.

After assessment of the severity of the disease by polysomnography it is of equal importance to determine the level of obstruction(s) in the upper airway.

Mallampati et al. developed the *Mallampati clinical scoring system* in the mid-1980s to predict difficulty in tracheal intubation based on the ability to visualize the faucial pillars, soft palate and uvula base.[7] The Mallampati score has been modified by Friedman et al. who then studied the value of this type of assessment in patients with obstructive sleep apnea.

Friedman modified the original Mallampati score in the following ways.

1. Anesthesiologists assess the palate by asking the patient to protrude their tongue. The tongue position during sleep is not protruded, so we ask the patient only to open their mouth and not protrude their tongue.
2. Mallampati had three positions and Friedman expanded to four positions and, most recently, has expanded it to five positions.
3. It really describes the position of the tongue more than the palate. The analysis, as used to assess OSAS, is therefore called the Friedman tongue position (see Chapter 16).

The Friedman staging system represents a clinical, anatomical staging system, independent of disease severity. Friedman et al. found patients classified with stage 1 disease had an 80.6% chance of successful cure with UPPP as opposed to success rates of respectively 38% and 8% in stage 2 and stage 3. The major advantage of this system is its easy use in various settings and its ability to predict which patients are most likely to fail (stage 3).[8]

*Sleep(naso)endoscopy* (sedated endoscopy) is another way of determining the levels of obstruction during induced sleep. This approach attempts to simulate the natural situation during snoring. Although this is a relatively time-consuming and costly method it is also the best option for topical preoperative dynamic diagnostic work-up for an ENT practice.[9]

Despite reports that each method is capable of good preoperative work-up, it is intriguing that the correlation between Friedman tongue position (or Friedman staging system) and findings with sleep endoscopy is low.[10]

The importance of determining the level of obstruction or collapsibility of the pharynx is increasingly recognized. Globally one way of describing the level of pharynx anatomy involves the subdivision into retropalatal and retrolingual obstruction. This has led to the following, much applied, preoperative classification: Type 1 refers to collapse at retropalatal level, Type 2 indicates collapse at both retropalatal and retrolingual level and Type 3 means collapse at the retrolingual area.[11]

## 3 OUTLINE OF PROCEDURE

UPPP targets obstructions at the oropharyngeal level by removing and tightening excess pharyngeal tissue and shortening an elongated uvula and soft palate. These interventions are often combined with tonsillectomy to increase the oropharyngeal lumen (see Chapter 29: Uvulopalatopharyngoplasty).

## 4 POSTOPERATIVE COMPLICATIONS

There are roughly three major groups of complications regarding UPPP.

1. **Perioperative complications:** such as edema and hemorrhage can lead to life-threatening situations in an already compromised upper airway. Kezirian et al. investigated the perioperative mortality rate of UPPP in a large prospective cohort study and found a 30-day mortality rate of 0.2%, mostly due to unsuccessful upper airway management.[12]
2. **Short-term complications:** may comprise transient velopharyngeal incompetence apparent by wound dehiscence, hemorrhage, wound infection, mild nasal regurgitation and is some cases hypernasal speech. In addition severe postoperative pain and poor intake can add to overall morbidity.
3. **Long-term complications:** include pharyngeal discomfort, dryness and tightness, postnasal secretions, dysphagia, prolonged angina, inability to initiate swallowing, speech and taste disturbances and numbness of the tongue, permanent velopharyngeal incompetence and nasopharyngeal stenosis.

In addition, there have been reports that tolerance to nasal continuous positive airway pressure (NCPAP) was diminished after UPPP, which compounds treatment failure because other options are now less successful too.[13]

## 5 SUBJECTIVE AND OBJECTIVE TREATMENT OUTCOMES

A distinction should be made between subjective and objective treatment outcome. Although a reasonable correlation usually exists between objective and subjective outcome, unexplained discrepancies still occur in many circumstances. A clinical reality is that a rise in AHI or RDI can occur with subjective improvement and vice versa. One of the consequences is that repeated polysomnography should be performed in all OSAS patients after surgery. Unresolved ethical issues occur for instance in a happy (e.g. reduced snoring and/or improvement of hypersomnolence) patient after surgery who in repeated PSG is shown to have a rise in AHI or an unhappy patient with no subjective improvement but a distinctively lower AHI in repeated PSG recordings. Concerning these discrepancies between objective and subjective UPPP outcome, Lu et al. noted a long-term subjective improvement in 80% of their cases which was not correlated with the polysomnographic results.[14] This raises the following question: if help-seeking behavior is mostly symptom driven and the patient now feels these symptoms no longer exist, how to motivate the patient for additional treatment to prevent long-term negative effect on health? The importance of treatment in (severe) OSAS is underlined by findings by Keenan et al. who showed that UPPP increases long-term survival in OSAS patients.[15]

# SECTION N  POSTOPERATIVE MANAGEMENT AND COMPLICATIONS

## 5.1 OBJECTIVE DEFINITIONS OF OUTCOME

These can be defined as:

- success.
- response.
- no change.
- deterioration.

*Success* is most commonly objectively assessed by polysomnography. Over the past decades various cut-off points have been used in different studies estimating UPPP outcome of which a brief review follows. Fujita was the first to define the cut-off value for success as an AI reduction of 50%. Other variables taken into account included the level of oxygenation ($SaO_2$ >85%) and the number of arousals.[3] The large meta-analysis of Sher et al. used an AI reduction with an absolute AI of 10 and/or an RDI reduction of 50%, with an RDI of less than 20 to evaluate treatment outcome.[11] Larsson et al. also used an RDI reduction of 50% together with a reduced RDI of 20 or less for their long-term evaluation of UPPP outcome.[16] A 50% reduction of the AHI was also used by Janson et al. and combined with an absolute AI value of 10 or less.[17]

Another frequently used outcome measure is the Oxygen Desaturation Index (ODI) where responders are defined as having a postoperative ODI of <20 with an ODI reduction of at least 50% compared to preoperative values.[16,18]

*Response* can be defined as improvement of AHI of between 20% and 50%.
*No change* can be defined as an increase or decrease in AHI of <20%. Variations (decrease and increase) of less than 20% can be regarded as falling within the normal night-to-night variability.
*Deterioration* is an increase of AHI of more than 20%.
*Treatment failure* comprises both *no change* in outcome as well as *deterioration*.

We propose this subdivision into responders (success and response) and non-responders (comprising both no change and deterioration) to achieve a simplified subdivision in treatment outcome and ease study comparison.

Issues that require attention in patient classification by PSG measurements are night-to-night variability and the influence of different types of leads when interpreting PSG values close to the cutoff point between responders and non-responders.[5]

For UPPP, another *clinical distinction* can be proposed:

1. There are no negative alterations visually present showing a typical, normal post-UPPP situation on examination, but there is a persistent negative outcome as measured by PSG (Figure 60.1). This may implicate that the indication for UPPP, as an isolated procedure, was incorrect; apparently the level of obstruction was not Type 1 (retropalatinal only). The other possibility is

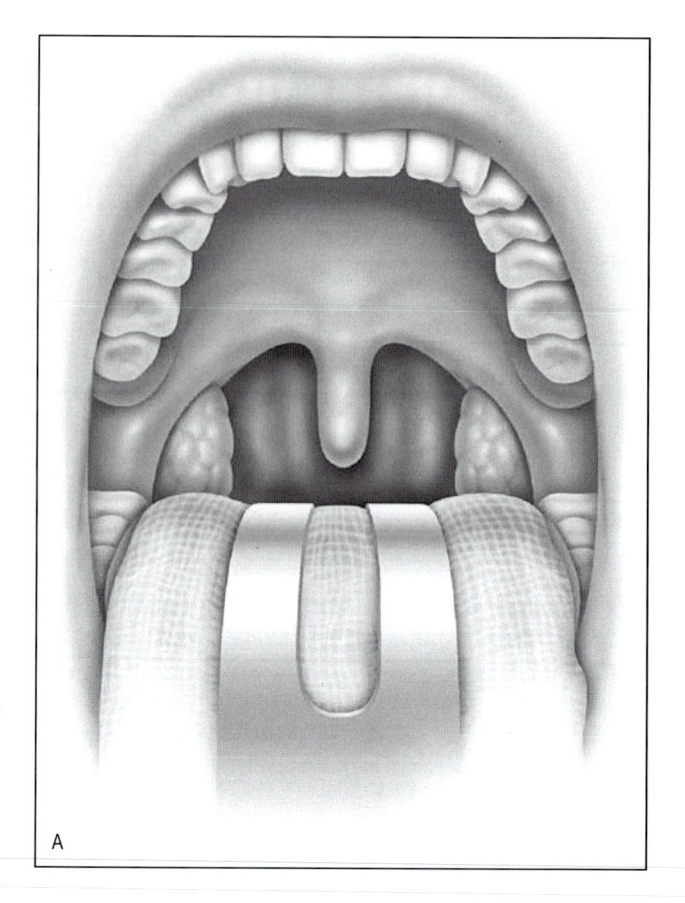

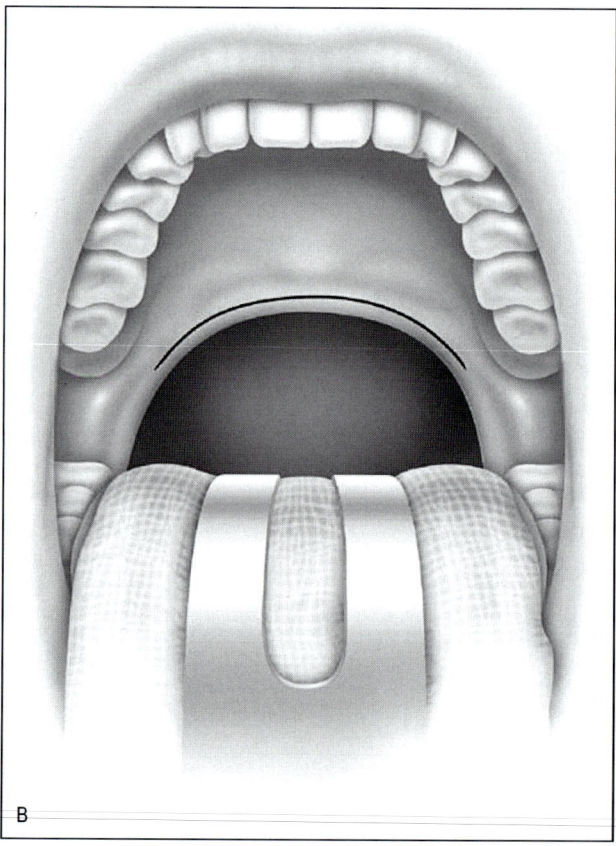

**Fig. 60.1** A, Situation before UPPP. B, Clinically desired situation after UPPP.

CHAPTER 60

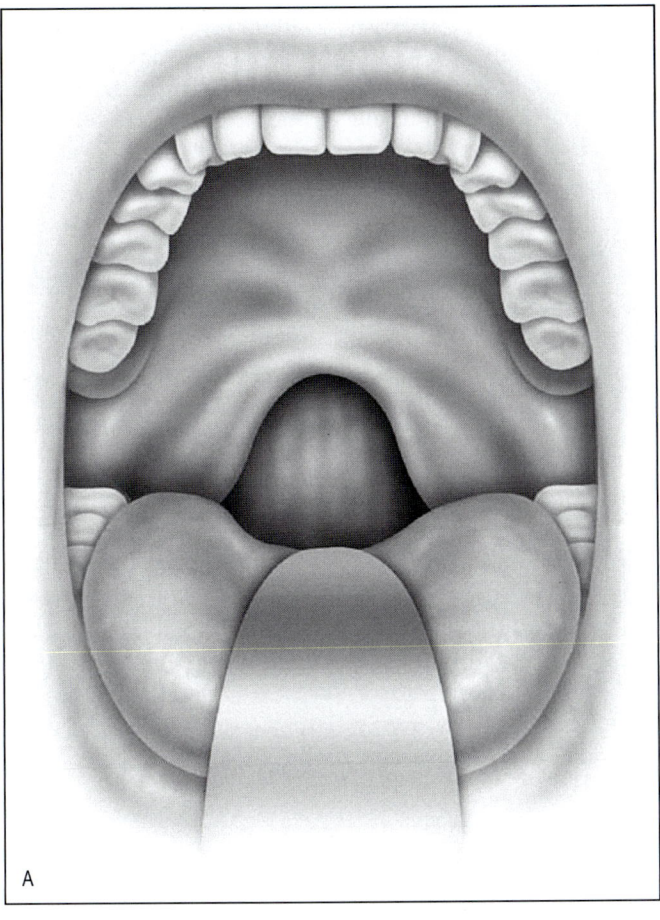

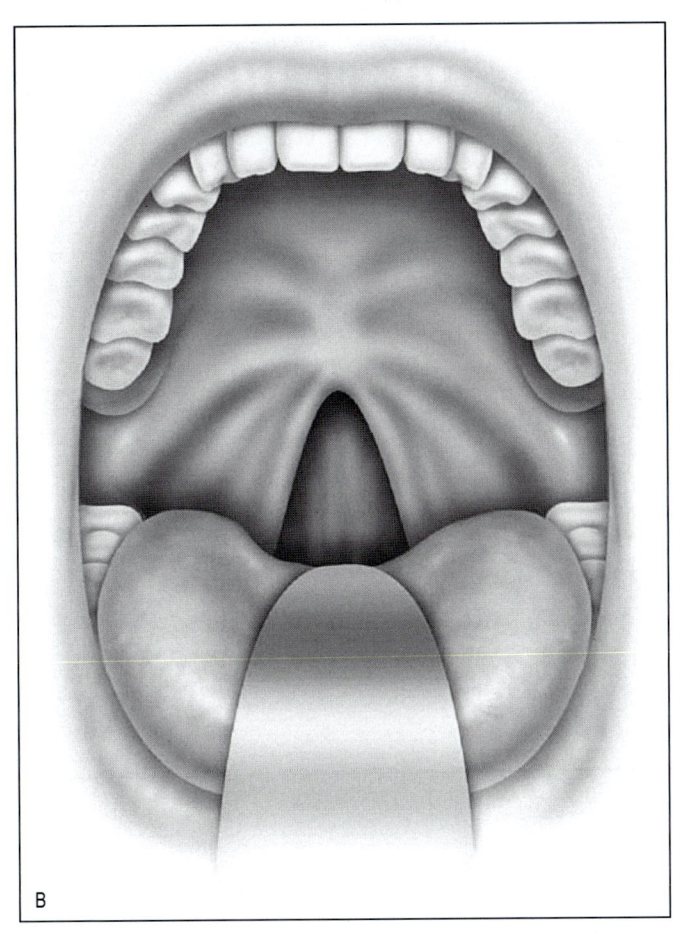

Uvulopalatopharyngoplasty: analysis of failure

**Fig. 60.2** A, Mild to moderate stenosis after UPPP; clinically undesired situation. B, Severe stenosis after UPPP; clinically undesired situation.

that the resection was inadequate. Very often the site of failure after UPPP is the retropalatinal area.
2. Treatment failure with distinct negative features such as nasopharyngeal stenosis (NPS) (Figure 60.2).

Nasopharyngeal stenosis is a much feared iatrogenic complication of UPPP. Severe stenosis is estimated to occur in less than 1% of post-UPPP cases.[19] Based on the degree of severity, nasopharyngeal stenosis can be divided into mild/moderate stenosis (Figure 60.2A) or severe stenosis (Figure 60.2B), each requiring a different approach. Mild to moderate stenosis can be managed with Z-palatoplasty according to Friedman.[20] In severe cases of NPS, Krespi and Kacker found that the use of $CO_2$ laser combined with a custom-made nasopharyngeal obturator gives satisfactory long-term results in severe NPS management.[19]

## 6 DISCUSSION: ANALYSIS OF UPPP FAILURE

The most cited meta-analysis is definitely that of Sher et al.,[11] showing an overall UPPP success rate of 40.7% in unselected patients. Sher et al. used as definition of success an AHI drop of >50% and AI <10. These data were early results in unselected patients, and since then it has become clear that level of obstruction determination is of paramount importance in improving success rates of any form of OSAS surgery. Better UPPP results can be expected in Type 1 patients (retropalatinal obstruction only), less good in Type 2 (both retropalatinal and retrolingual) and least satisfactory in Type 3 (retrolingual level only). Based on this rational approach definitive improvements of UPPP success percentages have been reported by, among others, Friedman et al.[8] (using the Friedman staging system), and by Hessel and de Vries (after the use of sleep endoscopy) for patient selection.[9]

In the case of OSAS, Fujita et al. were the first to select the polysomnographic cut-off point of an AI drop of 50% to evaluate a group of UPPP patients.[3] Fujita's definition of success was used in the meta-analysis of Sher et al. and adjusted to include an AI <10 to provide more strict criteria.[11] So far, this has been the most widely used way of attempting to evaluate UPPP outcome in an objective manner, although as discussed earlier many variations have been made and/or additional criteria added, leading to a confusing plethora of objective outcome measures. Hopefully the definitions recommended by the AASM

# SECTION N: POSTOPERATIVE MANAGEMENT AND COMPLICATIONS

in 2005 will lead to universal criteria and the formulation of uniform outcome measures to ease study comparison.[5]

A summary of some of the major short- and long-term studies on UPPP outcome for SUS and OSAS follows.

## 6.1 UPPP FOR SOCIALLY UNACCEPTABLE SNORING

Simple snoring is often the result of soft palate vibration. UPPP targets this area and it is therefore no surprise that initial success rates in this situation are high at approximately 87%. Unfortunately this percentage is almost reduced to half after long-term follow-up.[23] A retrospective review of snoring surgery by Jones et al. cites a wide range in success rate of 45% (at 2 years) to even 90% (at 5 years) but the general trend is a regression of positive outcome with time. The estimated overall failure rate of snoring surgery (including UPPP and irrespective of type of surgery) is ~66% at 2 years.[24]

Of equal importance is the level of partner satisfaction after UPPP. Prasad et al. found a significant reduction in sleep disturbance and an improved quality of life as measured by a questionnaire-based survey with a minimum of a 1-year follow-up.[25]

## 6.2 UPPP FOR OSAS

The range of success rates reported in various studies has a wide variation of 25–85%.[26]

In 1981 Fujita described the first cohort to be treated with UPPP and arbitrarily defined criteria for success which have since been widely applied. However, this value was based on the study group as a whole with large variation among the individuals. Even in this first study, two out of the total of 12 patients had an increase in apneas, although none indicated subjective worsening after UPPP. (Objective) UPPP 'failure' has been described from the beginning.[3] Sher et al. did the first meta-analysis which showed a success rate of 50% when using the criteria defined by Fujita. This rate dropped to 40.7% in unselected patients when adjusted to include an AI of <10. The success rate was 52.3% in the group of patients clinically suspected of unilevel oropharyngeal obstruction, indicating the importance of anatomical staging.[11]

The first long-term follow-up (46 months) was by Larsson et al. in a group of 50 UPPP patients. Using a postoperative RDI <20 and a RDI reduction of at least 50% as the criteria for success, they found 60% of patients to be responders at 6 months. This amount decreased to 38.8% by 21 months but climbed back to 50% at a mean of 46 months.[16] Janson et al. found a positive response of 64% 6 months postoperatively but a similar percentage of responders (48%) to other studies after a 4 to 8-year follow-up using a 50% or more decrease in AHI and a postoperative AI of less than 10 as criteria for success.[17] In 2000 Boot et al. published results of another long-term follow-up in unselected patients. Using ODI as criterion for success, this study showed that only ~20% remained as responder over time.[18]

Senior et al. found UPPP to be effective in 40% of their cohort of mild OSAS patients. Their study supported the increasing evidence of sub-optimal UPPP treatment outcome. However, the non-responders showed objective worsening on polysomnographic evaluation combined with lack of subjective symptom improvement.[21] This finding drew attention to an underreported aspect of UPPP outcome in the literature. Deterioration after UPPP was also noted by Hessel and de Vries who even found some failures in the Type 1 and 2 groups despite preoperative selection by sleep endoscopy. They reported better than average results of UPPP with use of sedated endoscopy for patient selection but encountered failures (deterioration) in approximately 10–15%. Results were negatively influenced by previous tonsillectomy (with relative short anterior–posterior diameter at retropalatal level) and simultaneous obstruction at tongue base level (Type 2 does worse than Type 1).[22]

## 6.3 COMPLICATIONS

Another aspect of UPPP failure is the occurrence of complications. Grontved and Karup administered a questionnaire to 69 patients 2 years post-UPPP. They found that 42% had complaints.[27] Although the majority of these were minor, it shows that patient satisfaction deserves ample attention and underlines the importance of both objective and subjective rating of surgical success.

This aspect was studied by Walker-Engstrom and colleagues who assessed quality of life after treatment of mild to moderate OSAS patients with either a dental appliance or UPPP over a 1-year follow-up period. They found that although both interventions led to significant improvement in quality of life (evaluated by the dimensions vitality, contentment and sleep), the subjective improvement was greater for UPPP. However, the AI and AHI rate (<5 resp. <10) was more normalized in the dental appliance group than the UPPP group (78% vs. 51%), underlining once again the frequent discrepancy between subjective and objective treatment outcomes.[28]

It is concerning to discover that long-term outcome of UPPP on OSAS shows a high level of relapse.[17,18,21] Furthermore, there are increasing reports of disease deterioration after surgical intervention.[21,22] This raises the question whether it is justified to put patients at risk of surgery for an intervention that in the long run is likely to give minimal to no improvement and possibly even worsening of the situation. UPPP indeed appears not to be the single-step answer but it does prove sufficient therapy for a specific group of patients. The subsequent question therefore is: which patients are these and how do we identify them preoperatively?

## 6.4 WHICH FACTORS ARE ASSOCIATED WITH THE VARYING RESPONSE RATE TO UPPP?

When understanding the factors associated with OSAS, it is first of all important to appreciate the multifactorial pathophysiology of this disease. The complex interplay between numerous factors gives way to varying degrees of OSAS in different individuals.

*Multilevel involvement* is probably one of the most complicating factors in OSAS management. UPPP targets the oropharyngeal level but collapse at the hypopharyngeal level, if present, is not altered.[21,26]

The influence of preoperative weight or *Body Mass Index* is a much debated issue. Riley et al. found that morbidly obese patients had less successful UPPP outcome.[29] However, there are conflicting results, as Sher et al. found no significant effect of BMI on UPPP outcome in their large meta-analysis.[11] On the other hand, Larsson et al.[6] found a significant lower preoperative BMI in their responder group but this was not confirmed by Boot et al.[30] Larsson et al. also found a negative influence of postoperative weight gain on UPPP efficacy which was partly reversed in the same group after weight reduction.[16]

As for the *severity of the disease*, Sher et al. found that UPPP is less successful in more severe cases of OSAS and this relationship remained apparent despite stricter adjustment of the definition of success.[11] Using the same criteria for success, Senior et al. found no difference in UPPP outcome between mild and severe OSAS patients.[21] This finding was also supported by Friedman et al. who showed that their clinical anatomical staging system is superior to disease severity in predicting UPPP outcome.[26]

The influence of *gender* is interesting, foremost because of the significant difference in the pattern of SDB between the sexes, such as presenting symptoms, the severity of disease and the association with BMI. This is an area that needs further research, as does the role of ethnicity, which shows differences in the distribution of risk factors among various ethnic groups without a clear explanation. *Age* shows a tendency to increase the prevalence of snoring and OSAS up until middle age after which there is no further change.[1] Once again the exact mechanism is unknown.

Other comorbidities such as disproportionate anatomy, allergy and hypoventilation syndrome have been observed but their precise contribution as potential risk factors is less studied.[1]

Polysomnographic recordings are the most frequently used way of obtaining objective data on pre- and postoperative outcome. An aspect that until recently was not fully recognized and included in these recordings is the so-called 'positional sleep apnea'. These so-called position-dependent OSAS patients have an AHI in a supine position that is twice the AHI in other positions. Awareness of this positional sleep apnea phenomenon and correction for it, if necessary, when interpreting polysomnographic results can influence overall UPPP outcome.[31,32]

## 6.5 THE VALUE OF PREOPERATIVE PATIENT SELECTION FOR UPPP

Over the years various patient selection methods have been developed to influence the likelihood of surgical success. The majority are based on the above-mentioned risk factors thought to influence UPPP outcome. It is imperative to take these factors into account when considering UPPP as a surgical treatment option.

Patient selection methods can be divided into subjective and objective measurement tools. It needs emphasizing that the majority of assessment tools are in some way subjective due to symptom scoring by the patient and/or partner or inter-investigator variability. This not only leads to difficulty in developing (objective) diagnostic measures but also complicates comparison of different studies.

The growing insight into the pathophysiology of OSAS places high demands on preoperative selection methods. Especially the multilevel involvement combined with alteration in dynamic circumstances necessitates the use of multiple selection modalities, as no single test has proved to cover the vast area of OSAS physiology so far.

To date, *polysomnography* remains the backbone of the OSAS diagnostic work-up for disease severity and the most frequently used way of selecting patients for surgery and evaluating postoperative outcome. Although polysomnography is a valuable instrument in obtaining objective data it does not give information on the levels involved in upper airway collapse. *Topical diagnostic work-up* is presently either done by clinical examination only (e.g. using the Mallampati–Friedman staging) or (in combination) with sleep endoscopy. Sleep endoscopy is in our own experience the most feasible and promising technique to address this issue, but the subject is highly controversial in whether all patients in whom surgery is considered should have sleep endoscopy routinely performed. Hessel and de Vries showed that UPPP success rate (defined as an AHI drop <20) almost doubles by preoperatively combining PSG and sleep endoscopy in the diagnostic work-up.[9] This study revealed two interesting findings. The first and only statistically significant finding is that UPPP is less successful in patients with prior tonsillectomy as many of these patients have a relatively shorter anterior–posterior diameter between posterior pharyngeal wall and soft palate. This has led to an important change in our policy. Currently we more frequently perform ZPP than simple UPPP in these cases.

The other important finding in this study confirmed that cases of combined retropalatal–retrolingual obstruction did worse than sole palatal obstruction. Therefore we now manage Type 2 cases with a relatively low AHI by combined UPPP and radiofrequency of the tongue base, while in more severe obstruction (as assessed by sleep endoscopy and higher AHI) we prefer to combine UPPP, radiofrequency of the tongue base and hyoid suspension as primary surgery, instead of UPPP only (see Chapter 50: Multilevel surgery). Continuing on our experience with multilevel surgery, we found that secondary hyoid suspension after UPPP failure is less successful than primary hyoid suspension for patients with obstruction at tongue base level and moderate to severe OSAS (see Chapter 49: Hyoid suspension as the only procedure). In addition, a respectively relative or functional post-UPPP stenosis at palatal level can often not be salvaged by hyoid suspension.[33]

Once again we emphasize the importance of careful preoperative assessment. Our preference remains the combination of PSG and sleep endoscopy despite understandable criticism over sleep endoscopy (the primary question being: is artificially induced sleep a reliable representation of natural sleep?). We feel that at present there are no better methods to preoperatively (dynamically) diagnose the level of obstruction in OSAS especially as recent investigation of the correlation of the Mallampati/Friedman staging system with sleep endoscopy showed a low correlation.[10]

In general, when attempting to evaluate UPPP outcome (and failure) the ongoing difficulty with the available literature is the lack of uniform definitions of success and the use of modified UPPP techniques with adjunctive measures, which makes comparison difficult and inconclusive and at times yields conflicting results.[34]

of OSAS calls for a shift in thinking on the role of UPPP in surgical OSAS management. It should not necessarily always be regarded as a first-step, stand-alone treatment, but should also be seen as part of a multistep intervention plan tailored to the individual need of the patient.

As knowledge about the pathophysiology of OSAS increases, uniformity in definitions and reporting is crucial to provide the clarity needed to improve current practice and develop new methods of assessment and treatment.

UPPP research has led to various useful guidelines but the exact indications for UPPP in the management of OSAS remain to be defined. Based on our present knowledge, the ideal patients for UPPP are Type 1 patients with tonsils in situ, either assessed by the Mallampati–Friedman staging system or (in our own experience) by sleep endoscopy. Type 1 patients with prior tonsillectomy do less well. Z-palatoplasty should be considered in these patients who have a short anterior–posterior diameter at retropalatinal level. Type 2 patients are often successful too, but definitively less successful than Type 1 individuals. In these patients either a simultaneous or staged tongue base procedure (e.g. radiofrequent tongue base ablation, hyoid suspension or genioglossal advancement) depending on level of AHI and severity of obstruction (ideally, in our experience assessed during sleep endoscopy) should be offered to the patient. Type 3 patients should not have UPPP at all. However, UPPP on good indication remains the workhorse of OSAS surgery.

Much remains to be elucidated in the exact mechanisms of UPPP failure. However, the above considerations have been shown to contribute to UPPP success and should be taken into account when determining which patients in the spectrum of sleep disordered breathing are candidates for this surgical intervention.

## 7 CONCLUSION

In the field of SDB, understanding OSAS and optimizing its treatment continues to be a challenge. Given the complex pathophysiology, it seems only logical to have a holistic approach to OSAS treatment. Components of this treatment aimed at optimizing outcome include thorough preoperative screening but also equal efforts in reducing other contributing factors such as rigorous weight control programs and life-style changes. Patients should be well informed about treatment success rates to give realistic expectations and ensure patient compliance for possible adjunctive measures.

In the case of UPPP, it appears that technically most has been achieved. Focus should now be aimed at preoperative assessment to optimize application in the individual patient. Topical diagnostic work-up seems to be the key. In addition, realization of the multilevel pathophysiology

## REFERENCES

1. Boehlecke BA. Epidemiology and pathogenesis of sleep-disordered breathing. Curr Opin Pulm Med 2000;6:471–78.
2. Ikematsu T. Study of snoring 4th report Therapy [in Japanese]. J Jpn Otol Rhinol Laryngol Soc 1964;64:434–35.
3. Fuijta S, Conway W, Zorick F, Roth T. Surgical correction of anatomic abnormalities in obstructive sleep apnoea syndrome: uvulopalatopharyngoplasty. Otolaryngol Head Neck Surg 1981;89:923–34.
4. Standards of Practice Committee of the American Sleep Disorders Association. Practice parameters for the indications of polysomnography and related procedures. Sleep 1997;20:406–22.
5. Kushida CA, Littner MR, Morgenthaler T, et al. Practice parameters for the indications for polysomnography and related procedures: an update for 2005. Sleep 2005;28:499–21.
6. Johns MA. new method for measuring daytime sleepiness: the Epworth Sleepiness Scale. Sleep 1991;14:540–45.
7. Mallampati SR, Gatt SP, Gugino LD, et al. A clinical sign to predict difficult tracheal intubation: a prospective study. Can Anaesth Soc J 1985;32:429–34.
8. Friedman M, Ibrahim H, Lee G. Clinical staging for sleep-disordered breathing: a guide to surgical treatment. Oper Tech Otolaryngol Head Neck Surg 2002;13:191–5.

9. Hessel NS, de Vries N. Results of UPPP after diagnostic work-up with PSG and sleep endoscopy; a report of 136 snoring patients. Eur Arch Otorhinolaryngol 2003;260:91–5.
10. den Herder C, van Tinteren H, de Vries N. Sleep endoscopy versus modified Mallampati score in sleep apnea and snoring. Laryngoscope 2005;115:735–9.
11. Sher AE, Schechtman KB, Piccirillo JF. The efficacy of surgical modifications of the upper airway in adults with obstructive sleep apnea syndrome. Sleep 1996;19:156–77.
12. Kezirian EJ, Weaver EM, Yueh B, et al. Incidence of serious complications after uvulopalatopharyngoplasty. Laryngoscope 2004;114:450–53.
13. Mortimore IL, Bradley PA, Murray JAM, Douglas NJ. Uvulopalatoplasty may compromise nasal CPAP therapy in sleep apnea syndrome. Am J Respir Crit Care Med 1996;154:1759–62.
14. Lu SJ, Chang SY, Shiao GM. Comparison between short-term and long-term postoperative evaluation of sleep apnoea after uvulopalatopharyngoplasty. J Laryngol Otol 1995;109:308–12.
15. Keenan SP, Burt H, Ryan CF, Fleetham JA. Long-term survival of patients with obstructive sleep apnea treated by uvulopalatopharyngoplasty or nasal CPAP. Chest 1994;105:155–59.
16. Larsson LH, Carlsson Nordlander B, Svanborg E. Four year follow-up after uvulopalatopharyngoplasty in 50 unselected patients with obstructive sleep apnea syndrome. Laryngoscope 1994;104:1362–8.
17. Janson C, Gislason T, Bengtsson H, et al. Long-term follow-up of patients with obstructive sleep apnea syndrome treated with uvulopalatopharyngoplasty. Arch Otolaryngol Head Neck Surg 1997;23:257–62.
18. Boot H, Wegen van R, Poublon RML, et al. Long-term results of uvulopalatopharyngoplasty for obstructive sleep apnea syndrome. Laryngoscope 2000;110:469–75.
19. Krespi YP, Kacker A. Management of nasopharyngeal stenosis after uvulopalatoplasty. Otolaryngol Head Neck Surg 2000;123:692–5.
20. Friedman M, Ibrahim HZ, Vidyasagar R, et al. Z-palatoplasty (ZPP): a technique for patients without tonsils. Otolaryngol Head Neck Surg 2004;131:89–100.
21. Senior BA, Rosenthal L, Lumley A, et al. Efficacy of uvulopalatopharyngoplasty in unselected patients with mild obstructive sleep apnea. Otolaryngol Head Neck Surg 2000;123:179–82.
22. Hessel NS, de Vries N. Increase of apnoea–hypopnoea index after uvulopalatopharyngoplasty: analysis of failure. Clin Otolaryngol 2004;29:682–5.
23. Hicklin LA, Tostevin P, Dasan S. Retrospective survey of long-term results and patient satisfaction with uvulopalatopharyngoplasty for snoring. J Laryngol Otol 2000;114:675–81.
24. Jones TM, Earis JE, Calverley MA, Swift AC. Snoring surgery: a retrospective review. Laryngoscope 2005;115:2010–15.
25. Prasad KR, Premraj K, Kent SE, Reddy KTV. Surgery for snoring: are partners satisfied in the long run? Clin Otolaryngol Alli Sci 2003;28:497–502.
26. Friedman M, Vidyasagar R, Bliznikas D, Joseph N. Does severity of obstructive sleep apnea/hypopnea syndrome predict uvulopalatopharyngoplasty outcome?. Laryngoscope 2005;115:2109–13.
27. Grontved AM, Karup P. Complaints and satisfaction after uvulopalatopharyngoplasty. Acta Otolaryngol Suppl. 2000;543:190–92.
28. Walker-Engstrom ML, Wilhelmsson B, Tegelberg A, et al. Quality of life assessment of treatment with dental appliance or UPPP in patients with mild to moderate obstructive sleep apnoea. A prospective randomized 1-year follow-up study. J Sleep Res 2000;9:303–8.
29. Riley RW, Powell NB, Guilleminault C. Obstructive sleep apnea syndrome: a review of 306 consecutively treated surgical patients. Otolaryngol Head Neck Surg 1993;108:117–25.
30. Boot H, Poublon ML, van Wegen R, et al. Uvulopalatopharyngoplasty for the obstructive sleep apnoea syndrome: value of polysomnography, Mueller manoeuvre and cephalometry in predicting surgical outcome. Clin Otolaryngol 1997;22:504–10.
31. Oksenberg A, Silverberg D, Arons E, Radwan H. Positional vs. non positional obstructive sleep apnea patients: anthropomorphic, nocturnal polysomnographic and multiple sleep latency test data. Chest 1997;112:629–39.
32. Richard W, Kox D, Herder den C, et al. The role of sleep position in obstructive sleep apnea syndrome. Eur Arch Otorhinolaryngol 2006; 263(10):946–50.
33. Den Herder C, van Tinteren H, de Vries N. Hyoidthyroidpexia: a surgical treatment for sleep apnea syndrome. Laryngoscope 2005;115:740–45.
34. Schechtman MB, Sher AE, Piccirillo JF. Methodological and statistical problems in sleep apnea research: the literature on uvulopalatopharyngoplasty. Sleep 1995;18:659–66.

# SECTION N — POSTOPERATIVE MANAGEMENT AND COMPLICATIONS

## CHAPTER 61

# Salvage of failed palate procedures for sleep-disordered breathing

*David J Terris and Manoj Kumar*

## 1 INTRODUCTION

Surgical procedures designed to shorten or otherwise modify the palate may provide relief of upper airway collapse at the palatal level in patients with sleep disordered breathing (SDB). For patients who fail, or suffer a relapse after an initial surgical success, salvage surgical techniques may be appropriate. Although the principles of these salvage techniques are similar to the commonly performed primary surgical procedures, subtle modifications of the approach are sometimes required, and these are emphasized in this chapter.

The uvulopalatopharyngoplasty (UPPP) procedure has become a mainstay in the management of palatal collapse for patients with SDB. A review of literature has shown that 40.7% of patients who have undergone this procedure have a favorable response. A favorable response is defined as either an Apnea/Hypopnea Index (AHI) of less than 10 episodes per hour or an AHI <20 per hour as well as a 50% decrease in the AHI from the base line.[1] In addition, in an effort to decrease the morbidity of surgical treatment, several office-based surgical interventions have been developed and implemented for the treatment of obstruction at the palate level, including laser-assisted uvulopalatoplasty (LAUP), and radiofrequency ablation of the palate (RFAP). While these procedures have proven effective in treating mild SDB in short-term analyses, the long-term evaluation of these procedures has revealed a substantial rate of recurrence of both the snoring and daytime sleepiness, and in some cases a steady trend toward recurrence has been shown over time.[2] In patients with severe sleep apnea, however, it was demonstrated that UPPP has virtually no place in its management.

The salvage of patients who have undergone these procedures and either failed at the palate or suffered long-term recurrence of symptoms has received relatively little attention in medical literature. Re-treatment has been considered, and reports of successful series of patients have been documented. Li et al. showed that patients who have relapsed after successful RFAP treatment may be rescued with subsequent RFAP procedures with improvement in both snoring and sleepiness. The potential for long-term recidivism following UPPP, LAUP and RFAP procedures with a second palate procedure, emphasizes the need for technical knowledge in surgically managing patients who have failed initial palate surgery for SDB. We describe the implementation of well-known palatal intervention in patients who have been previously treated with a palatal procedure. We have found that many of these patients who have either failed initial treatment with prior palatal surgery or suffered a long-term recurrence may be successfully salvaged.

We consider here the use of four basic palatal surgical interventions: UPPP, LAUP, RFAP and palatal advancement, while recognizing that there are a number of other effective treatments. Although all these procedures are designed to enlarge the velopharyngeal isthmus and to decrease the vibration of the soft palate, they achieve this goal in different ways. We acknowledge that virtually any permutation of primary procedure and secondary salvage procedure can be considered. To illustrate the essential possibilities, however, we have focused on five typical circumstances that lend themselves, primarily because of the post-surgical anatomy, to one or other of the salvage strategies.

## 2 SALVAGING LAUP WITH RFAP

### 2.1 PATIENT SELECTION

Patients who have had their snoring successfully mitigated with LAUP but have experienced a relapse may be appropriate candidates for re-treatment with LAUP. If they are reluctant to suffer the discomfort associated with this procedure, or if they are experiencing any type of dysphagia symptoms or occasional aspiration as a result of the prior treatment, it may be preferable to consider a trial of RFAP. Radiofrequency energy causes a low-temperature molecular disintegration, resulting in volumetric tissue removal with minimal collateral tissue damage.[3]

## 2.2 PROCEDURE

The treatment is performed as previously detailed with the patients seated in the office. After achieving local anesthesia, a commercially available RFAP hand-piece connected to a 465 kHz radiofrequency device (Somnus, Inc., Sunnyvale, CA) is introduced submucosally in a midline (600 J) and two lateral locations (300 J) for three separate sequences of energy, delivering a total of 1200 J at a target temperature of 85°C and 10 watts of power. The intended effect is the shrinkage of the soft tissues, resulting in tightening and modest shortening of the palate (Fig. 61.1).

## 2.3 COMPLICATIONS

RFAP is not associated with any major complications. The salvage operation may involve the risks of attaining suboptimal results as in primary surgery. RFAP, although intended to be mucosa sparing, is nevertheless associated with a high incidence of mucosal injuries, many of which are occult.[4] Mucosal edema, if it happens, settles by itself. Superficial ulceration of the soft palate was also reported.[5]

## 3 SALVAGING UPPP WITH LAUP

### 3.1 PATIENT SELECTION

The failed UPPP may present particular challenges in treatment because of the diminished palatal tissue (raising the

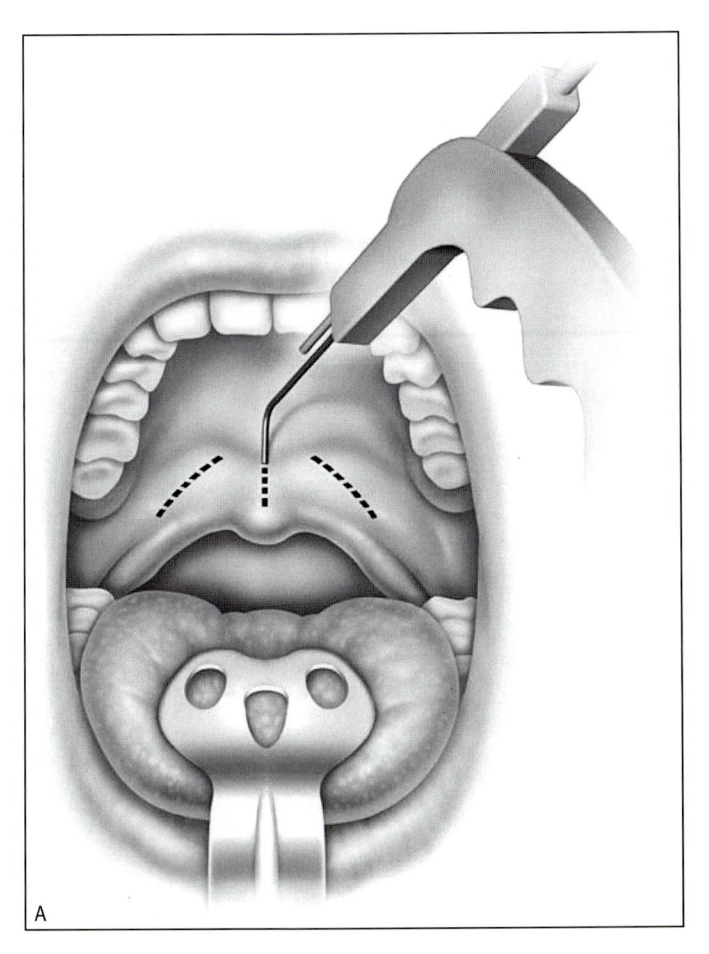

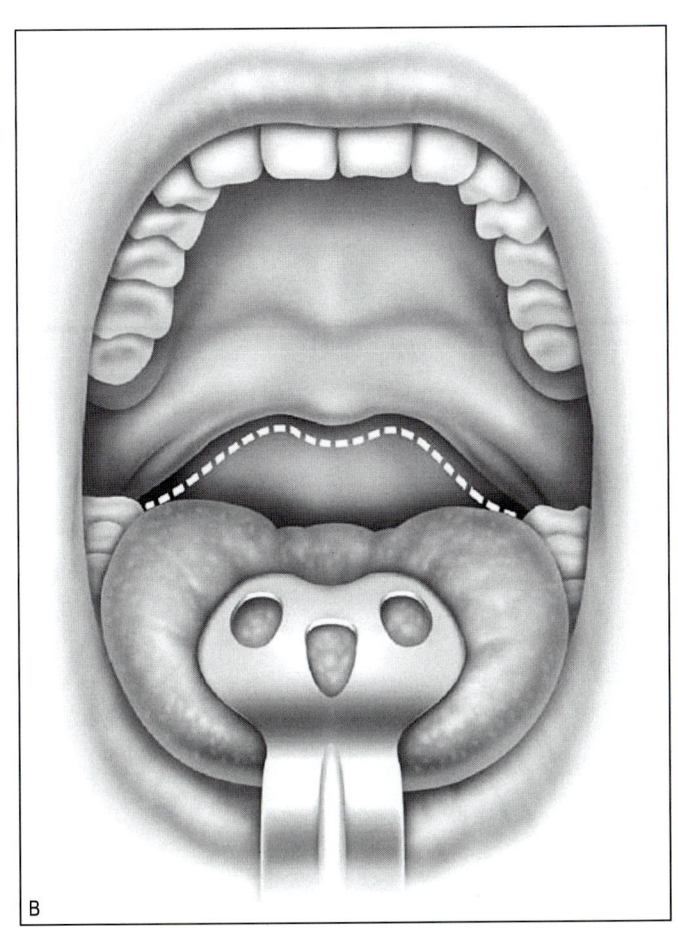

**Fig. 61.1** View of the palate of a patient who underwent laser-assisted uvulopalatopharyngoplasty (LAUP) previously (A), but has recurrence of symptoms. The patient elects to undergo rescue with radiofrequency ablation of the palate (RFAP) which is performed with multiple energy delivered sites as indicated (dotted lines). The intended effect is depicted in (B); note the modest shortening/tightening of the palate that results.

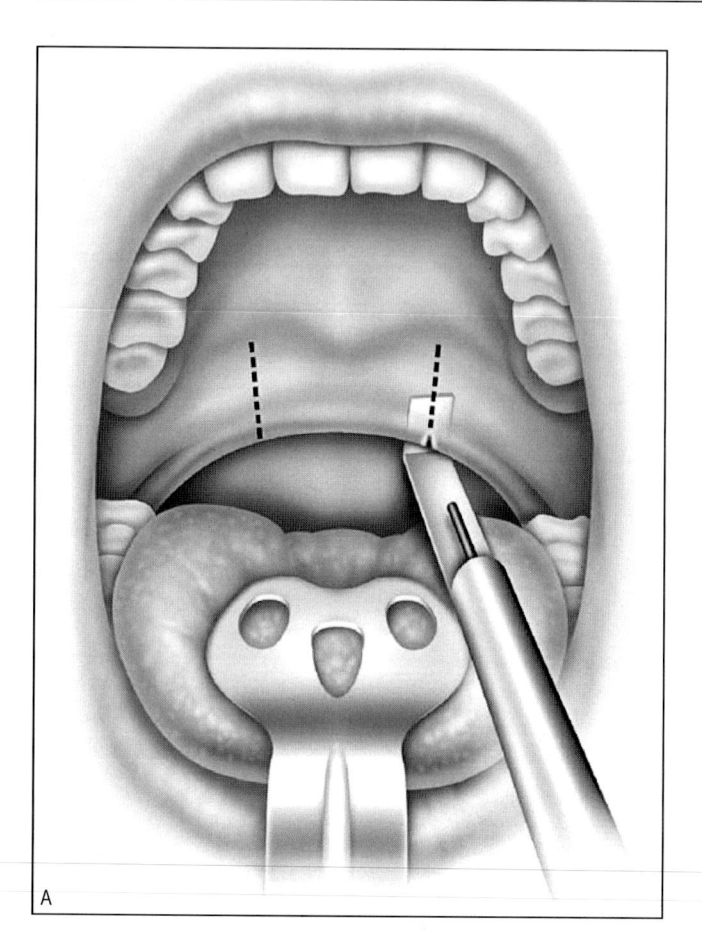

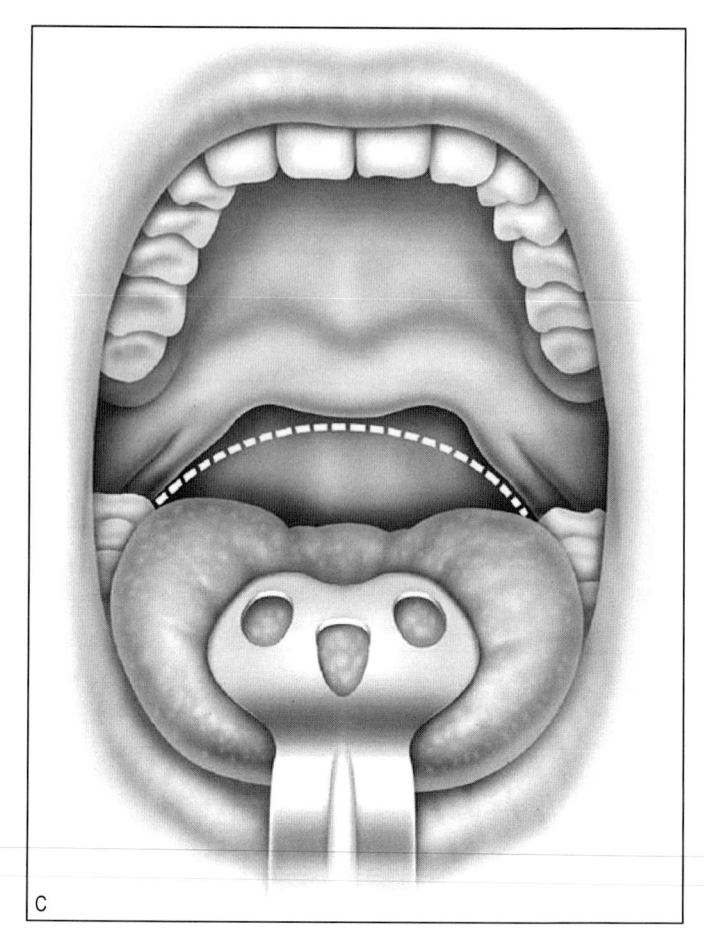

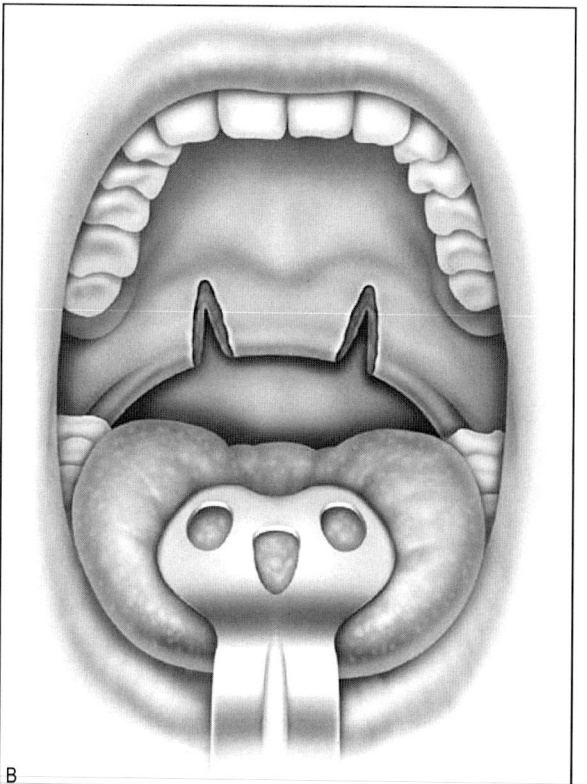

SECTION N — POSTOPERATIVE MANAGEMENT AND COMPLICATIONS

**Fig. 61.2** This patient has undergone successful uvulopalatopharyngoplasty with long-term return of symptoms. The surgical objectives will include not only retightening of the palatal tissue, but restoration of some of the function lost by prior complete resection of the uvula. Vertical through-and-through trenches are created bilaterally utilizing a $CO_2$ laser with a back-stop hand-piece. The wounds are allowed to heal secondarily over a period of 1–3 weeks (A & B). The intended results include a 'neo-uvula' in addition to tightening of the lateral palate (C).

risk of velopharyngeal insufficiency) and the substantial scar tissue that may be present. Therefore the midline palate must be treated with respect, and operated on only rarely, and with caution. This procedure is especially suitable when the palate remains somewhat low-lying and the relapse of symptoms is felt to be related to softening of scar tissue.

## 3.2 PROCEDURE

Lateral through-and-through trenches are accomplished with $CO_2$ laser at a relatively high setting (20 W) to minimize the lateral thermal injury. Some degree of the restoration of the uvular function may be accomplished along with modest shortening and substantial tightening of the free edge of the palate (Fig. 61.2).

## 3.3 COMPLICATIONS

Prolonged pain and impaired healing may happen, though rarely. Postoperative hemorrhage, temporary palatal incompetence and temporary loss of taste are reported as complications for primary laser-assisted palatal surgeries but are rare with revision procedures.[6]

## 4 SALVAGING UPPP WITH REVISION UPPP

### 4.1 PATIENT SELECTION

The patient who manifests significant SDB after failed UPPP, and who exhibits more severe palatal retraction may require a more aggressive surgical strategy.

### 4.2 PROCEDURE

Generally performed in the operating room under general anesthesia, a revision UPPP is accomplished without the removal of additional palatal tissue. Vertical incisions are made through the lateral palate and the edges of the incisions are carefully sutured, approximating the mucosal edges in such a way as to prevent cicatricial healing (Fig. 61.3).

### 4.3 COMPLICATIONS

In spite of careful and atraumatic surgical technique, unimpeded wound healing typically results in some degree of lateral retraction. Nevertheless restoration of some uvular function is usually possible, and desirable palatal tightening is the rule.

## 5 SALVAGING RFAP WITH LAUP

### 5.1 PATIENT SELECTION

Patients with bothersome snoring who are successfully treated with RFAP but suffer a relapse may be salvaged by re-treatment with RFAP. Those that never achieve satisfactory reduction of symptoms are probably better served by LAUP or UPPP. Because the degree of scar tissue in the palate is typically modest, the LAUP is usually straightforward.

### 5.2 PROCEDURE

The procedure can be performed in the usual manner, under local anesthesia in the office. Vertical lateral trenches are accomplished with a $CO_2$ laser, and the uvula is shortened using a fishmouth technique to minimize mucosal resection. Satisfactory healing is typical and a high rate of success can be expected.

### 5.3 COMPLICATIONS

Prolonged pain and impaired healing may occur but are rare.

## 6 SALVAGING UPPP WITH PALATAL ADVANCEMENT

### 6.1 PATIENT SELECTION

Palatal advancement has been offered as an alternative to surgeries described above in patients with failed UPPP. This technique enlarges and stabilizes the upper pharyngeal airway not by aggressive resection or modification of soft tissues, but by altering soft tissue attachments of the hard palate. Favorable posterior airway changes come at the expense of the oro-palatal airway and therefore this technique is not suitable for patients with a large tongue.

### 6.2 PROCEDURE

A palatal flap, medial to the greater palatine foramen, is created with its margin approximately 1.5 cm anterior to

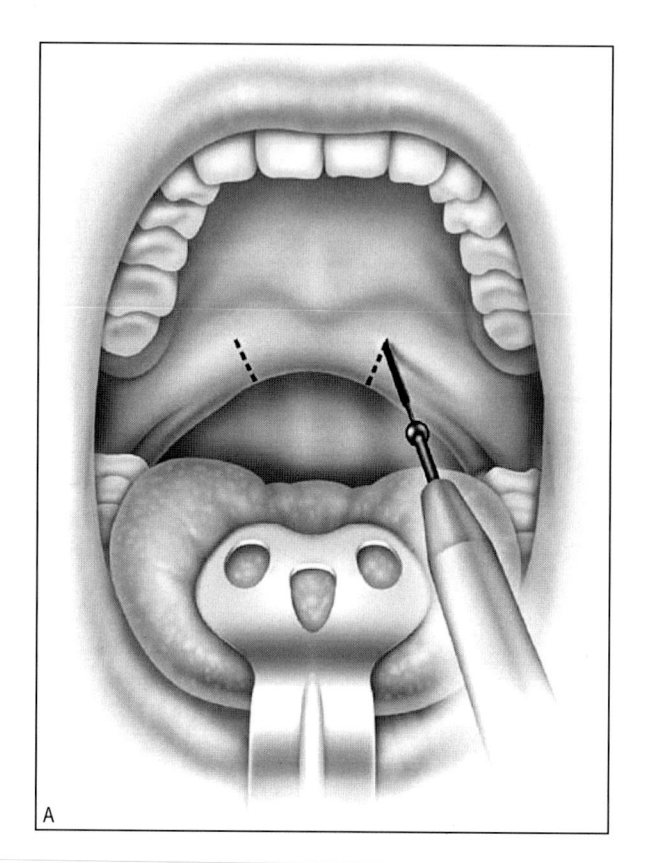

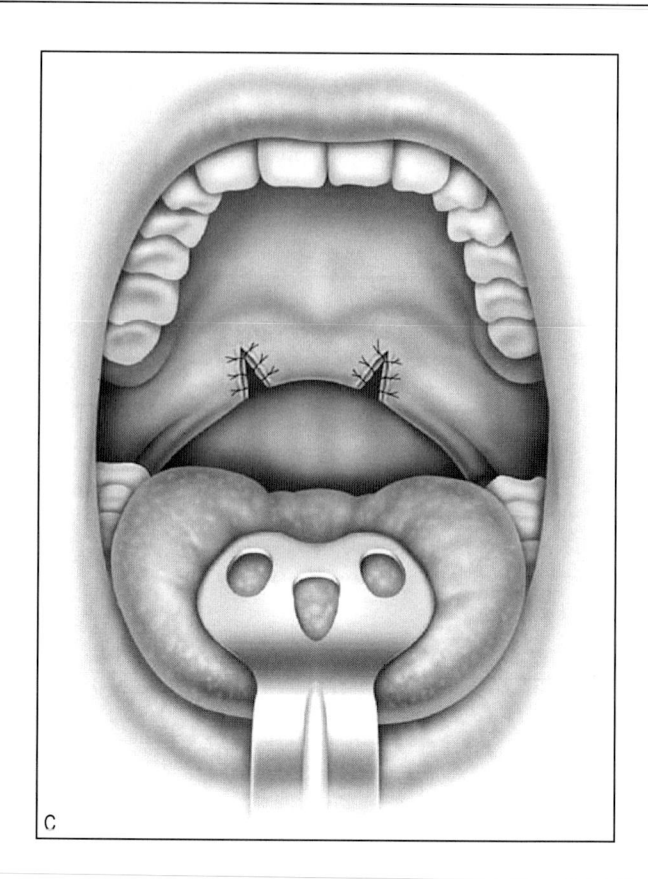

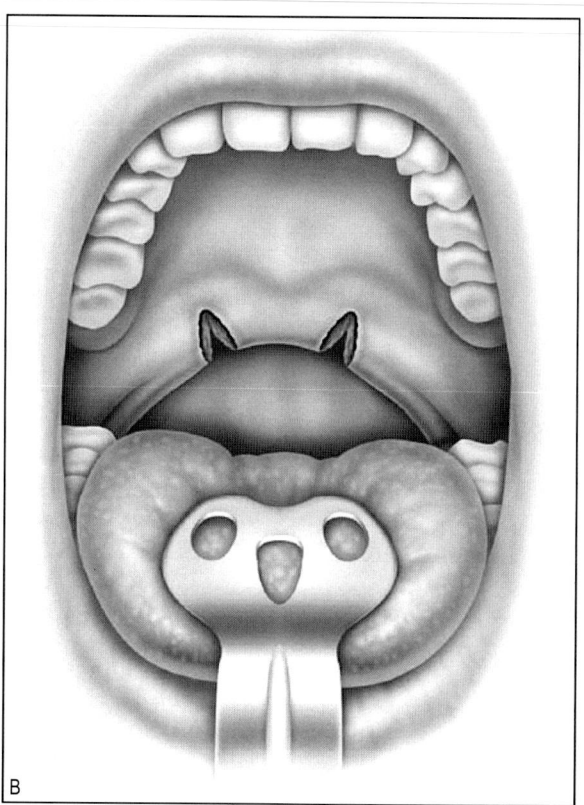

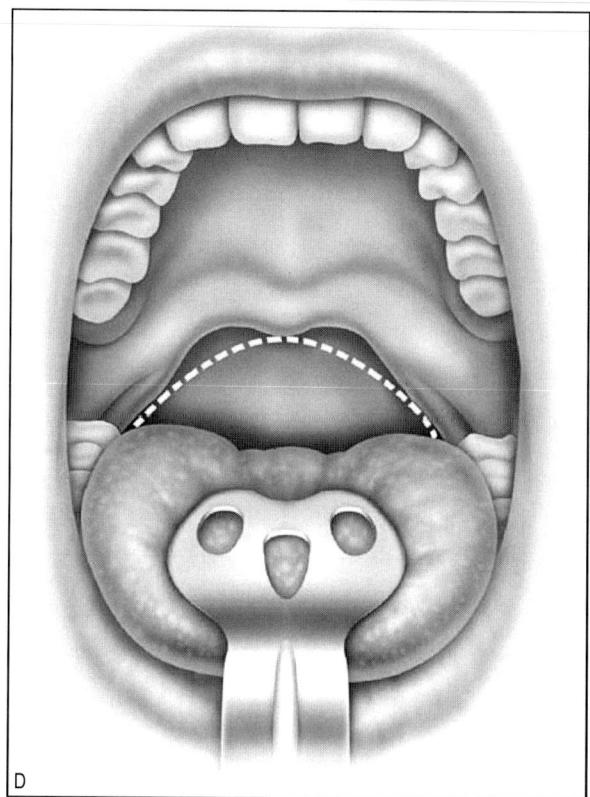

# SECTION N
## POSTOPERATIVE MANAGEMENT AND COMPLICATIONS

**Fig. 61.3** The higher arched palate visible in this patient is reflective of a more aggressive palatopharyngoplasty, and therefore a more sophisticated and cautious approach is necessary. An electrocautery or other instrument is used to divide the palate laterally (A), with care taken to avoid injury to the central palatal mucosa. A typical intraoperative appearance is depicted (B). To avoid cicatricial healing, each edge of each incision is closed primarily with absorbable sutures (C). The final result should not lead to any further shortening of the central palate, but rather yields stiffening and tightening of the lateral palate only, with some restoration of a 'neo-uvula' (D).

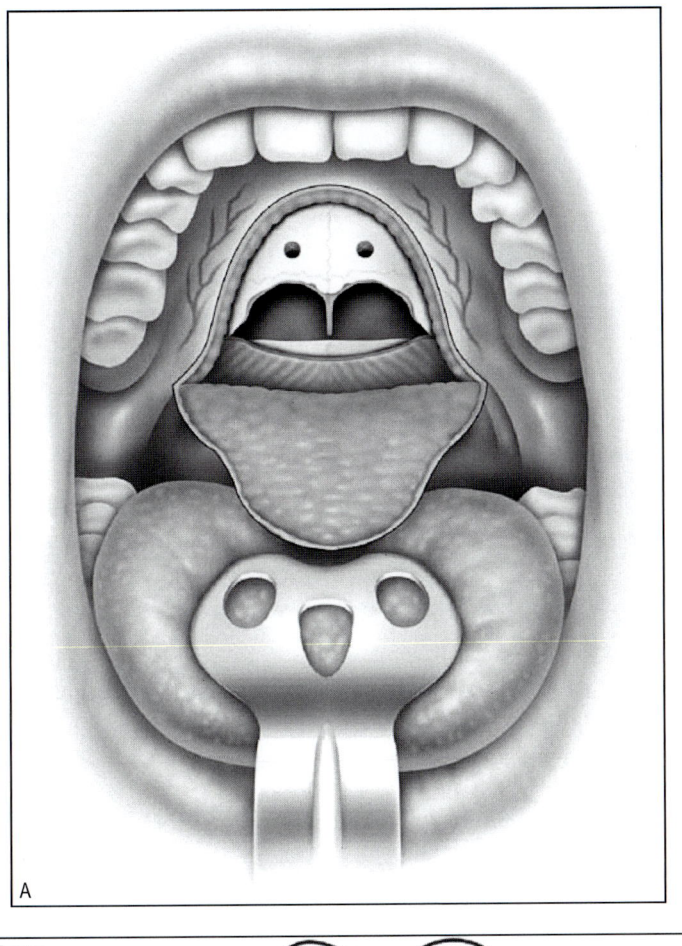

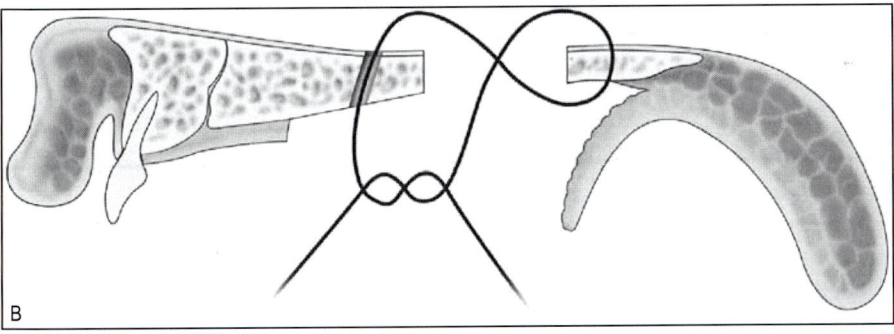

# CHAPTER 61
## Salvage of failed palate procedures for sleep-disordered breathing

**Fig. 61.4** A palatal flap, medial to the greater palatine foramen, is elevated off bone, staying superficial to the tensor aponeurosis (A). An osteotomy of the posterior hard palate is performed, and up to 1 cm of posterior hard palate bone is removed. Drill holes are placed, for subsequent placement of sutures to approximate the osteotomized segment with the hard palate (B).

the junction of hard and soft palate. The flap is elevated off bone, staying superficial to the tensor aponeurosis, which is identified and its attachments preserved. An osteotomy of the posterior hard palate is performed, leaving 2–3 mm of bone to which the tensor aponeurosis remains attached. Up to 1 cm of posterior hard palate bone is then removed with a rotary drill. Drill holes are placed, proximal to this osteotomy, through the palate for subsequent placement of sutures. These sutures approximate the osteotomized segment with the hard palate. The palatal flap is closed in layers (Fig. 61.4).

## 6.3 COMPLICATIONS

The most common complication of palatal advancement pharyngoplasty is oro-antral fistula and it is reported in

391

12% of cases.[7] Because of the risk of fistula, a soft diet is recommended for at least 2 weeks.

## 7 POSTOPERATIVE MANAGEMENT

Some of these procedures, especially revision UPPP, are essentially as painful as the primary procedure. Non-steroidal anti-inflammatory drugs or a combination of paracetamol and codeine are prescribed along with antiseptic mouthwash.

## 8 SUCCESS RATE

All five of these procedures have been successfully performed to salvage patients who have either failed prior palate surgery or suffered a long-term relapse after initially successful treatment. The success rate is lower in patients who have never achieved control of their symptoms than in those who enjoyed successful treatment at some point, but then experienced a relapse.

While a number of potential mechanisms for the relapse of symptoms following palatal surgery have been postulated, it is likely that, as with other surgical scars, the gradual maturation and softening of the palatal scar tissue may lead to failure of the procedure and return of objectionable snoring. This softened palatal tissue may be re-operated. The additional scar tissue created by the salvage procedure may enhance the effective stiffening of the palate induced by the original procedure. Methods of rescue with reduced surgical trauma may be appropriate, resulting in less pain and faster recovery. Finally, the salvage palate procedure can frequently be done in the office, and repeated as necessary.

## 9 INJECTION SNOREPLASTY (SCLEROTHERAPY)

Injection sclerotherapy can also be safely employed as a salvage technique in patients who have either failed an initial palatal procedure or suffered a long-term recurrence. Sclerotherapy is performed in outpatient office settings after topical anesthesia with lidocaine oral spray. Routinely, no injection of local anesthesia is given. Multiple sclerotherapy agents are available with excellent safety records and documented efficacy.[8] Sotradecol®, a trade name for sodium tetradecyl sulfate, is the most common hardening agent used in injection snoreplasty. During the treatments, 2 ml of the sclerosing agent is injected with a single needle penetration into the midline soft palate using a 27 G needle bent at a 30–45° angle. The patient is advised to return to the office 4 weeks after the first injection treatment. The decision to proceed with a second injection is based on lack of acceptable response to the first treatment, as judged by subjective questionnaire and clinical evaluation. The second injection on the palate is given on either side of the midline. In the absence of any improvement, the treatment is terminated and no further injections are given.

## REFERENCES

1. Sher AE, Schechtman KB, Piccirillo JF. The efficacy of surgical modifications of the upper airway in adults with obstructive sleep apnea syndrome. Sleep 1996;19(2):156–77.
2. Hicklin LA, Tostevin P, Dasan S. Retrospective survey of long-term results and patient satisfaction with uvulopalatopharyngoplasty for snoring. J Laryngol Otol 2001;114(9):675–81.
3. Rombaux P, Hamoir M, Bertrand B, Aubert G, Liistro G, Rodenstein D. Postoperative pain and side effects after uvulopalatopharyngoplasty, laser-assisted uvulopalatoplasty, and radiofrequency tissue volume reduction in primary snoring. Laryngoscope 2003;113(12):2169–73.
4. Terris DJ, Chen V. Occult mucosal injuries with radiofrequency ablation of the palate. Otolaryngol Head Neck Surg 2001;125(5):468–72.
5. Fischer Y, Khan M, Mann WJ. Multilevel temperature-controlled radiofrequency therapy of soft palate, base of tongue, and tonsils in adults with obstructive sleep apnea. Laryngoscope 2003;113(10):1786–91.
6. Walker RP, Gopalsami C. Laser-assisted uvulopalatoplasty: postoperative complications. Laryngoscope 1996;106(7):834–38.
7. Woodson BT, Robinson S, Lim HJ. Transpalatal advancement pharyngoplasty outcomes compared with uvulopalatopharyngoplasty. Otolaryngol Head Neck Surg 2005;133(2):211–17.
8. Brietzke SE, Mair EA. Injection snoreplasty: investigation of alternative sclerotherapy agents. Otolaryngol Head Neck Surg 2004;130(1):47–57.

SECTION N  POSTOPERATIVE MANAGEMENT AND COMPLICATIONS

# CHAPTER 62

# Revision uvulopalatopharyngoplasty (UPPP) by Z-palatoplasty (ZPP)

*Michael Friedman and Paul Schalch*

## 1 INTRODUCTION

Uvulopalatopharyngoplasty (UPPP) is the single most common surgical procedure performed for the correction of retropalatal obstruction causing or contributing to the obstructive sleep apnea/hypopnea syndrome (OSAHS). Although its success rate has been reported at only 40% (when objective success is defined as a 50% reduction in the Apnea/Hypopnea Index (AHI) with a postoperative AHI of less than 20),[1] when appropriate patient selection criteria are applied its success rate can be as high as 80%[2] (see Chapter 16: Friedman tongue position and the staging of obstructive sleep apnea/hypopnea syndrome).

UPPP's effectiveness also increases dramatically when performed in combination with several adjunctive procedures that address the hypopharynx, like radiofrequency tongue base reduction.[3] Many studies, however, still show a considerable failure rate.

UPPP failure is multifaceted, as is OSAHS. Causes of persistent obstruction range from morbid obesity with pan-airway obstruction to inadequate palatal resection with a variable position and amount of the remaining soft palate. A significant number of patients are often treated with a form of minimal or conservative UPPP for a variety of reasons. These patients may present with persistent or recurrent OSAHS due to a long segment of palate that causes persistent obstruction. Persistent retropalatal obstruction after UPPP has been extensively studied by several authors.[4,5] Up to 75% of patients exhibit persistent obstruction localized to the level of the palate after manometric analysis of the retropalatal airway. In fact, sleep endoscopic studies on patients who had a failed UPPP procedure have shown that in 50% of patients, persistent obstruction at the retropalatal level is the cause of failure. In other cases, patients present with nasopharyngeal stenosis due to postoperative scarring.

When patients are not willing to accept CPAP as a form of permanent treatment, they often seek a surgical alternative. A modified version of UPPP for patients without tonsils, Z-palatoplasty (ZPP),[6] is presented in Chapter 33. In this chapter, we present further modifications of this technique for patients requiring revision of a previously performed UPPP due to persistent or recurrent symptoms.

## 2 PATIENT SELECTION

Selection criteria follow the classification guidelines already described by Friedman et al.[7] Patients with Friedman tongue position (FTP) III or IV must have adjunctive treatment to increase the retrolingual airway, in addition to revision palatal surgery. Candidates for revision UPPP may have had a history of previous UPPP or laser-assisted uvulopalatoplasty with tonsillectomy. It is important that before undergoing UPPP revision by ZPP (as is true for all surgical procedures aimed at the treatment of OSAHS), the patient undergoes a 30-day CPAP trial, in order to document failure of this alternative as a permanent form of management, based on compliance issues. Physical exam should focus on documenting the presence of an obstruction at the level of the soft palate, and it should assess the likelihood of retrolingual obstruction by means of FTP. In addition, it should either confirm or rule out the presence of nasopharyngeal stenosis by means of fiberoptic nasopharyngolaryngoscopy and Mueller maneuver. Sleep endoscopy may provide additional evidence of persistent retropalatal obstruction.[8] Even if not routinely performed, sleep endoscopy is especially valuable for evaluation of revision surgery patients. Adequate medical clearance and a thorough review of the procedure and its complications, such as temporary velopharyngeal incompetence (VPI) and, most importantly, the risk of permanent VPI, should be conducted with the patient before obtaining consent.

## 3 SURGICAL TECHNIQUE (OUTLINE OF PROCEDURE)

The concept of revision UPPP is similar to ZPP, with modifications based on the presenting anatomy, and on scar tissue from previous interventions. The underlying principles, as well as the goals, remain the same: (1) excision of mucosa only; (2) splitting of the soft palate in the midline, in order to create two Z-plasty flaps for reconstruction; and (3) a very meticulous two-layered closure. The goal is to increase the retropalatal space in both the anterior–posterior dimension, as well as in the lateral dimension. In addition, the procedure often corrects significant nasopharyngeal stenosis, when present.

The surgical technique is illustrated in Figures 62.1–62.6. Two adjacent flaps are outlined on the palate (Fig. 62.1). The flaps for revision surgery will generally be smaller than in primary ZPP, depending on the length of the previously resected soft palate. Only mucosa of the anterior aspect of the two flaps is removed (Fig. 62.2). The two flaps are then separated from each other by splitting the palatal segment down the midline (Figs 62.3 and 62.4). A two-layered closure that brings the midline all the way to the anterolateral margin of the palate is accomplished (Figs 62.5 and 62.6). The final result creates a distance of 3–4 cm between the posterior pharynx and the palate. Additionally, the lateral dimension of the palate is usually doubled to approximately 4 cm. The exact dimensions of the flaps, which extend in a butterfly pattern, are illustrated in Figure 62.1. The anterior midline margin of the flap is halfway between the hard palate and the free edge of 'a normal' soft palate. The distal margin is the free edge of the palate, and the lateral extent is posterior to the midline, and all the way to the lateral extent of the palate.

Friedman anatomical stage II and III patients concomitantly undergo radiofrequency tongue base reduction, based on previously published protocols.[3] The Somnus Somnoplasty™ system (Gyrus ENT, Memphis, TN) double-probed hand piece with rapid lesion technique is used to deliver 600 joules to each of five sets of points outlined to the right and left of the midline, posterior to the circumvallate papillae. A total of 3000 joules (rapid lesion technique) is delivered during the procedure. Patients with residual

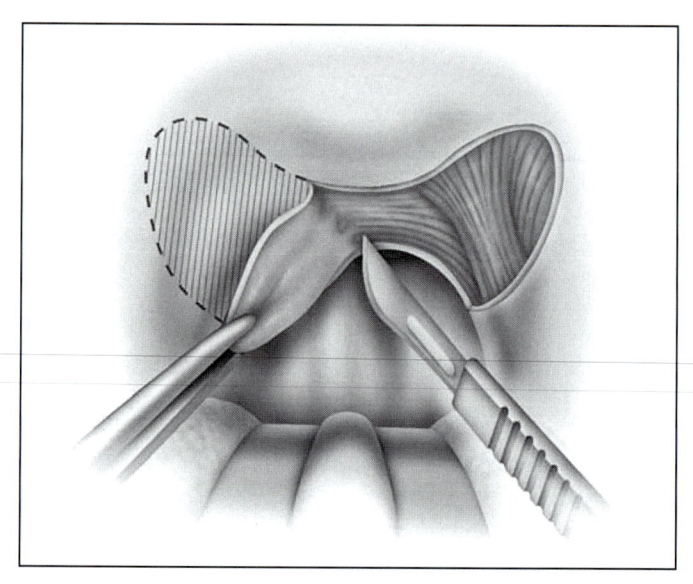

**Fig. 62.2** Removal of anterior mucosa without muscle by means of sharp dissection.

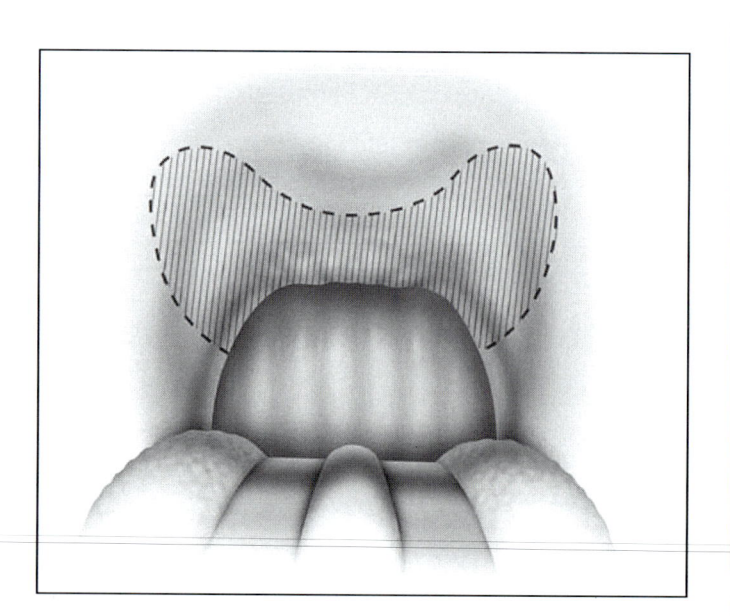

**Fig. 62.1** Palatal mucosa, outlined before excision.

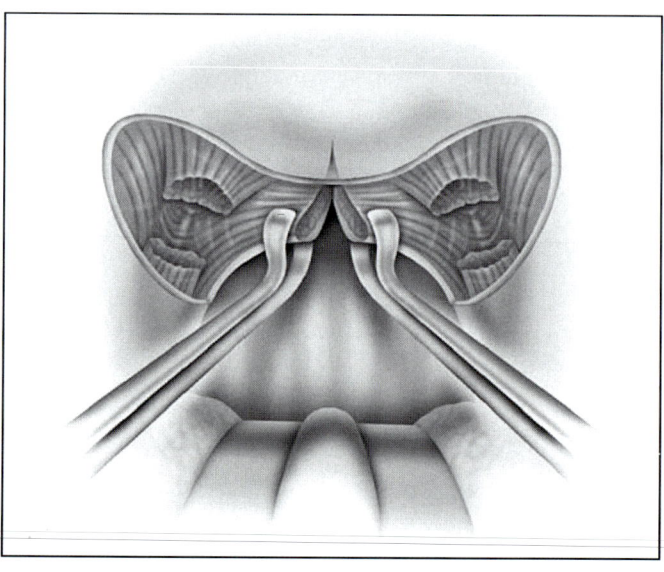

**Fig. 62.3** The soft palate is split in the midline. If the palatoglossus muscles are still present, they are divided.

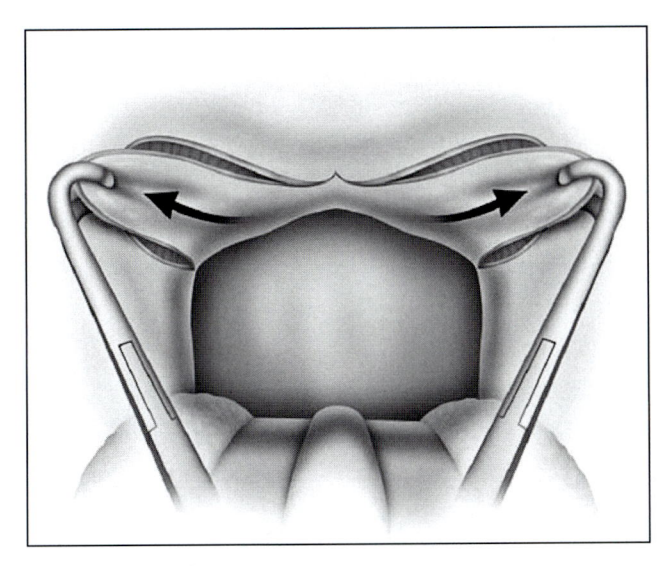

Revision uvulopalatopharyngoplasty (UPPP) by Z-palatoplasty (ZPP) **CHAPTER 62**

**Fig. 62.4** Z-plasty flaps, retracted anteriorly and laterally into position.

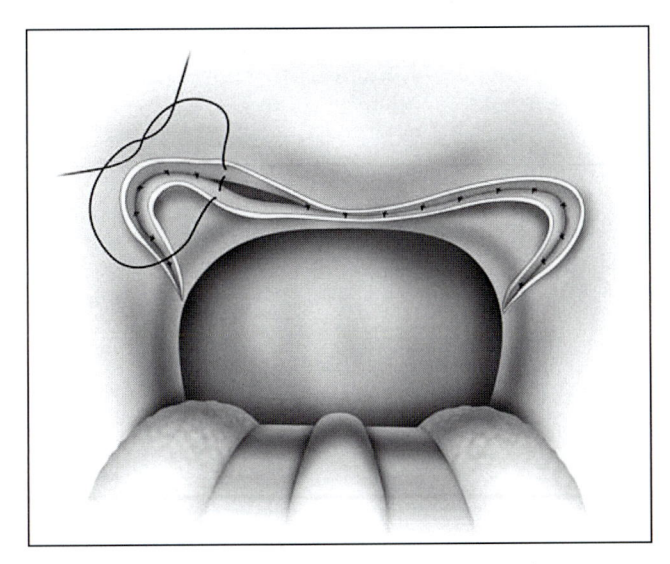

**Fig. 62.5** Meticulous submucosal closure with 2-0 Vicryl™ (Ethicon, Inc., Somerville, NJ).

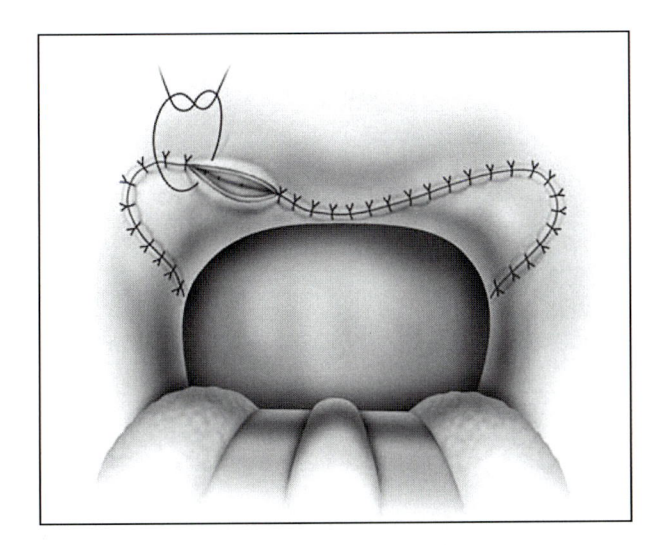

**Fig. 62.6** Second layer closure of mucosa with 3-0 chromic.

snoring after surgery can be treated with additional tongue base reduction in the office, under local anesthesia.

## 4 POSTOPERATIVE MANAGEMENT AND COMPLICATIONS

All patients receive preoperative antibiotics and pre- and postoperative steroids. Patients are usually discharged after one or two postoperative days, upon tolerance of a liquid or soft diet, and once pain is controlled with oral analgesics. Patients are also discharged on a tapered dose of oral methylprednisolone and antibiotics. Significant morbidity is observed in the first 24–48 hours postoperatively in the form of pain and dysphagia. Narcotic medication use averages 10 days, as does a return to normal diet.[9] Immediate or delayed postoperative bleeding is rare. Airway complications after surgery in patients with OSAHS usually occur in the immediate postoperative period. Often, patients with OSAHS wake up with excellent muscle strength, and are combative and confused. If these patients are extubated before they are alert enough to follow instructions, upper airway obstruction can secondarily cause postobstructive pulmonary edema. Reintubation may be necessary but, even in the most controlled conditions, is extremely difficult. Placement of a nasopharyngeal airway can often bypass the area of obstruction and eliminate the need for reintubation. By appropriately delaying extubation until the patient is fully able to follow commands, airway complications can be avoided.

Temporary VPI is an expected consequence the patient should be aware of. Its duration varies between 1 and 14 weeks, with a mean of 4 weeks. Clinically significant, permanent VPI is rare, but it is a potential complication that needs to be addressed appropriately. Patients frequently report a persistent sensation of 'phlegm' in the throat, and a 'change' in swallowing. An appropriate preoperative discussion with the patient, as mentioned before, will provide the patient with realistic expectations regarding postoperative symptoms and time of recovery.

Other complications are related to the adjunctive procedures performed, specifically tongue base reduction. Tongue base infection is related to TBRF. It requires antibiotic treatment, and in rare cases, tongue base abscess incision and drainage.

## 5 SUCCESS RATE OF THE PROCEDURE

### 5.1 SUBJECTIVE AND OBJECTIVE SYMPTOM ELIMINATION

Subjective success is based on comparative improvements in snoring levels, from both the patient's and the bedpartner's perspective, as well as on overall daytime sleepiness and well-being. When comparing snoring levels and ESS scores obtained before the original UPPP with data obtained after revision ZPP in a series of 31 patients, Friedman et al. found statistically significant improvement in both parameters. When applying strict criteria of snoring improvement (that is 50% decrease in snoring level with a postoperative snoring level of 5), improvement was found in 100% of the patients.[9] Quality of life parameters were also significantly improved in all eight domains of the validated SF-36v2™ Health Survey (QualityMetric, Lincoln, RI) assessment tool, which is translated into an improvement in physical functioning, role limitation as a result of physical health problems, bodily pain, general health, vitality, social functioning, role limitation as a result of emotional problems, and mental health.

When focusing on objective success, ZPP shows considerable improvement over UPPP. Objective cure rates based on polysomnographic data consistently show improvement in the mean values of delta and REM sleep, as well as improvement in the Apnea Index, Apnea/Hypopnea Index, and minimum oxygen saturation. Using the classic definition of objective cure proposed by Sher et al.[1] (50% reduction in AHI, with a final postoperative value of less than 20), 68% of patients had successful treatment of their OSAHS, and none of the remaining 32% worsened with the revision procedure.

While morbidity is comparable to classic UPPP, the radical nature of the procedure makes it prone to several complications. Temporary VPI occurs in virtually 100% of the patients, and it also persists longer and is more severe than in UPPP. While permanent VPI did not occur in the original series of patients, the frequency of temporary VPI suggests that its incidence might be higher than in UPPP in a large enough patient population. Should permanent VPI ensue, this procedure is not reversible. This procedure should therefore only be considered for very select patients with severe disease, in whom other forms of treatment are not an option. Patients must be willing to accept the morbidity and the significant risk of failure, as well as reasonable chance for improvement, if not an actual cure.

## 5.2 WHAT TO DO IF THE PROCEDURE FAILS

Failure in this procedure, as in any other procedure, can be defined as the persistence of symptoms. Failure also occurs when symptoms of snoring and daytime sleepiness are eliminated but polysomnographic data indicate persistent disease, often with a pattern of elimination of apneas, but with persistent hypopneas. Sleep endoscopy is a valuable tool for assessing failure, and should be performed to identify the anatomic site of persistent obstruction. Failure in achieving satisfactory results requires the resumption of CPAP therapy by the patient. Other surgical options for patients unwilling to accept CPAP as a permanent form of management include techniques that focus on the hypopharynx, like genioglossal advancement, thyrohyoid suspension, hyomandibular suspension, and tongue base suspension. Salvage surgery in the form of maxillomandibular advancement, as described by Li et al.,[10] is likely the best option, due to its expanding effect on the entire upper airway. Transpalatal advancement pharyngoplasty may be considered if retropalatal obstruction persists.[11]

## 6 CONCLUSION

In spite of considerable advances in appropriate patient selection for UPPP, a significant number of patients still fail to show improvement after surgery. For patients who refuse to accept CPAP as a permanent form of management, revision surgical options are limited. Confirmation of persistent retropalatal obstruction is crucial in planning a revision procedure. Rerouting the scarred portion of the residual soft palate in an attempt to enlarge the retropalatal space is the key element in revision by ZPP, together with radiofrequency reduction of the base of the tongue, which addresses the hypopharynx concomitantly. ZPP revision for UPPP failure entails significant postoperative pain and temporary VPI. It should, therefore, be limited to select patients with severe disease. Patients who wish to proceed with surgery must accept the potential for significant morbidity, and risk of failure. There is, however, a high likelihood of subjective and objective improvement, with a reasonable chance for cure.

## REFERENCES

1. Sher AE, Schechtman KB, Piccirillo JF. The efficacy of surgical modifications of the upper airway in adults with obstructive sleep apnea syndrome. Sleep 1996;19:156–77.
2. Friedman M, Vidyasagar R, Bliznikas D, et al. Does severity of obstructive sleep apnea/hypopnea syndrome predict uvulopalatopharyngoplasty outcome? Laryngoscope 2005;115:2109–13.
3. Friedman M, Ibrahim H, Lee G, et al. Combined uvulopalatopharyngoplasty and radiofrequency tongue base reduction for treatment of obstructive sleep apnea/hypopnea syndrome. Otolaryngol Head Neck Surg 2003;129:611–21.
4. Woodson B, Wooten M. Manometric and endoscopic localization of airway obstruction after uvulopalatopharyngoplasty. Otolaryngol Head Neck Surg 1994;111:38–43.
5. Metes A, Hoffstein V, Mateika S, et al. Site of airway obstruction in patients with obstructive sleep apnea before and after uvulopalatopharyngoplasty. Laryngoscope 1991;101:1102–8.
6. Friedman M, Ibrahim H, Vidyasagar R, et al. Z-palatoplasty (ZPP): a technique for patients without tonsils. Otolaryngol Head Neck Surg 2004;131:89–100.
7. Friedman M, Ibrahim H, Joseph N. Staging of obstructive sleep apnea/hypopnea syndrome: a guide to appropriate treatment. Laryngoscope 2004;114:454–59.

8. Pringle M, Croft C. A grading system for patients with obstructive sleep apnoea – based on sleep nasendoscopy. Clin Otolaryngol Allied Sci 1993;18:480–84.
9. Friedman M, Duggal P, Joseph N. Revision uvulopalatoplasty by Z-palatoplasty. Otolaryngol Head Neck Surg 2007; 136:638–43.
10. Li K, Riley R, Powell N, et al. Maxillomandibular advancement for persistent obstructive sleep apnea after phase I surgery in patients without maxillomandibular deficiency. Laryngoscope 2000;110:1684–88.
11. Woodson B, Toohill R. Transpalatal advancement pharyngoplasty for obstructive sleep apnea. Laryngoscope 1993;103:269–76.

# SECTION O PEDIATRIC OSAHS

## CHAPTER 63

# Management of sleep-related breathing disorders in children

*David H. Darrow and Kaalan E. Johnson*

## 1 INTRODUCTION

Sleep-related breathing disorders (SRBD) are a common occurrence in children. While such events may be central in etiology, most affected children experience obstructive sleep disorders, caused by anatomic variations and complicated by the diminished pharyngeal muscle tone and neurophysiologic changes that typically accompany sleep. Hyperplasia of the tonsils and adenoid is the most common cause of such obstruction, but infants and toddlers may be affected at a variety of sites in the upper respiratory tract. Causes of SRBD in children may be grouped on the basis of age, simplifying the differential diagnosis for a given patient (Table 63.1). In small children, caliber of the airway may be reduced due to nasal obstruction, compromised skeletal anatomy, hyperplastic pharyngeal or laryngeal soft tissues or neuromuscular compromise. In addition, in older children, obstruction due to obesity has been encountered with increasing frequency over the last two decades.[1,2]

Successful management of SRBD in children depends on accurate identification of the site of obstruction and assessment of the severity of obstruction. Only then can appropriate surgical and non-surgical remedies be considered.

**Table 63.1 Causes of sleep-related breathing disorders in children**

| Neonates and infants |
|---|
| Nasal aplasia, stenosis, or atresia |
| Nasal or nasopharyngeal masses |
| Craniofacial anomalies: |
|     Hypoplastic mandible (Pierre Robin, Nager's, Treacher Collins) |
|     Hypoplastic maxilla (Apert's, Crouzon's) |
| Macroglossia (Beckwith–Wiedemann) |
| Vascular malformations of tongue and pharynx |
| Congenital cysts of the vallecula and tongue |
| Neuromuscular disorders |
| **Toddlers and older children** |
| Rhinitis, nasal polyposis, septal deviation |
| Syndromic narrowing of nasopharynx (Hunter's, Hurler's, Down's, achondroplasia) |
| Adenotonsillar hyperplasia |
| Obesity |
| Macroglossia (Down's) |
| Vascular malformations of tongue and pharynx |
| Neuromuscular disorders |
| **Iatrogenic** |
| Nasopharyngeal stenosis |

## 2 DIAGNOSIS OF SRBD IN CHILDREN

In most children with SRBD, the presenting symptom is *stertor*, a term used to describe sonorous breathing in the upper airways, including snoring. The prevalence of snoring during sleep has been reported as 3–12% in children,[3] although some studies suggest the rate may be as high as 27%.[4] Primary snoring is generally not considered a form of SRBD, although some studies do suggest the possibility of associated morbidity such as elevated blood pressure and reduced arterial distensibility.[5]

In its mildest form, SRBD presents as upper airway resistance syndrome (UARS). Affected children demonstrate episodic arousals resulting from partial obstruction of the upper airway, associated with symptoms of heroic snoring, mouth-breathing, sleep pauses or breath-holding, gasping, perspiration, and enuresis. Daytime manifestations of sleep disturbance include morning headache, dry mouth, halitosis, and most significantly behavioral and neurocognitive disorders.[6] Hypersomnolence may occur in older children and adolescents. Other signs and symptoms include audible breathing with open mouth posture, hyponasal speech, and chronic nasal obstruction with or without rhinorrhea.

# Management of sleep-related breathing disorders in children

Approximately 40% of children who snore demonstrate more significant degrees of obstruction characteristic of obstructive hypopnea syndrome (OHS) or obstructive sleep apnea syndrome (OSAS) as defined below.[3] The most severely affected patients may develop cor pulmonale, right ventricular hypertrophy, congestive heart failure, alveolar hypoventilation, pulmonary hypertension, pulmonary edema, or failure to thrive, and are at risk for permanent neurological damage and even death.

Physical examination is critical in establishing the site of obstruction and will ultimately determine the most appropriate surgical intervention. The examination should include assessment of the patient's weight and body habitus, a complete examination of the head and neck with attention to potential sites of obstruction, and auscultation of the patient's heart and lungs. Friedman tongue position (FTP), described in Chapter 16 on clinical staging, should be assessed. Children with FTP III or IV have significant retrolingual obstruction in addition to possible tonsillar and adenoid obstruction. Postoperative PSL and follow-up is essential in those patients since they are likely to have residual or recurrent OSAHS after tonsillectomy and adenoidectomy. Findings of nasal dyspnea or mouth-breathing, hyponasal speech, mandibular hypoplasia, drooling, neuromuscular deficit, and tonsillar hyperplasia all suggest some degree of upper airway obstruction. In many cases, such as infants in whom the jaw is extremely micrognathic or toddlers in whom the tonsils are massively enlarged, office examination alone may suffice. Ancillary studies such as high kilovoltage radiography of the adenoid pad and/or lingual tonsils and direct fiberoptic assessment of the nasal vault, adenoid pad, and distal pharynx and larynx may be useful in selected cases. In severely obstructed children, chest radiography and electrocardiography should be considered as well. In cases of nasal obstruction in infants and young children, CT scanning may be desirable in order to define the bony anatomy and to assess the relationship of nasal masses to the sinonasal tract and the central nervous system. At some institutions, cross-table lateral fluoroscopy, drug-induced sleep endoscopy, or cine MRI may be performed during sleep to aid in localizing the site of obstruction.

When a history of severe symptoms of sleep disturbance correlates with obvious physical findings of airway obstruction, additional studies to establish a patient's candidacy for surgical intervention may be superfluous. However, studies suggest that in most cases accurate diagnosis of SRBD cannot be established solely on the basis of a history and physical examination.[7] SRBD occurs primarily during REM sleep when children are less likely to be observed by their parents,[8] and in many cases of UARS and OHS parents may misinterpret the symptoms only as snoring in the absence of obstruction. In addition, airway dynamics during sleep cannot be determined by static examination in the office setting, and fiberoptic assessment of the airway is often deceptive due to the distorted wide-angle view.

Similarly, radiographic assessment of the adenoid tissue and tongue base may be difficult to interpret. In such cases, polysomnography (PSG) remains the gold standard for objective correlation of ventilatory abnormalities with sleep disordered breathing.[7] However, the severity of obstruction for which intervention is recommended remains controversial, with most authors advocating aggressive management of children whose Respiratory Distress Index (RDI; obstructive apneas + hypopneas per hour) is between 1 and 5. Furthermore, the expense and scheduling difficulties associated with PSG make this a cumbersome method of assessment in many otolaryngology practices. Other techniques of assessment including audiotaping, videotaping, and home and abbreviated PSG have demonstrated favorable results, but require further study.

## 3 MANAGEMENT OF SRBD IN CHILDREN

### 3.1 NON-SURGICAL MANAGEMENT

Treatment of SRBD in children is tailored to the etiology of the airway obstruction. Medical management, such as thioxanthines and methylphenidate, may be useful in cases of central apnea. Pharmacotherapy may also be considered in less severe cases of obstructive apnea, or when surgical intervention does not address the pathology. Examples of such disorders include neonatal rhinitis, allergic rhinitis, and acute tonsillitis. Systemic steroids are effective in reducing lymphoid hyperplasia, but the results are often transient. In cases of chronic upper airway obstruction, positive airway pressure has demonstrated high efficacy in treating SRBD in children; however, the dropout rate is high and the rate and duration of nightly use are relatively low even among compliant children.[9] Other alternatives, such as mechanical correction by prostheses, orthodontia, or weight loss, may be worth consideration as well, although these interventions are rarely tolerated in children and are often ineffective. As a result, even in cases of SRBD due to obesity and neuromuscular impairment, surgical management is generally considered as first-line therapy and other modalities are entertained postoperatively to address residual obstruction.

### 3.2 SURGICAL MANAGEMENT

#### 3.2.1 PREOPERATIVE PLANNING

Preoperative planning is an essential component of the surgical management of patients with SRBD. Such individuals are prone to airway embarrassment during induction of anesthesia, and the surgeon and anesthetist should discuss emergency intervention for the airway should the patient become acutely obstructed. In most cases, dynamic airway collapse may be overcome by bag/mask ventilation used with an oral airway. In patients with severe micrognathia, macroglossia, or lingual tonsil hyperplasia, visualization of the larynx may be compromised. In such cases, the operating team should preoperatively assemble those items necessary for intubation with a Bullard laryngoscope, flexible fiberoptic bronchoscope, or fiberoptic intubation wand, and patients should be intubated under conditions of maximal topical and minimal systemic anesthesia, preferably in the sitting position.

Postoperative respiratory distress is common after surgery for SRBD due to effects of anesthesia, bleeding, edema, and residual airway compromise. Patients at greatest risk include those with severe OSAS, diminished neuromuscular tone (i.e. cerebral palsy), morbid obesity, skeletal and craniofacial abnormalities such as hypoplasia of the midface and/or mandible or nasopharyngeal vault, and very young children (under age 2–3).[10,11] As a result, high-risk individuals who are undergoing even routine procedures such as adenotonsillectomy should be admitted to a high-visibility bed in the hospital with continuous cardiac and oxygen saturation monitoring. Intraoperative use of steroids and postoperative placement of nasopharyngeal airways and tongue sutures for anterior traction may reduce the risk of airway compromise after surgery. Narcotics and sedatives should be used sparingly in severely obstructed children. Obese patients and those with reduced neuromuscular tone may benefit from airway support with positive airway pressure. In the most extreme cases, overnight endotracheal intubation may be desirable. If it is suspected that the airway may be difficult to reintubate should obstruction occur after extubation, the tube should be remove in the operating room setting.

### 3.2.2 NASAL AND NASOPHARYNGEAL OBSTRUCTION

SRBD due to nasal and nasopharyngeal masses is best addressed by removal of the mass. Depending on the pathology, the procedure may be as simple as a transoral, retropalatal approach for adenoidectomy or marsupialization of nasolacrimal duct cysts, or as complex as an anterior craniofacial approach for encephalocele. In most cases, microdebriders fitted with blades of appropriate size can be used to resect such lesions (see Adenotonsillectomy section below). Some nasal and nasopharyngeal neoplasms may require aggressive resection, as well as preoperative embolization (juvenile nasopharyngeal angiofibroma) or postoperative radiation therapy or chemotherapy (malignancies).

Choanal stenosis or atresia and stenosis of the piriform aperture are common causes of obstructive apnea in neonates. While unilateral disease is often well tolerated until school age years, bilateral cases usually require early intervention due to the dependence of neonates on nasal breathing. Affected infants present with cyclic cyanosis relieved by crying, and the diagnosis is further established by inability to pass a 6-French suction catheter through the nasopharynx. Respiratory distress can typically be relieved using an oropharyngeal airway; the diagnosis is then confirmed and characterized by CT scanning. Such babies should not otherwise leave an intensive care setting until a secure airway is established by tracheotomy or repair of the bony defect. Timing of surgery is controversial; early repair with avoidance of tracheotomy is always desirable, but children several weeks to several months old will better tolerate bleeding and will better accommodate instruments used in the nasal cavity.

While choanal atresia may be approached by either the transpalatal or the transnasal route, improvements in endoscopic and powered instrumentation have made the transnasal approach the first choice for most otolaryngologists. Our preferred approach is as follows.

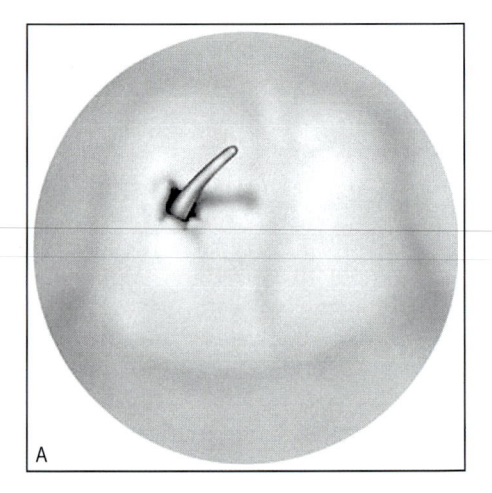

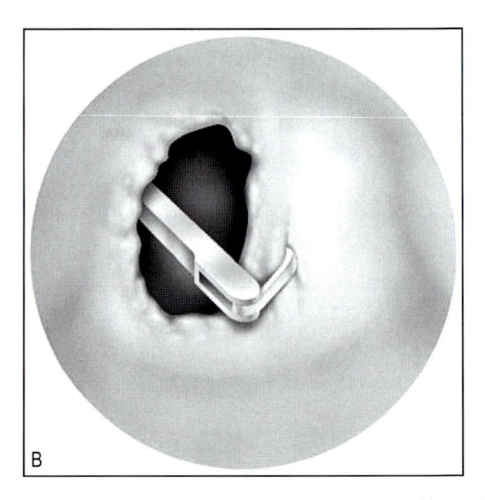

**Fig. 63.1** Endoscopic transnasal repair of choanal atresia. Viewed through a 120° telescope in the oropharynx, the atretic plate is perforated with a Van Buren sound (A). After dilating the perforation to the largest sound, backbiting forceps are introduced transnasally and used to resect the nasopharyngeal end of the nasal septum (B). After initial resection of bone, the endoscope may be placed transnasally to remove bone with greater precision.

1. Anatomy of the nasal cavity is confirmed endoscopically using a small rigid nasal endoscope. The mucosa overlying the atresia plate is injected with 1% lidocaine with 1:100,000 epinephrine and the nose is briefly packed with pledgets of oxymetazoline.
2. The patient's head is placed in extension and a Malek mouth gag (Stryker-Leibinger; Kalamazoo, MI) suspended on a stack of towels is used to facilitate exposure of the nasopharynx. A 3-0 silk suture placed through the uvula is secured cranially outside the patient to improve the exposure.
3. A 120° rod lens telescope (Karl Storz; Culver City, CA) is placed in the oral cavity with the palate retracted to directly visualize the atresia plate(s) via the nasopharynx.
4. A 6-French Van Buren urethral sound is passed into the nasal cavity on one side. Contact between the sound and the atresia plate is confirmed endoscopically by visualizing the sound through the thin plate, or by observing mucosal movement if the plate is thicker.
5. The atresia plate is perforated with the sound (Fig. 63.1A), and the perforation is dilated as much as possible using progressively larger sounds. This procedure is duplicated on the opposite side.
6. A backbiting forceps is introduced into one side of the nose and passed closed through the perforated atresia plate. The forceps are then opened and used to excise the posterior portion of the vomer (Fig. 63.1B).
7. Once the vomer has been considerably reduced, the mouth gag is removed and the procedure is completed transnasally using a 0° telescope. A 2.9 mm or 3.5 mm microdebrider blade is used in oscillating mode to remove any loose or undesirable soft tissue or cartilage. If necessary, the microdebrider may also be fitted with a 2.9 mm round burr used at high speed to drill down any remaining bony prominences.
8. Mitomycin C, which has been reported to reduce the risk of restenosis, may be applied topically to the choanal mucosa at a concentration of 0.4 mg/ml.
9. Stenting of the choanae is not usually necessary, but may be considered in some cases. Our preference is to use individual endotracheal tube stents for each side of the nose, trimmed to keep one end just inside the nasal introitus and the other just beyond the choana. The tube length is measured and recorded so caregivers can suction the appropriate distance. The tubes are rotated to place the beveled end facing anteriorly; a 2-0 silk sutures is then placed transseptally between the tubes and an additional suture is placed through the inferior tip on each side, securing the tube sublabially.

In cases of piriform aperture stenosis, the offending bone may be approached through a sublabial approach (Fig. 63.2), and the aperture is widened using the 2.9 mm round burr at high speed. Stents may be placed as in choanal atresia repair if desired.

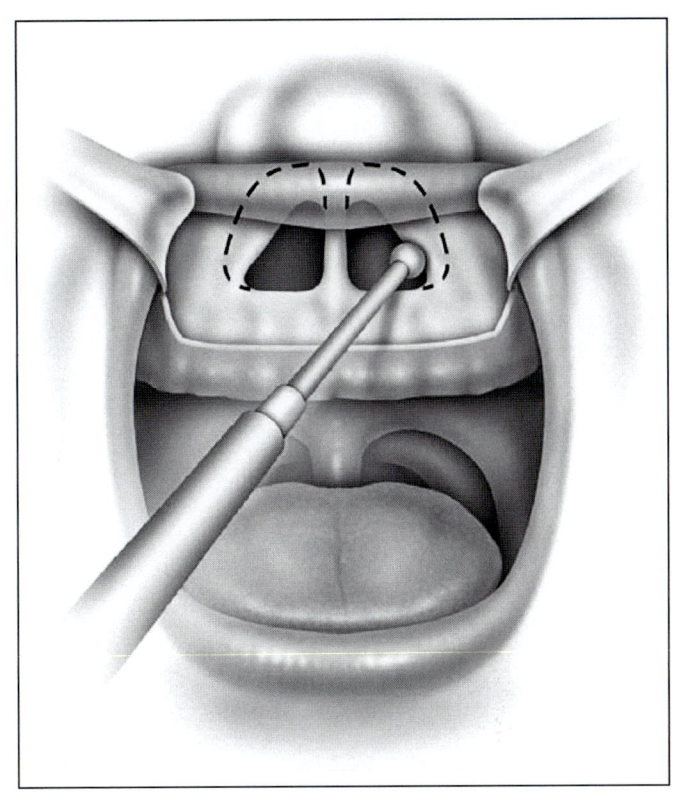

**Fig. 63.2** Transoral repair of piriform aperture stenosis. Piriform aperture is exposed by a sublabial approach. Intranasal degloving incisions may be added if necessary. A drill or microdebrider fitted with a small cutting burr is used to widen the aperture bilaterally.

Patients return to the office 2–4 weeks postoperatively for reassessment and stent removal if placed, and again 8 weeks postoperatively. Steroid-containing ototopical drops may be used to reduce the risk of infection and granulation tissue. Should respiratory distress return, a trip to the operating room for dilation and/or revision should be considered.

Restenosis is the most common complication of these procedures. Success rates (permanent patency) in recent studies are quoted as 78% to 95% with 1–3 year follow-up; number of required revisions is very variable.[12,13]

Nasopharyngeal stenosis, once a common complication of syphilis, may result as a complication of adenotonsillectomy, uvulopalatopharyngoplasty, or surgery for cleft palate or velopharyngeal insufficiency. This disorder often causes obstruction of the upper airway that is even more significant than the disorder the original surgery was intended to correct. Typically, cicatrix forms circumferentially in the velopharynx as a result of excessive removal of mucosa from opposing surfaces.

In mild cases, lysis of the scar with some combination of steroid injection, topical application of mitomycin C, and nasopharyngeal stenting may be sufficient to re-establish adequacy of the nasopharyngeal airway. However, frequently simple release of the scarred area results in recurrence, and treatment must therefore include the movement of fresh, well-vascularized tissue to cover the denuded bed.

SECTION 0 PEDIATRIC OSAHS

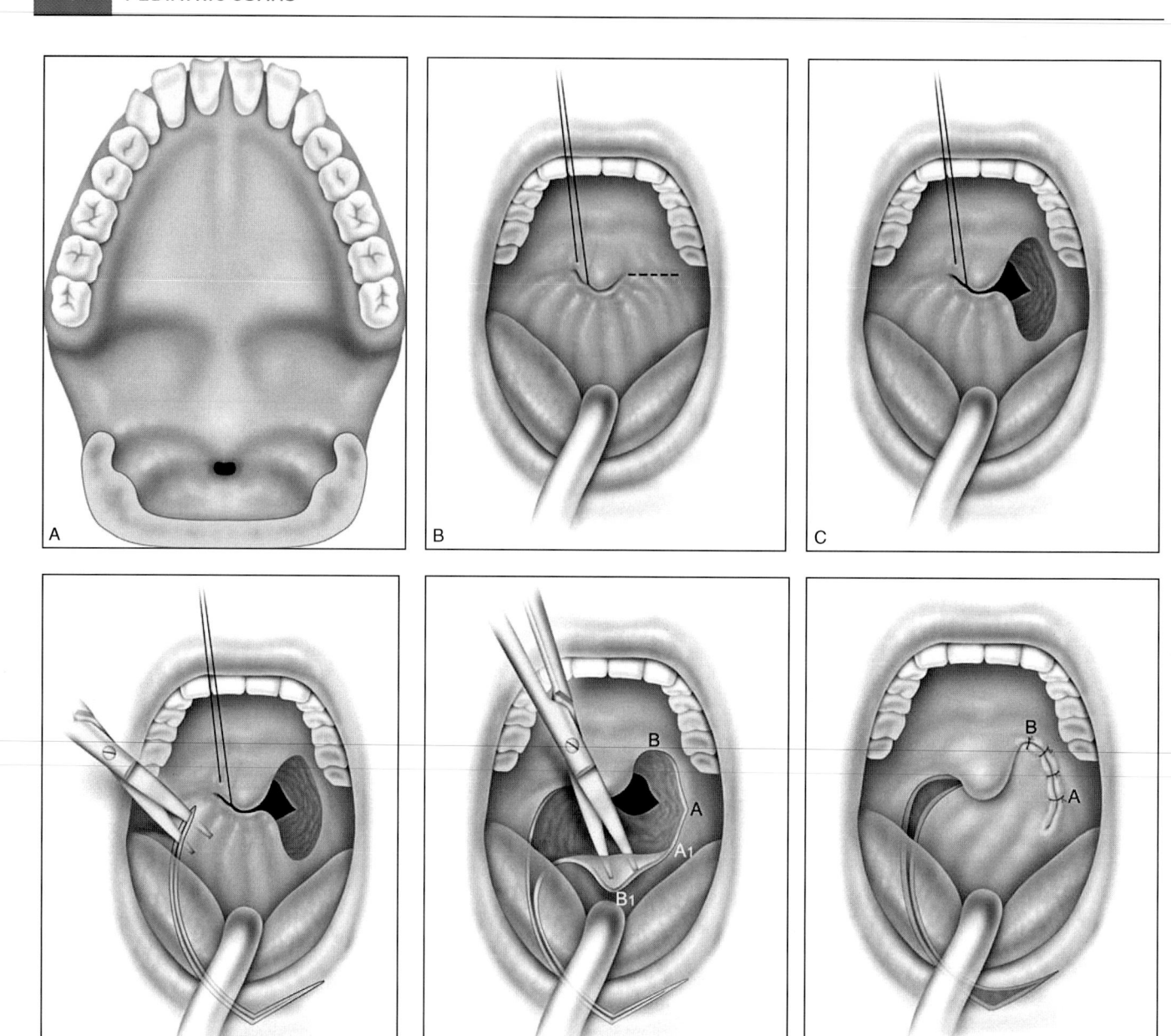

Fig. 63.3 Laterally based pharyngeal flap for correction of nasopharyngeal stenosis. A, The velopharyngeal port is circumferentially narrowed. B and C, A retraction suture is placed in the uvula and a lateral incision is made from velopharyngeal opening into lateral scar on one side and deepened. D, The mucosa is elevated from the scar inferolaterally; excess scar may be excised. A laterally based posterior pharyngeal flap is incised incorporating a back cut. E, The flap is elevated along with the underlying muscle. F, Points ($A_1$) and ($B_1$) are closed to points (A) and (B) respectively, covering the denuded area. (After Cotton RT, Nasopharyngeal stenosis. Arch Otolaryngol 1985;111:146–8, Copyrighted 1985, American Medical Association.)

A variety of techniques has been recommended, including Z-plasty, laterally based pharyngeal flaps, other advancement and rotation flaps, and radial forearm and jejunal free flaps. In most cases, the unilateral laterally based pharyngeal flap described by Cotton[14] results in an adequate nasopharyngeal airway without restenosis. The procedure is as follows (Fig. 63.3).

1. The pharynx is exposed using a tonsil/adenoid mouth gag of the surgeon's choosing (Fig. 63.3A). A 3-0 silk suture is placed through the uvula for purposes of retraction. The pharyngeal wall is injected with 1% lidocaine with 1:100,000 epinephrine lateral to the remaining velopharyngeal port.
2. The stenosis is released using a scalpel and scissors if necessary (Fig. 63.3B). The incision is carried through the underlying muscle and as far lateral as possible.
3. Flaps are developed submuscularly superior, inferior, and lateral to the incision (Fig. 63.3C).
4. A laterally based posterior pharyngeal flap is incised including an inferior back cut. The flap is elevated with the underlying muscle (Fig. 63.3D and E).

5. The area denuded by release of the stenosis is covered by advancing the pharyngeal flap. Closure is performed with 4-0 Vicryl and chromic gut sutures (Fig. 63.3F).
6. The entire area is injected with triamcinolone 40 mg/ml to reduce the risk of restenosis. Application of mitomycin C may also be considered.
7. Stents are placed, consisting of soft nasopharyngeal airways, endotracheal tubes, or prefabricated prostheses. We prefer to leave the stents for 8 weeks or as long as tolerated, although the necessary duration of such stenting is controversial.

In refractory cases, more distal flaps such as the facial artery myomucosal (FAMM) flap or the sternocleidomastoid myocutaneous flap may be necessary considerations. Patients should be followed for at least 12 months postoperatively for surveillance of restenosis and compromise of vocal resonance.

## 3.2.3 ADENOTONSILLAR HYPERPLASIA AND OROPHARYNGEAL OBSTRUCTION

Adenotonsillectomy is generally the first intervention considered for most patients with SRBD, providing they have at least mild adenotonsillar hyperplasia. Improvements in snoring and polysomnography may be anticipated postoperatively in such patients, including those in whom obesity exacerbates their airway obstruction.[15–18] Improvement following adenotonsillar surgery has also been demonstrated in children with preoperative enuresis, orthodontic abnormalities, and behavioral issues prior to surgery. Validated surveys suggest an overall improvement in quality of life after adenotonsillectomy.[19,20]

Over the past century, there has been an evolution in tonsillectomy and adenoidectomy indications, techniques, and devices. In the age of ether anesthesia, clinicians emphasized expedience and efficiency at the expense of complete dissection of the tissues. As improvements in anesthesia permitted more methodical dissection, new techniques were developed in an effort to reduce pain and bleeding associated with the procedure. Several new devices for tonsillectomy and adenoidectomy have been proposed in recent years as technology has evolved.

With the report by Krespi and Ling of serial tonsillectomy with $CO_2$ laser in the outpatient setting came the notion that partial tonsillectomy was safe and less painful than traditional tonsillectomy for patients with tonsil hyperplasia.[21] It is theorized that the exposure of muscle resulting from removal of the tonsil capsule is the cause of pain associated with tonsillectomy, and that leaving some small portion of the tonsil behind may vastly diminish this sequela.[22] Proposed many years ago, the technique had been abandoned due to the risk of tonsil regrowth at a time when most such procedures were performed for recurring infection. Initially studied using the $CO_2$ laser, intracapsular tonsillectomy is now more commonly performed using the microdebrider given its greater efficiency and lower cost (Fig. 63.4). Randomized studies comparing microdebrider intracapsular tonsillectomy to complete electrocautery tonsillectomy generally suggest a modest advantage in pain reduction, particularly otalgia, and return to normal activity; other outcomes yielded less consistent results.[23–26] The procedure involves a slight increase in duration and blood loss. Devices for traditional tonsillectomy developed over the last 20 years, such as the harmonic scalpel (Ethicon Endo-Surgery; Cincinnati, OH), radiofrequency devices (Somnoplasty, Somnus Medical Technologies, Sunnyvale, CA), and Coblation® (Fig. 63.5; ArthroCare Corp., Sunnyvale, CA) have been studied in small trials that suggest modest reduction in pain compared with electrocautery, with further decrease in postoperative pain when the tonsil is reduced rather than excised.

Techniques of adenoidectomy include curettage, suction electrocautery ablation (Fig. 63.6), Coblation® (Fig. 63.7) and removal by power-assisted devices (Fig. 63.8). Traditional curettage is inexpensive but is the least precise of these techniques and is associated with hemorrhage that must be controlled before leaving the operating room. Electrocautery dissection, by definition, is associated with less bleeding and is also a precise and inexpensive device.

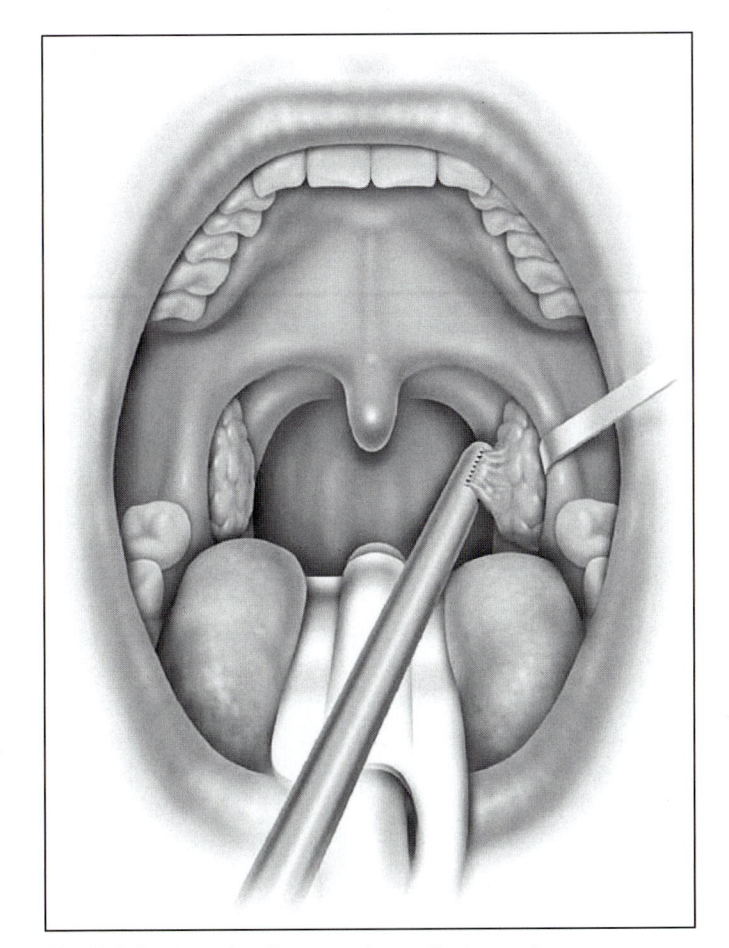

**Fig. 63.4** Power-assisted intracapsular tonsillectomy using a microdebrider. The microdebrider is used at 2000 rpm.

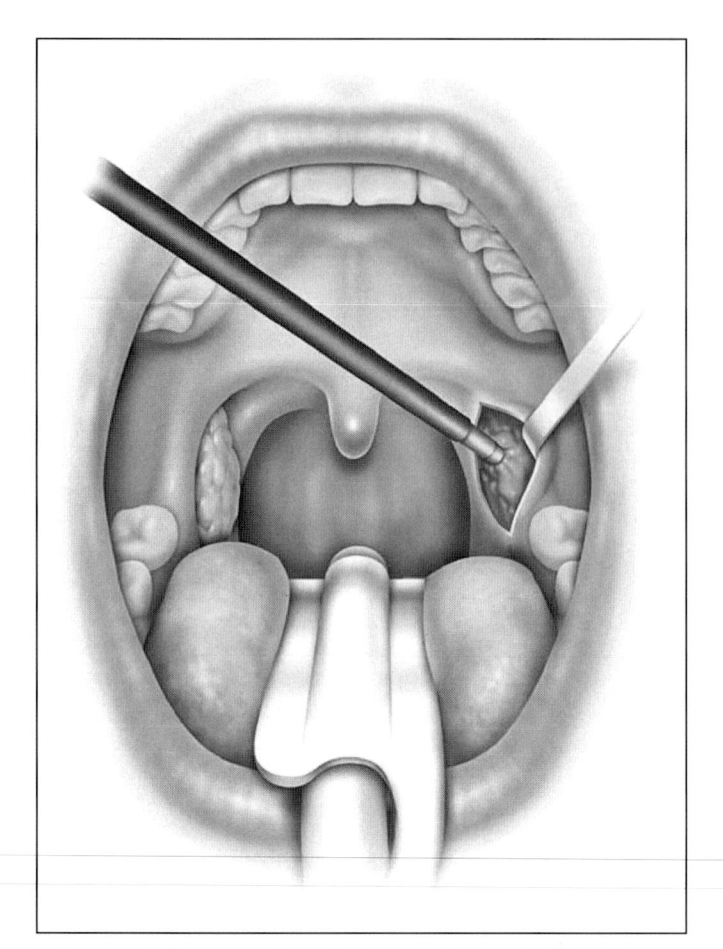

**Fig. 63.5** Tonsillectomy performed using Coblation® (ArthroCare Corp., Sunnyvale, CA). The procedure may be used to excise the entire tonsil along the capsule or in a tonsil-sparing, intracapsular technique.

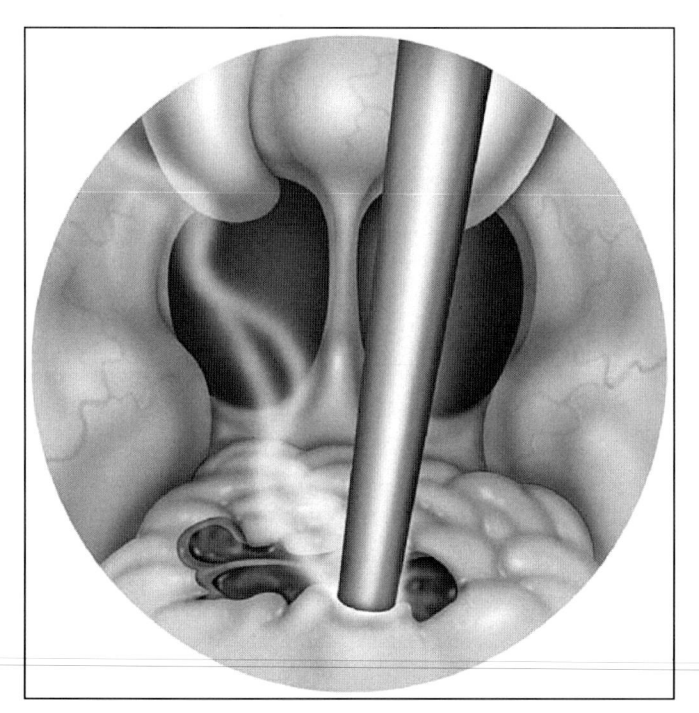

**Fig. 63.6** Suction cautery adenoidectomy. High cautery settings (40 watts or more) are used to fulgurate the tissue, and suction facilitates its removal.

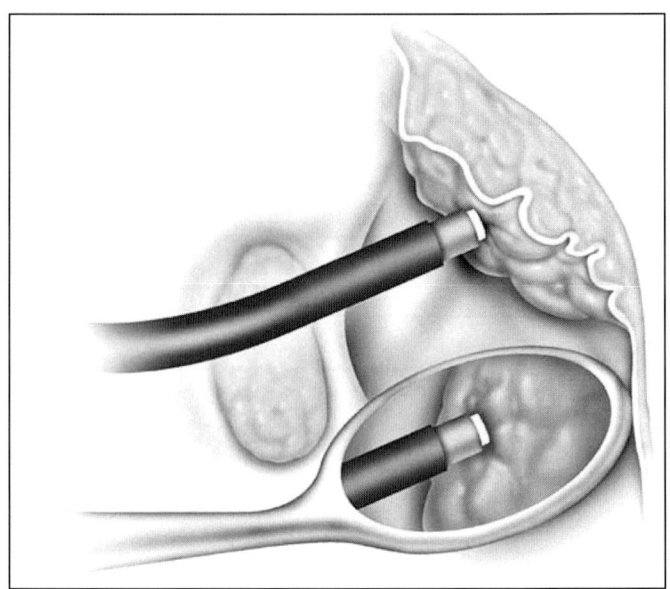

**Fig. 63.7** Adenoidectomy performed using Coblation® (ArthroCare Corp., Sunnyvale, CA). The wand is bent for application in the nasopharynx.

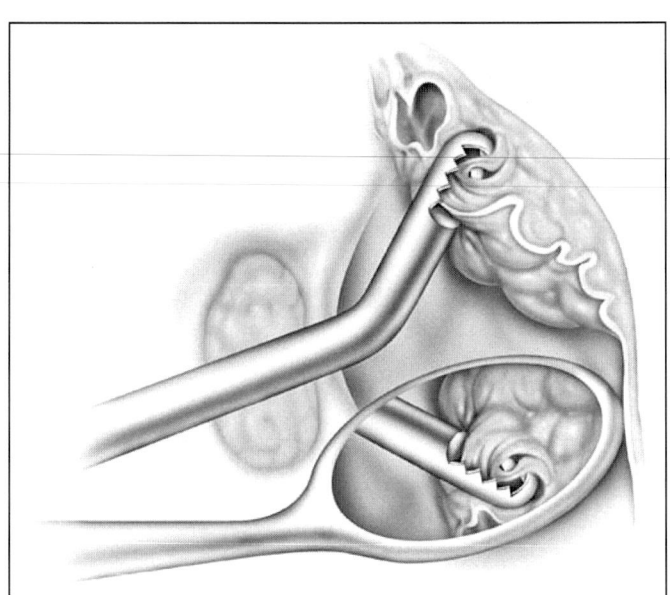

**Fig. 63.8** Power-assisted adenoidectomy using the Straight Shot® microdebrider (Medtronic/Xomed; Jacksonville, FL) fitted with the RADenoid® blade. The microdebrider is used at 2000 rpm.

However, high settings are required on the cautery device, with the potential for thermal injury to deep structures, and surgical times have been variable. Studies of power-assisted (microdebrider) techniques have demonstrated excellent precision with rapid removal of tissue and minimal additional time for cautery, but the disposable blades add significant expense.

Uvulopalatopharyngoplasty is not commonly performed in children, perhaps since most children with sleep apnea do not demonstrate the redundant tissue found in adults with similar symptoms. Several studies have demonstrated that the procedure is efficacious in the most difficult-to-treat patients with SRBD, particularly those with obesity, neurological impairment, or Down syndrome. However, these reports are retrospective, and it remains unclear whether resection of the palate and uvula adds significantly to tonsillectomy with plication of the tonsil pillars. In addition, nasopharyngeal stenosis remains a significant risk when the procedure is performed at the same time as adenoidectomy.

### 3.2.4 MACROGLOSSIA AND THE PTOTIC TONGUE

Children with macroglossia generally have Beckwith–Wiedemann syndrome (macroglossia, omphalocele, visceromegaly, cytomegaly of the adrenal cortex), Down syndrome, or a vascular malformation of the tongue. Complications of macroglossia include aberrant dental eruption and malocclusion, maldevelopment of the maxilla and mandible, excessive drying of the tongue with ulceration, and airway obstruction. Unfortunately, surgical reduction of the tongue is generally effective only for the first three indications, and less so for airway obstruction. The procedure usually consists of a resection of the lingual margin or a wedge resection with or without aggressive resection at the foramen cecum, and therefore fails to address obstruction at the distal oropharynx and tongue base. As a result, airway obstruction persists in many children undergoing tongue reduction for macroglossia.

Other methods of managing macroglossia include suture suspension of the tongue, genioglossus advancement, and radiofrequency ablation. The tongue suspension suture technique (Repose®, InfluENT, Concord, NH) in children has been reported only in individual cases, and recently in a series of 16 patients refractory to treatment with adenotonsillectomy.[27] The procedure is performed as follows (Fig. 63.9).

1. The procedure is performed under general anesthesia with nasotracheal intubation. The patient is placed in tonsillectomy position, with the oral cavity exposed using a Molt mouth prop. A 2-0 silk retraction suture is placed at the tip of the tongue.
2. After injection of 1% lidocaine with 1:100,000 epinephrine, a small midline incision is made in the floor of the mouth medial and posterior to the submandibular ducts. Through this incision, a disposable battery-operated screw inserter is used to place a 3 mm mini-screw attached to a #1 polypropylene suture in the midline of the mandible below the level of the incisor roots (Fig. 63.9A). Firm placement of the screw is confirmed by gently pulling on the suture.
3. A preloaded proprietary suture passer with a suture loop is passed through the floor of mouth incision posteriorly toward the base of tongue. The suture is passed out the tongue base approximately 1.0–1.5 cm lateral to the midline (to the right of the midline if the surgeon is right handed), caudal to the foramen cecum (Fig. 63.9B). Care is taken not to injure the neurovascular bundle of the tongue laterally. The suture loop is then grasped as the suture passer is removed.
4. The suture passer is loaded with a strand of the polypropylene suture attached to the screw and passed

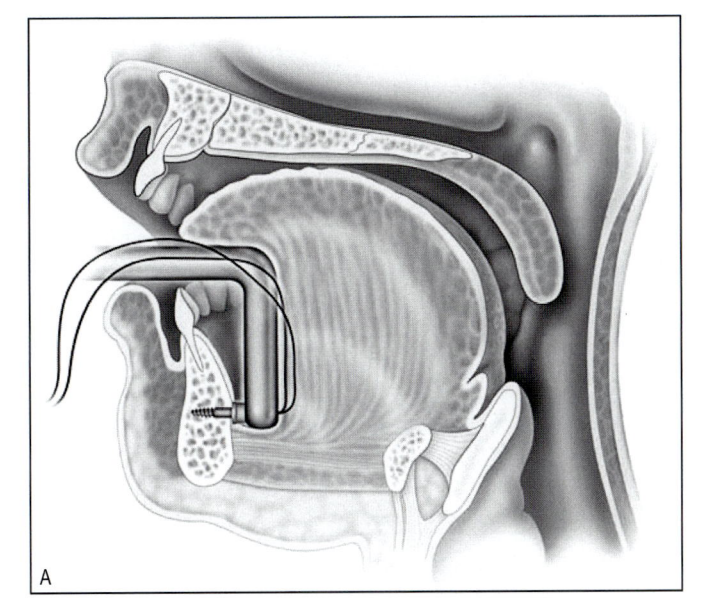

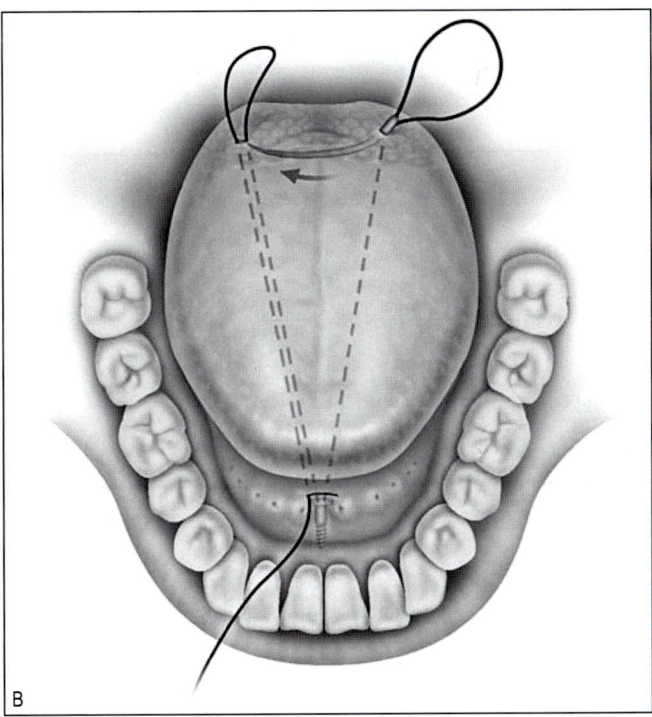

**Fig. 63.9** Tongue base suspension using the Repose® system (InfluENT, Concord, NH). A, A disposable battery-operated screw inserter is used to place a 3 mm mini-screw attached to a #1 polypropylene suture in the midline of the lingual mandibular surface below the roots of the incisor teeth. B, After passing a suture loop through the floor of mouth and out the tongue base on one side, the polypropylene suture attached to the screw is passed through the floor of mouth and out the tongue base symmetrically on the opposite side. The polypropylene suture is loaded on a large curved Mayo needle and passed submuscularly into the contralateral suture loop.

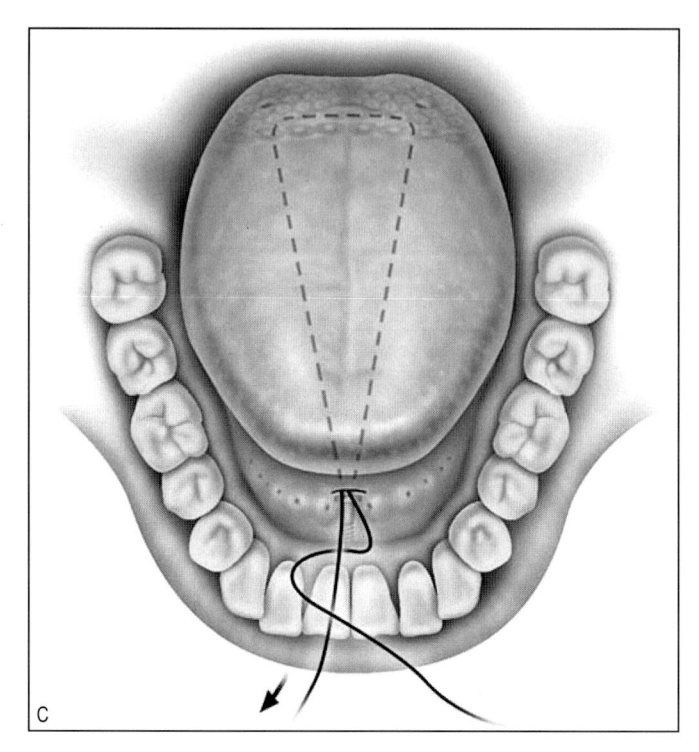

**Fig. 63.9** (Continued) C, The loop is then pulled anteriorly through the floor of mouth and into the incision, dragging along the polypropylene suture and pulling the tongue base anteriorly. The suture is then tied to a second anchor suture pre-attached to the screw.

through the floor of mouth and out the tongue base symmetrically on the opposite (left) side.

5. The polypropylene suture exiting at the tongue base is loaded on a large curved Mayo needle. The suture is inserted and tunneled submuscularly from its origin (left) to the exit point of the contralateral (right) suture loop. After removing the needle the single polypropylene strand is passed through the loop.
6. The loop is pulled anteriorly through the floor of mouth and into the incision, dragging along the polypropylene suture from the screw (Fig. 63.9C). The suture is then knotted to a second anchor suture attached to the screw, pulling the tongue base anteriorly. Care must be taken not to break the suture or cause necrosis of the tissue at the tongue base. Executed correctly, tightening the suture creates an indentation in the tongue base. The knot is then buried submucosally in the floor of mouth, and the incision site is closed with chromic suture.

Overall success of tongue suspension was reported as 63%, but only 50% among children with Down syndrome.[27]

Genioglossus advancement through advancement of the genial tubercle is rarely performed in young children due to the risk of injury to the developing mandibular incisors. However, the procedure may be considered for older children whose mandibles are well developed (Fig. 63.10).

1. A preoperative panoramic/tomographic radiograph of the mandible is performed to establish the anatomy of the mandibular incisors and the anterior mandible. The patient is anesthetized and intubated nasotracheally or orotracheally. The anterior vestibule (gingivobuccal sulcus) is infiltrated with 1% lidocaine with 1:100,000 epinephrine.
2. An incision is made in the sulcus, leaving a cuff of mucosa on the mandibular side to facilitate closure. The incision is carried subperiosteally until the inferior border of the mandible is exposed. The location of the genial tubercle is estimated based on the preoperative radiograph and confirmed by palpation of the lingual surface of the mandible.
3. Using a sagittal saw, a rectangular osteotomy is performed through the outer cortex such that the genial tubercle is included. In the fully developed mandible, the center of the osteotomy is approximately 5 mm below the incisor root tips. An outer cortex screw placed in the center of the osteotomy assists in manipulation of the bone segment.
4. Cuts are made through the inner cortex, freeing the osteotomy segment. Once hemostasis is obtained, the segment is advanced and rotated 90° (Fig. 63.10A), pulling the base of tongue anteriorly (Fig. 63.10B).
5. The outer cortex and bone marrow are removed from the segment and the bone is contoured with fluted and diamond burrs.
6. The segment is fixed in position using a screw placed through the inferior aspect of the osteotomy segment into the inferior mandibular border. The mucosa is reapproximated using absorbable suture.

Patients may generally be discharged within 24 hours after surgery. Complications of genioglossus advancement are unusual, but include dental injury, hematoma, and hypesthesia of the teeth and chin. The procedure has not been reported in any large series of children; however, adults usually undergo simultaneous procedures such as uvulopalatopharyngoplasty and hyoid advancement since genioglossus advancement alone will rarely correct severe sleep apnea. When performed with adjunctive procedures, studies demonstrate a widened retrolingual airway, improvement in oxygen saturation, and a 70% reduction in Respiratory Distress Index.[28]

Radiofrequency ablation of the tongue has not been reported in children except for those with lymphatic malformations.[29] In adults with sleep apnea, only modest results have been obtained, and the improvement has been shown to deteriorate over time.[30] The device (Somnoplasty; Somnus Medical Technologies, Sunnyvale, CA) uses radiofrequency to create a submucosal coagulum that results in tissue contracture and reduction in tissue volume. The tongue handpiece consists of two prongs with retractable needles. After infiltration of local anesthesia, the handpiece

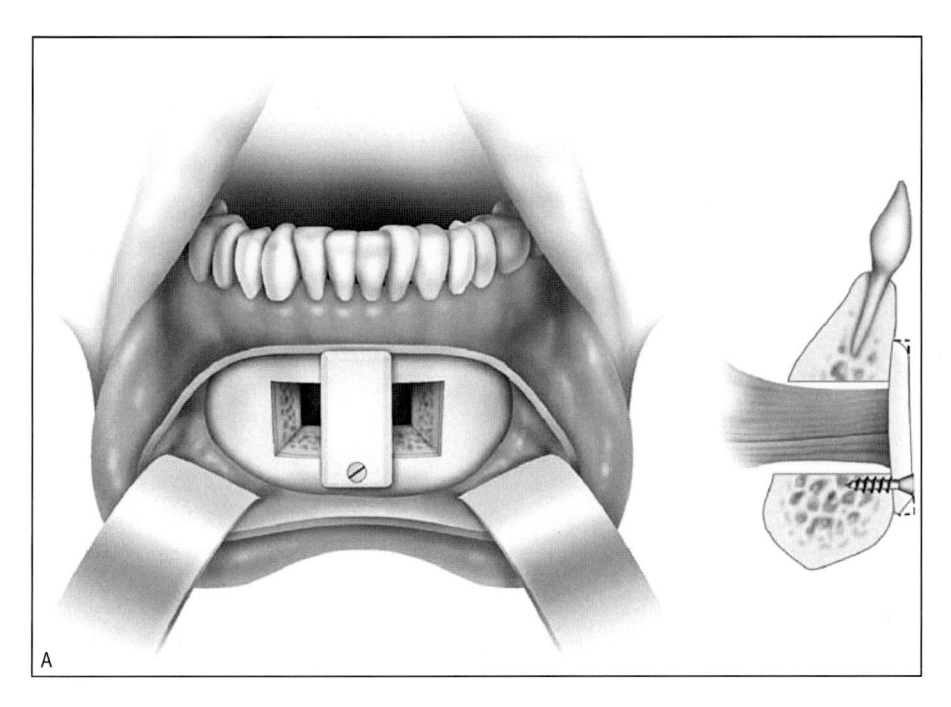

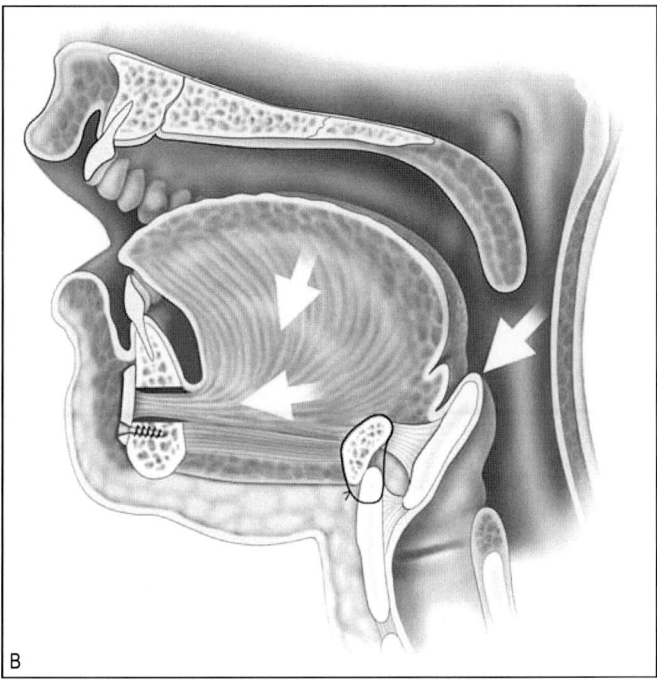

**Fig. 63.10** Genioglossus advancement. A, Through a mandibular sulcus incision, a rectangular osteotomy is performed 5 mm below the incisor root tips. Initial cuts are made through the outer cortex so as to include the genial tubercle. After placing an outer cortex screw in the center of the osteotomy, cuts are made through the inner cortex freeing the osteotomy segment which is then rotated 90°, pulling the base of tongue anteriorly (B).

is placed in contact with the mucosa and the needles are then advanced into the muscle. The needles are placed no further than 2 cm from the midline to avoid injury to the neurovascular pedicles. Complications include postoperative edema, abscess formation and tissue necrosis.

Submucosal minimally invasive lingual excision (SMILE) has recently been described as a novel method of reducing tissue of both the anterior tongue and the tongue base.[31] The procedure uses ultrasound and endoscopically guided Coblation® reduction of lingual tissue through a small incision in the anterior tongue (Fig. 63.11).

1. General anesthesia is administered through either a nasotracheal tube or a previously placed tracheotomy. Preoperative administration of intravenous steroids and antibiotics is recommended. The oral cavity is gently brushed with antiseptic oral rinse and a retraction suture is placed through the anterior midline tongue tip.

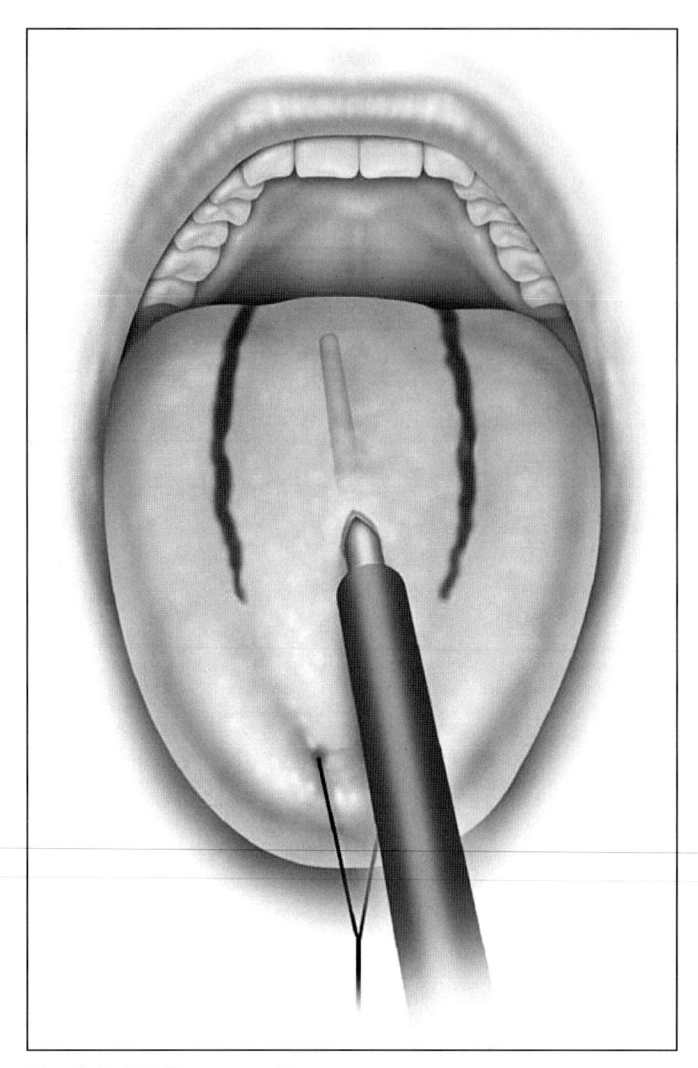

**Fig. 63.11** SMILE technique. After delineating the course of the lingual arteries with a hand-held ultrasound probe, a midline incision is made ending 2 cm from the tongue tip and opened bluntly. The Coblator® wand (ArthroCare Corporation, Austin, Texas) is inserted into the incision and advanced in the posterior direction. Tissue is excised in a dorsal to ventral fashion by alternating anterior and posterior movements of the wand.

2. A hand-held ultrasound probe is used to delineate the course of the lingual arteries bilaterally and the vessels are marked. A midline incision is made approximately 2 cm from the tongue tip with blunt dissection to open the incision.
3. The EVAC 70 T&A Plasma Wand attached to the Coblator II Surgery System (ArthroCare Corporation, Austin, TX) is inserted into the incision and programmed for ablation at a setting of 9. The wand is advanced in the posterior direction with care to stay medial to the marked courses of the lingual arteries. Tissue is excised in a dorsal to ventral fashion by alternating anterior and posterior movements of the wand. The non-operating hand palpates the tip of the wand through the tongue mucosa. Progress may be monitored by intermittently removing the wand and inserting a 0° irrigating endoscope into the surgical cavity.
4. The anterior tongue incision is left open to reduce the risk of hematoma.

After surgery, the patient is either extubated and monitored or intubated for less than 24 hours. Intravenous steroid and antibiotics are continued. Once extubated, the patient is started on a regular, soft diet. Children are observed for less than 72 hours and discharged home with 7 days of oral antibiotics, steroids, and analgesics. We suggest the procedure is better tolerated and more effective than other means of tongue reduction.

Vascular malformations of the tongue are generally of lymphatic or venous origin. Microcystic lymphatic malformation causing the tongue to be both wide and thick is extremely difficult to treat. Surgical resection may be performed transorally or transcervically and is tailored to sites of obstruction and dentofacial deformity. Regardless of approach or technique, recurrence is exceedingly common. Limited success has been reported using radiofrequency and Coblation® technology. Many such patients retain a tracheotomy indefinitely. Conversely, lymphatic malformations that are macrocystic may be virtually eliminated by sclerotherapy with OK-432, alcohol, bleomycin, or tetracycline.[32] All of these sclerosants are known to cause significant inflammation; hence all patients with involvement of the neck, pharynx, or larynx who are not already tracheotomized should be monitored for postoperative airway obstruction. Venous malformations of the tongue may be reduced considerably using a combination of superficial and intralesional Nd:YAG laser therapy, alcohol sclerosis, and/or excision.[33]

Ductal cysts of the vallecula may present with sleep disordered breathing in neonates. Occasionally, the presentation may also be consistent with laryngomalacia. These lesions are thought to result from mucous gland obstruction, but the etiology has not been definitively elucidated. The diagnosis may be difficult to make endoscopically due to the position of the mass, and lateral radiograph of the upper airway may be useful when the diagnosis is suspected. The lesion is managed surgically as follows (Fig. 63.12).

1. The patient is nasotracheally intubated and the head is positioned for suspension laryngoscopy. A Parsons or other slotted laryngoscope facilitates instrumentation, but any operating laryngoscope may be utilized. The tongue is suspended and the cyst visualized.
2. The dome of the cyst is grasped with small cup forceps and a laryngeal scissors is used to open the cyst cavity.
3. Once the cyst has been decompressed, the cyst wall is removed using the microdebrider (Fig. 63.12). The blade is inserted into the cyst cavity, and initial excision of the cyst wall is performed on the side opposite the forceps. The remaining cyst wall is then regrasped so as to permit completion of the excision.
4. $CO_2$ laser applied to the base helps to control hemorrhage and theoretically reduces the risk of recurrence.

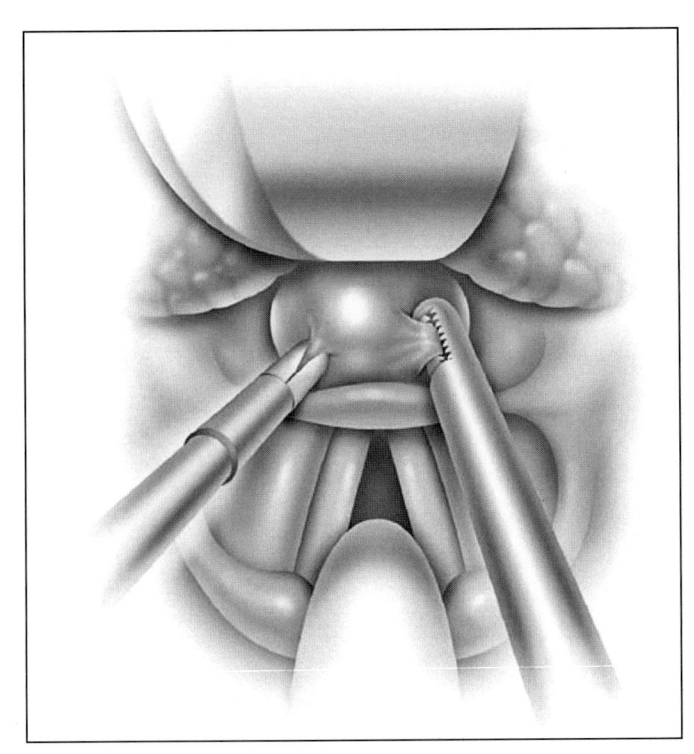

# Management of sleep-related breathing disorders in children

## CHAPTER 63

**Fig. 63.12** Excision of vallecular cyst. After nasotracheal intubation and suspension laryngoscopy, the cyst is aspirated and/or opened with microscissors. The cyst wall may then be grasped with microcup forceps and excised using the microdebrider. We prefer to treat the cyst base with $CO_2$ laser to lessen the risk of recurrence.

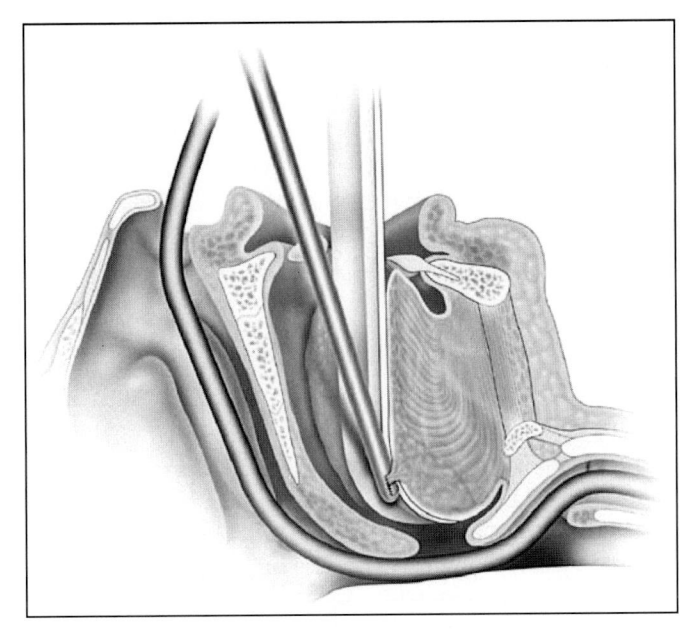

**Fig. 63.13** Lingual tonsillectomy. After nasotracheal intubation, an operating laryngoscope is suspended with the tip just cranial to the vallecula. Lingual tonsil tissue may then be excised using the microdebrider with a straight sinus blade as shown; alternatively, the $CO_2$ laser or Coblator® may also be used.

In most cases, results are excellent immediately after surgery. Recurrence and complications are rare and extended follow-up is not necessary.

Hyperplastic lingual tonsil tissue can also occupy the tongue base and vallecula, causing obstruction and retroflexion of the epiglottis. Excision of this tissue may occasionally be necessary in patients with diffuse lymphoid hyperplasia, such as those with Down syndrome or post-transplantation lymphoproliferative disorder, if symptoms are not relieved by adenotonsillectomy alone. Candidacy for the procedure is established by direct and fiberoptic assessment of lingual tonsil size and by lateral neck radiography. The procedure is performed as follows.

1. After induction of general anesthesia, the patient is nasotracheally intubated. In the most severe cases of lingual tonsil hyperplasia, fiberoptic intubation may be necessary. Preoperative steroid medication is administered.
2. With the table rotated 90° and the head in the Rose position, a 2-0 silk retraction suture is placed in the anterior tongue. The tongue base is infiltrated with 1% lidocaine with 1:100,000 epinephrine.
3. An operating laryngoscope is introduced transorally and suspended with the tip just above the vallecula (Fig. 63.13). We prefer the Parsons laryngoscope for this so that instruments can easily be introduced through the slide slot; a Lindholm scope can also be used if the procedure is to be performed with a $CO_2$ laser. The operating microscope is fitted with a 400 mm lens and focused on the surgical field. Alternatively, particularly when hand-held instruments are used, a Jennings mouth gag may be used to keep the mouth open while the field is exposed with a 70° telescope.
4. Lingual tonsil tissue may be excised using a variety of techniques. Coblation performed using the EVAC 70 T&A Plasma Wand attached to the Coblator II Surgery System (ArthroCare Corporation, Austin TX) causes minimal bleeding and results in efficient removal of tissue. The microdebrider fitted with a 3.5 mm tricut straight sinus blade can be used in the oscillating mode at 2000 revolutions per minute with even greater efficiency but with increased bleeding (Fig. 63.13). $CO_2$ laser may also be used for the dissection, offering the advantage of less bleeding and the disadvantage of less efficiency. Settings depend on the laser used; if a flash-scanner is available, excellent results are obtained using the laser in this mode at 6–10 watts with a spot size of 3 or 4 mm. When a scanner is not used, the beam should be defocused and the power increased. Suction cautery is also an alternative modality.

In all cases, the dissection is kept above the muscle layer, intermittently controlling bleeding with oxymetazoline packs and suction electrocautery. The telescope or laryngoscope is periodically relocated to keep the level of dissection even.

Patients are monitored overnight on the floor or in the intensive care unit depending on their preoperative degree of obstruction. Two to three doses of steroid are given postoperatively and pain is managed appropriately. A regular diet may be taken. Complications include taste disturbance, scarring or injury to the neurovascular bundle if the dissection is excessive, and bleeding. Patients should be monitored for at least a year for evidence of tissue regrowth. There are no large-scale studies of the efficacy of the procedure in children or adults.

### 3.2.5 HYPOPLASIA OF THE MIDFACE AND MANDIBLE

Upper airway obstruction due to hypoplasia of the midface and mandible is usually associated with craniofacial syndromes. Micrognathia due to Pierre Robin sequence often improves within the first 2 years of life without surgical intervention for the mandible. In cases of mild airway obstruction, children with competent caretakers may be managed by prone positioning and nasopharyngeal stenting via nasal trumpet or similar device. When symptoms are more severe, airway obstruction may be relieved by temporary repositioning of the ptotic tongue through labioglossopexy. The surgical technique is as follows (Fig. 63.14).

1. If the patient is not already intubated, preparation is made for intubation by flexible fiberoptic bronchoscopy or Bullard laryngoscopy in the event the larynx cannot be visualized using a standard anesthesia laryngoscope. After being taken to the operating room, the patient is anesthetized via mask and subsequently intubated by one of these techniques with an age-appropriate tube. Nasal intubation can be performed; however, our experience has been that an oral endotracheal tube does not interfere with the surgery. A weight-appropriate dose of cefazolin or clindamycin is given. A small amount of 1% lidocaine with 1:100,000 epinephrine is then injected for hemostasis into the soft tissues of the ventral tongue, the anterior floor of mouth, and the lingual surface of the anterior mandibular alveolus. The patient's lower face and chin are sterilely prepared and draped.
2. A Molt mouth prop is opened laterally between the upper and lower alveolus to expose the anterior oral cavity. A 2-0 silk suture placed through the dorsal tongue facilitates manipulation of the tongue during the procedure. The lingual frenulum may need to be released by transection or Z-plasty. A long T-shaped incision is made on the anterior ventral tongue and carried vertically from the tongue tip to the frenulum. An opposing incision is made in similar fashion along the lower lip to the anterior mandibular alveolus. The wound edges on both incisions are undermined to create mucosal flaps and the underlying tongue and orbicularis oris muscles are exposed.
3. The vertical lip-to-alveolus incision is carried down to the bone and a small periosteal elevator is used to tunnel along the anterior and posterior aspects of the mandible.

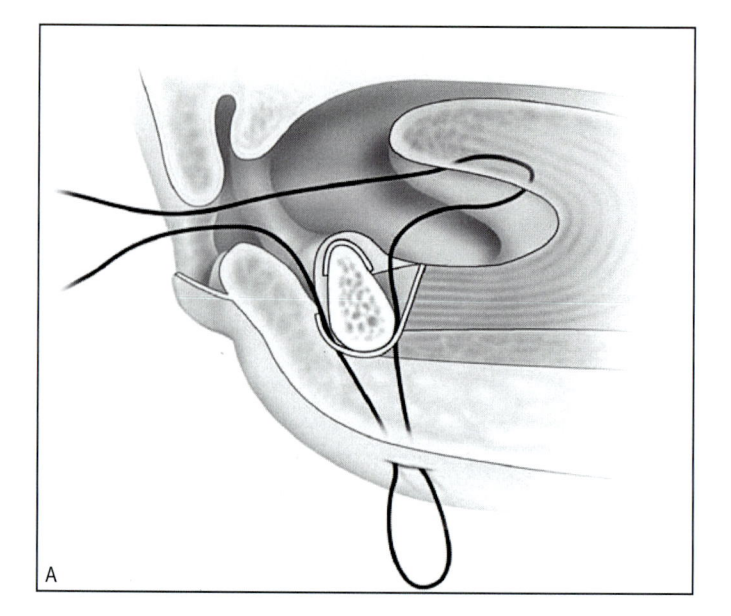

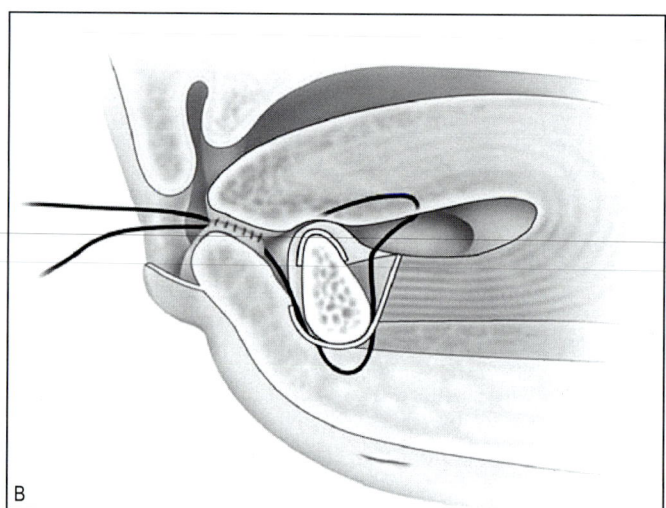

**Fig. 63.14** Labioglossopexy for glossoptosis. A, After T-shaped incisions are made on the anterior ventral tongue and lower lip exposing the underlying tongue and orbicularis oris muscles, a periosteal elevator is used to tunnel along the anterior aspect of the mandible and to detach the genioglossus muscle. A spinal needle passed through the soft tissue along the anterior and posterior surfaces of the mandible through the skin of the mentum facilitates placement of a 0 or 2-0 Prolene circummandibular stay suture passed through muscle. The two ends of the suture are then placed into the tongue muscles in a location that will allow approximation of the muscle directly to the alveolar ridge incision (B). The ventral tongue mucosal flaps are then matched to the flaps of the lower lip and approximated using a 4-0 chromic gut suture.

The genioglossus muscle is gently detached from the genial tubercle using blunt dissection.
4. An 18 or 20-gauge spinal needle is passed through the soft tissue along the posterior surface of the mandible and through the skin of the mentum; a small skin incision is made at the exit site. Dissection of the subcutaneous tissue deep to the incision allows the suture to pass close to the mandible and reduces slippage. A non-absorbable

suture without needle (i.e. 0 or 2-0 Prolene) is placed through the spinal needle and retrieved at the mentum. The spinal needle is then withdrawn and passed from the mouth through the skin incision a second time, this time along the anterior surface of the mandible. The suture tail is threaded through the needle and the needle is withdrawn.

5. The posterior end of the non-absorbable suture is placed through a free or traumatic needle. The needle is buried deep into the tongue musculature adjacent to the foramen cecum and brought back into the oral cavity at the caudal end of the tongue incision. The suture is tied while drawing the 2-0 silk suture anteriorly to take tension off the tongue. The knot is positioned submucosally.
6. The ventral tongue mucosal flaps are then matched to the flaps of the lower lip and approximated using a 4-0 chromic gut suture. Prophylactic placement of a nasopharyngeal airway reduces the risk of postoperative obstruction after extubation and facilitates suctioning of the airway.

Postoperative management includes nasogastric feeding to prevent aggressive sucking. The nasopharyngeal airway can be discontinued several days postoperatively and oral feedings are usually attempted in about 1 week. Oral feeding is usually unaffected by the procedure. The child can be discharged home once the airway is deemed adequate and the patient is able to obtain adequate nutrition by mouth. Dehiscence of the adhesion is the most common complication of labioglossopexy, but fewer than 5% require a return to the operating room for revision. Other reported complications include tongue lacerations, Wharton duct injury, wound infection, and scarring. Some authors feel that syndromic patients tend to be more difficult to manage due to numerous anomalies or conditions contributing to airway obstruction and impaired feeding. Kirschner et al.[34] had an 83% rate of conversion to tracheostomy in syndromic children.

The child should be closely monitored as an outpatient to ensure appropriate growth and development. The patient should be evaluated at about 1 month postoperatively and then at 2–3 month intervals. Tongue mobility should be closely monitored, although the effect on speech development is minimal. Takedown of labioglossopexy is usually performed at 6–9 months of age, often coinciding with repair of the palate. Adequacy of the airway should be confirmed endoscopically prior to takedown.

When symptoms are too severe for labioglossopexy, multiple sites of obstruction are present, or the patient's medical situation is exceedingly grave, tracheotomy remains the most reliable and least morbid means of airway management. However, patients should show signs of mandibular 'catch-up' growth within the first few months; when this is not the case, distraction osteogenesis should be considered.

First described for the treatment of limb length discrepancies, osteotomy with distraction of bone is now widely accepted as the procedure of choice in the early management of airway obstruction due to craniofacial disproportion.[35–38] The procedure takes advantage of the rapid healing and capacity for growth in the pediatric skeleton. Distraction osteogenesis has been used for over a decade to advance the mandible in cases of retrognathia and micrognathia, but indications have expanded to include neuromuscular disorders. With modifications to the expansion devices, distraction of the midface is also beginning to replace Le Fort osteotomies with bone grafting.[37,38]

Distraction osteogenesis is divided into four phases: surgery, distraction, consolidation, and removal. Prior to surgery, all candidates for mandibular distraction undergo airway endoscopy and craniofacial assessment by three-dimensional CT scanning. The scans are used to determine whether the distraction vector will be horizontal, vertical, or both, and where the osteotomies are made. Airway patency may also be estimated in relaxed and jaw-thrust positions, and precise bony measurements are taken from the scan. The surgeon usually determines preoperatively whether intraoral or external devices are to be used. While external devices permit multivector control of the distraction and are more easily applied to small mandibles, intraoral distractors may leave a more acceptable facial scar. In addition, intraoral devices have some mechanical advantage since their point of application is closer to the point of distraction resistance.

The operative technique is as follows.

1. Intubation for the procedure may be nasotracheal or orotracheal. Candidates for the procedure are often difficult to intubate using traditional direct laryngoscopy, and plans should be made preoperatively for possible intubation using the flexible or Bullard laryngoscopes.
2. After infiltration of 1% lidocaine with 1:100,000 epinephrine into the mucosa overlying the ascending ramus of the mandible, an initial internal incision is made along the oblique line. Alternatively, an external submandibular incision may be made in infants in whom intraoral exposure is limited. Subperiosteal dissection is performed both medially and laterally, exposing approximately 2 cm of bone on either side of the mandibular angle. The buccal surface of the mandible is marked for osteotomy anterior or posterior to the angle as determined by the preoperative CT scan. The lingula is identified and the lingual cortex osteotomy is marked so as to avoid injury to the inferior alveolar nerve (Fig. 63.15A).
3. For internal devices, the device plates are applied to either side of the planned osteotomy using at least four screws in each plate (Fig. 63.15B). A stab incision is made at the exit point of the activation arm through the skin. A reciprocating saw or a fissure burr is used to perform the osteotomy, with care to remain well

the osteotomy. Holes are hand-drilled so that the hole size is carefully controlled. After both cortices have been drilled, the bit is removed and pins are screwed in without moving the guide. The desired depth is obtained by palpating the pin lingually. The external distractor is adjusted to fit onto the pins. A small gap is left between the device and the skin to facilitate pin care and to accommodate swelling. The position of the device is marked on the pins to facilitate replacement. The distractor is again removed. The osteotomy is completed using osteotomes on the inferior and superior borders and on the lingual aspect to avoid injury to the nerve. The distractor is replaced and tightened. At this point, activation is attempted to ensure movement of the proximal and distal segments. The device is then returned to its starting position. The incision is closed except for the pin sites and the pins are cut flush with the device.

5. The procedure is repeated on the opposite side. We prefer to treat the two sides sequentially so as to avoid destabilizing the anterior mandible and subsequent loss of contour.

After a lag phase of 48–72 hours, distraction is started at a rate of 1–2 mm per day, with adjustments every 12 hours. Once the desired length of the mandible has been achieved, adequacy of the airway is verified by flexible or rigid laryngoscopy prior to consolidation. In children who already have a tracheostomy, downsizing and bedside occlusion can be performed. The consolidation phase is usually about 4–10 weeks during which the hardware may be left in place. The final stage is removal of the hardware and minor scar revision.

Avoidance of or decannulation from tracheotomy in appropriately selected patients undergoing distraction of the mandible is >80%.[35–38] Complications include pin site infections, injury to the inferior alveolar and marginal nerves, damage to tooth buds, resorption and ankylosis of the temporomandibular joint, and failure to maintain distraction. Complication rates are difficult to quantify since most series are small and follow-up is limited.

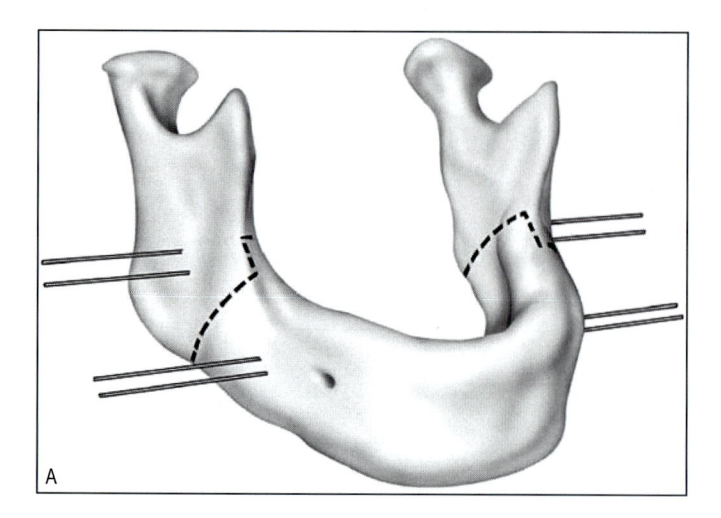

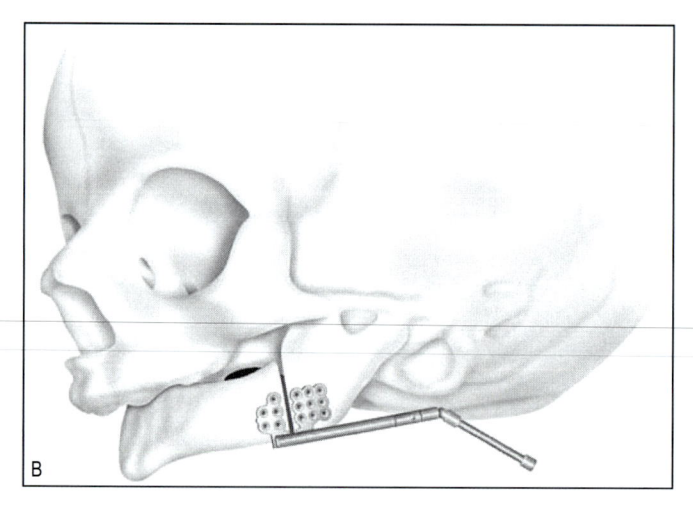

**Fig. 63.15** A, Technique of mandibular distraction. Planned bone cuts and pin placement for mandibular distraction. Bone cuts are designed as in a bilateral sagittal split osteotomy. For external distractor, two pins are placed on either side of the osteotomy. The medial osteotomy is prepared by scoring the bone, and the bone is released with a gentle twist of the osteotome. (From Darrow DH, Weiss DD. Management of sleep-related breathing disorders in children. Oper Tech Otolaryngol Head Neck Surg 2002;13:111–18.) B, Application of an intraoral mandibular distractor. (From Allen GC. Mandibular distraction osteogenesis for neonatal airway obstruction. Oper Tech Otolaryngol Head Neck Surg 2005;16:187–93.)

away from the inferior alveolar nerve bundle. Lateral, superior, and inferior aspects of the mandible are cut, leaving the mid portion of the lingual cortex intact. An osteotome placed into the cuts and gently twisted completes the medial osteotomy.

4. For external devices, one or two pins are placed on either side of the osteotomy, depending on the distractor used (Fig. 63.15A). A 25-gauge needle is used to mark the insertion sites on the skin, which is injected with local anesthetic. A 5–10 mm incision is made for the pin(s) through which blunt dissection is performed parallel to the marginal nerve until the exposed mandible is encountered. A drill guide is placed through the incision until it is in contact with the bone 5–8 mm from

## REFERENCES

1. O'Brien LM, Sitha S, Baur LA, Waters KA. Obesity increases the risk for persisting obstructive sleep apnea after treatment in children. Int J Pediatr Otorhinolaryngol 2006;70:1555–60.
2. Tauman R, Gozal D. Obesity and obstructive sleep apnea in children. Paediatr Respir Rev 2006;7:247–59.
3. Schechter MS. Section on Pediatric Pulmonology. Subcommittee on Obstructive Sleep Apnea Syndrome. Technical report: diagnosis and management of childhood obstructive sleep apnea syndrome. Pediatrics 2002;109:e69.
4. Owen GO, Canter RJ, Robinson A. Snoring, apnoea, and ENT symptoms in the paediatric community. Clin Otolaryngol 1996;21:130–34.
5. Kwok KL, Ng DK, Cheung YF. BP and arterial distensibility in children with primary snoring. Chest 2003;123:1561–6.
6. Gozal D. Sleep disordered breathing and school performance in children. Pediatrics 1998;102:616–20.

7. Section on Pediatric Pulmonology. Subcommittee on Obstructive Sleep Apnea Syndrome. Clinical Practice Guideline: Diagnosis and Management of Childhood Obstructive Sleep Apnea Syndrome. Pediatrics 2002;109:704–12.
8. Goh DY, Galster P, Marcus CL. Sleep architecture and respiratory disturbances in children with obstructive sleep apnea. Am J Respir Crit Care Med 2000;162:682–6.
9. Marcus CL, Rosen G, Ward SL, et al. Adherence to and effectiveness of positive airway pressure therapy in children with obstructive sleep apnea. Pediatrics 2006;117:e442–51.
10. Biavati MJ, Manning SC, Phillips DL. Predictive factors for respiratory complications after tonsillectomy and adenoidectomy in children. Arch Otolaryngol Head Neck Surg 1997;123:517–21.
11. Rosen GM, Muckle RP, Mahowald MW, et al. Postoperative respiratory compromise in children with obstructive sleep apnea syndrome: can it be anticipated?. Pediatrics 1994;93:784–8.
12. Van Den Abbeele T, Francois M, Narcy P. Transnasal endoscopic treatment of choanal atresia without prolonged stenting. Arch Otolaryngol Head Neck Surg 2002;128:936–40.
13. Kubba H, Bennett A, Bailey CM. An update on choanal atresia surgery at Great Ormond Street Hospital for Children: preliminary results with Mitomycin C and the KTP laser. Int J Pediatr Otorhinolaryngol 2004;68:939–45.
14. Cotton RT. Nasopharyngeal stenosis. Arch Otolaryngol 1995;111:146–48.
15. Suen JS, Arnold JE, Brooks LJ. Adenotonsillectomy for treatment of obstructive sleep apnea in children. Arch Otolaryngol Head Neck Surg 1995;121:525–30.
16. Mora R, Salami A, Passali FM, et al. OSAS in children. Int J Pediatr Otorhinolaryngol 2003;67(Suppl 1):S229–31.
17. Mitchell RB, Kelly J. Outcome of adenotonsillectomy for severe obstructive sleep apnea in children. Int J Pediatr Otorhinolaryngol 2004;68:1375–79.
18. Mitchell RB, Kelly J. Adenotonsillectomy for obstructive sleep apnea in obese children. Otolaryngol Head Neck Surg 2004;131:104–8.
19. Stewart MG, Glaze DG, Friedman EM, et al. Quality of life and sleep study findings after adenotonsillectomy in children with obstructive sleep apnea. Arch Otolaryngol Head Neck Surg 2005;131:308–334.
20. De Serres LM, Derkay C, Sie K, et al. Impact of adenotonsillectomy on quality of life in children with obstructive sleep disorders. Arch Otolaryngol Head Neck Surg 2002;128:489–96.
21. Krespi YP, Ling EH. Laser-assisted serial tonsillectomy. J Otolaryngol 1994;23:325–7.
22. Koltai PJ, Solares CA, Mascha EJ. Xu M. Intracapsular 'partial' tonsillectomy for pediatric tonsillar hypertrophy. Laryngoscope 2002;112(8 Pt 2):17–19.
23. Derkay CS, Darrow DH, Welch C, Sinacori JT. Post-tonsillectomy morbidity and quality of life in pediatric patients with obstructive tonsils and adenoid: microdebrider vs. electrocautery. Otolaryngol Head Neck Surg 2006;134:114–20.
24. Lister MT, Cunningham MJ, Benjamin B, et al. Microdebrider tonsillotomy vs. electrosurgical tonsillectomy: a randomized, double-blind, paired control study of postoperative pain. Arch Otolaryngol Head Neck Surg 2006;132:599–604.
25. Mixson CM, Weinberger PM, Austin MB. Comparison of microdebrider subcapsular tonsillectomy to harmonic scalpel and electrocautery total tonsillectomy. Am J Otolaryngol 2007;28:13–17.
26. Sobol SE, Wetmore RF, Marsh RR, et al. Postoperative recovery after microdebrider intracapsular or monopolar electrocautery tonsillectomy: a prospective, randomized, single-blinded study. Arch Otolaryngol Head Neck Surg 2006;132:270–74.
27. Shott SR. Suspension or Repose® genioglossus advancement – surgical treatment of OSA beyond T&A. Presented at the Annual Meeting of the American Society of Pediatric Otolaryngology, San Diego, CA, April 2007.
28. Miller FR, Watson D, Boseley M. The role of the Genial Bone Advancement Trephine system in conjunction with uvulopalatopharyngoplasty in the multilevel management of obstructive sleep apnea. Otolaryngol Head Neck Surg 2004;130:73–9.
29. Grimmer JF, Mulliken JB, Burrows PE, Rahbar R. Radiofrequency ablation of microcystic lymphatic malformation in the oral cavity. Arch Otolaryngol Head Neck Surg 2006;132:1251–6.
30. Li KK, Powell NB, Riley RW, Guilleminault C. Temperature-controlled radiofrequency tongue base reduction for sleep disordered breathing: long-term outcomes. Otolaryngol Head Neck Surg 2002;127:230–34.
31. Maturo SC, Mair EA. Submucosal minimally invasive lingual excision: an effective, novel surgery for pediatric tongue base reduction. Ann Otol Rhinol Laryngol 2006;115:624–30.
32. Alomari AI, Karian VE, Lord DJ, et al. Percutaneous sclerotherapy for lymphatic malformations: a retrospective analysis of patient-evaluated improvement. J Vasc Interv Radiol 2006;17:1639–48.
33. Waner M, Suen JY. Treatment options for the management of vascular malformations. In: Hemangiomas and Vascular Malformations of the Head and Neck. Waner M, Suen JY, eds. New York: Wiley-Liss; 1998, pp. 315–47.
34. Kirschner RE, Low DW, Randall P, et al. Surgical airway management in Pierre Robin sequence: is there a role for tongue–lip adhesion? Cleft Palate Craniofac J 2003;40:13–18.
35. Sidman JD, Sampson D, Templeton B. Distraction osteogenesis of the mandible for airway obstruction in children. Laryngoscope 2001;111:1137–46.
36. Imola MJ, Hamlar DD, Thatcher G, Chowdury K. The versatility of distraction osteogenesis in craniofacial surgery. Arch Facial Plast Surg 2002;4:8–19.
37. Imola MJ, Tatum SA. Craniofacial distraction osteogenesis. Facial Plast Surg Clin North Am 2002;10:287–301.
38. Mandell DL, Yellon RF, Bradley JP, et al. Mandibular distraction for micrognathia and severe upper airway obstruction. Arch Otolaryngol Head Neck Surg 2004;130:344–48.

SECTION O   PEDIATRIC OSAHS

CHAPTER 64

# Obstructive sleep apnea in children with adenotonsillar hypertrophy

*Soichiro Miyazaki and Min Yin*

Obstructive sleep apnea (OSA) is a common and serious cause of morbidity during childhood. It affects 1–3% of children of 2–8 years old. However, habitual snoring during sleep is a much more frequent occurrence and affects up to 27% of children, with a decrease in frequency in 9 to 14 year olds. OSA in children presents some characteristics which differ from those in adults. Adenotonsillar hypertrophy (Fig. 64.1) is the most frequent causative disease according to our recent experience (Table 64.1). In addition, OSA results in some specific features (Table 64.2), which may only be observed in children. Furthermore, the correlation between OSA and sudden infant death syndrome (SIDS), and ALTE (apparent life-threatening event) in infants should be addressed further.

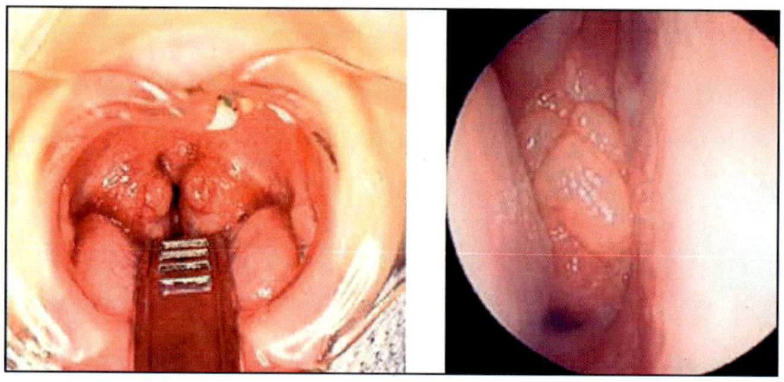

## 1 DIAGNOSIS OF DYSPNEA IN CHILDREN

Polysomnographic diagnosis is usually necessary for adults, in whom clinical symptoms will be presented when there are more than five apneas per hour, or over 30 times in 7 hours of sleep. In the case of children, apnea-like symptoms may be observed even when there is continuous hypoventilation, but not a typical apnea. We measured the esophageal pressure (Peso) to evaluate the respiratory efforts in children with adenotonsillar hypertrophy and OSA, and discovered that the degree of Peso increased even without apnea when in deep sleep (Fig. 64.3). Therefore, because the measurement of polysomnography (PSG) in a child is difficult, and also because of the specific characteristic of children's OSA, the diagnostic criterion of PSG is still unclear in children, especially in infants.

Monitoring oxygen saturation during sleep seems to be valid. The degree of stenosis in airways can be detected by profile roentgen film (Fig. 64.4), or by direct observation

**Fig. 64.1** Adenotonsillar hypertrophy observed by fiberscope.

| Table 64.1 The causative diseases of obstructive sleep dyspnea in children | |
|---|---|
| Hypertrophy of tonsil and adenoid | 88.9% |
| Habitual angina | 3.7% |
| Nasal allergy | 2.5% |
| Sudden infant death syndrome | 1.2% |
| Hunter–Hurler syndrome | 1.2% |
| Niemann–Pick's disease | 1.2% |
| Prader–Willi syndrome | 1.2% |

| Table 64.2 Typical features of OSA in children |
|---|
| Adenoid face |
| Mouth-breathing |
| Chest deformity (Fig. 64.2) |
| Snoring and apnea |
| Supraclavicular and intercostals retractions |
| Sweating |
| Late awaking, or forced awaking |
| Longer daytime sleep, sleepiness |
| Late asleep |
| Sudden awakening |
| Bed wetting or its recurrence |
| Abnormal behavior |
| Poor academic achievement |

CHAPTER 64

Obstructive sleep apnea in children with adenotonsillar hypertrophy

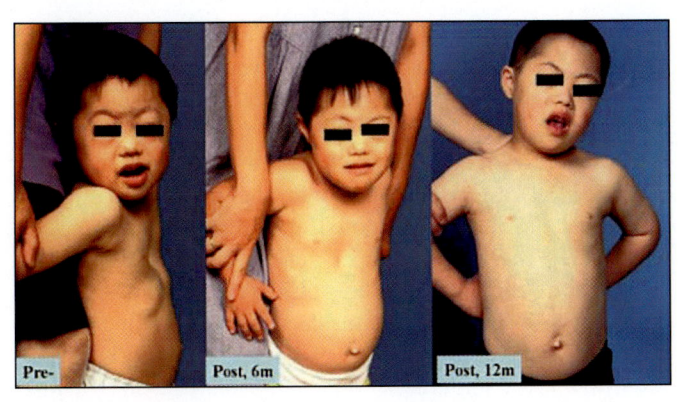

**Fig. 64.2** Chest deformity pre- and post-adenoidectomy. A case of a 5-year-old boy (preoperation) with severe obstructive sleep apnea. The chest deformity improved obviously after 6 months and 12 months of adenotonsillectomy.

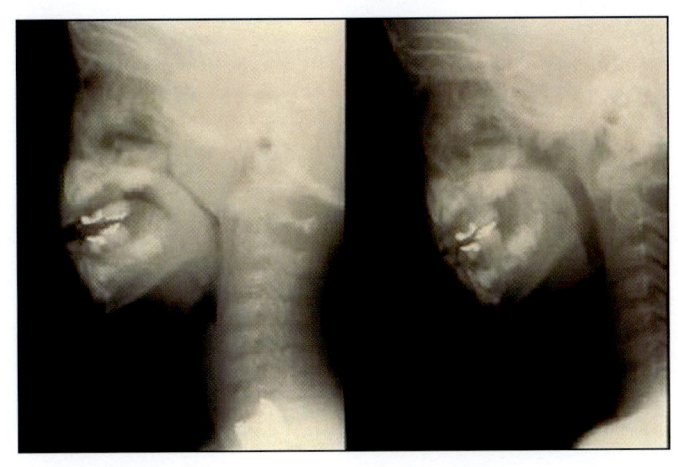

**Fig. 64.4** Profile roentgen film of upper airway in children pre- and post-adenotonsillectomy.

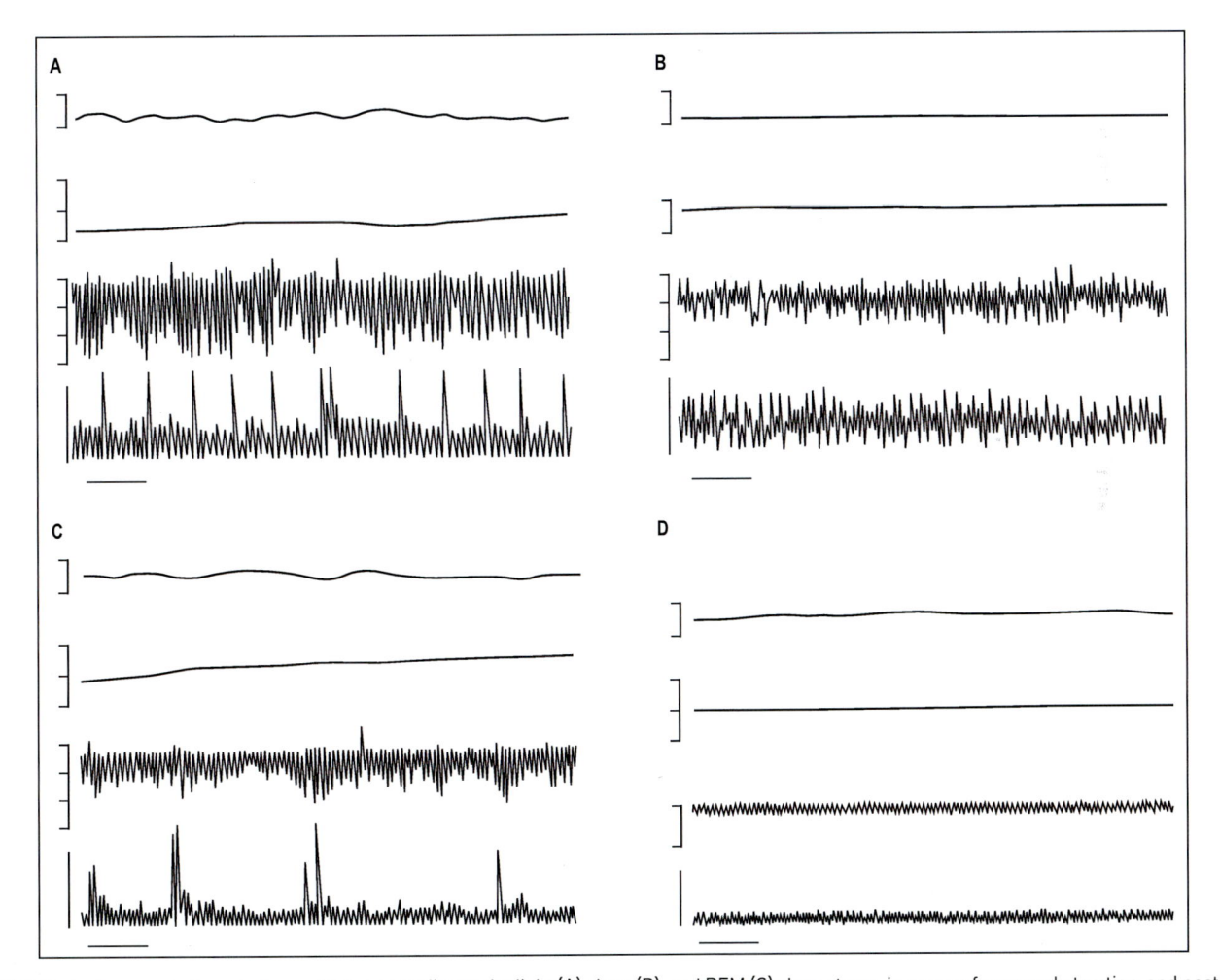

**Fig. 64.3** Typical presurgical respiratory patterns according to the light (A), deep (B), and REM (C) sleep stages in a case of severe obstruction, and postsurgical respiratory pattern during light sleep (D).

under a thin flexible fiberscope. A video camera is nowadays available in many families. A video record is also useful in observing respiratory situations, and even in cases without obvious desaturation, apnea could be found.

In 37 children with adenotonsillar hypertrophy, we inv estigated the thickness of adenoid, size of the airway space, and the lowest saturation during sleep. The lowest saturation was correlated to neither adenoid thickness nor airway

415

space (Fig. 64.5). The grade of upper airway stenosis by adenoid or tonsillar hypertrophy on profile roentgen films could not predict the severity of apnea during sleep. For precise diagnosis of respiratory severity caused by adenoid–tonsillar hypertrophy, video observation with simultaneous $SpaO_2$ monitoring is necessary. However, this result did not suggest that roentgenic measurement of stenosis is meaningless. When severe hypertrophy of the tonsil and adenoid is recognized, the possible existence of respiratory impairment should be investigated out of caution. Even in cases with moderate hypertrophy, severe apnea could be a possible accompaniment.

On the other hand, the adenoid and tonsil keep growing after birth until around 8 years old. Although the airway space in the pharynx also becomes larger, the ratio of adenotonsillar thickness to airway space reaches its peak at 4–6 years old. A previous study pointed out that children with OSA showed severe hypertrophy at younger ages (less than 3 years), which differed significantly compared to physiological hypertrophy of normal children (Fig. 64.6). Earlier surgical treatments are necessary for these cases.

## 2 TREATMENTS

Antibiotics and other anti-inflammatory medicines are sometimes applied, only for acute nasal obstruction. Anti-allergic treatment is also necessary. We experienced a case of apnea cured by controlling a nasal allergy in a 4-year-old boy with 3–10 second apnea, observed from 2 years old. Nasal allergic signs could be inspected, with the tonsil of 1°, and moderate adenoid. His bedroom was north-facing and relatively damp. After changing the bedroom to the south side with more sunshine, the allergic symptoms improved and the episodes of sleep apnea disappeared.

In cases of repeated upper airway inflammation, tonsil hypertrophy and adenoid face, positive surgery can be considered. Adenoidectomy and tonsillectomy are the first choices for children with OSA. These procedures are relatively simple with a low complication rate, and usually result in a cure. However, the decision to operate should be made not according to the roentgen degree of adenotonsillar hypertrophy, but based on good observation of sleep situations, as well as saturation monitoring. Mandibular distraction osteogenesis is applicable only for children with craniofacial deformities, for which it has better long-term effects. Tracheotomy is also appropriate for some children with severe obesity.

Nasal continuous positive airway pressure (CPAP) is usually the second-line treatment for children who do not respond to adenoidectomy and tonsillectomy, or when adenoidectomy and tonsillectomy are not indicated. In children with heavy obesity, weight reduction should be tried before surgical treatment. Lateral and prone positions are helpful in the relief of apnea. It is important to give instruction on sleep position in addition.

## 3 RECENT ADVANCEMENTS IN ADENOIDECTOMY AND TONSILLECTOMY

Traditional adenoidectomy is performed by the Le Force method or Beckmann method. These approaches were well applied for decades, and were recognized as useful. However, some complications were observed, such as the difficulty in total resection, injuries to the soft tissues of the Eustachian tube orifice, the posterior wall of the epipharynx and the soft palate, and bleeding during and after the operation. In order to improve these problems, new procedures have been developed.

### 3.1 MICRODEBRIDER ADENOIDECTOMY

The microdebrider system (Fig. 64.7) was applied in adenoidectomy. The probe of the microdebrider is curved about 30° ahead and is inserted through an oral approach, with access to the adenoid from behind the soft palate. The operation is carried out under direct vision using an endoscope from a nasal approach. Numerous advantages of microdebrider over traditional techniques have been cited, including reduced operation time (by nearly 5 minutes), decreased intraoperative and postoperative bleeding,

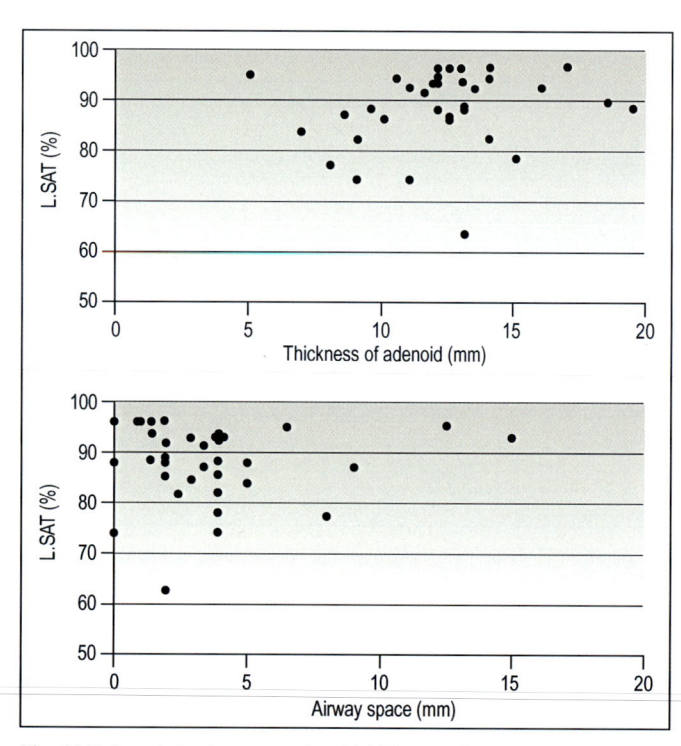

**Fig. 64.5** Correlation between adenoid thickness, airway space and lowest saturation. No significant relationship was recognized.

Obstructive sleep apnea in children with adenotonsillar hypertrophy

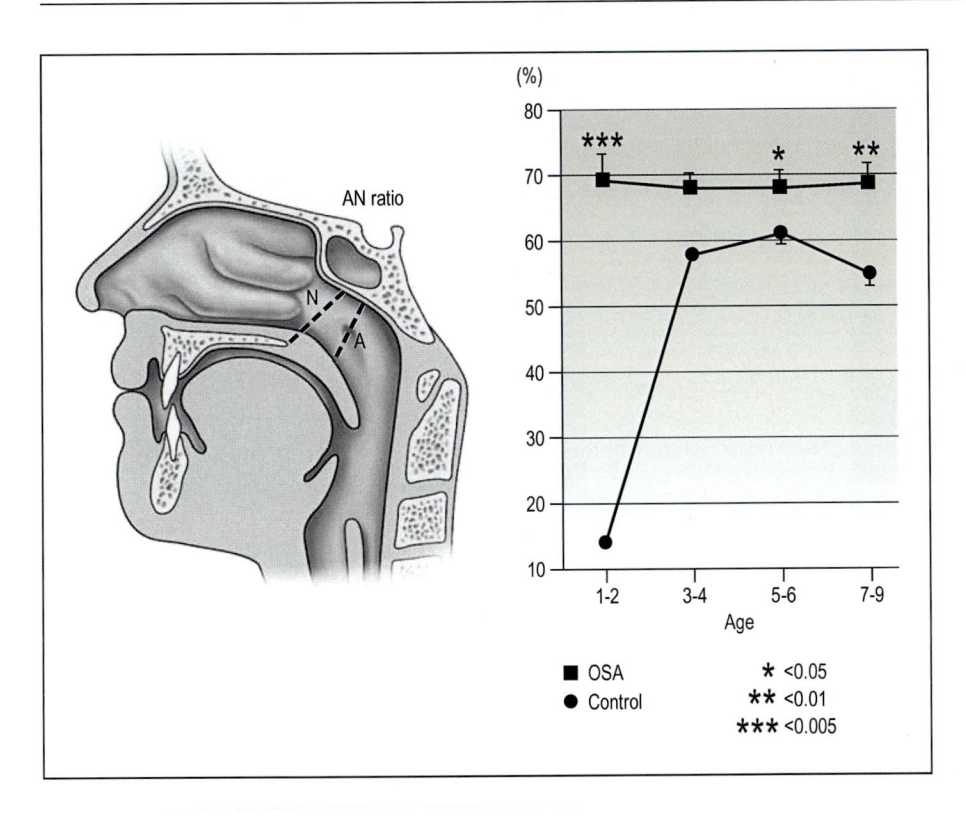

CHAPTER 64

**Fig. 64.6** Adenoid size was already large enough to induce sleep dyspnea in sleep apnea children less than 3 years old compared with a control group (Shintani et al. 1997).

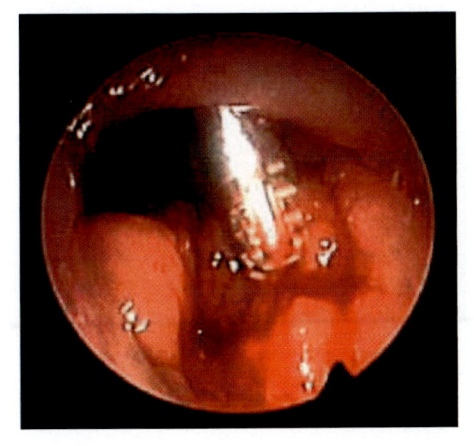

**Fig. 64.7** Microdebrider system in adenoidectomy.

improved visualization and precision for tissue removal, and an overall faster wound healing. The soft tissues around the torus tubalis and posterior nasal aperture could be ablated more easily and safely than in the traditional approach.

## 3.2 SUCTION COAGULATOR ADENOIDECTOMY

The suction coagulation system was another recommended method. In this approach, the soft palate should be elevated first by a catheter. The operation is under direct observation by 70° endoscope. The probe is appropriately angled in the tip (Fig. 64.8), and is inserted into the adenoid from an oral approach. After several seconds of electrification (with output being regulated between 30 and 45 W), the adenoid tissue is then coagulated and sucked out. The probe is pulled out after stopping the electrical charge, and then inserted again for coagulation. Coagulation should be performed from lateral to midline when around the torus tubalis, and from superior to inferior when near the posterior nasal aperture. Thus, a thorough removal of the adenoid can be ensured with little injury to the surrounding tissue. The operation may be completed when the epipharynx can be viewed from the posterior nasal aperture after careful hemostasis.

## 3.3 COBLATION TONSILLECTOMY

The conventional management of tonsillectomy was performed. Nowadays, intracapsular tonsillectomy can be performed by a variety of technical means, such as cold dissection, electrocautery, microbipolar and radiofrequency. Coblation tonsillectomy has been recently introduced in clinical practice. Using this method, only the mucosa at the superior pole is to be incised by a surgical knife. Afterwards, dissection of the tonsil can be performed by alternatively applying dissection and coagulation models of the coblation system (Fig. 64.9).

## 4 EFFICACY OF SURGICAL TREATMENT

We use a sleep diary to evaluate the efficacy of the treatment. Figure 64.10 is a typical sleep diary of a boy with

SECTION 0 PEDIATRIC OSAHS

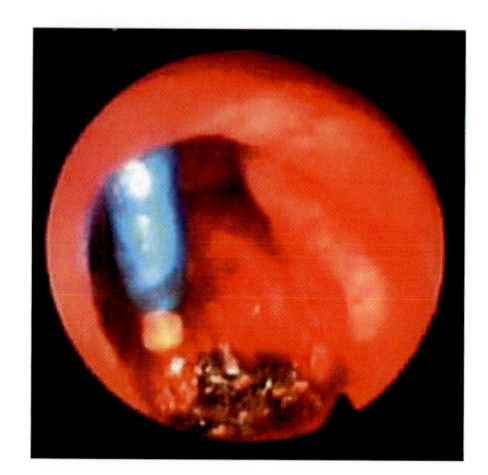

Fig. 64.8 Suction coagulation system.

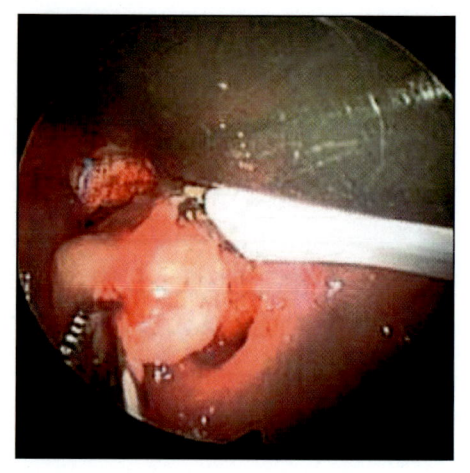

Fig. 64.9 Coblation-assisted tonsillectomy.

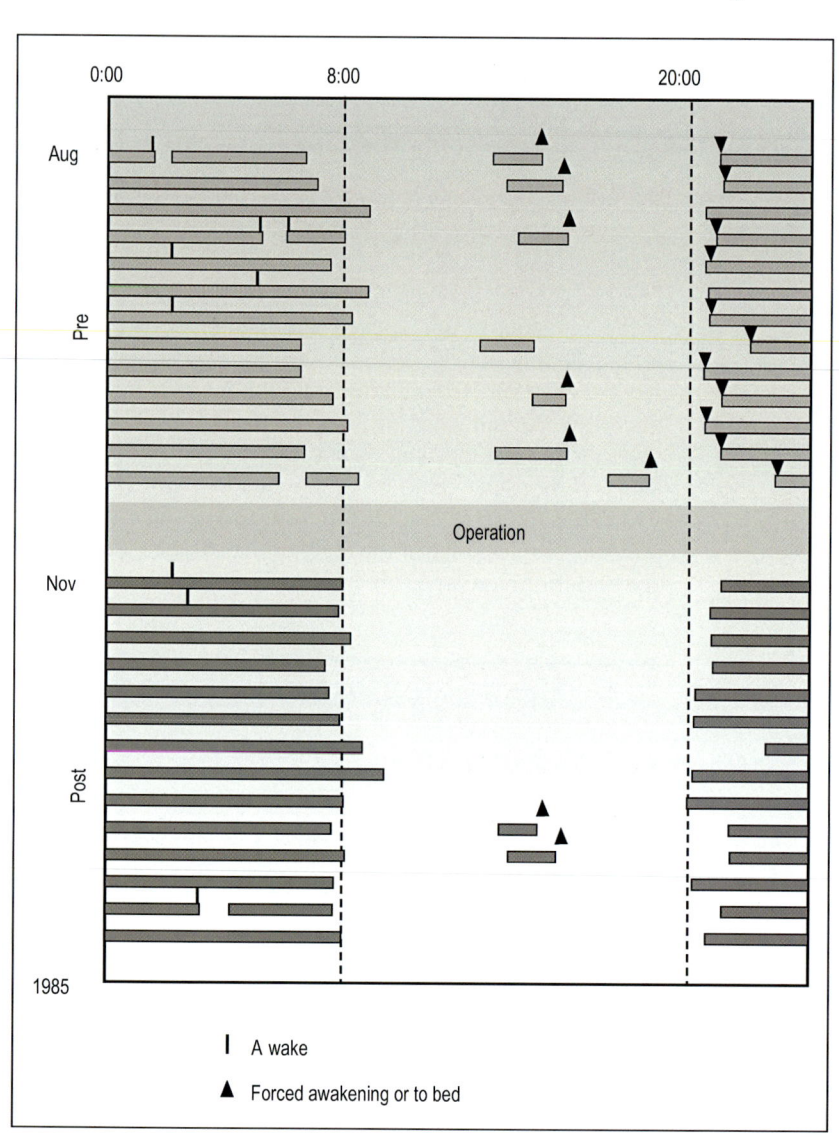

Fig. 64.10 A typical sleep diary of a boy with a moderate OSA pre- and postoperation.

moderate OSA, pre- and postoperation. Before surgery, the boy consistently avoided going to bed at night, fighting desperately against sleep. As a consequence, his mother usually had to force him to go to bed at night. He sometimes awoke during the night. His time of awakening was very irregular in the morning. In the day time, he often took long naps. After surgery, many of these problems disappeared and his night sleep became undisturbed.

418

Obstructive sleep apnea in children with adenotonsillar hypertrophy

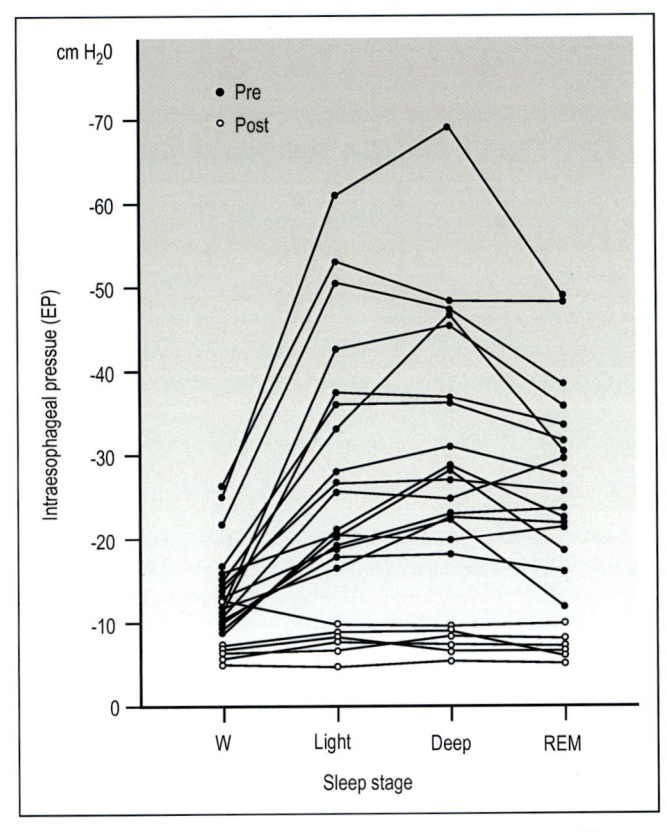

**Fig. 64.11** Esophageal pressure levels before and after adenotonsillectomy.

**Table 64.3** Surgical effects on sleep in adenoid–tonsillar hypertrophy (n = 15)

| | Preoperation (%) | Postoperation (%) 6 months | 12 months | 2–5 years |
|---|---|---|---|---|
| Snoring | 100 | 7 | 14 | 8 |
| Difficulty of sleep onset | 60 | 0 | 7 | 15 |
| Intermittent awakenings | 67 | 0 | 0 | 0 |
| Body movement | 80 | 28 | 28 | 38 |
| No spontaneous awakenings | 93 | 14 | 15 | 15 |
| Somnolence | 57 | 7 | 7 | 8 |

Figure 64.11 shows the Peso pattern according to sleep stages in 15 cases of adenoid–tonsillar hypertrophy. Six of them underwent tonsillectomy adenoidectomy. Their postoperative Peso levels decreased significantly in comparison with preoperative levels. Figure 64.3 shows typical changes of respiratory dynamics in different sleep stages in a boy with severe OSA.

Long-term surgical effects in the sleep situation were noted (Table 64.3). Before the operation, 90–100% of patients showed difficulty in spontaneous awakening, reporting snoring or impaired breathing. These symptoms decreased to 10–20% after surgery. Improvement of chest deformity could also be observed (see Fig. 64.2).

## FURTHER READING

Abou-Jaoude PM, Manoukian JJ, Daniel SJ, et al. Complications of adenotonsillectomy revisited in a large pediatric case series. J Otolaryngol 2006;35:180–85.

Anand A, Vilela RJ, Guarisco JL. Intracapsular versus standard tonsillectomy: review of literature. J La State Med Soc 2005;157:259–61.

Bellosa A, Chidambaram A, Morar P, et al. Coblation tonsillectomy versus dissection tonsillectomy: postoperative hemorrhage. Laryngoscope 2003;113:450–52.

Cohen SR, Simms C, Burstein FD. Mandibular distraction osteogenesis in the treatment of upper airway obstruction in children with craniofacial deformities. Plast Reconstr Surg 1998;101:312–18.

Coticchia JM, Yun RD, Nelson L, Koempel J. Temperature-controlled radiofrequency treatment of tonsillar hypertrophy for reduction of upper airway obstruction in pediatric patients. Arch Otolaryngol Head Neck Surg 2006;132:425–30.

Friedman M, LoSavio P, Ibrahim H, Ramakrishnan V. Radiofrequency tonsil reduction: safety, morbidity, and efficacy. Laryngoscope 2003;113:882–7.

Hoffmann HJ, Damus K, Hillman L, et al. Risk factors for SIDS: results of the National Institute of Child Health and Human Development SIDS cooperative epidemiological study. Ann NY Acad Sci 1988;533:13–30.

Hultcrantz E, Linder A, Markstrom A. Long-term effects of intracapsular partial tonsillectomy (tonsillotomy) compared with full tonsillectomy. Int J Pediatr Otorhinolaryngol 2005;69:463–9.

Koltai PJ, Solares CA, Koempel JA, et al. Intracapsular tonsillar reduction (partial tonsillectomy): reviving a historical procedure for obstructive sleep disordered breathing in children. Otolaryngol Head Neck Surg 2003;129:532–8.

Lister MT, Cunningham MJ, Benjamin B, et al. Microdebrider tonsillotomy vs. electrosurgical tonsillectomy: a randomized, double-blind, paired control study of postoperative pain.. Arch Otolaryngol Head Neck Surg 2006;132:599–604.

Mandell DL, Yellon RF, Bradley JP, et al. Mandibular distraction for micrognathia and severe upper airway obstruction. Arch Otolaryngol Head Neck Surg 2004;130:344–8.

Miyazaki S. Sleep-induced respiratory disturbance in children with adenotonsillar hypertrophy: the obstructive sleep dyspnea syndrome. Operat Tech Otolaryngol Head Neck Surg 1991;2:69–72.

Miyazaki S, Itasaka Y, Yamakawa K, et al. respiratory disturbance during sleep due to adenoid–tonsil hypertrophy. Am J Oto 1989;10:143–9.

Nunez DA, Provan J, Crawford M. Postoperative tonsillectomy pain in pediatric patients: electrocautery (hot) vs. cold dissection and snare tonsillectomy – a randomized trial. Arch Otolaryngol Head Neck Surg 2000;126:837–41.

Shintani T, Asakura K, Kataura A. Evaluation of the role of adenotonsillar hypertrophy and facial morphology in children with obstructive sleep apnea. ORL 1997;59:286–91.

Temple RH, Timms MS. Paediatric coblation tonsillectomy. Int J Pediatr Otorhinolaryngol 2001;61:195–8.

Timms MS, Temple RH. Coblation tonsillectomy: a double blind randomized controlled study. J Laryngol Otol 2002;116:450–52.

Wynn R, Rosenfeld RM. Outcomes in suction coagulator adenoidectomy. Arch Otolaryngol Head Neck Surg 2003;129:182–5.

# SECTION O  PEDIATRIC OSAHS

## CHAPTER 65

# The effect of polysomnography on pediatric adenotonsillectomy postoperative management

*Anthony A. Rieder, Stacey L. Ishman and Valerie Flanary*

## 1 INTRODUCTION

Sleep disordered breathing (SDB) often presents in the pediatric population with loud snoring, respiratory pauses and mouth-breathing. For those with enlarged adenoids or tonsils, adenotonsillectomy can be curative. The decision for surgery is based upon the clinical history and physical examination. The polysomnogram is the gold standard for diagnosis of SDB, however, it is costly, time limiting and often not readily available and it is unclear which patient groups require or benefit from its use preoperatively.[1,2] Several studies have identified populations at high risk for postoperative complications including children with craniofacial disorders, failure to thrive, neurological impairment, Down syndrome, obstructive sleep apnea and children age 3 or less.[3–7] Because of the increased risk, preoperative polysomnography and postoperative overnight observation have been recommended for these patients to differentiate primary snoring from obstructive sleep apnea.[8,9] In addition, several authors have concluded that polysomnographic results are predictive of postoperative complications and postoperative course.[3–5,7] A recent retrospective study is summarized here which reviewed the postoperative course of children 3 years of age and younger and correlated these findings with the severity of obstruction as measured by preoperative polysomnogram.

## 2 PATIENT SELECTION

Children 3 years of age and younger who underwent tonsillectomy or adenotonsillectomy at The Children's Hospital of Wisconsin from July 1997 to July 2002. Procedures were performed by attending surgeons or by a resident with attending supervision.

## 3 OUTLINE OF METHODS

Data were extracted from each patient's medical chart and included: preoperative polysomnography results, admitting diagnosis, surgeon, medical co-morbidities, length of stay, postoperative complications and associated interventions. In addition, postoperative progress notes were reviewed to identify the general postoperative course for each patient as well as any information that could be attributed to the medical decision-making process. Patients were grouped based on whether or not they had undergone preoperative polysomnography (PSG). The average length of stay (LOS) was used as an objective indicator for evaluating the postoperative course in subject groups.

## 4 RESULTS

The charts for 305 children age 3 years of age or younger were reviewed. Twenty-three children were excluded from the study for the following: incomplete chart ($n = 8$), procedure miscoded ($n = 2$), additional procedures performed ($n = 5$), or procedure performed during period of acute illness ($n = 8$). The remaining 282 sets of patient data were included in the statistical analysis. The average age was 30 months. Table 65.1 summarizes the age distribution. Upper airway obstruction was identified as the primary indication for surgery in 271 of the patients.

Sleep studies, including complete 16-channel ($n = 38$), 4-channel ($n = 3$), or hardcopy pulse oximetry ($n = 2$), were performed preoperatively in 43 patients. The average age of patients that had a preoperative PSG was significantly younger at 25.9 months, compared to 31.1 months in the non-PSG group ($P < 0.0001$). Twenty-seven patients were classified to have obstructive sleep apnea (OSA) (Respiratory Disturbance Index [RDI] ranged from 1 to 52) and

11 were classified to have upper airway resistance syndrome (UARS). UARS was defined as abnormally increased upper airway resistance during sleep that led to increased respiratory effort and sleep fragmentation without defined apneic or hypopneic episodes or notable oxygen desaturations.[10] Sleep studies without a calculated RDI or UARS were classified as normal, mildly abnormal, or significantly abnormal by the pulmonologist reading the study.

When the subjects were grouped using their RDI as a measure of OSA severity, there was no statistical difference between the average length of stay (LOS) for OSA patients. The average LOS for patients with UARS (2.2 days) was significantly longer when compared to the average LOS stay (1.57 days) for patients with OSA ($P = 0.0448$). The average LOS, when calculated by age group in the non-PSG and PSG groups, was less in the non-PSG group at 1.06 days compared to 1.98 days in the PSG group ($P < 0.0001$). The shortest average LOS occurred in the 37–47 month age distribution in both groups. The average LOS for both groups is listed in Table 65.2. The discharge criteria for patients typically required that the patients not require any supplemental oxygen and were able to maintain oxygen saturations above 90% without periods of sustained desaturation attributed to upper airway obstruction.

Complications were identified in 62 patients (21.9%). For this study, a complication was defined as any documented desaturation event (regardless of $SaO_2$ nadir) or any other event/complication that required medical intervention or readmission, or prolonged the patient's LOS. Complications occurred in 43 of 239 patients (17.9%) in the non-PSG group, and in 19 patients of 43 (44.2%) in the PSG group. Of those 62 patients, the most common complication identified was oxygen desaturation representing 65.1% of the total complications in the non-PSG group and 57.9% in the PSG group. Overall, desaturation events occurred in 13.8% ($n = 39$) of the entire study population. Complications for each group are listed in Table 65.3.

Table 65.4 lists the total complications and LOS by age group for the 62 patients with complications. The highest complication rate (32.8%) was found in children of 24 months and younger, while the lowest rate (8.1%) occurred in the group aged 37–47 months. There was no statistical difference in the mean age of the patients who had complications in the PSG group (26.5 months) compared to the non-PSG group (27.2 months) ($P = 0.7279$). The average LOS for patients with complications in the non-PSG group was 1.74 days compared to 2.63 days in the PSG group. A trend toward a longer average LOS was identified in the PSG group but the difference did not reach statistical significance ($P = 0.0997$).

Co-morbidities and associated medical conditions were identified in 88 patients. The most common conditions are listed in Table 65.5. Fifty-seven (23.8%) of the non-PSG patients were found to have co-morbidities, compared to 31 (72%) patients in the PSG group. Notably, 11 of 43 patients (25.5%) with complications in the non-PSG had co-morbidities compared to 14 of 19 patients (73.6%) with complications in the PSG group.

## 5 DISCUSSION

Sleep disordered breathing and habitual snoring are common in the pediatric population with a reported prevalence

Table 65.1 Age distribution

| Age (months) | Total study group | Sleep study | No sleep study |
|---|---|---|---|
| 0–24 | 67 | 18 | 49 |
| 25–36 | 141 | 20 | 121 |
| 37–47 | 74 | 5 | 69 |
| Total | 282 | 43 | 239 |
| Average age (months) | 30.2 | 25.9 | 31.1 |

From Rieder AA, Flanary V. The effect of polysomnography on pediatric adenotonsillectomy postoperative management. Otolaryngol Head Neck Surg 2005;132(2):263–7.

Table 65.2 Average length of stay

| Age distribution (months) | Sleep study group — No. of patients | Sleep study group — Average length of stay (days) | No sleep study group — No. of patients | No sleep study group — Average length of stay (days) | P value |
|---|---|---|---|---|---|
| 0–24 | 18 | 2.0 | 49 | 1.3 | 0.0048 |
| 25–36 | 20 | 2.1 | 121 | 1.1 | 0.0018 |
| 37–47 | 5 | 1.4 | 69 | .81 | 0.0126 |
| Total | 43 | 1.98 | 239 | 1.06 | 0.0001 |

From Rieder AA, Flanary V. The effect of polysomnography on pediatric adenotonsillectomy postoperative management. Otolaryngol Head Neck Surg 2005;132(2):263–7.

between 4–11% and 10–15% respectively.[11,12] Upper airway obstruction (UAO) secondary to adenotonsillar hypertrophy is noted to be the primary cause of sleep disordered breathing in children, and has replaced recurrent tonsillitis as the most common indication for pediatric adenotonsillectomy.[13] Adenotonsillectomy is considered the primary surgical treatment option for children with obstructive sleep disorders, having been shown to improve sleep, breathing, PSG results, enuresis and patient quality of life.[14,15]

Several studies have compared formal PSG to the clinical diagnosis of OSA.[16,17] These studies showed that the two correlate poorly; however, they were completed before there was a clear consensus on the definition of pediatric OSA and prior to recognition of UARS, making it hard to draw any conclusions. In actual practice, the decision to perform an adenotonsillectomy is often made based upon clinical history and physical exam without the benefit of a diagnostic sleep study. This is consistent with the findings of our study in which only 15% of the patients ($n = 43$) had a formal preoperative sleep study of any type. In children suspected of having OSA, these sleep studies have been shown to have a high predictive value.[22] Sleep studies are typically ordered for patients with co-morbidities, for patients whose clinical diagnosis is unclear or are considered to be at increased surgical risk. This trend is reflected in the data from this study in which 72% of the patients with sleep studies had other co-morbidities compared to 24% of the patients without sleep studies.

PSG has also been advocated to assist with postoperative planning and monitoring and as a method to predict the likelihood of postoperative respiratory complications after adenotonsillectomy. Several studies have looked at the risk factors associated with postoperative complications.[3–5,7] All of these studies identify age younger than 2 or 3 years of age as a significant risk factor for postoperative respiratory compromise. Other risk factors identified include craniofacial anomalies, failure to thrive, hypotonia, morbid obesity, Apnea/Hypopnea Index greater than 5 (or 10) and low preoperative oxygen saturation nadir. These are all retrospective studies which used a number of different inclusion/exclusion criteria for patients along with a variety of definitions and complication classifications.

Pediatric post-adenotonsillectomy complication rates have ranged from 0% to 32% in published series with airway issues or compromise representing 0–16% of the overall complications.[6,18–20] Those studies that were limited to younger children (3 years of age and younger) demonstrated a rate of airway complications ranging from 0% to 5%.[6,18,19] Our study compares similarly with an overall complication rate of 22%, but our rate of airway complications was higher with a rate of 14% ($n = 39$). However, it is misleading to directly compare complication rates between these studies as different airway complication definitions were used. For this study, a complication was defined as any documented desaturation event (regardless of $SaO_2$ nadir) or any other event or complication that required medical intervention or readmission, or prolonged the patient's length of hospital stay. Some studies have identified minor and major complications depending upon the intervention required[7] while other studies

**Table 65.3 Complications**

| Complication | Group with sleep study (43) No. of patients | Group without sleep study (239) No. of patients |
|---|---|---|
| Desaturation event | 11 (26%) | 28 (12%) |
| Poor oral intake | 6 (14%) | 10 (4%) |
| Pneumonia/atelectasis | 0 | 3 (1%) |
| Seizure | 0 | 1 (0.4%) |
| Bleeding | 1 (2%) | 1 (0.4%) |
| Death | 1 (2%) | 0 |
| Total no. of patients with complications | 19 (44%) | 43 (18%) |

From Rieder AA, Flanary V. The effect of polysomnography on pediatric adenotonsillectomy postoperative management. Otolaryngol Head Neck Surg 2005;132(2):263–7.

**Table 65.4 Age distribution of complications by group**

| | Total study group | | Group with sleep studies | | Group without sleep studies | |
|---|---|---|---|---|---|---|
| Age distribution (months) | No. of patients | Fraction of total complications (%) | No. of patients | Average length of stay (days) | No. of patients | Average length of stay (days) |
| 0–24 | 22 | 22/67 (32.8) | 7 | 2.28 | 15 | 1.87 |
| 25–36 | 34 | 34/141 (24.1) | 10 | 3.00 | 24 | 1.75 |
| 37–47 | 6 | 6/74 (8.1) | 2 | 2.00 | 4 | 1.25 |
| Total | 62 | | 19 | 2.63 | 43 | 1.74 |

From Rieder AA, Flanary V. The effect of polysomnography on pediatric adenotonsillectomy postoperative management. Otolaryngol Head Neck Surg 2005;132(2):263–7.

| Table 65.5 Co-morbidities | |
|---|---|
| Co-morbidity | No. of patients |
| Asthma/reactive airway disease | 25 |
| Neurologic impairment (Down syndrome, developmental delay, cerebral palsy) | 18 |
| Prematurity | 10 |
| Craniofacial anomaly or syndrome | 9 |
| Neurologic impaired swallow | 8 |
| Laryngomalacia | 6 |
| Platelet dysfunction | 6 |
| Seizure disorder | 4 |
| Other (recurrent croup, cardiac anomalies, recurrent pneumonia, reflux) | 10 |

From Rieder AA, Flanary V. The effect of polysomnography on pediatric adenotonsillectomy postoperative management. Otolaryngol Head Neck Surg 2005;132(2):263–7.

have attempted to identify complications based on the degree of airway obstruction or oxygen saturation nadir.[4,5] Furthermore, the significance of postoperative desaturations is controversial. Theoretically, a decrease in oxygen saturation may increase the postoperative patient risk; however, no stratification of desaturation events was used and no formal studies currently support this conclusion.

In this study, the correlation of SDB or UAO severity, identified on preoperative PSG, was examined versus a patient's postoperative course using average LOS as an indicator. There was no statistical difference found in average LOS when stratified by OSA severity. However, there was a statistically significant difference in the average LOS for UARS patients (2.2 days) when compared to patients with OSA (1.5 days) ($P = 0.0424$). UARS has generally been considered to be a milder form of SDB as compared to OSA; therefore, it is difficult to explain these findings. Additionally, the patients that underwent preoperative PSG had a statistically significant longer average LOS at 1.98 days compared to the patients in the non-PSG group at 1.06 days ($P < 0.0001$). This is consistent with the finding that the PSG group had a higher percentage of co-morbidities (72%) when compared to the non-PSG group (24%).

These data are tempered by the limitations intrinsic to retrospective review. It is often not possible to determine the rationale for many of the postoperative decisions that were made for each subject. The classification of respiratory complications is also difficult because the oxygen saturation nadir and duration of each desaturation event were not always recorded in the medical chart. Next, surgical technique and adjuvant therapies, such as anesthetic methods, intraoperative medications including steroids and postoperative analgesia were not controlled for and are not addressed by this study. Additionally, the local complication rate for children greater than 3 years of age was not evaluated, but instead reported complication rates from other studies were used for comparison.

## 6 CONCLUSION

This study reinforces previous data suggesting that the complication rate in children 3 years of age and younger may be higher than that in older children. However, the nature of the complications does not appear to have a large impact on the LOS of these children. This study also suggests that the 3 year old and younger group, in the absence of other co-morbidities, can safely undergo adenotonsillectomy without undergoing preoperative PSG provided these patients have close postoperative monitoring. Furthermore, the relative utility of PSG in the pediatric population is closely related to issues of cost, timing, and interpretation expertise. The average cost of overnight PSG at a qualified institution is $600–2800.[21] In addition, while home studies are valuable in the evaluation of adults, these studies have not been validated in young children and thus they continue to require overnight stays for PSG. Given this information, it may be impractical to consider performing PSG on all pediatric patients prior to adenotonsillectomy. Higher risk, as indicated by the increased LOS, for patients with co-morbidities does appear to exist and we would reserve the use of preoperative PSG for these patients and for patients with ambiguous clinical history.

The data in this study are inconclusive with regards to which medical co-morbidities and which immediate postoperative findings would mandate an overnight inpatient stay. In addition, it is unclear whether LOS is the most reliable measure of postoperative course. Also, the very conservative definition of a respiratory complication as any documented desaturation event (regardless of $SaO_2$ nadir) or any other event/complication that required medical intervention, readmission, or prolonged the patient's LOS may also have minimized the respiratory differences between the PSG and non-PSG patient groups. A prospective study that controls for the previously mentioned surgical variables, and clearly defines the timing, degree, and duration of respiratory complications and their interventions is necessary to determine if preoperative PSG is necessary for all children 3 years of age or younger. Clearly, however, preoperative PSG findings had little influence on the postoperative management of patients in this study when using patient LOS as a measure.

## REFERENCES

1. Leach J, Olson J, Hermann J, Manning S. Polysomnographic and clinical findings in children with obstructive sleep apnea. Arch Otolaryngol Head Neck Surg 1992;118:741–4.
2. Messner AH. Evaluation of obstructive sleep apnea by polysomnography prior to pediatric adenotonsillectomy. Arch Otolaryngol Head Neck Surg 1999;125:353–6.
3. Biavati MJ, Manning SC, Phillips DL. Predictive factors for respiratory complications after tonsillectomy and adenoidectomy in children. Arch Otolaryngol Head Neck Surg 1997;123:517–21.

4. McColley SA, April MM, Carroll JL, et al. Respiratory compromise after adenotonsillectomy in children with obstructive sleep apnea. Arch Otolaryngol Head Neck Surg 1992;118:940–43.
5. Rosen GM, Muckle RP, Mahowald MW, et al. Postoperative respiratory compromise in children with obstructive sleep apnea syndrome: can it be anticipated?. Pediatrics 1994;93(5):784–8.
6. Slovik Y, Tal A, Tarasiuk A, et al. Complications of adenotonsillectomy in children with OSAS younger than 2 years of age. Int J Pediatr Otorhinolaryngol 2003;67:847–51.
7. Wilson K, Lakheeram I, Morielli A, et al. Can assessment for obstructive sleep apnea predict post adenotonsillectomy respiratory complications. Anesthesiology 2002;96:313–22.
8. Section on Pediatric Pulmonology/Subcommittee on obstructive sleep apnea syndrome. Clinical practice guideline: diagnosis and management of childhood obstructive sleep apnea. Pediatrics 2002;109:704–12.
9. American Thoracic Society. Standards and indications for cardiopulmonary sleep studies in children. Am J Respir Crit Care Med 1996;153:866–78.
10. Guilleminault C, Chowdhuri S. Upper airway resistance syndrome is a distinct syndrome. Am J Respir Crit Care Med 2000;161:1412–16.
11. Messner A, Pelayo R. Pediatric sleep-related breathing disorders. Am J Otolaryngol 2000;21:98–107.
12. Guilleminault C, Pelayo R. Sleep-disordered breathing in children. Ann Med 1998;30:350–56.
13. Ross AT, Kazahaya K, Lawrence WC. Revisiting outpatient tonsillectomy in young children. Otolaryngol Head Neck Surg 2003;128(3):326–31.
14. Goldstein NA, Fatima M, Campbell TF, et al. Child behavior and quality of life before and after tonsillectomy and adenoidectomy. Arch Otolaryngol Head Neck Surg 2002;128:770–75.
15. Serres LM, Derkay C, Sie K, et al. Impact of adenotonsillectomy on quality of life in children with obstructive sleep disorders. Arch Otolaryngol Head Neck Surg 2002;128:489–96.
16. Goldstein NA, Sculerati N, Walsleben JA, et al. Clinical diagnosis of pediatric obstructive sleep apnea validated by polysomnography. Otolaryngol Head Neck Surg 1994;111(5):611–17.
17. Wang RC, Elkins TP, Keech D, Wauquier A, Hubbard D. Accuracy of clinical evaluation in pediatric obstructive sleep apnea. Otolaryngol Head Neck Surg 1998;118:69–73.
18. Berkowitz RG, Zalzal GH. Tonsillectomy in children under 3 years of age. Arch Otolaryngol Head Neck Surg 1990;116:685–6.
19. Helmus C. Tonsillectomy and adenoidectomy in the one and two-year-old child. Laryngoscope 1979;89:1764–71.
20. Postma DS, Folsom F. The case for an outpatient 'approach' for all pediatric tonsillectomies and/or adenoidectomies: a 4-year review of 1419 cases at a community hospital. Otolaryngol Head Neck Surg 2002;127:101–8.
21. Leach J, Olson J, Hermann J, Manning S. Polysomnographic and clinical findings in children with obstructive sleep apnea. Arch Otolaryngol Head Neck Surg 1992;118:741–4.
22. Brouillette RT, Morielli A, Leimanis A, et al. Nocturnal pulse oximetry as an abbreviated testing modality for pediatric obstructive sleep apnea. Pediatrics 2000;105:405–12.

# SECTION O  PEDIATRIC OSAHS

# CHAPTER 66
# Current techniques of adenoidectomy

*Peter J. Koltai and Christopher M. Discolo*

## 1 INTRODUCTION

The clinical significance of adenoid hypertrophy was not truly appreciated until the mid-19th century. This was due to their relatively inaccessible location given the technology available at that time. Once discovered, various techniques for the removal of the adenoids were developed. Some of these basic techniques have remained with us since that time.

Although commonly known for causing chronic sinonasal symptoms or influencing chronic ear disease, enlargement of the adenoids can play a prominent role in obstructive sleep apnea.

## 2 PATIENT SELECTION

Children with signs and symptoms of obstructive sleep apnea, or those with polysomnogram-proven disease, should have their adenoids evaluated as part of a routine work-up. This can be done in a number of ways. In children of just about any age, flexible fiberoptic nasopharyngoscopy provides the most direct means of evaluation. A camera and monitor attached to the scope can provide families with visual reinforcement. Alternatively, a lateral plain film of the nasopharynx can demonstrate adenoid hypertrophy and resultant compromise of the nasal air column. Although not routinely obtained to evaluate for adenoid hypertrophy, CT scans and MRIs can also demonstrate enlargement of the adenoid pad.

Adenoidectomy is usually inappropriate in children with a history of cleft palate, overt or submucous, or those with a history of velopharyngeal insufficiency. A balance between relief of obstruction and the creation of velar incompetence is crucial. Families must be counseled as to the increased risk for this important complication, even if a limited procedure is performed.

Very commonly, adenoidectomy is performed in concert with tonsillectomy as the most common surgical procedure to treat obstructive sleep apnea in children.

## 3 OUTLINE OF PROCEDURES

Various options for airway management exist and it is important for the surgical and anesthesia teams to decide on this before the procedure begins. A straight endotracheal tube, laryngeal mask airway (LMA) or oral RAE tube (Ring–Adair–Elwyn) may be used. The surgeon must consider factors such as other procedures (i.e. tonsillectomy) being performed when deciding on the type of airway management.

Historically, adenoidectomy was performed with the surgeon facing the patient, who was sitting upright. Some surgeons still currently employ an orientation similar to that of endoscopic sinus surgery. Today, the Rose position is commonly used in which the patient's head and neck are extended and the surgeon sits behind the patient. The eyes are protected and the patient is sterilely draped. A mouth gag, such as the Crowe–Davis or McGyver, is then carefully inserted into the mouth and the oropharynx is exposed. The mouth gag can be suspended per surgeon preference. The soft palate should then be visually inspected and palpated to ensure that a submucous cleft is not present. Visualization of the nasopharynx can be easily achieved using a defogged #5 laryngeal mirror and a headlight. Exposure can be enhanced using either one or two red rubber catheters. These are placed transnasally, retrieved from the oropharynx and then clamped back on themselves, effectively retracting the soft palate.

### 3.1 CURETTE ADENOIDECTOMY

The use of a curette to remove the adenoids dates back to some of the earliest attempts at this procedure and remains an incredibly popular technique worldwide. The original design of Jacob Gottenstein has been modified and many different lengths, widths and curvatures are available. The basic principle is that of a sharp horizontal knife-edge that is designed to cut through the base of the adenoid bed. The instrument is designed to follow the natural curvature of the nasopharyngeal skull base (Fig. 66.1).

The curette may be passed blindly into the nasopharynx, or the laryngeal mirrors may be used to guide the cutting edge into position. Visualization of the fossa of Rosenmuller helps guide appropriate curette size. The curette is placed against the vomer and then pushed through the adenoid tissue to the more resistant deeper layers. The handle is pulled toward the head and the surgeon's other hand acts as a fulcrum at approximately the level of the incisors. The curette is swept in an arc through the adenoid tissue until the level of Passavant's ridge, which is the inferior aspect of the dissection. After the initial pass, the adenoid bed is inspected for the completeness of the procedure. If there is residual adenoid tissue left behind, it must be removed using either a smaller curette or St Claire-Thompson forceps. A tonsil sponge is then generally placed into the nasopharynx to aid in hemostasis. These sponges may contain medications such as oxymetazoline or can be used alone. It is our preference to finalize hemostasis using a suction monopolar cautery using mirror guidance although other techniques including pressure packing, bismuth subgallate and silver nitrate have been described. Once final hemostasis is achieved, the nasopharynx and oropharynx should be irrigated and the stomach emptied of its contents prior to extubation.

## 3.2 ABLATION ADENOIDECTOMY

The widespread use of the suction monopolar cautery unit to achieve hemostasis after adenoidectomy naturally led to its use as a primary means of reducing adenoid tissue. With the patient in the Rose position, as described above, the adenoid pad is viewed with a mirror. The monopolar cautery unit, generally set at 30–40 watts, can then be shaped to fit the patient's unique anatomy. Starting at the choana and working inferiorly, the adenoids are sequentially ablated using the cautery unit (Fig. 66.2). As the tissue fluid is vaporized there is dramatic reduction in the size of the adenoid tissue. Care is taken to avoid inadvertent cautery of non-adenoidal tissue. Bleeding tends to be minimal using this technique and can be controlled with any of the methods described above.

Proponents of this technique cite its low technical difficulty, lower intraoperative blood losses, reduced operating room times and reduced cost compared to other techniques as rationale for its widespread use.

## 3.3 TRANSNASAL ADENOIDECTOMY

Essentially, two types of transnasal procedures exist. Both utilize rigid nasal endoscopes as in endoscopic sinus surgery. In traditional transnasal techniques the adenoids are

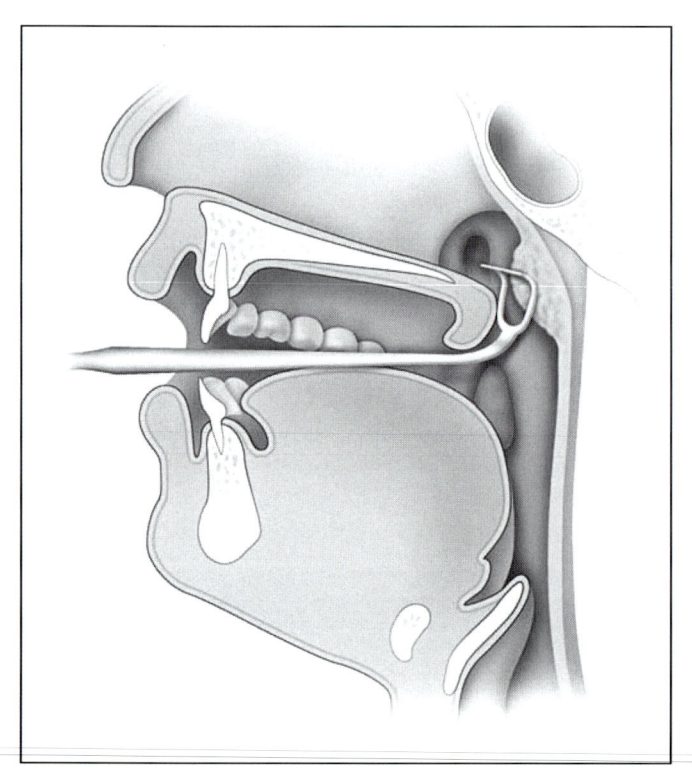

**Fig. 66.1** Placement of adenoid curette. Note how curve of instrument approximates contour of skull base for effective removal of tissue without damage to underlying structures.

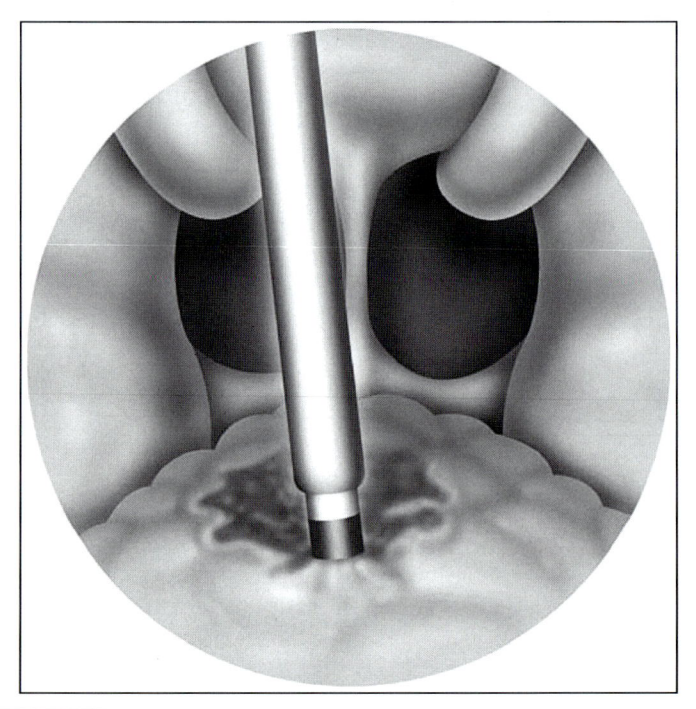

**Fig. 66.2** Ablation adenoidectomy. Under mirror visualization the adenoid pad is ablated using the suction monopolar cautery. Note ability to adequately view the choana and Eustachian tube region with this technique to avoid inadvertent injury to these structures.

removed using sinus instruments such as Blakesley forceps. More recently the soft tissue shaver has been advocated to allow more rapid removal of the adenoid tissue.

These techniques are particularly useful for adenoid tissue that prolapses into the nasal cavity or for residual adenoidal tissue in the choana that cannot be removed via a transoral route. Another potential indication for this technique would be in the child with cervical instability who cannot have the neck extended, such as in certain cases of Down syndrome. Still others have advocated this technique for use in children with submucous cleft palate, where only limited amounts of tissue are to be removed.

During a powered transnasal adenoidectomy, the child is maintained in neutral position and the nasal cavities are decongested. Our preference is to use topical 0.05% oxymetazoline on neurosurgical pledgets. Once the nasal cavity is decongested, a 0° telescope is introduced and used to visualize the adenoids. Anatomic factors can limit visualization such as a markedly deviated nasal septum or hypertrophy of the inferior turbinate. The microdebrider can then be introduced into either the ipsilateral or contralateral nostril and the adenoids can be removed. Bleeding can be controlled using bipolar or monopolar cautery passed transnasally or using techniques described above.

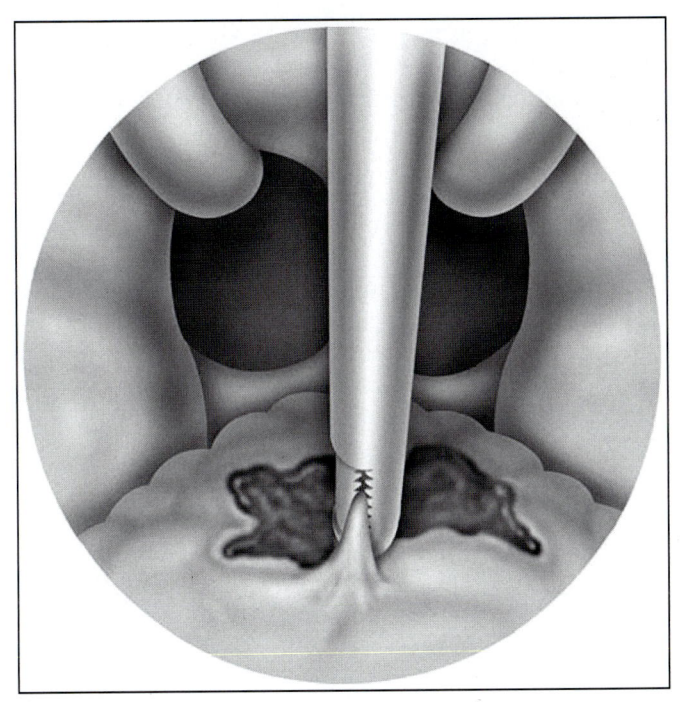

**Fig. 66.3** Powered transoral adenoidectomy. Note excellent visualization afforded by this procedure. Precise control of the tip of the microdebrider is possible to optimize adenoid removal and minimize risk of injury to surrounding structures.

## 3.4 POWERED TRANSORAL ADENOIDECTOMY

Practiced in the United States for well over a decade now, the transoral use of a microdebrider has gained widespread popularity because of its ease of use, safety and proven efficacy. One criticism of this technique is the slightly higher cost associated with the microdebrider blades. It is our procedure of choice for removal of the adenoids.

With the patient in the Rose position with transnasal catheters and a mouth gag in place, the mirror is used to visualize the nasopharynx. Various pre-curved blades exist on the market and these allow for continued visualization during removal (Fig. 66.3). Starting in the region of the choana, the adenoid tissue is removed in a side-to-side manner that progresses inferiorly. The microdebrider is generally set on oscillating mode at 1500 rpm and tissue is removed only at the location of the blade, which is kept under vision at all times. This allows for precise control during removal of tissue. By angling the blade, the Eustachian tube orifice can be cleared of any adenoid tissue without injury. Furthermore, the depth of dissection can be more effectively monitored compared to the curette technique to avoid inadvertent injury to the underlying musculature. This technique also allows the surgeon to very precisely leave adenoid tissue inferiorly to minimize the risk of postoperative velopharyngeal insufficiency, especially in the child with a developmental anomaly of the palate.

Once the adenoids are removed bleeding is controlled as described above.

## 3.5 RADIOFREQUENCY ADENOIDECTOMY

This technology, which has been in use for tonsillectomy, uses radiofrequency energy to excite the sodium ions in saline, which creates a plasma that disintegrates tissue bonds at temperatures around 80°. The result is similar to cautery adenoidectomy but without the tissue char from 400° temperatures of the cautery. A suction wand that bends easily into the nasopharynx but does not clog during resection remains a challenge.

## 3.6 POSTOPERATIVE MANAGEMENT AND COMPLICATIONS

Upon arrival in the recovery room, patients should be adequately monitored with continuous pulse oximetry. Once the child is fully awake, oral diet may be resumed. Initially this is in the form of clear liquids and diet may then be advanced to soft foods. Adenoidectomy performed without concurrent tonsillectomy generally has a quicker recovery time with much less postoperative pain. The use of narcotics is generally not necessary and should probably be avoided in the child with sleep apnea. Following adenoidectomy, we favor the use of non-steroidal anti-inflammatory drugs, such as ibuprofen, alternating every 3 hours with acetaminophen. The best literature available suggests that this regimen is more effective for control of pain, and does not pose an increased risk of bleeding.

Adenoidectomy performed alone is generally an outpatient procedure and most patients are able to go home the day of surgery. Temporary observation can be considered in patients with craniofacial abnormalities, obesity, bleeding disorders, significant obstructive sleep apnea or other medical co-morbidities.

Fortunately, complications after adenoidectomy are rare. The most common complication of adenoid surgery is regrowth of tissue causing recurrence of symptoms. A recent large series by Stewart and colleagues found a 1.6% rate of secondary adenoidectomy. Postoperative hemorrhage is rare and is usually associated with concurrent tonsillectomy. Torticollis is known to occur after adenoidectomy from irritation of the paravertebral muscles. A more severe form of a post-adenoidectomy inflammatory process in the upper cervical region is Grisel syndrome, a non-traumatic atlantoaxial subluxation. It has been postulated that the risk of Grisel syndrome increases with increasing use of monopolar cautery in the nasopharynx.

The problem most otolaryngologists fear following adenoidectomy is velopharyngeal incompetence (VPI); in most cases it is temporary and resolves in 4–6 weeks. However, there is a small percentage of children, reported to range from one per 1500 to one per 10,000 patients, who will have persistence of the VPI. While the adenoid pad is not part of the velopharyngeal sphincter, it may assist in closure in children with structural or functional abnormalities of the soft palate. Children at risk of developing persistent VPI after adenoidectomy often can be identified preoperatively by presence of repaired cleft palate, submucous cleft palate, high arched palate, or palatal hypotonia. When it is necessary to open up the nasopharyngeal airway for these children, performing a very high, perichoanal adenoidectomy can be safely done with a variety of techniques all of which demand close visualization of the site of resection.

Perhaps the worst complication is nasopharyngeal stenosis. Depending on the severity, surgical correction is difficult and unpredictable with a high rate of failure. A cluster of cases in Texas following use of the potassium titanyl phosphate (KTP) laser for adenoidectomy highlighted this otherwise rare complication.

## 4 SUCCESS RATE OF PROCEDURE AND WHAT TO DO IF THE PROCEDURE FAILS

Adenoidectomy, usually combined with tonsillectomy in cases of sleep apnea, has an excellent success rate. Studies have demonstrated long-term improved quality of life for these patients. Newer data suggest that sleep apnea may negatively contribute to certain conditions such as attention deficit hyperactivity disorder (ADHD) and correction of the apnea leads to lower disease severity and reduced medication usage. The most critical aspect of early success is the complete removal of obstructing tissue. Because of this, the authors recommend visual inspection of the adenoid bed even if the technique to remove the adenoids was a blind one. In patients whose symptoms return several months to years after the initial procedure, adenoid regrowth must be considered. An article by Emerick and Cunningham sheds light on a potentially overlooked cause of recurrent symptoms, hypertrophy of the tubal tonsils. Tubal tonsils, also known as Gerlach tonsils, are found beneath the mucosa in the region of the torus tubarius. Hypertrophy of this tissue has been shown to cause symptoms similar to those of adenoid hypertrophy. In this study, tubal tonsils were ablated using suction cautery.

If symptoms do not resolve following successful surgery, obstruction at other anatomic locations must be entertained.

## FURTHER READING

Clemens J, McMurry JS, Willging JP. Electrocautery versus curette adenoidectomy: comparison of postoperative results. Int J Pediatr Otorhinolaryngol 1998;43:115–22.

Elluru RG, Johnson L, Myer CM. Electrocautery adenoidectomy compared with curettage and power-assisted methods. Laryngoscope 2002;112:23–25.

Emerick KS, Cunningham MJ. Tubal tonsil hypertrophy: a cause of recurrent symptoms after adenoidectomy. Arch Otolaryngol Head Neck Surg 2006;132:153–56.

Giannoni C, Sulek M, Friedman EM, et al. Acquired nasopharyngeal stenosis: a warning and review. Arch Otolaryngol Head Neck Surg 1998;124:163–7.

Heras H, Koltai PJ. Safety of powered instrumentation for adenoidectomy. Int J Pediatr Otorhinolaryngol 1998;44:149–53.

Koltai PJ, Kalathia AS, Stanislaw P. Power assisted adenoidectomy. Arch Otolaryngol Head Neck Surg 1997;123:685–8.

Stewart MG, Glaze DG, Friedman EM, et al. Quality of life and sleep study findings after adenotonsillectomy in children with obstructive sleep apnea. Arch Otolarynger Head Neck Surg 2005;131(4): 308–14.

Yanagisawa E, Ho SY, Mirante JP. Powered transnasal adenoidectomy. In: Yanagisawa E, Christmas DA, Mirante JP, eds. Powered Instrumentation in Otolaryngology: Head and Neck Surgery. Canada: Thomson Learning; 2001, p. 247.

# SECTION O  PEDIATRIC OSAHS

## CHAPTER 67
# Radiofrequency tonsil reduction: safety, morbidity and efficacy

*Michael Friedman and Paul Schalch*

## 1 INTRODUCTION

Tonsillectomy remains one of the most popular surgical procedures performed worldwide. Its role as a surgical strategy to widen the pharyngeal space for the treatment of obstructive sleep apnea/hypopnea syndrome (OSAHS) in pediatric patients still remains widely accepted, whereas its utility as a sole procedure for the same purpose in adults is quite limited.[1] Tonsillectomy remains, however, an important adjunct procedure and an essential component of uvulopalatopharyngoplasty (UPPP). Over the years, many different techniques besides the classic cold knife dissection have arisen, all with variable results when it comes to decreasing the major morbidities of the procedure, such as pain, reduced activity level, hemorrhage, and postoperative decrease in fluid intake, leading to dehydration.

Pain after tonsillectomy is a result of the disruption of the tonsil capsule, thereby exposing the pharyngeal muscle and nerve fibers of both the glossopharyngeal and vagus nerves that supply the tonsillar bed. Once these are exposed to the pharyngeal environment, these tissues become inflamed, which leads to muscle spasm. Inflamed constrictor muscles are a source of intense pain, due to the role these muscles play during swallowing. The intense heat produced by the electrocautery, when used for hemostasis or dissection, causes further tissue damage.

This mechanism is the rationale for developing techniques aimed at performing tonsil reduction without disrupting the capsule: the concept of *subtotal capsule-sparing* tonsil reduction. In pediatric patients, subtotal tonsil resection showed an earlier decrease in postoperative pain, decreased pain medication requirements, and an earlier return to diet, when compared to traditional total tonsillectomy.[2] More recently, temperature-controlled radiofrequency was introduced as a much more effective and safe device for tonsil reduction. The underlying principle of temperature-controlled radiofrequency is the generation of a plasma field at the probe's surface, which allows for tissue ablation at relatively low temperatures (40–70°C). This plasma field consists of highly ionized particles that break down the molecular bonds of local tissue with a reduction in heat dissipation to surrounding structures, as opposed to coagulation by diathermic methods, which generates temperatures greater than 500°C. The other advantage of the radiofrequency generator is that it can be used for bipolar coagulation, in order to achieve hemostasis during the procedure. The versatility of this technique consists of the ability to design different wands that can generate varying amounts of energy, depending on the need to ablate, to reduce the volume of tissue, or a combination of both. This is determined by the primary indication for tonsillectomy and the anatomical characteristics of the patient. The device can be used as a cutting tool to dissect along the capsular plane of the tonsil, much like a traditional tonsillectomy. It can also be used to create small channels in the tonsil in order to dissipate ionizing energy to the surrounding tissue, thereby causing tissue death days to weeks later. This then leads to shrinkage and tissue volume reduction due to the ensuing fibrosis. This variant, known as radiofrequency ablation, is not frequently performed any more, due to comparatively better results with coblation techniques. When the objective is to perform subtotal tonsil reduction, the instrument can be used to remove tonsillar tissue layer by layer, beginning at the exposed surface while avoiding the underlying capsule (radiofrequency coblation or cold ablation), thus causing significantly decreased morbidity. The difference between ablation and coblation lies in the mechanism of tissue destruction. Coblation primarily shrinks tissue by molecular disintegration (as opposed to heat-induced necrosis), operates at lower frequencies and voltage, and requires a conductive fluid (isotonic saline), which becomes ionized. Coblation of soft tissue produces immediate results, without the need for resorption of necrotic tissue. For this reason, coblation has largely replaced ablation techniques for the purpose of tonsil reduction.

In this chapter, we describe the techniques of total radiofrequency-assisted tonsillectomy and radiofrequency subtotal (capsule-sparing) tonsillectomy. Radiofrequency tonsillar ablation is also briefly mentioned.[3]

## 2 PATIENT SELECTION

In general, indications for tonsillectomy are updated on a regular basis by the American Academy of Otolaryngology–Head and Neck Surgery. The procedure is indicated for the reduction of chronically enlarged tonsils, when they are associated with obstructive sleep disordered breathing, particularly in children with associated failure to thrive.[4] Other indications for tonsillectomy include recurrent streptococcal infection, peritonsillar abscess, and chronic cryptic tonsillitis. Relative contraindications for radiofrequency reduction techniques are asymmetrical tonsillar hypertrophy, clinical diagnosis or high suspicion of lymphoma, history of peritonsillar abscess, and repeated streptococcal infections (recurrent infectious tonsillitis). Such patients should undergo traditional total tonsillectomy, due to the need for complete removal of tonsillar tissue. Patients with chronic or recurrent non-streptococcal inflammatory cryptitis may also benefit from subtotal tonsil coblation.

## 3 SURGICAL TECHNIQUE (OUTLINE OF PROCEDURE)

### 3.1 TOTAL RADIOFREQUENCY-ASSISTED TONSILLECTOMY

Coblation can be used for the traditional complete excision of the tonsils. Electrolyte solution is not injected, as coblation is a surface technique in which saline irrigation is utilized. Optimal coblation is achieved with an abundant flow of saline solution. The device used by our group is the Coblator II Surgery System with the EVAC™ 70 Plasma Wand (Arthrocare ENT, Sunnyvale, CA) (Fig. 67.1). Small vessels are sealed as the tissue is dissected, so hemostasis is very effective and efficient. More aggressive hemostasis can be performed if necessary, by operating the wand in the cautery mode. The coagulation setting used is usually 3 to 5. If larger vessels are exposed during total subcapsular excision, the conventional monopolar or bipolar cautery can be used, with a significant increase in postoperative pain due to more extensive tissue injury, and a higher risk for postoperative hemorrhage.

The dissection for total tonsillectomy is similar to the traditional technique. The capsule is identified by blunt dissection. The tonsil is retracted inferiorly and medially with an Allis clamp, and once the capsule is exposed, the wand is used to dissect it from the tonsillar fossa musculature in a superior-to-inferior and a lateral-to-medial direction (Fig. 67.2). Dissection is facilitated by retracting the tonsil inferomedially, due to the creation of a plane under tension. The power is set at a moderate coblation level (6 to 7) and the tip of the instrument is directed towards the capsule, leaving a small space over the tissue, which allows a plasma layer to form. As the dissection proceeds, the fibrous tissue will be preferentially excised. Small blood vessels are fused as they are encountered, by applying more pressure with the tip of the wand.

### 3.2 CAPSULE-SPARING SUBTOTAL TONSILLECTOMY

With the subtotal, capsule-sparing technique, about 90–95% of the tonsil can be removed. The tonsillar tissue is ablated from the surface inward with retraction of the pillar, which helps avoid the capsule and the surrounding extratonsillar structures. We use the coblation system by Arthrocare. The highest power settings are used while removing the tissue layer by layer, using brush-like motions (Fig. 67.3). The ensuing tonsillar reduction is immediate. Bleeding is usually controlled with coblation because it comes from small-caliber vessels. Meticulous care in preserving the anterior and posterior pillars is essential in order to achieve the best results. A thin layer of tissue is left in situ, which ensures that the surgeon will avoid penetrating the tonsillar capsule

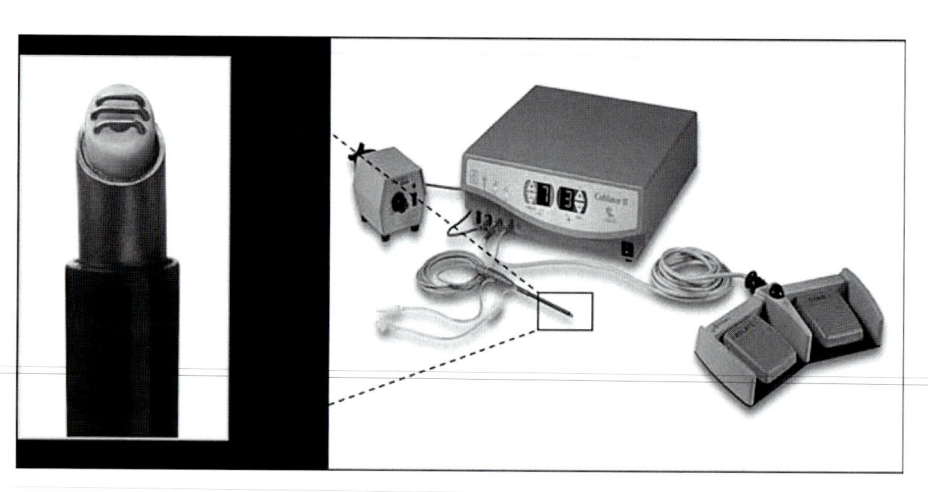

**Fig. 67.1** Coblator II Surgery System with the EVAC™ 70 Plasma Wand.

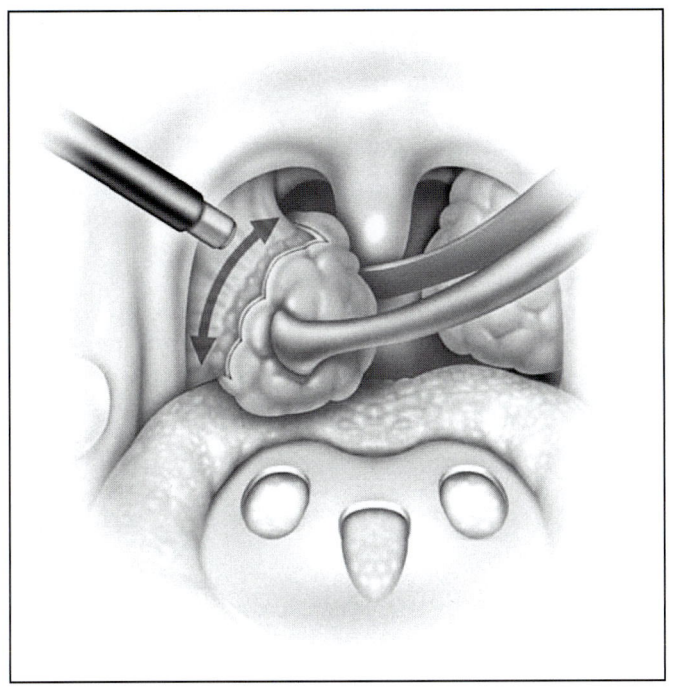

**Fig. 67.2** Total tonsillectomy (radiofrequency assisted). A plane is created by retracting the tonsil inferomedially, and the wand is used to dissect it from the tonsillar fossa musculature in a superior-to-inferior and a lateral-to-medial direction.

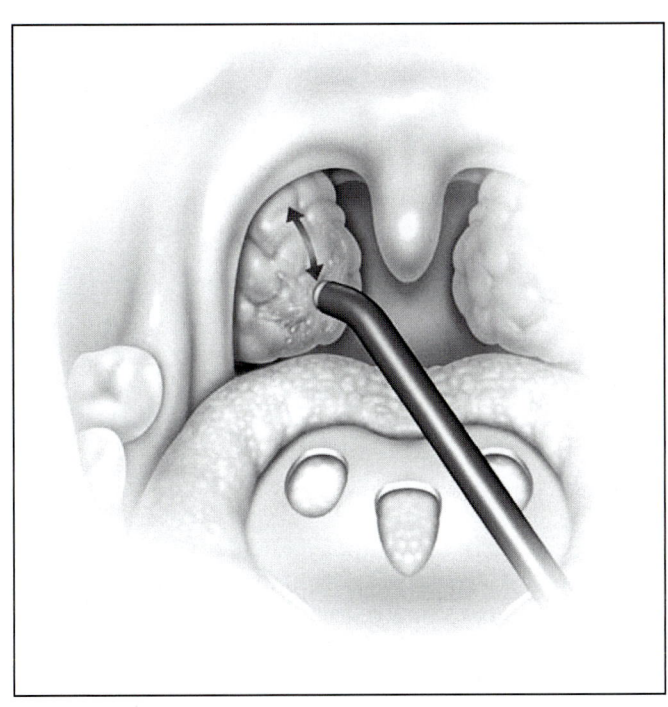

**Fig. 67.3** Subtotal tonsillectomy. The tonsillar tissue is ablated from the surface inward, thus sparing the capsule.

and exposing the underlying pharyngeal muscle. This allows for faster healing, reduced scarring, and a decreased incidence of postoperative bleeding.[5] As the surgeon approaches the point where most of the tissue has been removed, the power setting is reduced and careful palpation is performed, in order to determine the need for carefully removing any additional tissue. Penetrating the capsule or injuring the pillars will result in increased bleeding, which might require the use of electrocautery. The electrodes at the tip of the wand should be periodically wiped off, and if the tip of the wand becomes clogged, it should be rinsed in saline solution by dipping it into a basin while activating the pedal to flush the suction port.

## 3.3 RADIOFREQUENCY TONSIL ABLATION

Tonsil ablation requires the injection of fluid or electrolytes into the tissue before treatment. Channels are created by inserting the wand into the tissue and ablating. The wand will leave a lesion of about 4 mm in diameter and about 10–12 mm in length, depending on how deep the wand is inserted. In the immediate postoperative period, the amount of swelling actually exceeds the total tissue volume reduction, but shrinkage progressively occurs between the first and third weeks post procedure and the tonsillar tissue volume is effectively reduced.

## 4 POSTOPERATIVE MANAGEMENT AND COMPLICATIONS

In general, five parameters can be used to assess the patient, whether adult or pediatric, in the immediate postoperative period: mean pain level on the first postoperative day; the number of days the pain is greater than 1 out of 10 (based on the visual analog scale: 0 being no pain, 1 being the lowest, and 10 the highest pain experienced); number of days narcotic medications are used for pain control; number of days before resumption of a normal diet; and number of days until a return to normal activity.

Radiofrequency-assisted total tonsillectomy can result in significant postoperative pain, swelling, and a delayed return to regular diet, much like traditional, electrocautery-assisted tonsillectomy. The liberal use of electrocautery during the procedure is probably responsible, at least in part, for such comparable morbidity,[6] particularly when larger vessels are exposed and more tissue injury is caused by the efforts to achieve hemostasis. Timms and Temple[7] demonstrated, however, that by minimizing the use of electrocautery during total, coblation-assisted tonsillectomy in pediatric and adult patients, the mean duration of postoperative pain was 2.4 and 5 days respectively, compared to 7.6 and 9 days for electrocautery-assisted tonsillectomy.

Pediatric patients undergoing capsule-sparing tonsillectomy experience an average intensity of pain of 2.5 (on a scale of 0 to 10) after coblation, with an average duration of 2.7 days postoperatively. Adults experience about 2.5 days at an average pain intensity of 2.8. By postoperative day 3, virtually all patients who undergo subtotal, capsule-sparing tonsil coblation are pain free, which represents a remarkable improvement when compared with classic, cold dissection tonsillectomy, which averages 9–10 days. Narcotics are rarely needed beyond day 1, and a return to normal activity level and regular diet occurs, on average, by postoperative day 2.[5] Consistent with these figures, Arya did not find any difference between intra- and subcapsular tonsillectomies when analyzing postoperative pain scores by means of visual analog pain scales in a double-blind, randomized, controlled study.[8]

Similar morbidity can be described for radiofrequency tonsil ablation, where pediatric patients experience an average 1.5 pain intensity level, for a mean of 1.7 days, and adults complain of 1.6 days of pain, at a mean intensity of 1.5.[5]

Coblation-assisted total tonsillectomy has been associated with an increased risk of postoperative hemorrhage. In 2003, the National Prospective Tonsillectomy Audit of England and Northern Ireland was initiated in order to determine the magnitude of this increased risk.[9,10] After reviewing 11,796 tonsillectomies, we found that 4.4% of the 684 patients who underwent coblation-assisted tonsillectomy had either primary hemorrhage (leading to prolonged hospital stay, blood transfusion, or return to the OR) or secondary hemorrhage (within 28 days, leading to readmission). We concluded that the main factor in this increased risk of hemorrhage, when compared to traditional, cold dissection tonsillectomy (where only 1.28% of 1327 patients had postoperative hemorrhage), was an inappropriate use of coblation and/or electrocautery, in order to stop intraoperative bleeding. Significant thermal damage to the surrounding tissue is likely responsible for delayed-type hemorrhage. A learning curve is therefore crucial in attaining the best results and in minimizing complications when using radiofrequency-assisted total tonsillectomy. Other authors, however, have described a decreased incidence of delayed hemorrhage in patients who underwent coblation tonsillectomy, when compared to blunt dissection or electrocautery diathermy tonsillectomies.[11,12]

Subtotal radiofrequency tonsil coblation, on the other hand, is safer because of the underlying principle of capsule sparing, and intraoperative and postoperative complications are very rare. Intraoperative blood loss is usually minimal, and while postoperative hemorrhage should always be considered a potential complication, it is also an extremely rare occurrence. Due to an early return to normal diet, IV fluids are usually not required, and because tonsillectomy opens the previously obstructed pharynx, the risk of airway obstruction is usually not a concern.

Radiofrequency tonsil ablation is also safe in terms of postoperative hemorrhage, but may cause significant postoperative edema. This may temporarily result in more airway obstruction than the obstruction caused by the tonsils themselves, possibly requiring an overnight admission for observation. Airway obstruction is, nevertheless, very rare.

## 5 SUCCESS RATE OF THE PROCEDURE

The efficacy of radiofrequency tonsil reduction can be compared to classic tonsillectomy in terms of its efficacy, under the assumption that classic tonsillectomy removes 100% of the tonsillar tissue. In a series of adult and pediatric patients published by Friedman et al.,[5] it was found that tonsillar ablation achieved a volumetric reduction ranging between 30% and 70%, with a mean reduction of about 51% in pediatric patients, whereas tonsillar radiofrequency coblation achieved shrinkage ranging between 75% and 95%, with a mean of about 86%. Adult patients showed similar results, ranging from 40% to 70% and averaging about 54% for tonsillar ablation, and 75–95% with an average of 90% for tonsillar coblation. The coblation group was statistically more effective in terms of tonsil removal in both patient populations, with the additional advantage of yielding more consistent results.

When comparing tonsillar tissue ablation with coblation, it becomes evident that coblation has three distinct advantages over ablation. First, the amount of tonsil reduction is unpredictable when using ablation, with a significantly spread range of 30–70%, despite identical techniques by the same surgeon. Coblation enables the surgeon to have more control and more precision, as well as consistency in results. Second, ablation causes significant edema in the immediate postoperative period in many instances. This requires close monitoring of the airway in an intensive care setting during an overnight stay, especially in the pediatric group. Third, the use of ablation is limited to treating airway obstruction, not chronic tonsillitis. The technique achieves shrinkage of the tissue, rather than effective en bloc removal of diseased tissue, as coblation. The partial, rather than total resection is an inherent disadvantage of these techniques, considering that there is a small risk of regrowth of tonsillar tissue comparable to adenoidectomy, where subtotal resection is the standard of practice. A learning curve is necessary in spite of the simplicity of these techniques, and results are proportional to the experience of the surgeon.

When coblation is used to perform total tonsillectomy, as opposed to subtotal tonsillectomy, very similar results in terms of morbidity are achieved when compared to classic tonsillectomy. The wand is basically used as a dissection tool that removes the tonsil along the capsular plane, thereby exposing underlying muscle and nerves. The disruption of the capsule underlies the main source of morbidity, which is pain, and in this setting, coblation does not offer a distinct advantage over cold dissection tonsillectomy. As noted earlier, the key and common mistakes that can increase morbidity of the subcapsular technique are the

Table 67.1  Causes of sleep-related breathing disorders in children

| Neonates and infants |
|---|
| Nasal aplasia, stenosis, or atresia |
| Nasal or nasopharyngeal masses |
| Craniofacial anomalies |
|     Hypoplastic mandible (Pierre Robin, Nager's, Treacher Collins) |
|     Hypoplastic maxilla (Apert's, Crouzon's) |
| Macroglossia (Beckwith-Wiedemann) |
| Vascular malformations of tongue and pharynx |
| Congenital cysts of the vallecula and tongue |
| Neuromuscular disorders |
| *Toddlers and older children* |
| Rhinitis, nasal polyposis, septal deviation |
| Syndromic narrowing of nasopharynx (Hunter's, Hurler's, Down's, achondroplasia) |
| Adenotonsillar hyperplasia |
| Obesity |
| Macroglossia (Down's) |
| Vascular malformations of tongue and pharynx |
| Neuromuscular disorders |
| *Iatrogenic* |
| Nasopharyngeal stenosis |

inadvertent contact of the active wand with the oropharyngeal mucosa, overly aggressive tonsil coblation that exposes muscle and causes potential bleeding, and incomplete coblation of tissue that leaves more than 10% of the tonsil intact. Subtotal tonsillectomy should not be performed on patients undergoing classic uvulopalatopharyngoplasty, since tonsillar tissue would be buried under the pillars after closure.

## 5.1 WHAT TO DO IF THE PROCEDURE FAILS

Should the volumetric reduction of the tonsillar tissue be suboptimal, a repeat procedure to remove more tissue in the subcapsular plane can be attempted. This can be done either under local anesthesia in an office-type setting, or in the operating room under sedation or general anesthesia, depending on the magnitude of resection needed. There is always the option of converting a subcapsular tonsillectomy to a total tonsillectomy, whether it is done by means of radiofrequency coblation, or by the traditional, cold-knife dissection with additional morbidity.

## 6 CONCLUSION

Tonsillectomy, either alone or, most frequently, in combination with other procedures, remains one of the most common surgical procedures performed for the management of OSAHS, in both the pediatric and adult population. Subcapsular radiofrequency coblation shows distinct advantages over classic tonsillectomy, including early elimination of pain, early return to normal diet and activity, and precise removal of tonsillar tissue. This technique is ideal for hypertrophic tonsils in the context of airway obstruction in sleep apnea.

## REFERENCES

1. Sher AE, Schechtman KB, Piccirillo JF. The efficacy of surgical modifications of the upper airway in adults with obstructive sleep apnea syndrome. Sleep 1996;19:156–77.
2. Hultcrantz E, Linder A, Markstrom A. Tonsillectomy or tonsillotomy? A randomized study comparing postoperative pain and long-term effects. Int J Pediatr Otorhinolaryngol 1999;51:171–76.
3. Morris L, Lee K. Coblation techniques for sleep disordered breathing. In: Terris D, Goode R, eds. Surgical Management of Sleep Apnea and Snoring. Location?: Informa Healthcare; 2005.
4. Darrow D, Siemens C. Indications for tonsillectomy and adenoidectomy. Laryngoscope 2002;112:6–10.
5. Friedman M, LoSavio P, Ibrahim H, et al. Radiofrequency tonsil reduction: safety, morbidity, and efficacy. Laryngoscope 2003;113:882–7.
6. Bäck L, Paloheimo M, Ylikoski J. Traditional tonsillectomy compared with bipolar radiofrequency thermal ablation tonsillectomy in adults: a pilot study. Arch Otolaryngol Head Neck Surg 2001;127:1106–12.
7. Timms M, Temple R. Coblation tonsillectomy: a double blind randomized controlled study. J Laryngol Otol 2002;116:450–2.
8. Arya A, Donne A, Nigam A. Double-blind randomized controlled study of coblation tonsillotomy versus coblation tonsillectomy on postoperative pain in children. Clin Otolaryngol 2005;30:226–9.
9. Lowe D, van der Meulen J, Cromwell D, et al. Key messages from the National Prospective Tonsillectomy Audit. Laryngoscope 2007;117:717–24.
10. Hopkins C, Ajulo P, Krywawych M, et al. The impact of the interim report of the National Prospective Tonsillectomy Audit. Clin Otolaryngol 2005;30:475–6.
11. Belloso A, Chidambaram A, Morar P, et al. Coblation tonsillectomy versus dissection tonsillectomy: postoperative hemorrhage. Laryngoscope 2003;113:2010–3.
12. Divi V, Benninger M. Postoperative tonsillectomy bleed: coblation versus noncoblation. Laryngoscope 2005;115:31–3.

SECTION O  PEDIATRIC OSAHS

CHAPTER 68

# Microdebrider-assisted tonsillectomy

*Peter J. Koltai and Christopher M. Discolo*

## 1 INTRODUCTION

Tonsillectomy remains one of the most common surgical procedures performed on children. In contrast to several decades ago when infectious indications were common, the reason most children undergo tonsillectomy today is to relieve upper airway obstruction. Traditional 'extracapsular' tonsillectomy remains a fairly morbid procedure. Children routinely require several days off from school and parents are often forced to take time off from work. Despite advances in surgical technology a significant reduction in postoperative pain following this procedure has eluded surgeons. This is evidenced by the wide array of techniques available to the surgeon. Furthermore, the rate of postoperative hemorrhage has remained fairly stable despite the technique practiced. Partial 'intracapsular' tonsillectomy seeks to significantly reduce postoperative pain and hemorrhage risk while effectively treating upper airway obstruction.

## 2 PATIENT SELECTION

Patients suffering from upper airway obstruction secondary to tonsil hypertrophy are candidates for partial tonsillectomy. Caregivers are fully informed of the differences between total and partial tonsillectomy and the rationale for each procedure. The potential for tonsil regrowth and the risk for development of chronic streptococcal tonsillitis need to be addressed (see Postoperative management and complications) during the informed consent process.

Relative contraindications to the performance of intracapsular tonsillectomy include a history of chronic tonsillitis and tonsil regrowth following a previous partial tonsillectomy.

The safety of intracapsular tonsillectomy in the young patient has been studied. Bent et al. found no significant difference in the rate of readmission, pain, oral intake or analgesic requirements in patients younger than 3 years of age who underwent partial tonsillectomy compared to a control group.[1]

## 3 OUTLINE OF PROCEDURE

After general anesthesia is achieved, the patient is placed in the Rose position. According to surgeon preference the airway may be managed with a straight endotracheal tube, an oral RAE (Ring–Adair–Elwyn) tube or a laryngeal mask airway (LMA). The jaw is opened using a mouth gag, which can then be suspended. If concurrent adenoidectomy is to be performed, the soft palate is first inspected and palpated for the presence of a submucous cleft and then retracted using catheters that are placed through the nasal cavities and retrieved from the oropharynx. This maneuver also helps to stabilize the tonsillar pillars and pulls the uvula out of the surgical field.

With the microdebrider set at a rate of 1500 rpm on oscillating mode, dissection of the tonsil begins at the inferior pole (Fig. 68.1). This helps prevent blood from obscuring visualization of the anterior and posterior pillars. Dissection proceeds from a lateral to medial direction until the plane of the pillars is reached. At this point it is generally helpful to further stabilize and control the anterior pillar to maximize tissue removal and minimize injury to mucosa. A Hurd elevator is particularly helpful in this circumstance as it can also help to medialize the remaining tonsil tissue, making dissection easier. Dissection is carried down to but not through the capsule of the tonsil. The use of a mirror can facilitate dissection of the superior pole. Care is taken to avoid inadvertent injury to the uvula, which can occur rapidly given the suction associated with the microdebrider. After dissection is completed, hemostasis is achieved using suction cautery with settings generally between 20 and 40 watts according to surgeon preference (Fig. 68.2). The contralateral tonsil is then dissected in an identical fashion. Once the procedure is completed the pharynx is irrigated with sterile normal saline and the mouth gag is allowed to relax. After approximately one minute the gag is reopened and hemostasis is confirmed. A suction catheter is then passed under direct vision and the stomach and hypopharynx are suctioned free of any blood or irrigation fluid that may cause post-extubation laryngospasm. The mouth gag and nasal catheters (if present) are removed

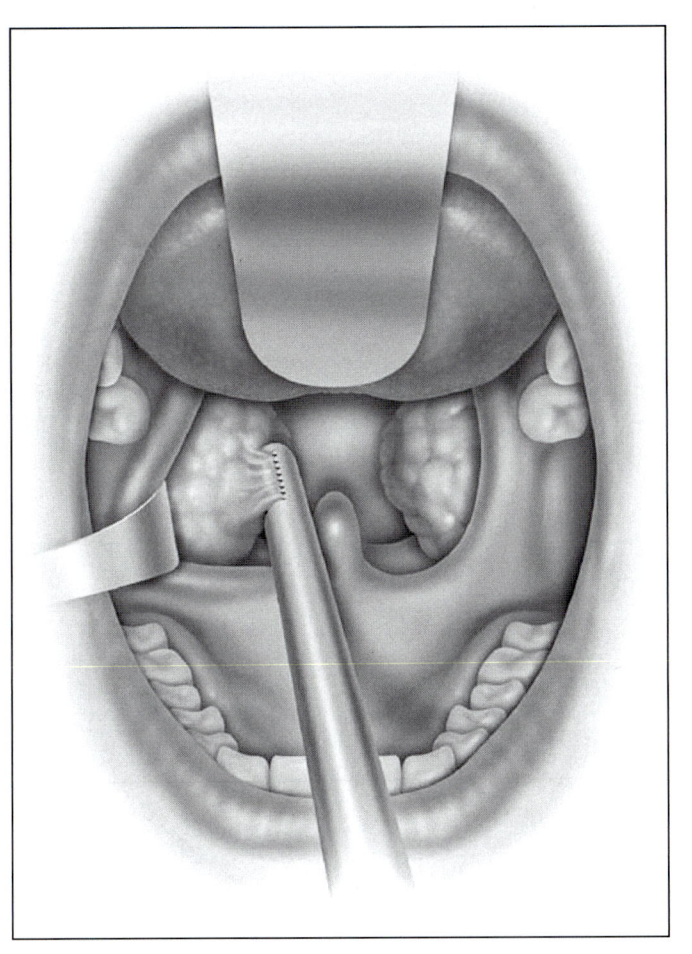

**Fig. 68.1** With the mouth gag in place and the anterior tonsillar pillar secured, the microdebrider is used to begin dissection.

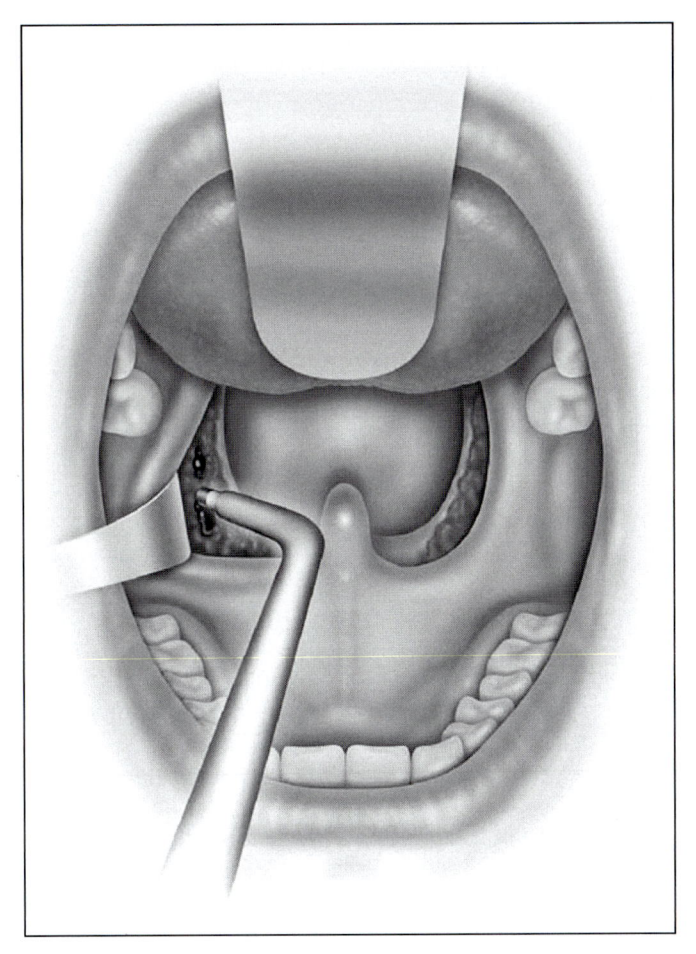

**Fig. 68.2** Final hemostasis is achieved using a suction electrocautery unit. Note tonsil capsule which remains intact at end of dissection.

and the patient is turned over to anesthesia personnel for extubation.

Studies have shown that, when compared to total tonsillectomy, intracapsular tonsillectomy may produce slightly increased intraoperative blood loss and require slightly more operative time. A recent study of 300 patients found that intracapsular tonsillectomy was performed on average in 10 minutes while electrocautery tonsillectomy took 8 minutes.[2] This study also found no significant difference in overall blood loss but 15% of the intracapsular group lost more than 25 milliliters of blood compared to only 4% in the electrocautery group.

In the pediatric patient, adenoidectomy is routinely combined with tonsillectomy in an attempt to remove potentially obstructing lymphoid tissue. Various techniques exist to remove the adenoids (see Chapter 66: Current techniques of adenoidectomy). Our preference is to perform microdebrider-assisted adenoidectomy. The addition of adenoidectomy does not add significantly to the overall morbidity of the operation. As children age, the adenoids undergo regression and so in the older child performance of both procedures may not be necessary. Obviously, each procedure must be tailored to the individual patient's needs

and direct visualization of the adenoid pad to assess its size is recommended. This may be performed either preoperatively in the office setting or during surgery at the time of tonsillectomy. Lateral plain films of the nasopharynx may also be used to assess the size and degree of obstruction produced by the adenoids.

## 4 POSTOPERATIVE MANAGEMENT AND COMPLICATIONS

In the recovery room patients are appropriately monitored. Oral diet is resumed, generally in the form of clear liquids, once an adequate level of consciousness is reached. Pain medicine may be administered either via an intravenous route or orally. The use of non-steroidal anti-inflammatory drugs in the postoperative period is controversial and may lead to an increased risk of postoperative hemorrhage. It is our practice to use either acetaminophen or acetaminophen/narcotic combinations. The use of narcotic medication in the child with sleep apnea must be carefully considered. This population may have reduced respiratory drive in the presence of even low doses of narcotics. Patients who are observed in the hospital overnight should have continuous pulse oximetry. Consideration can also be given to temporary observation in an intensive care unit setting for patients with craniofacial abnormalities, severe preoperative sleep apnea, young age, history of bleeding disorder or other significant medical co-morbidities. It is our practice to routinely observe healthy patients less than 4 years of age overnight prior to discharge following tonsillectomy.

The most common and potentially life-threatening complication of tonsillectomy is hemorrhage. Generally bleeding will occur at two distinct time periods after surgery. Rarely patients will hemorrhage within the first 24 hours following surgery and this is generally ascribed to incomplete hemostasis at the time of the operation. More commonly hemorrhage occurs several days after surgery. Management of post-tonsillectomy hemorrhage varies and depends on multiple factors including the age and co-operativeness of the child, degree of hemorrhage, and hemodynamic stability of the patient, among others. Cautery in the awake and co-operative patient is certainly an option but in the young or unco-operative patient this may prove an impossible task. In that case, general anesthetic is required. In patients who have had minor bleeding without an obvious source, observation may be a viable option. Children are generally observed for approximately 12–24 hours prior to discharge home following a minor episode of bleeding.

One potential advantage of intracapsular tonsillectomy is a potentially decreased risk of postoperative hemorrhage compared to traditional procedures. A recent multi-center retrospective review of 870 patients found a 0.7% rate of delayed postoperative hemorrhage.[3]

As mentioned earlier in this text, the risk of potential tonsil regrowth must be discussed with patients and their families preoperatively. A recent study reviewed 278 children who underwent intracapsular tonsillectomy.[4] Nine patients (3.2%) experienced regrowth of tonsil tissue associated with snoring and two of these required revision surgery. We are currently in the process of reviewing a large series of patients who are several years removed from their intracapsular procedures to better understand the rate and severity of regrowth that does occur.

Because the intracapsular procedure does leave tonsil tissue behind it should have no influence on the future development of streptococcal tonsillitis.

## 5 SUCCESS RATE OF PROCEDURE AND WHAT TO DO IF THE PROCEDURE FAILS

Fortunately, in children, tonsillectomy with or without adenoidectomy to treat obstructive sleep apnea has an excellent success rate. Intracapsular procedures appear to have equally effective results when compared to traditional methods.

As with adults, children can have obstruction at multiple levels of the upper aerodigestive tract. This is especially true for children with associated craniofacial malformations. If symptoms do not resolve in the postoperative period, a sleep study is recommended as snoring can exist without apnea. Recalcitrant apnea needs to be addressed based on the anatomic level of obstruction occurring. Tracheotomy remains the gold standard to treat sleep apnea.

In patients who experience recurrent symptoms in a delayed fashion after undergoing partial tonsillectomy with or without adenoidectomy, one must consider the possibility of regrowth at either of these anatomic locations.

## REFERENCES

1. Bent JP, April MM, Ward RF, et al. Ambulatory powered intracapsular tonsillectomy and adenoidectomy in children younger than 3 years. Arch Otolaryngol Head Neck Surg 2004;130:1197–200.
2. Derkay CS, Darrow DH, Welch CW, et al. Post-tonsillectomy morbidity and quality of life in pediatric patients with obstructive tonsils and adenoid: microdebrider vs. electocautery. Otolaryngol Head Neck Surg 2006;134:114–20.
3. Solares CA, Koempel JA, Hirose K, et al. Safety and efficacy of powered intracapsular tonsillectomy in children: a multi-center retrospective case series. Int J Pediatr Otorhinolaryngol 2005;69:21–6.
4. Sorin A, Bent J, April M, et al. Complications of microdebrider-assisted powered intracapsular tonsillectomy and adenoidectomy. Laryngoscope 2004;114(2):297–300.

## FURTHER READING

Hultcrantz E, Linder A, Markstrom A. Long-term effects of intracapsular partial tonsillectomy (tonsillotomy) compared with full tonsillectomy. Int J Pediatr Otorhinolaryngol 2005;69(4):463–9.

Koltai PJ, Solares CA, Mascha EJ, et al. Intracapsular partial tonsillectomy for tonsillar hypertrophy in children. Laryngoscope 2002;112(8 part 2) Suppl No. 100:17–19.

Koltai PJ, Solares CA, Koempel JA, et al. Intracapsular tonsillar reduction (partial tonsillectomy): reviving a historical procedure for obstructive sleep disordered breathing in children. Otolaryngol Head Neck Surg 2003;129(5):532–8.

Ray RM, Bower CM. Pediatric obstructive sleep apnea: the year in review. Curr Opin Otolaryngol Head Neck Surg 2005;13(6):360–65.

Sobol SE, Wetmore RF, Marsh RR, et al. Postoperative recovery after microdebrider intracapsular or monopolar electrocautery tonsillectomy: a prospective, randomized, single-blinded study. Arch Otolaryngol Head Neck Surg 2006;132(3):270–74.

# SECTION O  PEDIATRIC OSAHS

# CHAPTER 69

# Laryngomalacia

*Peggy E. Kelley*

## 1 INTRODUCTION

Laryngomalacia is the term most widely used to describe the 'inward collapse of supraglottic structures during inspiration', as originated by Jackson and Jackson in 1942. The inward collapse of the epiglottis or arytenoids results in stridor that is typically inspiratory and high-pitched. Laryngomalacia is often cited as the most common congenital laryngeal anomaly and most frequent cause of stridor in infants. The stridor is often present at birth, and is usually noticed by 2 weeks of age. Laryngomalacia is usually positionally dependent and is worse at times of increased work of breathing. Older children and adults may be diagnosed with laryngomalacia occurring particularly during exercise. This brings into question the idea that laryngomalacia is only a congenital problem.

## 2 PATIENT SELECTION

The stridor of laryngomalacia is well described and the diagnosis can be easily made with fiberoptic laryngoscopy, but the pathogenesis is still unknown. The first proposed mechanism of pathogenesis was floppiness of the airway secondary to infantile cartilage abnormalities, but histological study did not support this.[1] Others suggest that there is poor neuromuscular control with relative hypotonia of the supraglottic dilator muscles.[1] The cause of the hypotonia is presumed to be central in nature but the pathophysiology is not understood.

Research of decades ago and again more recently has looked at pathways of chemosensory reflexes in the larynx causing apnea as a means of understanding laryngeal function.[2,3] Others looking at the larynx more directly found that the laryngeal adductor reflex elicited by a calibrated puff of air to the larynx could be used as a diagnostic tool correlated with airway patency control, swallowing and apnea.[4,5] Recent work by Thompson et al.[6] found that children with laryngomalacia also have altered laryngeal sensation. The larynx of a child with laryngomalacia requires a more intense puff of air to activate the laryngeal adductor reflux than children without laryngomalacia. Thompson also found that those with severe laryngomalacia (children requiring surgical management) have a more elevated reflex level than children with mild to moderate laryngomalacia. The children with severe laryngomalacia were also relatively hypoxic with a mean $SaO_2$ of 88.6% vs. 98–99% in children with moderate or mild laryngomalacia.[6] The cause of the altered laryngeal sensation is currently under investigation and should shed light on the etiology of laryngomalacia.

There is a subset of children with laryngomalacia who have additional diagnoses[7,8] but laryngomalacia is usually isolated and children with isolated laryngomalacia are developmentally normal. Many studies cite reflux disease as being at least a comorbid factor in explaining the symptoms of laryngomalacia.[9–11] It is not clear whether the reflux is the primary problem or if reflux occurs secondary to the changes in intrathoracic pressure with the increased work of breathing that occurs with more significant laryngomalacia. A third option is to consider reflux as either primary or secondary.

To that end, it may be helpful to consider the diagnosis of laryngomalacia as having two subsets: *primary laryngomalacia* (Fig. 69.1), in which there is actual anatomic variation such as the shortening of the aryepiglottic folds[12] or a more pronounced omega-shaped epiglottis, and *secondary laryngomalacia* (Fig. 69.2) in which reflux disease is the inciting factor. In primary laryngomalacia, the anatomic anomaly narrows the laryngeal inlet. Venturi principles of airflow then describe the resulting 'floppy airway'[8] such as described in obstructive sleep apnea when the soft palate and tongue base are sucked against the posterior pharyngeal wall as a result of tonsils and/or adenoids narrowing the airway. Primary laryngomalacia may result in enough airway distress to induce secondary reflux which then exacerbates the edema and swelling of the tissues that are being sucked into the airway with each breath as seen on fiberoptic evaluation. Secondary laryngomalacia then is when the airway is anatomically normal to begin with but in the

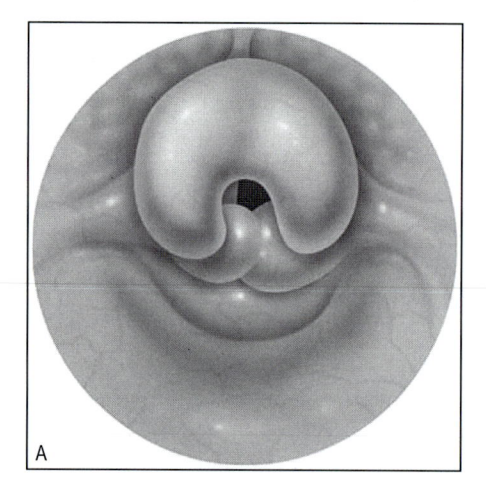

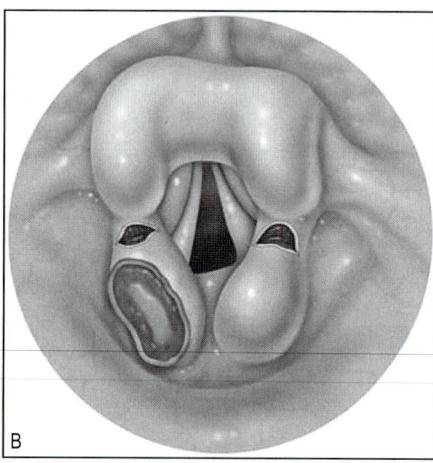

**Fig. 69.1** A, Primary laryngomalacia: anatomic anomaly such as shortened aryepiglottic folds causes narrowing of the laryngeal inlet. Venturi principles describe forces that result in infolding of the arytenoids or epiglottis with inspiration. B, Primary laryngomalacia after supraglottoplasty with division of aryepiglottic folds.

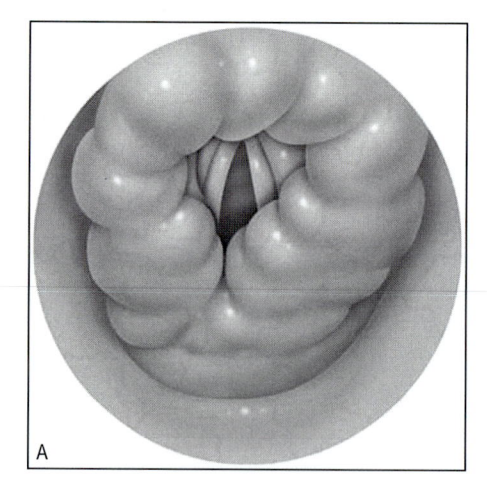

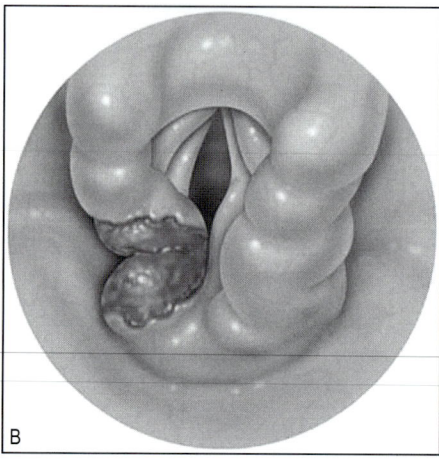

**Fig. 69.2** A, Secondary laryngomalacia: narrowing of the laryngeal inlet caused by edema of the supraglottic structures secondary to reflux disease. B, Secondary laryngomalacia with failure of medical therapy for reflux after supraglottoplasty with mucosal removal.

child with reflux disease, the airway becomes edematous which begins the process of narrowing and the resulting airway collapse with inspiration.

## 2.1 PREOPERATIVE EVALUATION

The preoperative evaluation of the patient with stridor begins with a history that includes how well the patient is eating, growing and developing. This gives a sense as to how significant the stridor is and what management options may be necessary. The diagnosis of laryngomalacia is made when viewing the larynx during inspiration and expiration and correlating the noise heard with infolding of the supraglottic structures. It is sometimes helpful to perform laryngoscopy with the patient in both sitting and lying positions. The evaluation of laryngeal dynamics is most directly made in the awake patient as general anesthesia may affect the dynamics of the airway.[13] The size of the flexible laryngoscope may also influence the airway dynamics by obstructing the nasal cavity and thus increasing the force for inspiration so the smallest scope that affords good visualization should be chosen for each patient. Another consideration is the positioning of the infant as there can be differences in the airway dynamics if the child is in a sitting or lying position.[14] Laryngoscopy in both positions may be considered particularly if what is seen in one position is not what was expected.

When performing laryngoscopy, the surgeon is evaluating the airway for edema, erythema, anatomic structure and movement. Rotation of the epiglottis posteriorly, the arytenoids anteriorly and areas of inward collapse of the supraglottic structure are identified. In addition to noting the static endpoints of inspiration and expiration, evaluation should include where the larynx is positioned in the airway and if the larynx rotates as a whole up toward the tongue base into a protective position away from the esophagus. Shaker described the esophagoglottal closure reflex that occurs when the airway is exposed to reflux.[15] This reflex may account for the neuromuscular abnormalities and inco-ordinate swallowing seen in the infant with laryngomalacia. If the airway is sufficiently swollen, it may be impossible to determine if there is underlying anatomic anomaly or if the obstruction is secondary only to edema.

A medical trial with a proton pump inhibitor for mild to moderate airway erythema and edema in the child who is not growing well or having feeding difficulties may result in improvement or resolution of the stridor.[10,16] If the child is then able to consistently feed and gain weight, surgery may be avoided, particularly for secondary laryngomalacia. For severe airway obstruction a burst of steroid for 2–5 days is often helpful to relieve acute symptoms and allow more precise evaluation of the underlying anatomy upon repeating the laryngoscopy 1–2 weeks later. If the child presents in airway distress before 1 month of age medical therapy is unlikely to succeed and supraglottoplasty is offered. Supraglottoplasty is the term used to describe the division or removal of any supraglottic tissue for the relief of airway obstruction in the patient with laryngomalacia.[13] Approximately 10% of infants with laryngomalacia require surgical intervention. Infants requiring surgery are those with significant primary laryngomalacia and those with secondary laryngomalacia in whom reflux therapy has been inadequate to relieve airway obstruction or feeding difficulties.

Debate exists concerning the need for the evaluation of synchronous airway lesions with a full microlaryngoscopy and bronchoscopy in every child with laryngomalacia. It has been shown that the majority of secondary airway problems are found in patients who have progressive symptoms unresponsive to medical therapy or observation. Microlaryngoscopy and bronchoscopy should be performed on any child being taken to the operating room for possible supraglottoplasty, but may not be necessary for every child with laryngomalacia.[17]

## 3 SURGICAL PROCEDURE

Any airway surgery should begin with a discussion between the surgeon and anesthesiologist of the anesthetic plan for the procedure even *before* the patient is brought into the operating room. Options for ventilation include spontaneous ventilation, apneic anesthesia or supraglottic jet ventilation. Intubation is recommended for the specific technique described below for ary epiglottic (AE) fold division with microlaryngeal instruments. The use of proximal jet ventilation is previously described.

Airway surgery in children is performed under general anesthesia. This typically begins with a mask induction as the child may not yet have intravenous access. Once the patient is induced by mask inhalation and IV access is obtained, the patient is maintained with a spontaneous breathing technique of inhalational gases often supplemented with propofol as needed. Paralysis is avoided at least until the airway evaluation is completed and the exact surgical plan is outlined.

Topical lidocaine without epinephrine is applied to the supraglottic and laryngeal mucosa as a mucosal anesthetic and to reduce reflex laryngeal adduction induced by laryngeal stimulation. Microlaryngoscopy/bronchoscopy is performed to elucidate the anatomic areas of concern in each patient with laryngomalacia and to rule out any additional airway anomalies. With adequate control of active reflux disease, the patient who remains symptomatic usually has a specific anatomic anomaly such as shortened AE folds. Based on the areas of anatomic narrowing found on preoperative evaluation and the microlaryngoscopy and bronchoscopy performed at the beginning of the procedure, the surgical plan is made for division of AE folds only or also for removal of unilateral inward collapsing mucosa.[18,19] Bilateral mucosal excision may result in supraglottic stenosis.[20] While this is a rare complication, stenosis of the supraglottic structure is a very difficult complication to treat. Often a tracheostomy is required, at least temporarily. Unilateral supraglottoplasty is highly successful and avoids the risk of circumferential stenosis. The opposite side may require supraglottoplasty at a future date 15%[19] to 17%[18] of the time. Bilateral supraglottoplasty also carries a reoperation rate of 5.1%.[19] Therefore, unilateral supraglottoplasty is recommended.

Once the surgical plan has been made, the larynx is then exposed. Options for laryngeal exposure include suspension laryngoscopy with a laryngoscope holder and a microscope for visualization or hand-held suspension laryngoscopy and the endoscope for visualization. Suitable laryngoscopes for traditional suspension include the Cherry Jako, Jako-Cherry, Benjamin, Lindholm or Weerda operating laryngoscopes. The latter laryngoscopes provide superior binocular vision and a broad inlet to facilitate instrument manipulation.[17] Hand-held laryngoscopy is accomplished using the anesthesiology intubating laryngoscope with a straight blade. A Wisconsin or Wis-Hipple blade is ideal as the larger posterior opening allows easier access for the endoscope and instrumentation needed to perform supraglottoplasty. The laryngoscope tip may be placed in the vallecula or against the laryngeal surface of the epiglottis depending on the portion of the larynx needing exposure and manipulation. Tissue can be divided or resected using microlaryngeal instruments, the microdebrider,[21] or the carbon dioxide laser.

Consistent success has been experienced using the Wisconsin anesthesia blade in the valleculae to expose the larynx. Typically only the epiglottic tip and the posterior edge of the cricoid are seen. The 4 mm Hopkins rod telescope can maneuver between the epiglottis and the arytenoids. If the patient is breathing spontaneously, bilateral respiratory movement of the vocal folds can rule out vocal cord paresis as this may be the first good look at the vocal folds. Flexible laryngoscopy preoperatively may see only the arytenoids moving and no view of the true vocal folds as the epiglottis is tilted posteriorly covering the folds. Once microlaryngoscopy and bronchoscopy are complete and any additional airway lesions or malacia are noted, the patient is intubated. It is not uncommon that a half size smaller than expected endotracheal tube is all that will fit through the constricted supraglottic opening until the aryepiglottic folds have been released. Once the aryepiglottic folds are released, there is a large air leak around the small tube. In severe aryepiglottic shortening, the patient may only be able to be intubated by inverting the epiglottis into the trachea. The epiglottis is then teased out of the airway using the endoscope at the epiglottic edge or by pressing gently on the pediole of the epiglottis. With the assistant then holding the Wisconsin blade (Fig. 69.3) the aryepiglottic fold is divided using a microlaryngeal scissor, first on one side and then, after repositioning around the endotracheal tube, the other. The endotracheal tube can be used to lever open the narrowed laryngeal inlet by using the endoscope and pushing down on the endotracheal tube to expose the aryepiglottic fold for division. The endoscope is used for the dual purpose of exposure of the aryepiglottic fold and the visualization of the fold to be divided. The fold is cut until the larynx springs open. Typically this is just after a small blood vessel is encountered. Bleeding is controlled with oxymetazoline on a $\frac{1}{4} \times \frac{1}{4}$ inch surgical sponge. At the beginning of the procedure the arytenoids and the epiglottis are parallel. After dividing the aryepiglottic folds, the epiglottis and arytenoids are nearly perpendicular. The patient is then extubated at the end of the procedure

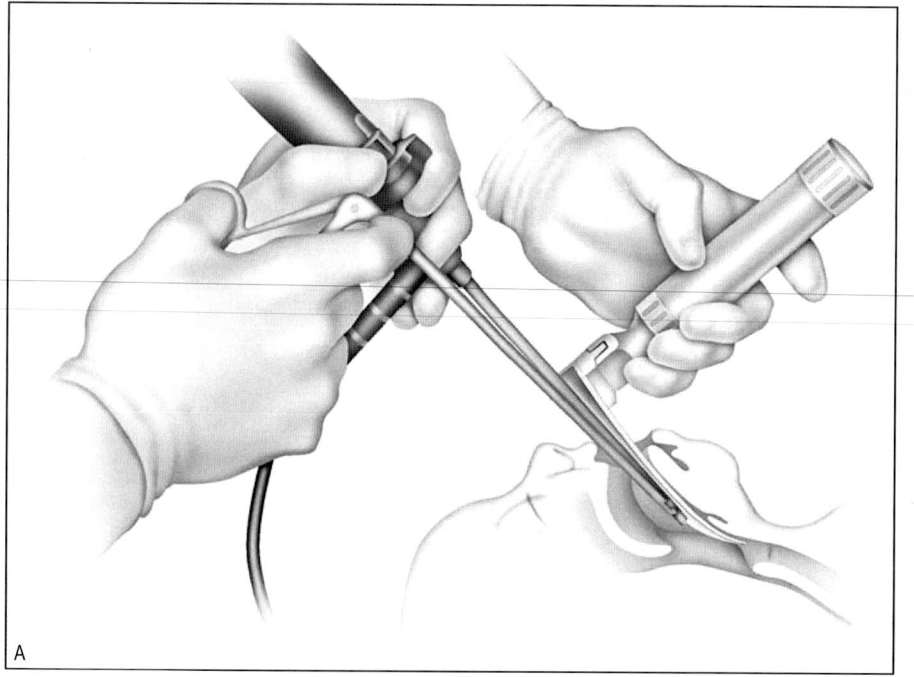

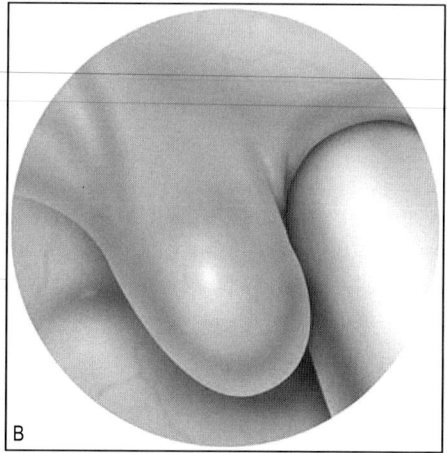

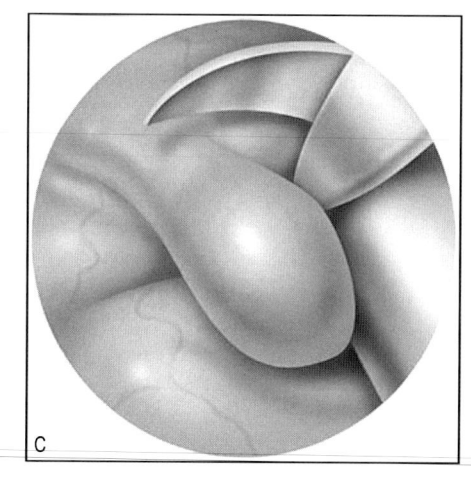

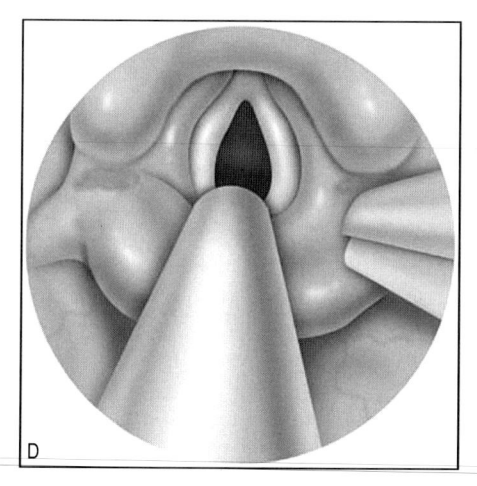

**Fig. 69.3** A, Use of intubating laryngoscope and endoscope instead of suspension laryngoscopy and microscope. B, View of left shortened aryepiglottic fold before division. C, Microlaryngeal scissors in position to clip shortened left aryepiglottic fold. D, View after releasing left and right aryepiglottic folds with scissors just finishing on the right.

# Laryngomalacia — CHAPTER 69

if possible. It is rare that mucosa and submucosal tissue need to be removed from the arytenoids if good preoperative medical control of the edema is accomplished with proton pump inhibitors and/or steroids. Mucosal resection, only if required as determined in the preoperative evaluation, is accomplished using cup forceps and scissors (Fig. 69.4).

If instead of microlaryngeal instruments, the $CO_2$ laser is chosen to perform supraglottoplasty, the typical settings for the $CO_2$ laser are superpulse mode at 6–8 watts for a spot size of 0.5 mm. The use of the $CO_2$ laser requires patient protection from divergent laser beams with moist eye pads and towels to cover any exposed skin. The $CO_2$ laser is used to divide the aryepiglottic folds and remove edematous mucosa overlying the arytenoids. It is important to remove the minimal amount of tissue necessary to relieve the airway obstruction seen at the beginning of the case as overreduction of mucosa and submucosal tissue can lead to supraglottic stenosis. It is important to base the amount of mucosal and submucosa reduction on the beginning laryngoscopy as manipulation of the larynx and time in suspension apparatus can result in acute swelling that, if removed, may result in removing more tissue than needed or stenosis.

The microdebrider wand can also be used to divide the aryepiglottic folds and to remove redundant arytenoids mucosa. This is described by Zalzal and Collins.[21]

In the young infant, suspension laryngoscopy is easily accomplished with the anesthesia intubating laryngoscope (Fig. 69.3). The laryngoscope is lightweight and can be easily maneuvered but does require an assistant to hold the instrument so the surgeon can operate bimanually. The advantage of the laryngoscope being hand held exists only when microlaryngeal instrumentation and the endoscope, or microdebrider with endoscope is the chosen technique. If the $CO_2$ laser is used for the procedure, the static suspension laryngoscopy is preferred for stability. For the very small infant, the weight of the suspension laryngoscope can be problematic and the manipulation of the $CO_2$ laser equipment cumbersome.

Using the endoscope and hand-held laryngoscope instead of the microscope with full suspension laryngoscopy reduces surgical time because the microscope and suspension apparatus do not need to be positioned. The shorter duration also minimizes the length of time the larynx is traumatized with suspension instruments. Using the endoscope and anesthesia laryngoscope, the patient is routinely extubated at the end of the procedure. The extubated patient is monitored in an airway unit or pediatric intensive care unit until feeding well without supplemental oxygen and is discharged in 1–3 days. The intubated patient is usually extubated the day following the procedure and feeding is begun. Hospital discharge is common in 2–5 days.[18] Overnight stays are becoming more common and of 70 cases reported in Leeds, UK, 85% were discharged the following day.[22] Discharge can be based on good oral intake and airway improvement.

## 4 COMPLICATIONS

Complications of supraglottoplasty are rare (10 [7.4%] of 136).[20] While few in number, the complications of supraglottoplasty carry significant morbidity, often requiring repeat surgical procedures or prolonged intensive care and hospitalization. It is therefore incumbent on the surgeon to prevent and avoid as many of the complications as possible. Complications cited include granulomas,[20] sepsis,[13] need for further procedures[18–20] and supraglottic stenosis.[19,20] Supraglottic stenosis is the most feared complication as it is very difficult to correct once it develops. Whereas reconstructing the subglottis is based on a cartilage ring, there is no solid structure in the supraglottis on which to base a reconstruction. Surgery to repair the supraglottic stenosis may only, therefore, result in restenosis or worsening stenosis necessitating a tracheotomy for airway control. Many authors now agree that the complication of supraglottic stenosis is more onerous than the risk of a second surgery when performing a unilateral supraglottoplasty with mucosal

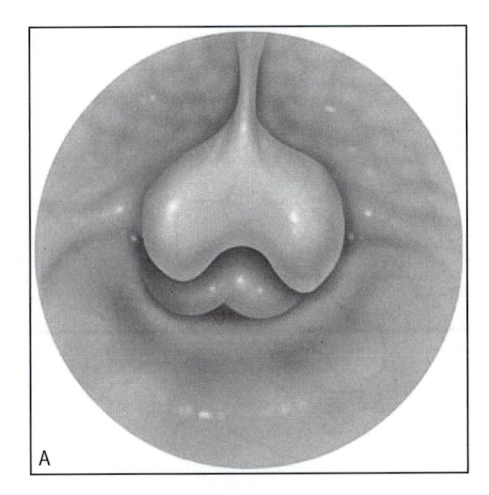

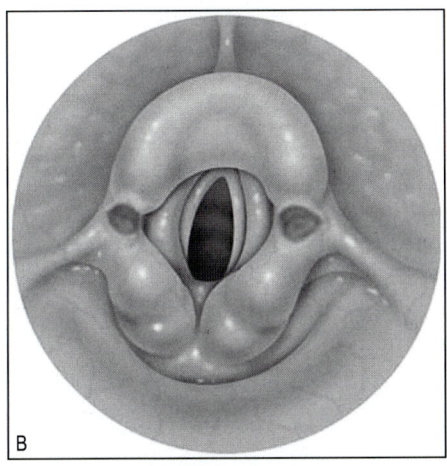

**Fig. 69.4** View of larynx with Wis-blade laryngoscope and 4 mm Hopkins rod laryngoscope, (A) before and (B) after division of aryepiglottic folds.

441

ablation.[18–20] It is therefore recommended to begin conservatively and remove only that mucosa which is necessary, and to avoid bilateral mucosal removal at the initial operation.

## 5 POSTOPERATIVE CARE

Postoperative care is chosen to minimize the chance of surgical complication. Empiric treatment with a proton pump inhibitor for the possible negative effects of reflux on airway healing should be considered for at least the first 6 weeks following supraglottoplasty.[19,23] Steroids are helpful in the control of airway edema and the modulation of healing. Steroids are given for 5 days postoperatively. If stridor returns at the conclusion of the steroids a longer tapering dose over 2 weeks may be helpful early in the postoperative course. Antibiotics are given for 1–2 weeks depending on the length of time a steroid is used. Follow-up in the office with flexible laryngoscopy is performed at the 2-week postoperative visit to monitor healing and assess the potential for supraglottic stenosis. Parents should be counseled to call if the stridor returns before the scheduled postoperative visit so that medical adjustment is possible. Early repeat flexible laryngoscopy may be indicated for a return of the patient's stridor. Often all that is needed is an adjustment of the proton pump inhibitor dosing as the patient may start to grow quickly following airway surgery.

## 6 SUCCESS RATE

The success rate for the procedure is reported between 80%[20] to 100%[18,19] of the time. It may be noted that the lower success rate was recorded in patients with additional airway abnormalities[8,20] and before proton pump inhibitors were widely used (Table 69.1). Poor outcome is usually in those patients with a secondary airway abnormality or significant neurological involvement. Patients with isolated laryngomalacia should expect improvement of their stridor with a single procedure.[22]

### 6.1 FURTHER THERAPY

If clipping the aryepiglottic folds or unilateral mucosal resection is unsuccessful in relieving the airway obstruction that results in poor patient growth and development, the patient may be returned to the operating room for revision surgery. Preoperative evaluation with awake flexible laryngoscopy is critical in planning the revision surgical procedure. The laryngoscopy may be performed in the office or can be performed in the operating room just before anesthesia is induced. Revision surgery may consist of the removal of unilateral mucosa when only AE fold division has been performed and postoperative flexible laryngoscopy shows infolding arytenoids or epiglottic edges or, in the case of previous mucosal removal, the opposite side can undergo mucosal ablation or removal. Care should still be taken not to remove mucosa bilaterally at this stage as supraglottic stenosis can result.

Should supraglottic surgery be unsuccessful in managing the airway a tracheotomy can be performed. Decannulation will be dependent on the patient's growth increasing the radius of the airway and/or resolution of laryngeal edema and erythema that is causing airway obstruction. At times, the pending need for a tracheotomy may herald the need for a Nissen fundoplication with or without gastrostomy tube as proton pump inhibitors do not successfully treat all patients with gastroesophageal reflux. Another consideration for patients whose airway edema persists is an evaluation for eosinophilic esophagitis.[23,24] For certain patients correction of this problem can be dramatic.

**Table 69.1 Supraglottoplasty**

| Indications | Contraindications | Special instrumentation | Tips and pearls |
|---|---|---|---|
| Failure to thrive Airway obstruction Cyanosis with feeds Cor pulmonale Apneic spells Bradycardic spells | Other uncorrectable airway anomalies Multiple levels of anomalies Uncontrollable edema of the airway | Microlaryngeal scissors – straight and side opening $CO_2$ laser | Control reflux first Use antibiotics, steroids, and proton pump inhibitors postoperatively |

Kelley PE. Surgical treatment of laryngomalacia. Operative techniques in otolaryngology. Head Neck Surg 2005;16:198–202.

### 6.2 LONG-TERM FOLLOW-UP

Once outside the initial healing period, it is uncommon for symptoms to recur. Laryngomalacia generally resolves within the first year or two of life, even in children with additional diagnoses. Long-term follow-up is therefore expectant as it is with the children who have milder laryngomalacia not requiring surgical therapy.

## REFERENCES

1. Chandra RK, Gerber ME, Holinger LD. Histological insight into the pathogenesis of severe laryngomalacia. Int J Pediatr Otorhinolaryngol 2001;61:31–38.

2. Goding GS, Pernell KJ. Effect of second laryngeal stimulation during recovery from the laryngeal chemoreflex. Otolaryngol Head Neck Surg 1996;114(1):84–90.
3. Richardson MA, Adams J. Fatal apnea in piglets by way of laryngeal chemoreflex: postmortem findings as anatomic correlates of sudden infant death syndrome in the human infant. Laryngoscope 2005;115(7):1163–9.
4. Thompson DM, Rutter MJ, Rudolph CD. Altered laryngeal sensation: a potential cause of apnea of infancy. Ann Otol Rhinol Laryngol 2005;114(4):258–63.
5. Thompson DM. Laryngopharyngeal sensory testing and assessment of airway protection in pediatric patients. Am J Med 115 Suppl 2003; 3A: 166S–68S.
6. Thompson DM, Rutter MJ, Myer CM, Cotton RT. Hypoxia and altered laryngeal reflexes: a correlation of laryngomalacia disease severity. IXth International Congress of the European Society of Pediatric Otorhinolaryngology, Abstract 2006.
7. Portier F, Marianowski R, Morrisseau-Durand MP, Zerah M, Manac'h Y. Respiratory obstruction as a sign of brainstem dysfunction in infants with Chiari malformations. Int J Pediatr Otorhinolaryngol 2001;57:195–205.
8. Sichel JY, Dangoor MB, Eliashar R, Halperin D. Management of congenital laryngeal malformations. Am J Otolaryngol 2000;21:22–30.
9. McClurg FLD, Evans DA. Laser laryngoplasty for laryngomalacia. Laryngoscope 1994;104:224–52.
10. Roger G, Denoyellle F, Triglia JM, et al. Severe laryngomalacia: surgical indications and results in 115 patients. Laryngoscope 1995;105:1111–17.
11. Burton LK, Murray JA, Thompson DM. Ear, nose, and throat manifestations of gastroesophageal reflux disease. Complaints can be telltale signs. Postgrad Med 2005;117(2):39–45.
12. Manning SC, Inglis AF, Mouzakes J. Laryngeal anatomic differences in pediatric patients with severe laryngomalacia. Arch Otolaryngol Head Neck Surg 2005;131(4):340–43.
13. Holinger LD, Konior RJ. Surgical management of severe laryngomalacia. Laryngoscope 1999;99:136–42.
14. Yellon RF, Borland LM, Kay DJ. Flexible fiberoptic laryngoscopy in children: effect of sitting versus supine position. IXth International Congress of the European Society of Pediatric Otorhinolaryngology, Abstract 2006.
15. Shaker R, Dodds WJ, Ren J, Hogan WJ, Arndorfer RD. Esophagoglottal closure reflex: a mechanism of airway protection. Gastroenterology 1992;102:857–61.
16. Polonovski JM, Contencin P, Francois M. Aryepiglottic fold excision for the treatment of severe laryngomalacia. Ann Otol Rhinol Laryngol 1990;99:624–7.
17. Yuen HW, Tan HK, Balakrishnan A. Synchronous airway lesions and associated anomalies in children with laryngomalacia evaluated with rigid endoscopy. Int J Pediatr Otorhinolaryngol 2006;70(10):1779–84.
18. Kelly SM, Gray SD. Unilateral endoscopic supraglottoplasty for sever laryngomalacia. Arch Otolaryngol Head Neck Surg 1995;121:1351–4.
19. Reddy DK, Matt BH. Unilateral vs. bilateral supraglottoplasty for severe laryngomalacia in children. Arch Otolaryngol Head Neck Surg 2001;127:694–9.
20. Denoyelle F, Mondain M, Gresillon N, et al. Failures and complications of supraglottoplasty in children. Arch Otolaryngol Head Neck Surg 2003;129:1077–80.
21. Zalzal GH, Collins WO. Microdebrider-assisted supraglottoplasty. Int J Pediatr Otorhinolaryngol 2004;69(3):305–306.
22. O'Donnell S, Murphy J, Bew S, Knight, L.C. Aryepigolottoplasty: The Leeds perspective. IXth International Congress of the European Society of Pediatric Otorhinolaryngology, Abstract 2006.
23. Rudolph CD. Gastroesophageal reflux and airway disorders. In: The Pediatric Airway: An Interdisciplinary Approach. Myer CM, Cotton RT, Shott SR, eds. Philadelphia: JB Lippincott; 1995, pp. 327–57.
24. Thompson DM, Arora AS, Romero Y, Dauer EH. Eosinophilic esophagitis: its role in aerodigestive tract disorders. Otolaryngol Clin North Am 2006;39(1):205–21.

# Index

## A

acetaminophen, 92, 103
acoustic rhinometry (AR), 126, 132–3
acromegaly, 292
adenoidectomy, 416–17, 425–8
  ablation/suction cautery, 403–4, 417, 418, 426
  complications, 366, 428
  curette, 425–6
  patient selection, 425
  postoperative management, 427–8
  power-assisted/microdebrider, 403, 404, 416–17, 427, 435
  radiofrequency, 427
  success rate, 428
  techniques, 403–4, 416–17, 425–7
  transnasal, 426–7
  in velopharyngeal insufficiency, 376
  *see also* adenotonsillectomy
adenoids
  enlarged, 65, 125, 403–5, 425
  sphincter pharyngoplasty and, 374–5
adenotonsillar hyperplasia, 403–5, 414–19
  diagnosis of dyspnea, 414–16, 417
  efficacy of surgery, 417–19
  non-surgical management, 416
  surgical treatment, 416–17
adenotonsillectomy, 403–4
  complications, 421, 422–3
  predictive value of polysomnography, 420–3
  *see also* adenoidectomy; tonsillectomy
adjustable positive airways pressure (APAP), 60, 61–2
  *see also* positive airway pressure (PAP) therapy
Aethoxysklerol (AES), 166
age differences
  adenotonsillectomy complications, 421, 422, 423
  uvulopalatopharyngoplasty outcome, 383
AHI *see* Apnea Hypopnea Index
airflow
  assessment, 27, 30
  nasal, evaluation, 126
airway (upper)
  clinical examination, 11
  difficult intubation/ventilation, 90–1, 102
  edema, postoperative, 83, 92, 101–2
  evaluation, 11–20, 81
  mechanism of maintenance, 78
  morphologic abnormalities, 6–7
  obese patients, 96, 97
  PAP-associated changes, 66
  $P_{crit}$ *see* critical closing pressure
  preoperative assessment, 98
  pressure recordings *see* pressure recordings
  resistance, contribution of nose, 121–2, 124
airway obstruction
  evaluation, 11–20, 42–4, 81
  Fujita classification *see* Fujita classification of obstruction
  Mueller maneuver *see* Mueller maneuver
  multilevel *see* multilevel airway obstruction
  postoperative, 101–2
    maxillofacial procedures, 332, 337
    uvulopalatopharyngoplasty, 180, 214, 362, 395
    velopharyngeal insufficiency surgery, 371, 376
  severity *see* severity of OSA/OSAHS
alar batten graft, external nasal valve repair, 137
alcohol consumption, 45, 48
aliasing, 27, 28
allergic rhinitis, 65, 140, 143, 416
Alloderm®, posterior pharyngeal wall augmentation, 375
American Academy of Sleep Medicine (AASM)
  oral appliances, 72
  polysomnography guidelines, 22–3, 33–4
American Board of Medical Specialties (ABMS), 1–2
American Board of Sleep Medicine, 1
American College of Sports Medicine (ACSM), 55
American Society of Anesthesiologists (ASA), 94, 97
analgesia, postoperative, 91–2, 103
  adenoidectomy, 427–8
  lateral pharyngoplasty, 231
  minimally invasive palatal procedures, 150–1, 156, 162–3, 166
  nasal surgery, 146
  Powell–Riley protocol, 332
  tongue base surgery, 289, 298
  tonsillectomy, 435–6
  uvulopalatopharyngoplasty, 193, 199
  zetapalatopharyngoplasty, 204
  *see also* pain, postoperative
anesthesia, 88–94, 96–103
  choice of technique, 89
  clearance, 90
  emergence, 100–1
  increased risks, 88
  intraoperative management, 90–1, 99–101
  monitoring during, 98–9
  pediatric patients, 399–400
  postoperative management, 91–4, 101–3
  preoperative assessment, 97–8
  preoperative management, 88–90, 97–9
  risk scoring, 97
  team, communication with, 90
angina, postoperative, 363
anorexiants, 56
anti-obesity medications, 55–7
antibiotics, perioperative, 92
antihypertensive therapy *see* blood pressure control
anxiolytics, 89, 93, 98
apnea, 4, 33
  central, 34
  mixed, 34
  obstructive, 34
Apnea Hypopnea Index (AHI), 19, 45–6
  after nasal surgery, 126–7
  benefits of weight loss, 54
  defining surgical success, 113, 380
  OSAHS score and, 107
  treatment thresholds, 46, 49–50, 61, 80
Apnea Index (AI), 46, 380
apparent life-threatening events (ALTE) in infants, 24, 414
appetite-suppressing drugs, 56
arousals (respiratory effort-related; RERA), 33, 88
  definition, 34
  Respiratory Disturbance Index, 46
  subcortical, 37–8
arrhythmias *see* cardiac arrhythmias
aryepiglottic (AE) folds
  shortened, 439, 440
  surgical division, 440–1
Asian faces, modified maxillomandibular advancement osteotomy, 334–7
aspiration of gastric contents, 89, 98
atherosclerosis, 85
attention deficit hyperactivity disorder (ADHD), 428
awakenings, frequent, 4, 5

## B

barbiturates, 98
bariatric surgery, 49, 57–8
  benefits, 54
Beckwith–Wiedemann syndrome, 405
behavioral effects, obstructive sleep apnea, 46
behavioral modification, obstructive sleep apnea, 47–8
benzodiazepines, 89, 98
Bernoulli principle, 116, 120
bi-level positive airways pressure (BI-PAP), 60, 66
  *see also* positive airway pressure (PAP) therapy
bimaxillary protrusion, 334, 335
bipolar polysomnographic recordings, 25, 26
bipolar radiofrequency surgery, 235, 236
bit depth, polysomnographic recordings, 27
bleeding, postoperative
  coblation inferior turbinate reduction, 146
  laser-assisted uvulopalatoplasty, 151–2
  maxillomandibular advancement osteotomy, 337
  snare uvulectomy, 156
  tongue base surgery, 255–6, 290, 298
  tonsillectomy, 432, 436
  uvulopalatopharyngoplasty, 181, 199, 363
  zetapalatopharyngoplasty, 204
bleeding disorders, 255
blood pressure control, 93, 102–3
  maxillofacial surgery, 332, 337
  submucosal glossectomy, 255, 297
  *see also* hypertension
body mass index (BMI), 51
  laser-assisted uvulopalatoplasty and, 148, 152
  multilevel surgery and, 117
  OSAHS score, 107
  table, 52
  treatment thresholds, 54, 55–6
  uvulopalatopharyngoplasty outcome and, 383
  *see also* obesity
body movements, 4
bone anchoring device
  hyomandibular suspension with hyoid distraction, 321, 322
  nasal valve repair, 130, 131, 138
  tongue base resection with hyoepiglottoplasty, 284–5
  tongue suture suspension, 259–60, 274, 405–6
bone grafts, maxillomandibular advancement osteotomy, 331, 335–6
Breathe Right™ nasal strips, 125–6, 129–30
bronchoscopy, in laryngomalacia, 439
bruxism, 4, 7

## C

C-reactive protein (CRP), 85–7
cannabinoid receptors, 56–7
capnometry *see* end tidal $CO_2$
CAPSO *see* cautery-assisted palatal stiffening operation
carbonization, tissue, 240
cardiac arrhythmias, 24, 97
  postoperative, 363
cardiology clearance, 90
cardiovascular complications, postoperative, 363

445

# INDEX

cardiovascular disease, 46, 85
  preoperative assessment, 97–8
cardiovascular risk factors
  PAP therapy and, 66, 86
  surgical treatment and, 85–7
carotid intima-media thickness (IMT), 86
cartilage spanning graft, internal nasal valve repair, 136–7
cautery-assisted palatal stiffening operation (CAPSO), 159–63
  patient selection, 159–61
  postoperative care and complications, 162–3
  success rate, 163
  surgical technique, 159, 160, 161–2
Celon AG Medical Instruments, 237
cephalometry, lateral X-ray, 13–14, 81, 187
  Asians *vs* Caucasians, 334
  open tongue base resection, 280
certification, sleep medicine, 1–2
chest
  funnel, 79, 415
  negative pressure, 78–9
Cheyne–Stokes breathing, 66
children
  adenotonsillar hyperplasia, 403–5, 414–19
  adenotonsillectomy *see* adenoidectomy; adenotonsillectomy; tonsillectomy
  craniofacial abnormalities, 77, 410–12
  distraction osteogenesis, 341, 411–12
  laryngomalacia, 437–42
  macroglossia and ptotic tongue, 405–10
  magnetic resonance imaging, 15
  mandibular growth pattern, 78–9
  nasal and nasopharyngeal obstruction, 125, 400–3
  obstructive sleep apnea, 39–41, 399, 414–19
  oropharyngeal obstruction, 403–5
  polysomnography *see* polysomnography (PSG), children
  postoperative management, 400
  preoperative planning, 399–400
  sleep-related breathing disorders, 398–412, 421–2
    causes, 398
    diagnosis, 398–9
    non-surgical management, 399
    surgical management, 399–412
  submucosal glossectomy, 256, 407–8
  tracheostomy, 359, 411
  velopharyngeal insufficiency, 370, 371
choanal atresia, 400–1
cholesterol, 53, 66
chronic obstructive pulmonary disease (COPD), 66
claustrophobia, 64, 66
cleft palate
  adenoidectomy and, 427, 428
  surgery, 224, 371
clinical assessment, 3
co-morbid conditions, 3, 49
  PAP therapy, 61, 66
  preoperative clearance, 90
coagulation
  necrosis, 234
  submucous, 233, 234, 235–7, 241
coblation *see* radiofrequency cold ablation
Coblator system (Arthrocare), 237, 430
columelloplasty, 138
compliance
  nasal CPAP, 70
  PAP therapy, 48, 63–5
computed tomography (CT), 14–15, 292, 399
continuous positive airways pressure (CPAP), 48, 60–7, 80
  analysis of failures, 69–70
  benefits, 66, 86
  children, 416
  nasal obstruction and, 65, 121
  nasal surgery and, 65, 127, 128
  oral appliances with, 75
  polysomnographic titration, 23, 61
  postoperative, 89, 92, 214
  preoperative, 81–2, 89
  provision, 61–2, 65–6
  rare cases with difficulty, 66
  *see also* positive airway pressure (PAP) therapy
Cook airway exchange catheter, 101
coronary artery disease (CAD), 24, 33
corticosteroids
  intranasal, 125
  laryngomalacia, 439, 442
  postoperative airway edema, 83, 92, 102
cost analysis, polysomnography, 34
Cottle maneuver, 125, 130
COX-2 non-steroidal anti-inflammatory drugs, 92
CPAP *see* continuous positive airways pressure
craniofacial abnormalities, 6, 77
  chronic mouth breathers, 125
  congenital, 24–5
  distraction osteogenesis, 339–41, 411–12
  hypothesis, 78–9
  orthodontic treatment and, 76–7
  surgical management, 410–12
  X-ray cephalometry, 13
craniopharyngioma, 39
critical closing pressure ($P_{crit}$), 19–20, 184–7
  effects of UPPP, 186–7
CT scanning *see* computed tomography
cyanosis, 4
cytokines, pro-inflammatory, 85–6

## D

daytime sleepiness, excessive *see* excessive daytime sleepiness
daytime symptoms, 5, 6, 7
deep vein thrombosis (DVT), prophylaxis, 93
dehiscence, wound *see* wound dehiscence
dehydration, postoperative, 364
dental abnormalities, 6–7
dental overjet, 7
dentures, 222
depression, 5
descending palatine arteries, 332
device therapy, 48
dexamethasone, postoperative airway edema, 92, 98, 102
diabetes mellitus, 66, 90
diet therapy, 55
discharge, postoperative, 94
distraction osteogenesis (DO), 339–41, 411–12
dolichofacial pattern, 77, 78–9
Down syndrome, 405, 406, 427
doxapram, 101
drains, surgical, 254–5, 285
drooling, 4
dry mouth, 4
durable medical equipment (DME) providers, 61, 62, 65
dynamic range, polysomnographic recordings, 27
dysphagia
  hypertrophic lingual tonsils, 265
  postoperative
    expansion sphincter pharyngoplasty, 224, 226
    external submucosal glossectomy, 298
    lateral pharyngoplasty, 231
    radiofrequency tongue base reduction, 245
    submucosal uvulopalatopharyngoplasty, 199
    zetapalatopharyngoplasty, 204
dyspnea
  diagnosis in children, 414–16
  paroxysmal nocturnal, 4

## E

ear, nose and throat (ENT) medicine *see* otolaryngology
economics, polysomnography, 34
edema
  postoperative airway, 83, 92, 101–2
  postoperative tongue, 245, 297–8
electro-oculogram (EOG), 25, 27
electrocardiogram (ECG), 25, 26, 27
electrocautery ablation
  adenoidectomy, 403–4
  *see also* cautery-assisted palatal stiffening operation (CAPSO)
electrocoagulation, 235–7, 241
  *see also* coagulation
electroencephalogram (EEG), 22
  case study, 39–41
  polysomnographic recordings, 25, 27
electrolytic effect, radiofrequency surgery, 238
electromyogram (EMG), 25–6, 27
electrotomy, 233, 234, 240–1
  tissue resection, 234
empty nose association, 65
end tidal $CO_2$ ($ETCO_2$), 22, 26, 27
endocannabinoid system (ECS), 56–7
endoscopic coblation lingual tonsillectomy, 265–7
endoscopy, upper airway
  awake, 11, 187–8
  minimally invasive submucosal glossectomy (SMILE), 249–52
  sleep, 12, 17–18, 42–4
    description of findings, 17, 43
    multilevel obstruction, 43, 111
    patient selection, 42
    specificity and sensitivity, 43–4
    technique, 42–3
    uvulopalatopharyngoplasty, 379
    value, 383
endotracheal intubation, 90–1, 99–100
  difficult, algorithm, 102
  extubation, 91, 100–1
  predicting difficult, 90, 98
  preoxygenation, 99
  preparation for, 90
  techniques, 90–1, 100
endotracheal tube (ETT), 100
epidemiology, OSAHS, 3
epiglottic obstruction
  methods of evaluation, 12
  nasendoscopic evaluation, 18, 43
  submucosal glossectomy failure, 257
epileptiform activity, 40
Epworth Sleepiness Scale (ESS), 5, 46, 47, 378
Eschmann tube exchange catheter, 101
Esmarch appliance, 73
Esmarch–Heiberg manipulation, 72
esophageal pressure (Peso) recordings, 18, 22
  children, 414, 415, 419
esophagoglottal closure reflex, 438–9
eszopiclone (Lunesta®), 63
ethanol, palatal sclerotherapy, 166
excessive daytime sleepiness (EDS), 5
  indicating surgery, 80–1
  measurement, 23–4
exercise, 55
expansion sphincter pharyngoplasty, 224–6
extubation, tracheal, 91, 100–1

## F

face masks, 62
Fairbanks uvulopalatopharyngoplasty technique *see under* uvulopalatopharyngoplasty
Faradic effect, 238
fascia lata, hyomandibular suspension, 295–7, 299
fat
  pharyngeal deposition, 15, 96
  visceral, 54
fatigue, daytime, 7
Friedman surgical staging system, 11, 107–9
  multilevel pharyngeal surgery, 269
  uvulopalatopharyngoplasty, 107–9, 188, 379
  zetapalatopharyngoplasty, 201, 202
Friedman tongue position (FTP), 6, 104–10, 378–9
  children, 399
  determination, 104–5, 106
  laser-assisted uvulopalatoplasty, 148
  original and new systems compared, 104, 105
  OSAHS score, 105–7
Fujita classification of obstruction, 321
  multilevel surgery and, 111, 306–7
Fujita's procedure *see* uvulopalatopharyngoplasty
functional somatic syndromes, 7
fungal infections, postoperative, 152
funnel chest, 79, 415
Furlow double opposing Z-plasty, 371–3

# INDEX

## G

gastric banding surgery, 54, 57
gastric bypass, Roux-en-Y (RYGB), 57
gastroesophageal reflux (GER), 4
  causing laryngomalacia, 437, 438–9
  management, 89, 442
gender differences
  sleep-disordered breathing, 3, 4, 8
  uvulopalatopharyngoplasty outcome, 383
genioglossus advancement (GA), 271–2, 301–3
  complications, 332
  hyoid suspension with, 276–7
  one-stage multilevel surgery with/without, 312–20
  pediatric patients, 406, 407
  postoperative management, 302
  Powell–Riley phase I, 327–8
  presurgical evaluation, 301
  rationale, 83, 301
  success rates, 276–7, 303, 332–3
  surgical technique, 271–2, 273, 301–2, 303
geniohyoid muscles, 282
genioplasty, 335
George gauge, 72
Gerlach tonsils, hypertrophy, 428
glossectomy
  external submucosal, 281, 292–300
    complications, 298
    outcomes, 298–9
    patient selection, 292–3
    postoperative management, 297–8
    salvage options, 299–300
    surgical procedure, 293–7
  midline laser (MLG), 287–91
    complications, 289–90
    patient selection, 287
    postoperative management, 289
    results, 290–1
    surgical procedure, 287–9, 290
  minimally invasive submucosal, 248–57
    complications, 255–6
    endoscopically assisted *see* submucosal minimally invasive lingual excision
    outcomes, 256
    patient selection, 248
    pediatric patients, 407–8
    percutaneous approach, 248–9, 256
    postoperative management, 255
    procedures, 248–55
    salvage options, 256–7
    *vs* open tongue base resection, 285–6
  submucosal midline (local), 248, 252
  *see also* tongue base resection
glossoptosis, 410–11
glycopyrrolate, 98, 101
Grass polysomnography systems, 22, 23, 24
Grisel syndrome, 428
Gyrus ENT system, 237, 244–5

## H

Han-uvulopalatopharyngoplasty *see* uvulopalatopharyngoplasty (UPPP), Han modification
headache, 5
heart failure, 24
heart rate, 37–8
hemorrhage, postoperative *see* bleeding, postoperative
hemostasis, intraoperative, 103
  genioglossus advancement, 302
  submucosal glossectomy, 249
Herbst device, 75
hiccups, postoperative, 290
history, clinical, 4–5, 7, 47
home sleep testing, 60
humidification, 64, 66
hyoglossus muscles, 280, 282–3
hyoid suspension (hyothyroidopexy), 269
  alone, 305–11
  complications, 310, 332

genioglossus advancement with, 276–7
one-stage multilevel surgery with, 312–20
operative technique, 269, 270–1, 307, 308
patient selection, 305–7
postoperative management, 307
Powell–Riley phase I, 328, 329
rationale, 83, 305
results, 307–10, 332–3
*see also* hyomandibular suspension
hyolingual complex, preoperative evaluation, 280
hyomandibular suspension, 269
  external submucosal glossectomy with, 295–7, 298, 299
  and hyoid distraction–expansion, 321–4
  open tongue base resection with, 279, 284–5
hyothyroidopexy *see* hyoid suspension
hypertension, 6
  benefits of PAP therapy, 66
  preoperative assessment, 90, 98
  sibutramine and, 56
  submucosal glossectomy and, 255
  uvulopalatopharyngoplasty and, 363
  *see also* blood pressure control
hypnotic agents, 63–4, 89, 93
hypoglossal nerve, 279, 280
  external submucosal glossectomy, 293, 294
  injury, 245, 256, 310, 318
  intraoperative monitoring, 281
  open tongue base resection, 283, 284
  ultrasound detection, 248
hypopharyngeal obstruction
  combined with obstruction at other levels, 111
  Friedman tongue position, 104–5, 107
  genioglossus advancement, 301, 302
  maxillofacial surgical techniques, 326–33
  surgical techniques, 83, 112, 117
  uvulopalatopharyngoplasty (UPPP) efficacy and, 107–9
hypopharyngeal procedures, minimally invasive *see* minimally invasive hypopharyngeal procedures
hypopnea, 33, 34
hypotension, 7
hypoxemia, cardiovascular effects, 85–6

## I

implants, palatal Pillar® *see* palatal implants
infants
  polysomnography, 24–5
  sleep-related breathing disorders, 398
infections, postoperative
  laser-assisted uvulopalatoplasty, 152
  nasal valve repair, 132
  open tongue base resection, 281, 285
  tongue base reduction by radiofrequency, 204, 245, 395
  tracheotomy/tracheostomy, 352
inferior alveolar nerve, 330, 332
inflammatory markers, 85–6
infraorbital nerve, nasal valve repair, 131, 132
injection snoreplasty (IS), 165–7
  as salvage technique, 392
insomnia, chronic, 7
intensive care unit (ICU), postoperative monitoring, 83, 92, 101
interleukin-1 (IL-1), 85
interleukin-6 (IL-6), 85–6
interleukin-18 (IL-18), 85, 86
intermaxillary fixation (IMF)
  intraoperative, 329, 330–1
  postoperative, 336
intraoperative management, 90–1, 99–101
intubation *see* endotracheal intubation

## J

Joule's law, 238–9

## K

Klearway, 74, 75

## L

labioglossopexy, 410–11
laparoscopic adjustable silicone gastric banding (LASGB), 57, 58
laryngeal mask airway (LMA), 90, 100
laryngomalacia, 437–42
  preoperative evaluation, 438–9
  primary, 437, 438
  secondary, 437–8
  surgical management, 439–42
laryngoscopy, 100
  laryngomalacia, 438–9, 440, 441, 442
  lingual tonsillectomy, 265
laryngospasm, postoperative, 101, 364
laryngotracheal deformities, tube-related, 352–3
laser-assisted uvulopalatoplasty (LAUP), 148–53, 163, 184
  British method, 149, 150, 151
  complications, 151–2
  failed radiofrequency ablation of palate (RFAP), 389
  failed uvulopalatopharyngoplasty, 387–9
  patient selection, 148–9
  postoperative management, 150–1
  procedure, 149–50
  results, 152–3
  salvage of failed, 386–7
laser midline glossectomy *see* glossectomy, midline laser
laser supraglottoplasty, 441
lateral pharyngeal wall
  collapse, 43, 224, 227
  fat deposition, 15, 96
lateral pharyngoplasty (LP), 184, 224, 227–31
  patient selection, 227
  postoperative care and complications, 231
  results, 226, 231
  surgical technique, 227–31
lateral X-ray cephalometry *see* cephalometry, lateral X-ray
LAUP *see* laser-assisted uvulopalatoplasty
Le Fort I osteotomy, 329, 330, 335, 336
lifestyle management, 54–5
lingual artery
  external submucosal glossectomy, 293, 294
  minimally invasive submucosal glossectomy, 248, 250, 253
  open tongue base resection, 279, 280, 283, 284
  small branches, 254, 255, 298
lingual tonsil hypertrophy, 15, 257, 265
  midline laser glossectomy and, 288
  non-surgical treatment, 266
  pediatric patients, 409
  preoperative evaluation, 266
lingual tonsillectomy
  endoscopic coblation, 265–7
  operative techniques, 266, 409
  patient selection, 265–6
  pediatric patients, 409–10
  submucosal glossectomy failure, 257
  uvulopalatopharyngoplasty, 192
lingual veins, 279, 280
  external submucosal glossectomy, 293, 294
lingualplasty, submucosal, 248, 253–5
linguoplasty, midline laser glossectomy (MLG) with, 287–91
lipectomy, during tracheostomy, 344
lipids, plasma, 53
local anesthesia
  cautery-assisted palatal stiffening operation, 161
  inferior turbinate reduction procedures, 140, 144, 145
  injection snoreplasty, 165
  laser-assisted uvulopalatoplasty, 149
  palatal implants, 171
  postoperative analgesia, 91, 101
  radiofrequency tongue base reduction, 244
  snare uvulectomy, 154, 155
  uvulopalatal flap, 207
lymphatic malformations, microcystic, tongue, 408

## M

macroglossia, 6, 248
  contraindicating tongue suture suspension, 262

447

# INDEX

macroglossia, (Continued)
  pediatric surgery, 405–10
  pediatric syndromal, 256, 405
  preoperative evaluation, 280, 292–3
  retrognathia with, 257
  vs lingual tonsil hypertrophy, 265
  see also retrolingual (retroglossal) obstruction
magnetic resonance imaging (MRI), 15–17
  before tongue reduction surgery, 280, 292
Maintenance of Wakefulness Test (MWT), 23–4
majority of epoch (MOE) rule, sleep staging, 37, 39
Mallampati score, 6, 17, 378–9
  vs Friedman tongue position, 104, 105
mandible
  distraction osteogenesis, 340, 411–12
  growth effects of negative thoracic pressure, 78–9
  hypoplasia, 410–12
  postoperative fractures, 332
mandibular advancement devices, 48, 72, 73–5
  non-titratable, 73–4
  titratable, 74–5
mandibular osteotomy with genioglossus advancement see genioglossus advancement
mandibular plane to hyoid distance, 280
mandibular repositioner, 74
Marfan's syndrome, 339
masks
  PAP therapy, 62
  side effects, 66
maxillofacial skeletal deficiency, 410–12
  distraction osteogenesis, 339–41, 411–12
  labioglossopexy, 410–11
maxillofacial surgery, 326–33
  complications, 332
  patient selection, 326–7
  postoperative management, 332
  success rate, 332–3
  techniques, 327–31 see also specific techniques
maxillomandibular advancement, distraction osteogenesis, 340, 341, 410–11
maxillomandibular advancement osteotomy (MMO; MMA)
  complications, 332
  modified for Asian faces, 334–7
  patient selection, 327
  postoperative management, 332
  Powell–Riley phase II, 82, 328–31
  rationale, 83, 339
  success rates, 84, 333, 334
  uvulopalatopharyngoplasty failures, 187
maxillomandibular widening, by distraction osteogenesis, 340, 341
meal replacements, 55
meals, before bedtime, 48
medical clearance, 90
medical conditions, associated see co-morbid conditions
metabolic syndrome, 53–4
microarousals, 37–8
microdebrider (power-assisted)
  adenoidectomy, 403, 404, 416–17, 427, 435
  tonsillectomy, 434–6
micrognathia, 410
microlaryngoscopy, in laryngomalacia, 439
micronutrient supplements, 58
midazolam, 98
midface hypoplasia, 410–12
midline laser glossectomy (MLG), 287–91
minimally invasive hypopharyngeal procedures
  lingual tonsillectomy, 265–7
  radiofrequency applications, 233–42
  radiofrequency tongue base reduction, 243–6
  submucosal glossectomy, 248–57
  tongue base stabilization, 258–63
minimally invasive palatal procedures
  cautery-assisted palatal stiffening, 159–63
  injection snoreplasty, 165–7
  laser-assisted uvulopalatoplasty, 148–53
  palatal implants, 169–75
  snare uvulectomy, 154–8
minimally invasive single-stage multilevel surgery (MISSMLS), 113
minimally invasive surgical treatment, 112–13

mitomycin-C, topical, 366, 369, 401
MMA, MMO see maxillomandibular advancement osteotomy
monitoring
  postoperative see postoperative monitoring
  during surgery, 98–9
monopolar radiofrequency surgery, 234–5
Montgomery tracheal cannula, 345, 347
mouth breathers, obligate, 65
mouth breathing
  chronic childhood, 125
  instability, 122
Mueller maneuver (MM), 11–13, 81, 104, 224
  multilevel pharyngeal surgery, 269
multilevel airway obstruction, 80
  incidence, 111
  methods of evaluation, 12
  sleep nasendoscopy, 43
  uvulopalatopharyngoplasty, 112, 276–7, 383, 384
multilevel surgery, 111–17, 268–77
  conceptual basis, 111–12
  history, 112
  minimally invasive, for mild/moderate OSAHS, 112–13
  patient selection, 268–9
  postoperative care and complications, 274–6
  risk management and complications, 117
  role of nasal surgery, 116, 127, 269
  short- vs long-term results, 115
  single stage procedure, 312–20
    complications, 318
    patient selection, 312
    patients and methods, 312–15
    pre- and postoperative care, 315–18
    results, 318, 319–20
  single stage vs multi-staged, 115–16
  success rates, 276–7
  systematic review of literature, 113–15
  techniques, 116–17, 269–74
Multiple Sleep Latency Test (MSLT), 23–4
muscle relaxants, 91, 100
mylohyoid muscle, 282
myocardial infarction, 85

# N

Nager's syndrome, 376
narcotic agents
  postoperative analgesia, 91–2, 103
  preoperative use, 89, 98
nares, 120
nasal congestion, 125
nasal continuous positive airways pressure (NCPAP) see continuous positive airways pressure
nasal decongestant test, 125, 143–4
nasal masks, 62
nasal masses/neoplasms, 400
nasal obstruction, 120–3
  anatomical basis, 120–1, 124
  benefits of treatment, 122–3
  causes, 124–5
  CPAP therapy and, 65, 121
  diagnostic evaluation, 7, 81, 125–6
  inferior turbinate hypertrophy, 140, 143
  at nasal valve, 129
  pediatric patients, 125, 400–3
  postoperative, 92
  sleep-disordered breathing and, 121–2, 124
  surgical therapy see nasal surgery
  velopharyngeal insufficiency, 376
nasal packing, postoperative, 92
nasal polyps, 125
nasal pressure transducers, 30
nasal septal deviation, 121, 124, 125
  inferior turbinate hypertrophy with, 143
  nasal valve collapse, 129, 130, 135
nasal septum, 120
nasal strips, Breathe Right™, 125–6, 129–30
nasal surgery, 124–8
  CPAP and, 65, 127, 128
  impact on snoring and OSAHS, 122–3, 126–7
  inferior turbinate hypertrophy, 140–2, 143–7
  nasal valve collapse, 129–33, 135–8

preoperative evaluation, 125–6
rationale, 82–3, 124
role in multilevel treatment, 116, 127, 269
single vs multi-stage, 115–16
nasal turbinate, inferior
  bipolar radiofrequency coblation reduction, 143–7
  obstructive hypertrophy, 140, 143
  radiofrequency volumetric reduction, 140–2
nasal turbinectomy, 65, 140
nasal valve, 120–1, 129
  collapse, 124–5, 129, 134–8
    evaluation, 126, 129–30, 135
    surgical techniques, 135–8
  external, 120, 134–5
    reconstruction techniques, 137–8
  internal, 120–1, 124, 134
    reconstruction techniques, 135–7
  obstruction, 129
  suspension (repair), 129–33, 138
    complications, 132
    patient selection, 129–30
    postoperative management, 132
    success rate, 132–3
    surgical technique, 130–2, 138
nasal vestibule, 120
nasendoscopy see endoscopy, upper airway
nasometry (nasalence testing), 370
nasopharyngeal airway, 90, 101
nasopharyngeal masses/neoplasms, 400
nasopharyngeal obstruction, pediatric patients, 400–3
nasopharyngeal obturator, 366, 367–9
nasopharyngeal stenosis (NPS)
  after adenoidectomy, 366, 428
  after uvulopalatopharyngoplasty, 181–2, 199, 366–9
    grading, 366, 367, 381
    surgical techniques, 366, 367, 368
    treatment options, 367–9
  pediatric patients, 401–3
neck circumference, 6, 51–3, 98
neonates
  choanal atresia or stenosis, 400–1
  polysomnography, 24–5
  sleep-related breathing disorders, 398
Nernst equation, 238
neurocognitive impairment, 5
neuromuscular blockade, 91, 100
nocturia, 5
nocturnal airway patency appliance (NAPA), 73, 74
nocturnal symptoms, 4–5, 6, 7
non-steroidal anti-inflammatory drugs (NSAIDs), 92, 103
nose
  airflow evaluation, 126
  airway resistance, 121–2, 124
  anatomic changes, 7
  cross-sectional area (CSA), 126, 132–3
  functional valvular anatomy, 120–1, 124
  ventilatory reflexes, 122
Nyquist's theorem, 27

# O

obesity, 51–8
  abdominal, 53–4
  airway changes, 96, 97
  anesthesia management, 89
  association with OSAHS, 6, 51, 96
  bariatric surgery, 49
  causes, 53
  childhood, 399
  evaluation, 51–3
  history taking, 53
  lifestyle management, 54–5
  management, 48, 51–8
  pharmacotherapy, 55–7
  preoperative assessment, 97–9
  risk assessment, 53–4
  surgery see bariatric surgery
  tracheostomy, 343
  treatment, 54–8
  uvulopalatopharyngoplasty outcome and, 383
obstructive sleep apnea (OSA), 3
  adenotonsillectomy, 420–1, 423

# INDEX

airway evaluation, 11–20
clinical presentation, 4–7
decision making and treatment algorithm, 45–50
definitions, 45–6
effects, 33, 46
evaluation and diagnosis, 46–7
with intact sleep architecture, 37–9
pediatric, 39–41, 399, 414–19
polysomnography, 33–41
position-dependent, 33–7, 383
severity *see* severity of OSA/OSAHS
sleep state dependent, 36–7
treatment, 47–50
obstructive sleep apnea/hypopnea syndrome (OSAHS), 3
adverse effects, 80
children, 399
clinical assessment, 3
clinical presentation, 4–7
definition, 45–6
epidemiology, 3
score, 105–7
severity *see* severity of OSA/OSAHS
surgical staging *see* Friedman surgical staging system
*vs* upper airway resistance syndrome, 8
occlusion, dental
effects of oral appliances, 75, 76
maxillomandibular advancement osteotomy and, 330–1, 332, 335
operating tables, 99
opioids *see* narcotic agents
oral appliances (OA), 48, 72–7
CPAP with, 75
patient evaluation, 13, 14, 72
postoperative management, 75–7
practical procedures, 72–3
side effects, 75, 76
types, 73–5
oral breathing *see* mouth breathing
oral seal, 77–9
orlistat, 56
oronasal fistula, 220, 222
oropharyngeal airway, 101
oropharyngeal obstruction
combined with obstruction at other levels, 111
pediatric patients, 403–5
sleep nasendoscopy, 43
surgical treatment, 83, 111–12
orthodontic treatment, 76–7, 335
orthostatic intolerance, 7
OSA *see* obstructive sleep apnea
OSAHS *see* obstructive sleep apnea/hypopnea syndrome
OSAHS score, 105–7
osteotomy
Le Fort I, 329, 330, 335, 336
sagittal split, 329–30, 336
transpalatal advancement pharyngoplasty, 220, 221
otolaryngology (ENT), 1–2
positive airway pressure therapy, 60, 61–6
outpatient surgery, 88–9
overweight, 51–8
evaluation, 51–3
history taking, 53
risk assessment, 53–4
treatment, 54–8
*see also* obesity
oximeter, 27
oxygen desaturation, postoperative
adenotonsillectomy, 421, 423
uvulopalatopharyngoplasty, 362–3
oxygen desaturation index (ODI), 380
oxygen saturation
impact of nasal surgery, 127
as measure of disease severity, 46
postoperative monitoring, 92
oxygenation, postoperative, 92

## P

pain, postoperative
cautery-assisted palatal stiffening operation, 163
hyoid suspension and expansion, 324
injection snoreplasty, 166
laser-assisted uvulopalatoplasty, 151
nasal valve repair, 132
submucosal glossectomy, 256, 298
submucosal uvulopalatopharyngoplasty, 198–9
tonsillectomy, 429, 431–2
uvulopalatopharyngoplasty, 195, 364
Z-palatoplasty, 204
*see also* analgesia, postoperative
palatal advancement with pharyngoplasty *see* transpalatal advancement pharyngoplasty
palatal flutter snoring, 43, 159, 165, 169
palatal implants (Pillar®), 169–75
combined with other procedures, 170
extrusion, 172–3
failure, 175
patient selection, 170
postoperative management, 172
procedure outline, 170–2
success rate, 173, 174
palatal obstruction *see* retropalatal obstruction
palatal obturator, velopharyngeal insufficiency, 370
palatal sclerotherapy, 165–7, 392
palatal stiffening procedures, 159
cautery-assisted *see* cautery-assisted palatal stiffening operation
implants, 169–75
injection snoreplasty, 165–7
palatal surgery
expansion sphincter pharyngoplasty, 224–6
multilevel techniques, 116
salvage procedures for failed, 386–92
transpalatal advancement pharyngoplasty, 217–23
uvulopalatal flap, 206–10
zetapalatopharyngoplasty, 201–5
*see also* minimally invasive palatal procedures; uvulopalatopharyngoplasty
palate
avascular necrosis, 332
cleft *see* cleft palate
high arched, 6
PAP *see* positive airway pressure
parasomnias, 7
paresthesia, lips, 337
P$_{crit}$ *see* critical closing pressure
pectus excavatum, 79, 415
pedometers, 55
percutaneous submucosal glossectomy, 248–9, 256
perioperative management, 88–94, 96–103
perioperative risk scoring, 97
pharyngeal flap
pediatric nasopharyngeal stenosis, 402–3
velopharyngeal insufficiency, 371, 373–4
pharyngocutaneous fistula, 281, 285
pharyngoplasty
expansion sphincter, 224–6
lateral *see* lateral pharyngoplasty
posterior wall augmentation, 375
sphincter, 371, 374–5
transpalatal advancement *see* transpalatal advancement pharyngoplasty
*see also* uvulopalatopharyngoplasty; zetapalatopharyngoplasty
pharynx
classification system (types 1–3), 187–8, 379
fat deposition, 15, 96
lateral wall *see* lateral pharyngeal wall
morphologic abnormalities, 6, 15
multilevel surgery *see* multilevel surgery
physical activity, 55
physical examination, 5–7, 47
Pickwickian syndrome, 47
Pierre Robin syndrome, 24–5, 78, 410
piezoelectric respiratory sensors, 27, 31
Pillar® implants *see* palatal implants
piriform aperture stenosis, 400, 401
plasma surgery, 241–2
*see also* radiofrequency cold ablation (coblation)
plethysmography, respiratory inductive (RIP), 27, 30, 31
Poiseuille's law, 121
polysomnography (PSG), 22–31, 33–41
airflow and respiratory signals, 30

analog systems, 25, 26–7
children, 24–5, 399, 414
before adenotonsillectomy, 420–3
case review, 39–41
cost analysis, 34
CPAP titration, 23, 61
digital, 25, 26–7
guidelines, 22–3, 33–4
interpretation, 35–41
measures of disease severity, 45–6
montage channels, 25–7
montages, 25, 26
postoperative, 24
Powell–Riley two-phase protocol, 82
uvulopalatopharyngoplasty, 187, 379, 380
preoperative, 24, 81
adenotonsillectomy, 420–3
uvulopalatopharyngoplasty, 378, 383
recording systems, 22, 23, 24
special populations, 24–5
split night, 23
units of sensitivity, 27
position
dependent obstructive sleep apnea, 33–7, 383
sensors, 26, 27
positioning
postoperative, 91, 101
during surgery, 99, 100
positive airway pressure (PAP) therapy, 48, 60–7
analysis of failures, 69–70
auto-titrating machines, 61–2
benefits, 66, 86
objectives, 60
practice model, 61–6
risks, 66
surgical procedures to improve use, 49, 64–5
therapeutic indications, 60–1
*see also* continuous positive airways pressure
posterior pharyngeal wall augmentation, 375
postobstructive pulmonary edema (POPE), 352, 363–4
postoperative assessment, 24
postoperative complications, increased risk, 88
postoperative management, 83, 91–4, 101–3
pediatric patients, 400
uvulopalatopharyngoplasty, 179, 361–5 *see also* under specific procedures
postoperative monitoring, 83, 92
need for, 88, 89
pediatric patients, 400
Powell–Riley two-phase surgical protocol, 80, 326–33
complications, 332
patient selection, 326–7
postoperative management, 332
rationale, 82
success rate, 332–3
surgical techniques, 327–31
premedication, 98
preoperative assessment, 24, 97–8
children, 399–400
preoperative management, 88–90, 93, 97–9
preoxygenation, 99
pressure flow diagrams, 19, 20
pressure recordings, 12, 18–19, 22
children, 414, 415, 419
nasal pressure transducers, 30
propofol
pharmacokinetics, 43
sleep nasendoscopy, 17, 42–4
proton pump inhibitors, 439, 442
PSG *see* polysomnography
psychomotor impairment, 5
psyllium mucilloid, 56
pulmonary edema, postobstructive (POPE), 352, 363–4
pulse oximetry, 92

## Q

quality of life, 5, 152

## R

radiofrequency ablation of palate (RFAP)
LAUP salvage with, 386–7

449

# INDEX

radiofrequency ablation of palate (RFAP) (Continued)
  minimally invasive multilevel surgery, 113
  salvage of failed, 386, 389
radiofrequency adenoidectomy, 427
radiofrequency cold ablation (coblation)
  adenoidectomy, 403, 404
  inferior turbinate reduction, 143–7
    complications, 146
    patient selection, 143–4
    postoperative management, 146
    procedure outline, 144–6
    success rate, 146–7
  lingual tonsillectomy, 265–7
  submucosal glossectomy, 248, 249–50, 252, 254
  tonsil reduction, 429, 430–1, 432
  tonsillectomy see tonsillectomy, coblation
radiofrequency surgery, 233–42
  basics, 237–42
  bipolar, 235, 236
  defined, 237
  equipment technology, 234–7
  history, 237–8
  monopolar, 234–5
  physical and technical basics, 238–9
  therapeutic effects, 234
  tissue effects, 239–40
  types of application, 233, 240–2
radiofrequency tongue base reduction (TBRF or RFTB), 243–6
  complications, 204, 245
  hyoid suspension with, 311
  minimally invasive multilevel surgery, 113
  one-stage multilevel surgery, 312–20
  patient selection, 243
  pediatric patients, 406–7
  postoperative management, 245
  preoperative evaluation, 243
  procedure, 243–5
  results, 245–6
  revision uvulopalatopharyngoplasty, 394
  uvulopalatopharyngoplasty with, 198, 246
  zetapalatopharyngoplasty with, 201, 203
  see also glossectomy
radiofrequency tonsil ablation, 431, 432
radiofrequency tonsil reduction, 429–33
  patient selection, 430
  postoperative management, 431–2
  success rate, 432–3
  surgical technique, 430–1
radiofrequency volumetric reduction for turbinate hypertrophy, 140–2
ramped position, 99, 100
referential polysomnographic recordings, 25, 26
reflux see gastroesophageal reflux
REM sleep, obstructive sleep apnea during, 36, 37
Repose® bone anchoring system
  hyomandibular suspension with hyoid distraction, 321, 322
  tongue base resection with hyoepiglottoplasty, 284–5
  tongue suture suspension, 259–60, 274, 275–6, 405–6
Respiratory Disturbance Index (RDI), 46
respiratory effort-related arousals see arousals
respiratory inductive plethysmography (RIP), 27, 30, 31
respiratory signals, polysomnographic assessment, 30, 31
retrognathia, 6, 257
retrolingual (retroglossal) obstruction
  evaluation, 12, 14, 43
  external submucosal glossectomy, 292–3
  hyoid suspension, 305–6
  hyomandibular suspension and hyoid expansion, 321–3
  lingual tonsillectomy, 265
  midline laser glossectomy, 291
  minimally invasive submucosal glossectomy, 248, 256, 257
  minimally invasive treatment, 112–13
  multilevel surgery, 312, 313–15
  UPPP failure, 112, 187
  see also macroglossia
retropalatal obstruction
  cautery-assisted palatal stiffening, 163
  evaluation, 12, 14

expansion sphincter pharyngoplasty, 224
  multilevel surgery, 312, 313
  transpalatal advancement pharyngoplasty, 217
  uvulopalatopharyngoplasty, 83, 184, 187, 199–200
rhinitis, 125
  allergic, 65, 140, 143, 416
  vasomotor, 140
rhinomanometry (RM), 126
rhinometry, acoustic (AR), 126, 132–3
rimonabant, 57
risk scoring, perioperative, 97
rocuronium, 100
Rose position, 425
Roux-en-Y gastric bypass (RYGB), 57

## S

sagittal split osteotomy, 329–30, 336
saturation, polysomnographic recordings, 27, 29
scar formation, after coagulation necrosis, 234
sclerotherapy
  palatal, 165–7, 392
  vascular malformations of tongue, 408
sedation, sleep nasendoscopy, 17–18, 42–4
sedatives, 48
  postoperative, 93
  preoperative, 89, 98
seizures, nocturnal, 40
sella-nasion-subspinale (SNA) angle, 280
sella-nasion-supramentale (SNB) angle, 280
severity of OSA/OSAHS
  adenotonsillectomy postoperative course and, 421, 423
  clinical assessment, 11–13, 269
  multilevel treatment and, 112, 114–15, 116–17
  OSAHS score, 105–7
  $P_{crit}$ and, 19, 20, 187
  pediatric assessment, 413–15, 417
  polysomnographic measures, 45–6
  treatment options by, 49–50
  uvulopalatopharyngoplasty outcome and, 383
  see also Apnea Hypopnea Index; polysomnography
sexual dysfunction, 5
sibutramine, 56
signs, clinical, 5–7
sinus cones, 65
sinusitis, chronic, 65
sleep, 4
sleep-disordered breathing (SDB)
  clinical assessment, 3
  definitions of disease, 45–6
  effects, 46, 61
  in women, 8
Sleep Heart Health Study, 46
sleep medicine, 1–2
sleep position therapy, 48
sleep-related breathing disorders (SRBD)
  children, 398–412, 421–2
  polysomnography, 22–4, 33–41
sleep-related symptoms, 4–5, 6, 7
sleep staging, majority of epoch (MOE) rule, 37, 39
sleep studies
  home testing, 60
  recommended tests, 22–3
  see also polysomnography
sleeping pills, 63–4
SMILE see submucosal minimally invasive lingual excision
snore guard, 74
snoreplasty, injection, 165–7, 392
snoring, 4, 33
  after nasal surgery, 126–7
  children, 398–9, 414, 421–2
  endoscopic evaluation, 17, 43–4
  palatal flutter, 43, 159, 165, 169
  social effects, 46
  surgery, 65
snoring sound test, 72
social effects, obstructive sleep apnea, 46
sodium tetradecyl sulfate (STS), injection snoreplasty, 165–6, 392
Sotradecol® see sodium tetradecyl sulfate
space problem, orofacial complex, 77–8

speech problems
  hypernasality, 370, 376
  postoperative changes, 181
  see also velopharyngeal insufficiency
speech therapy, 370
sphenopalatine nerve block, 144, 145
sphincter pharyngoplasty, 371, 374–5
splay conchal graft, internal nasal valve repair, 137
spreader graft, internal nasal valve repair, 135–6
Starling model of airway resistance, 121–2
steroids see corticosteroids
stertor, 398
stoma buttons, 345–6
strain gauges, 30
stridor, 437, 438
stroke, 24, 85
submucosal glossectomy see under glossectomy
submucosal lingualplasty, 248, 253–5
submucosal minimally invasive lingual excision (SMILE), 248, 249–52, 256
  pediatric patients, 407–8
submucosal uvulopalatopharyngoplasty see under uvulopalatopharyngoplasty
submucous coagulation, 233, 234, 235–7, 241
submucous vaporization, 233
succinylcholine, 100
sucralfate, 151
suction coagulator adenoidectomy, 403–4, 417, 418, 426
sudden infant death syndrome (SIDS), 414
superficial vaporization, 233, 234
superior pharyngeal constrictor (SPC) muscles, lateral pharyngoplasty, 227, 228–30
supraglottic stenosis, 439, 441–2
supraglottoplasty, 439–42
  complications, 441–2
  postoperative care, 442
  success rate, 442
  surgical procedure, 439–41
surgical facility, selection, 88–9
surgical staging system, Friedman see Friedman surgical staging system
surgical treatment, 48–9, 80–4
  generic patient care protocols, 93
  impact on cardiac risk factors, 85–7
  indications, 80–1
  intraoperative management, 90–1, 99–101
  multilevel see multilevel surgery
  patient selection, 81–2
  perioperative management, 88–94, 96–103
  polysomnography before/after, 24, 81, 82
  postoperative management, 83, 91–4, 101–3
  preoperative management, 88–90, 93, 97–9
  procedures, 82–3
  rationale, 80
  success rates, 70, 84
  supporting PAP use, 49, 64–5
swallowing
  difficulties see dysphagia
  preoperative evaluation, 217
sweating, nocturnal, 4
symptoms
  daytime, 5, 6, 7
  sleep-related (nocturnal), 4–5, 6, 7
Syndrome Z, 54

## T

taste disturbances, postoperative, 181, 226, 290
teeth, maxillomandibular advancement osteotomy, 335, 336
temporomandibular joint (TMJ) clicking, 6
thermal effect, radiofrequency surgery, 238–9
thermisters, airflow, 27, 30
thermocouples, airflow, 27, 30
Thornton adjustable positioner (TAP), 75
throat discomfort
  after uvulopalatopharyngoplasty, 181, 199
  after zetapalatopharyngoplasty, 204
  see also pain, postoperative
tissue
  ablation, by vaporization, 234
  effects, radiofrequency surgery, 239–40

# INDEX

resection, by electrotomy, 234
resistance (impedance), 236
temperature, 236
volume shrinkage, coagulation necrosis, 234
tongue
　advancement *see* genioglossus advancement
　neurovascular bundle, 248, 253, 279
　postoperative edema, 245, 297–8
　postoperative hematoma, 255, 297, 298
　postoperative infections, 204, 245, 395
　ptosis, 410–11
　size estimation, 280, 292–3
　suture, postoperative airway obstruction, 371, 376
　vascular malformations, 408
　*see also* macroglossia
tongue base
　obstruction *see* retrolingual (retroglossal) obstruction
　radiofrequency reduction *see* radiofrequency tongue base reduction
　stabilization, 258–63
tongue base resection with hyoepiglottoplasty (TBRHE) (open), 279–86
　anatomy, 279–80
　complications, 281
　presurgical evaluation, 280
　procedure, 281–6
　results, 280–1
　*see also* glossectomy
tongue retaining device (TRD), 72, 73
tongue suspension suture, 259–63
　complications, 262, 263, 276
　multilevel surgery, 272–4
　patient selection, 261–2
　pediatric patients, 405–6
　pros and cons, 263
　rationale, 258–9
　results, 262, 263, 277
　technique, 259–61, 274, 275–6
tonsillar pillar hypertrophy, 6
tonsillectomy
　coblation, 417, 418, 430, 431, 432
　Han-uvulopalatopharyngoplasty, 212
　indications, 430
　lateral pharyngoplasty with, 228
　lingual *see* lingual tonsillectomy
　microdebrider-assisted, 434–6
　pediatric patients, 403, 404, 416–17
　previous
　　palatal surgery, 201
　　uvulopalatopharyngoplasty outcome and, 383–4
　radiofrequency ablation, 431, 432
　submucosal uvulopalatopharyngoplasty with, 196
　subtotal capsule-sparing, 429, 430–1, 432, 434–6
　uvulopalatal flap with, 209, 210
　uvulopalatopharyngoplasty with, 178, 184, 191
　velopharyngeal insufficiency, 376
　*vs* radiofrequency tonsil reduction, 429, 432–3
tonsils
　enlarged, 6, 403–5
　　magnetic resonance imaging, 15
　　multilevel surgery, 117
　　nasal obstruction, 125
　lingual, hypertrophy *see* lingual tonsil hypertrophy
　radiofrequency reduction, 429–33
　size
　　grading, 105, 108
　　OSAHS score, 107
　tubal, hypertrophy, 428
topical anesthetics, 92
torticollis, postoperative, 428
tracheal deformities, tube-related, 352–3
tracheal intubation *see* endotracheal intubation
tracheo–innominate artery fistula, 352
tracheostomy, 49, 91, 349–59
　Bjork flap, 351
　closure, 359
　H-flap, 344–5, 351
　laryngomalacia, 442
　long-term tube-free (LTTFT), 349, 353–7
　　closure, 358, 359
　patient selection, 350
　pediatric, 359, 411
　routine method, 343

semantics, 349–50
speech-ready, long-term tube-free, 354–7
　benefits, 356, 357
　postoperative care, 356
　supplementary sling procedure, 357
　surgical technique, 354–6
stoma buttons, 345–6
tube-dependent, 343–8, 350–3
　complications, 352–3
　efficacy in OSA, 346–7, 351–2
　surgical techniques, 343–5, 346
tube-free, 350, 353–7
U-flap technique, 345
tracheostomy tubes, 345, 347
　complications, 352–3
tracheotomy, 49, 91, 350–1
　complications, 350–1, 352–3
　efficacy in OSA, 351–2
　open tongue base resection, 280, 281, 286
　patient selection, 350
　preoperative, 326–7
　semantics, 349–50
tramadol, 92
tranquillizers, 63–4
transient ischemic attacks, 24
transpalatal advancement pharyngoplasty (TPAP), 178, 217–23
　complications, 222, 391–2
　failed uvulopalatopharyngoplasty, 187, 200, 389–92
　postoperative care, 222
　preoperative evaluation, 217–18
　results, 222
　surgical technique, 218–22
Treacher Collins syndrome, 24–5
tubal tonsils, hypertrophy, 428
tumour necrosis factor-α (TNF-α), 85
turbinate, inferior nasal *see* nasal turbinate, inferior

## U

ultrasound guidance, submucosal glossectomy, 248, 249, 253
upper airway *see* airway
upper airway resistance syndrome (UARS), 3
　adenotonsillectomy, 421, 423
　children, 398
　clinical presentation, 7
　epidemiology, 3
　snare uvulectomy, 154–8
　*vs* OSAHS, 8
UPPP *see* uvulopalatopharyngoplasty
uvula
　effects of removal, 181
　erythema and edema, 6
　uvulopalatopharyngoplasty preserving, 211–15
uvulectomy
　cautery-assisted palatal stiffening operation, 160, 161
　expansion sphincter pharyngoplasty, 226
　snare, 154–8
　　complications, 156–7
　　patient selection, 154
　　postoperative management, 156
　　procedure, 154–6
　　results, 157
　techniques compared, 157–8
uvulopalatal flap (UPF), 206–10
　advantages, 206–7
　complications, 210
　extensions, 207, 209, 210
　postoperative management, 209–10
　rationale, 83
　technique, 207–8
　*see also* zetapalatopharyngoplasty
uvulopalatopharyngoplasty (UPPP), 176–83
　complications, 180–2, 195, 361–4, 379, 382–3
　effects on airway, 184–7
　external submucosal glossectomy with, 298, 299
　factors affecting response, 383
　failures
　　analysis, 378–84
　　causes, 187, 393
　　salvage procedures, 187, 386, 387–92
　　Z-palatoplasty revision, 200, 393–6

Fairbanks technique, 190–4
　objectives, 190
　patient selection, 190
　postoperative management, 193–4
　results, 194
　surgical procedure, 190–3
Friedman staging system, 107–9, 188
Han modification (uvula preservation) (H-UPPP), 211–15
　outcomes and complications, 214–15
　patient selection, 211
　postoperative management, 214
　preoperative care, 211–12
　techniques, 212–13
history, 184
midline laser glossectomy with, 287–91
modifications, 178, 184, 201
multilevel airway obstruction, 112, 276–7, 383, 384
nasopharyngeal stenosis after *see under* nasopharyngeal stenosis
one-stage multilevel surgery with, 312–20
open tongue base resection with, 281
outcomes
　long-term polysomnography, 187, 379, 380
　subjective and objective, 379–81
patient selection, 176–7, 187–8, 378–9
　clinical examination/scores, 11, 187–8
　CT scanning, 15
　lateral cephalometry, 13, 187
　Mueller maneuver, 12–13
　pharyngeal pressure measurements, 19
　sleep videoendoscopy, 18
　value, 383–4
pediatric patients, 404–5
postoperative management, 179, 361–5
radiofrequency tongue base reduction with, 198, 245
rationale, 83
repeat, 389, 390
submucosal, 195–200
　complications, 198–9
　failures, 199–200
　patient selection, 195–6
　postoperative management, 198–9
　success rate, 199
　surgical technique, 196–8
success rates, 70, 83, 182, 381
technique, 178–9, 184, 185–6
*vs* uvulopalatal flap, 206, 207
*vs* zetapalatopharyngoplasty, 201, 204
uvulopalatoplasty, laser-assisted *see* laser-assisted uvulopalatoplasty (LAUP)

## V

vallecular cysts, congenital, 408–9
vaporization
　plasma surgery, 241–2
　submucous, 233
　superficial, 233, 234
　tissue ablation, 234
vascular malformations, tongue, 408
velocardiofacial syndrome, 371, 376
velopharyngeal insufficiency (VPI), 370–7
　postoperative
　　adenoidectomy, 428
　　expansion sphincter pharyngoplasty, 226
　　Han-uvulopalatopharyngoplasty, 214
　　laser-assisted uvulopalatoplasty, 152
　　lateral pharyngoplasty, 231
　　transpalatal advancement pharyngoplasty, 222
　　uvulopalatal flap, 206, 207, 210
　　uvulopalatopharyngoplasty, 180–1, 199
　　Z-palatoplasty, 202, 204, 395, 396
　surgical treatment, 181, 370–7
　　operative techniques, 371–5
　　patient selection, 370–1
　　postoperative management and complications, 375–6
　　results, 376
velopharyngeal stenosis, postoperative, 152
venous malformations, tongue, 408
venous thromboembolism prophylaxis, 93
ventilating catheter, 101

451

# INDEX

ventilation
  difficult, 90–1, 102
  see also endotracheal intubation
vibrissae, 120
videoendoscopy, upper airway see endoscopy, upper airway
vigilance, decreased, 5
visceral adipose tissue (VAT), 54
vitamin supplements, 56, 58
voice, postoperative changes, 181

## W

waist circumference, 51, 53–4
waist-to-hip ratio, 51

weight loss, 48, 54–8
Wharton's duct injury, 276
women, sleep-disordered breathing, 8
wound dehiscence
  lateral pharyngoplasty, 231
  submucosal glossectomy, 256
  submucosal uvulopalatopharyngoplasty, 199
  transpalatal advancement pharyngoplasty, 222
  uvulopalatal flap, 210
  uvulopalatopharyngoplasty, 181, 195
wound infections see infections, postoperative

## Z

Z-plasty, Furlow double opposing, 371–3

zaleplon, 93
zetapalatopharyngoplasty (Z-palatoplasty; ZPP), 178, 196, 201–5
  complications, 204
  patient selection, 202
  postoperative management, 204
  success rate, 204–5
  surgical technique, 202–3, 204
  uvulopalatal flap and, 207
  uvulopalatopharyngoplasty failures, 200, 393–6
    patient selection, 393–4
    postoperative care and complications, 395
    success rate, 395–6
    surgical technique, 394–5
zolpidem (Ambien®), 63, 93

Edwards Brothers Malloy
Ann Arbor MI. USA
January 25, 2016

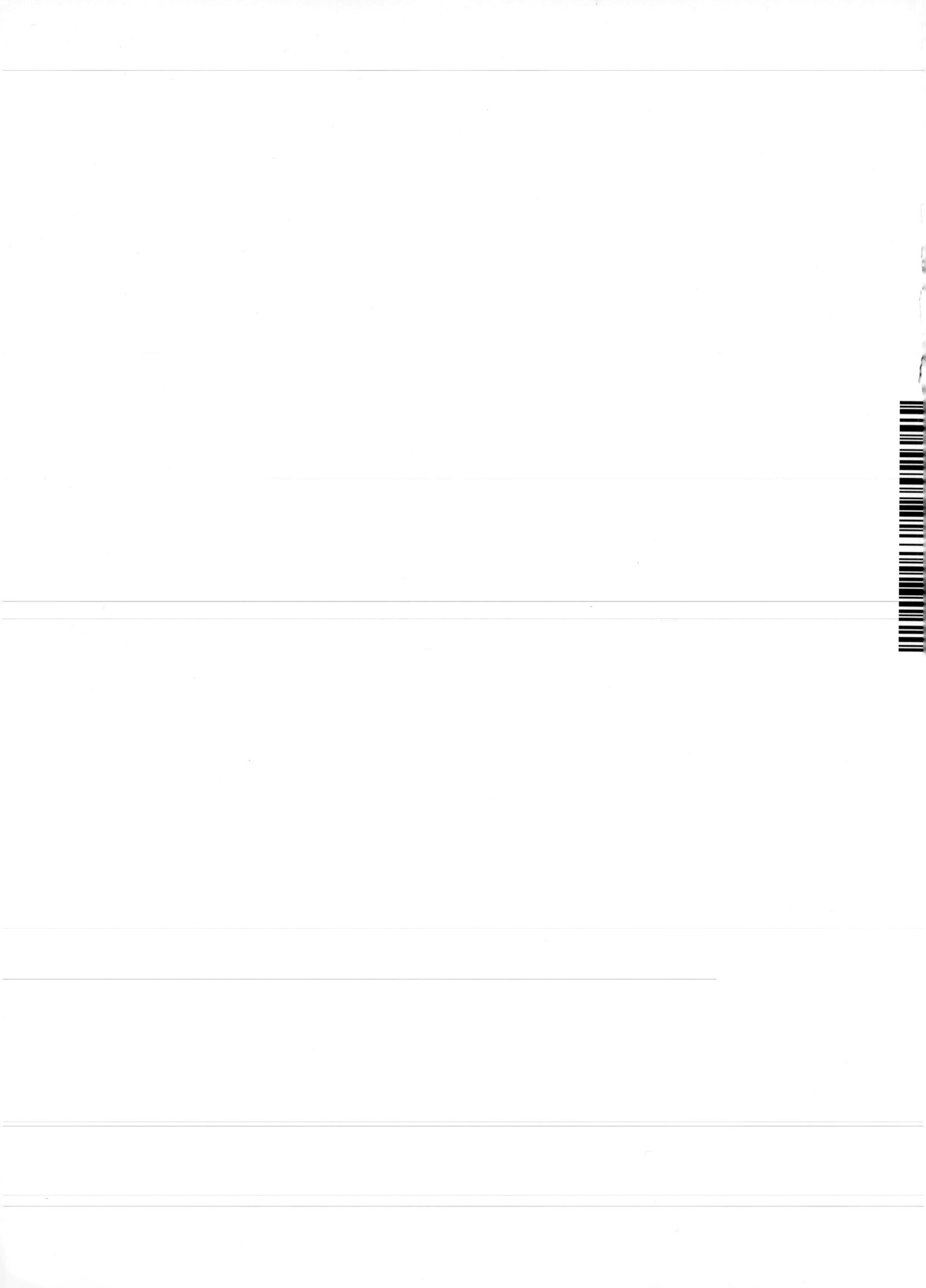